PROCEDURES FOR PRIMARY CARE PHYSICIANS

OTHER PRIMARY CARE SERIES TITLES

Fleming and Barry/ADDICTIVE DISORDERS
Goldstein and Goldstein/PRACTICAL DERMATOLOGY
Mercier/PRACTICAL ORTHOPEDICS

Procedures for Primary Care Physicians

EDITED BY

JOHN L. PFENNINGER, M.D.
Director
The National Procedures Institute
Midland, Michigan;
Associate Clinical Professor
Department of Family Practice
Michigan State College of Human Medicine
East Lansing, Michigan

GRANT C. FOWLER, M.D.
Residency Director
Hermann/LBJ Family Practice Program;
Assistant Professor
Department of Family Practice and Community Medicine
University of Texas Houston Health Science Center-Medical School
Houston, Texas

Illustrated by Theodore G. Huff and Associates

With 925 illustrations

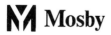 Mosby

St. Louis Baltimore Berlin Boston Carlsbad Chicago London Madrid
Naples New York Philadelphia Sydney Tokyo Toronto

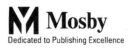
Mosby
Dedicated to Publishing Excellence

Editors: Stephanie Manning, Susie Baxter
Developmental Editor: Anne Gunter
Project Manager: Barbara Bowes Merritt
Editing and Production: Carlisle Publishers Services
Cover Design: G.W. Graphics
Manufacturing Supervisor: John Babrick

A NOTE TO THE READER
The authors and publisher have made every attempt to check content for accuracy, but it is not the intention of this book to make the reader an expert at the procedure. New technology, new investigations, and broader experience may alter recommended drugs, techniques, and procedures.

Printed in the United States of America

Composition by Carlisle Communications, Ltd.
Printing/Binding by Maple-Vail Book Mfg. Group, York

Mosby–Year Book, Inc.
11830 Westline Industrial Drive
St. Louis, Missouri 63146

Library of Congress Cataloging-in-Publication Data

Procedures for primary care physicians / edited by John L. Pfenninger,
  Grant C. Fowler ; illustrated by Theodore G. Huff and associates.
      p. cm.
    Includes bibliographical references and index.
    ISBN 0-8016-6384-9
    1. Primary care (Medicine) 2. Surgery, Minor.   I. Pfenninger,
John L.   II. Fowler, Grant C.
    [DNLM: 1. Primary Health Care—methods.   W 84.6 P963 1994]
  RC48.P76 1994
  617—dc20
  DNLM/DLC
  for Library of Congress   94-9013
                                                                 CIP

95 96 97   /   9 8 7 6 5 4 3 2

CONTRIBUTORS

Barbara S. Apgar, M.D.
Clinical Associate Professor
Department of Family Practice
University of Michigan Medical School
Ann Arbor, Michigan

Richard J. Bakeman, D.D.S.
Private Practice
Midland, Michigan

John M. Boltri, M.D.
Private Practice
Union Camp Family Medical Center
Savannah, Georgia

David B. Bosscher, D.O.
Associate Clinical Professor
College of Osteopathic Medicine
Michigan State University
East Lansing, Michigan;
Assistant Director
Family Practice Residency Program
MidMichigan Regional Medical Center
Midland, Michigan

Michael L. Brown, M.D.
Clinical Instructor
Department of Family Medicine
University of Washington School of Medicine;
Clinical Faculty
Emergency Department and Department of Family
  Medicine
Swedish Hospital Medical Center
Seattle, Washington

Richard E. Brunader, M.D.
Residency Director
Department of Family Practice
University of California, San Francisco
School of Medicine
San Francisco, California;
Department of Family Practice
Natividad Medical Center
Salinas, California

Fred D. Catrett, M.D., Ph.D.
Private Practice
Houston, Texas

Richard C. Cherkis, M.D.
Associate Professor
Department of Obstetrics and Gynecology
University of Rochester
School of Medicine & Dentistry;
Assistant Director
Department of Obstetrics and Gynecology
Highland Hospital of Rochester
Rochester, New York

Mark E. Clasen, M.D., Ph.D.
Chairman
Department of Family Practice
Wright State University School of Medicine
Dayton, Ohio

Lori Crago, M.D.
Highline Medical Group
Seattle, Washington

Timothy A. Curran, M.D.
Department of Family Practice
John Peter Smith Hospital
Fort Worth, Texas

George C. Denniston, M.D.
Clinical Assistant Professor
Department of Family Medicine
University of Washington School of Medicine
Seattle, Washington

Daniel J. Derksen, M.D.
Assistant Professor
Department of Family and Community Medicine
University of New Mexico School of Medicine
Albuquerque, New Mexico

William H. Dery, M.D.
Associate Professor
Department of Family Practice
Michigan State University
East Lansing, Michigan;
Associate Director
Family Practice Residency
MidMichigan Regional Medical Center
Midland, Michigan

Marvin A. Dewar, M.D., J.D.
Director
Family Practice Residency Program
Department of Community Health and Family
  Medicine
University of Florida College of Medicine
Gainesville, Florida

Donald E. DeWitt, M.D.
Clinical Professor and Procedural Skill
  Coordinator
Department of Family Medicine
East Carolina University School of Medicine
Greenville, North Carolina

John F. Donnelly, M.D.
Assistant Professor and Clerkship Director
Department of Family Practice and Community
  Medicine
University of Texas Houston Health Science
  Center–Medical School
Houston, Texas

Susan Shevaun Duiker, M.D.
Assistant Professor
Department of Family Practice and Community
  Medicine
University of Texas Houston Health Science
  Center–Medical School;
Medical Director
UT Hermann Center for Family Practice
Houston, Texas

Scott W. Eathorne, M.D.
Department of Family Practice and Sports
  Medicine
Providence Hospital
Southfield, Michigan

Steven H. Eisinger, M.D.
Associate Professor of Obstetrics/Gynecology and
  Family Medicine
Department of Family Medicine
University of Rochester School of Medicine and
  Dentistry
Rochester, New York

Joseph Ellis, D.P.M.
Private Practice
La Jolla, California

William Jackson Epperson, M.D.
Family Medicine and Office Gynecology
Waccamaw Neck Medical Center
Murrells Inlet, South Carolina

Steven Fettinger, M.D.
Associate Clinical Professor
Department of Obstetrics and Gynecology and
  Reproductive Biology
Michigan State University College of Human Medicine
East Lansing, Michigan;
Women's Obstetrics & Gynecology
Saginaw, Michigan

Gregory J. Forzley, M.D.
Medical Director
Priority Health
Holland Community Hospital
Grand Rapids, Michigan

Grant C. Fowler, M.D.
Residency Director
Hermann/LBJ Family Practice Residency;
Assistant Professor
Department of Family Practice and Community
  Medicine
University of Texas Houston Health Science
  Center–Medical School
Houston, Texas

Donald M. Gelb, M.D.
Associate Clinical Professor
Department of Family Medicine
College of Medicine
University of California, Irvine;
Professor
California Medical School of the Pacific
Irvine, California

Ken Grauer, M.D.
Professor and Assistant Director
Family Practice Residency Program
University of Florida College of Medicine
Gainesville, Florida

Lee Green, M.D.
Department of Family Practice
University of Michigan Medical School
Ann Arbor, Michigan

Fred M. Hankin, M.D.
Department of Orthopedic Surgery
St. Joseph Mercy Hospital
Ypsilanti, Michigan

Peter Hanson, M.D.
Professor of Medicine and Co-director
Preventive Cardiology Program
University of Wisconsin Clinical Science Center
Madison, Wisconsin

John Harlan Haynes III, M.D.
Assistant Clinical Professor
Department of Family and Community Medicine
University of Texas Southwestern Medical Center
Dallas, Texas;
Medical Director
Hospital Corporation of America Medical Alliance
Fort Worth, Texas

Scott T. Henderson, M.D.
Assistant Professor
Department of Family Practice
University of Wyoming College of Health Sciences
Cheyenne, Wyoming

John E. Hocutt, Jr., M.D.
Clinical Assistant Professor
Department of Family Medicine
Thomas Jefferson University Medical College
Philadelphia, Pennsylvania;
Instructor of Family Medicine
Medical Center of Delaware
Wilmington, Delaware

Hugh H. Hogle, M.D.
Medical Director
HCA St. Mark's Breast Care Services
Salt Lake City, Utah

J. Christopher Hough, M.D.
Medical Director
Geriatric Services
MidMichigan Regional Medical Center
Midland, Michigan

Edward A. Jackson, M.D.
Assistant Clinical Professor
Department of Family Practice
Michigan State University College of Human Medicine
East Lansing, Michigan;
Associate Director of Family Practice
Saginaw Community Hospital
Saginaw, Michigan

Robert E. James, M.D.
Instructor
Department of Urology
University of California, San Francisco
School of Medicine
San Francisco, California;
Chairman
Department of Surgery
Santa Rosa Memorial Hospital
Santa Rosa, California

Raymond E. Jarris, Jr., M.D.
Clinical Instructor
Department of Family Medicine
University of Washington School of Medicine;
Emergency Department
Swedish Medical Center
Seattle, Washington

Dietrich Jehle, M.D.
Associate Professor
State University of New York at Buffalo;
Director of Emergency Medicine
Erie County Medical Center
Buffalo, New York

Jeffrey R. Kovan, D.O.
Assistant Professor
Department of Family Practice
Michigan State University College of Human
* Medicine*
East Lansing, Michigan;
Assistant Director of Family Practice
Kalamazoo Center for Medical Studies
Kalamazoo, Michigan

Diane Lillis, R.N.
Administrative Manager
Preventive Cardiology Program
University of Wisconsin Clinical Science Center
Madison, Wisconsin

Kelly T. Locke, M.D.
Eau Claire Family Medicine Clinic
Eau Claire, Wisconsin

Gailen D. Marshall, M.D., Ph.D.
Director
Division of Allergy and Clinical Immunology
Department of Internal Medicine
University of Texas Houston Health Science
* Center–Medical School*
Houston, Texas

Donald N. Marquardt, M.D., Ph.D.
Staff Physician and Consultant
Waterloo Family Practice Residency Program
Northeast Iowa Medical Education Foundation
Waterloo, Iowa

Malcolm L. Mazow, M.D.
Professor of Ophthalmology and Pediatrics
University of Texas Houston Health Science
* Center–Medical School*
Houston, Texas

Douglas B. McKeag, M.D.
Professor of Family Practice
Coordinator of Sports Medicine
Michigan State University College of Human Medicine
East Lansing, Michigan

Terrence L. Meece, M.D.
Medical Director
Preferred Health Partnership, Inc.
Knoxville, Tennessee

Lewis E. Mehl, M.D.
Medical Center Hospital
Department of Psychiatry
Burlington, Vermont

Julie Graves Moy, M.D.
Clinical Assistant Professor
Department of Family Medicine
Baylor College of Medicine
Houston, Texas

Gary R. Newkirk, M.D.
Associate Clinical Professor
Department of Family Medicine
University of Washington School of Medicine
Seattle, Washington

Daniel A. Norman, M.D.
Assistant Clinical Professor of Medicine
University of Nevada School of Medicine
Reno, Nevada;
Chief, Gastroenterology
Barton Memorial Hospital
South Lake Tahoe, California

John M. O'Brien, M.D.
Clinical Assistant Professor and Director of Graduate
*   Education*
Department of Family Practice
University of Michigan Medical School
Ann Arbor, Michigan

Nelly A. Otero, M.D.
Private Practice
Orlando, Florida

James R. Palleschi, M.D.
Assistant Clinical Professor
Department of Urology
University of California, San Francisco
School of Medicine
San Francisco, California;
Chief, Section of Renal Transplantation
Santa Rosa Memorial Hospital
Santa Rosa, California

John M. Passmore, Jr., M.D.
Assistant Clinical Professor
Department of Family Practice and Community
*   Medicine*
University of Texas Houston Health Science
*   Center–Medical School;*
Staff Cardiologist
Diagnostic Cardiology of Houston
Houston, Texas

James F. Peggs, M.D.
Clinical Associate Professor of Family Practice
Associate Chairman for Clinical Affairs
Department of Family Practice
University of Michigan Medical School
Ann Arbor, Michigan

John R. Pfeifer, M.D.
Adjunct Professor
Health Sciences Oakland University;
Associate Clinical Professor of Surgery
Wayne State University School of Medicine;
Director
Surgical Research Providence Hospital
Southfield, Michigan

John L. Pfenninger, M.D.
Director
The National Procedures Institute
Midland, Michigan;
Associate Clinical Professor
Department of Family Practice
Michigan State College of Human Medicine
East Lansing, Michigan

Gregg K. Phillips, M.D.
Emergency Department
John Peter Smith Hospital
Fort Worth, Texas

Gayle M. Randall, M.D.
Assistant Professor
Department of Medicine
UCLA School of Medicine;
Director, Gastrointestinal Endoscopy
West Los Angeles Veterans Administration
Los Angeles, California

James E. Rasmussen, M.D.
Professor of Dermatology and Pediatrics
University of Michigan Medical School
Ann Arbor, Michigan

Stephen Ratcliffe, M.D.
Division Chief of Family Medicine
Department of Family and Preventive Medicine
University of Utah School of Medicine
Salt Lake City, Utah

Ralph M. Richart, M.D.
Professor of Pathology
College of Physicians and Surgeons
Columbia University
New York, New York

Elizabeth A. Roaf, B.S.
University of Vermont College of Medicine
Burlington, Vermont

Terry S. Ruhl, M.D.
Assistant Clinical Professor
Department of Family Medicine
Michigan State University College of Human Medicine
East Lansing, Michigan;
Associate Director
Family Practice Residency Program
MidMichigan Regional Medical Center
Midland, Michigan

Gary E. Ruoff, M.D.
Clinical Professor
Department of Family Practice
Michigan State University College of Human Medicine
East Lansing, Michigan;
Director of Clinical Research
Westside Family Medical Center
Kalamazoo, Michigan

Len Scarpinato, D.O.
Instructor
Community Medicine and Family Practice
Medical College of Wisconsin;
Critical Care Curriculum Coordinator for Family
 Practice Residency
Departments of Family Medicine, Internal Medicine,
 and Critical Care
St. Mary's Hospital
Milwaukee, Wisconsin

Nancy V. Schantz, M.D.
Associate Director
St. Joseph Family Medicine Residency Program
St. Joseph Medical Center
Stamford, Connecticut

Clark B. Smith, M.D.
Associate Professor and Program Director
Department of Family Medicine
University of Tennessee College of Medicine
Memphis, Tennessee

George F. Snell, M.D.
Associate Professor
Department of Family and Preventive Medicine
University of Utah School of Medicine
Salt Lake City, Utah;
Residency Director
Department of Family Practice
McKay-Dee Hospital Center
Ogden, Utah

James A. Sterling, M.D.
Assistant Professor
Department of Family Medicine
Texas A&M University Health Science Center College of
 Medicine
College Station, Texas;
Clinical Faculty
Department of Family Medicine
Scott and White Hospital
Temple, Texas

James A. Surrell, M.D.
Assistant Clinical Professor of Surgery
Michigan State University
East Lansing, Michigan;
Colorectal Surgeon
Ferguson-Blodgett Digestive Disease Institute
Grand Rapids, Michigan

James T. Telfer, M.D.
Department of Orthopedic Surgery
St. Joseph Mercy Hospital
Ypsilanti, Michigan

Jay R. Varma, M.D.
Associate Professor
Department of Family Medicine
Medical College of Georgia
Augusta, Georgia

George Villanueva, D.O.
Department of Family Practice
Pacific Hospital
Long Beach, California

Lydia A. Watson, M.D.
Assistant Clinical Professor
Department of Obstetrics and Gynecology
Michigan State University College of Human Medicine
East Lansing, Michigan

Barry D. Weiss, M.D.
Professor
Department of Family and Community Medicine
University of Arizona College of Medicine
Tucson, Arizona

Robert L. Williams, M.D.
Assistant Professor
Department of Family Medicine–Research Division
Case Western Reserve University School of Medicine;
Director
Department of Family Practice
MetroHealth Clement Center
Cleveland, Ohio

Thomas C. Wright, M.D.
Assistant Professor of Pathology
College of Physicians and Surgeons
Columbia University
New York, New York

George G. Zainea, M.D.
Surgeon
MidMichigan Regional Medical Center
Midland, Michigan

Thomas J. Zuber, M.D.
Assistant Clinical Professor
Michigan State College of Human Medicine
Saginaw, Michigan;
Associate Director
The National Procedures Institute
Midland, Michigan

To our families.

To Kay Pfenninger, the wife who encouraged, prodded, supported, sacrificed, and consoled through these three years.

To Stacey, Dana, and Matthew Pfenninger, the children who had to forgo many fun weekends and evenings but continued to give the "pat on the back" and encouragement to complete this text.

To "Grandma Rose" Pfenninger, who rode the horse and buggy through all types of weather to assist a general practitioner in the early 1920s while she was only a teenager. It is Grandma Rose who began the dream of medicine as a career.

To our parents, Ann and Bernard Pfenninger, and Jack and Frances Fowler, who were the role models of hard work, dedication, and love.

To "Pops" Feinauer and Vernice ("Guinevere"), the Pfenninger in-laws, who "covered" on many occasions and were substitute parents, not just grandparents, to allow work to progress on this book.

A special dedication to Matthew Pfenninger. Our hopes, dreams, and prayers are always with you.

To these belong the laurels of this text.

FOREWORD

In 1930, more than 80% of the physicians in the United States were general family doctors, providing comprehensive health care at a reasonable cost. By 1980, the self-reported percentage of family doctors in the United States was 15%. Along with this trend of dwindling numbers has been a gradual decline of diagnostic and therapeutic skills held by those physicians who do practice general family medicine.

One definition of a generalist physician (formerly a general practitioner) is a family physician who can provide a breadth and continuity of commonly needed health care services. These physicians care for children, deliver babies, manage simple fractures, counsel single parents, go to the hospital, maintain an office, and, when all else fails, comfort the dying. Their goal is to provide health care from the nursery to the nursing home, without taking the patient to the poor house along the way.

Today, of the 625,000 physicians in the United States, fewer than 10% comprehensively wield the clinical skills needed to provide such care. The headlong rush to subspecialize in medicine has left family physicians in the minority. Still, they are an important minority whose number is now growing in response to the projected needs of the twenty-first century American health care system.

Since 1983, a group of family physicians, supported by the American Academy of Family Physicians (AAFP), has constructed a series of demonstration projects to propagate diagnostic and therapeutic skills in family medicine. Many of the procedural pioneers in family practice have quietly and unselfishly contributed their professional energies to the resuscitation of full-service family practice within a medical education system gone far, far astray. This book stands as a contribution to that effort. Although some may view the teaching and learning of clinical skills as "proceduralism," the skills that are depicted in this book represent the desire of physicians to remain clinically excellent. No amount of psychosocial expertise can overcome the credibility lost when a physician cannot perform basic clinical services on behalf of his or her patient.

Recently, a prominent dean of a well-known medical school asked me why the residency programs at my institution, the University of Tennessee, persisted in teaching a comprehensive set of procedural clinical skills when, in his opinion, managed care organizations and health maintenance organizations would effectively amputate these skills from the day-to-day practice of family physicians. I disagree with this vision of the future, but it is true that some family physicians voluntarily relinquish many of the clinical skills described in this book. It is my hope that the skills described in its pages will become required curriculum, not only for residents, but, particularly, for faculty. One of the major challenges for the success of this book (and the specialty of family practice) is the development of accountability in a health care system that has become overly fragmented, costly, and inaccessible.

Are these skills needed? During the past 20 years, family physicians have been manipulated, exploited, and oppressed in a variety of ways that makes study of their actual needs very complex. For example, a lack of reported interest in obstetrical care cannot be used to justify the tremendous void that exists in women's health care as provided by family physicians. Residents are not likely to acquire clinical skills that family physician faculty members cannot themselves demonstrate in their positions as role models. A lack of procedural skill among family practice faculty and practitioners is particularly troubling in rural and underserved communities. These communities cannot afford platoons of various subspecialized physicians.

Although excellent health care is available from a combination of obstetricians, pediatricians, and internists, a well-trained, comprehensive-care family physician should be able to deliver continuing health care unrestricted by age, sex, organ system, and pregnancy. The physician should be skilled in many of the procedures described here to screen for, prevent, and treat common disease entities. If family practice simply becomes synonymous with "generic primary care," there will be very little need for many of the skills described in this book. My compliments to the editors and the authors for executing a labor of love in an outstanding fashion. They have chosen the road less traveled.

WM. MACMILLAN RODNEY, M.D.
Professor and Chairman
Department of Family Medicine
The University of Tennessee, Memphis;
Residency Director
UT-Healthplex Family Practice Residency Program

PREFACE

The inspiration for this text came from busy primary care physicians across the country. Medicine in the 1990s is changing rapidly. The high cost of hospital care, emergency room visits, and even the expenses of freestanding day surgery centers have created a forceful impetus for physicians to perform previous hospital-based procedures and surgeries in the office. Fast-paced lifestyles have added performance pressure: the patient's time is at a premium. No longer will they accept referrals for simple procedures or the subsequent inconvenience. Patients expect their physician to perform most routine procedures. In certain areas of the country, competition for patients has increased, resulting in the need for physicians to master certain procedural skills to enhance their status and desirability. Overwhelmed with paperwork and other responsibilities, primary care physicians have little time to spend preparing for or performing a procedure (much less orienting their staff), and yet some procedures in the office are becoming more complex. Thus, among other things, physicians are pressured from patients, health care plans, greater competition, paperwork, and their own staff. It was at the urge and cry of these pressured physicians for a concise and yet all-encompassing reference for procedures that this book was created.

Coupled with these pressures, there has been a parallel explosion in new technology. There has also been a clarification and refinement in techniques and indications for older technology. Safer medications and monitoring units are also available to facilitate performing procedures in the office. However, few primary care physicians have the time to stay up-to-date with the changes in technology. New technology or new applications of old technology allow definitive care for conditions in a simpler fashion with less risk and expense than ever before. Radiofrequency loop cervical conization, which is now done in the office setting, has or will soon replace the majority of in-hospital cervical conizations. This procedure may cost as little as 20% of in-hospital costs. Fiberoptic diagnoses allow for a more comprehensive evaluation and earlier diagnosis of cancer. More importantly, these diagnoses can now be made by the same physician who cares for the patient most of the time. These technological advances save lives, add to the quality of life, are cost effective, and decrease liability.

Interestingly, there is a wide variety of procedures currently being performed by primary care physicians. However, there is a large individual and geographic variation. These variations will no doubt diminish with the advent of managed care. It is well known that it is very cost effective to keep procedures in the hands of primary care physicians, yet there is no comprehensive text detailing the performance of these procedures. With our first attempt, this text is not yet perfect. We relied on authors from all over the country, and more than 80 authors contributed.

There is a wide range of style and practicality. The intent of the text is to give direction and to serve as a resource and brief review for a particular procedure—not to be all-inclusive in a single text.

The chapters in this book in no way intend to make the reader an expert at any procedure. It is a rare procedure that can be safely "learned from the book." The majority of procedures will be mastered by attending courses and then followed by a preceptor arrangement. The text merely combines and lists those procedures that primary care physicians perform, sometimes on a daily basis. The text may serve as a review for physicians and staff on those procedures that are not performed on a day-to-day basis.

Procedures for Primary Care Physicians will not be a static document. It will grow and change with time. The chapters will be refined and the contents revised to be more concise and direct. This can only happen through feedback from the readers. Suggestions from you, the reader, would be most appreciated. Submissions of new or even alternatives to current chapters are most welcome.

As the title states, this text is directed to primary care physicians—family and general practitioners, emergency physicians, pediatricians, obstetricians, internists, house officers, medical students, military medics, paramedics, nurse practitioners, and all other "primary care" providers. It is hoped that the contents will enhance the performance of procedures, improve patient care and satisfaction, and lead to greater physician self-fulfillment.

JOHN L. PFENNINGER, M.D.
GRANT C. FOWLER, M.D.

ACKNOWLEDGMENTS

The number of people to be thanked in a text of this magnitude is too great to allow mention of them all. Each, in his or her own way, has added greatly to its value. The special people who provided their support and encouragement include: Grant Fowler, M.D., for giving large blocks of his time and expertise—without his assistance, the text would be nowhere near completion; Len Scarpinato, D.O., for his editorial assistance; Barbara Apgar, M.D., for the moral support needed when the "going got rough"; Don DeWitt, M.D., for encouraging the vision; Pat Wolfgram, the hospital librarian, for retrieving the voluminous number of reference articles; Joan Haddix, Joi Henton, and Shirley Marsh, for their typing assistance; and Beth Moe, Denise Willard, and Linda Hallman for their secretarial skills. To Ted Huff, I give my sincere thanks for developing educational diagrams out of what were sometimes mere scratchings of the pen. A sincere thanks goes to Cindy Trickel of Carlisle Publishers Services, who provided invaluable editorial guidance in converting thoughts into words.

A special thanks also goes to all the family physicians in Midland, Michigan. They not only provided after-hours coverage for me, but also provided the encouragement to continue on through many personal crises. My office staff and nurses also deserve my gratitude.

Each and every author of this book also deserves special recognition. There were many refusals to assist in this project because of over-commitment and lack of belief in the project. For those authors who did contribute, it meant extra sacrifice and dedication. They participated in a dream that has now come to fruition.

To all of these, a sincere thank-you.

JOHN L. PFENNINGER, M.D.

A special thanks to the residents, faculty, and staff of the Hermann/LBJ Family Practice Program and the Department of Family Practice and Community Medicine at the University of Texas Houston Health Science Center–Medical School for their contributions, patience, and encouragement—without which this book might not have happened.

GRANT C. FOWLER, M.D.

CONTENTS

PART ONE   DERMATOLOGY   1

1 / **Suture Selection   3**
William Jackson Epperson

2 / **Needle Selection for Laceration and Incision Repair   7**
William Jackson Epperson

3 / **Laceration Repair   12**
George Snell

4 / **Skin Biopsy   20**
George Snell

5 / **Approach to Various Skin Lesions   27**
John L. Pfenninger
Thomas J. Zuber

6 / **Treatment of Ingrown Toenails   38**
James F. Peggs

7 / **Nail Plate and Nail Bed Biopsy   44**
James F. Peggs

8 / **Subungual Hematoma Evacuation   47**
James F. Peggs

9 / **Incision and Drainage of an Abscess   50**
Daniel J. Derksen

10 / **Acne Therapy   54**
Thomas J. Zuber
John L. Pfenninger

11 / **Treatment of Hypertrophic Scars and Keloids   58**
Thomas J. Zuber
John L. Pfenninger

12 / Sclerotherapy   63
John R. Pfeifer

13 / Unna Paste Boot   78
Donald E. DeWitt

14 / Wood's Light Examination   81
Donald E. DeWitt

15 / Laser Therapy   84
James E. Rasmussen
John L. Pfenninger

16 / Radiofrequency Surgery   91
Donald E. DeWitt
John L. Pfenninger

17 / Cryosurgery   102
John E. Hocutt, Jr.

18 / Ring Removal from an Edematous Finger   121
John Harlan Haynes III

19 / Tick Removal   125
John Harlan Haynes III

20 / Fishhook Removal   128
John Harlan Haynes III

PART TWO   ANESTHESIA   133

21 / Local Anesthesia   135
Daniel J. Derksen
John L. Pfenninger

22 / Topical Anesthesia   141
William Dery

23 / Peripheral Nerve Blocks and Field Blocks   145
Julie Graves Moy
John L. Pfenninger

24 / Pediatric Sedation   156
David B. Bosscher

25 / Bier Block   160
Robert Williams

26 / Technique of Trigger Point Injection   164
Gary E. Ruoff

27 / Oral/Facial Anesthesia   168
Richard J. Bakeman

PART THREE   EYES, EARS, NOSE, AND THROAT   177

28 / Audiometry   179
Gregory J. Forzley

29 / Auricular Hematoma Evacuation   184
Gregory J. Forzley

30 / Myringotomy   188
Gregory J. Forzley

31 / Cerumen Impaction Removal   192
Gregory J. Forzley
Gary R. Newkirk

32 / Tympanometry   197
Gregory J. Forzley

33 / Ear Piercing   202
Gregory J. Forzley

34 / Removal of Foreign Bodies from the Ear and Nose   206
John Harlan Haynes III
Gary R. Newkirk

35 / Chalazion and Hordeolum Therapy   214
Lewis E. Mehl

**36 / Corneal Abrasions and Removal of Corneal or Conjunctival   221
Foreign Bodies**
Grant C. Fowler

37 / Visual Function Evaluation   231
Fred D. Catrett
Malcolm L. Mazow

38 / **Tonometry**   237
John M. Boltri

39 / **Management of Epistaxis**   242
Nancy V. Schantz

40 / **Flexible Fiberoptic Rhinolaryngoscopy**   249
Grant C. Fowler

41 / **Indirect Laryngoscopy**   260
Grant C. Fowler

42 / **Nasogastric Tube and Salem Sump Insertion**   264
Julie Graves Moy

43 / **Emergency Cricothyroidotomy and Tracheostomy**   270
Nancy V. Schantz

44 / **Reduction of Dislocated Temporomandibular Joint**   279
Richard J. Bakeman
Grant C. Fowler

45 / **Reimplantation of an Avulsed Tooth**   283
Richard J. Bakeman
Grant C. Fowler

46 / **Tongue-Tie Snipping (Frenotomy) for Ankyloglossia**   287
Gary R. Newkirk

PART FOUR   CARDIOVASCULAR AND RESPIRATORY   291

47 / **Percutaneous Arterial Line Placement**   293
Grant C. Fowler

48 / **Central Venous Catheter Insertion**   300
John F. Donnelly
John M. Passmore, Jr.

49 / **Swan-Ganz Catheterization**   319
Len Scarpinato

50 / **Venous Cutdown**   332
Grant C. Fowler

51 / **Arterial Puncture**   340
Grant C. Fowler

52 / Noninvasive Venous and Arterial Studies of the Lower Extremities   348
Grant C. Fowler

53 / Ambulatory Blood Pressure Monitoring   369
Peter Hanson
Diane Lillis

54 / Holter Monitoring   378
Ken Grauer

55 / Office Electrocardiograms   408
Mark E. Clasen
Grant C. Fowler

56 / Stress Testing   413
Terrence L. Meece

57 / Cardioversion   437
Thomas J. Zuber
John L. Pfenninger

58 / Chest Tube Insertion   444
Nelly A. Otero

59 / Endotracheal Intubation   452
Len Scarpinato

60 / Temporary Pacing   464
Len Scarpinato

61 / Thoracentesis   477
Terry S. Ruhl

62 / Pulmonary Function Testing   485
Edward A. Jackson

PART FIVE   URINARY AND MALE REPRODUCTIVE   493

63 / Bladder Catheterization   495
Robert E. James
James R. Palleschi

64 / Suprapubic Catheter Insertion/Change   500
Robert E. James
James R. Palleschi

65 / Suprapubic Taps or Aspirations   504
Robert E. James
James R. Palleschi

66 / Basic Urodynamic Studies for Urinary Incontinence   508
J. Christopher Hough

67 / Androscopy   514
John L. Pfenninger

68 / Vasectomy   520
George C. Denniston
John L. Pfenninger

69 / Prostate Massage   541
Robert E. James
James R. Palleschi

70 / Adult Circumcision   544
Donald E. DeWitt

71 / Self-Injection Therapy for the Treatment of Impotence   550
Robert E. James
James R. Palleschi

PART SIX   GYNECOLOGY AND FEMALE REPRODUCTIVE   557

72 / Diagnostic Hysteroscopy   559
Barbara S. Apgar

73 / Endometrial Biopsy   563
Barbara S. Apgar

74 / Hysterosalpingography   571
Steven Fettinger

75 / IUD Insertion   578
John L. Pfenninger

76 / IUD Removal   586
John L. Pfenninger

77 / Culdocentesis (Colpocentesis)   588
Steven H. Eisinger

78 / Bartholin's Cyst/Abscess: Word Catheter Insertion   596
Barbara S. Apgar

79 / The Pap Smear: Screening for Cervical Cancer   601
Gary R. Newkirk

80 / HPV-DNA Testing of the Cervix   613
Gary R. Newkirk

81 / The Colposcopic Examination   616
Gary R. Newkirk

82 / Cervical Conization   640
Lydia A. Watson

83 / Crycone of the Cervix   645
John E. Hocutt, Jr.

84 / Treatment of Vulvar, Perianal, Vaginal, Penile, and Urethral Condyloma Acuminata   653
Barbara S. Apgar
John L. Pfenninger

85 / Postcoital Examination Test or Sims-Huhner Test   666
Barbara S. Apgar

86 / Wet Smear and KOH Preparation   669
Barbara S. Apgar

87 / Dilation and Curettage   672
Timothy A. Curran

88 / Permanent Female Sterilization (Tubal Ligation)   678
Gary R. Newkirk

89 / First-Trimester Abortion   699
Steven H. Eisinger

90 / Breast Biopsy   714
Hugh H. Hogle

91 / Contraceptive Implants (Norplant)   718
John L. Pfenninger

92 / Loop Electrosurgical Excision Procedure (LEEP) for Treating CIN   729
Thomas C. Wright
Ralph M. Richart

93 / Barrier Contraceptives: Cervical Cap, Condom, and Contraceptive Sponge   742
Barry D. Weiss

94 / Diaphragm Fitting   750
Barbara S. Apgar

95 / Cervicography   757
Richard C. Cherkis

PART SEVEN   OBSTETRICS   763

96 / Amniocentesis   765
Clark B. Smith

97 / Spontaneous Fetal-Movement Counting   773
Steve Ratcliffe

98 / The Nonstress Test   776
Steve Ratcliffe

99 / Contraction Stress Test   781
Steve Ratcliffe

100 / Episiotomy   785
Donald N. Marquardt

101 / Pudendal Anesthesia   794
Donald N. Marquardt

102 / Paracervical Block   799
Scott T. Henderson

103 / Cervical Ripening/Vaginal Prostaglandins   803
Scott T. Henderson

104 / Obstetric Ultrasound   807
Richard Brunader

PART EIGHT   **PEDIATRICS**   **829**

105 / **Intraosseous Venous Access**   **831**
Kelly T. Locke

106 / **Neonatal Resuscitation**   **841**
Marvin Dewar

107 / **Umbilical Artery Catheterization**   **847**
James A. Sterling

108 / **Suprapubic Bladder Aspiration**   **852**
Marvin Dewar

109 / **DeLee Suctioning**   **855**
David B. Bosscher

110 / **Pediatric Arterial Puncture and Venous Cutdown**   **858**
Gregg K. Phillips

111 / **Newborn Circumcision**   **863**
S. Shevaun Duiker
Grant C. Fowler

112 / **Dorsal Penile Nerve Block**   **874**
Grant C. Fowler
S. Shevaun Duiker

PART NINE   **GASTROINTESTINAL**   **879**

113 / **Inguinal Hernia Reduction**   **881**
George G. Zainea

114 / **Gastric Lavage**   **884**
John Harlan Haynes III

115 / **Abdominal Paracentesis and Peritoneal Lavage**   **892**
Michael L. Brown

116 / **Clinical Anorectal Anatomy and Examination**   **898**
James A. Surrell

117 / **Anoscopy**   **902**
Jay R. Varma

118 / Flexible Sigmoidoscopy   907
Jay R. Varma
John L. Pfenninger

119 / Office Treatment of Hemorrhoids   929
George Zainea
Gayle Randall
Daniel A. Norman
John L. Pfenninger

120 / Perianal Skin Tags (External Hemorrhoidal Skin Tags)   954
James A. Surrell

121 / Anal Fissure/Lateral Sphincterotomy   958
James A. Surrell

122 / Pilonidal Cyst/Abscess Incision and Drainage   964
James A. Surrell

123 / Perianal Abscess Incision and Drainage   969
James A. Surrell

124 / Diagnostic Esophagogastroduodenoscopy (EGD)   974
Donald M. Gelb
John L. Pfenninger
George Villanueva
Elizabeth A. Roaf

125 / Colonoscopy   992
James A. Surrell

PART TEN   ORTHOPEDICS   1001

126 / Ankle Splinting, Taping, and Casting   1003
Jeffrey R. Kovan
Douglas B. McKeag

127 / Cast Immobilization   1014
Scott W. Eathorne
Douglas B. McKeag

128 / Shoulder Dislocations   1028
Fred M. Hankin

129 / Nursemaid's Elbow: Subluxation of the Radial Head   1033
Fred M. Hankin
James L. Telfer

130 / Joint and Soft Tissue Aspiration and Injection   1036
John L. Pfenninger

131 / Extensor Tendon Repair   1055
Thomas J. Zuber
John L. Pfenninger

132 / Orthoses, Plantar Warts, Corns, and Calluses   1060
Joseph Ellis

PART ELEVEN   MISCELLANEOUS   1065

133 / Antibiotic Prophylaxis for Bacterial Endocarditis   1067
John L. Pfenninger

134 / Informed Consent   1071
Julie Graves Moy

135 / Anaphylaxis   1076
Daniel J. Derksen

136 / Heimlich Maneuver   1080
Raymond E. Jarris, Jr.

137 / Topical Hemostatic Agents   1084
Thomas J. Zuber
John L. Pfenninger

138 / Wound Dressing   1090
William Dery

139 / Allergy Testing   1096
Gailen D. Marshall

140 / Fine-Needle Aspiration Cytology and Biopsy   1102
Lee Green

141 / Lumbar Puncture   1109
John O'Brien

142 / Bone Marrow Aspiration and Biopsy   1115
John O'Brien

143 / Muscle Biopsy   1120
Lori Crago

144 / Emergency Department Ultrasound   1123
Grant C. Fowler
Dietrich Jehle

PART ONE

Dermatology

CHAPTER 1

Suture Selection

William Jackson Epperson

Numerous suture types have been developed that are best suited for a variety of tissue properties in the body. The qualities most important for suture include flexibility, strength, secure knotting, and low propensity for contribution to infection. The goal of suturing is to maintain the approximation of tissues securely until healing allows for tissue strength to be maintained alone.

The two main categories of suture are *absorbable* and *nonabsorbable*. All types of suture are foreign to the body; therefore, the degree with which the body reacts against the suture is an important consideration in suture choice.

Suture size is indicated by using a "0," with the more "0s" designating smaller-sized suture (e.g., 4-0 is smaller than 3-0). Suture materials are standardized by specific regulations, which assures consistent width and tensile strength.

Absorbable suture is a sterile strand of synthetic polymer or mammalian-derived collagen. The rate of absorption and the duration of tensile strength are important considerations. For example, the suture may lose effective strength long before it has been absorbed. Various coatings and materials have been developed to prolong the tensile-strength retention of absorbable suture. These coatings also aid in the passage of suture through tissue by decreasing friction.

The *natural absorbable suture* (*mammalian collagen* or *"gut" sutures*) are derived mainly from the submucosa of sheep intestine, the serosa of beef intestine, or the flexor tendons of beef. They are available in plain or chromic (coated with chromic salts to help delay reabsorption). Tensile strength is determined by the percent of collagen in the gut suture. Any noncollagen materials within the gut suture can cause severe tissue reactions, so purity of the protein is very important.

Common *synthetic absorbable* suture materials include polyglactic acid (Vicryl), polyglycolic acid (Dexon), and polydioxanone (PDS). These materials have the desirable property of extended time of tensile strength (Fig. 1-1).

Nonabsorbable suture is used for skin and also for permanent internal placement such as in cardiovascular, orthopedic, and plastic surgery. Many raw materials

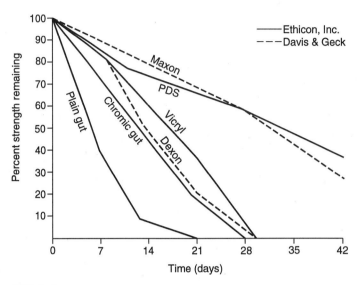

FIG. 1-1.
In vivo strength retention of absorbable sutures.

are used, including silk, cotton, stainless steel, nylon, polyester, and polypropylene. Table 1-1 reviews the various features of each of these sutures.

Nonabsorbable sutures are removed from the skin when no longer needed. With vascular and orthopedic applications there is often a need for more permanent materials that retain their tensile strength for a longer time. Tendon repair requires prolonged healing time and needs long-term tensile strength to give adequate time for self-repair. Vascular grafts must have the support of suture for an indefinite period of time. The anastamosis of the graft and a blood vessel is never secured by the fibroblast and collagen of the body alone.

Braided suture adds strength and helps to secure the knotting, but the negative side is it is more likely to harbor infection. *Monofilament* is better to use in the presence of infection, but its knots are less dependable. Tissue reaction is very important in delicate tissues where scar and fissure formation may be a problem, which is why gut suture may not be a good choice for use on the face.

Knots are an important consideration in terms of whether they remain tied and, therefore, do not cause a significant reduction in the strength of the suture material. The knot is the weakest part of the completed suture ligature. Proper knotting technique requires the application of a square knot or double loop followed by a square knot tie. Oftentimes knots are accomplished as half-hitches that are weak and do not remain secure. The more friction a suture has, the less likely it is to incur slippage and loss of the knot's integrity. Braided suture knots rarely slip, while monofilament often comes untied in the absence of proper knotting technique.

Each surgeon will have his or her own choice of suture based on training and individual preferences. No one type of suture choice is always correct. Through

TABLE 1-1.
Common Suture Materials

Suture	Types	Make-up	Usage	Tissue Reaction	Absorption Rate	Tensile Strength Retention
Absorbable						
Gut	Plain	Mammalian collagen	Superficial vessels and quick healing subcutaneous tissues	Moderate	70 days	7 to 10 days
Gut	Chromic	Mammalian collagen	Versatile; also good in the presence of infection; do not use on skin because of reaction	Moderate	90 days	21 to 28 days
Polyglycolic acid (Dexon*)	Mono	Synthetic polymer	Buried sutures; good tensile and knot strength	Mild	40% 7 days	20% in 15 days 5% in 28 days
Polydioxanone (PDS†)	Mono	Polyester polymer	Versatile; body cavity closure, bowel	Mild	210 days	70% in 14 days 50% in 28 days
Polyglactic acid (Vicryl†)	Braided	Coated polymer	Subcutaneous skin; buried sutures	Mild	60 to 90 days	60% in 14 days 30% in 21 days
Polyglyconate (Maxon)	Mono	Polyester	Smoother knot and excellent first-throw holding	Mild	180 to 210 days	81% in 14 days 59% in 28 days
Nonabsorbable						
Cotton	Twisted fibers	Cotton fiber	Ligating, some skin but generally too reactive	Minimal	Never; encapsulated in the body	50% in 6 months 30% in 2 years
Silk	Braided	Silkworm spun fiber	Ligating, some skin but rarely used	Moderate	2 years	Gone in one year
Steel	Mono	Alloy Fe-Ni-Cr	Tendons, sternum, abdominal wall	Low	Never; encapsulated in the body	Indefinite
Nylon (Ethilon, Dermalon)	Mono	Synthetic polymer	Skin	Very low	20% a year	Loses 20% a year
Polyester (Mersilene)	Braided	Polyester	Cardiovascular, general, and plastic surgery	Minimal	Never; encapsulated in the body	Indefinite
Polypropylene (Prolene†)	Mono	Synthetic polymer	Skin, vascular, plastic surgery	Minimal	Never; encapsulated in the body	Indefinite

*Dexon Plus has a synthetic coating to facilitate knot tying and passage through tissue.
†Vicryl, Prolene, and PDS are registered trademarks of Ethicon, Inc.

TABLE 1-2.

Common Suture Use

	Skin (Interrupted)	Skin (Subcuticular)	Buried	Removal
Face	5-0 or 6-0 nylon	4-0 or 5-0 Prolene	4-0 or 5-0 synthetic absorbable or 6-0 clear nylon	4 to 7 days
Extremities, trunk	4-0 or 5-0 nylon	3-0 or 4-0 synthetic absorbable	4-0 Prolene or 3-0 or 4-0 synthetic absorbable	7 to 14 days

application of the appropriate suture characteristics to the various applications in the body's tissues, the ease of operation will lead to an acceptable result.

Table 1-2 generalizes some recommendations for suture commonly used in an office setting.

CPT/BILLING CODES

CPT codes for dermatologic procedures involving the use of suture are numerous and must be reviewed carefully for appropriate reimbursement. For excision of benign lesions, code numbers 11200 through 11471 are used. Malignant lesions are coded from 11600 to 11646. Laceration repair is coded based on length and severity. Simple lacerations are coded 12001 to 12021, intermediate lacerations are coded 12031 to 12057, and complex cases are coded from 13100 to 13300. The use of skin flaps and graft repairs and for surgery on specific areas of the skin, such as the eyelids, will require other more specific codes for proper documentation.

BIBLIOGRAPHY

Moy RL, Waldman B, Hein DW: A review of sutures and suturing techniques, *J Dermatol Surg Oncol* 18:785, 1992.

Moy RL, Lee A, Zolka A: Commonly used suture materials in skin surgery, *Am Fam Physician* 4(6):2123, 1991.

Postlethwait RW et al: Human tissue reaction to suture, *Ann Surg* 181(2):144, 1975.

Schwartz SI et al, editors: *Principles of surgery,* ed 4, New York, 1984, McGraw-Hill.

Van Winkle W, Hastings JC: Considerations in the choice of suture materials for various tissues, *Surg Gynecol Obstet* 135:114, 1972.

Way LW: *Current surgical diagnosis & treatment,* ed 9, Norwalk, Conn, 1991, Appleton & Lange.

Wound closure manual, Somerville, N.J., 1985, Ethicon.

CHAPTER 2

Needle Selection for Laceration and Incision Repair

William Jackson Epperson

There are dozens of needle types that have been developed for specific surgical needs. The needle facilitates the appropriate placement of suture. Inappropriate needle selection can damage the tissues, causing poor results and delayed healing. For example, a tapered point is needed in suturing the bowel, where prevention of leakage is imperative. A cutting needle would never be appropriate in the reanastomosis of bowel or blood vessels.

Most needles are made of noncorrosive stainless steel. Through a process of heating the metal, maximal strength and ductility (the ability to bend under pressure without breaking) are achieved. Each needle type is sharpened to a varying degree depending on its usage. Also, to assist with passage through tissue, most needles receive a thin silicone coat.

NEEDLE DESIGN

The surgical needle is composed of an eye, a body, and a point (Fig. 2-1). There are three types of needle eyes—the closed eye, the French (split or spring) eye, and the swaged eye.

The *closed eye* is that commonly seen in the sewing needle. The closed-eye needle may be round, square, or oval. *French-eyed* needles have a longitudinal slit at the eye with internal ridges that catch and hold the suture in place. Both closed-eyed and French-eyed needles must be threaded. This threading is time consuming, and the unthreading of needles may often occur at an inopportune moment during a procedure. Tying the suture to a closed-eye needle increases the diameter of the eye being pulled through tissue, which can lead to unwanted results (Fig. 2-2). A *swaged eye,* where the metal is literally molded around the suture, alleviates most needle-to-suture problems and prevents the repeated use of a dull or contaminated needle.

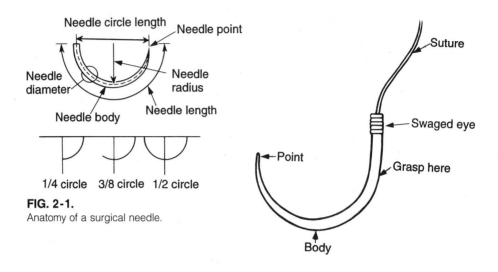

FIG. 2-1.
Anatomy of a surgical needle.

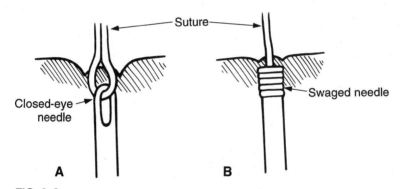

FIG. 2-2.
A, Tissue disruption caused by double-suture strand with closed-eyed needle. **B,** Tissue disruption minimized by single-suture strand swaged to needle.

The *body* of the needle is important for both strength and grasping by the needle holder. Various shapes of the body are important for added strength as well as for matching the flow of the needle through the tissues as directed by the point. A flattened body with concave or convex surfaces helps to reduce unwanted needle rotation when suturing. The shape of the body of the needle allows for a variety of uses (Fig. 2-3).

Needle *points* are the most important needle consideration. The basic types include cutting, tapered, and blunt, and most needles have a mixed variety of these features (Fig. 2-4).

The two opposing edges of a cutting needle allow for easy passage through tough tissues. This makes cutting needles ideal for suturing skin, with its dense supporting structures. However, these cutting edges have their drawbacks when it

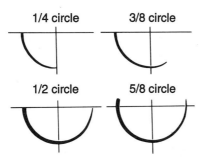

FIG. 2-3.
Needle body shapes.

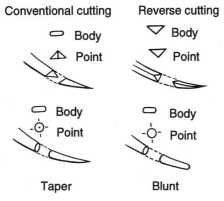

FIG. 2-4.
Needle points and body shapes.

comes to tendons and oral mucous membranes, which are easily damaged by overcutting.

The *conventional cutting* needle has a cutting edge on its inside or concave curvature. The inside cutting in the direction of force is a negative characteristic of this needle. The suture force tends to concentrate at the apex of the triangle, and tissues outside of the desired suture channel are cut. For this reason, it is used less frequently than the reverse cutting needle.

The *reverse cutting* needle has its cutting edge on the outer curvature of the needle. This gives a flat surface along the inner edge, thereby reducing the incidence of suture pulling through tissues into the margin of the wound. Unless specified otherwise, a "cutting needle" now refers to a "reverse cutting" design.

Taper cut or *round needles* have an oval body to reduce twisting in the needle holder. These points are useful in less dense tissues that require small holes and minimal tissue injury, such as in fascia and bowel.

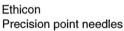

Ethicon
Precision point needles

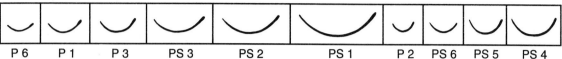

P 6   P 1   P 3   PS 3   PS 2   PS 1   P 2   PS 6   PS 5   PS 4

Precision cosmetic needles

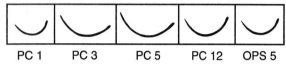

PC 1   PC 3   PC 5   PC 12   OPS 5

Davis & Geck

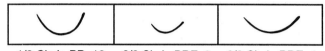

1/2 Circle PR–13   3/8 Circle PRE–2   3/8 Circle PRE–4

FIG. 2-5.
Ethicon and Davis and Geck needle nomenclature for facial closures (actual sizes).

The *blunt point* needle is used in friable parenchymal tissue, such as tissues of the liver and kidney. This point allows for dissection through tissue, avoiding the trauma of cutting.

Many terms have been developed by suture manufacturers to categorize their products for different purposes and to denote their size. For skin (FS) and cutting (CE) needles should be used on thick skin. On cosmetic areas, plastic (P), plastic skin (PS), premium (PRE), or precision cosmetic (PC) needles are recommended. Generally, a three-eighths curvature is adequate for most cutaneous procedures (Fig. 2-5).

Generally, a larger needle is used for deep buried sutures, while a smaller needle can be used to close the skin. Location of closure is also important. For instance, facial closures are often done with a P-3 needle, while other areas with thicker skin will require an FS-2 or FS-3. It is important to review the descriptions on the suture packet. Oftentimes, a picture of the needle can aid in proper selection.

Needles should be handled only with needle holders, otherwise damage to the needles may occur. The needle holder size must match that of the needle. The needle should be grasped below the swaged eye, but beyond the middle body region (Fig. 2-1). The swaged metal must be sufficiently soft to wrap around the suture; therefore, if it is grasped here, it bends easily. The body of the needle is firm, not malleable, and is less likely to bend. The tip of the needle holder should just cover the needle, and the handle should be closed only to the first or second ratchet. During needle placement, the force must be advanced in the direction of the curvature of the needle.

CONCLUSION

Often, one may find that an ordinary suturing procedure becomes more difficult than expected. This difficulty can often be improved by reassessing the appropriateness of the instruments being used. Needle selection is often a key factor in facilitating the ease of the operation and ultimate good surgical results.

BIBLIOGRAPHY

Moy RL, Waldman B, Hein DW: A review of sutures and suturing techniques, *J Dermatol Surg Oncol* 18:785, 1992.

Schwartz SI et al, editors: *Principles of surgery,* ed 4, New York, 1984, McGraw-Hill.

Tier WC: Considerations in the choice of surgical needles, *Surg Gynecol Obstet* 149:84, 1979.

Way LW: *Current surgical diagnosis & treatment,* ed 9, Norwalk, Conn, 1991, Appleton & Lange.

Wound closure manual, Somerville, N.J., 1985, Ethicon.

CHAPTER 3

Laceration Repair

George Snell

Lacerations are a commonly seen problem in physicians' offices, urgent-care centers, and hospital emergency rooms. They are seldom life-threatening, but since most are sustained traumatically they are often associated with substantial emotional upset on the part of the patient, parent, or accompanying party. Calmness, as well as competent and thorough treatment, is often the best management course for both the tissue and emotional trauma.

There are four goals of primary wound closure:

1. Stop bleeding
2. Prevent infection
3. Preserve function
4. Restore appearance

These goals should be kept in mind by the physician who is handling tissues and assisting nature's healing processes. The stages of wound-healing should be known by the physician providing care for lacerations; discussions can be found in references at the end of the chapter.

EQUIPMENT

- Prep pack containing eight to ten 4 × 4 inch gauze sponges in metal prep basin wrapped for sterilization
- Suture pack (double wrap for sterilization) containing: sterile drape (to be placed under lesion if needed); fenestrated drape (applied over the lesion); 6-inch plastic needle holder (Fig. 3-1); curved dissecting scissors (Fig. 3-1); two mosquito hemostats—one curved, one straight; suture scissors; six 4 × 4 inch gauze sponges; Adson toothed forceps (Fig. 3-1); and medicine cup
- Skin hooks (Fig. 3-2): Used for atraumatic tissue handling, "homemade" from a 1 cc insulin syringe plus a 25-gauge needle (A commercially manufactured instrument is also available.)

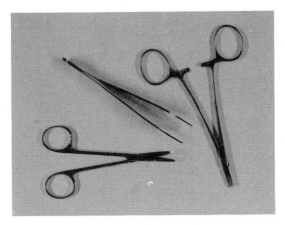

FIG. 3-1.
Suture pack items:

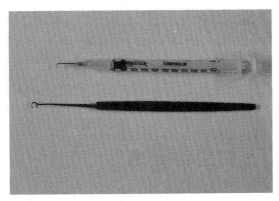

FIG. 3-2.
Homemade and commercial skin hooks.

INITIAL ASSESSMENT AND LOCAL ANESTHESIA

Many wounds can be examined and cleansed without anesthesia. However, to provide the patient prompt comfort and allow for a thorough examination, it is often helpful to anesthetize the wound before treatment. (See Chapter 21, Local Anesthesia.) The initial evaluation before anesthesia, however, should include an assessment of any peripheral nerve damage and motor function disturbance.

WOUND PREPARATION

Following the initial assessment and administration of local anesthetic, wounds should be thoroughly inspected for foreign bodies, deep tissue layer damage, and

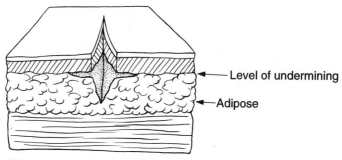

FIG. 3-3.
Site to undermine skin.

injury to nerve, vessel, or tendon. Cleansing of the wound can be accomplished by mechanical and chemical means. Mechanical methods include wiping, brushing, and irrigation. Copious saline irrigation is probably best accomplished by forcing saline through a 18- to 22-gauge needle with a 25 cc syringe. Chemical cleansing is less important, but it is often accomplished with antiseptic soaps that contain hexachlorophene (pHisohex), chlorhexidine gluconate (Hibiclens), or povidone-iodine (Betadine).

Following the cleansing process, wounds should be examined for devitalized tissue that needs removal or debridement. This debridement may convert a jagged, contaminated wound into a clean surgical one and can be accomplished with a scalpel or sharp tissue scissors.

After debridement, wound edges should be held together to see if they are under any tension. Skin mobility can be increased by undermining. A scissors or scalpel should be used for undermining, which is done in the subcutaneous plane beneath the dermis to allow the skin to glide together. (See Fig. 3-3 and the section on excisional skin biopsy in Chapter 4, Skin Biopsy.)

TECHNIQUE

Ideally, there are three principles that should be incorporated in the process of closing any wound (see Figs. 3-4 and 3-5).

1. Eliminate dead space where tissue fluid and blood can accumulate.
2. Accurately approximate tissue layers to each other, including fat/fascial junction, dermal/fat junction, and epidermal margins.
3. Approximate the wound with minimal tension. Lacerations are approximated using a variety of suturing techniques:
   Simple interrupted dermal suture (Fig. 3-6). Keep the skin margins level or slightly everted. The needle should enter the skin surface at a right angle. The final stitch should be as wide as the suture is deep. The opposite skin margin is approximated using the mirror image of the placement of the first part of that suture, and the distance from the suture's exit to the wound margin should

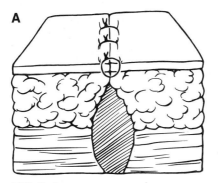
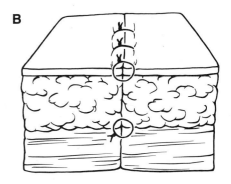

FIG. 3-4.
A, Improper and **B,** proper wound closures.

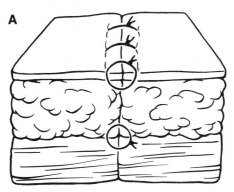
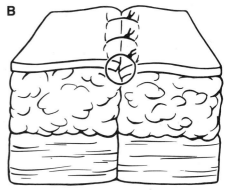

FIG. 3-5.
A, Proper tissue apposition and **B,** inappropriate excess tightness.

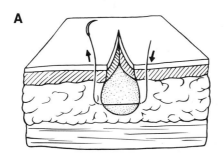
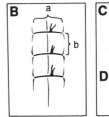
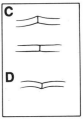

FIG. 3-6.
Interrupted dermal suture. **A,** Proper depth; **B,** Proper spacing (a=b); **C,** Proper final appearance; **D,** Improper final appearance.

equal the distance from the suture's point of entry to the wound margin. The final shape should appear like an Erlenmeyer flask. As a general rule, these sutures need to be no closer than 2 mm apart in a fine plastic closure and can be substantially farther apart in other types of closures. Avoid tying the knots too tight. The distance between sutures should equal the total distance across the incision (Fig. 3-6, *B*).

Subcutaneous suture with inverted knot or "buried stitch" (Fig. 3-7). Deeper wounds or wounds under tension are best closed by not relying solely on dermal sutures. A well-placed subcutaneous suture can do much to aid in closing a wound and removes tension from the skin sutures. Absorbable sutures are usually used for this purpose; however, for facial wounds, a clear monofilament synthetic suture material can be used and will help eliminate an inflammatory reaction or subsequent rejection of the suture. The inverted knot technique places the bulk of the knot below the skin margins to be approximated. To start the stitch, begin at the bottom of the wound and come up. Go straight across the incision then down to the base once again and tie (thus placing the knot most inferior in the wound). The wound may need to be closed in multiple layers as shown in Fig. 3-7.

Vertical mattress suture (Fig. 3-8). This suture promotes eversion of the skin and is helpful when considerable skin tension is present or where the skin is very thick, such as in the palms and soles. It is also useful where the natural tendency of the loose skin is to promote inversion of the wound margins.

Intracuticular running suture (Fig. 3-9). This suture is used to close linear wounds that are not under much tension and yields an excellent cosmetic result. The ends of the suture do not need to be tied; taping under slight tension will preserve approximation.

Three-point or half-buried mattress suture (Fig. 3-10). This suture is designed to permit closure of the acute corner of a laceration without impairing blood flow to the tip. It is an intradermal stitch in which the needle is inserted initially into the skin on the nonflap portion of the wound at the mid-dermis

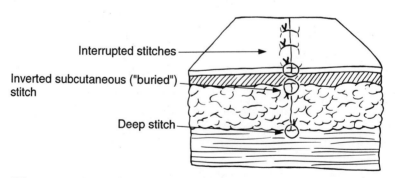

Interrupted stitches

Inverted subcutaneous ("buried") stitch

Deep stitch

FIG. 3-7.
Inverted subcutaneous suture. Also shown is layered closure.

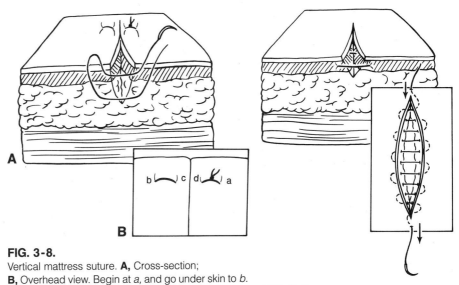

FIG. 3-8.
Vertical mattress suture. **A,** Cross-section;
B, Overhead view. Begin at *a,* and go under skin to *b.*
Come out, go in at *c,* and exit at *d.*

FIG. 3-9.
Intracuticular running suture.

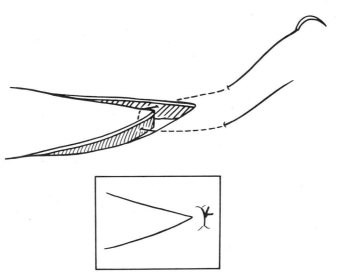

FIG. 3-10.
Three-point or half-buried mattress.

level; and then at the same level, the suture is passed transversely through the tip and returned on the opposite side of the wound paralleling the point of entrance. The suture is tied, drawing the tip snugly into place in good opposition. This same approach can be utilized in closing a stellate 4- or 5-point laceration, drawing the tips together in a purse-string fashion.

POSTPROCEDURE CARE

Most wounds are best protected with some sort of dressing during the first 24 to 48 hours after closure. Continued oozing might be expected or pressure might be needed. For hemostasis, a pressure dressing should be applied over a nonstick type of gauze dressing. Trade names for such dressings include Xeroderm, Adaptic, and Telfa. It is not usually necessary to keep a wound dry until the time of suture removal. Suggestions for the timing for suture removal are as follows:

Facial wounds: 3 to 5 days
Scalp and extremity wounds (not over mobile joints and chest): 7 to 8 days
Palms, soles, back, and skin over mobile joints, such as knees and elbows: 10 to 14 days

Wounds under considerable tension that are repaired may need to be splinted for optimal healing. Some wounds, such as those on the face or scalp, need not be covered at all. A quick check to inspect for evidence of infection or subcutaneous bleeding is sometimes necessary 2 or 3 days following closure and may serve as an indicator of the physician's concern and care. A wound instruction handout can be given; a sample one is seen in Box 3-1.

**BOX 3-1. PATIENT EDUCATION HANDOUT
CARE OF SUTURED LACERATIONS**

1. Keep wound and dressing clean. You may shower. Do not expose the wound to moisture for prolonged periods of time.
2. **Wet Dressing:** If the dressing gets wet, remove it, blot the wound dry with a sterile gauze pad, and reapply a clean, dry dressing, e.g., a sterile gauze pad.
3. **Dressing Changes:** Remove the dressing applied after two days and reapply a sterile dressing. Repeat this procedure every day until the stitches are removed, unless instructed otherwise.
4. **Signs of Infection:** If any of the following signs of infection appear, contact a physician immediately:
   a. Wound becomes red, swollen, tender or warm.
   b. Wound begins to drain or fester.
   c. Red streaks appear around the wound.
   d. Tender lumps appear in the groin or under the arm.
   e. Chills or fever occur.
5. **Infection Check:** Because of the nature of your injury, the possibility of infection is increased. Please return to be checked in____days.
6. **Stitch Removal:** The physician suggests that the stitches be removed in about ____days.
7. **Tetanus Immunization:** For your records, you/your child received the following:
   a. Tetanus Toxoid____
   b. DT (Diptheria-Tetanus)____
   c. DPT (Diptheria-Pertussis-Tetanus)____
   d. Other____

TABLE 3-1.

Summary Guide to Tetanus Prophylaxis in Routine Wound Management

History of absorbed tetanus toxoid (doses)	Clean, minor wounds		All other wounds*	
	Td[†]	TIG	Td[†]	TIG
Unknown or < three	Yes	No	Yes	Yes
≥ Three[‡]	No[§]	No	No[‖]	No

Source: Centers for Disease Control *MMWR* 1991:40, No. Rr-10, 1-28.

*Such as, but not limited to, wounds contaminated with dirt, feces, soil, and saliva; puncture wounds; avulsions; and wounds resulting from missiles, crushing, burns and frostbite.

[†]For children <7 years old; DTP (DT, if pertussis vaccine is contraindicated) is preferred to tetanus toxoid alone. For persons ≥7 years of age, Td is preferred to tetanus toxoid alone.

[‡]If only three doses of *fluid* toxoid have been received, then a fourth dose of toxoid, preferably an absorbed toxoid, should be given.

[§]Yes, if >10 years since last dose.

[‖]Yes, if >5 years since last dose. (More frequent boosters are not needed and can accentuate side effects.)

CONCURRENT TREATMENT

- Tetanus prophylaxis: Table 3-1 is a summary guide to tetanus prophylaxis. "TIG" is tetanus immune globulin.
- Prophylactic antibiotics are indicated in the following circumstances:
    Probable contamination from trauma source
    Animal or human bite wounds
    A preexisting medical condition that subjects the patient to increased risk of infection and possible bacteremia; e.g., valvular heart disease, diabetes
- Analgesic medication may need to be administered for a few days depending upon the extent of the trauma, the pain threshold of the patient, and the concerns of the family.

CPT/BILLING CODES

Billing codes for this procedure are too varied and beyond the scope of this text. The code depends on location, size, and type of closure. If undermining is done, and buried sutures are placed along with a cosmetic closure (multiple close interrupted or running subcuticular), the procedure should be charged as an intermediate or a complex closure.

BIBLIOGRAPHY

Breitenbach K, Bergera J: Principles and techniques of primary wound closure, *Prim Care* 13(3):411, 1986.

Moy RL et al: Commonly used surgical techniques in skin surgery, *Am Fam Physician* 44(5):1625, 1991.

Snell G: Surgical problems. In Taylor RB, editor: *Family medicine principles and practice,* ed 3, New York, 1994, Springer-Verlag.

CHAPTER 4

Skin Biopsy

George Snell

Most diagnoses of skin problems can be resolved with careful inspection and palpation. However, invasive biopsy may be needed for questionable diagnoses or for treatment. Biopsies can include partial dermal thickness procedures, such as shave or curettage biopsy, or full thickness sampling with punch or excisional biopsy. There are three important considerations:

1. The procedure needs to be done with the use of local anesthetic.
2. Sufficient tissue must be obtained for an accurate diagnosis. This often requires complete removal of the lesion.
3. Minimal scarring with little interference with function should be the end result.

INDICATIONS

- To make or confirm a diagnosis for definitive treatment
- To excise and thus cure the lesion
- To perform elective removal for cosmetic reasons

CONTRAINDICATIONS

- Infection at the site of proposed biopsy
- Bleeding disorder (or coagulopathy of sufficient consequence that hemostasis would be difficult)
- Allergy to local anesthetics (see Chapter 21)

EQUIPMENT

The prep pack and suture pack outlined in Chapter 3, Laceration Repair, may be needed in addition to the following:

- For punch biopsy: Although permanent punch biopsy instruments (2 mm through 10 mm) are available (Fig. 4-1, A), disposable punches are recom-

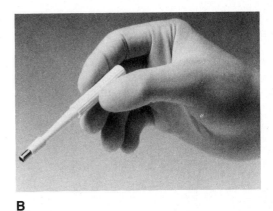

A

B

FIG. 4-1.
Permanent (**A**) and disposable (**B**) punch biopsy instruments. (**B,** Courtesy of Zinnanti Surgical Instruments, 21540-B Prairie St., Chatsworth, CA 91311, 800-223-4740.)

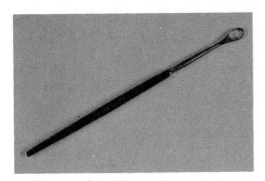

FIG. 4-2.
Fox dermal curette.

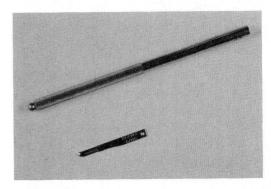

FIG. 4-3.
Beaver blade and handle.

mended (Fig. 4-1, *B*); pickups; sharp fine-tissue scissors (The most commonly used punch instrument sizes are 3 and 4 mm.)
- Fox dermal curette for curettage (Fig. 4-2)
- Beaver knife handle and blade No. 65 or No. 67 for excisional biopsies (Fig. 4-3) **or** BardParker blade No. 15c, a modification of the No. 15 BardParker blade (This blade makes finer excisions and can be used with the standard reusable BardParker scalpel handle.)

TECHNIQUE

Shave Biopsy

This technique removes elevated skin lesions in which a complete thickness of the skin is not necessary for either diagnosis or treatment. After an anesthetic wheal has been created intradermally, shave the lesion with a scalpel or excise it with dissecting scissors. When removing large lesions, it is best to go from one end to the

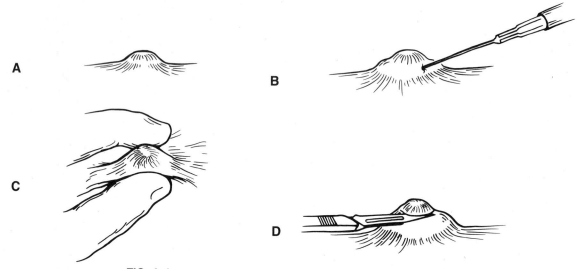

FIG. 4-4.
One technique of shave biopsy. **A,** Color the lesion to demarcate it clearly. **B,** Inject a local anesthetic to elevate the lesion. **C,** Roll the skin between thumb and forefinger to create a flat cutting surface and a tamponade effect on the surrounding blood vessels. **D,** With a No. 15 blade held parallel to the skin or at a slight downward angle, shave the lesion flush with or slightly below the surrounding skin.

center, then from the other end to center. This avoids a possible complication of cutting too deeply, which tends to occur when the lesion is removed all in one direction. Preserve the partial thickness of tissue for pathologic examination. The base of the wound can be treated with light electrodesiccation or chemical cautery with Monsel's solution. No suturing is necessary, and the wound should heal without scarring if only superficial layers of the dermis have been involved. (Also see Chapter 16, Radiofrequency Surgery.)

Biopsies of obviously benign intradermal or compound nevi, epithelial tags, and small basal cell carcinomas can be performed easily in this fashion. If melanoma is suspected, determining the depth of lesion is important, and *shave biopsies are contraindicated* (Fig. 4-4).

Curettage Biopsy

Curettage is another method for removing lesions that do not require full thickness skin sampling. After creating the anesthetic wheal, use the Fox curette to scrape away the tissue to be removed. Once again, electrodesiccation or chemical cautery can be applied to the base of the wound. Lesions amenable to this form of therapy include seborrheic keratoses, superficial basal cell carcinomas, and crusting actinic keratoses. Repeat curettements can be used if recurrences of the lesion occur.

Punch Biopsy

This method for taking full-thickness skin for examination can be used for excisional biopsy of skin lesions less than 5 mm in diameter. It can also be used as an incisional (partial removal) biopsy to obtain a diagnosis. Punch biopsies are not suitable for eyelids, lips, or penile lesions. If one is attempting to diagnose a systemic disease, the most recently developed lesions are more likely to yield a diagnosis than those that have been present for weeks or those that have developed secondary lesions such as excoriation or infection.

After cleansing and anesthetizing the area, select a properly sized punch, and apply tension to the skin perpendicular to the natural skin tension lines (Fig. 4-5). Rotate the punch in a single direction through the skin to the subcutaneous tissue. A slight decrease in resistance will be appreciated. Lift the skin with forceps or a skin hook and remove it by cutting the subcutaneous base with sharp tissue scissors (Fig. 4-6). Apply pressure for hemostasis. Punch biopsies with diameters of 2 and 3 mm seldom need suturing, while most 4 mm samples will need closure with a suture. Steri-Strips are adequate in most cases or the skin edges can be approximated with a simple interrupted dermal suture. A single vertical mattress

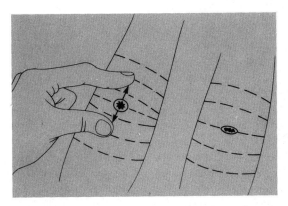

FIG. 4-5.
Proper stretching of skin tension lines before punch biopsy. Upon release, the tendency will be to make the circular biopsy more elliptical and more cosmetically pleasing.

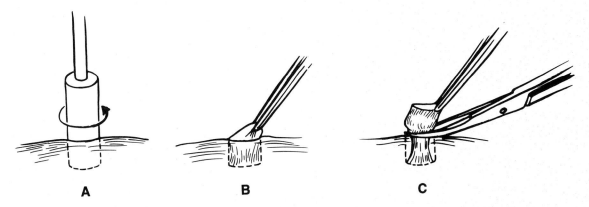

A **B** **C**

FIG. 4-6.
Punch biopsy technique. **A,** Twisting the punch; **B,** Picking up the loosened piece; **C,** Cutting with scissors.

suture will provide optimum closure. Wound management is then similar to that for sutured lacerations.

The specimen should be properly prepared for appropriate studies, which may include placing it in saline, 10% formalin, or in a sterile container for culture. For immunofluorescent studies, the tissue may need to be frozen in liquid nitrogen.

Elliptical Excision Biopsy

This technique removes the entire lesion with full dermal thickness and is commonly used. Draw an outline of the planned excision with a skin marking pen *before* placement of local anesthetic. This preserves the natural skin lines and allows proper placement and size for the excision. The ellipse should be three times as long as it is wide and should lie parallel to the skin tension lines. The corner angle of the ellipse should be approximately 30 degrees. Greater than 30-degree angles are more likely to produce a "dog ear" of excessive tissue after the wound is closed (Fig. 4-7).

Cleanse, anesthetize, and drape the area in a sterile fashion. Incise following the outline made with the marking pen. Free one corner of the ellipse and excise the full thickness of tissue. To prevent going too deep, excise from end to center, then from opposite end to center. Hemostasis should be attained before closure.

Frequently, after removing the specimen, there is a significant gap between tissue margins. If there is pronounced tension when the margins are brought together, undermine the edges to release this tension. Failure to do so will lead to spreading of the scar over time and to poor cosmetic results. Approximately one third to one half of the undermined tissue will be available to pull to the center. Undermining is done in the subcutaneous tissue on both sides of the wound (Fig. 4-8). Undermine each edge the width of the excised tissue.

A simple single-layer closure may be satisfactory for small lesions without tension. Otherwise, the wound should be undermined and closed in layers utilizing a subcutaneous suture (absorbable Vicryl or Dexon) with inverted knot (Fig. 4-9).

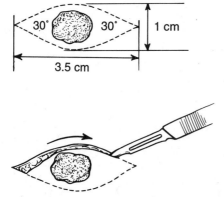

FIG. 4-7.
Elliptical excision biopsy technique. See text for details.

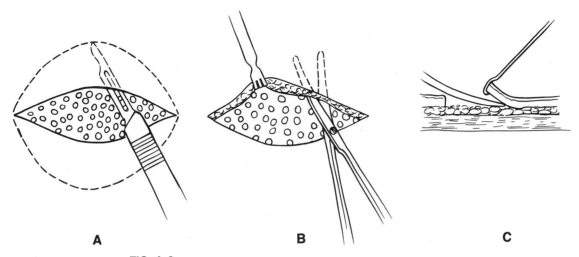

A **B** **C**

FIG. 4-8.
Subcutaneous undermining to release tension on wound margins with scalpel (**A**) and scissors (**B**). This also aids eversion of edges during closure. Proper level for undermining within subcutaneous fat (**C**).

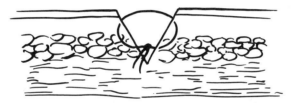

FIG. 4-9.
Deep inverted sutures to close dead space.

With this technique, pressure on the skin margins is reduced. After placement of the deep sutures, the skin margins should be nearly apposed even without the final skin stitches. This is followed by dermal closure with an interrupted or running suture.

Appropriate suture material for closure includes: 6-0 nylon for the face, 5-0 for upper extremities and chest, and 4-0 for back, scalp, and lower extremities. Buried suture generally should be absorbable. Most commonly used is Vicryl (3-0 or 4-0) and Dexon (3-0 or 4-0). Chromic catgut is too inflammatory and loses tensile strength too quickly for skin repair.

Management of Excess Tissue After Biopsy

Excess tissue may "pooch out" at the ends of the wound, forming a "dog ear." Place a skin hook in the corner of the wound, making a tent of the excess skin. Incise along one side of the tent, creating a triangular flap. Draw the flap to one side

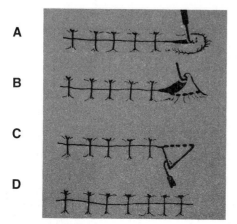

FIG. 4-10.
Management of excess tissue after closure (the "dog ear"). The principle to be remembered is that some tissue must be removed. **A,** The excess tissue is "tented up." **B,** An extension of the incision is made. **C,** The tissue is folded over the newly extended incision and the excess removed with scissors or scalpel. **D,** The final wound is longer but now lies flat.

and incise in a straight line, matching the first incision, and remove the flap. Close the extension of the wound, which should now lie flat (Fig. 4-10).

POSTPROCEDURE CARE

Postprocedure care of biopsies is similar to that of the closure of primary clean lacerations (see Chapter 3, Laceration Repair).

CPT/BILLING CODES

The CPT codes are too numerous for the scope of this text. Coding varies in terms of site, technique, and whether or not the lesion is malignant. The number of biopsies also alters billing codes.

BIBLIOGRAPHY

Breitenbach K, Bergera J: Principles and techniques of primary wound closure, *Prim Care* 13(3):411, 1986.

Moy RL et al: Commonly used surgical techniques in skin surgery, *Am Fam Physician* 44(5):1625, 1991.

Snell G: Surgical problems. In Taylor RB, editor: *Family medicine principles and practice,* ed 3, New York, 1994, Springer-Verlag.

Zuber TJ, DeWitt D: The fusiform excision, *Am Fam Physician* 49(2):371, 1994.

CHAPTER 5

Approach to Various Skin Lesions

John L. Pfenninger

Thomas J. Zuber

This chapter provides guidelines for the diagnosis and treatment of common skin lesions. Table 5-1 can be used as a guide for proper biopsy and treatment techniques. Many of the techniques are reviewed elsewhere in this text. These guidelines are not intended to be all-inclusive, but they do provide a framework for the approach to common skin lesions.

All excised skin lesions are best sent to the pathologist for definitive diagnosis. With selected lesions, such as skin tags or sebaceous cysts, many physicians will rely on their clinical judgment and avoid the added laboratory expense. However, in today's litigious society, the physician must be absolutely certain of the diagnosis when deciding not to send tissue to the pathologist for evaluation.

ACHROCHORDON (SKIN TAG)

Although many physicians prefer to use electrosurgery to remove achrochordons, the most direct and simple approach is to elevate the tag with pickups and excise it with sharp tissue scissors at the level of the surrounding skin. If it has a broad base, a local anesthetic may be required. Monsel's solution (ferric subsulfate) or aluminum chloride may be used for hemostasis.

BASAL CELL CARCINOMA

Basal cell carcinoma lesions typically have small central depressions and raised pearly borders. However, their actual appearance can vary markedly from the classic description. Sclerosing basal cell cancers may manifest as flat lesions with nondescript borders. Others are nonhealing ulcerations that never do become elevated. Some are pigmented and may be confused with seborrheic keratoses,

TABLE 5-1.

Surgical Diagnosis and Management of Common Skin Lesions

Procedure

Lesion	Punch biopsy	Shave biopsy	Shave removal	Fusiform excision	Incisional biopsy	Cautery/curettement	Cryotherapy	Electrosurgery (Radiofrequency)	85% Trichloroacetic acid	Laser ablation	Radiation	Fluorouracil 5% or masoprocol 10%	Other
Achrochordon (Skin tags)		X*	X*				X	X					
Cancer, basal cell	X	X		X	X	X*	X	X		X	X	X	
Cancer, squamous cell	X			X*	X	X		X		X	X	X	
Condyloma acuminata†	X	X	X	X‡		X	X	X	X	X		X§	X
Dermatofibroma	X	X	X	X*	X		X	X		X			
Hemangiomas, cherry	X‡	X	X				X	X		X			
Keratoacanthoma	X	X	X	X*	X	X	X	X		X		X	
Keratosis, actinic	X	X	X	X	X	X	X	X	X			X	
Keratosis, seborrheic	X	X	X*	X‡	X	X	X	X	X				
Lentigo	X	X	X				X*			X			
Lentigo maligna	X			X*	X								
Lipomas				X	X								
Melanoma	X			X*	X								
Molluscum contagiosum	X‡	X	X			X	X	X	X				X
Pyogenic granuloma	X	X	X	X	X	X	X	X	X	X			
Nevi, acquired	X		X‖	X	X			X‖	X‖	X			
Nevi, atypical	X			X*	X								
Nevi, giant congenital	X			X	X					X‖			
Paronychia¶													X
Rashes	X												X
Sebaceous hyperplasia	X	X	X	X‡		X	X	X					
Sebaceous cysts				X¶									X
Telangiectasias								X		X			X
Warts (Verruca vulgaris)	X	X	X		X‡	X	X	X	X	X			X
Warts, plantar	X	X	X			X	X	X	X	X			X
Xanthalasma		X	X	X		X		X		X			X

*Procedure of choice.
†See Chapter 84.
§Not approved by the FDA.
¶See special comments in text.
‖ An exception; used only if certain that lesion is benign.
‡Used only if cancer is a possibility or nature of lesion unknown.

nevi, or even melanomas. They may appear erythematous and bleed easily, mimicking a pyogenic granuloma. A flat and scaly lesion may look like a squamous cell carcinoma.

A biopsy should be taken of all nonhealing, changing, or enlarging skin lesions. Once a diagnosis is made, the proper approach for treatment can be planned.

When a biopsy is taken of a suspected basal cell carcinoma, almost any area of the lesion is appropriate for sampling. Biopsy of ulcerated lesions are best obtained at the border, which may not be involved in the ulceration process.

Basal cell carcinomas can be very aggressive in the nasolabial folds and in the preauricular areas. The inner canthal area can be an especially difficult area to excise and treat because of tearduct involvement. In these locations, Moh's chemosurgery may be indicated as a primary excisional method, because it ensures complete removal. Careful follow-up is needed to detect early recurrences.

There are many approaches to the treatment of basal cell cancers. Radiation therapy is rarely used, but it may be necessary when the lesions are located in areas such as the lid margins or the inner canthal areas, and in large lesions found on elderly patients.

Basal cell cancers generally involve the upper portions of the skin and only very rarely metastasize. For the majority of lesions that are smaller than 1 cm, treatment with cautery and curettement is a rapid and effective solution. Cure rates approach 92% to 95%, and scarring is usually minimal.

With cautery and curettement, scoop out the lesion with a large dermal curette. Scrape the base of the lesion until a gritty feeling is encountered. Then fulgurate or cauterize the entire base to destroy remaining cells and to control bleeding. After the first cauterization, again vigorously curette the site to remove any of the char. Again perform fulguration or cauterization. Carry out the third and final curettement with a smaller dermal curette that more easily enters any tiny crevices in the wound site. Be careful not to penetrate too deeply and pass through the entire dermis. Should this happen, a small window of fatty tissue will be visible in the bottom of the wound. After the third curettement, fulgurate or cauterize the lesion once again, and place a dressing. Although the wound appears significantly ulcerated, the long-term cosmetic results of this procedure are generally very acceptable.

Encourage the patient to wash the area three or four times a day with soap and water to prevent an eschar from forming. Immediately after washing, have the patient apply an antibiotic ointment to keep the area moist. The ointment can be applied six or eight times a day, not so much to prevent infection, but rather to aid the reepithelization of the wound.

Lesions in younger patients, larger-sized lesions, lesions in more aggressive locations, sclerosing-type basal cell cancer lesions, and lesions with ill-defined margins may require *complete excision* to enable the pathologist to examine the margins. Margins can be marked to aid in the histologic evaluation. Some physicians feel that excision is more cosmetically acceptable than cautery and curettement. All the various clinical factors should be weighed when selecting the method of lesion removal.

After being treated for a basal cell carcinoma, the patient must be observed closely, because 50% of patients will develop new basal cell cancers within 5 years.

SQUAMOUS CELL CARCINOMA

Squamous cell carcinoma often presents as a diffuse, nonhealing, crusted lesion. It frequently occurs at the base of an actinic keratosis. The lesions may be multifocal in origin and, like actinic lesions, are due to solar damage. Since the margins of these lesions are not very clear, many prefer to excise squamous cell carcinomas. If 5-flurouracil (Efudex) or masoprocol (Actinex) are used to treat actinic changes, any posttreatment residual lesions should be removed for biopsy to rule out squamous cell carcinoma. When taking a specimen of a suspected squamous cell cancer, try to include portions of the central area as well as the edge. A deep punch biopsy into subcutaneous fat is preferred by many pathologists.

CONDYLOMA ACUMINATA

Many therapeutic interventions are available to treat condyloma acuminata. See Chapter 84, Treatment of Vulvar, Perianal, Vaginal, Penile, and Urethral Condyloma Acuminata.

DERMATOFIBROMA

Dermatofibromas frequently occur on the anterior surface of the lower leg. The etiology is unknown, but dermatofibromas may represent a fibrous reaction to trauma, viral infection, or insect bites. They are frequently confused with verrucae or nevi. Dermatofibromas do not progress to cancers, and once the diagnosis of dermatofibroma is confirmed, the physician can often merely observe the lesions. They are generally deep-seated lesions, and many physicians prefer complete excision if removal is desired. Cryotherapy can be attempted, but dermatofibromas are generally quite cryoresistant.

KERATOACANTHOMA

Keratoacanthoma is a common, benign epithelial tumor found with elderly patients. This lesion may have a viral etiology. Keratoacanthoma is often confused with squamous cell carcinoma, but it is a distinct entity.

The lesion begins as a dome-shaped papule that continues to enlarge rapidly. A fully developed tumor is a round, dome-shaped mass with a central keratin-filled crater. The lesion stops growing after six weeks, and then it may slowly regress over the next twelve months.

Since these lesions leave a considerable scar, most physicians do not advocate simply observing their resolution. Topical or intralesional injection of flurouracil, cryotherapy, blunt dissection, electrodesiccation and curettage, or conventional excision all provide acceptable results. Keratoacanthomas can recur, and patients should be followed closely during and after treatment. The major differential diagnoses include basal and squamous cell cancer.

ACTINIC KERATOSES

Actinic keratoses are sun-induced, premalignant lesions. When multiple lesions are present, they can be treated with flurouracil or masoprocol. Lesions that do not resolve require surgical sampling for biopsy. The risk that actinic keratoses will progress to squamous cell carcinoma is probably less than 1% in early lesions, and as high as 10% to 20% for persistent hypertrophic lesions. The patient should be counseled that both flurouracil and masoprocol can cause significant erythema and tenderness in the areas treated. Steroid creams may be used to reduce the inflammatory response. Alternatively, daily application of retinoic acid (Retin-A) 0.025% or 0.05% may resolve the lesions.

SEBORRHEIC KERATOSES

Seborrheic keratoses are benign, hyperkeratinized, superficial epidermal lesions that are common with aging. Their size ranges from 2 mm to 3 cm, but they have no malignant potential. The typical lesion can be easily lifted off with a fingernail. Patients often say that they have removed the lesion or rubbed it off with a towel, only to have it recur. Seborrheic keratoses are occasionally confused with basal cell carcinomas, squamous cell carcinomas, nevi, and verrucous lesions.

Most seborrheic keratoses can be easily removed, after anesthesia, with radio-frequency (electrosurgery) technique. Alternatively, shave excision with mild curetting of the base can be performed. Hemostasis can be accomplished with Monsel's solution or aluminum chloride. Minimal scarring should result, since the lesion is superficial. Some physicians prefer cryotherapy; however, this treatment may cause more discomfort, it precludes histologic assessment, and multiple treatments may be required. It is essential that the clinician be absolutely sure of the diagnosis if cryotherapy is to be used. One study showed a correct preoperative diagnosis in only 49% of cases. (Stern, 1991)

LENTIGO

Lentigos, or liver spots, are frequently encountered brownish or tan macules that occur on the sun-exposed areas of the face, shoulders, arms, and hands. Lentigos increase in number during childhood and adult life, and occasionally they fade. Biopsy of lesions with irregular borders should be performed to rule out malignant melanoma. Cryotherapy is the treatment of choice, although bleaching and depigmenting creams may be used.

LENTIGO MALIGNA (MELANOMA IN SITU)

Lentigo maligna is a sun-associated precursor of lentigo maligna melanoma, a type of invasive melanoma. These lesions can grow to be several centimeters in diameter, and usually occur on the face. They are slow-growing macules with irregular borders and pigmentation. These lesions are often confused with liver spots, which are smaller, have a homogeneous color, and appear mainly over the dorsae of the hands and forearms. The estimated lifetime risk of transformation to melanoma is only 4.7%, and some physicians prefer close observation as the treatment of choice.

LIPOMAS

Lipomas generally present as a palpable mass under the skin. Most lesions are nontender, move freely, and have a soft, irregular consistency. Lipomas generally do not progress to malignancy, but rapidly growing or changing lesions should be removed. Removal may also be necessary when lipomas occur in areas of pressure or when they cause pain or discomfort. Lesions are removed by making an incision through the dermis following the skin lines, and by using hemostats or curved tissue scissors to dissect the lesion from the surrounding adhering tissue. Pressure on the base of the lesion will often extrude the lipoma through the incision. Some lipomas are encapsulated, but often the edges are obscure; it may be difficult to determine whether all of the lesion has been removed. Once the diagnosis of lipoma has been made in one area, other similar lesions do not necessarily require removal unless they are symptomatic.

MELANOMA

The major caveat regarding melanomas is that the depth of lesion is very important in determining appropriate definitive treatment. Primary care physicians should not feel uncomfortable about performing a biopsy of any lesion with characteristics that may be consistent with a melanoma. Use the mnemonic "A,B,C,D,E" to remember the clinical features of malignant melanoma:

Asymmetry
Border irregularity
Color variegation
Diameter > 6 mm
Elevation above skin surface

Since it is so important to determine the depth of the lesion, *never* perform a shave biopsy or shave removal if melanoma is a consideration. When choosing a site for punch or incisional biopsy within a pigmented lesion, choose the area that is most nodular or atypical (darkest in color, inflamed, or irregular). Recent National Institutes of Health (NIH) guidelines indicate that with lesions that penetrate less than 1 mm, 1 cm excisional margins should be adequate. An extensive workup for metastases is not indicated for the minimal depth lesions (see Table 5-2).

MOLLUSCUM CONTAGIOSUM

Molluscum are small, 2 to 3 mm, papular, wartlike excrescenses with central umbilication. They usually appear as a crop of multiple lesions. Expectant observation is certainly acceptable, but many patients desire to have these viral lesions removed. Table 5-1 describes the treatments that are possible. Curettement with a dermal curette is the treatment of choice, and it rarely requires anesthesia. These lesions frequently occur in children; a topical anesthetic such as 20% benzocaine (Hurricaine gel) or EMLA (eutectic mixture of local anesthetic) may increase patient cooperation during treatment. See Chapter 22, Topical Anesthesia.

TABLE 5-2.

Treatment of Suspicious Pigmented Lesions and Melanomas

Stage	Recommended Treatment	Survival
Suspicious pigmented lesion	Punch, incisional, or excisional biopsy down to subcutaneous fat	Not affected by biopsy procedure
Early melanoma		
Melanoma in situ (limited to epidermis)	Excision with margin of 0.5 cm normal skin, and layer of subcutaneous tissue	Not affected
Depth < 1 mm	Excision with margin of 1.0 cm normal skin, and subcutaneous tissue down to fascia	95% (8 year)
Intermediate melanoma		
Depth 1.0 to 4.0 mm	After diagnostic biopsy, wide-margin excision and adjunctive therapy should be considered (Refer)	Poor
High-risk melanomas		
Depth > 4.0 mm	After diagnostic biopsy, wide-margin excision and adjunctive therapy should be considered (Refer)	Poor

Adapted from National Institutes of Health Consensus Conference: Diagnosis and treatment of early melanoma, *JAMA* 268(10):1314-19, 1992. Used with permission.

PYOGENIC GRANULOMAS

Pyogenic granulomas are small, rapidly growing, nodular, friable, vascular lesions that often bleed when touched. They occur at sites of trauma or previous surgery. Because of their vascular nature, pyogenic granulomas are best treated with curettement followed by cautery of the base. These lesions will recur if any tissue remains, and some physicians advocate complete excision.

ACQUIRED NEVI

Acquired nevi are benign, melanocytic nevi that are absent at birth, and first appear in early childhood. The lesions become more numerous until middle age, and the majority of white adults have at least one acquired nevus. Lesions are often found on sun-exposed areas.

Common acquired nevi follow a predictable developmental progression. The earliest lesions are junctional nevi, with the nevus cells at the junction between the dermis and epidermis. By late adolescence, the growths develop into compound nevi, with nevus cells in both the dermis and epidermis. Compound nevi may develop hairs. By late adulthood, the lesions regress into intradermal nevi.

If the lesions lose their pigment, they may turn pink or flesh-colored. At all stages, common benign acquired nevi have smooth, distinct, symmetric borders. Patients with large numbers of acquired nevi should be monitored closely, because they are at higher risk for developing melanoma.

Raised or pedunculated benign nevi can often best be excised with a shave removal technique (frequently radiofrequency technique is used). *There should be no suspicion whatsoever of melanoma.* If malignancy is even suspected, either a full-thickness biopsy of the lesion should be performed prior to removal, or the lesion should be treated by complete excisional removal rather than shave removal. Superficial lesions generally do not recur, but the deeper compound nevi frequently do unless the full depth of the lesion is excised. It is difficult to determine when the entire lesion has been removed using a shave technique. The deeper dermal lesions are generally flat, while the superficial epidermal lesions are raised or pedunculated.

DYSPLASTIC NEVI

Dysplastic nevi, or atypical moles, are acquired nevi that become dysplastic over time. The lesions are generally larger than common acquired nevi, and may have irregular margins, variable pigmentation, and irregular surface contour. Because the risk for melanoma is increased in patients with atypical moles, and because melanoma can develop from an atypical lesion, some physicians advocate full excision of suspicious lesions.

GIANT CONGENITAL NEVI

Giant congenital nevi, or "bathing trunk nevi," are larger than 20 cm in diameter, and often extend over large portions of the body. The lesions grow proportionally with the anatomic site, their surfaces may be irregular, and they may contain coarse hairs. Their management is very controversial. The lifetime risk of developing into melanoma is 5% to 20%; therefore, some physicians advocate early removal and grafting. Others advocate close monitoring. Melanoma can develop at any site within the lesion, and biopsies of the most irregular portions of the lesions may not detect malignant change. Efforts to completely eradicate these lesions must be tempered by the potential for treatment-induced scarring and disfigurement.

PARONYCHIA

Paronychia are infections of the distal phalanx along the proximal and lateral edges of the nail. Paronychia produce signs of local infection, including redness, tenderness, and swelling. Mild paronychia can be treated with soaks and antibiotics. More significant infections may develop into abscesses. As with all abscesses, they are best incised and drained. A digital block is often needed, and the incision technique is described in Fig. 5-1. Occasionally packing may be used to keep the abscess from reaccumulating.

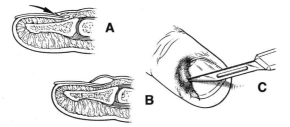

FIG. 5-1.
A separation of the cuticle from the nail (*arrow*) (**A**) can lead to a paronychia (**B**). In acute paronychia, drain any pus and consider a culture. A simple nick (**C**) through the most translucent area of the abscess is usually all that is required. (From Steck W: *Modern Medicine* 55:51, 1987. Used with permission.)

RASHES (EXANTHEMS, DERMATOSES)

In many cases, biopsy of a "rash" or ill-defined dermatologic lesion is not very helpful. Unless the clinical diagnosis is fairly clear, the primary care physician may be wise to obtain a dermatology consultation. Biopsies of these lesions may be indicated for clarification of a fairly discrete differential diagnosis (as with inflammatory dermatoses), or for ruling out a cutaneous neoplasm.

When multiple sites are involved, the following simple guidelines may be followed for selecting a lesion for a biopsy specimen: It is best to select those areas that have the primary inflammatory changes, but that are free from secondary changes such as crusting, fissuring, erosion, ulceration, and infection. Choose sites where the scars will not be obvious and where hypertrophic scarring is generally not a problem.

If the primary lesion is a *macule,* select a "fresh" lesion that is more abnormal in color. Generally, perform a punch biopsy, advancing the punch into the subcutaneous fat. *Papules* should be removed completely, if possible. Select a mature lesion without secondary changes. If the lesion is a *plaque,* the biopsy specimen should consist of the thickest area through the full depth into the subcutaneous fat. The same technique is used for *nodular* lesions and *suspected neoplastic* lesions. For *vesicles,* choose an intact lesion whenever possible. Rupturing a sac makes histologic interpretation more difficult. If *bullae* are present, sample the lesion at the margin where the blister roof is attached to the remainder of the specimen.

SEBACEOUS HYPERPLASIA

Sebaceous adenosum, or senile sebaceous hyperplasia, are small growths composed of enlarged sebaceous glands. These very small 2 to 3 mm lesions can often mimic early basal cell cancer. If numerous lesions are present in the temporal and forehead areas, they are unlikely to be cancerous. Treatment consists of removal of the elevated portions of the papule with shave or electrosurgical technique. Biopsy is indicated if the nature of the lesion is uncertain; however, treatment can generally be carried out on the basis of the clinical diagnosis.

SEBACEOUS CYSTS

The epidermal cyst, or sebaceous cyst, is a round, tense, keratinizing cyst that is freely mobile and very superficial. Most patients present with a slowly growing lesion, which on physical examination is subcutaneous, smooth, and nontender. A history of drainage or inflammation with purulent discharge may or may not be present, but it does help solidify the diagnosis.

In the past, a surgeon's adeptness was often judged by whether or not he or she could remove the lesion intact without rupturing the capsule. This requires a fairly generous incision over the area and judicious removal of the entire sac, which decreases the likelihood of any recurrence. The cavity is then irrigated and closed with sutures. Maintaining an intact sac during removal is no longer felt to be required.

In an alternative approach, a small incision is made into the cyst, the contents are expressed, and iodoform gauze is packed into the cavity. Healing occurs from the inside out as the iodoform gauze is gradually removed over 10 to 14 days. Several visits to the physician's office are often required. Healing is encouraged by having the sac scar shut, which prevents recurrence. This technique is still used for an infected sebaceous cyst.

A more recent technique preferred by patient and physician alike is an adaptation of these approaches. After anesthesia, a small 3 to 4 mm incision is made directly into the cyst using a No. 11 blade. All contents are expressed using external pressure. Frequently (especially in scalp cysts), this external pressure will not only extrude the sebaceous material of the cyst, but the sac itself. If the sac is not produced, then curved hemostats are inserted into the wound and repeated attempts are made to grasp the sac and pull it out in its entirety. The wound is irrigated, but because of the limited length of the incision, it does not require suturing. The patient is told to express the area once or twice a day until there is no fluid drainage. Up to 95% of all sebaceous cysts can be treated with this method without recurrence. Average time for removal is less than 15 minutes. This technique should not be used for cysts larger than 2 cm in diameter or for cysts with a history of infection. Should the sac adhere or not be entirely removed, either full excisional removal can be performed or iodoform gauze can be placed within the cavity and gradually removed over 10 to 14 days with the hope that sufficient scarring will take place to occlude the sac and prevent recurrence.

TELANGIECTASIAS

Small cherry hemangiomas, a type of telangiectasia, are benign, small, red, vascular lesions that do not require treatment. If irritated or bleeding, they can be cauterized. Malignancy is not a consideration. Spider veins, another type of telangiectasia, are best treated with sclerotherapy and occasionally with radiosurgery. Spider veins on the leg can produce significant pain and paresthesias if left untreated. See Chapter 12, Sclerotherapy.

COMMON AND PLANTAR WARTS (VERRUCA VULGARIS AND PLANTARIS)

The recurrence rates associated with all treatments of common warts are 30% or higher. Most over-the-counter and prescription preparations are acidic, caustic solutions. In time, 60% of warts will resolve spontaneously. Vitamins enhance the immune system and may aid wart resolution. Numerous treatment methods are used and noted in Table 5-1.

Plantar warts are treated with methods similar to those used with common warts. Physicians should avoid surgical excisions on the bottom of the feet since the scar tissue often remains painful after healing. A patient may suffer with the irritated scar, which produces an effect not unlike a pebble in a shoe. Soaking followed by paring of callous tissue will improve the efficacy of any treatment. Cryotherapy is effective without resulting in scarring.

WARTS (CONDYLOMA ACUMINATA)

See the previous section, Condyloma Acuminata.

XANTHELASMA

Xanthelasma, the most common form of xanthoma, is a yellow-white plaque on the eyelids. The diagnosis of xanthelasma can be made clinically. The goal of all treatments is to stay within a very superficial layer. Light fulguration or cauterization is often sufficient. With radiofrequency excision, it is easier to control depth. Often an incision can be made with an 18-gauge needle and the lesion can be expressed. Recurrences, because of the nature of the lesion, are common.

BIBLIOGRAPHY

Drake LA et al: Guidelines of care for cutaneous squamous cell carcinoma, *J Am Acad Dermatol* 28(4):628, 1993.

Drake LA et al: Guidelines of care for malignant melanomas, *J Am Acad Dermatol* 28(4):638, 1993.

Habif TP: *Clinical dermatology,* ed 2, St Louis, 1990, Mosby.

Klin B, Ashkenazi M: Sebaceous cyst excision with minimal surgery, *Am Fam Physician* 41:1746, 1990.

Kuflik AS, Janniger CK: Basal cell carcinoma, *Am Fam Physician* 48(7):1273, 1993.

Kurban RS, Kurban AL: Skin disorders of aging: diagnosis and treatment, *Geriatrics* 48:30, April 1993.

NIH Consensus Conference: Diagnosis and treatment of early melanoma, *JAMA* 268:1314, 1992.

Pariser RJ: Skin biopsy: lesion selection and optimal technique, *Modern Med* 57:82, 1989.

Stern RS, Boudreaux C, Arndt K: Diagnostic accuracy and appropriateness of care for seborrheic keratoses, *JAMA* 265:74, 1989.

CHAPTER 6

Treatment of Ingrown Toenails

James F. Peggs

An ingrown toenail is a common affliction that can result from a variety of conditions and that can produce a good deal of discomfort and disability. The great toe is virtually the only toe involved, and either the medial or lateral border of the nail may be affected.

Several palliative measures are available to relieve painful symptoms of ingrown toenail. These include elevation of the involved nail edge with a small cotton wick; selective trimming of the affected nail edge (though this usually provides only temporary relief at best); frequent soaking; and the use of loose-fitting footwear. Unfortunately, resolution of the problem is rare without an operative approach.

Removal of the toenail, either partial or total, remains the definitive treatment for bothersome ingrown nails. For recurrent episodes, ablation of the germinal nail tissue can be used to prevent regrowth of the nail.

INDICATIONS

- Onychocryptosis (ingrown nail)
- Onychomycosis (fungal infection of the nail)
- Chronic, recurrent paronychia (inflammation of the nail fold)
- Onychogryposis (deformed, curved nail)

CONTRAINDICATIONS

- Allergy to local anesthetics (see Chapter 21, Local Anesthesia)
- Bleeding diathesis

EQUIPMENT

- 3 ml or 5 ml syringe with long (1 or 1.5 inch) needle (25- or 27-gauge)
- Local anesthetic *without* epinephrine (see Chapter 21)
- A narrow periosteal elevator (nail elevator)
- Sterile scissors with straight blades (or an English nail splitter)

- Rubber band or small Penrose drain
- Two straight hemostats
- Alcohol swabs
- Sterile gauze and tubular gauze dressing
- Antibiotic ointment (Mycitracin, Bactroban)
- Phenol solution (88%) for permanent ablation of the nail, if desired
- As an alternative to phenol, the Ellman Surgitron (radiofrequency unit) with specially designed Teflon-insulated matrix tip (less inflammation and excellent results)

— Post procedure instructions
— Dressing

TECHNIQUE

Removal of Partial or Full Nail

1. With the patient supine, scrub and drape the toe in a sterile fashion.
2. Administer local anesthetic (5 ml total) in ring-block fashion. Raise a wheal at the base of the toe on the dorsal surface on the affected side (medial or lateral) and direct the injection toward the plantar surface to envelop both the extensor and plantar branches of the digital nerve on that side, depositing 1 ml at each site. Perform a second puncture at the corresponding site of the other side and advance the needle in the plantar direction to allow delivery of 1 ml of anesthetic to each branch of the digital nerve (Fig. 6-1).
3. When anesthesia is achieved (5 to 10 minutes), use a straight hemostat to firmly secure a wide rubber band around the base of the toe to serve as a tourniquet.
4. Loosen and lift the nail (at least 25% of the nail for partial removal) from the nail bed by using the flat, pointed blade of the scissors, a single jaw of a straight hemostat, or a narrow periosteal elevator (the elevator works best to decrease the likelihood of injury to nail bed). Introduce and advance the instrument with continued upward pressure against the nail and away from the

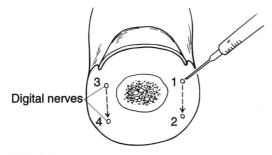

Digital nerves

FIG. 6-1.
Ring-block technique for digital nerve block. *Step 1:* Raise a wheal at the base of the toe on the dorsal surface. *Step 2:* Direct the needle toward the plantar surface, delivering 1 ml of anesthetic to the extensor and plantar branches of the digital nerve. *Step 3:* Perform a second puncture at the corresponding site of the other side and advance the needle in the plantar direction to allow delivery of 1 ml of anesthetic to each branch of the digital nerve.

nail bed to minimize injury and bleeding (Figs. 6-2 and 6-3). It is important to completely free the proximal nail at its base under the edge of the cuticle to allow removal and to expose the germinal tissue of the nail bed. Loosen the entire nail in this fashion if the entire nail is to be removed.

5. If a nail is to be partially removed, use scissors or a nail splitter to completely split the nail in a longitudinal direction to include the base of the nail that rests beneath the cuticle. Grasp that portion of the nail to be removed lengthwise with a straight hemostat and remove it, using a steady pulling motion with a simultaneous upward twist of the hand toward the affected side (Fig. 6-4). This twisting action will ensure that the nail will be rolled out from beneath the affected nail margin instead of rolling over it. If the entire nail is to be removed, the nail may be removed in two halves or in its entirety following a thorough loosening and lifting of the nail. In removing the entire nail, the forceps should produce lifting and distal traction on the nail as it separates from the nail bed.

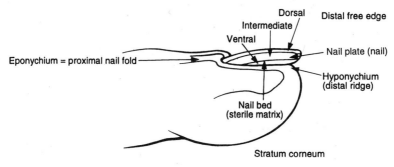

FIG. 6-2.
Nail bed anatomy and terminology.

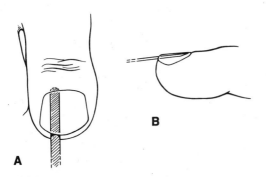

FIG. 6-3.
A, Periosteal elevator (advanced all the way under the cuticle). **B,** Periosteal elevator (upward pressure, forward motion toward base of nail).

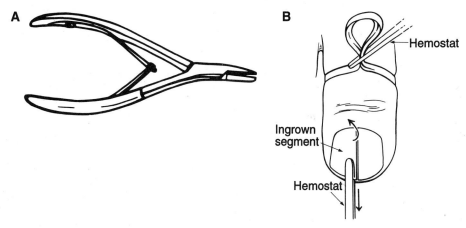

FIG. 6-4.
A, Nail splitter. **B,** Technique for nail removal after nail has been split. Grasp that portion of the nail to be removed lengthwise with a straight hemostat, and remove it using a steady pulling motion with a simultaneous upward twist of the hand toward the affected side.

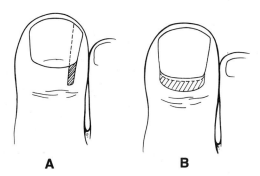

FIG. 6-5.
Area of nail bed to be cauterized in partial (**A**), and total nail removal (**B**).

Nail Plate Ablation

In the case of recurrent problems with the regrowing toenail (pain or infection), permanent ablation of the germinal tissue is recommended.

1. Remove total or partial nail as described previously.
2. With cotton swabs, sponge the exposed nail bed dry and then cauterize the germinal tissue, including that under the cuticle, by application of phenol on a cotton swab to the nail bed tissues (Fig. 6-5). Use caution to avoid phenol contact with normal skin. Hold the phenol-dampened cotton swab in place for 3 minutes.
3. Swab the area with isopropyl alcohol to neutralize the phenol.

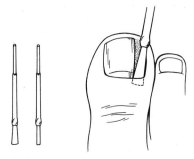

FIG. 6-6.
Application of nail matrixectomy electrode with coated side up. The lateral 25% of the nail has been removed. Two sizes of electrodes are available (2 or 4 mm).

Alternatively, the Ellman Surgitron radiofrequency unit (see Chapter 16, Radiofrequency Surgery) can be used. The inflammatory response is markedly reduced.

1. Remove whole or partial nail as described previously.
2. Place antenna lead under the heel of foot.
3. Turn unit to "Hemo-part rect" (hemostasis/coagulation setting) and set the power at 2.
4. Insert wide or narrow insulated matrixectomy tip over nail matrix, insulated side up (Fig. 6-6). These electrodes are insulated with Teflon on one surface to prevent damage to the undersurface of the proximal nail fold while ablating the nail matrix with the uninsulated surface. A slight upward pressure should be exerted against the undersurface of the nail fold to ensure that no pressure is exerted on the underlying matrix. The field must be free of blood. For proper effect, there should be a slight gap between electrode and matrix.
5. Apply power and slowly withdraw the electrode. Contact should be for only 5 to 6 seconds. A sizzling sound should be heard. This step can be repeated once after a 15-second cooling period. Multiple applications are necessary to ablate the entire nailplate.

POSTPROCEDURE CARE

Apply antibiotic ointment to the nail bed, cover with a sterile gauze pressure dressing, remove the tourniquet, and wrap with tubular gauze dressing.

The foot should be rested and preferably elevated during the first 12 to 24 hours. Because phenol ablates the nerve endings of the nail plate, pain should be absent when it is used. There is minimal pain with the radiofrequency unit. Nonsteroidal antiinflammatory drugs (NSAIDs) may be used for discomfort.

The dressing should be changed in 24 hours, at which point ambulation can be encouraged. The toe should be soaked in warm water for 20 minutes twice daily for four days. Topical antibiotics are recommended by some physicians. Tell the patient to expect a sterile exudate from the nail bed for several weeks. Emphasize proper nail hygiene to prevent further recurrences (Fig. 6-7).

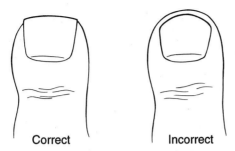

Correct   Incorrect

FIG. 6-7.
Proper nail care prophylaxis. Trim the nail flat but not too short.

COMPLICATIONS

- Infections (Treat with soaks and appropriate antibiotics.)
- Regrowth of nail and return of symptoms (Regrowth rate following phenol cauterization is 4% to 25%; for radiofrequency, less than 5%.)

CPT/BILLING CODES

11730	Nail removal, partial or complete
11750	Permanent nail removal (matrixectomy), partial or complete

BIBLIOGRAPHY

Freiberg A, Dougherty S: A review of management of ingrown toenails and onychogrypo-sis, *Can Fam Physician* 34:2675, 1988.

Hettinger DF et al: Nail matrixectomies using radio wave technique, *J Podiatric Med* 81(6): 317, 1991.

Hill GJ: *Outpatient surgery*, ed 2, Philadelphia, 1980, W.B. Saunders.

Robb JE, Murray WR: Phenol cauterization in the management of ingrowing toenails, *South Med J*:236, July 1982.

CHAPTER 7

Nail Plate and Nail Bed Biopsy

James F. Peggs

The presence of melanocytes in the germinal tissue of the nail matrix makes this a possible site for development of malignant melanomas. Primary subungual malignant melanomas frequently appear as pigmented bands or streaks in the nail plate, and account for up to 3.5% of all cutaneous malignant melanomas (15% to 20% in blacks). Distinction between the numerous benign causes of pigmented streaks (trauma, malnutrition, and normal occurrence in many blacks and Asians) and malignant lesions is frequently difficult. Biopsy is often recommended to confirm the diagnosis.

The *nail plate* is the hard structure composed of keratinized squamous cells, which is commonly called the nail itself. The *nail bed* refers to the softer tissue beneath the nail which provides germinal tissue for the nail plate and to which the nail plate is attached (see Fig. 6-2).

INDICATIONS

- Thickened, distorted nail plate with a negative evaluation for fungal infection (potassium hydroxide [KOH] scraping, culture)
- Longitudinal pigmented linear streak in the nail plate suspicious for malignancy

CONTRAINDICATIONS

- Allergy or sensitivity to local anesthetics (see Chapter 21, Local Anesthesia)
- Bleeding diathesis

EQUIPMENT

- 3 mm disposable punch biopsy
- Local anesthetic *without* epinephrine
- Sterile scissors with straight blades (or a narrow periosteal elevator)

- Sterile rubber band or small Penrose drain
- Two sterile straight hemostats
- Sterile gauze and tubular gauze dressing
- Antibiotic ointment (Mycitracin, Bactroban)
- 5-0 or 6-0 nylon sutures
- Needle holders
- Suture scissors

TECHNIQUE

Nail Plate (Nail) Biopsy

1. With steady pressure, hold the punch perpendicular to the nail; rotation of the punch will painlessly produce a round biopsy specimen. No anesthetic is required.
2. Elevate the biopsy sample and lyse the underlying nail bed tissue with the scissors or scalpel.

Nail Bed Biopsy

1. Employ digital anesthetic using the ring-block technique (Fig. 7-1).
2. Partially remove the nail plate according to the procedure in Chapter 6, Treatment of Ingrown Toenails.
3. When the affected nail bed has been exposed, use a 3 or 4 mm punch to obtain the biopsy specimen as close to the proximal origin of the pigmentation as possible. The biopsy specimen should be 2 to 3 mm in thickness. (See Chapter 4, Skin Biopsy.)

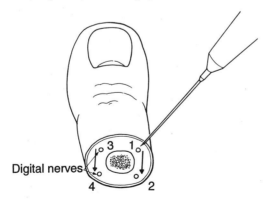

Digital nerves

FIG. 7-1.
Ring-block technique for digital nerve block. *Step 1:* Raise a wheal at the base of the toe on the dorsal surface. *Step 2:* Direct the needle toward the plantar surface, delivering 1 ml of anesthetic to the extensor and plantar branches of the digital nerve. *Step 3:* Perform a second puncture at the corresponding site of the other side and advance the needle in the plantar direction to allow delivery of 1 ml of anesthetic to each branch of the digital nerve.

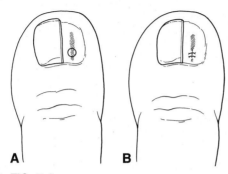

FIG. 7-2.
Nail bed biopsy. **A,** 3 mm biopsy specimen obtained. **B,** Sutured nail bed.

4. Close the biopsy site with one or two 5-0 or 6-0 nylon sutures oriented along the longitudinal plate (Fig. 7-2).
5. Apply a dressing of antibiotic ointment and sterile gauze.

COMPLICATIONS

- Bleeding
- Infection

CPT/BILLING CODE

11100   Nail biopsy

BIBLIOGRAPHY

Baran R, Kechijian P: Longitudinal melanonychia, *J Am Acad Dermatol* 21:1165, 1989.
Daniel CR III, editor: Symposium on the nail, *Dermatol Clin* 3:371, 1985.
Stone OJ, Barr RJ, Herten RJ: Biopsy of the nail area, *Cutis* 21:257, 1978.
Tom DWK, Scher RK: Melanoychia striata in longitudinem, *Am J Dermatopathol* (suppl 7):161, 1985.

CHAPTER 8

Subungual Hematoma Evacuation

James F. Peggs

Injuries to the nail bed and fingertip are the most common injuries to the upper extremity. Most common among these is a subungual hematoma, which results from a direct blow to the fingernail causing bleeding into the space between the nail bed and the fingernail itself. Intense pain can result from the pressure generated by such a hematoma. Evacuation of the hematoma can produce significant relief and can be safely performed in the outpatient setting. Toenails can be treated in the same fashion.

INDICATIONS

- Visible, painful hematoma beneath the involved nail

CONTRAINDICATIONS

- Crushed or fractured nail
- Hematomas involving greater than 50% of the nail *may* indicate laceration of the underlying nail bed (Removal of the nail and repair of the laceration is recommended by some experts to avoid a posttraumatic nail deformity. Others recommend leaving the nail in place as a splint. The patient should be warned that the nail *may* be deformed unless the nail bed is examined and treated.)

EQUIPMENT

- Alcohol lamp or Bunsen burner, metal paper clip, and forceps or hemostat
- *Or* battery-operated cautery unit
- *Or* radiofrequency or electrocautery unit with needle or pointed electrode

TECHNIQUE

1. Wash the digit as thoroughly as possible with an antibacterial soap to decrease the possibility of contamination of the hematoma and subsequent infection.
2. Create a hole in the nail directly over the hematoma to allow decompression.

   Paper-clip method. Partially straighten a metal paper clip, grasp it with the forceps, and heat it over the lamp. Place the heated clip firmly on the nail, allowing it to melt the tissue for a few seconds until the nail is completely perforated (Fig. 8-1).

   Cautery method. In similar fashion, apply an electric cautery tip to the nail and create a hole in the nail bed (Fig. 8-2).

In both of these procedures, the heated tip will be cooled by the hematoma upon perforation of the nail, thereby preventing injury to the nail bed. The hole created in the nail should be of sufficient size so as not to self-close within a few hours (adequate size is 1 to 2 mm). Elevation of the finger, cool compresses, and a simple bandage are recommended during the first 12 hours.

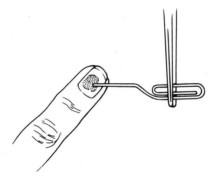

FIG. 8-1.
A heated paper clip is placed directly over the hematoma to create a perforation of the nail.

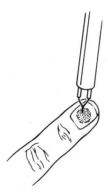

FIG. 8-2.
A cautery unit may be used to perforate the nail and evacuate the subungual hematoma.

COMPLICATIONS

- Infection of the remaining hematoma

CPT/BILLING CODE

11740   Subungual hematoma evacuation

BIBLIOGRAPHY

Simon RR, Wolgin M: Subungual hematoma: association with occult laceration requiring repair, *Am J Emerg Med* 5:302, 1986.
Van Beek AL: Management of acute fingernail injuries, *Hand Clinics* 1:23, 1990.
Zook EG: Nail bed injuries, *Hand Clinics* 1(4):701, 1985.

CHAPTER 9

Incision and Drainage of an Abscess

Daniel J. Derksen

An abscess is a localized infection characterized by a collection of pus surrounded by inflamed tissue. When a sweat gland or hair follicle forms an abscess, it is called a *furuncle,* or *boil.* When the furuncle extends into the subcutaneous tissue, it is referred to as a *carbuncle. Paronychia* are abscesses that involve the nail.

Most often, *Staphylococcus aureus* is the causative agent in abscesses, but some abscesses are due to *Streptococcus* species or a combination of microorganisms, including gram-negative and anaerobic bacteria. Perianal abscesses are usually caused by enteric organisms. Abscesses can occur in any location, but they are commonly found on the extremities, buttocks, breast, or in hair follicles.

A small abscess may respond to warm compresses or antibiotics and drain spontaneously. As the abscess enlarges, the inflammation, collection of pus, and walling off of the abscess cavity render such conservative treatments ineffectual. The treatment of choice for an abscess is incision and drainage (I & D), and if this treatment is done properly, antibiotics are usually unnecessary. In a nonlactating woman, a breast abscess that is not subareolar is rare, and should prompt a biopsy in addition to I & D of the abscess.

INDICATIONS

- A localized collection of pus that is tender and not spontaneously resolving

CONTRAINDICATIONS

Facial furuncles should not be incised or drained if they are located within the triangle formed by the bridge of the nose and the corners of the mouth. These infections should be treated with antibiotics and warm compresses, as the risk of septic phlebitis with intracranial extension can follow I & D of a furuncle in this area.

Patients with diabetes, debilitating disease, or compromised immunity should be observed following I & D of an abscess. A culture should be obtained by aspiration or swab of the abscess cavity, because the abscess may have been caused by unusual organisms. The infection may also warrant the administration of antibiotics.

EQUIPMENT

- Local anesthetic (1% to 2% lidocaine) or diphenhydramine (Benadryl) 50 mg/cc
- Syringe with 25- to 30-gauge needle
- Possibly a cryo freeze unit or ethyl chloride
- Alcohol or povidone-iodine (Betadine) wipe
- 4 × 4 inch gauze
- No. 11 blade
- Curved hemostats
- Possibly iodoform gauze (⅜- to 1-inch width, depending on abscess size)
- Possibly culture materials
- Bandage scissors
- Dressing of choice

TECHNIQUE

1. Prep the abscess area with povidone-iodine and drape in a sterile fashion.
2. Administer a field block with local anesthetic (see Chapter 21) to allow an adequate incision to be made. Avoid infiltrating the abscess cavity; rather, concentrate on anesthetizing the perimeter of the tissue around the abscess. Local anesthetics usually work poorly in the acidic milieu of an abscess. More anesthetic than usual may be needed to relieve pain. Alternatively, diphenhydramine (Benadryl) 10 to 25 mg can be injected into the area for anesthesia. Dilute a 50 mg (1 cc) vial in a syringe with 4 cc of normal saline. Cryocautery can be used to freeze the roof of the abscess. This can be done with a nitrous oxide unit, liquid nitrogen, or ethyl chloride. The incision is then made through the cooled skin, which is now anesthesized.
3. Make a sufficiently wide incision with a No. 11 blade to allow drainage of the abscess cavity and to prevent premature closure of the incision.

   Note: Protective eyewear should be worn if the abscess contents appear to be under enough pressure to cause expulsion of material upon incision. Recurrence of the abscess is most often due to an inadequate incision. Paronychia can be treated following digital block by partial or complete removal of the offending nail if recurrent.

4. If a culture is obtained, it should be from the abscess cavity and not from the superficial skin over the abscess. Alternatively, the abscess cavity can be aspirated with a large-bore (18-gauge) needle before the incision is made. The aspirated contents can then be sent for the appropriate cultures in more complicated cases. Rarely is this helpful in the routine superficial abscesses.
5. The abscess cavity should be thoroughly explored. This can be accomplished with a sterile cotton-tipped applicator or with hemostats. Attempts should be made to break down any walled-off pockets or possible septa. The cavity

can be packed with a rubber drain or with packing material, such as iodoform gauze (see Fig. 9-1). The length and width depends on abscess size.

6. Depending on the location and the size of the abscess, the drain can be slowly advanced over several days, or the packing material can be changed daily or several times per day.

7. A sterile dressing can be applied over the area. Healing should progress from the inside out; that is, epithelialization of the abscess cavity should occur before healing of the incision site to minimize the chance of recurrence.

Usually I & D is sufficient treatment to cure an abscess. When surrounding cellulitis is present, or when the patient has risk factors mentioned previously, dicloxacillin (250 mg to 500 mg every 6 hours) can be used. Alternative antibiotics can be used, but must cover *Staphylococcus* organisms until the culture results have returned and a more specific antibiotic treatment is determined. If the packing is tight in the abscess cavity, the pain can be sufficient to warrant the use of acetaminophen or nonsteroidal antiinflammatory drugs (NSAIDs). Rarely are narcotics ever needed. The I & D alone may provide sufficient pain relief from a tense abscess such that no pain medication is needed.

In a patient with a tooth abscess, penicillin therapy should be started, and the patient should be referred to a dentist. For perianal abscess, see Chapter 123, Perianal Abscess Incision and Drainage. For paronychia, see Chapter 6, Treatment of Ingrown Toenails.

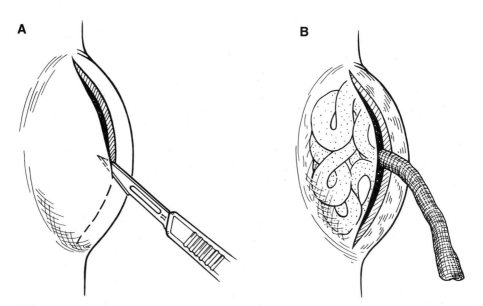

FIG. 9-1.
Incision and drainage of an abscess. **A,** Prep and drape the area. Inject 1% to 2% lidocaine around the perimeter of the abscess, taking care not to infiltrate the abscess cavity. Make an incision sufficiently wide to allow drainage and prevent premature closure, which could result in recollection of pus and recurrence of the abscess. **B,** Place a drain. In this case, iodoform gauze is used.

POSTPROCEDURE PATIENT EDUCATION

Some patients can be taught to change their own packing, replace the dressings, and advance the drain. Other patients may require home nursing visits or may have to return to clinic to have this done. Patients should be instructed to watch for signs of recurrence of the abscess, or for evidence of further infection such as cellulitis. Patients should be instructed to notify the clinician immediately if any of the following occur:

- Recollection of pus in the abscess
- Fever and chills
- Increased pain or redness
- Red streaks near the abscess
- Increased swelling in the area

COMPLICATIONS

Following I & D of any abscess, the site should be watched for signs of cellulitis or recollection of pus. Bacteremia and septicemia are complications of an inadequately treated abscess. In patients with diabetes or diseases that interfere with immune function, an abscess on an extremity can be complicated by severe cellulitis or gangrene, with subsequent loss of the affected extremity.

Perianal abscess I & D frequently results in a chronic anal fistula up to 50% of the time in adults (see Chapter 123, Perianal Abscess Incision and Drainage). This complication usually requires fistulectomy by a surgeon. An abscess in the palmar aspect of the hand can extend from superficial to deep tissue via the palmar fascia. Deep infection is suspected when the simple I & D fails to reduce the erythema, pain, pus, or swelling. More extensive surgical debridement, hospitalization, and intravenous antibiotics may be necessary in a patient with a deep palmar abscess, which is a surgical emergency.

CPT/BILLING CODES

Incision and drainage codes vary by complexity and site. Consult the CPT Code book for specific numbers.

CHAPTER 10

Acne Therapy

Thomas J. Zuber

John L. Pfenninger

Acne is a disease of the pilosebaceous follicle that commonly afflicts adolescents and adults. The disease involves increased sebum production, obstruction of the pilosebaceous unit, bacterial proliferation, and inflammation. Many topical and systemic medications have been developed to treat acne. When these medications fail to control the disease, or when significant lesions develop, several procedures may be utilized to intervene. This chapter will focus on the procedures a primary care physician might consider in the office treatment of acne.

COMEDO REMOVAL

The removal of open comedones (blackheads, noninflamed plugged pores) enhances the patient's appearance while preventing the development of inflamed acne lesions. Instruments, such as the round loop extractor (Fig. 10-1) or the Schamberg extractor, effectively extract the plug by allowing uniform, smooth pressure to encircle the pore (Fig. 10-2). Many physicians discourage this maneuver if the comedo is closed and presenting as an uninflamed papule with pasty white material under the keratinized surface. Cystic acne can be worsened by attempted treatment with a comedo extractor.

Open comedones that offer resistance to the comedo extractor can sometimes be loosened and removed with a No. 11 blade. Use the blade or extractor tip or a needle to stretch the walls of the pore opening without cutting into tissue. Then

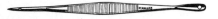

FIG. 10-1.
Comedo extractor.

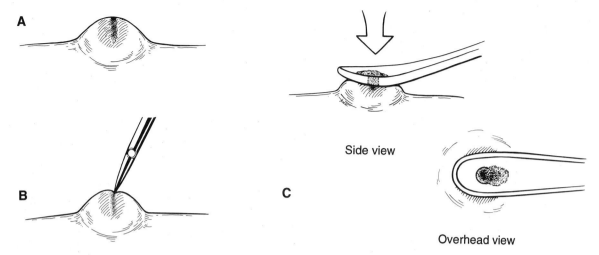

Side view

Overhead view

FIG. 10-2.
Use of comedo extractor to express cystic contents. **A,** Comedo; **B,** Incising lesion with sharp point;
C, Expressing contents through central hole. Using an extractor forces the contents out through the
central opening, preventing material from being forced into normal tissue.

insert the scalpel point 1 mm into the comedo, following the angle of the follicle
opening. Angle the tip to bring the plug upward through the enlarged pore
opening. If there is still resistance, hold the comedo extractor in the other hand and
apply lateral pressure to the base as the blade lifts the plug through the center of
the extractor. A large amount of sebaceous material may be found beneath the plug.

ACNE SURGERY FOR PUSTULES AND CYSTS

When performed correctly, the surgical drainage of acne pustules and cysts speeds
resolution of the lesions, prevents subdermal rupture, and enhances cosmetic
appearance. Closed comedones can also be opened to prevent their progression to
inflammatory lesions.

Enter the head of a white pustule with a small (25-gauge) needle or with the tip
of a No. 11 blade. Drain the pustule with lateral pressure or with the assistance of
an extractor. Superficial cysts that have thin roofs and easily palpated fluid can be
drained by making a small incision that is less than 4 mm long. Some physicians
advocate that the base of a drained superficial cyst be gently curetted to dislodge
any necrotic debris. Deep cysts often respond more favorably to intralesional
corticosteroid injection.

INTRALESIONAL CORTICOSTEROID INJECTION

Individual nodular or cystic acne lesions often dramatically decrease in size
following an intralesional injection of a corticosteroid. It is reassuring to patients to
know that a fast, relatively painless procedure is available when lesions arise.

Patients with severe acne often require repeated injections every 2 to 3 weeks. Multiple cysts can be treated in one session.

Several steroid preparations may be used, such as triamcinolone acetonide 10 mg/cc, triamcinolone diacetate 25 mg/cc, or betamethasone suspension 6 mg/cc. Triamcinolone acetonide 10 mg/cc (Kenalog-10) is frequently employed, diluted 1:1 with saline. Saline is the preferred diluent because injections of local anesthetics, such as lidocaine, are painful.

When preparing for an injection, shake the steroid vial to disperse the suspension. First draw the saline into a tuberculin syringe, followed by an equal amount of triamcinolone. An air bubble can be moved through the syringe to mix the two. Then insert a 30-gauge needle through the thinnest portion of the cyst roof and deliver 0.1 to 0.3 cc of the resulting 5 mg/cc triamcinolone acetonide mixture. Some physicians advocate using a maximum volume of 0.2 cc to reduce the risk of skin atrophy. The injection usually blanches the cyst.

Inject into the upper portion of the cyst. Skin atrophy can follow injections if the steroid is deposited below the cyst or if the steroid concentration is too high. Counsel patients that skin depression may occur, but in most cases it is temporary and gradually resolves in 4 to 6 months.

CRYOSLUSH THERAPY

Some physicians advocate the use of cryotherapy to produce superficial erythema and desquamation in the treatment of acne. A slush produced by mixing solid carbon dioxide and acetone can be lightly painted on the skin. Cryogenic sprays have also been developed. Mopping the face with large cotton applicators dipped in liquid nitrogen may achieve the same result and also reduces skin oiliness—while utilizing materials readily available in many primary care offices. Facial cryotherapy has become less popular in recent years with the advent of newer therapies.

SCAR REVISION

A variety of procedures can be utilized to remove or revise acne scars. Deep, "ice-pick" scars can be excised, using a punch biopsy, and immediately replaced with a full-thickness punch graft of normal skin. The physician must remove the *entire* scar pit with this technique. If the pit is angled and the punch biopsy leaves a portion of pit below the new skin, a cyst may later develop. Extensive shallow pits, superficial scarring, or irregular skin contour can be smoothed with chemical peels or dermabrasion. Collagen injections can also be used to smooth the skin surface.

Many physicians feel that the risks of the scar-revision procedures are significant. Dermabrasion results are unpredictable; frequently hypopigmentation can occur. When performed by dermatosurgeons expert in the techniques, scar-revision procedures can provide a benefit to carefully selected patients.

CPT/BILLING CODES

10040	Acne surgery, opening of multiple cysts, comedones, or pustules
10060	Incision and drainage of abscess
11900	Intralesional injection of up to 7 lesions
11901	Intralesional injection of more than 7 lesions
15780-87	Dermabrasion
15790-91	Chemical peel
17340	Cryotherapy (CO_2 slush)
17360	Chemical exfoliation for acne

BIBLIOGRAPHY

Cunliffe WJ: Acne vulgaris: pathogenesis and treatment, *Br Med J* 5:1394, 1980.

Domonkos AN, Arnold HL, Odom RB: *Andrew's diseases of the skin: clinical dermatology,* ed 7, Philadelphia, 1982, W.B. Saunders.

Habif TP: *Clinical dermatology: a color guide to diagnosis and therapy,* ed 2, St Louis, 1990, Mosby.

Lowney ED et al: Value of comedo extraction in treatment of acne vulgaris, *JAMA* 189:1000, 1964.

Quan M, Strick RA: Management of acne vulgaris, *Am Fam Physician* 38:207, 1988.

Strauss JS: Sebaceous glands. In Fitzpatrick TB et al, editors: *Dermatology in general medicine,* ed 3, New York, 1987, McGraw-Hill.

Tolman EL: Acne and acneiform dermatoses. In Moschella SL, Hurley HJ, editors: *Dermatology,* ed 2, Philadelphia, 1985, W.B. Saunders.

CHAPTER 11

Treatment of Hypertrophic Scars and Keloids

Thomas J. Zuber

John L. Pfenninger

The skin of predisposed individuals may respond to injury or surgery by developing excessive scar growths known as hypertrophic scars or keloids. *Hypertrophic scars* are self-limited growths that enlarge within the boundaries of a wound and then frequently regress. The natural history for most hypertrophic scars is spontaneous involution within two years. *Keloids* are benign, hard, fibrous proliferations of collagen that expand beyond the original size and shape of a wound. They tend to persist and frequently invade surrounding tissue, extending in a clawlike fashion.

Hypertrophic scars and keloids both represent abnormalities in the synthesis and degradation of collagen. Hypertrophic scars have a threefold increase in collagen-synthesis enzymes over normal scars, while keloids exhibit 20 times the normal levels.

Hypertrophic scars can occur at any site of skin injury. Those that follow surgical incisions usually remain linear. Hypertrophic scars frequently result after burns, producing an unsightly, pink scar that may contract. They may itch, but generally they do not produce the pain and hyperesthesia seen with keloids.

The incidence of keloids in dark-skinned individuals is 15 to 20 times that found in light-skinned people. Keloids appear frequently in anatomic sites that are subject to motion or increased skin tension, such as the shoulders, upper back, and presternal areas. Keloids may develop on the face after acne, or on the earlobe following ear piercing.

This chapter will focus on the office techniques used in the treatment of hypertrophic scars and keloids. Because of the natural regression of hypertrophic scars, therapy for these lesions is generally limited to injections alone. Although radiation therapy for keloids has been advocated, this therapy will not be reviewed at length. The malignancy potential of radiation in the treatment of a benign disease makes this therapy less desirable. Malignant transformation of keloids, if it occurs at all, is very rare.

The location, size, and duration of a keloid determines the most appropriate therapy. Cryotherapy, corticosteroid injection, surgical excision, pressure therapy, or a combination of these modalities may be chosen for the treatment of keloids.

CRYOTHERAPY

Tissue-destruction techniques used for treating keloids often incite further keloid formation, so cryotherapy is not generally advocated as a single therapeutic modality. Cryotherapy can be valuable for softening hard keloids before injection. Edema of the skin allows better dispersal of the steroid and minimizes its deposition into the subcutaneous or surrounding normal tissue. Light cryotherapy improves keloid regression, allows for lower injection pressures, and decreases the pain associated with injections.

A 10- to 15-second freeze with liquid nitrogen (−189°C) is usually required for earlobe keloids and keloids on most sites other than the midsternal region. Freezing for more than 25 seconds with liquid nitrogen frequently produces persisting posttreatment hypopigmentation. A 30- to 45-second freeze is usually adequate for most keloids when using a closed-probe, nitrous oxide temperature-controlled cryotherapy system (−89°C).

After cryotherapy, wait 20 to 60 minutes for tissue edema to develop before injecting corticosteroids. Patients may leave the office, return to the waiting room, or review patient education tapes while waiting.

CORTICOSTEROID INJECTIONS

Hypertrophic scars and keloids may be softened and flattened by intralesional corticosteroid therapy. Corticosteroids represent effective monotherapy for hypertrophic scars and small keloids, and are frequently employed as the initial therapy for large keloids.

Early, small, or narrow lesions are initially treated with intralesional injection every 4 weeks. Early keloids are softer and more responsive to injection than older inactive lesions. Avoid injecting into surrounding normal skin to prevent perilesional atrophy. When a lesion flattens too near the skin surface, decrease the frequency and concentration of an injection. Overaggressive therapy often results in excessive skin thinning and telangiectasias.

Injections are frequently performed with a 25- or 27-gauge needle and a Luer-Lok syringe. Very small needles (30-gauge and smaller) may be unable to penetrate dense lesions effectively. Locked syringes are necessary to prevent needle disengagement when injecting under pressure.

Many medication regimens have been developed. Triamcinolone acetonide 10 mg/cc (Kenalog-10) is a popular choice of steroid preparation. Although undiluted steroid can be used for unresponsive or dense lesions, many physicians prefer to dilute the triamcinolone 1:3 with physiologic saline or 1% lidocaine to create a 2.5 mg/cc solution. This dilute concentration limits postinjection hypopigmentation.

Administer the corticosteroid as the needle tracts through the lesion. Firm lesions limit the amount of medication that can be administered. Frequently, no more than 0.4 cc can be placed. The lesion often blanches with the injection.

Systemic effects from the corticosteroids are rare—but possible with repeated injections of higher concentrations. Local effects include hypopigmentation, hyperpigmentation, perilesional atrophy, and perilymphatic linear atrophy. These effects often improve over time, and this therapy is generally considered safe and effective.

SURGICAL EXCISION

Therapy of keloids limited to surgical excision and primary skin closure leads to a recurrence rate greater than 50%. Corticosteroid injections combined with surgical removal provide good results. The corticosteroid therapy may be initiated 2 months before surgery, at the time of surgery, or 2 to 4 weeks postoperatively.

Proper surgical technique during the excision reduces the recurrence of keloids. Because tissue trauma may incite further growth, the wound bed and surrounding tissues must be handled gently. Avoid using instruments that crush the tissue.

When an excision is performed, close the skin under minimal tension. Some surgeons avoid subcuticular absorbable sutures, which may increase tissue reaction. Skin closure should be accomplished with a very fine nonabsorbable suture material, such as 6-0 nylon.

A 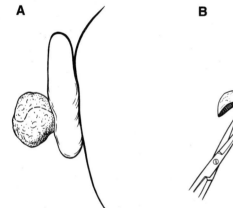   **B** 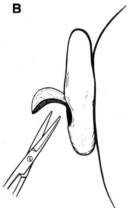   **C**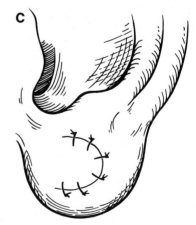

FIG. 11-1.
Resection of a keloid on an ear lobe. The skin overlying a keloid can be used to create a low tension wound closure. **A,** Half the skin is selected for the flap. **B,** The skin is sharply dissected from the underlying keloid, and the subcutaneous keloid is totally excised. **C,** The wound is closed with simple interrupted nonabsorbable small suture.

Some surgeons advocate removal of every vestige of a keloid; however, wide excision of normal skin around keloids does not reduce the rate of recurrence. Other surgeons advocate leaving a rim of incompletely excised keloid in place to serve as a barrier to further keloid growth. It is unclear whether this technique provides significant benefit over standard excisions.

Local advancement flaps can be employed to limit the wound tension after excision. Fig. 11-1 shows a low-tension flap created after the removal of a globular earlobe keloid. While some surgeons advocate skin grafting to provide low-tension skin closure, this therapy has been complicated by large donor-site keloids.

Before attempting surgical excision of keloids, effectively counsel the patient. A detailed informed consent procedure must create appropriate patient expectations. Postoperative results vary widely, and patients must understand that keloids may recur regardless of the treatment method employed.

PRESSURE THERAPY

Pressure applied to burn sites often prevents hypertrophic scar formation, or it induces regression of early hypertrophic scars. Similarly, pressure bandaging following keloid surgery reduces the rate of recurrence. Pressure bandaging is employed until the scar is no longer red; however, patient compliance may be poor if months of therapy are required. Many physicians prefer to use postoperative injections to ensure adequate therapy.

Following earlobe keloid excision, a pressure earring can be worn beginning 2 weeks after surgery. A spring-loaded, light-pressure earring prevents the complication of skin necrosis. Hypoallergenic pressure earrings with a self-adjusting clasp may be purchased from Padgett Instruments, Inc. (800-842-1029). These earrings cost about $40 and are available in a variety of styles and colors that encourage prolonged use.

ALTERNATIVE METHODS

Carbon dioxide (CO_2) laser removal of keloids has not been shown to reduce keloid recurrence when used as the only treatment modality. Using concurrent corticosteroid injection and allowing healing by second intention provides better results. Some investigators are injecting hyaluronidase with steroids after cryotherapy with good results (84% control). Although the mechanism of action is unknown, silastic gel sheeting is being used with success. Positive polarity electrical stimulation is the latest approach being reviewed.

BIBLIOGRAPHY

Apfelberg DB, Maser MR, Lash H: The use of epidermis over a keloid as an autograft after resection of the keloid, *J Dermatol Surg* 2:409, 1976.

Cheng LH: Keloid of the ear lobe, *Laryngoscope* 82:673, 1972.

Domonkos AN, Arnold HL, Odom RB: Andrews' diseases of the skin. In *Clinical dermatology,* ed 7, Philadelphia, 1982, W.B. Saunders.

Golladay ES: Treatment of keloids by single intraoperative perilesional injection of repository steroid, *South Med J* 81:736, 1988.

Habif TP: *Clinical dermatology: a color guide to diagnosis and therapy,* ed 2, St Louis, 1990, Mosby.

Hirshowitz B, Lerner D, Moscona AR: Treatment of keloid scars by combined cryosurgery and intralesional corticosteroids, *Aesth Plast Surg* 6:153, 1982.

Kelly AP: Keloids and hypertrophic scars. In Parish LC, Lask GP, editors: *Aesthetic dermatology,* New York, 1991, McGraw-Hill.

Maguire HC: Treatment of keloids with triamcinolone acetonide injected intralesionally, *JAMA* 192:325, 1965.

Nemeth AJ: Keloids and hypertrophic scars, *J Dermatol Surg Oncol* 19:738, 1993.

Pierce HE: Keloids: enigma of the plastic surgeon, *J Nat Med Assoc* 71:1177, 1979.

Pollack SV, Goslen JB: The surgical treatment of keloids, *J Dermatol Surg Oncol* 8:1045, 1982.

Stegman SJ, Tromovitch TA, Glogau RG: *Basics of dermatologic surgery,* Chicago, 1982, Year Book Medical.

Stucker FJ, Shaw GY: An approach to management of keloids, *Arch Otolaryngol Head Neck Surg* 118:63, 1992.

Weimar VM, Ceilley RI: Surgical gems: treatment of keloids on earlobes, *J Dermatol Surg Oncol* 5:522, 1979.

CHAPTER 12

Sclerotherapy

John R. Pfeifer

Large, bulging varicose veins are best treated surgically using small incisions and sparing the great saphenous vein when possible. Although injection of cutaneous spider veins, or *telangiectasia,* of the lower extremity is generally done for cosmetic reasons, most of these lesions also produce symptoms ranging from numbness, or paresthesia, to pain (either aching or burning). The procedure is tedious and time consuming, and there is a significant incidence of recurrence. However, because of the unattractive appearance of telangiectasia and the associated discomfort, there is a high patient demand for sclerotherapy. This chapter outlines the current office management of these patients and a description of the sclerotherapy technique.

INDICATIONS

- Small bulging varicose veins
- Dilated venules
- Telangiectasia (spider veins)

Although the treatment of larger bulging varicose veins is controversial and many sclerotherapists do inject them, these veins should probably be surgically excised using ¼-inch phlebectomy incisions. The results are cosmetically very good, and the recurrence rate is lower. The injection of large veins is often complicated by skin pigmentation, which can be distressing to the patients.

CONTRAINDICATIONS

The multicenter Food and Drug Administration trial on Sotradecol/aethoxyscklerol has established excellent exclusion criteria for the study. A partial list of these exclusion criteria serves as a commendable list of relative and absolute contraindications to injection.

- Patients with large varicose veins (greater than 6 mm in diameter)—best treated with surgery since they are often in communication with a source of venous reflux
- Pregnant women
- Elderly and sedentary patients (older than 65 years of age)
- Generalized systemic disease (cardiac, renal, hepatic, pulmonary, and collagen diseases, and malignancies) (*relative contraindication,* depending on nature and severity)
- Advanced rheumatic disease, osteoarthritis, or any disease that interferes with patient mobility
- Arterial insufficiency of lower extremities
- Bronchial asthma or demonstrated allergies to sclerosant (except with hypertonic saline)
- Acute superficial or deep thrombophlebitis
- Acute febrile illness
- Obesity
- Patients on anticoagulants

PATIENT EVALUATION

A complete preliminary history and physical should be performed, and special attention given to the arterial and venous system. In addition to a general history questionnaire, a specific encounter form is used to evaluate the patient for sclerotherapy (Box 12-1). The patient may have one or two laboratory studies to complete the assessment of the venous system.

Examine the patient in the erect position (after 5 to 10 minutes of standing to allow for maximum inflation of bulging varicosities). Accurately mark bulging varicosities and spider veins on leg diagrams (Fig. 12-1). A copy of this diagram should be on the chart at the time of each injection treatment to facilitate an accurate record of injection locations.

Measure the patient for support hose. A variety of brands are available. Discourage the use of over-the-counter support hose since the patient needs a stocking specific to his or her measurements. The patient should bring the stockings to the first injection visit.

LABORATORY STUDIES

Initially, photoplethysmography (PPG) is used to evaluate venous valve function and the degree of venous insufficiency. With proper technique, superficial and deep insufficiency can be identified and corrected before injection therapy. If there is any question of deep vein thrombosis, the phleborrheograph (PRG) is used to rule out a recent venous occlusion. Duplex scanning is the best method of precisely assessing deep venous occlusion, either acute or chronic. The presence of chronic

BOX 12-1. PATIENT EVALUATION FORM
SCLEROTHERAPY

DATE _____ NAME _____

AGE _____ SEX _____

HEIGHT _____ WEIGHT _____

REFERRED BY _____

1. How many years have you noticed this problem? _____

2. Have you ever been previously treated for this problem?

   Yes _____ No _____

   By whom and when? _____

   _____

   With what method?

   Injection   _____
   Electrocautery   _____
   Laser   _____
   Surgery   _____

3. When did the problem with your veins occur?

   Age   _____
   Before pregnancy?   _____
   After pregnancy?   _____
   After trauma?   _____
   After birth control
      or Premarin therapy?   _____
   Other   _____

4. Is there a family history of varicose or spider veins?

   Mother   _____
   Father   _____
   Sister   _____
   Brother   _____
   Children   _____
   Aunts   _____
   Uncles   _____

5. Do you have a history of:

   Smoking   _____
   Blood clots _____

Lupus   _____
Bleeding disorders   _____
Easy bruisability   _____
Dark spots after
   skin injury or surgery   _____
Easy scarring   _____

6. Are you developing new veins?   _____

7. Are your present veins getting bigger?   _____

8. After prolonged standing or sitting do your legs ache?   _____

9. Do your legs or veins ache before menses?   _____

10. Does walking or exercise relieve or aggravate the pain?   _____

11. Describe any symptoms you have from your veins:

    _____

    _____

12. Are you required to be on your feet for long periods?   _____

13. Do you jog, run, jump rope, or do aerobics?   _____

    How often per week?   _____

14. Are you pregnant or planning a pregnancy soon?   _____

15. Did you read and understand the patient education materials given to you?   _____

16. Do you understand the risks and benefits as well as possible complications to vein injection?   _____

17. Are you prepared to wear support hose on a regular basis as described?   _____

Comments: _____

_____

Continued.

BOX 12-1.–cont'd
SCLEROTHERAPY: PHYSICAL EXAM

VARICOSITIES: R   L

Vulvar   ____ ____
Groin   ____ ____
Thigh   ____ ____
Below knee   ____ ____

PULSES: R   L

Femoral   ____ ____
Popliteal   ____ ____
Dorsalis pedis   ____ ____
Post tibial   ____ ____

PRESENCE OF: R   L

Edema   ____ ____
Stasis pig   ____ ____
Cellulitis   ____ ____
Active ulcer   ____ ____
Healed ulcer   ____ ____
Venules   ____ ____
Tenderness   ____ ____

PPG   ____ ____

PRG   ____ ____

IMPRESSION: _____

_____

PLAN: Discussed: Measurements:

             • method   Ankle _____

             • cost

             • complications   Thigh _____
                 hyperpigmentation
                 blistering   Length _____
                 recurrence
                 pain   Shoe   _____
                 phlebitis
                                            _____
             • stockings   Nurse Initials

_____

_____

cc: _____ _____ _____
                      Physician Signature   Date

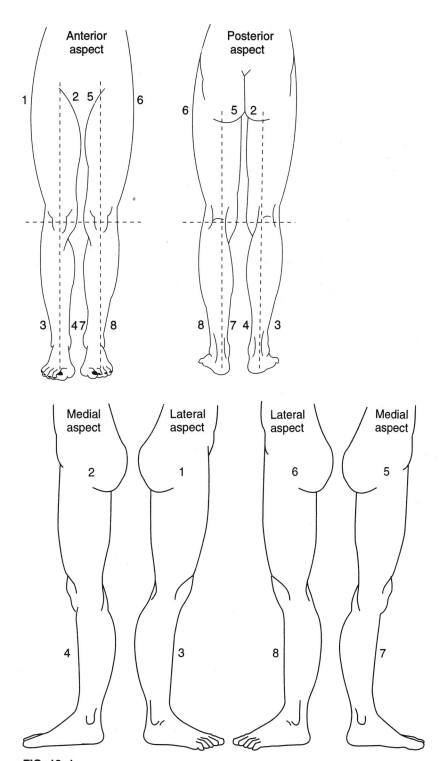

FIG. 12-1.
Leg diagrams for documentation of veins and location of injections.

deep vein occlusion is not a contraindication for sclerotherapy. However, the presence of *acute deep vein thrombosis* (DVT) is an *absolute* contraindication for sclerotherapy. If acute DVT is detected, sclerotherapy should be postponed for six months.

PREPROCEDURE PATIENT EDUCATION

A signed permit should be obtained, even though this is an office procedure. Written permission to photograph the patient also should be obtained. A single "Consent to Treatment" form, which includes permission for both injection and photography, can be used (Box 12-2).

Before performing injection sclerotherapy, give a verbal and written comprehensive explanation of the procedure, and its attendant risks to the patient (Box 12-3).

**BOX 12-2. CONSENT TO TREATMENT
INJECTION THERAPY FOR SPIDER VEINS**

I have been informed by the doctor of the nature of injection treatment of my veins. I understand the possible side effects, which include recurrence, skin pigmentation, skin ulcers, and localized clotted veins. I have read over the handouts provided and understand the risks and benefits. I have been given the opportunity to have all my questions answered.

I authorize the doctor to take photographs of me before and after treatment, and to permit such photographs to be used at the doctor's discretion for purposes of medical lecturing, research, or scientific publication, with the provision that I will not be identified.

Fees and Payment

Injections are billed individually at $_____ each. Most treatments will not exceed twenty injections per appointment. Due to the costs of providing this treatment and the variability of insurance coverage, payment is expected at the time this service is rendered. A deposit of $_____ is required no later than (10) days prior to my scheduled appointment. This deposit confirms my appointment time and will be credited to my balance on my treatment day. All future scheduled appointments will also require a deposit in advance. The balance at the time of treatment will then be that which exceeds the deposit. (Payment by cash, check, Visa, or Mastercard will be accepted.) I understand all terms as written above, and I authorize the doctor to administer such treatment to me.

_____   _____
WITNESS   PATIENT'S SIGNATURE

                                                      _____
                                                      DATE

BOX 12-3. PATIENT EDUCATION HANDOUT
INJECTION THERAPY FOR SPIDER VEINS

As you begin a program of sclerotherapy for your spider veins, there are some things that you should be aware of.

1. **Certain veins require three or four treatments before they disappear.**
   The principle of injection therapy for small skin veins is to inject a sclerosing (scarring) agent into the vein, which causes the vein wall to become inflamed and seal together. When the vein can no longer carry blood, it is no longer visible through the skin. Certain veins require three or four treatments before they disappear.

2. **There is occasional skin pigmentation (brown spots).**
   When the tiny needle is inserted into the vein and the salt solution is injected, occasionally the vein will rupture allowing this solution to leak into the surrounding tissue. This may result in a brown pigmented spot in the skin, which rarely is permanent and usually disappears with time. It is usually small and no more obvious than the vein that was initially treated. However, you should be aware that this is a possible complication of injection sclerotherapy, although it only occurs in approximately 10% of the cases.

3. **There is a rare occurrence of small skin ulcers after an injection.**
   Very rarely, an injection will be irritating enough to cause a small area of skin loss (or ulcer). In more than 70,000 injections, this complication has occurred 37 times. These ulcers are the size of a pencil eraser, and can heal without incident, leaving just a small white scar.

4. **Flare formation ("matting").**
   Occasionally, immediately following injection, a new cluster of veins may form in proximity of the vein just injected. This has the appearance of a "blush" in the skin. These can usually be controlled by repeat injection.

5. **Pain.**
   Very small needles are used, and the discomfort during injection is minimal.

6. **You will be required to wear support hose after treatment.**
   After injection, your legs will be compressed with small gauze pads and a compression stocking (either calf high or a pantyhose). This compression support must stay in place for three days and two nights, during which time you will not be able to shower or have a complete bath. Then the stocking alone is used (except during sleep) for an additional two weeks, during which you may resume your normal bathing routine. Cool baths or showers are advised.

7. **Activities after injection.**
   During the injection treatments, your daily activities are not restricted. You may continue to work and perform your daily activities. However, aggressive exercising (such as jogging, tennis, or high-impact aerobics) should be avoided one to three weeks following treatment.

8. **New spider veins may form, requiring subsequent treatment.**
   Because humans function and work in the erect position, there is extra pressure on the veins of the leg. Thus, there is a tendency for new spider veins to form. Even after most of your veins have been removed by sclerotherapy, be aware that *new spider veins can develop*. We ask all our patients to return for periodic reevaluation so that any new veins can be injected before they become too large or too numerous. Use of compression hose on a regular basis can reduce the likelihood of recurrence.

PRESCLEROTHERAPY PHOTOGRAPHY

Evaluation of sclerotherapy results is highly subjective. Frequently, as the series of sclerotherapy treatments progresses, patients will forget how extensive their veins were before injection. Therefore, it is important to photograph all areas of planned injection before beginning sclerotherapy.

Keep the prints in the patient file and periodically review them with the patient. This photographic record allows the treating physician to evaluate improvement objectively as treatment progresses.

COMPRESSION STOCKINGS

Faria and Morales have pointed out that many spider telangiectasia are related to venous insufficiency, and there is direct communication between telangiectatic channels and the deep venous system. Observations have supported this finding: a leg that is not supported with a compression stocking following injection has a more rapid rate of recurrence of spider veins. Goldman et al. noted improvement in sclerotherapy results when compression was used.

Author's note: In my experience, the use of an adequate compression stocking has reduced recurrence by approximately 50%.

If only below-knee injections are carried out, then 30 to 40 mm Hg below-knee stockings can be used. If thigh injections are performed, a 20 to 30 mm Hg pantyhose is fitted. If larger veins are injected, 4- or 6-inch Ace bandages are snugly applied to the leg, and the compression stocking is worn over the Ace bandages for the first three days. Over-the-counter hose do not provide the support necessary for these patients.

Instruct the patient to wear the compression stocking for three days and two nights after treatment and to avoid strenuous exercise. For the first three days, the injection sites are padded with gauze compression pads under the compression hose. After the first three days, the patient may take daily showers but must wear the support stocking during the day for two weeks, removing it only at night. When breast lesions are treated, they are compressed with elastic bandages overnight only.

Author's note: I recommend that patients wear compression stockings on a long-term basis for most of their standing activities.

EQUIPMENT

- Electric table: needs only vertical motion and does not need to flex
- Headlamp
- 3-power ocular magnification loupes
- Air-Tite syringes: 1 cc (high quality, and the least expensive)

- Hypertonic saline 23.4%, 30 cc vials
- 4- or 6-inch Ace bandages for selected patients
- Compression hose (measured for the patient)
    Below knee
    Pantyhose
    Sheer support
- 30-gauge needles, 0.5 inch
- Non-sterile 4 × 4 inch gauze
- Paper tape
- Antiseptic solution (Zephiran)
- Nonsterile physician gloves
- *Optional:* rubber gloves for patient or nurse to pull on stockings

PATIENT PREPARATION

It is important to realize that although sclerotherapy is done to alleviate symptoms of pain, paraesthesia, etc., the majority of patients also are motivated by cosmetic concerns. Therefore, results are not based on the usual physician parameters of clinical improvement. Rather, the patient's own assessment of results is important. In fact, the patient's decision to proceed with treatment depends on his or her reaction to the degree of pain during the procedure, and on his or her assessment of the result. In sclerotherapy, patient comfort and patient satisfaction become critical factors in determining whether to continue with treatment. The physician's preinjection preparation of the patient becomes an important component of the procedure. A supportive physician is important, but supportive and kind office personnel are equally important, since it is they who handle the many questions posed by sclerotherapy patients.

Occasionally patients are injected on the day of preliminary evaluation. However, the majority are scheduled for a separate sclerotherapy appointment on another day. Instructions on what to do to prepare for injection are given to patients so they are adequately prepared for the injection procedure (Box 12-4).

BOX 12-4. PATIENT INSTRUCTIONS
PREPARATION FOR INJECTION TREATMENT

1. On the day of your injections, bring your compression stockings.
2. Do not use bath oil, lotion, or powder on your legs the night before or the day of your injection treatment.
3. Wear loose slacks, sweat pants, a dress, or a skirt, and wear comfortable, loose shoes to accommodate the dressing.
4. If possible, bring loose-fitting shorts to wear during the injection procedure.
5. Please call your insurance company to check the extent of insurance coverage for this procedure.

SCLEROSANTS

Hypertonic saline is recommended in this text because of the low risk of complications and generally excellent outcome associated with its use. However, there is a variety of other solutions available. Goldman's *Sclerotherapy: Treatment of Varicose and Telangiectatic Veins* is highly recommended for the interested reader.

TECHNIQUE

1. Have the patient lie flat in a horizontal position on the treatment table (either supine or prone, depending on location of venous lesion). Trendelenburg position and tourniquets are not necessary. A high-intensity light (preferably a headlamp) is an absolute necessity.
2. Photograph the legs and record it in the log book. Photos may show patients in a standing or horizontal position.
3. Prepare the leg with aqueous Zephiran or a similar colorless antiseptic solution. Infection after sclerotherapy is rare, and thus the site is prepped mainly to render the skin more transparent so that the veins are easier to see.
4. Use an injection solution of 23.4% saline (0.47 cc) plus 2% plain lidocaine (0.03 cc) mixed in a 1 cc tuberculin syringe. (This solution is prepared in advance by injecting 2 cc of 2% plain lidocaine into a 30 cc multiple-dose vial of 23.4% saline. This dilutes the saline to 18.7%.) Five to ten syringes should be preloaded by the assistant before entering the room.
5. Each injection is limited to 0.5 cc of solution to minimize the risk of traversing the communicating vein and reaching the deep venous system.
6. Use a 30-gauge needle to enter the vein. A 3-power ocular loupe will facilitate accurate entry of the vein. *Injection must be intraluminal.* Perivenous injection leads to pigmentation. You should bend the needle to 30 degrees to allow easier entry into the vein.
7. The injection should be made slowly. Watch the tip of the needle as you inject. The appearance of a small bleb suggests extravasation and means that that individual injection should be terminated. If you watch carefully and stop immediately when extravasation occurs, these small blebs should subside without leaving a blemish. It is not necessary—and may in fact be harmful—to attempt to dilute small extravasation blebs.
8. Proper injection will result in blanching along the course of the injected vein. Erythema around the injected vein appears immediately after injection and indicates that the saline solution has been injected correctly throughout the distribution of the vein. Veins refill rapidly.
9. After injection, withdraw the needle and apply pressure directly over the area with three stacked 4 × 4 inch gauze squares folded once. Use paper tape to secure the gauze pad in place.
10. Each needle is only used for 3 to 4 injections because a sharp needle is necessary.

Author's note: On the average, I administer 15 injections per session, and the patient typically has three sessions. I have injected as many as 80 sites in a single session if the patient has distance or time constraints. An area should not be reinjected a second time before four weeks have elapsed.

POSTPROCEDURE CARE

During the course of the sclerotherapy treatment, compress the sites with gauze pressure pads (three 4×4 inch pads folded once and secured with paper tape). Apply the compression hose over these pads *before* the patient gets off the treatment table. Thus the patient's legs are not permitted in the dependent position until the compression stocking is in place. The office nurse, compression therapist, or a trained office assistant should put the stocking on the patient and instruct him or her in proper application and removal of the hose. Rubber gloves aid in this process.

Patients are then given a list of instructions to follow for the first two weeks after treatment (Box 12-5).

COMPLICATIONS

- Recurrence is not a complication of sclerotherapy; however, patients view recurrence as a complication. Remember, this is a gravity-related disorder and all varicose veins and spider veins tend to recur. If patients are warned prior to injection, they are less concerned and less hostile.

BOX 12-5. INSTRUCTIONS TO FOLLOW AFTER INJECTION TREATMENT

Days 1 to 3. The stockings should remain in place for three days (no bathing; wear them to bed). The compression stockings are an important part of the treatment because they minimize the amount of blood reentering the injected vein. Elevate your legs as much as possible. No jogging or high-impact aerobics are allowed at this time. At the end of the three days, you may remove the stockings and discard the gauze pads. (You may find standing in the shower a convenient way to loosen the tape that holds the gauze pads; this also reduces the irritation to sensitive skin.) Do not be surprised if injected areas appear bruised at this time; that is normal with many skin types. You may resume normal activity.

Days 4 to 14. Continue to wear the compression stockings daily. Remove them at night to sleep. You may resume daily cool showers. Avoid jogging or high-impact aerobics during this time.

Days 15 on. Continue to wear the compression stockings whenever you can, as this will reduce the rate of recurrence of spider varicose veins.

- Pigmentation is seen in 3% to 5% of patients and usually disappears in a few months, but may last as long as a year.
- Telangiectatic matting (flare formation) is seen in 1% to 3% of patients. These small venous blush formations near the site of injection are very distressing to the patient. They can be eliminated by subsequent injection of dominant veins within the blush formation.
- Ulceration occurs in 37 per 70,305 injections (or 1 per 1900 injections). These are usually small, full-thickness ulcers less than 1 cm in diameter. They all heal within 1 to 3 months.
- Superficial phlebitis is occasionally seen in veins adjacent to the injection site.
- Deep-vein thrombosis may occur. This is very rare, and the risk is minimized if the volume of injection is limited.

  Author's note: In my experience, this occurred in only one patient who, after treatment with anticoagulants and hospitalization, experienced no long-term sequelae.

- Anaphylaxis can occur with nearly all agents except hypertonic saline.

SUPPLIERS

- *Support Hose:*

Sigvaris
P.O. Box 570
Branford, CT 06405
800-322-7744

Jobst Institute, Inc.
P.O. Box 652
Toledo, OH 43694
800-537-1063

Medi USA
76 W. Seegers Road
Arlington Heights, IL 60005

- *Luxtec Headlamp and Ocular Loupes:*

Plagens Associates, Inc.
9408 Maltby Road
Brighton, MI 48116
800-722-7713

United Surgical Inc.
3101 Davison
Flint, MI 48506
313-736-5707

- *Syringes and Needles:*

Air-Tite Syringes
423 S. Lynnhaven Road, #104
Virginia Beach, VA 23452
800-231-7762

- *Hypertonic Saline:*

  Dermatologic Lab and Supply, Inc.   Ivenex
  201 Ridge   Gibcol Ivenex Division
  Council Bluffs, IA 51501   The Dexter Corporation
  800-831-6273   Chagrin Falls, OH 44022

- *Venous Noninvasive Diagnostic Equipment (PPG, Doppler, etc.) and Assistance with All Sclerotherapy Supplies:*

  Sam Wagner
  P.O. Box 431
  202 Dodd Street
  Middlebourne, WV 26149
  304-758-2370

- *Patient Education Materials:*

  American Academy of Dermatology   Contemporary Communications
  930 North Meacham Rd.   P.O. Box 17985
  P.O. Box 4014   Marietta, GA 30007
  Schaumburg, IL 60168-4014   404-434-1406
  708-330-0230

CONCLUSION

Injection sclerotherapy using hypertonic saline solution is a safe, relatively painless method of ablating small varicose veins, reticular venules, and spider telangiectasia, with a minimum of complications. The attending physician will have better results and happier patients if he or she remembers several important concepts:

1. Although spider veins are symptomatic, most patients seek treatment because they are unhappy with the appearance of their legs. Be cautious and conservative so that you do not create a blemish worse than what the patient already has.
2. Sclerotherapy should be viewed as a semicosmetic procedure, and the patient's high degree of expectation must be carefully considered.
3. Careful preinjection discussion of risk must occur with patients so that they are fully aware of the protracted and tedious nature of sclerotherapy, as well as the potential complications.
4. The effect of gravity and incompetent venous valves must always be remembered. Varicose veins and spider veins tend to recur. The wearing of compression hose in the immediate postinjection period is mandatory. Compression hose worn on a long-term basis will significantly reduce recurrence.

5. Meticulous technique is essential in sclerotherapy:

- Be sure your needle is in the vein.
- Inject slowly.
- Inject only 0.5 cc *maximum* per injection; avoid large bolus injections.
- Watch the needle tip; stop injecting if there is extravasation.

With careful and precise technique, the majority of small telangiectatic (spider) veins can be eliminated. Patient satisfaction with the procedure is high.

CPT/BILLING CODES

To bill for a single injection, the CPT code is 36470. To bill for multiple injections (more than one), the CPT code is 36471 and the number of injections is placed in the quantity box. If both legs are injected on the same day, the procedure must be billed as a bilateral procedure. Blue Cross Blue Shield of Michigan has a bilateral modifier (50) that is put in the modifier box. Medicare is billed on two separate claim lines, one for each leg. Private insurance could be billed on two separate lines, indicating left leg and right leg, or if billed on one line the number of injections for each leg could be listed in the remarks section.

BIBLIOGRAPHY

Bergan JT, Yao JST: *Venous problems*, Chicago, 1978, Year Book.

Browse, Burnand, Thomas: *Diseases of the veins*, London, 1988, Edward Arnold.

Faria JL, Morales IN: Histopathology of the telangiectasia associated with varicose veins, *Dermatologica* 127:321, 1963.

Fegan WG: Continuous compression technique of injecting varicose veins, *Lancet* 2:109, 1963.

*Goldman MP: *Sclerotherapy: treatment of varicose and telangiectatic veins*, St Louis, 1991, Mosby.

Goldman MP et al: Compression in the treatment of leg telangiectasia: a preliminary report, *J Dermatol Surg Oncol* 16:4, 1990.

Goldman MP et al: Treatment of facial telangiectasias with sclerotherapy, laser surgery, and/or electrodessication: a review, *J Dermatol Surg Oncol* 19:899, 1993.

Green D: Sclerotherapy for varicose and telangiectatic veins, *Am Fam Physician* 46(3):827, 1992.

Hobbs JT: The treatment of varicose veins: a random trial of injection compression therapy versus surgery, *Br J Surg* 55:777, 1968.

Pfeifer JR, Hawtof GD: Injection sclerotherapy and CO_2 laser sclerotherapy in the ablation of cutaneous spider veins of the lower extremity, *Phlebology* 4:231, 1989.

Ricci S, Georgieu M: Office varicose vein surgery under local anesthesia, *J Dermatol Surg Oncol* 18:55, 1992.

Editor's note: This text by Goldman is "the bible" on sclerotherapy for the novice and the experienced alike. It is very practical, has numerous diagrams and color photographs, and is a resource and reference for all topics relating to sclerotherapy.

Sigg K: Treatment of varicosities and accompanying complications; ambulatory treatment of phlebitis with compression bandage, *Angiology* 3:355, 1952.

Sodick NS: Predisposing factors for varicose and telangiectatic leg veins, *J Dermatol Surg Oncol* 18:883, 1992.

Weiss MA, Weiss RA, Goldman MP: How minor varicosities cause leg pain, *Contemp OB/Gyn:*113, August 1991.

Williams RA, Wilson SE: Sclerosant treatment of varicose veins and deep vein thrombosis, *Arch Surg* 119:1283, 1984.

CHAPTER 13

Unna Paste Boot

Donald E. DeWitt

The Unna paste boot is used primarily when a semiimmobilizing soft-pressure dressing or gradient-pressure dressing over a joint or extremity is needed. It is commonly available in a 4-inch roll or bandage that is impregnated with a calamine/gelatin/zinc oxide compound.

INDICATIONS

- Usage has varied over the years; however, at present, one of the best uses of the Unna boot is for the initial treatment of an *acute ankle sprain with severe swelling,* where immobilization and non-weight bearing are needed until other means of treatment are appropriate. It can be used on any extremity sprain with soft tissue swelling as a first approach, using an air-inflated splint after the swelling has subsided.
- The Unna boot can be used as a symmetrical gradient pressure dressing for *venous stasis ulcers* to help reduce venous hypertension, control edema, and prevent delayed venous return. It is a very effective part of overall therapy. Debridement should be carried out first (if indicated) and then the ulcer should be covered with a permeable dressing, such as Tegaderm (pouched or regular).
- In *acute and chronic tendonitis,* the Unna boot acts as a soft immobilizer.

CONTRAINDICATIONS

- Acute sprains with fractures
- Venous stasis ulcers that are infected and need debridement and cleaning; e.g., ulcers with heavy exudate and crusted ulcers with associated cellulitis
- Active phlebitis

TECHNIQUE

The Unna boot is easy to apply, change, and remove, and it is not as cumbersome as a splint. For the lower extremity, roll the bandage on like a cast, beginning at the distal part of the foot and going up to just below the tibial tuberosity. It is important that the gradient pressure applied with this technique be uniform without any constricting bands (no tourniquet effect). Place the greatest pressure over the area of concern, and then less pressure as the bandage application proceeds proximally. Change the boot weekly. The number of changes is dictated by response to therapy, such as the gradual reduction in swelling, but there is no limitation.

Make sure the skin is completely dry before application. The boot may be applied directly over the skin but most physicians place a *smooth* snug layer of Kerlex or Kling over the entire area first. For the lower extremity, cut the bandage frequently during the application, and symmetrically cover the entire heel. Do not use any reverse turns as might be done in casting. Keep the foot at a 90-degree angle to the tibia. Overlap successive layers 50% and make the boot three layers thick. Cover the outside with any of four materials: elastic roller bandage, Coban, Kling, or Tube Gauze. Such a dressing can usually be left on seven days without being changed. The Unna boot really never dries as does a cast. Rather, it remains soft and compressible (Figs. 13-1 and 13-2).

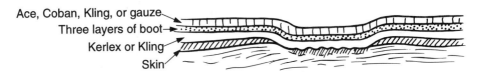

Ace, Coban, Kling, or gauze
Three layers of boot
Kerlex or Kling
Skin

FIG. 13-1.
Layered method of applying Unna boot for a decubitus ulcer.

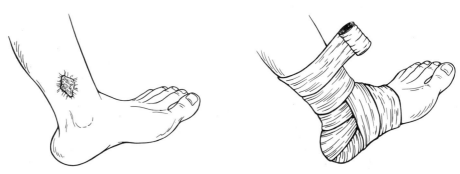

FIG. 13-2.
Technique of rolling on the Unna boot.

POSTPROCEDURE CARE

The boot must be kept dry. Remove the boot with a large bandage scissors. Cleanse and dry the skin thoroughly. When the boot is used for stasis ulcers, inspect the foot carefully for the presence of infection, and debride again if necessary before applying a second boot. To obtain good results, the patient must comply with all other aspects of medical therapy as well. For sprains, as the swelling subsides, the compression advantage will be lost. A second boot will have to be applied or more appropriate therapy, such as an inflated splint, will have to be utilized. Teach the patient to check for signs of impaired circulation and to report any paresthesia or unusual discomfort.

COMPLICATIONS

When the Unna boot is used repeatedly over a long period, there are occasional skin reactions to the bandage. The bandage does not adhere to the skin even if the skin was not covered before application. If the patient complains of pain, or if there is a lot of drainage soaking through or a bad odor, remove and inspect the ulcer. If applied too tightly, it may cause neurovascular complications.

SUPPLIER

Dome paste bandage: Miles Inc., Pharmaceutical Division

CPT/BILLING CODE

29580   Unna paste boot application

Or use a specific code for joint immobilization (e.g., ankle-29540).

CHAPTER 14

Wood's Light Examination

Donald E. DeWitt

The Wood's lamp is a dermatological instrument that makes use of invisible, long-wave ultraviolet radiation and visible blue/white fluorescence (Fig. 14-1). The Wood's light, long-wave ultraviolet energy from a Wood's lamp, is converted to visible light after it interacts with various molecules in or on the skin specimen being examined. The color of this secondary (fluorescent) light, seen best in a darkened room, is usually characteristic of a disease or condition. A magnifying lens may be interposed between the surface being examined and the light source. For many conditions, however, this is not necessary since the color result is used for the diagnosis.

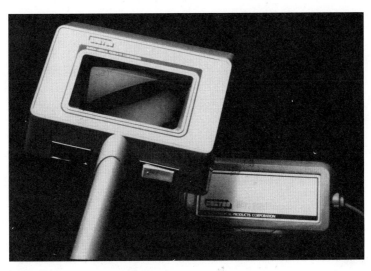

FIG. 14-1.
The Wood's lamp (ultraviolet light).

DIAGNOSTIC USES

- Tinea capitis
- Erythrasma
- Vitiligo, albinism, tuberous sclerosis, and other pigmentary conditions
- *Pseudomonas* infections
- Porphyria cutanea tarda
- Tinea versicolor
- Scabies
- Detection of some chemicals that are applied to the skin or taken systematically
- Adjunct in finding corneal abrasions or herpetic corneal lesions

INDICATIONS

- Any dermatitis in body folds such as the inguinal, perianal, interdigital, axillary, or inframammary area (for example, erythrasma, *pseudomonas* infections)
- Patches of scalp scaling and partial hair loss, especially when the hairs are broken or shorter than normal (tinea capitis)
- Pigmentary conditions
- Pruritic papules on the glans penis, areolae, volar aspect of the wrist, and the finger web areas (scabies)
- Blisters or punctated erosions on the exposed portions of the hands and forearms, with follow-up urine examination (porphyria cutanea tarda)
- Patches of scaling and altered pigmentation of the skin (tinea versicolor)

TECHNIQUE

The instrument is simply turned on and held 8 inches above the surface being examined.

MOST COMMON FINDINGS

Condition	Color
1. Tinea capitis (three varieties)	1. Bright yellow green to pale green
2. Erythrasma	2. Coral red to pink
3. *Pseudomonas aeruginosa* infections	3. Aqua green or white green
4. Tinea versicolor	4. Golden yellow

DRUGS AND MISCELLANEOUS

- Tetracycline: Systemic tetracycline can create yellow fluorescence in *some* inflammatory lesions such as acne papules, areas of ulceration, and granulation tissue. Dried urine on hospital gowns or filter paper also will appear fluorescent yellow when it contains tetracyclines and can be used to confirm that patients are taking their medications.

- Fluorescein: When given intravenously, this dye will produce yellow fluorescence in the skin. The most common use of fluorescein is to help identify corneal abrasions and infection. The dye is used topically usually by moistening a small strip of impregnated paper. A drop is allowed to fall in the conjunctival sac. The Wood's light is then used to detect the areas of staining.
- Miscellaneous: Many cosmetics, topical medications, and industrial chemicals may be detected on the skin by their fluorescence.

SUPPLIER

Burton Medical Products Corporation
7922 Haskell Avenue
Van Nuys, CA 91406
818-989-4700

BIBLIOGRAPHY

Brophy et al: Intertriginous dermatoses; common puzzling problems, *Post Grad Med* 78(7):105, 1985.

Frieden IJ: Diagnosis and management of tinea capitis, *Pediatr Ann* 16(1):39, 1987.

Ginsburg CM: Superficial fungal and microbacterial infections of the skin, *Pediatr Infect Dis*:19, 1985.

Jerdan et al: Cutaneous manifestations of *Corynebecterium* Group JK sepsis, *J Am Acad Dermatol* 16:444, 1987.

Pembroke AC: Fungal infections of the skin, *Practitioner* 230:229, 1986.

Sindhuphak W et al: Erythrasma—overlooked or misdiagnosed? *Int J Dermatol* 24:95, 1985.

CHAPTER 15

Laser Therapy

James E. Rasmussen

John L. Pfenninger

With the widespread acceptance of radiofrequency surgery, laser dermatologic and gynecologic surgery has been limited more and more to vascular lesions. This chapter covers both carbon dioxide and pulsed tunable dye lasers.

Lasers are expensive (see Table 15-1), and their price sharply curtails the number of primary care physicians using them in the office. It is possible to obtain the necessary training and to use the more expensive units available within hospitals, but the likelihood of having sufficient patient volume to maintain competency is small.

Thus, practicality may limit the primary care physician to the carbon dioxide laser. For office procedures, the units with the lower power and lower cost are generally adequate.

CO$_2$ LASER METHOD

Indications and Uses

- When a bloodless field is essential
- For removal of extensive lesions in patients with pacemakers
- When electrosurgery is contraindicated
- Periungual or extensive verrucae or condyloma
- Patients with bleeding disorders
- When other techniques have failed
- Actinic chelitis
- Rhinophyma
- Tattoos (Q-switched ruby laser is better.)
- Bowenoid papulosis or squamous cell carcinoma of the penis
- Hemorrhoids
- Cervical dysplasia

TABLE 15-1.

Cost of Laser Units

Laser Type	Cost*
Carbon dioxide	$ 15,000-60,000
Argon	25,000-30,000
Argon tunable dye	125,000
Flashlamp-pumped pulsed dye	165,000
Copper vapor	115,000

*Add smoke evacuator ($2,000 to $5,000) and maintenance costs for each unit.

Although the laser can be used on a myriad of other lesions, this list of indications is narrowed to those clinical situations where the carbon dioxide laser may actually produce better outcomes than other modalities.

Contraindications

- Known HIV-positive status (*relative contraindication*)
- Large vascular lesions (Other laser modalities are preferred.)

Advantages

- Precision in cutting, vaporizing, or coagulating tissue
- Better hemostasis (improves visibility)
- Reduced scarring (in most instances)
- Infection is rare
- Perhaps less pain, since sensory nerve endings are cauterized
- Can be performed on an outpatient basis

Disadvantages

- Costly, cumbersome, space-occupying equipment
- HPV/HIV may be present in smoke plume, and there is a risk of inhalation
- May actually be associated with more prolonged healing times
- Safety issues
- Noxious odor

Complications

- Hypertrophic scarring (especially with tattoos)
- Postprocedural cutaneous texture changes
- Eye injury to personnel (if not properly protected)
- Fire/explosions
- Excessive granulation tissue
- Unintentional burns to patients, personnel, operator

Considering all of the complications, most physicians conclude that the majority of nonvascular cutaneous lesions can be treated with much less expensive modalities that are effective and safe, and that produce acceptable cosmetic results.

Training

For the clinician interested in further laser education, contact one of the following:

The American Society for Laser Medicine and Surgery
2404 Stewart Square
Wausau, WI 54401
715-845-9283

Circadian, Inc.
3942 North First St.
San Jose, CA 94134
408-954-1808

Coherent Laser
6522 Timbermill Way
Reynoldsburg, OH 43068
614-759-4463

Laser Institute of America
12424 Research Parkway, Suite 130
Orlando, FL 32826
407-380-1553

Marshfield Clinic
1000 North Oak Avenue
Marshfield, WI 54449
715-387-9460

Wenske Laser Center
Ravenwood Hospital
Corner of Damen and Wilson
Chicago, IL
312-878-4300 Ext. 4505

PULSED TUNABLE DYE LASER METHOD

A variety of lasers have been used to treat flat, vascular lesions (port-wine stains) since the late 1970s. The early lasers used an argon lasing medium. These machines are difficult to use because the treatment field is limited to 1 to 2 mm, and the relatively long pulse duration does not allow selective photothermolysis. A much more useful laser, termed the *pulsed tunable dye,* became available in the mid-1980s. This machine has a substantial advantage of a 5 mm treatment spot size, and a very short pulse duration, which allows the interior of the blood vessel to be destroyed without much heating of the surrounding tissue. Consequently, blood vessels are destroyed in preference to the surrounding dermis. This reduces the incidence of scarring to nearly zero.

Indications

Currently available pulsed tunable dye lasers use a wavelength of 585 nm and penetrate approximately 1.5 mm into the dermis. This limits their utility to flat, or nearly flat, vascular lesions such as port-wine stains, spider telangiectasias, and small hemangiomas (cherry angiomas, pyogenic granulomas). This laser is not useful for larger hemangiomas (strawberry hemangiomas, cavernous hemangiomas).

Equipment

- Pulsed tunable dye laser (Candela or others)
- Protective goggles for patient, observers, medical assistants, and operator

Preprocedure Patient Education

Patient and parents need to be given a thorough discussion of the results, side effects, and cost of therapy. It is important for patients to realize that successful therapy will require multiple treatment sessions for each specific site. Published averages range from three to seven treatments per area. Treatment is usually given in half-hour sessions of about 350 to 450 pulses. An area of approximately 125 to 250 cm^2 may be treated during this time period. Each pulse produces a moderately painful sensation on the skin and an immediate bruising effect. Patients should be shown preprocedure photos, immediately postprocedure photos, and results as seen at 2- to 4-month intervals. This clearly details the gross bruising that accompanies this procedure and the lid swelling when it is done around the eyes.

Patients should also be aware that the treatment is expensive, and that it may be considered a cosmetic procedure by certain insurance companies, which consequently will not reimburse for it. The method of payment should be clarified before the patient begins therapy. Each session will cost $400 to $600, depending on local charges, surgical room fees, operating room nurses, and type of anesthesia (general or local).

Technique

The procedure is moderately painful, but it can usually be tolerated by most adults. Children, as well as some adolescents and a few adults, require oral sedation or general anesthesia. Eutectic mixture of local anesthetic (EMLA) will help reduce skin pain by 25% to 75%, depending on the patient and the degree of anxiety.

After showing the patient the appropriate photographs and answering all questions, perform a test patch on several sites. Try to pick those areas most sensitive and least sensitive to the laser. If a port-wine stain occupies a large area of the face, do three or four test patches including one on the upper lid, as well as the forehead, the cheek, and the lip. Specific techniques of test patching vary. Some physicians prefer to use four separate energy levels within a single test patch. Others prefer to fill an area of about 1 cm² on a certain body site with laser pulses at a certain energy level, and then increase or decrease the energy levels on other body sites as needed. The patient is then seen again after two to four months, a sufficient amount of time for complete healing. It is important to emphasize that during this time the patient should use sunscreens and wear protective clothing.

On the patient's second visit, treat a larger area with the energy level that has produced the best results with the fewest side effects. As a general rule, the forehead requires 5.5 to 6.5 J; the lids, 4.5 to 5.5 J; the nose, 6.5 to 8.5 J; the upper lip, 6.5 to 7.5 J; the ear, 5.5 to 6.5 J; the sides of the neck, 5.5 to 6.5 J; the upper extremity, 5.5 to 7.0 J; and the lower extremity, 5.5 to 7.5 J. Children require lower energy levels (4.5 to 6.0 J).

Most laser operators use the 5 mm pulse with 10% to 15% overlap to produce a uniform decrease in color. Other operators prefer the furnace-filter technique, or the open-grid technique, in which a small amount of space is left between each laser pulse.

Author's note: In my experience, this often produces very objectionable irregular decreases in vasculature, which is often upsetting to patients.

Postprocedure Care

It is crucial that the patient keep the area lubricated with a topical antibiotic ointment. In addition, the patient must avoid sun exposure and local trauma. This advice is particularly pertinent in the case of children, who must be told to refrain from all forms of contact sports for the next 5 to 10 days. The skin is extremely fragile and can easily be peeled off. Sun exposure should be avoided because the laser has a tendency to produce hyperpigmentation in deeply tanned areas. Patients should be encouraged to use ice as a local anesthetic.

Complications

If used at the proper energy level, the flashlamp-pumped tunable dye laser has little tendency to scar the face and neck. Nevertheless, tell patients that there is a 5% chance of scarring, to cover the possibility for the informed consent. In over two years of laser use, not a single scar has occurred on the head or neck. However, on the lower extremities, scarring occurs in 5% to 20% of patients. This may be caused by local trauma from factors such as clothing, but some of it remains unexplainable. In addition, the lower extremities commonly develop hyperpigmentation, which is almost invariable when larger areas are treated. This pigmentation resolves in two to eight months, but it can be very distressing to patients if not explained in advance. Blistering is commonly seen, particularly on the eyelids, if the energy level is set too high. Consequently, it is better to begin at a lower energy level if you are not sure of the patient's response. For children and for adults with extensively sun-damaged skin, it is best to start with energy levels 0.5 to 1.0 J lower than you think may be necessary. In addition, the laser may remove much of a patient's natural tan and freckles in the treated area. This change is usually not permanent, but it can be distressing if not explained in advance. It is possible to produce hypertrophic scars, but this is a rare complication.

Documentation

To document the procedure, complete a surgical note that indicates the site of treatment and the total number of pulses to be delivered. Take photographs immediately before and after the procedure (these are then kept in a permanent collection). Also note the patient's response to the procedure and, for future reference, describe whether analgesia was adequate. This is particularly important as it relates to children. (For oral sedation and analgesia, try diazepam 10 mg orally or sublingually for adults, and chloral hydrate 50 to 100 mg/kg orally for very young children [maximum 1 g]. Chloral hydrate has not proved nearly as useful a sedative or anxiolytic as diazepam. The advantage of sublingual diazepam is that the dose can be titrated during the operative procedure.)

CPT/BILLING CODES

The billing codes for laser therapy of vascular lesions depend on the size of the area being treated.

17106	Destruction of cutaneous vascular proliferative lesions less than 10 cm^2
17107	Destruction of cutaneous vascular proliferative lesions 10.0 to 50.0 cm^2
17108	Destruction of cutaneous vascular proliferative lesions over 50.0 cm^2
57513	Laser ablation of the cervix

The codes used for most other lesions are the usual codes for "destruction by any method," 17000-17286.

BIBLIOGRAPHY

Ashinoff R, Geronemus R: Port-wine stains in infants treated with a tunable dye laser, *J Am Acad Dermatol* 24:467, 1991.

Bailin PL, Ratz JL, Wheeland RG: Laser therapy of the skin: a review of principles and applications, *Dermatol Clin* 5:259, 1987.

Gregory RO, Roenigk RK, Wheeland RG: When and when not to use cutaneous laser therapy, *Patient Care* 67: November 1991.

Olbricht SM: Use of the carbon dioxide laser in dermatologic surgery: a clinically relevant update for 1993, *J Dermatol Surg Oncol* 19:364, 1993.

Olbricht SM, Arndt, KA: Carbon dioxide laser treatment of cutaneous disorders, *Mayo Clin Proc* 63:297, 1988.

Reyes AL, Geronemus R: Treatment of port-wine stains in children using the flashlamp-pumped tunable dye laser, *J Am Acad Dermatol* 23:1142, 1990.

Tan OT, Sherwood K, Gilcrest B: Treatment of children with port-wine stains using the flashlamp-pulsed tunable dye laser, *N Engl J Med* 320:416, 1989.

Editor's note: The entire April 1993 issue of the *Journal of Dermatologic Surgery and Oncology* (Vol. 19, No. 4) is dedicated to laser surgery.

CHAPTER 16

Radiofrequency Surgery

Donald E. DeWitt

John L. Pfenninger

Radiofrequency surgery—modern electrosurgery—has become a versatile tool for the primary care physician in the practice of dermatology and gynecology. It is both time- and cost-effective, and it is an efficacious treatment for a multitude of lesions. Tissue can either be delicately removed with excellent cosmetic results, or tissue can be totally ablated. Appropriate selection of waveform and current intensity allows either excision, ablation, coagulation, or fulguration. The technique can be used for both benign and malignant lesions. The Ellman Surgitron electrosurgical unit is essentially a portable generator that creates high frequency current of 3.8 to 4.0 MHz, which is comparable to radiowave frequency for broadcasting (Figs. 16-1 and 16-2). Many other units have recently been introduced into the market. The Surgitron, however, has a long successful history, and can be used with a multitude

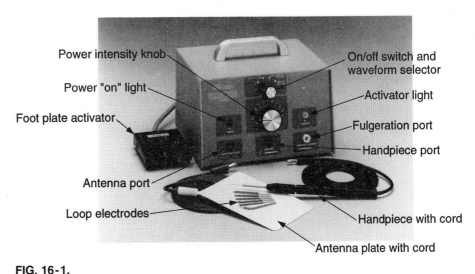

FIG. 16-1.
The Ellman Surgitron radiofrequency unit with foot pedal, antenna plate, and hand wand tip holder. A variety of electrode tips are lying on the white antenna plate.

of electrode tips for a large variety of applications. Various manufacturer units may vary in the frequency output from 250,000 to 4.0 million cycles per second. Unless otherwise noted, discussion here will be in reference to the Ellman Surgitron.

There are three choices of electrical waveforms plus a fulguration current (four models). By changing waveforms, one obtains different effects. The settings of the Ellman unit are described as *filtered fully rectified, fully rectified,* and *partially rectified.* These correspond with a *pure cutting* effect (90% cutting, 10% coagulation), a *blended* current to allow 50% cut and 50% coagulation, and a 90% *coagulation* (hemostasis) effect, respectively. A separate outlet also provides a spark-gap fulgurating current (referred to as "hyfercation") for very superficial cautery (Fig. 16-3).

Advantages of using radiofrequency technique include rapidity of treatment, a nearly bloodless field, minimal postoperative pain, and rapid healing. Local anesthetic is used except in rare instances. Since the frequency is so high, the current from this unit passes through the body without causing painful muscle contractions or nerve stimulation (Faraday effects). Radiosurgery using the *cutting wave* cuts without pressure, needing only a featherlike touch and thus minimizes tissue damage. The tissue damage that does occur is very superficial and comparable to that which occurs with laser. This is in contrast to true cautery, which causes damage similar to third-degree burns. Additionally, radiosurgery avoids the risk of electrical burns to the patient. Instead of a ground plate, an *antenna* is used to focus the "radio waves." In contrast to electrical units, this antenna does not have to be in skin contact with a patient, rather it only needs to be under the patient near the operating field. (Some radiofrequency generators, however, do require grounding pads or plates. Be sure to follow the manufacturer's recommendations.)

The high-frequency energy of this unit is concentrated at the tip of each electrode. During each procedure, the electrode itself remains cold; however, the highly concentrated electrical energy creates molecular energy inside each cell it contacts, thereby creating tissue heat and actually vaporizing the cell much the

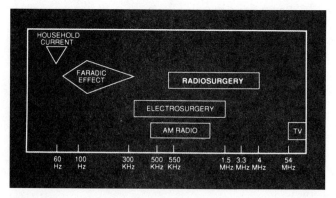

FIG. 16-2.
Comparison of uses and effects of various electrical frequencies.

Mode or function	Waveform	Configuration
Electrocoagulation Hemostasis Cautery	Partially rectified	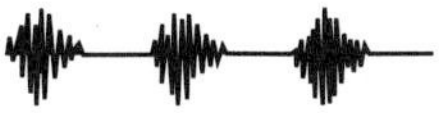
Blend Cut and coag	Fully rectified	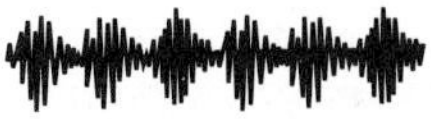
Cutting Electrosection	Fully filtered and fully rectified	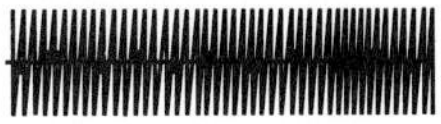
Fulgeration Electrodessication	Markedly damped	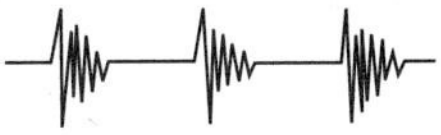

FIG. 16-3.
Common terminology for various modes, waveform characterization, and waveform configuration for the outputs of the radiofrequency unit.

same as laser does. It is important to remember that the amount of heat generated is dependent on the amount of time the tip is in contact with the tissue, the size of the electrode, the power setting, the type of waveform selected, and the radiowave frequency.

Proper technique is accomplished when the loop electrodes pass through the tissue smoothly, like cutting through butter. Generally, a motion of 5 to 8 mm per second is appropriate. If there is sparking, the power setting is too high. If the flow is not smooth, either the operator is going too fast, the power setting is too low, or the electrode is dirty (debris or carbon buildup).

INDICATIONS

Radiofrequency surgery can be used for a variety of skin and mucosal lesions. It is especially helpful when good cosmetic results are essential. Common uses and lesions treated include the following:

Incisions

Excisions

Electro-epilation

Cauterization of "bleeders"

Nail plate ablation (ingrown toenails)

Skin tags

Verruca

Condyloma

Pyogenic granulomas

Nevi (benign)

Mucosal lesions and seborrheics

Hemangiomas

Basal cell cancers

Squamous cell carcinomas

Actinic keratoses, seborrheic keratoses

Sebaceous hyperplasia

Syringomas

Cervical biopsies

Cervical conizations

Chalazions

Telangiectasias (spider veins)

Hemorrhoids (especially tags)

Rhinophyma

Xanthelasma

CONTRAINDICATIONS

- Cardiac pacemakers (*relative contraindication,* need to follow precautions)
- Uncooperative patient

TECHNIQUES

There are a multitude of applications possible with the variety of tips available (Fig. 16-4). There are loop and straight wire electrodes for excising, incising, or shaping tissue; ball electrodes for coagulation; and rod electrodes for fulguration and desiccation. More specific electrodes are available for nail matrixectomies and large-loop electrical excision procedures of the cervix. Most applications are accomplished with simple local anesthesia, regional field blocks, or digital blocks. Radiosurgery is relatively atraumatic when correctly applied; consequently, the risks of scar tissue formation are minimal compared with those associated with scalpel surgery. For the majority of cases, the handpiece is inserted into the "hand piece" port to enable selection of various output modes. (If inserted into "fulgeration port," that will be the only output.)

The Ellman company provides a large chart with each instrument, which summarizes the proper mode and tip to use with each specific lesion or procedure.

Biopsies or excisions of lesions may be accomplished with the standard ellipse technique utilizing the *vari-tip electrode* (Fig. 16-5), or a scalpel blade

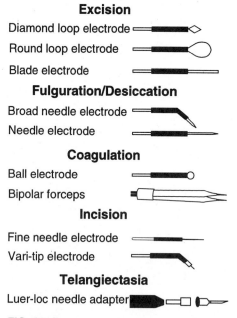

Excision

Diamond loop electrode

Round loop electrode

Blade electrode

Fulguration/Desiccation

Broad needle electrode

Needle electrode

Coagulation

Ball electrode

Bipolar forceps

Incision

Fine needle electrode

Vari-tip electrode

Telangiectasia

Luer-loc needle adapter

FIG. 16-4.
Multiple electrode tips available for the Ellman Surgitron radiofrequency unit.

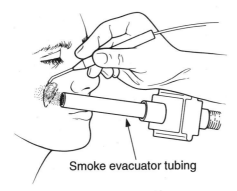

Smoke evacuator tubing

FIG. 16-5.
Use of the vari-tip wire electrode to carry out an elliptical excision.

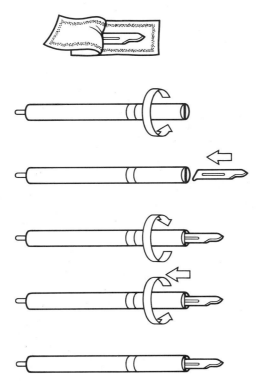

FIG. 16-6.
Technique of inserting scalpel blade into handle for radiofrequency surgery. Most surgery is carried out with the loop electrodes or vari-tip wire. The scalpel is most frequently used for "bloodless" undermining.

inserted into a *chuck adaptor* (Fig. 16-6). The unit is set at *filtered-cut*. The proper power setting is between tissue drag and tissue spark, usually between 2 and 3. The thickness and dryness of skin may cause some variation in this latter setting. Remove any hyperkeratinized tissue, and be sure the skin is moist. The vari-tip electrode is denoted as such because its length can be adjusted to the depth of cut desired by pulling it out or pushing it back into the plastic insulated cuff. These two electrodes can also be used to undermine skin and control the bleeding (cut/coag or blended mode).

If the lesion to be removed is large and elevated, a biopsy specimen may be obtained by simply using the loop electrodes to remove the sample (Fig. 16-7). However, with smaller, flatter lesions, using the loop to obtain a shave biopsy specimen may cause sufficient artifact in the tissue specimen to obscure pathology. For smaller lesions, then, use a regular scalpel blade (without current) to obtain a shave biopsy specimen. Follow this with the loop electrode to smooth out the base and control bleeding. Remember, when obtaining a biopsy sample for suspected melanoma, the depth of lesion penetration is *very important*. Do *not* do simple shave biopsies.

Basal cell cancers may be treated using a combination of curettement and desiccation or fulguration. For this, a *pointed rod* or *ball electrode* is used in the end piece with the cord plugged into the right-hand fulgeration port (*white*) (Fig. 16-1), and the power should be set at approximately 5. This works especially well with nodular lesions and lesions on and around the nose. Cautery and curettement is generally carried out three times (see Chapter 5, Approach to Various Skin Lesions).

Condyloma acuminata may be excised using a loop electrode with the unit set at *cut and coag (rectified)* and power set at approximately 2. For larger lesions, "debulk" them with the initial pass, then feather out the edges with a very light touch. (Alternatively, any residual after the initial pass may be removed with

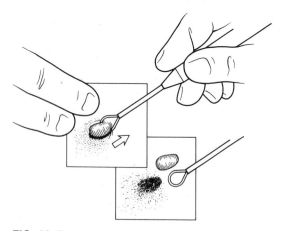

FIG. 16-7.
Technique of removing a raised skin lesion with a broad base.

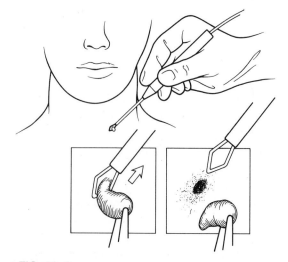

FIG. 16-8.
Technique of removing a lesion with a pedunculated base.

fulguration/desiccation of the bases.) Small warts on all parts of the body may be easily destroyed using a fine needle or ball electrode and the unit set at *hemo-part-rect,* with electrode cord in the white fulguration receptacle, and a power setting just strong enough to produce a slight spark.

Xanthelasma may be easily destroyed using the same technique described previously for condyloma. Use the least power necessary.

Fibroepithelial skin tags may be simply removed, usually without anesthesia, with the loop electrode, the cut and coag rectified setting, and power setting at slightly less than 2 (Fig. 16-8).

Seborrheic keratoses are successfully treated using the same technique described for large condyloma or as described for shave excisions. Remember, the lesion is very superficial, so deep removal is not necessary. This will minimize scarring.

Sebaceous cysts may be uncovered for intact removal or extraction of the capsule by using a small ellipse around the central pore. The length and depth of the ellipse is obviously dependent on the size of the cyst and thickness of the skin. The vari-tip electrode is set at skin thickness (estimate). With an Allis clamp, put slight traction on the ellipsed area of skin over the cyst wall itself. The lesion is bluntly dissected free and removed. The dial is set at *cut coag* and the power dial at no more than 2.

Telangiectasias are effectively treated using the electrocoagulation technique. The upper dial is set on *cut coag,* the power set at less than 1, and a fine-tip needle is used. There is a hypodermic needle adaptor available for the handpiece; a short 33-gauge hypodermic needle can be attached to the adaptor for this procedure (Fig. 16-4). An assortment of insulated needles can be purchased from the manufacturer as well (Fig. 16-9). Treatment lasts a fraction of a second. Generally, anesthetic is not used, and the unit is activated before touching the lesion. Vessels should be penetrated at approximately 1 mm intervals. *Spider angiomas* can be treated similarly; however, larger lesions may require canalization of the feeder

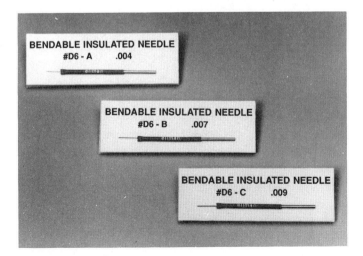

FIG. 16-9.
Insulated needles available for treatment of telangiectasia.

vessel with the needle electrode. *Senile angiomas* are best treated using light electrode desiccation. Facial lesions respond the best. Spider veins on the lower extremity do not respond well. There is often prolonged pigmentation and recurrence of the lesions.

Actinic keratoses are easily treated with a desiccation technique; however, those lesions that do not respond appropriately should be studied further to rule out neoplastic changes. If there is any doubt, a shave biopsy sample should be obtained before treatment.

Plantar warts are treated in a multitude of ways. However, for small and new lesions, the desiccation technique with curettement works well once the lesion has been pared down to the rete pegs.

For ingrown toenail surgery, where ablation of part or all of the growth center is desired, the *matrixectomy* electrodes perform superbly (Fig. 16-10). (See Chapter 6, Treatment of Ingrown Toenails.)

Other lesions: *tattoos, sebaceous hyperplasia, eccrine hydrocystomas, milia, verrucae plana, verrucae vulgaris, venous lakes,* and *trichoepitheliomas.* For those doing laparoscopy, radiosurgical techniques can be used for endometriosis, pelvic inflammatory disease, myomectomy, and, in skilled hands, ectopic pregnancy. The vari-tip has also been used for blepharoplasties.

Cervical dysplasia (CIN): For those trained in colposcopy and treatment of cervical intraepithelial neoplasia (CIN), this unit can be adapted to the LLETZ (large loop excision of the transformation zone) procedure with a special set of electrodes designed for this specific purpose (Fig. 16-11). This office procedure allows a "tailored" cervical conization. (See Chapter 92, Loop Electrosurgical Excision Procedure [LEEP] for Treating CIN.)

Warning: As with laser, there has been documentation of vaporization of viral particles (HPV and HIV) in the smoke plume that accompanies destruction and/or excision of tissues with this technique. Those present in the room should wear protective masks, and a smoke-evacuation system is mandatory (Fig. 16-12). The suction should be at a distance

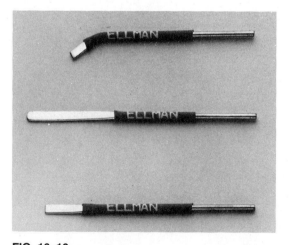

FIG. 16-10.
Teflon-coated tips used for nail matrixectomies. Upper Teflon side is applied against eponychium.

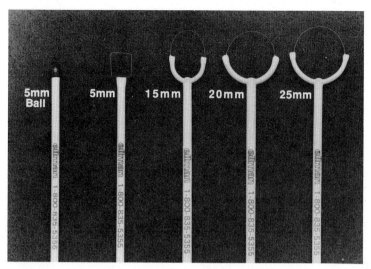

FIG. 16-11.
LLETZ electrodes used to perform office cervical conizations.

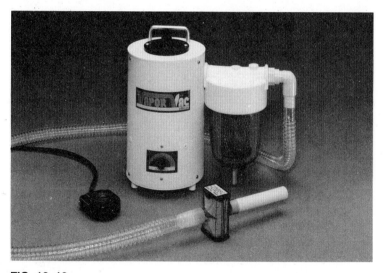

FIG. 16-12.
Smoke evacuator with both viral and charcoal filters.

no greater than 2 cm from the operative site. Proper vacuums have a viral filter as well as a charcoal filter to limit the offensive odor. Some physicians have created their own vacuum exhaust systems leading to the exterior of the building. However, a compact portable unit is available from the various manufacturers.

The techniques utilizing this unit are easily mastered and are best accomplished by attending a workshop on radiosurgery or by following the instructions given in Pollock's *Electrosurgery of the Skin*. Practice these instructions at home on a piece of beefsteak. Simplicity, economy, and versatility are unique to this instrument. The lesions that can be removed using it are myriad, depending on one's scope of practice and versatility.

POSTPROCEDURE CARE

Several approaches are acceptable in the postprocedure care of these lesions (Box 16-1). To decrease the likelihood of scarring, moist healing and prevention of eschar are essential.

Although not always adaptable, moist healing can occur when the lesion is simply covered with a small piece of synthetic material. A wound check in 3 to 4 days may be advised. Leave the covering in place for a total of one week, providing there is not an excessive accumulation of serum. If serum does accumulate, simply change the dressing. Usually, after 7 days, the wound can be left open to continue its healing process without any covering unless it is in an area that may be irritated by clothing. This method is not practical in hair-bearing sites or if multiple lesions are removed.

The second method is to wash the areas that were treated lightly 4 times per day with mild soap and water. Use a washcloth for light debridement to prevent eschar formation. Apply a topical antibiotic ointment as frequently as necessary to keep the lesion moist. A dressing is not needed except at bedtime, to assure that the area stays moist.

BOX 16-1. POSTPROCEDURE PATIENT EDUCATION HANDOUT RADIOFREQUENCY SURGERY

The radiofrequency unit that was used to remove your skin lesions causes very little residual damage. Patients occasionally report a feeling as if they were burned. Usually two tablets of ibuprofen 200 mg taken 4 times per day for 2 or 3 days will help relieve this discomfort. Please treat all the areas as follows:

1. For the next 7 days, wash the areas that were treated at least 4 times per day with soap and water. (Sometimes the physician will want you to use a special type of covering for a week. If so, follow those special instructions.)
2. After washing, apply a thin layer of antibiotic ointment on them. This will not only be soothing, but will also help the areas heal.
3. You will note redness around the area where the lesion was removed. This is to be expected. However, streaks of red leading away from the area might signal an infection. If you see these streaks, please call the doctor right away. The area must be kept moist and may require 8 to 10 applications per day.
4. Remember that any and all lesions can return. If a particular abnormality was removed and appears to come back or looks changed or different, please return to the physician for a follow-up examination. You never know when cancer can start!

COMPLICATIONS

- Broken wire causing laceration (Discard worn tips.)
- Too deep an excision causing excessive scarring
- Destruction of tissue for pathologic review, caused by improper technique
- Handpiece in wrong port or unit in wrong mode to obtain desired effect
- Pacemaker dysfunction
- Inadvertent burns either on the patient or operator due to unintended activation of handpiece
- Poor healing, due to improper use of equipment

Although some of these complications can be avoided, they still, on occasion, do occur. Removing a lesion on someone who is on aspirin or anticoagulant therapy may be accompanied by increased bleeding, necessitating heavier use of the coagulation waveform. Another complication that may be seen in diabetic patients or in older patients with thin, poorly nourished skin is slow or delayed healing. In this case, patients can often be instructed in self-care of the wound, with periodic inspections by the physician. Performing any procedures with these techniques on the lower extremities of diabetics can certainly be fraught with problems related to healing delay and possibly secondary infection. Scarring must also be considered a complication; however, once proper technique is established, a scar by this method of treatment is often less pronounced than those produced by other surgical techniques. Excising too deeply increases the likelihood of scars.

CPT/BILLING CODES

Billing codes for radiofrequency surgery are very complex; codes vary with the lesion size, benign or malignant characteristics, location, and type of removal. Some lesions would be billed out as true "excision." Others would be billed as "shave excision." Still others would be termed "destruction" or "biopsy." The reader is advised to consult the most recent CPT coding manuals.

BIBLIOGRAPHY

Brown CD, Zitelli JA: A review of topical agents for wounds and methods of wounding: guidelines for wound management, *J Dermatol Surg Oncol* 19:732, 1993.

Hainer BL: Fundamentals of electrosurgery, *JFP* 4:419, 1991.

*Pollock SV: *Electrosurgery of the skin*, New York, 1991, Churchill Livingstone.

Zuber TJ, Purvis JR: Coding and reimbursement of primary care biopsy and destruction procedures, *JFP* 35:433, 1992.

> *Editor's note:* This is a comprehensive, concise, small text that provides a thorough practical review of radiosurgery.

CHAPTER 17

Cryosurgery*

John E. Hocutt, Jr.

Cryosurgery is the deliberate destruction of diseased tissue by freezing in a controlled manner. It is critically important that the art and technique of cryosurgery be mastered by all primary care physicians. The procedure is often a better alternative than cold-knife surgery, especially when convenience, healing, disability during healing, discomfort, and scar formation are considered.

After careful study of this chapter and participation in a quality clinical course, physicians not yet using cryosurgery can rapidly master the proper technique with minimal personal proctoring. Begin with a few basic commonly used procedures, and then increase capabilities by assimilating additional techniques one at a time.

GENERAL CONSIDERATIONS

- Lesions treated with cryosurgery usually heal with minimal or no scar formation. Even if excessive freezing is done, scarring is rarely significant.
- Complete healing may take more than 6 to 8 weeks in extreme cases, but the results are usually excellent. Selective destruction of cells occurs during the freeze, while the collagen and fibroelastic tissue matrix is preserved; therefore, there is no great demand for fibroblasts to create extensive new scarlike tissue. Since the fibroelastic matrix is preserved, normal cells can grow back in an organized fashion.
- The procedure is safe, simple, and easy to learn. It usually takes less time than conventional surgery. Patients usually prefer to avoid injections of local anesthetic, and they can essentially ignore the lesion between treatments. They appreciate the omission of suture insertion and (especially) removal. Patients also welcome being able to bathe and swim while the lesion is healing.
- The freezing itself has an anesthetic effect, although a burning sensation is experienced initially, more so on initial thawing. Explain to patients that it will

*Much of the contents of this chapter was previously published in *American Family Physician* (volume 48, issue 3, pp. 445-456, 1993). It is revised and adapted here with permission.

feel like an ice cube stuck to the skin; this often reassures them enough to cope with the minimal amount of pain experienced. However, very young children often will not accept the procedure without crying. Their fear of the unknown increases when the unpleasant cold sensation starts. They have difficulty trusting that the burning feeling will actually improve in a very short time instead of continually getting worse.

- Secondary infection simply has not been a problem. Even with overfreezing, and with cryosensitive patients who overreact with excessive tissue destruction, infection occurs rarely. Excessive freezing may result in wound weeping for longer than 6 to 8 weeks, but infection should not be expected unless the area receives repetitive friction or poor skin care.

ADVANTAGES OF CRYOTHERAPY

- Local anesthetic and needles are not required.
- Freezing produces minimal pain.
- Final healing is cosmetically excellent, with minimal or no scarring.
- Minimal physician time is required.
- Preoperative skin preparation is not required.
- Multiple lesions can be treated in one setting.
- Postoperative infection is rare; cases are reportable.
- The procedure is ideal for patients with light-complexioned skin.

DISADVANTAGES OF CRYOTHERAPY

- A second office visit is required in one or two days after freezing if surgical debridement is done (usually it is not).
- Use is limited in patients with darker skin because of pigment changes. Even with brief partial thickness–freeze technique, some melanocytes are destroyed and the healed cryolesion may be slightly lighter in color than the surrounding skin.
- Use is limited in areas of hair growth, such as around the eyebrows and eyelashes, and on scalps with thin hair, because even brief freezing tends to destroy hair follicles.
- Healed cryolesions will not tan sufficiently, are more susceptible to sunburn, and require sunscreen protection.

PRINCIPLES

The nitrous oxide–powered cryosurgery tip is effective and very safe. Nitrous oxide is quite unstable, and once it is released from the probe, it immediately breaks down to molecular nitrogen and oxygen. The physical characteristics of the nitrous oxide gas enable the cryotip's temperature to be easily lowered to −89°C. A carbon dioxide–powered tip generally does not get cold enough to effect a quality freeze (−65°C). Alternative methods include liquid nitrogen applied with a cotton-tipped applicator or through a closed system (Brymill Cryogun). Verruca-Freeze is a compressed gas that freezes tissue on vaporization.

At −2.2°C, cells begin to freeze. At −5°C, cells will supercool, but often they recover. Tissue destruction occurs between −10°C and −20°C. A deeper freeze with temperatures between −40°C and −50°C ensures that malignant cells are completely destroyed.

The size of the ice ball that forms around the tip of the probe provides a good estimate of the depth of the freeze. The *lethal zone* (tissue temperature less than −20°C) is 2 to 3.5 mm inward from the outer margin of the ice ball. This is especially crucial to remember in cases of premalignant or malignant lesions. The size of the ice ball is the most important factor in determining the freeze time. Factors prolonging the freeze time include low tank pressure, increased tissue vascularity, excessive keratin covering (needs to be removed or moistened), and poor tip-to-lesion contact. The use of different systems (nitrous oxide, liquid nitrogen, carbon dioxide, etc.) dramatically affect the rapidity and depth of freeze. Liquid nitrogen can be applied with the cotton-tipped applicator, or in a spray fashion (Brymill Cryogun). This also affects freezing parameters.

PHYSIOLOGY

Erythema and hyperemia are immediate responses to effective freezing. Edema and exudation (blister formation) peak within 24 to 48 hours, and usually subside after 72 hours. The extracellular collagen structures are more resistant to freezing than the cells themselves.

Seventy-two hours after freezing, the lesion becomes bloodless. Crust formation begins, and this crust will slowly wither away over the next several days. Reepithelialization occurs from the outer margin inward. Fibroblasts lay down minimal new collagen along a preserved, well-formed collagen matrix, rather than along a random matrix, which would lead to scar formation.

The healed cryolesion is soft, with minimal to no scarring. Pigmentation is often decreased, and hair and sweat glands may be destroyed in the area of freezing. It is best to caution the patient *in advance* that although the area that was frozen will not develop much of a scar, the pigmentation may be decreased. The contrast does diminish with time, however. Occasionally the inflammatory response may result in the development of a transient halo of hyperpigmentation. This usually clears nearly completely over several months.

INDICATIONS

- Incision and drainage (I & D) of abscess (to anesthetize before incision)
- Actinic keratoses (full-thickness freeze)
- Basal cell cancer (full-thickness destructive freeze)

- Condyloma acuminata
- Cervical intraepithelial neoplasia (CIN, dysplasia), "cryoconization"
- Freckles (lentigo)
- Granulation tissue
- Hypertrophic scars
- Keloids
- Molluscum contagiosum
- Papular nevi (full-thickness freeze)
- Seborrheic keratoses (blister debridement)
- Skin tags and polyps
- Verrucae (including plantar)
- Hemorrhoids
- Sebaceous hyperplasia
- Small hemangiomas

ABSOLUTE CONTRAINDICATIONS

- Proven sensitivity or adverse reaction to cryosurgery
- Nonacceptance of the possibility of skin pigment changes
- Melanoma
- Areas of end-stage compromised circulation
- Lesions in which identification of tissue pathology is required

RELATIVE CONTRAINDICATIONS

- Immunoproliferative neoplasms (e.g., myeloma, lymphoma)
- Macroglobulinemia
- Active severe collagen vascular diseases
- Severe active ulcerative colitis
- Acute poststreptococcal glomerulonephritis (almost 100% of these patients have high levels of cryoglobulins)
- Active severe subacute bacterial endocarditis, syphilis, Epstein-Barr infection, cytomegalovirus infection
- Chronic severe hepatitis B
- High levels of cryoglobulins
- High-dose steroid therapy

These patients are likely to have an exaggerated response to cryosurgery, because they have high levels of circulating cryoglobulins. If cryosurgery is appropriate or necessary for any of these patients, be sure to obtain informed consent and perform a pretest on the axilla or thigh before treating a more prominent area. Proceed with caution, and greatly shorten the freezing times until the response can be predicted. You may be able to freeze lesions effectively and safely with a much shorter freeze time; with overfreezing, the risk of tissue slough and marked hypopigmentation increase. Therefore, start slowly and advise patients that extra visits and treatment sessions may be necessary. A conservative approach is best in light of their clinical situation.

LESIONS DIFFICULT TO TREAT WITH CRYOSURGERY

- Dermatofibroma
- Hidradenitis
- Flat nevi
- Squamous cell cancer
- Most vascular lesions (especially if extensive)

AREAS NOT RECOMMENDED FOR CRYOSURGERY

- Recurrent basal cell cancer
- Areas where hair loss is critical to the patient
- Areas where pigment changes are critical to the patient
- Feet, ankles, and lower legs, when circulation is in question (especially diabetics)
- Melanomas
- Basal cell cancers in nasolabial fold or preauricular areas (often more extensive and tendency to recur)
- Periorbital area (induces immediate swelling)
- Port-wine stain (use laser)

EQUIPMENT

- Nitrous oxide–powered cryoprobe unit (Fig. 17-1 and 17-2) **or** Brymill Cryogun (Fig. 17-3) **or** Verruca-Freeze Unit (Fig. 17-4) **or** liquid nitrogen in a special storage dewar (The storage dewar is also needed for the Brymill Cryogun.)
- Assorted cryoprobe tips or nozzles for dermatologic lesions for nitrous oxide and Brymill units (Fig. 17-5)
- K-Y jelly or Cryojel
- Cotton-tipped swabs
- Minute/second timer

SUPPLIERS

Brymill Cryogun
Brymill Corporation
P.O. Box 2392
Vernon, CT 06066
203-875-2460

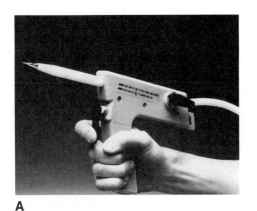
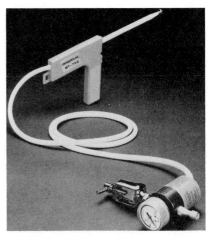

FIG. 17-1.
A, Cryosurgical hand gun with fine tip for dermatological applications. It can be used with nitrous oxide or carbon dioxide. **B,** Cryosurgical hand gun with cervical probe attached. Pressure gauge and attachment yoke are also shown.

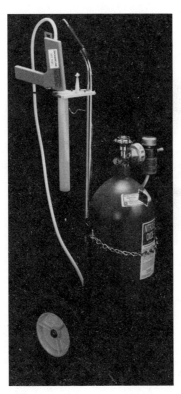

FIG. 17-2.
Cryosurgical unit. Handpiece is placed in holder, and connected to a 20-pound nitrous oxide tank.

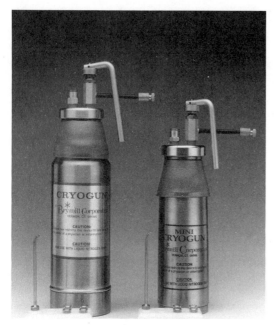

FIG. 17-3.
Brymill Cryogun is refillable with liquid nitrogen. (Courtesy of Brymill Corporation)

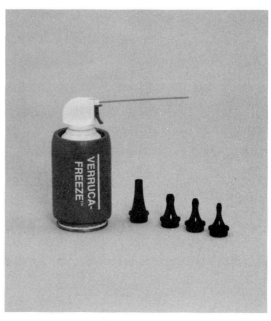

FIG. 17-4.
Self-contained Verruca Freeze unit with various sizes of specula. (Courtesy of CryoSurgery, Inc.)

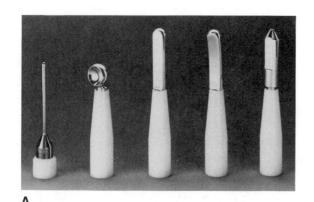

A

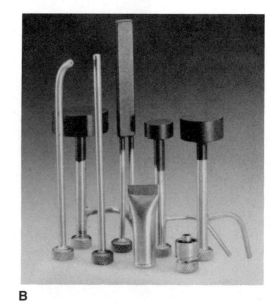

B

FIG. 17-5.
Various cryosurgical tips for treatment of a variety of dermatological lesions with nitrous oxide tank **(A)** and Brymill Cryogun **(B)**. **(B,** Courtesy of Brymill Corporation)

Brymill Cryogun
Olympus Corporation
4 Nevada Drive
Lake Success, NY
800-645-8160

Verruca-Freeze
CryoSurgery, Inc.
P.O. Box 50035
Nashville, TN 37205
800-729-1624

For companies supplying nitrous oxide units, see Chapter 83, Crycone of the Cervix. Liquid nitrogen dewars are available from most local oxygen and nitrogen supply firms.

PREPROCEDURE PATIENT EDUCATION

Before the procedure, the patient should be advised of the basic technique, the expected sensation during treatment, and the possible complications (Box 17-1). The advantages of and rationale for using cryosurgery should also be reviewed.

**BOX 17-1. PATIENT EDUCATION HANDOUT
WART REMOVAL**

The removal of warts in certain locations can be difficult—especially if they are on the bottom of the feet. With your cooperation, a combination of acid and cryosurgery (freezing) can be used to more effectively remove these viral infections without much disability during treatment or damage to the surrounding skin.

Every night for about two weeks, clean the lesion, and apply some Compound W (17% salicylic acid gel) on the wart. Then cover the wart and gel application with Mediplast (40% salicylic acid pads with adhesive backing) so that the pad slightly overlaps the wart.

Leave the pads on as long as possible. Remove them each evening, bathe, and then reapply. The treated wart should turn white and look fluffy. If the area becomes very sore or red, stop treatment and call our office. If the pad moves excessively during the day because of your activity, apply them in the evening when you come home or when you do not have to move around as much.

Once you have prepared the area well, it will be easy for the physician to remove the layer that covers the wart and to freeze the base where the root is. Cryosurgery leaves little or no scar, and usually only leaves the skin lighter in color. Most people can continue to do all their daily activities, including swimming and bathing, during treatment. No anesthesia is needed.

The freezing employed with cryosurgery can kill hair follicles, so it's not appropriate for treating large areas of the scalp. If you have an intense skin reaction to cold, please tell the doctor *before* the warts are removed.

METHOD OF APPLICATION

Brymill Cryogun (Figs. 17-3 and 17-5, *B*)

Either contact probes or spray-tipped nozzles may be used with liquid nitrogen. A perpendicular spray (versus a tangential direction) provides a more rapid, deeper freeze.

Verruca Freeze (Fig. 17-4)

Select a speculum size that will completely encompass the lesion. Hold the speculum securely against the skin to prevent leakage. Dispense enough liquid from the cannister to fill the speculum approximately 1/8 to 1/4 inch. Avoid splattering; use a gentle spray. Allow the fluid to evaporate (20 to 25 seconds). Remove the cone speculum.

Liquid Nitrogen

Pour the liquid into a cup. Use a small or large cotton-tipped applicator, insert it into the cup, then apply the liquid to the lesion. Freezing times are markedly shortened with liquid nitrogen. Size of applicator and amount of pressure applied also affect rapidity and depth of freeze.

Nitrous Oxide Unit

Place a thin layer of water-soluble gel on the lesion to hydrate the lesion and to enhance even contact with the cryoprobe. Select a probe with a size and shape that corresponds with the lesion size (Fig. 17-6). Hold the cryogun and trigger in one hand and guide the probe tip to a point adjacent to the site of freezing. Activate the

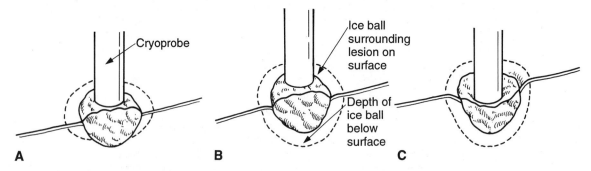

FIG. 17-6.
Cryosurgery of a deep but narrow lesion. **A,** If a wide cryoprobe tip is used, the deepest part of the lesion will not be frozen even though a 3 to 5 mm margin of ice ball is obtained. **B,** To ensure that the entire lesion is frozen, a tip smaller than the lesion may be used, thereby limiting the lateral spread of the ice ball; or **C,** The cryoprobe tip may be pressed down until the top of the lesion is below the skin surface, causing the lesion to form a hemisphere around the tip. The cold will penetrate deeper before too much normal tissue is frozen by lateral spread.

gun and quickly guide the probe into place on the lesion. The ice ball will immediately connect the skin to the probe tip (5 to 10 seconds).

TECHNIQUE: GENERAL GUIDELINES

1. Freeze the lesion until the ice ball extends 2 to 3 mm beyond the edge of diseased tissue. The depth of freeze is roughly equal to or slightly less than the size of the horizontal freeze. The most effective destruction technique is to freeze rapidly, thaw, then refreeze.
2. The time of freeze is important (Table 17-1). *Initial treatments should be conservative until the patient's response to freezing is identified.* Patients should be labeled "supersensitive," "sensitive," "normal," and "resistant" to freezing. Supersensitive patients (rarely encountered) may have elevated levels of cryoglobulins, and the possibility of an underlying lymphoma, malignancy, or immune deficit should be considered. These patients will exhibit the most marked hypopigmentation response and may slough large areas of skin.
3. A general rule for estimating freeze time is the 1-2-3 rule: one minute for the skin, two minutes for hemorrhoids, and three minutes for the cervix. These are approximate times that should be adjusted according to patient sensitivity, type of lesion, presence of malignancy, and lesion vascularity (see Table 17-1). Vascular lesions will involve longer freezing times. Any active bleeding will need to be controlled, and pressure from the probe will need to be applied to squeeze as much blood as possible out of the lesion.
4. Bandages are not necessary unless the lesion is continually irritated or begins to weep.

TABLE 17-1.

Freeze Time Guidelines for Nitrous Oxide Technique

Tissue	Lesion	Freeze Time*
Skin	Full-thickness benign	1-1.5 min
	Full-thickness, malignant	1.5-3 min[†]
	Plantar warts (after debridement)	40 sec
	Condyloma	45 sec
	Verrucae	1-1.5 min
	Vascular lesions (with pressure)	1.5 min
	Seborrheic keratoses (2 mm margin)	30 sec[†]
	Actinic keratoses (3 mm margin)	1.5 min[†]
	Basal cell cancer (3-5 mm margin)	1.5 min[†]
Hemorrhoids	Cryoligation	2 min
	Cryo without ligation	2-3 min[†]
Cervix	Cervicitis	3 min
	Cervical intraepithelial neoplasia I, II, III	3 min[†]
	Cervical intraepithalial neoplasia I, II (alternative method)	5 min

*Freeze times are approximate guidelines and should be adjusted to the size of the ice ball, which is far more important than the time.
[†]freeze-thaw-refreeze

TECHNIQUE: SPECIFIC PROCEDURES

Presurgical Keratin Preparation

Lesions with dense keratin coverings are extremely resistant to cryosurgery. The keratin must be debrided prior to freezing. Especially in the case of plantar warts, debridement plus freezing is necessary. The patient can help prepare the wart with two weeks of salicylic acid application: After bathing and cleaning the area, the patient should apply a 17% solution (Compound W) to the wart(s) and a piece of Mediplast (40% salicylic acid), or Trans-Ver-Sal, cut just a little larger than the wart. This is left in place 24 hours until the next day's application. (If the pad migrates significantly during the day, it may be used only at night.)

After two weeks, a soft white layer of keratin can be peeled away, revealing the base or root of the plantar wart lesion. A 40-second freeze is sufficient for such an exposed area. A longer freeze time is usually quite painful and may produce significant soreness for up to two weeks.

Alternatively, any lesion with significant keratin buildup can be surgically debrided with a No. 10 or 15 blade before cryotherapy. In the case of verrucae, excise in thin layers until the red punctate vasculature is seen. Try to avoid bleeding.

Blister Debridement Technique

The blister debridement cryosurgical technique is especially helpful in the removal of *seborrheic keratoses,* common, benign skin lesions frequently seen in the elderly. They are not premalignant, but occasionally they can be mistaken for a pigmented basal cell cancer. When in doubt, remove a sample for biopsy before doing cryosurgery. It is essential that the lesion be hydrated. Apply a water-soaked gauze pad to the area for 5 to 10 minutes and then water-soluble gel (or apply the

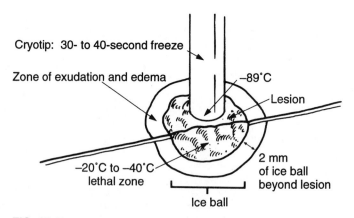

FIG. 17-7.
Partial thickness freeze used for removal of superficial lesions (e.g., seborrheic keratoses). Cryotip should cover or nearly cover entire lesion to limit depth of freeze.

gel alone for 5 to 10 minutes before the freezing). For superficial epidermal lesions, freeze for 30 to 40 seconds or until the ice ball reaches 2 to 3 mm beyond the cryotip (Fig. 17-7).

If indicated, surgically debride each treated lesion in 24 to 48 hours. Edema and exudation (vesiculation) peak at 24 to 48 hours and subside by 72 hours. During this time, the dermis and epidermis separate, lifting the lesion to the top of the blister. Removal of the prepared lesion with iris scissors is a painless procedure. After 72 hours, the lesion may sink like a graft and thereafter may bleed on attempts at removal. If left alone, the lesion will eventually slough spontaneously, but surgical debridement one or two days after freezing yields better results. A trained assistant may perform the debridement. Many physicians have the patient return in 24 to 48 hours for debridement only if the lesions have been resistent to previous treatment. A 2 to 3 mm freeze margin usually invokes enough lesion damage that seborrheic keratoses will slough after 2 to 3 weeks. If only a partial slough occurs, refreezing the remnant will resolve the problem.

A disadvantage of this technique is that a second office visit is needed for the debridement procedure.

Full-Thickness Freeze Technique

The full-thickness freeze technique may be used for benign and premalignant lesions (see Fig. 17-8). *Actinic keratoses* are very common premalignant skin lesions, often occurring in light-complexioned persons exposed to sunlight. They are most easily located by palpation of the skin and visual inspection. If the diagnosis is in question, confirm by obtaining a small punch biopsy specimen before treatment.

Follow debridement and moisturizing steps as previously outlined. Freeze for 1 to 1½ minutes or until the ice ball extends 3 mm beyond the lesion. The extent of the ice ball is more important than timing. When freezing is complete, activate the

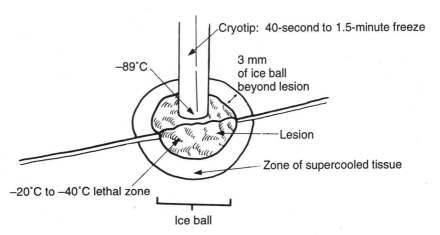

FIG. 17-8.
Full-thickness freeze technique. Cryotip should be slightly smaller than lesion to allow full depth freeze before extending too far into normal skin.

rapid thaw, or turn off the cryoprobe. Do not attempt to detach the cryoprobe until the rapid thaw releases it.

Full-Thickness Destructive Freeze Technique

This technique is used for treating malignant lesions such as basal cell carcinomas. Be sure to confirm the diagnosis by obtaining a punch biopsy specimen prior to treatment. Malignancies of tissues composed of anything but basal cells (e.g., melanomas and squamous cell carcinomas) should not be treated with this technique.

Follow preparation steps as above, but continue the freeze for at least 1½ minutes or until the ice ball is between 5 and 8 mm beyond the lesion (Fig. 17-9). When freezing is complete, activate the rapid thaw. Do not attempt to detach the cryoprobe until the rapid thaw has released the tip. Since a malignancy is being treated, it is wise to document the time *and* the extent of the freeze.

Allow 5 to 7 minutes for complete thawing, then *repeat the freeze*. Malignant cells are more cryoresistant and destruction requires temperatures of −40° to −50°C. The freeze, thaw, refreeze technique is recommended in all cases, and this should be documented.

Full-Thickness Freeze Technique for Anatomically Large or Irregular Skin Lesions

Some lesions are too large to be completely frozen by a cryoprobe in a single freeze. In such cases, note the central location of the cryoprobe. This spot will be the margin of the cryoprobe placement for the next adjacent freeze. This allows for a 50% overlap.

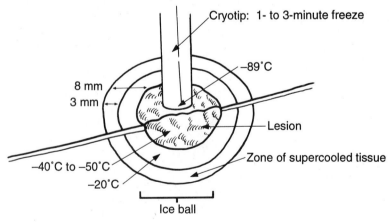

FIG. 17-9.
Full-thickness destruction freeze technique (malignant lesions).

After the first application, wait 5 to 7 minutes until the tissue has completely thawed. Begin the second sectional freeze, overlapping the first cryoprobe placement by 50% as noted above. Repeat this technique until the entire target tissue is covered. Freezing of extremely large lesions can begin on one side, then the opposite side can be frozen while the first is thawing. Progressing from opposite sides to the center will save time and still allow for a 50% freeze overlap.

Hypertrophic Scars and Keloids

The hyperemia and edema that immediately follow freezing and thawing soften the hypertrophic scar or keloid and allows a much more even distribution of intralesional steroid, as well as easy penetration by the needle into the tissue.

1. Select a cryotip slightly narrower than the scar. You do *not* want the ice ball to extend beyond the scar.
2. Apply a thin coat of water-soluble gel to the scar only. (Do not cover any of the surrounding skin.)
3. Moisten and warm the cryotip. Freeze until the ice ball progresses just to the edge of the scar, usually for 20 seconds to 1 minute, occasionally longer if necessary.
4. Wait approximately 10 to 15 minutes for mild tissue swelling, then proceed with intralesional injection of a steroid (such as triamcinolone diacetate [Aristrocort] or triamcinolone acetonide [Kenalog 10 mg/cc]) using a small, 30-gauge needle. Use very dilute solutions (0.1 cc diluted with 0.5 to 0.9 cc of 1% lidocaine *without* epinephrine) and a sufficient volume to infiltrate the entire scar.

Anesthesia for Incision and Drainage of Abscesses

1. Select a cryotip that will cover the intended area of incision. Apply a thin coat of water-soluble gel to the most dependent portion of the abscess.
2. Moisten and warm the cryotip. Make firm contact with the tissue and activate the gun.
3. Freeze until the ice ball covers an area slightly larger than the area that is to be opened. Make the incision through the ice ball along the skin tension lines. As the tissue is thawing, insert a hemostat and spread the tissue to promote drainage.
4. Obtain cultures of purulent drainage, if desired, after thawing has occurred.
5. Insert sterile iodoform gauze or a small Penrose drain if needed. Apply a bulky gauze dressing to absorb drainage. Arrange for a follow-up visit.

Condyloma Acuminata (See Chapters 83 and 84)

1. Find all the lesions. For women, examine the genitalia and the cervix with a colposcope to look for very small lesions, particularly in the vaginal introitus, on the vaginal walls, vulva, and cervix. Lesions in sensitive areas (e.g., vulva, vaginal introitus) should be anesthetized. If the lesions are on mucous mem-

branes, freezing is not recommended (chemical ablation, laser, or excision is more appropriate). A cryocone of the cervix is necessary if dysplastic lesions extend onto the cervix. A thorough work-up is necessary before treating the cervix or any external lesion. Women with external condyloma have a high incidence of cervical dysplasia.

2. Moisten the skin lesions with a water-soluble gel.

3. Touch the lesion(s) with the probe, activate the nitrous oxide–powered tip, and effect adherence after 3 to 5 seconds. Then apply gentle traction. Do not pull too hard, or you may tear the tissue being treated or the surrounding skin.

4. Freeze for approximately 45 seconds. Judge actual freezing time by the size of the ice ball, which should extend 2 mm beyond the margin of the lesion(s) (Fig. 17-10). Within minutes after freezing, the condyloma on skin will darken and then will turn black; they should slough within a few days. If they do not turn dark, refreezing may be necessary.

Thick clusters may need to be frozen in blocks, using cryotraction after the probe adheres to the surface of the lesions.

Penile, perianal, and vulvar areas are more sensitive. Individual lesions and small groups of condyloma can be frozen without anesthetic, or topical 5% lidocaine may be applied 3 to 5 minutes prior to freezing. Topical benzocaine 20% (Hurricaine) is more effective, especially if it is allowed enough time to take effect before freezing is attempted. EMLA cream may be appropriate in some situations. Massive lesions may require injections of local anesthetic or general anesthetic. Such extensive lesions are often best left to those who treat them frequently.

It is critical to treat every lesion, or recurrence is likely. Complete treatment is often difficult and requires extreme patience of the physician and extreme cooperation of the patient. Try your best not to freeze any normal skin between the

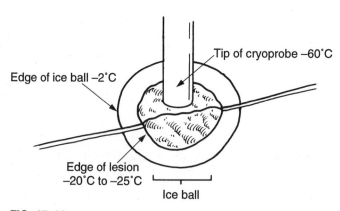

FIG. 17-10.
To ensure that all of the tissue of the lesion reaches the −20°C to −25°C necessary for destruction, the outer edge of the frozen area (the "ice ball") should extend at least 2.0 mm to 3.5 mm in all directions beyond the lesion.

lesions. Be sure to advise the patient to return quickly at the first sign of recurrence, so that thorough treatment may be resumed before extensive lesions regrow.

A combination of electrosurgery and cryosurgery may speed the treatment of extensive perianal, vulvar, or penile lesions. The cryosurgery component will allow preservation of the elastic tissue matrix and expandability of the anal canal, penis, and vulva after healing. The electrosurgery component is used for tissue debridement: First, superficially electrocoagulate multiple lesions, then debride with scissors, and then freeze the base for 20 to 30 seconds. Be sure not to cut too deep. Alternatively, you may use an electrosurgical loop to excise the condyloma, and then freeze the base for 20 to 30 seconds. This is excellent for treatment of large areas of condyloma often seen on the genitalia.

Mulloscum Contagiosum

Freezing is often an excellent, nearly painless treatment for mulloscum contagiosum. Advise your patients, particularly children, to protect the healing crust to decrease the chance of scar formation.

1. Prepare each lesion with a small amount of water-soluble gel.
2. Freeze each lesion for 30 seconds to 1½ minutes. Use very fine-tipped probes to avoid freezing normal skin.
3. Advise the patient or parent that the lesions should fall completely off within two weeks or less. If they do not, the patient should return soon for retreatment to prevent their spread.

Vascular Lesions (Especially Hemangiomas and Strawberry Hemangiomas)

As with malignant lesions, vascular lesions are more cryoresistant, and a freeze, thaw, refreeze technique is recommended (see Fig. 17-11). See Chapter 83, Crycone of the Cervix, for a detailed explanation.

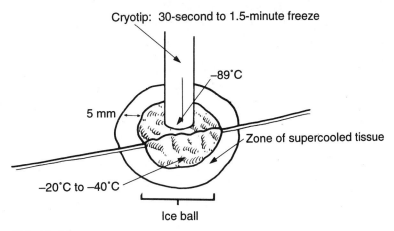

FIG. 17-11.
Full-thickness destructive freeze of vascular lesion.

1. Moisten and warm the cryotip in warm water, and apply water-soluble gel.
2. Make contact with the hemangioma and *exert firm pressure* to squeeze the blood out of the vascular channels.
3. Activate the cryogun, and hold pressure against the lesion throughout the freeze. Begin timing when the ice ball becomes visible. For larger lesions, freeze for 1½ minutes or until the ice ball extends out 5 mm. Allow 5 to 7 minutes for thawing, and then repeat the freeze.

POSTPROCEDURE PATIENT EDUCATION

The patient should be informed of the additional healing time, the anticipated excellent results, and the need to call the office when there is an overreaction to freezing. Document that the patient was told of permanent pigment changes, possible nerve involvement, and hair loss.

COMPLICATIONS

- Pigment cells and hair cells may be destroyed by cryosurgery.
- Vascular lesions are quite resistant to treatment and may recur.
- Areas of poor circulation may be susceptible to prolonged ulcer formation, especially in elderly diabetic patients (e.g., anterior tibia compartment).
- Tissue pathology documentation and verification of adequate destruction of malignant lesions is not possible with cryosurgery. Pretreatment biopsy is often required for actinic keratoses and basal cell carcinomas. Cryosurgery of more severe or critical cancers may best be left to those treating them frequently. A presumed "benign lesion" may be indeed malignant and thus inappropriately treated.
- Cryosurgery in the periorbital area may cause excessive swelling, in which the eyelid may be shut for several hours or days. However, cryosurgery of small, well-localized lesions on the eyelids is usually well tolerated. Be conservative on the freeze time until the individual patient's reaction is documented.
- Peripheral neuropathy can result when areas adjacent to nerves are frozen. The nerve sheath is cryoresistant, but the nerve tissue is somewhat more susceptible to damage. This side effect can be minimized by applying outward traction to the tip-lesion complex once good contact is achieved. The spread of cold is greatly decreased by traction and stretch on adjacent tissue. Also, the source of freeze is effectively removed from proximity to the nerve, significantly delaying nerve-damaging temperature drop.

    If the nerve is affected, recovery is usually complete within 4 to 6 weeks. Sensory nerves are most likely affected. If you are freezing an area that may be adjacent to a nerve (e.g., lateral aspect of finger), be sure to apply traction. Tell the patient that sensory loss may occur, and reassure that recovery is expected within 4 to 6 weeks. The patient will be much less concerned about it if it even occurs, and often will not bother calling you unless the sensory deficit remains for 3 months or longer, which is very unlikely.

- In general, the skin of infants and the elderly—as well as previously damaged skin—is more susceptible to necrosis and blistering than normal skin. Skin may be damaged as a result of sun exposure, radiation, and chronic topical steroid application. Reduce freeze times until the reaction of a damaged area is known. Written informed consent is suggested when freezing previously damaged skin.

CPT/BILLING CODES

10060	I & D, small abscess
10061	I & D, complicated or multiple
17000	Cryosurgery, face, single, benign*
17001	Cryosurgery, face 2, 3 lesions, each, benign
17002	Cryosurgery, face 4 or more, each, benign
17010	Cryosurgery, face, complicated lesions, benign
17100	Cryosurgery, other than face, single lesion, benign
17101	Cryosurgery, other than face, second lesion, benign
17102	Cryosurgery, other than face, 3 and up to 15, per lesion, benign
17104	Cryosurgery, other than face, 15 or more lesions, benign
17105	Cryosurgery, other than face, complicated lesions
17110	Destruction of molloscum contagiosum and flat warts, up to 15 lesions
40820	Destruction of lesion of mouth by cryotherapy, benign
46916	Destruction of lesions, anus, cryosurgery
46924	Destruction of lesions of anus extensive, any method
46934	Destruction of hemorrhoid, internal
46937	Destruction of rectal tumor, benign
54056	Destruction of lesions, penis, cryosurgery
56501	Destruction of lesion(s) of vulva; simple, any method
56515	Destruction of lesion(s) of vulva; extensive, any method
57061	Destruction of vaginal lesion(s); simple, any method
57065	Destruction of vaginal lesion(s); extensive, any method
57511	Cyrocone of cervix, initial or repeat

BIBLIOGRAPHY

Burke WA et al: Survival of herpes simplex virus during cryosurgery with liquid nitrogen, *J Dermatol Surg Oncol* 12(10):1033, 1986.

Domonkos AN, Arnold HL, Odom RB: *Andrews' diseases of the skin,* ed 7, Philadelphia, 1982, W.B. Saunders.

Elton RF: The appropriate use of liquid nitrogen, *Prim Care* 10(9):459, 1983.

Felmar E, Payton CE, Smietanka M: Primary care office procedures: treatment of genital lesions via cryocautery, *Prim Care:* June 1988.

---

*Coding of malignant lesions is very specific for location and size. Please refer to the coding manuals.

Ferris DG, Ho JJ: Cryosurgical equipment: a critical review, *JFP* 35:185, 1992.

Fitzpatrick TB: *Dermatology in general medicine,* ed 2, New York, 1979, McGraw-Hill.

Grealish RJ: Cryosurgery for benign skin lesions, *Fam Pract Recertification* 11(10):21, 1989.

Heidenheim M, Jemec GB: Side effects of cryotherapy, *J Am Acad Dermatol* 24:653, 1991.

Hocutt JE: Cryosurgery (parts 1, 2, 3), *Fam Pract Bulletin* 1(12):67, 1988; 1(16):91, 1989; 1(18):103, 1989.

Hocutt JE: Skin cryosurgery for the family physician, *Am Fam Physician* 48(3):445, 1993.

Jones SK, Darville JM: Transmission of virus particles by cryotherapy and multi-use caustic pencils: a problem to dermatologists? *Br J Dermatol* 121:481, 1989.

Torre D: Cutaneous cryosurgery: current state of the art, *J Dermatol Surg Oncol* 11(3):293, 1985.

Yliskoski M et al: Cryotherapy and CO_2 laser vaporization in the treatment of cervical and vaginal human papillomavirus (HPV) infections, *Acta Obstet Gynecol Scand* 68:619, 1989.

CHAPTER 18

Ring Removal from an Edematous Finger

John Harlan Haynes III

Soft tissue swelling of a finger occurs with trauma, fluid retention, weight gain, arthritis, allergic reaction, infection, or iatrogenic infusion infiltration. When the finger is constricted by circumferential banding, such as with ring jewelry, the patient may suffer neurovascular compromise, skin erosion, and severe pain.

If ring removal is not accomplished by lubrication and circular traction, the clinician may use the string-wrap method without harm to the patient or the ring. Alternatively, a conventional hand-operated circular saw or Steinmann pin cutter may be used to cut the ring. However, this damages jewelry and potentially could injure the patient. Caution should be taken to avoid implantation of metal filings, which may lead to foreign body granuloma and synovitis if the ring is cut.

INDICATIONS

- Acute or chronic finger edema with proximal band constriction

RELATIVE CONTRAINDICATIONS

- Open wound or fracture
- Deeply embedded ring erosion
- Lack of patient cooperation

STRING-WRAP METHOD

Equipment

- 2 to 3 yards of string, No. 1 silk or Mersilene, or umbilical tape—preferably on a spool
- Adhesive tape

- Small hemostat
- *Optional:* 1.5 ml 1% lidocaine *without* epinephrine
- *Optional:* 5 ml syringe with 27-gauge needle for digital nerve block
- Lubricating K-Y jelly

Technique

1. Some patients may require a digital block in case the pain increases from the compression and unwinding. If needed, 0.5 to 0.75 ml of 1% lidocaine is infiltrated deep into the neurovascular bundle on the proximal volar aspect of the affected finger bilaterally.
2. Lightly lubricate the finger near the ring. Pass the hemostat under the ring, grasp the end of the string, and thread it beneath the ring, pulling several inches of string through (Fig. 18-1, *A*). Tape the proximal end to the hand (Fig. 18-1, *B*).

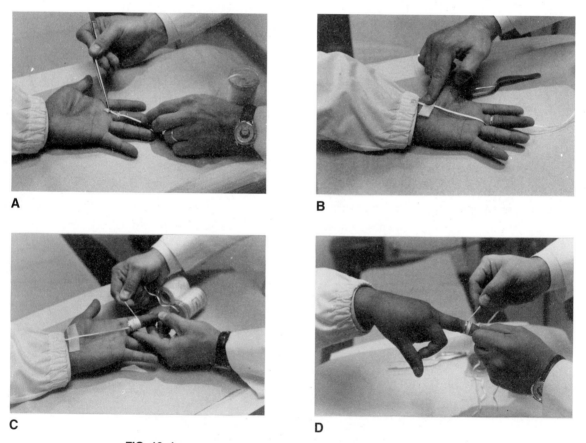

A

B

C

D

FIG. 18-1.
String-wrap method of removing ring from a swollen finger. See text for details.

3. Wrap the string circumferentially around the finger, beginning just adjacent to the ring margin. Wind the string in a smooth single layer distally using moderate tension until it encompasses the point of greatest swelling (Fig. 18-1, *C*).

4. Untape the proximal end of the string and pull distally toward the fingertip. Maintain tension along the long axis of the finger, moving the ring distally as the string unwinds beneath it. Force the ring over that portion of the finger that has been compressed by the wrap (Fig. 18-1, *D*). Once past the area of largest diameter, usually the proximal interphalangeal joint, the ring will slide off easily.

CIRCULAR SAW OR STEINMANN PIN CUTTER METHOD

Equipment

* Hand-held circular-blade ring cutter (e.g., Beaver) or Steinmann pin cutter with a McDonald elevator
* Large hemostats (e.g., Kelly clamps)
* 20 ml syringe filled with saline and 20-gauge intracath sheath

Technique

1. Slip the small hook of the ring cutter or elevator under the ring on the palmar surface to serve as a guide and barrier (Fig. 18-2).

2. Firmly grip the saw handle, and, using a 180-degree twisting motion, grind through the ring. Using the pin cutter, cut through the ring over the elevator.

3. The cut ends of the ring may be spread using hemostats with steady opposing forces.

4. Rinse the area with high-pressure saline to ensure evacuation of all metal filings.

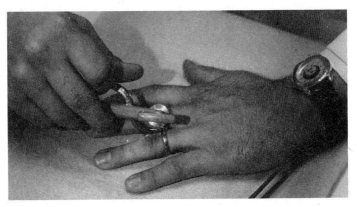

FIG. 18-2.
Hook of the ring cutter serves as a guide and barrier.

CPT/BILLING CODES

20670	Superficial removal of constricting metal band
20680	Deep removal of constricting metal band

BIBLIOGRAPHY

Fasano FJ, Hansen RH: Foreign body granuloma and synovitis of the finger: a hazard of ring removal by the sawing technique, *J Hand Surg* 12A:621, 1987.

Huss CD: Removing a ring from a swollen finger. In *Patient care: procedures for your practice,* Oradell, N.J., 1988, Medical Economics.

Mizrahi S, Lunski I: A simplified method for ring removal from an edematous finger, *Am J Surg* 151:412, 1986.

Roberts JR, Hedges JR: *Clinical procedures in emergency medicine,* Philadelphia, 1985, W.B. Saunders.

CHAPTER 19

Tick Removal

John Harlan Haynes III

Outdoor work and recreation in wooded areas is often accompanied by tick exposure. Although most bites are harmless, severe illness may result from microorganisms transmitted by the tick. Expedient and effective tick removal may be necessary to prevent illness.

Ticks are vectors of infectious human diseases, such as Rocky Mountain spotted fever, Q fever, and typhus (*rickettsia*); tick fever (*flavivirus*); tularemia (bacterium); babesiosis (Protozoa); and relapsing fever and Lyme disease (spirochetes). Envenomation of a neurotoxin secreted in the saliva of certain ticks may also result in progressive ascending neuromuscular paralysis. Tick bites can cause generalized allergic reactions, as well as local infection and induration.

There are two families of ticks that bite humans: soft (argasid) ticks and hard (ixodid) ticks. The hard ticks are most likely to be encountered by humans, and these ticks may hematogenously transmit microorganisms during all phases of development. In their larval stage, these are known as seed ticks and, with massive infestation, they can be removed with lindane shampoo.

Hard adult ticks are best removed mechanically. Care must be taken to remove the mouthpart and its surrounding, fleshlike "cement." If the "head" (mouthpart) is retained, it may be necessary to perform a punch biopsy in order to remove the surrounding skin and remnants. Empiric therapy with broad-spectrum antibiotics is usually a good prophylactic measure.

In the past, home remedies involved placing oil on the tick, which in effect would smother it, or using a hot match or cautery to get the tick to release itself. Both methods tend to cause the tick to regurgitate into the site and may promote disease transmission. Neither technique is currently recommended.

EQUIPMENT

- Blunt curved forceps or tweezers
- Rubber gloves

- Povidone-iodine scrub and solution
- Gauze and bandage

For difficult removal or retained mouthparts (in addition):

- Punch biopsy equipment for 3 to 6 mm size punch as appropriate
- Iris scissors
- Lidocaine 0.5 ml in syringe with 30-gauge needle
- *Optional:* aluminum chloride solution 6.25% on a cotton-tip swab
- *Optional:* nylon suture 5-0

TECHNIQUE

1. Gently paint the surrounding area with povidone-iodine solution.
2. Using blunt forceps, tweezers, or gloved fingers, grasp the tick as close to the skin surface as possible and pull upward and perpendicular, with steady even pressure.
3. Do not twist or jerk the tick, as this may break off mouthparts.
4. *Never* squeeze, crush, or puncture the body of the tick, because its fluids may contain infectious agents.
5. With protected hands, place the tick in a container of alcohol and freeze (in case subsequent identification is warranted).
6. Disinfect the bite site with povidone-iodine scrub or antibacterial soap.

In cases of a particularly tenacious tick or retained mouthparts:

1. Disinfect the area with antibacterial soap. Infiltrate the area beneath the bite with lidocaine.
2. Apply the punch biopsy instrument perpendicular to the skin so that it encompasses the tick. Stretch the skin on each side of the lesion. Advance the biopsy punch downward with moderate pressure using a clockwise-counterclockwise twisting motion. Penetration through the epidermis and dermis is confirmed with a marked decrease in resistance.
3. Remove the punch. Lift the biopsy specimen with forceps and cut the pedicle with iris scissors. Submit the tissue for histological study.
4. Disinfect the area again and apply pressure with gauze. If adequate hemostasis is not accomplished, cauterize with aluminum chloride solution or close with suture. Apply bandage.

COMPLICATIONS

Patients should be advised of the possibility of local or systemic infection. Excessive bleeding may be encountered but should be effectively stopped with pressure, cauterization, or suture.

CPT/BILLING CODES

10120	Removal of superficial foreign body, skin
10121	Incisional removal of foreign body, complex

BIBLIOGRAPHY

Jones BE: Human "seed tick" infestation, *Amblyomma americanum* larvae, *Arch Dermatol* 117:812, 1981.

Munns R: Punch biopsy of the skin. In *Patient care: procedures for your practice,* Oradell, N.J., 1988, Medical Economics.

Needham G: Evaluation of five popular methods for tick removal, *Pediatrics* 75(6):997, 1985.

Patterson J, Fitzwater J, Connell J: Localized tick bite reaction, *Cutis* 24(8):168, 1979.

Pearn J: Neuromuscular paralysis caused by tick envenomation, *J Neurol Sci* 34:37, 1977.

CHAPTER 20

Fishhook Removal

John Harlan Haynes III

The method used to remove a fishhook depends on the anatomical location of the injury and the conditions under which the removal is to take place. The first and best method described is the *string-yank* method, which may be used without anesthesia by anglers on the water. It is best used on the more resilient skin surfaces with underlying bone and muscle. For more embedded hooks, or for hooks in flaccid areas such as the earlobe, the *barb-sheath* or the *pull-through* technique may be more applicable. Local anesthesia with 1% lidocaine is well received by the anxious patient in an emergency setting. If the shank has already been clipped by a well-meaning first-aider, a strong needle driver or hemostat may be clamped over the exposed shank tip to facilitate removal.

INDICATIONS

• Fishhook embedded in subcutaneous tissue

CONTRAINDICATIONS

• Penetration into the eye with scleral perforation (dictates ophthalmology referral)

ANGLER'S STRING-YANK METHOD

Equipment

• Silk suture (0 or larger diameter), umbilical tape, or ordinary string, 2 to 3 feet in length

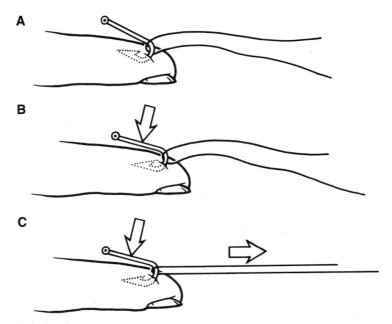

FIG. 20-1.
Angler's string-yank method of fishhook removal. See text for details.

Technique

1. Tie the midpoint of the string around the curve of the fishhook. Securely wrap the other ends several times around your index and middle finger (Fig. 20-1, *A*).
2. Place the involved extremity on a flat surface to provide stabilization. Depress the shank of the hook against the skin with the index finger of your free hand until it meets resistance. The shaft of the hook is then lifted approximately parallel to the underlying skin by grasping the eye with the thumb and middle fingers (Fig. 20-1, *B*). This maneuver will disengage the barb from the subcutaneous tissue.
3. With the shank depressed and the barb disengaged, firmly and quickly jerk the string, with follow-through, in one forceful move parallel to the shank (Fig. 20-1, *C*). Bystanders should stand clear from the flightpath. This method is effective and produces no additional wounds.

BARB-SHEATH METHOD

Equipment

- 0.5 ml lidocaine 1% in a syringe with 30-gauge needle
- 18-gauge needle

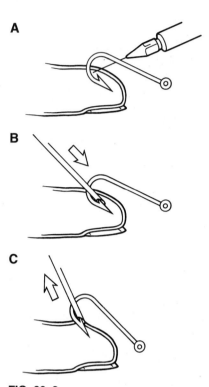

FIG. 20-2.
Removing fishhook using anesthetic when the hook is large and not too deep in the skin. See text for details.

Technique

1. After local anesthesia, introduce the 18-gauge needle through the entrance track along the inside curvature of the hook, parallel to the shank, with the bevel toward the inside of the curve so that the needle opening can engage the barb (Fig. 20-2, *A-B*).
2. Advance the hook slightly to dislodge the barb from the tissue. Gently pull and twist the hook so that the barb is firmly sheathed by the lumen of the 18-gauge needle.
3. Then back the hook and needle out together as a unit (Fig. 20-2, *C*).

TRADITIONAL PULL-THROUGH METHOD

Equipment

- 0.5 ml lidocaine 1% in syringe with 27-gauge needle
- Wire clipper

Technique

1. Provide local anesthesia over the point of the hook (Fig. 20-3, *A*).
2. Force the point through the anesthetized skin (Fig. 20-3, *B*).
3. When the barb tip is fully exposed, clip it off (Fig. 20-3, *C*).
4. Back the hook out along the direction of entry (Fig. 20-3, *D*).
5. Alternatively, if the shank has multiple barbs, clip off the eye of the hook and pull on the sharp end of the hook until the entire hook is removed (Fig. 20-4).

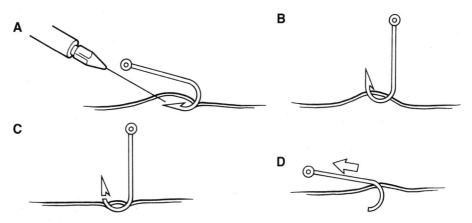

FIG. 20-3.
Traditional method for removing small fishhook. See text for details.

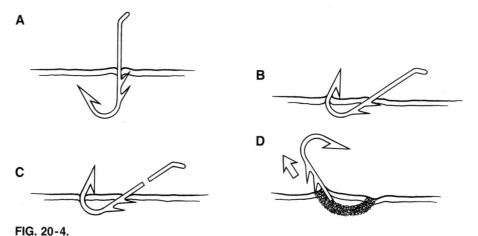

FIG. 20-4.
Removal of a barbed fishhook. **A,** The hook embedded in soft tissue. **B,** Twist the hook forward until the sharp end is visible. **C,** Cut off the eye of the hook. **D,** Pull on the sharp end to remove.

POSTPROCEDURE CARE

- Administer tetanus toxoid if more than 5 years have elapsed since its last administration.
- Empiric antibiotics and nonsteroidal antiinflammatory agents are good preventive measures.
- Soak the area in warm saline three times daily for two days.
- Warn the patient of the possibility of infection.

CPT/BILLING CODES

10120	Removal of subcutaneous foreign body, simple
10121	Incisional removal, foreign body, complex

BIBLIOGRAPHY

Cooke T et al: A few ways to unsnag a fishhook, *Emerg Med:*223, July 1981.

Roberts JR, Hedges JR: *Clinical procedures in emergency medicine*, Philadelphia, 1985, W.B. Saunders.

Simon RR, Brenner BE: *Emergency procedures and techniques*, Baltimore, 1984, William & Wilkins.

PART TWO

Anesthesia

CHAPTER 21

Local Anesthesia

Daniel J. Derksen

John L. Pfenninger

Local anesthetics are extremely useful in a wide variety of clinical settings. From simple laceration repair to abscess incision and drainage, local anesthetics are critical to patient comfort and physician ability to perform the necessary procedure. Local anesthetics prevent the generation and conduction of nerve impulses by several mechanisms: they increase the electrical excitation threshold, slow the propagation of nerve impulses, and disrupt the action potential and sodium permeability of nerve fibers. For the practicing physician, it is important to know that the progression and the duration of a local anesthetic is related to many factors, including the size of the area to be anesthetized; the nerve fiber diameter, myelination, and conduction velocity; the presence of infection; the blood supply in the area; the presence of chronic disease (e.g., diabetes); and the patient's pain threshold and anxiety level.

INDICATIONS

Any clinical procedure causing pain that could be eliminated by the use of a local anesthetic is sufficient to warrant the use of a local anesthetic (Tables 21-1 and

TABLE 21-1.

Commonly Used Local Anesthetics in the Office Setting (Also see Table 23-1)

Local Anesthetic	Onset(min)	Duration(hr)	Equivalent Conc.(%)
Lidocaine (Xylocaine)	1	0.5-1	1
Lidocaine w/epinephrine	1	2-6	1
Mepivacaine (Carbocaine)	3-5	0.75-1.5	1
Dibucaine (Nupercaine)	15	3-4	0.25
Dibucaine w/epinephrine	15	6	0.25
Bupivacaine (Marcaine)	5	2-4	0.25
Bupivacaine w/epinephrine	5	3-7	0.25
Etidocaine (Duranest)	3-5	3-7	0.5

Modified from Olin BR, editor: *Drug facts and comparisons*, St Louis, 1993, Mosby. Used with permission.

TABLE 21-2.

Maximum Dosages of Commonly Used Local Anesthetics (Also see Table 23-1)

Anesthetic	Concentration	Maximum Dose
Lidocaine (Xylocaine)	1%	4.5 mg/kg not to exceed 300 mg (30 cc in adult)
Lidocaine (Xylocaine) w/epinephrine	1%	7 mg/kg not to exceed 500 mg (50 cc in adult)
Bupivacaine (Marcaine)	0.25%	3 mg/kg not to exceed 175 mg (50 cc per average adult)
Bupivacaine (Marcaine) w/epinephrine	0.25%	3 mg/kg not to exceed 225 mg

21-2). Some of the outpatient procedures in which local anesthetics are used include incision and drainage of an abscess, laceration repair, biopsy (diagnostic or excisional), digital block for treatment of paronychia, aggressive treatment of warts (such as electrodiathermy or freezing), paracervical or submucosal block of the cervix, endometrial biopsy or curettage, and others. See Box 21-1 for selection criteria for local anesthetics.

CONTRAINDICATIONS

Local anesthetics should not be used in patients with a *known sensitivity*. However, this is very uncommon with amide anesthetics (lidocaine [Xylocaine], mepivacaine [Carbocaine], and bupivacaine [Marcaine]). The older anesthetics were esters (procaine [Novocaine] and tetracaine) and caused more allergic reactions. The two

---

BOX 21-1. SELECTION OF LOCAL ANESTHETICS/EFFECTS

Lidocaine (Xylocaine) without epinephrine
Can cause vasodilatation
0.5 to 1 hour duration depending on site/vascularity
Use in contaminated wounds
Use in fingers, nose, penis, toes, earlobes
Use if vascular disease is present or if patient is immunocompromised
Use if there are cerebrovascular or cardiovascular risks
Use for nerve blocks

Lidocaine (Xylocaine) with epinephrine
Causes vasoconstriction
Has longer duration
Use in highly vascular areas to improve visualization of field
Use in clean wounds
In general, do not use on fingers, nose, penis, toes, and earlobes

Bupivacaine (Marcaine)
For longer duration
For nerve blocks

groups do not cross-react, so a patient reporting an allergy to procaine can successfully use lidocaine. However, multidose vials also include paraben preservatives, which are chemically similar to ester anesthetics, and which may induce an allergic response in sensitive patients. Single-dose vials do not contain preservatives and may be indicated for the patient reporting allergy.

The employment of vasoconstrictors (i.e., epinephrine) along with local anesthetics is useful to decrease bleeding, reduce systemic absorption, and prolong the duration of action, but is contraindicated in several circumstances. Local anesthetics with vasoconstrictors should be used only with extreme caution where vasoconstriction could result in permanent destruction of tissue. In general, vasoconstrictors should not be used on the extremities—the nose, ear, penis, or ends of digits (fingers and toes). In addition, patients with known peripheral vascular disease may have an exaggerated vasoconstrictor response. Extreme care should be used if local anesthetics with vasoconstrictors are used in patients with diabetes, hypertension, arteriosclerosis, thyrotoxicosis, heart block, or cerebral vascular disease. If a skin flap has marginal viability or blood flow to a flap is compromised, do not use epinephrine.

APPROACHES FOR THE ALLERGIC PATIENT

- Use a cooling agent (ice cube, ethyl chloride, etc.).
- For small lesions, use no anesthetic.
- Use single-dose vials instead of multidose vials.
- Injecting normal saline can often provide enough relief to permit minor surgeries or suturing.
- Substitute an amide for an ester (if offending agent can be identified).
- Use diphenhydramine (Benadryl). Inject 10 to 50 mg in the usual fashion (50 mg per 1 cc diphenhydramine mixed with 4 cc of normal saline).

EQUIPMENT

- Sodium bicarbonate (Neutra-caine) 7.5% 5 ml vials
- 18-gauge needle to draw up solution
- 27- to 30-gauge needle for injection (various lengths)
- Alcohol swabs
- Various size syringes
- Anesthetic of choice

SUPPLIER

Sodium bicarbonate (Neutra-caine) 7.5% 5 ml vials
    MD, Inc.
    Suite 43, 408 State of Franklin Rd.
    Johnson City, TN 37604
    615-461-6185
    800-35-MDINC

TECHNIQUE

1. Using an alcohol swab, wipe the top of the vial of local anesthetic. Draw up the anesthetic with a large-bore needle (e.g., 18 gauge) into an appropriately sized syringe (most office procedures require less than 10 cc of local anesthetic). For most shave or biopsy excisions, 1 cc is sufficient. Discard the large-bore needle in an appropriate container (avoid recapping any needle, even if "sterile").

2. Depending on the tissue to be infiltrated, choose an appropriately sized needle. For most skin biopsies, a 1-inch, 27- to 30-gauge needle provides the necessary rigidity and causes minimal discomfort.

3. Inject either intradermally or subcutaneously, depending on the lesion and surgery intended. (Subcutaneous injection will take longer to take effect.) Before infiltration, draw back the syringe plunger. If there is blood return, do not

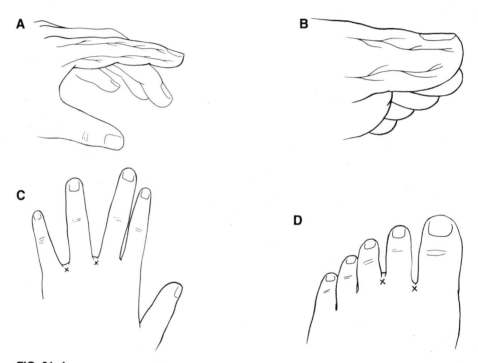

FIG. 21-1.
The anatomy of a digital block. In the finger (**A**) and toe (**B**) there are four nerves to block in order to obtain successful digital block. An anterior and posterior branch on each side of the digit needs to be blocked. If the proper site of infiltration is chosen, the four nerves of the finger (**C**) or toe (**D**) should be well anesthetized. The web space between each digit can be used to accomplish this. The needle should be moved to ensure that the anterior and posterior branch of the nerve on each side of the digit is blocked, infiltrating as the needle is withdrawn. A digital block may take several minutes to take effect. In the case of a severely inflamed paronychia, where the nail must be partially or entirely removed, additional local anesthetic may be necessary at the site of inflammation to eliminate pain and allow the removal to be done. It is best to avoid vasoconstrictor agents for local anesthetics for digital blocks. In addition, care should be taken to avoid systemic injection.

infiltrate; this will prevent systemic injection. Reposition the needle and draw the plunger back. If there is no blood return, infiltrate as the needle is withdrawn. Never infiltrate as the needle is advanced. This will help to prevent systemic injection. Before any digital or other block, a review of the related anatomy is recommended. In the case of digital blocks, it is important to remember the location and number of nerves supplying each digit (Fig. 21-1). *Inability to obtain adequate pain elimination is usually due to a failure to wait the necessary time for the local anesthetic to work.*

POSTPROCEDURE PATIENT EDUCATION

Instruct patients to watch for signs of infection or local reaction to the local anesthetic. Redness, pus, increased pain, red streaks up the extremity, or other problems should prompt a phone call or return visit to the physician.

REDUCING PAIN OF INJECTION

Injection of local anesthetics causes pain because of the needle and because of the acidity of the solution (pH 4.05 to 6.49), which causes a significant burning sensation. This short-lived pain can be eliminated by adding 1 ml of sodium bicarbonate 1 mg/ml solution to 10 cc of a 1% concentration of anesthetic. Patients, especially children, will note remarkable improvement in comfort. Infiltration with unbuffered solution has been found to be 2.8 to 5.7 times more painful than infiltration with buffered counterparts. There has been no significant difference detected in the time of onset or duration of anesthesia or in the surface area of skin anesthetized. Occasionally, the addition of bicarbonate can make the solution cloudy, but there are no known adverse effects from this.

Previously, it was recommended that the buffered solution be discarded after 24 hours. Bartfield, however, concluded that buffered lidocaine was stable for 1 week at room temperature. Refrigeration may nearly double that time.

TOPICAL ANESTHETICS

Certain clinical situations favor the use of a topical anesthetic. Examples include a combative child too large for the papoose board and too small to reason with, and patients with nosebleeds, eye injuries, corneal abrasions, or lesions on mucous membranes that need to be treated with painful modalities, such as liquid nitrogen or electrodiathermy. Mucous membranes (nose, mouth, throat, esophagus, and genitourinary tract) can be successfully anesthetized with many of the local anesthetics by direct topical application. It is best to use lidocaine (2% to 4%), cocaine (4% to 10%), or tetracaine (1% to 2%). Procaine and mepivacaine do not penetrate mucous membranes enough to be effective as topical anesthetics. Topical cocaine has the added advantage of vasoconstriction. However, many clinicians are hesitant to have cocaine preparations available in their clinic for security and other reasons. Vasoconstriction can also be obtained by using a low concentration of phenylephrine (0.005%) for topical anesthesia. Epinephrine does not penetrate mucous membranes well and is not useful in this setting. Topical application of cocaine or lidocaine has a peak effect within 2 to 5 minutes, while tetracaine requires 5 to 8 minutes. The effect lasts 30 to 45 minutes. Systemic effects are possible, especially in children. Consider using EMLA, a new topical anesthetic approach. For corneal abrasions or foreign body in the eye, the examination should be preceded by the administration of tetracaine 0.5%, 1 or 2 drops (see Chapter 22, Topical Anesthesia).

COMPLICATIONS

When a local anesthetic is used properly, complications are rare. Allergic reactions may occur (see Chapter 135, Anaphylaxis). Other complications are related to systemic absorption of the local anesthetic or to the effect of vasoconstriction when local anesthetics with epinephrine are used. If systemic absorption occurs, monitor cardiac and respiratory status carefully for the appropriate time, based on the half-life of the agent used. Anxiety, incoherent speech, lightheadedness, metallic taste, blurred vision, or drowsiness may be early signs of central nervous system toxicity and are difficult to differentiate from vasovagal effects. The use of epinephrine may cause arrhythmias or other cardiovascular or cerebrovascular changes, but this is very rare. Warm compresses to increase peripheral circulation can be used when excess vasoconstriction is observed (such as cyanosis, decreased pulse, or decreased capillary refill).

BIBLIOGRAPHY

Adriani J, Naraghi M: Local anesthetics: who should give them? *So Med Journal* 78(10): 1219, 1985.

Bartfield JM et al: Buffered lidocaine as a local anesthetic: an investigation of shelf life, *Ann Am Int Med* 21:16, 1992.

Doyle DJ: A closer look at local anesthetics, *Emerg Med* 23:147, April 1991.

Holmes HS: Options for painless local anesthesia, *Postgrad Med J* 89:71, 1991.

McKay W, Morris R, Mushlin P: Sodium bicarbonate alleviates pain on skin infiltration with lidocaine, with or without epinephrine, *Anesth Analg* 66:572, 1987.

Olin BR, editor: *Drug facts and comparisons,* St Louis, 1993, Mosby.

Trott A: Infiltration and nerve block anesthesia. In *Wounds and lacerations: emergency care and closure,* St Louis, 1991, Mosby.

CHAPTER 22

Topical Anesthesia

William Dery

Topical anesthesia offers patients with low pain threshold, needle phobia or superficial lesions an alternative to parenteral anesthesia. Various preparations and the intended area of use for topical anesthesia are listed in Table 22-1.

Other options for topical anesthesia include ice, ethyl chloride, TAC (tetracaine 2.5 mg; adrenaline 1:1000, 2.5 cc; cocaine 0.59 g; dissolved in sufficient sterile water to make 5 cc), and EMLA (eutectic mixture of local anesthetic).

TABLE 22-1.

Topical Anesthetic Preparations

Anesthetic	Concentration (%)	Form	Tissue
Benzocaine	1-5	Cream	Skin and mucous membrane
	20	Ointment	Skin and mucous membrane
	20	Aerosol	Skin and mucous membrane
Cocaine	4	Solution	Ear, nose, throat
Dibucaine	0.25-1	Cream	Skin
	0.25-1	Ointment	Skin
	0.25-1	Aerosol	Skin
	0.25	Solution	Ear
	2.5	Suppository	Rectum
Cyclonine	0.5-1	Solution	Skin, oropharynx, tracheobronchial tree, urethra, rectum
Lidocaine	2-4	Solution	Oropharynx, tracheobronchial tree, nose
	2	Jelly	Urethra
	2.5-5	Ointment	Skin, mucous membrane, rectum
	2	Viscous solution	Oropharynx
	10	Suppository	Rectum
	10	Aerosol	Gingival mucosa
Tetracaine	0.5-1	Ointment	Skin, rectum, mucous membrane
	0.5-1	Cream	Skin, rectum, mucous membrane
	0.25-1	Solution	Nose, tracheobronchial tree

From Covino BG, Vassallo HG: *Local anesthetics: mechanisms of action and clinical use,* New York, 1976, Grune & Stratton. Used with permission.

INDICATIONS

TAC

- Scalp, facial laceration repair (especially in children)

EMLA (Cream)

(Under occlusion on *intact* skin)

- Venipunctures (most frequently used in children)
- Lumbar puncture
- Arterial puncture
- Suture removal
- Dermabrasion
- Split thickness skin-graft donor sites
- Molluscum contagiosum—to anesthetize before curettage
- Venereal warts
- Intracutaneous allergy testing
- Epilation
- Meralgia paresthetica
- Superficial shave biopsy
- Removal of foreign body embedded in skin
- Nonsurgical uses for EMLA
    Postherpetic neuralgia
    Preputial adhesions in uncircumcised male

Ice/Ethyl Chloride

- Skin tag clipping
- Abscess incision and drainage

CONTRAINDICATIONS

TAC

- Hypersensitivity to tetracaine, adrenalin, or cocaine
- For use on mucous membranes or when direct contact with mucous membranes is unavoidable
- Patient with history of nonfebrile seizure disorder (*relative contraindication*)
- Compromised skin near wound, i.e., abraded, infected, burned (Epinephrine may cause excessive vasoconstriction.)
- Use on nose, penis, fingers, toes (*relative contraindication*)
- Patient with history of arrhythmia (*relative contraindication*)
- Lesions not on face or scalp: TAC less efficacious on these sites (*relative contraindication*)

EMLA

- Hypersensitivity to contents
- Thick epithelium: the efficacy diminishes as the thickness and vascularity of skin increases (*relative contraindication*)

TAC

Technique

1. After ruling out any absolute contraindications, ensure that wound characteristics are appropriate: Wound should be located on the face, scalp, or (possibly) a proximal extremity. Determine laceration size and depth; efficacy is usually unaffected by length and depth; however, early studies suggest that TAC be used only if the lesion is less than 5 cm long.
2. Remove any visible debris and fill the wound with 2 to 4 cc of TAC solution for 3 minutes. Follow this with cotton balls soaked in TAC for 10 minutes.
3. Observe the patient throughout application for signs and symptoms of toxicity: excessive drowsiness or excitation, seizure, arrythmia, vomiting, flushing, and urticaria.

Complications

No serious complications have been reported with this protocol.

- If a seizure occurs, it is likely caused by cocaine toxicity. Remove the TAC solution and provide supportive therapy.
- No increased rate of wound infections has been reported, although theoretically, a greater risk of infection is postulated because of vasoconstriction.
- The patient will subsequently have positive urine drug screen for cocaine for up to 72 hours.
- Adverse reactions have occurred after exposure to mucous membranes or large areas of compromised skin (burns, abrasions).

EMLA

Technique

1. Remove any oil, natural or otherwise, from the skin with soap, alcohol swab, and acetone.
2. Apply EMLA to intact skin and apply an occlusive dressing (Tegaderm, Opsite, Band-aid) for 60 to 90 minutes before the procedure. Depth of anesthesia should be 3 mm after 1 hour, and 5 mm after 2 hours. Duration of anesthesia is approximately 2 hours after removal. Diseased skin or mucous membranes will be penetrated more rapidly; therefore, decrease contact time to 5 to 30 minutes. EMLA is not approved for use on genital or mucosal surfaces, or on

open skin. One significant advantage of EMLA is that it does not distort the skin contour, such as seen with injection.

ICE

Technique

Rub the skin firmly with ice for 10 seconds. This technique offers approximately two seconds of anesthesia. Use with superficial skin tag clipping and venipuncture or prior to injection with local anesthetic.

ETHYL CHLORIDE

Technique

Spray the site for one to two seconds. This technique offers up to two seconds of anesthesia. Use with skin tag clipping and venipuncture or prior to injection with local anesthetic.

Complication

- Excessive freezing may lead to second-degree epidermolysis (blistering).

CONCLUSION

In the past, topical anesthetic options for dermatologic procedures were limited to ice and refrigerant sprays. These were extremely limited in efficacy because of their short duration of action. TAC has become the workhorse for topical anesthesia in children since 1980. Its efficacy and safety when used on the face or scalp are comparable to lidocaine. Its major disadvantage is its use is limited to few anatomic sites. Its advantage is patient acceptance of painless, needleless anesthesia. EMLA may prove to be an important preparation for painless administration of local anesthesia for procedures on intact skin (face, scalp, possibly proximal extremities).

BIBLIOGRAPHY

Bonadio WA, Wagner V: Efficacy of TAC topical anesthetic for repair of pediatric lacerations, *Am J Dis Child* 142:203, February 1988.

Covino BG, Vassallo H: *Local anesthetic: mechanisms of action and clinical use,* New York, 1976, Grune & Stratton.

Holmes HS: Options for painless local anesthetics, *Postgrad Med* 89(3): 1991.

Juhlin L, Evers H: EMLA: a new topical anesthetic, *Adv Dermatol* 5:75, 1990.

Thomas SH, Ray VG: Topical anesthesia for laceration repair in children, *Drug Therapy:* February 1992.

CHAPTER 23

Peripheral Nerve Blocks and Field Blocks

Julie Graves Moy

John L. Pfenninger

Many ambulatory procedures lend themselves well to local anesthesia with a field block or a peripheral nerve block. A *field block* is a method of providing anesthesia to a relatively small area by injecting a "wall" of anesthetic solution across the path of the nerves supplying the operative field. Instead of the injection being made directly into the area of the procedure, it is made into the soft tissue some distance away, where the nerves are situated. Advantages include longer duration of anesthesia than that with local infiltration, and no distortion of the operative field.

A *nerve block* is the infiltration of a local anesthetic near the nerve branch supplying sensation to a particular area. Blocking a nerve provides longer duration of anesthesia than that obtained with local cutaneous infiltration. Knowledge of the anatomy of peripheral nerves and scrupulous sterile technique are important for successful peripheral nerve blocks. Using this technique may reduce the amount of anesthetic needed, reduce distortion of tissues, and allow palpation of pathology to be excised.

In some sites (e.g., the breast), a nerve block cannot be obtained and thus the field block is the only reasonable alternative. However, where possible, the nerve block may be the procedure of choice. Also see Chapter 27, Oral/Facial Anesthesia.

INDICATIONS

Physicians may choose to use a field block or a nerve block for situations in which local anesthetic at the site of incision may not be effective (e.g., with infected tissue), or when the edema from the local anesthetic injection would distort anatomic landmarks and make approximation and repair difficult. The necessity to palpate deep tissue for excision would also be an indication for either type of block.

CONTRAINDICATIONS

Absolute

The need to inject through infected tissue, the presence of septicemia, and profound bleeding tendencies are contraindications.

Relative

A relative contraindication is any neurologic damage existing before the procedure. Document your findings before injection. Epinephrine-containing solutions should generally not be used in the hand, foot, penis, nose, or earlobes, nor should epinephrine be used in areas with poor vascular supply. History of allergy to local anesthetics would also contraindicate injections (see Chapter 21, Local Anesthesia).

EQUIPMENT

- Sterile field and agent for sterile preparation of skin
- Local anesthetic agent (see Table 23-1 and Chapter 21)
- 18-gauge needle to draw up solution
- 25- to 30-gauge needle for injection and appropriate size syringes (1 to 10 cc)
- Syringe
- Sterile gloves

PREPROCEDURE PATIENT EDUCATION

There are few complications with field and nerve blocks, so it is rare that the patient needs any extensive education. Depending on the agent used, the duration of anesthesia may be prolonged, and the patient should be informed of the expected length of action. In rare instances, a nerve could be traumatized, but long-term consequences are minimal. Any precautionary advice such as avoidance of heat or cold postprocedurely should be given to the patient. The possibility of paresthesia during the injection should be explained.

TECHNIQUE

Field Block

The technique of administering a field block is similar to the technique discussed under local anesthetics. In this instance, however, the area to be incised is spared from the injection. Rather, the area around the site is injected (Fig. 23-1). Repeat injections are made until the entire border of the field has been infiltrated. Allowing 5 to 10 minutes for the block to take effect will improve the resulting anesthesia.

TABLE 23-1.

Local Anesthetic Agents (Also see Tables 21-1 and 21-2)

Type	Name	Equivalent Concentration	Onset	Duration (minutes)	Maximum Dose
Amino esters					
	Procaine (Novocaine)	2%	Slow	15-30 min plain 30-90 min w/epi	600 mg
	Tetracaine (Pontocaine)	0.25%	Slow	120-240 min plain 240-480 min w/epi	100 mg plain 200 mg w/epi
	Chlorprocaine (Nesacaine)	2%	Fast	15-30 min plain 30-90 min w/epi	800 mg plain 1000 mg w/epi
Amino amides					
	Lidocaine (Xylocaine)	0.5-1%-2%	Fast	30-120 min plain 60-400 min w/epi	300 mg plain 500 mg w/epi
	Etidocaine (Duranest)	0.5%	Fast	120-240 plain	300 mg plain 400 mg w/epi
	Mepivacaine (Carbocaine)	1%	Moderate	30-120 min plain 60-400 min w/epi	300 mg plain 500 mg w/epi
	Bupivacaine (Marcaine)	0.25%	Slow	120-240 min plain 240-480 min w/epi	175 mg plain 225 mg w/epi

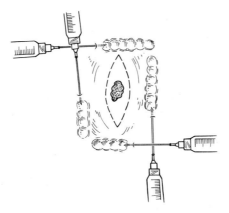

FIG. 23-1.
Field block technique.

Nerve Block

1. Before beginning any peripheral nerve block, perform a neurological examination of the area to be anesthetized and document this in the medical record. If any neurologic defect is present, include a description of it in the document of informed consent for the procedure, and have the patient sign a statement agreeing that the defect was present before the administration of the anesthetic.
2. Identify the appropriate nerve(s) and site to block.
3. Obtain informed consent.
4. Carefully clean and prepare the skin over the injection site in a sterile fashion.
5. Draw up the anesthetic. Usually a 25- to 30-gauge needle can be used to inject the anesthetic. The amount of anesthetic used will vary based on the location of the nerve.
6. Insert the needle into the site, withdrawing the plunger to avoid intravascular injection. If paresthesia is noted by the patient, withdraw the needle 2 mm and then inject the anesthetic. The goal is to inject perineurally, not into the nerve itself. If no paresthesia is noted at the expected site, confirm that there is no potential for intravascular injection and slowly inject the anesthetic. If the proper site has been identified, often as little as 1 or 2 cc will provide an excellent anesthetic field.
7. Allow 5 to 15 minutes for the block to take effect. Confirm anesthesia to pinprick before making an incision.

Common Nerve Blocks (Also See Chapter 27, Oral/Facial Anesthesia)

1. **Digital block of finger or toe.** Use 4 cc of 1% to 2% lidocaine *without* epinephrine for each finger, and 6 cc of the same for toes. Insert the 25-gauge ½-inch needle into the skin at the base of the finger or toe in the web space. Inject 1 cc into each lateral aspect of the finger, then 1 cc across the dorsal and the ventral surface of the finger in the subcutaneous space. For the toe, use 2 cc into each web space and 1 cc across the dorsal and the ventral surface of the toe. The dorsal digital nerves in both instances lie very close to bone. As the bone is touched with the needle tip, withdraw 1 or 2 mm and inject the solution (Fig. 23-2).
2. **Median nerve block.** The median nerve supplies sensation to the palmar aspect of the thumb, index, and middle fingers. In addition, the radial half of the palm is supplied by the median nerve. A nerve block may be indicated for extensive lacerations and incisions in these areas. The median nerve lies between the flexor carpi radialis and the palmaris longus. With flexion of the wrist, the palmaris longus stands out. The injection should be made at the flexor crease of the wrist just radial to the palmaris longus. Use 3 to 5 cc of 1% lidocaine *without* epinephrine (Figs. 23-3 and 23-6).
3. **Ulnar nerve block.** The ulnar nerve innervates the dorsal and palmar aspects on the ulnar side of the hand (fifth finger and ulnar side of the fourth finger). There are actually two branches of the ulnar nerve, which divides 4 to

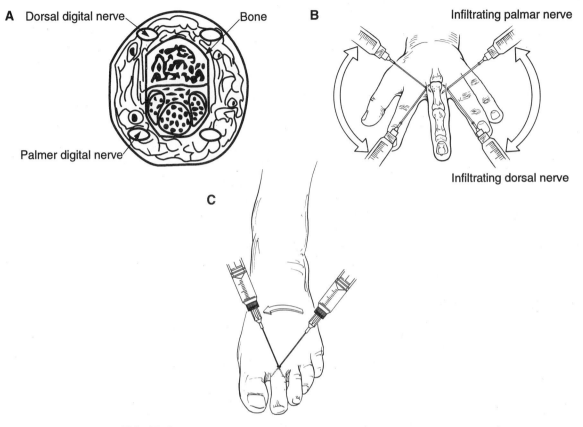

A Dorsal digital nerve — Bone

Palmer digital nerve

B Infiltrating palmar nerve

Infiltrating dorsal nerve

C

FIG. 23-2.
Anatomy and injection technique for digital nerve block. **A,** Four digital nerves of the finger. The bone is used as a landmark to find the proper plane of the dorsal digital nerve. **B,** Digital nerve block of the finger. The sites of the nerves are injected bilaterally. To obtain optimal effect, after blocking the nerves, place a "ring" of anesthetic entirely around the digit close to the bone. Inject superiorly over the bone and inferiorly under the bone in the subcutaneous plane. **C,** Digital nerve block of the toe showing an alternative method of injection. (**B** and **C** from Trott A: *Wounds and lacerations: emergency care and closure,* ed 2, St Louis, 1991, Mosby. Used with permission.)

5 cm proximal to the wrist. Therefore, the easiest way to obtain an ulnar block is to inject the ulnar nerve at the elbow where the nerve lies only 0.5 cm below the skin, between the medial epicondyle and the olecranon (Figs. 23-4 and 23-6). For all nerve blocks, it is best not to inject directly into the nerve, but around it; 2 to 3 cc of 1% lidocaine should be sufficient here.

4. **Radial nerve block.** The radial nerve innervates the dorsum of the thumb, index, and middle fingers, and the radial portion of the dorsum of the hand. Because of multiple divisions of the radial nerve, 10 cc of anesthetic is often required to obtain good results. Inject 3 cc of solution along the lateral border of the radial artery two finger breadths above the wrist. Then lay a superficial ring of solution from this point extending dorsally over the border of the wrist

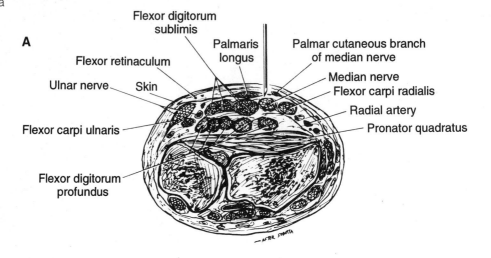

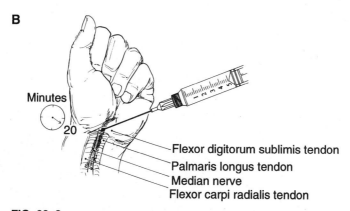

FIG. 23-3.
Median nerve block. **A,** Cross-sectional anatomy of the wrist. **B,** Location of injection. (From Trott A: *Wounds and lacerations: emergency care and closure,* ed 2, St Louis, 1991, Mosby. Used with permission.)

and into the snuff box area created by the tendons of the abductor pollicis longus and extensor pollicis brevis muscles. The nerve is in the superficial fascia just deep to the skin (Figs. 23-5 and 23-6).

5. **Supraorbital and supratrochlear nerve blocks (forehead block).** The supraorbital and supratrochlear nerves innervate the forehead and anterior scalp. The nerves exit at the supraorbital ridge. To assure that both nerves have been injected, infiltrate just above the bone beneath the entire medial two thirds of the eyebrow (Fig. 23-7, *A-B*).

6. **Infraorbital nerve block.** Palpate a notch in the infraorbital rim. The infraorbital nerve exits just beneath this small notch. Infiltrate directly over the infraorbital area, or use an intraoral technique. The latter approach requires a 1.5-inch needle, ideally 27-gauge. Introduce the needle at the gingival-buccal

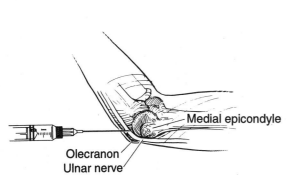

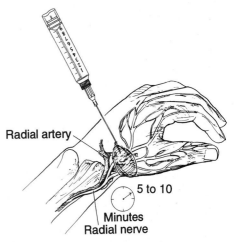

FIG. 23-4.
The site of an ulnar nerve block. (From Trott A: *Wounds and lacerations: emergency care and closure,* ed 2, St Louis, 1991, Mosby. Used with permission.)

FIG. 23-5.
The radial nerve block. (From Trott A: *Wounds and lacerations: emergency care and closure,* ed 2, St Louis, 1991, Mosby. Used with permission.)

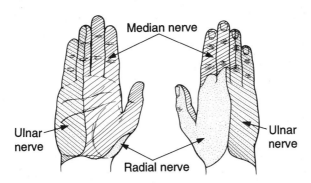

FIG. 23-6.
The distribution of cutaneous sensation by the radial, ulnar, and median nerves of the hand.

margin over the maxillary canine tooth. Advance it under the skin until the infraorbital foramen is reached. Use approximately 2 cc of anesthetic. This block is used especially to repair upper lip lacerations so that the vermilion border can be appropriately approximated. It can also be used for lacerations of the lower lateral nose and the lower eyelid (Fig. 23-7, *A-C*).

7. **Mental nerve block.** The mental nerve innervates the lower half of the lip. To avoid distortion that is inevitable with local injection around the vermilion border, inject the mental nerve. In adults, the nerve exits the mandible just

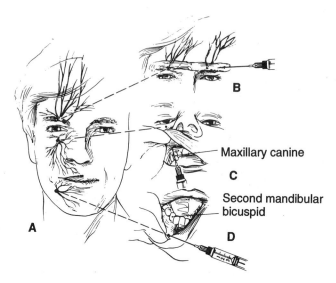

FIG. 23-7.
Locations of various nerves of the face and methods to obtain a nerve block. **A,** Position and course of the supraorbital, supratrochlear, infraorbital, and mental nerves. **B,** Technique for deposition of anesthetic to accomplish a supratrochlear and supraorbital (forehead) nerve block. **C,** Intraoral technique to anesthetize the infraorbital nerve. **D,** Intraoral technique to anesthetize the mental nerve. (From Trott A: *Wounds and lacerations: emergency care and closure,* ed 2, St Louis, 1991, Mosby. Used with permission.)

inferior to the second mandibular bicuspid, midway between the upper and lower edges of the mandible, and 2.5 cm from the midline of the jaw. As with the infraorbital nerve injection, introduce the needle at the gingival buccal margin inferior to the second bicuspid. After aspiration, inject 2 cc of anesthetic (Fig. 23-7, *A-D*).

8. **Ear block.**   Because of complex nerve innervations of the ear, it is impossible to infiltrate a solitary nerve. In addition, it is difficult to infiltrate *over* the cartilage since the skin here is so thin. One can obtain a complete block of the auricle by infiltrating completely around the ear with approximately 10 to 15 cc of 1% lidocaine *without* epinephrine (Fig. 23-8).

9. **Foot blocks.**   Foot blocks are indicated not so much to prevent distortion but rather to limit discomfort. The sole of the foot is exquisitely sensitive to injection, and it is often subject to puncture wounds, lacerations, and foreign bodies. Nerve blocks can actually be more comfortable than direct infiltration. The sural nerve runs behind the fibula and lateral malleolus to supply the heel and lateral aspect of the foot. The tibial nerve is found between the Achilles tendon and the medial malleolus, and its course is along the posterior tibial artery. The tibial nerve supplies the medial portion of the sole and the medial side of the foot. The two nerves do overlap innervation along the middle of the foot (Fig. 23-9). To block the sural nerve, insert the needle lateral to the Achilles tendon 1 to 2 cm proximal to the level of the distal tip of the lateral

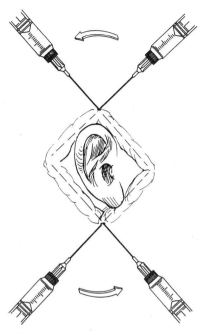

FIG. 23-8.
Technique to achieve field anesthesia of the ear. (From Trott A: *Wounds and lacerations: emergency care and closure,* ed 2, St Louis, 1991, Mosby. Used with permission.)

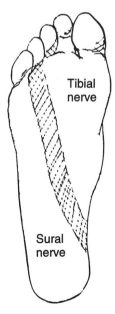

FIG. 23-9.
Distribution of sensory innervation to the foot. (From Trott A: *Wounds and lacerations: emergency care and closure,* ed 2, St Louis, 1991, Mosby. Used with permission.)

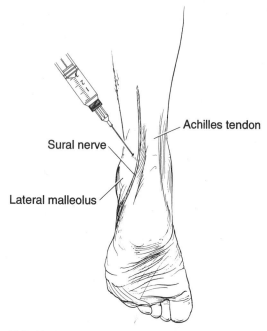

FIG. 23-10.
Location of the sural nerve block. (From Trott A: *Wounds and lacerations: emergency care and closure,* ed 2, St Louis, 1991, Mosby. Used with permission.)

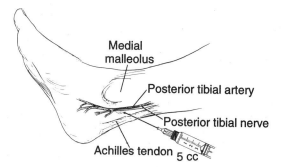

FIG. 23-11.
Location of the tibial nerve block. (From Trott A: *Wounds and lacerations: emergency care and closure,* ed 2, St Louis, 1991, Mosby. Used with permission.)

malleolus. To ensure that the entire nerve is infiltrated, introduce the needle several times in a fan-shaped motion, directing it to the posterior medial aspect of the fibula (Fig. 23-10).

To obtain a tibial nerve block, identify the posterior tibial pulsation. Pass the needle medial to the Achilles tendon toward the posterior tibial artery behind the medial malleolus. Infiltration is around the artery, but careful aspiration must be carried out to prevent intraarterial injection (Fig. 23-11).

CPT/BILLING CODES

64450   Introduction/injection of anesthetic agent (nerve block), diagnostic or therapeutic

Be sure to document both the diagnostic and procedural code for the local anesthesia. The CPT system allows separate billing for local anesthesia if it is administered by a physician different than the surgeon, but the CPT code includes local anesthesia for the surgical procedure in most cases. A code for the instrument tray is allowed if the procedure requires more than basic instruments. If the nerve blocks are being done for diagnostic reasons, they can be billed separately.

BIBLIOGRAPHY

Gilette RD: *Procedures in ambulatory care,* New York, 1987, McGraw-Hill.

Homes HS: Options for painless local anesthesia, *Postgrad Med J* 89(30):71, 1991.

Lebowitz PW, Newberg LA, Gilette MT, editors: *Clinical anesthesia procedures of the Massachusetts General Hospital,* Boston, 1982, Little, Brown & Co.

Mulroy MF: *Regional anesthesia: an illustrated procedural guide,* Boston, 1989, Little, Brown & Co.

Trott A: *Wounds and lacerations: emergency care and closure,* ed 2, St Louis, 1991, Mosby.

Wolcott MW, editor: *Ambulatory surgery and the basics of emergency surgical care,* ed 2, Philadelphia, 1988, J.B. Lippincott.

CHAPTER 24

Pediatric Sedation

David B. Bosscher

Anyone who performs minor procedures on pediatric patients knows the value of being able to safely and predictably sedate them. Children, especially preschool children, are often fearful of painful or unfamiliar techniques. When verbal reassurance does not allow the physician to perform the needed procedure safely, sedation is required. Sedation does not anesthetize the child sufficiently to perform a painful procedure, but it generates cooperation of the child, allowing proper anesthetics to be administered.

INDICATIONS

- Any necessary, minor procedure for which the cooperation of the child cannot be obtained using verbal reassurance

CONTRAINDICATIONS

- A medical condition that would cause respiratory compromise during sedation
- Sensitivity to one of the agents being used

EQUIPMENT

- The medication and the means to administer it (In most cases, this will mean a syringe and needle.)
- The means to support respiration if necessary (A bag and mask, an oral airway tube, and the equipment to administer oxygen are minimum respiratory support equipment required. Although intubation is rarely needed, appropriately sized endotracheal tubes and a laryngoscope should be available for emergency use.)

PRESEDATION CONCERNS

- Pediatric sedation does not relieve the practitioner of the need to explain the anticipated procedure to both the child (when appropriate) and the parent or guardian. Informed consent for both the sedation and the procedure should be obtained and documented.
- A trained nurse or other properly trained person should be present throughout the procedure to monitor the child and to assist with the procedure.
- The physician should be aware of the duration of action of the agent utilized for sedation. On the one hand, the duration of action should be sufficient to comfortably complete the procedure. On the other hand, if the duration of action is prolonged, the physician needs to ensure that the child will be properly monitored after the procedure is completed.

DOCUMENTATION

Documentation of any procedure should be scrupulous and complete. Obtain informed consent for both the contemplated sedation technique and the procedure itself. Document the issues discussed in obtaining informed consent in the patient record. Some medicolegal experts also recommend asking a parent or guardian to sign a form listing each procedure that the physician might perform. With regard to pediatric sedation, document how well the patient tolerated the method utilized. If side effects from the medication occur, document your approach to dealing with them. Finally, document that written instructions were provided covering the care of the child after discharge from the office or hospital.

TECHNIQUE

Be aware that many pediatric procedures can be done by simply gaining the child's confidence, offering basic information regarding the procedure, and then talking him or her through it. Be honest about when it might hurt. This strategy is most effective in children 6 years old or older.

With the preschool-aged child, when "verbal sedation" is not likely to be sufficient, several pediatric sedation techniques are available.

1. **The Lytic Cocktail.** This time-honored mixture of chlorpromazine (Thorazine), promethazine (Phenergan), and meperidine (Demerol) is given intramuscularly according to weight of the child: chlorpromazine 0.5 mg/kg, promethazine 0.5 mg/kg, meperidine 0.7 mg/kg. The lytic cocktail has undergone the test of time; many emergency department physicians still use it. However, many condemn its use because (*a*) the physician must be aware of the side effects of three medicines instead of one, and (*b*) its effect can be erratic and unpredictable.

2. **Chloral Hydrate (Noctec).** The wide margin of safety of this oral liquid has earned it a place among those who perform pediatric procedures. The dosage

for the child is 5 to 10 mg/kg. Chloral hydrate has an unpleasant smell and taste, making it difficult to entice a child to take much of it. After oral administration, it has an onset of action of around 60 minutes, making it relatively impractical for unplanned use. In addition, its sedative effects can be difficult to predict. An hour after ingesting chloral hydrate, the patient can be wide awake and unwilling to submit to the procedure. Chloral hydrate can be given intramuscularly or via rectal suppository, but these forms of the medication are often unavailable and have other disadvantages.

3. **Intranasal Midazolam (Versed).** This rapidly acting benzodiazepine is widely used by anesthesiologists who like its predictable onset of action, its low side-effect profile, and its amnestic effect. It is also now reversible. The medication causes children to become very cooperative, although it will not appear to sedate them. Intranasal midazolam dosage is 0.1 to 0.2 ml/kg of the injectable formulation. (Some researchers have used these dosages in subjects up to 18 years of age.) The solution is drawn up into a tuberculin syringe, the needle is removed, and the drug is then instilled in the child's nasal cavity. The onset of action is typically 10 to 15 minutes, and the duration of action is generally 15 to 20 minutes, with some effects lasting up to several hours. Midazolam can be utilized as a back-up strategy in instances where the physician unsuccessfully attempts to perform the procedure under "verbal anesthesia."

The medication has been utilized orally at a dosage of 0.5 to 0.75 mg/kg. Its onset of action is slower when this route is used, and some strong-tasting vehicle is required to overcome its bitter taste. Oral midazolam has a longer duration of action (up to 1 hour), but the recovery period is also prolonged with this route of administration.

With all administration routes, side effects are rare and are typical of benzodiazepines in general (occasional agitation, euphoria). Neither excessive drowsiness nor respiratory depression was seen in studies utilizing these dosages.

POSTSEDATION CONCERNS

- Respiratory depression is rare with any of these medications, but if it occurs, it is a significant problem. Flumazenil (Romazicon, formerly Mazicon) is an injectable antagonist of midazolam and can reverse any respiratory depression midazolam causes. Alert the parent or guardian to possible breathing problems. Naloxone (Narcan) can be used to reverse narcotic suppression.
- All of these medications can cause atypical or unexpected behaviors, ranging from acting drunk to making nonsensical statements or even agitation. Parents must be aware of the need to supervise the child constantly for several hours after the procedure. In addition, they should be prepared to protect the child and to reorient him or her as necessary until the medication effects wear off.

COMPLICATIONS

- Respiratory compromise is the most common complication. Remain alert for this possibility and be prepared to respond with appropriate measures.

- Children can experience unpredictable reactions to medications. Being familiar with the most common idiosyncratic reactions of the agent you are using is part of your minimum preparation. *AMA Drug Evaluations* or a similar text will offer more pertinent help than either the *Physician's Drug Reference* (PDR) or the drug package insert.
- The usual doses of medications will not always properly sedate some pediatric patients. At times, it may be impossible to perform the anticipated procedure.

BIBLIOGRAPHY

Kempe et al: *Current pediatric diagnosis and treatment,* East Norwalk, Conn, 1987, Appleton & Lange.

Niall et al: Preanesthetic sedation of preschool children using intranasal midazolam, *Anesthesiology* 69:972, 1988.

CHAPTER 25

Bier Block

Robert Williams

Intravenous (IV) regional anesthesia, also known as a Bier block, is a useful method of providing operative anesthesia to wide areas of the distal portion of an extremity. When executed with proper technique, the Bier block is a safe alternative to local or hematoma infiltration, and it provides superior anesthesia to these methods. At the same time, it has the advantage of being technically simpler to perform than other regional alternatives (e.g., axillary or brachial plexus infiltration).

INDICATIONS

Although the technique of IV regional anesthesia has been used on the lower extremity, it is most used in applications involving the upper extremity. Some experts suggest that one not consider a block of the lower extremity until sufficient experience with upper-extremity blocks is obtained. Any condition of a distal extremity requiring nonlocalized anesthesia would be a candidate for a Bier block. Examples include reductions of fractures or dislocations, repair of extensive lacerations, drainage of large abscesses, and tendon repair.

CONTRAINDICATIONS

Documented sensitivity to local anesthetics is an absolute contraindication (see Chapter 21, Local Anesthesia). Relative contraindications include the following:

- Injuries to the proximal extremity that would be adversely affected by application of a tourniquet
- Conditions predisposing to arterial thrombosis
- Difficulty in maintaining arterial occlusion with a tourniquet (e.g., inadequate cuff size in a massively obese patient)

EQUIPMENT

- Double-cuff automatic pneumatic tourniquet—available in models that can individually or simultaneously inflate or deflate both cuffs to preset pressures (As an alternative, ordinary blood pressure cuffs can be used if the dimensions of the arm can accommodate two appropriately sized cuffs between the axilla and the elbow without overlap.)
- Lidocaine, 1 cc/kg of the 0.5% solution for upper-extremity blocks, 2 cc/kg of the 0.25% solution for lower-extremity blocks
- Intravenous needle/cannula
- Sterile skin preparation solution (povidone-iodine)
- Tape
- Elastic bandage of sufficient size to wrap the entire extremity distal to the tourniquet

Although the risk of serious adverse reaction is very small when the procedure is followed correctly, it should be conducted only in facilities capable of managing serious local anesthetic toxicities. (See Complications.)

PREPROCEDURE PATIENT EDUCATION

Advise the patient that 95% of patients experience good or complete anesthesia with a Bier block; the remainder require additional analgesics or sedatives. Explain the potential for complications to the patient. Anesthesia will resolve within 30 minutes of tourniquet release.

TECHNIQUE

1. Measure the patient's blood pressure.
2. Test the pneumatic tourniquet or blood pressure cuffs for accuracy and maintenance of pressure, and then place on the proximal portion of the extremity.
3. After skin prep, place the intravenous needle/cannula in a vein in the distal portion of the extremity, preferably distal to the operative site. Attach the syringe with lidocaine and tape in place.
4. Have an assistant elevate the extremity above the heart, while you wrap the elastic bandage around it from fingers/toes to the distal cuff.
5. Rapidly inflate the proximal cuff to 50 mm Hg above the systolic blood pressure for upper-extremity blocks, and twice the systolic blood pressure for lower-extremity blocks. Assign an assistant to be responsible for continuously monitoring the maintenance of cuff pressures throughout the remainder of the procedure.
6. Lower the extremity, remove the elastic bandage, and check the distal pulses (Fig. 25-1). If no pulse is palpable, inject the appropriate dose of lidocaine. The IV may be removed.
7. After approximately 10 to 15 minutes, check the adequacy of anesthesia by gently manipulating the operative site. Additional time may be required to

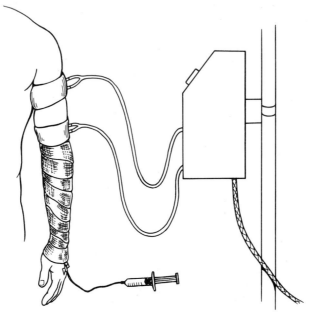

FIG. 25-1.
Bier block procedure, before removal of elastic bandage and injection of lidocaine, showing inflation of proximal cuff.

achieve full effect, though if after 20 to 30 minutes the anesthesia is inadequate, supplementary analgesia or sedation is advised.

8. After the initial 10 to 15 minutes, inflate the distal cuff to the same pressure as the proximal cuff, and then deflate the proximal cuff. This use of two cuffs reduces the pain associated with the occlusive tourniquet by allowing infusion of anesthetic under the proximal cuff before it is inflated.

9. When anesthesia is deemed adequate, the operation may proceed up to a maximum inflation time of two hours. Periodically monitor the blood pressure on the contralateral side to ensure proper tourniquet pressure. The tourniquet may remain inflated during intraoperative X-rays.

10. At completion of the procedure, but no sooner than 20 minutes after lidocaine injection (to permit diffusion of some of the lidocaine out of the vascular system), deflate and remove the distal cuff. Some physicians recommend cycles of deflation/inflation, but this has no advantage in lowering systemic plasma lidocaine levels.

11. Observe the patient for 10 to 15 minutes for signs of toxicity.

COMPLICATIONS

Minor adverse reactions to the lidocaine (dizziness, tinnitus, bradycardia, etc.) occur in less than 2% of patients after cuff deflation. Serious reactions (including seizures, cardiovascular collapse, and death) occur almost exclusively when the lidocaine is injected with the cuffs deflated—because of operator error or equipment malfunction—and are rare.

CPT/BILLING CODES

01995   Regional IV administration of local anesthetic agent (upper or lower extremity)

BIBLIOGRAPHY

Brown EM, McGriff JT, Malinowski RW: Intravenous regional anesthesia (Bier block): review of 20 years' experience, *Can J Anaesth* 36(3):307, 1989.

Farrell RG, Swanson SL, Walter JR: Safe and effective IV regional anesthesia for use in the emergency department, *Ann Emerg Med* 14(4):288, 1985.

Salo M et al: Plasma lidocaine concentrations after different methods of releasing the tourniquet during intravenous regional anaesthesia, *Ann Clin Res* 11:164, 1979.

CHAPTER 26

Technique of Trigger Point Injection

Gary E. Ruoff

Both myofascial pain syndromes and fibromyalgia demonstrate trigger-point involvement. Trigger points are tender spots or muscle hardenings located in different muscle groups often near bony attachments (Fig. 26-1). Interruption of the pain cycle by trigger-point injection, and spray-and-stretch manuevers may produce prolonged relief. Passive stretch following trigger-point therapy may provide additional benefit. Adjunctive therapies include acupressure, heat or ice massage, and electrical stimulation.

INDICATIONS

- Focal tender area identifiable by palpation without other identifiable neurologic or musculoskeletal findings or pathology

CONTRAINDICATIONS

- Infection at the site of the needle insertion
- Concomitant use of an anticoagulant
- A hemorrhagic syndrome
- Septicemia
- Resuscitation equipment not available

PREPROCEDURE PATIENT EDUCATION AND EVALUATION

- Provide the patient with a detailed explanation about the procedure and obtain written informed consent.
- Explain to the patient that the "area of pain reference" is caused by irritation of an area known as a "trigger point" and at times it may be somewhat distant from the site of pain.

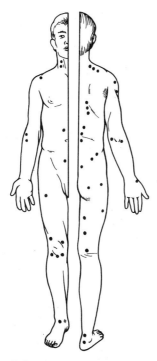

FIG. 26-1.
Common points of maximum tenderness. Note predominant locations at moving parts and sliding surfaces.

- Palpate the various muscle groups to locate the trigger point and the corresponding "area of pain reference" (point of maximal tenderness [PMT]).
- Explain to the patient that the periods of immediate relief that result from the treatment may be followed by pain greater than the original pain, and that follow-up injections may be necessary.

EQUIPMENT

- Alcohol wipes
- Sterile rubber gloves
- Several gauze pads
- Skin-marking pencil
- Antiseptic solution
- Lidocaine (0.25% to 1% *without* epinephrine) or bupivacaine (0.125% to 0.25%); steroid may also be used along with the local anesthetic (Dosage varies, depending on agent used, but generally a very small amount is needed.)
- 22-, 25-, or 27-gauge needles of varying lengths, depending on site to be injected
- 3 ml, 5 ml, or 10 ml syringes
- Resuscitation equipment (as for any injection)

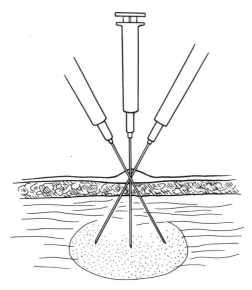

FIG. 26-2.
Injection of a trigger point.

TECHNIQUE

1. Place the patient in a comfortable or recumbent position to protect the patient in the event of a vasovagal reaction such as syncope.
2. Mark the precise site (trigger point or point of maximal tenderness) with a marking pencil.
3. Prepare the skin with an antiseptic solution or alcohol.
4. Use sterile gloves and sterile technique to identify the trigger point with your finger.
5. Use a 25-gauge needle, or even a 27-gauge needle when possible, for superficial muscle injections.
6. Begin with 5 ml of lidocaine (0.25% to 1%) or bupivacaine (0.125% or 0.25%).
7. Inject 0.25 ml to 0.50 ml of local anesthetic into the skin to produce a wheal (optional).
8. Slowly advance the needle perpendicular to the skin until the trigger point is identified.
9. Aspirate through the needle to determine if a blood vessel has been punctured.
10. Inject 0.5 ml to 2 ml of solution once the trigger point is located. The patient should experience immediate relief if the injection is properly located.
11. Withdraw the needle slightly and reinject the site two or three times as shown in Fig. 26-2.
12. Remove the needle and wipe the skin clean with a disinfectant.

Note: Never inject more than 10 ml of solution into any trigger-point area. No more than 4.5 mg/kg of lidocaine may be used at any one time (1% lidocaine is 10 mg/cc). Trigger point injection may be repeated as needed if no steroids are used. To break a cycle of pain, an injection may be needed every 3 to 4 days.

POSTPROCEDURE CARE

- Observe for a decrease in the patient's pain; it should be almost immediate.
- Observe for signs and symptoms such as lightheadedness, tinnitus, peripheral numbness, slurring of speech, drowsiness, evidence of seizure activity. These may indicate a toxic reaction to the local anesthetic.
- Observe for any bleeding into skin or muscle compartment.
- Assign stretching exercises, physical therapy, or rest as indicated.

COMPLICATIONS

- Vasovagal syncope
- Skin infection
- Toxic reactions to the local anesthetic
- Hematoma formation
- Neuritis
- Rebound pain
- Pneumothorax (if injecting over thorax)
- Compartment syndrome

CPT/BILLING CODE

20550   Injection, tendon sheath, ligament, trigger points or ganglion cyst

BIBLIOGRAPHY

Andres E, Sola AE, Bonica JJ: Myofascial pain syndromes. In Bonica JJ, editor: *The management of pain,* ed 2, Philadelphia, 1990, Lea & Febiger.

Bonica JJ: Management of myofascial pain syndromes in general practice, *JAMA* 146:732, 1957.

Simons DG, Travell JG: Myofascial origins of low back pain, *Postgrad Med* 73(2):1983.

Sola AE: Trigger point therapy. In Roberts JR, Hedges JR, editors: *Clinical procedures in emergency medicine,* Philadelphia, 1985, W.B. Saunders.

CHAPTER 27

Oral/Facial Anesthesia

Richard J. Bakeman

Tissues of the face and mouth have an enormous amount of sensory innervation. It is therefore understandable that the patient may endure a great deal of pain due to trauma or odontogenic disease. Trigeminal nerve block is a simple technique that eliminates this pain. The ability to administer this block broadens the scope of services a physician can offer patients. Furthermore, one or more of these nerve blocks can provide easy and profound anesthesia for suturing oral and facial lacerations. Quite frequently, the primary care physician will be the first clinician to see a patient exhibiting pain in the mouth or facial areas. Using a nerve block prevents distortion of tissue, allowing for more appropriate approximation of tissue edges. It also limits the amount of anesthesia needed and the number of injection sites.

Anatomical considerations are always important when discussing anesthesia. The trigeminal nerve (fifth cranial nerve) provides most of the sensory innervation to the face and oral cavity. The sensory divisions of the trigeminal (V) nerve are the opthalmic branch (V_1), the maxillary branch (V_2), and the mandibular branch (V_3). The emphasis of this text will be on maxillary and mandibular nerve anesthesia.

SUPRAPERIOSTEAL INJECTION

Indications

Supraperiosteal injections (local infiltration) are indicated for pulpal or soft tissue anesthesia of maxillary teeth and their surrounding structures. This injection is used when one or two teeth require anesthesia. It is useful for localized trauma, pathologies, or surgeries. Local infiltration injections have a high rate of success, are technically easy to administer, and are usually atraumatic (particularly in posterior segments). This injection is not suitable for large areas (i.e., entire maxilla) because of the large volumes of anesthetic required and the need for multiple injection sites.

A

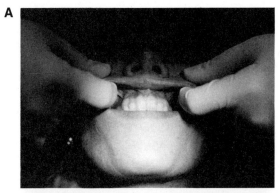

B

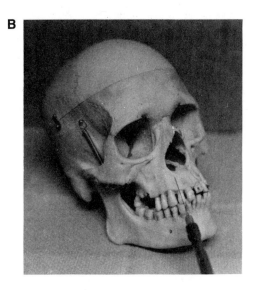

C

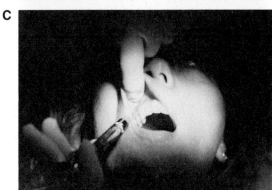

FIG. 27-1.
Supraperiosteal injection. See text for details.

Contraindications

- Infection at site of injection
- Dense bone overlying teeth so that the anesthetic solution cannot diffuse to the apices of teeth
- History of allergy or reaction to anesthetic (see Chapter 21, Local Anesthesia)

Equipment

- 25-, 27-, or 30-gauge short needles
- Syringe (Dental aspirating syringe with loops for fingers facilitates the procedure.)
- Anesthetic, such as 2% lidocaine with epinephrine 1:100,000 or 0.5% bupivacaine with epinephrine 1:200,000

Technique

1. Lift the lip, pulling tissue taught (Fig. 27-1, *A*).
2. The point of injection should be at the mucobuccal fold aiming at the apex of the tooth or region to be anesthetized (Fig. 27-1, *B-C*).

3. Aspirate.
4. If blood is aspirated, readjust the needle and reaspirate.
5. Upon negative aspiration, deposit 0.5 to 1.5 cc of anesthetic very slowly (over 45 seconds).
6. Anesthesia should be adequate in 2 to 5 minutes, depending on proper placement.

Complications

- Pain upon injection
- Hematoma (rare)
- Anesthetic reaction (rare)

POSTERIOR SUPERIOR ALVEOLAR NERVE BLOCK

Indications

Posterior superior alveolar (PSA) nerve block is used to achieve pulpal and soft-tissue anesthesia in the area of the first molar, second molar, and third molar, and their surrounding structures. This injection is indicated when two or more upper molars are affected or are involved in a procedure, and when local infiltration is ineffective or contraindicated (e.g., because of infection).

Contraindications

- History of allergy or reaction to anesthetic (see Chapter 21, Local Anesthesia)

Disadvantages

- Risk of hematoma
- Slightly more difficult target area

Equipment

- Equipment is same as that for supraperiosteal injection except that a long (1.25 or 1.5 inch) needle is used.

Technique

1. The target area is the infratemporal surface of maxilla, which is posterior to the maxilla and superior to the maxillary tuberosity (Fig. 27-2, *A*).
2. Position yourself at 10 o'clock for the left PSA and 8 o'clock for the right PSA.
3. Have the patient partly open his or her mouth. Move the mandible to the side of injection. Retract the cheek with your finger (Fig. 27-2, *B*).
4. Insert the needle at the height of vestibule over the second molar. Direct the needle superiorly, medially, and posteriorly, and advance it to the posterior border of the maxilla.

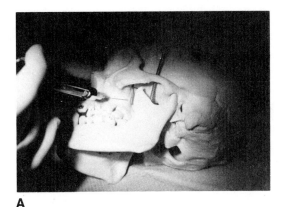

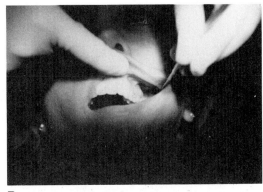

A   **B**

FIG. 27-2.
Posterior superior alveolar nerve block. See text for details.

5. Aspirate.
6. Turn the needle in a half turn and reaspirate.
7. If there is negative aspiration, deposit 1.0 to 1.8 cc of anesthetic slowly (over 60 seconds).
8. Wait 3 to 5 minutes for anesthesia to take effect.

INFRAORBITAL NERVE BLOCK

Indications

Infraorbital nerve block provides profound anesthesia for the maxillary incisors and cuspids for most patients, and for the area of the face below the eye, including the lip. Nerves that are blocked include the anterior superior alveolor nerve, inferior palpebral nerve, lateral nasal nerve, and superior labial nerve.

Advantages

- This injection is useful when the supraperiosteal nerve block is contraindicated or ineffective or if anesthesia of the face is needed.
- It is a simple and safe technique.

Disadvantages

- Hemostasis is not always adequately achieved.

Equipment

- Same as PSA injection

Technique

1. The target area is the infraorbital foramen (Fig. 27-3, *A*).
2. Identify the infraorbital notch on the infraorbital ridge.
3. Run your finger down from the notch to the infraorbital foramen to mark the target area.
4. Lift the lip and insert the needle in the mucobuccal fold over the maxillary second bicuspid, aiming at the marked infraorbital foramen (Fig. 27-3, *B*).
5. Aspirate.
6. Continue steps as in PSA injection.
7. Alternatively, inject directly over the infraorbital foramen.

Complications

- Hematoma (rare)

MAXILLARY (V₂) NERVE BLOCK

Indications

The maxillary nerve block provides profound anesthesia for the entire maxilla on the blocked side. This block is convenient when large areas of anesthesia are required and when the previously discussed injections are ineffective or contraindicated. It is very successful and reduces the amount of anesthetic and number of injection sites required.

Contraindications

- Pediatric patients

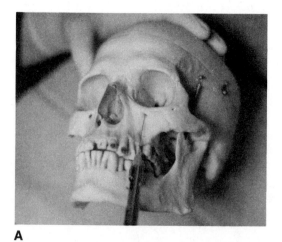

A

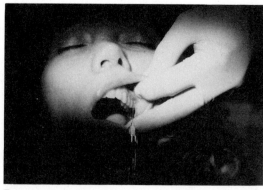

B

FIG. 27-3.
Infraorbital nerve block. See text for details.

Disadvantages

- Hematoma is common.
- Technique is more difficult.
- Hemostasis is not achieved as it would be with use of epinephrine locally.
- The injection can sometimes be painful.

Equipment

- Same as that for PSA and infraorbital injections

Technique

1. The target area is the maxillary nerve as it passes through the pterygopalatine fossa, superior and medial to the target area for the PSA block (Fig. 27-4, *A*).
2. Partially open the patient's mouth and position the mandible to the side of injection.
3. Retract the cheek with your index finger.
4. Place the needle in the height of the mucobuccal fold apical to the second molar (Fig. 27-4, *B*).
5. Advance the needle in the superior, medial, and posterior direction about 1.25 inches (this is slightly further than PSA injections).
6. Aspirate.
7. Continue steps as in PSA injection.

Complications

- Hematoma will develop quickly if maxillary artery or pterygoid venous plexus is punctured
- Intravascular injection

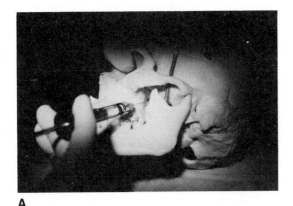

A

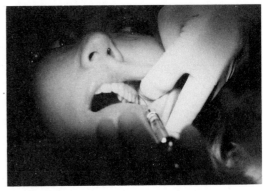

B

FIG. 27-4.
Maxillary nerve block. See text for details.

INFERIOR ALVEOLAR (V₃) NERVE BLOCK

The mandibular nerve block is one of the most useful nerve blocks for anesthesia of the lower third of the face. The inferior alveolar nerve block plus a supplementary buccal nerve block will provide profound anesthesia for the lower teeth to the midline, the body of the mandible, the anterior two thirds of the tongue, the floor of the mouth, and all soft tissue anterior to the mental foramen including that of the lower lip and chin.

Indications

- Appropriate when labial soft tissue anesthesia is needed (anterior to mental foramen)

Contraindications

- This block should not be done in the proximity of an infection or on patients with masochistic tendencies (i.e., mentally handicapped or young patients).

Advantages

- Well suited when anesthesia of lingual soft tissue is required
- One injection provides a wide area of anesthesia
- Can be used in all procedures involving lower teeth

Disadvantages

- High rate of failure (15% to 20%)
- Intraoral landmarks are not consistently reliable
- 10% to 15% positive rate of aspiration

Equipment

- Aspirating syringe (Dental aspirating syringe with loops for fingers facilitates the procedure.)
- 25- or 27-gauge long needle (1.25 inch)
- Local anesthetic of choice

Technique

1. Landmarks include the following:
   a. Greatest concavity of the anterior border of ramus
   b. Pterygomandibular raphe (formed by the posterior border of the buccinator muscle and the anterior border of the superior constrictor muscle) (Fig. 27-5, *A*)
   c. Occlusal plane of mandibular teeth
2. The target area is the mandibular nerve just before it enters the mandibular canal (Fig. 27-5, *B*).

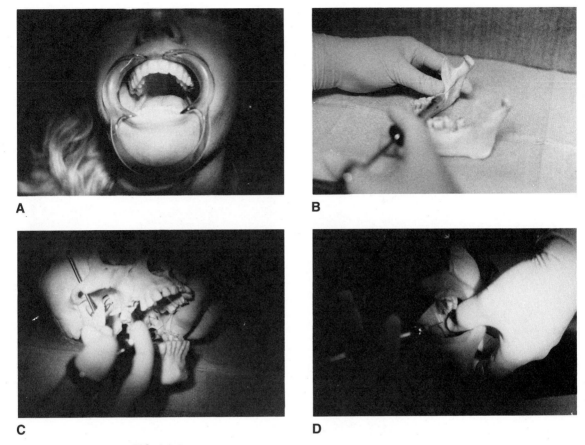

A

B

C

D

FIG. 27-5.
Inferior alveolar nerve block. See text for details.

3. The insertion point is the mucosa medial to the anterior border of the ramus but lateral to the pterygomandibular raphe.

4. The right-handed practitioner will administer the left block from the 10 o'clock position and the right block from the 8 o'clock position.

5. Place the patient in the supine position.

6. Place the thumb of your free hand on the anterior border of the ramus intraorally and determine the maximum concavity. Imagine a line running posteriorly from this point to the pterygomandibular raphe. This line indicates the vertical level of injection. It is between 6 and 10 mm above the posterior occlusal plane (Fig. 27-5, *C-D*).

7. The anterior-posterior dimension is estimated to be two thirds of the way posterior of the anterior border of the ramus on its medial surface. It falls on an imaginary line formed by the thumb in the concavity of the anterior border of the ramus and extraoral index finger on the posterior border of the ramus (Fig. 27-5, *D*).

8. Swing the barrel of the syringe so that it is positioned over the contralateral bicuspids.
9. Slowly penetrate the tissue until gentle bone contact is felt.
10. Aspirate.
11. If aspiration is negative, deposit 1.5 to 1.8 cc of anesthetic over a 60-second period.
12. Anesthesia will be in effect in 3 to 5 minutes.

Note: If the tip of the needle is inserted too far posteriorly, it may reach the parotid capsule. Injection here will cause a blocked seventh cranial nerve (facial) or temporary Bell's palsy.

Complications

- Hematoma (rare)
- Trismus
- Transient facial paralysis
- Intravascular injection

CPT/BILLING CODE

64400   Injection, anesthetic agent; trigeminal nerve, any division or branch

BIBLIOGRAPHY

Malamed SF: *Handbook of local anesthesia,* St Louis, 1980, Mosby.

PART THREE

Eyes, Ears, Nose, and Throat

CHAPTER 28

Audiometry

Gregory J. Forzley

Audiometry quantifies an individual's ability to hear sound through a range of intensities and frequencies. It can assist in diagnosis of the type of hearing disorder and assess the degree of impairment. Tuning-fork testing, utilizing the C-notes of the musical scale from low to high frequencies, is a common screening procedure. The pure-tone audiometer, in the tradition of tuning forks, is another way to test the auditory system by electronically sampling the octave series of the C-scale. The tones of the audiometer are "pure" in that they are relatively free of noise or overtones. The tone can be interrupted when desired, or the intensity (in decibels, dB) can be varied.

The pure-tone audiometer is made up of a variable-frequency oscillator that produces the sounds, an attenuator that permits variations of intensity (often in 5 dB steps), and a transducer, such as earphones or a bone vibrator, that converts electrical energy to acoustic energy. Through sounds produced in earphones held snugly to the head, each ear is tested separately and the results are then graphed as the *air conduction audiogram.* A separate test can be performed using a bone conduction oscillator or vibrator held against the mastoid or forehead by a headband to better evaluate for neural hearing loss. The vibrator sets the skull into oscillation with an associated disturbance of the fluid in the cochlea. These results are graphed as the *bone conduction audiogram,* which measures the response of the cochlea and the central auditory nervous system.

The goal of audiometry is to measure the lowest decibel intensity that can be heard for each frequency tested. This is defined as the threshold for that frequency. The individual's threshold is compared to the *audiometric zero,* a unit developed by the American National Standards Institute and derived from sampling a large population of ear-disease-free young adults.

The notations used to record the graphic results of the audiograms have been standardized by the American Speech-Language-Hearing Association (ASHA). The audiogram grid reflects the frequency in hertz (Hz) logarithmically on the horizontal axis, and the hearing level in decibels (dB) linearly on the vertical axis. The symbols used are noted in Fig. 28-1. In the past, the results for the right ear were

Response★

MODALITY	EAR		
	LEFT	UNSPECIFIED	RIGHT
AIR CONDUCTION-EARPHONES			
UNMASKED	X		O
MASKED	□		Δ
BONE CONDUCTION-MASTOID			
UNMASKED	>	∧	<
MASKED	]		[
BONE CONDUCTION-FOREHEAD			
UNMASKED	L	v	⌐
MASKED	Γ		⌐
AIR CONDUCTION-SOUND FIELD	✕	S	∅

★For NO RESPONSE, use a downward 45-degree arrow pointing to the left for the right ear symbols, and to the right for left ear symbols (e.g., ↙O for no response in the right ear unmasked).

FIG. 28-1.
Standardized symbols for recording audiogram results.

color-coded in red, and the left ear in blue. This is no longer recommended since color differences are lost when the results are copied.

INDICATIONS

- Subjective complaints of hearing loss, unilateral or bilateral
- Persistent serous otitis media, especially bilateral in children
- Initial evaluation of a failed hearing screen
- General screening in children at the earliest age possible and in the elderly with geriatric assessment
- Patient complaints of tinnitus, dizziness, or vertigo
- Speech delay in children
- Persistent behavioral problems or changes in children or the elderly
- Occupational screening and longitudinal evaluation with individuals in noisy work environments

CONTRAINDICATIONS

- Inexperienced technician
- Acute otitis media
- Local pinna infection causing pain from the earphone application
- Uncooperative patient
- Uncontrollable background noise in the room when testing

EQUIPMENT

- A pure-tone audiometer (A wide variety of models are available, including screening instruments testing only selected tones and decibel levels or alternatively, multiple-frequency, pure-tone air and bone conduction audiometers. The nonscreening instruments generally include frequencies of 125, 250, 500, 750, 1000, 1500, 2000, 3000, 4000, 6000, 8000 Hz in tone amplitudes ranging from −10 to +110 decibels.)
- An individual trained in proper techniques for obtaining reliable, reproducible, and valid test results (For industrial screening, the individual should be certified by the Council for Accreditation of Occupational Hearing Conservationists.)
- A quiet or sound-treated room, preferably tested (by an outside company) for acceptable ambient noise levels (Otherwise, thresholds may be artificially elevated, particularly in lower frequencies.)

SUPPLIERS

Beltone Electronics Corporation
4201 West Victoria Street
Chicago, IL 60646

Maico Hearing Instruments, Inc.
7375 Bush Lake Road
Minneapolis, MN 55435

Aussco-Vasc
3421 North Lincoln Avenue
Chicago, IL 60657

Singer Medical Products, Inc.
790 Maple Lane
Bensenville, IL 60106

Welch Allyn, Inc.
4341 State Street Road
P.O. Box 220
Skaneateles Falls, NY 13153

Handtronix
P.O. Box 21081
Salt Lake City, UT 84121

The last two manufacturers produce handheld, air-conduction screening devices even more portable than the traditional portable audiometer. They have been found to be very useful in screening.

Note: Handheld audiometers are very useful for screening purposes, such as the screenings done in school populations or in geriatric assessment. Their results are fairly reproducible by pure-tone audiometry.

TECHNIQUE

1. Seat the patient comfortably in such a way that he or she is looking neither at you nor at the control panel. The most common position of the patient is in a profile view to the examiner.

2. Large earrings, glasses, hats, and other items that may interfere with earphone application should be removed.
3. Instruct the patient to respond to the faintest detectable sound at each frequency. (The lowest level in decibels heard for each frequency is defined as the threshold.) Responses can consist of raising a hand or finger, or pressing a test button for the duration of audible sound. This step assists the examiner in determining false-positive responses.
4. Place the earphone speaker over the opening of the auditory canal, checking to be certain the tragus does not cover the opening.
5. Threshold testing is then initiated in the better ear (or the right ear if hearing is equal in both ears) with the following recommended sequence of frequencies: 1000 Hz, 2000 Hz, 4000 Hz, 8000 Hz, 1000 Hz (repeat), 500 Hz, and 250 Hz. Starting with 0-dB hearing levels and increasing in 10-dB increments, produce the tones for 1 to 2 seconds until the patient responds.
6. Increase the tone by 5 dB and, if the patient responds, reduce it by 10-dB increments until it is inaudible.
7. Continue repeated ascents in 5-dB increments and descents in 10-dB increments until a 50% reproducible response is obtained. Generally this requires 3 to 4 repetitions, with the patient attaining the same response at least half of the time. This result is then entered with the appropriate symbol on the audiogram.
8. Test the frequencies sequentially as previously noted, starting 15 to 20 dB below the threshold of the previously tested frequency. This is carried out until all frequencies have been tested.
9. If bone-conduction testing is planned, this same sequence can be applied and the results recorded with the appropriate symbols.
10. It may be necessary to mask or obscure one sound by another when the difference in hearing loss between two ears is great, such as a 50-dB difference. In that situation, crossover of sound to the better ear may occur and artificially lower the apparent threshold of the impaired ear. For more information on this technique, refer to Adams, Boies, and Hilger (1989).

INTERPRETATION

Air-conduction testing alone can approximate the degree of hearing loss, but the combination of air- and bone-conduction testing can be helpful in determining if the hearing loss is conductive, sensorineural, or both.

A threshold of up to 20 dB is considered normal, although subtle changes can be noted. Above that, hearing can be divided into degrees of hearing loss as follows: mild, 21 to 40 dB; moderate, 41 to 55 dB; moderately severe, 56 to 70 dB; severe, 71 to 90 dB; and profound, 91 dB or greater. Others have suggested slightly different ranges, but the degrees are quite similar. Further interpretation of results is beyond the scope of this text. Certain patterns of hearing loss, especially unilateral, can indicate disease.

CPT/BILLING CODES

92551	Screening test, pure-tone air only (An example of this is a single-decibel-level device with selected frequencies.)
92552	Pure-tone audiometry (threshold), air only
92553	Pure-tone audiometry, air and bone

BIBLIOGRAPHY

Adams GL, Boies LR Jr, Hilger PA: *Boies' fundamentals of otolaryngology,* Philadelphia, 1989, W.B. Saunders.

American Speech-Language-Hearing Association: Guidelines for audiometric symbols, *ASHA* 32(suppl 2):25, 1990.

Bluestone CD, Stool SE: *Pediatric otolaryngology,* Philadelphia, 1990, W.B. Saunders.

Bordley JE, Brookhouser PE, Tucker GF, Jr: *Ear, nose and throat disorders in children,* New York, 1986, Raven Press.

CHAPTER 29

Auricular Hematoma Evacuation

Gregory J. Forzley

An auricular hematoma can result from a direct or indirect blow to the external ear, such as commonly occurs in wrestling and boxing. Trauma may induce blood and serum to accumulate between the perichondrium and auricular cartilage, producing local pressure and interfering with the blood supply to the cartilage. Early treatment helps to prevent aseptic necrosis, loss of cartilage, and resultant distortion of the ear. With an auricular hematoma, there are also risks of secondary infection, perichondritis, and ultimately "cauliflower ear," which develops from fibrous organization of the clot. Primary care physicians, especially those involved in sports medicine, should be able to perform evacuations of auricular hematomas.

INDICATIONS

- Auricular hematoma
- A bluish, fluctulant swelling, usually involving the entire auricle

CONTRAINDICATIONS

- Hematoma accompanied by auricular laceration
- Injury beyond the abilities of the physician

EQUIPMENT

- Topical antiseptic, such as povidone-iodine (Betadine)
- For aspiration, 20-gauge needle and syringe
- Adhesive plastic ear drape or fenestrated drape
- Sterile gloves
- No. 15 scalpel blade and holder
- Curved hemostat
- Forceps

- 30-gauge needle and syringe
- Local anesthetic such as lidocaine 1% with 1:100,000 epinephrine
- Penrose drain or sterile rubber band and scissors
- Gauze dressing
- Petrolatum gauze or cotton balls soaked with petroleum jelly
- For alternate compression technique, add cotton dental roll or gauze, and silk or Vicryl suture (3-0) with needle and a needle holder
- Antibiotic ointment (Polysporin or Bactroban)
- Goggles

PREPROCEDURE PATIENT EDUCATION

Explain the indication for the procedure to the patient. Also explain the discomfort of injected local anesthetic and the necessity to remain immobile during the procedure. The patient should be prepared for mild discomfort.

TECHNIQUE

1. Position the patient comfortably in the supine position with the injured ear accessible.
2. Cleanse the helix with antiseptic solution.
3. Following universal blood and body fluid precautions for this portion as well as with the others, attempt aspiration of the hematoma (often successful by itself if the injury is quite recent).
4. If aspiration does not completely evacuate the hematoma, instill a small volume of local anesthetic anteriorly and posteriorly in the skin overlying the hematoma and into the hematoma itself. (The entire pinna can be anesthesized with several small injections into the soft tissue in the sulcus behind the ear. In this case, 1% lidocaine *without* epinephrine must be used.) See Chapter 23, Peripheral Nerve Blocks and Field Blocks.
5. While waiting for the anesthetic effect, drape the patient in order to keep hair away from the involved area.
6. With the No. 15 scalpel, make an incision over the hematoma, usually 4 mm to 5 mm in length. Multiple incisions may be needed.
7. Probe the cavity with the hemostat to ensure complete evacuation. Additional manipulation can be performed with digital pressure to assist in complete evacuation.
8. Insert a piece of the Penrose drain or rubber band through the incision.
9. Apply antibiotic ointment to the incision.
10. Fit the petroleum jelly-treated cotton externally to the contours of the ear. Apply a gauze compression dressing to the ear.
11. Prescribe prophylactic oral antibiotics and appropriate analgesia.
12. Instruct the patient to return in 48 hours for dressing removal and reevaluation. Redrain the ear or reapply the dressing as needed to maintain ear compression for 2 weeks.

ALTERNATIVE TECHNIQUE

Alternatively, a technique using cotton dental rolls for compression can be utilized. The technique is the same through Step 7.

8. Cut the dental roll to fit over most of the hematoma. The smaller remnant of cut roll will be stitched posteriorly.
9. After slightly straightening the suture needle, pass the needle through one end of the cut dental roll.
10. Pass the needle through the most cephalad end of the hematoma from anterior to posterior. With the intent to use the smaller remaining piece of dental roll as posterior compression, pass the needle back and forth through the smaller roll (Fig. 29-1).
11. Next, pass the needle through the inferior portion of the hematoma from posterior to anterior and then through the other end of the anterior dental roll.
12. Tie the suture, creating front and back compression of the hematoma.
13. Liberally apply antibacterial ointment over the dental rolls and the ear. Oral antibiotics are given.
14. Apply a gauze dressing.
15. Ask the patient to return in 24 hours, at which time the gauze dressing is removed. Instruct the patient to continue applying antibacterial ointment until the dental roll dressing is removed in 2 weeks.

POSTPROCEDURE PATIENT EDUCATION

Stress the importance of maintaining the compression for two weeks. The patient should understand the risk of complications, regardless of management, and should see a physician when there are signs of infection.

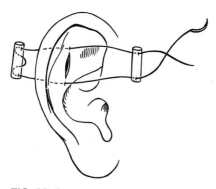

FIG. 29-1.
Alternative technique using cotton dental rolls for compression.

COMPLICATIONS

- Scar at the site of the incision
- Perichondritis (risk minimized by prophylactic oral antibiotics)
- Auricular deformity in spite of appropriate treatment, or if treatment of the hematoma is inadequate

CPT/BILLING CODES

69000   Simple auricular hematoma evacuation
69005   Complicated auricular hematoma evacuation

BIBLIOGRAPHY

Glasscock ME III, Shambaugh GE, Jr: *Surgery of the ear,* Philadelphia, 1990, W.B. Saunders.

Paparella MM, Shumrick DA: *Otolaryngology, vol 2, the ear,* Philadelphia, 1980, W.B. Saunders.

Schuller DE, Dankle SD, Strauss RH: A technique to treat wrestlers' auricular hematoma without interrupting training or competition, *Arc Otolaryngol Head Neck Surg* 115(2): 202, 1989.

CHAPTER 30

Myringotomy

Gregory J. Forzley

A myringotomy is an incision of the tympanic membrane that is made to allow ventilation of the middle ear, to permit drainage of middle ear fluid, or to obtain cultures from an infected middle ear. Generally, in children, it is an outpatient procedure performed under general anesthesia, in conjunction with tympanostomy tube placement. In a cooperative older child or adult, or in an infant who is appropriately restrained, it is possible to perform the procedure with local anesthesia. The procedure is often reserved for the otolaryngologist, but it may be appropriate for the experienced surgeon or primary care physician to perform myringotomy or diagnostic tympanocentesis in certain situations.

INDICATIONS

- Necessity of alleviation of conductive hearing loss from chronic middle ear effusion
- Necessity of immediate relief of pain and pressure from middle ear effusion or otitis media (Relief may be temporary unless a tympanostomy tube is placed.)
- To obtain a culture of the middle ear fluid (This may be warranted in situations, such as otitis media that has failed to respond to appropriate antimicrobial therapy; in complications such as mastoiditis, meningitis, paralysis of the facial nerve or others; or in otitis media in an immunocompromised patient, including neonates.)

CONTRAINDICATIONS

- Known anomolous positioning of the jugular bulb
- Uncooperative patient
- Permanent hearing loss in the opposite ear (In this situation, the procedure should be performed by an otolaryngologist if possible.)

- Acute external otitis
- An effusion associated with rheumatoid arthritis, although this is not clear in the current literature (*possible contraindication*)

EQUIPMENT

- Myringotomy knife (For tympanocentesis, a 20-gauge, short-beveled or spinal needle along with a collection device)
- Phenol solution; or, if preferred, 1% lidocaine with a 27-gauge needle and syringe
- Light source with magnification, such as an otoscope with an operating head, or an operating microscope and ear speculum (A head mirror can be used, but magnification is advantageous.)
- Small sterile ear forceps or bayonet forceps
- Sterile, small cotton-tipped applicator
- *Optional:* Baron suction tube (3 or 5 Fr.) with finger cut-off, if middle ear suctioning is desired
- Goggles

PREPROCEDURE PATIENT EDUCATION

As in all surgical cases, explain the indications for the procedure, the possible complications, and the general process of the procedure to the patient. Obtain signed informed consent and document it in the chart.

TECHNIQUE

1. Position the patient comfortably, either in the sitting position or supine with the head turned to one side. For the young infant, mild sedation, a restraining board, and an able assistant would be helpful. See Chapter 24, Pediatric Sedation. Universal blood and body fluid precautions should be observed.
2. Using the operating otoscope (or ear speculum and operating microscope), gently clean the ear canal of obstructing debris.
3. Using a small cotton-tipped applicator, carefully apply phenol to the exact location on the tympanic membrane for tympanocentesis or myringotomy. (Avoid contact of phenol with other tissue.) In most instances, the location is below an imaginary horizontal line through the inferior tip of the manubrium (Fig. 30-1), but often it is in the anterior or posterior inferior quadrant. Alternatively, although technically more difficult, anesthesia may be obtained by injecting the cartilaginous external auditory canal with the 27-gauge needle and 1% lidocaine at three to four points around the canal. The anesthetic is allowed to dissect down, blanching the ear canal and drum during the injection (see anesthesia for auditory canal in Chapter 34, Removal of Foreign Bodies from the Ear and Nose).

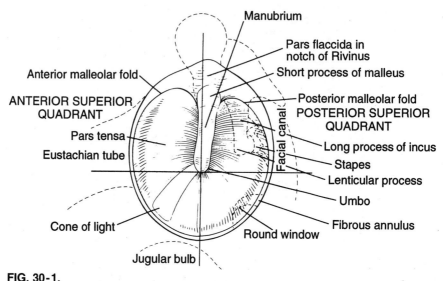

FIG. 30-1.
Anatomy of the middle ear. (From Miglets AW, Paparella MM, Saunders WH: *Atlas of ear surgery,* ed 4, St Louis, 1986, Mosby. Used with permission.)

4. Using the sharp myringotomy knife or tympanocentesis needle, incise the eardrum through the white spot produced by the phenol to a depth of no more than 2 mm (Fig. 30-2). A small opening is generally sufficient for thin mucoid or serous material, but a larger circumlinear incision may be necessary for suctioning purulent fluid or when an opening is needed for a longer time.

POSTPROCEDURE PATIENT EDUCATION

- Inform the patient not to allow water in the external auditory canal until the incision is closed (generally 2 to 4 weeks) and the patient is reevaluated.
- Instruct the patient to contact a physician if the ear canal becomes inflamed or painful, or if drainage persists.

COMPLICATIONS

- Chronic perforation of the tympanic membrane
- Pain and bleeding due to injury of the mucosal covering of the medial wall of the middle ear (promontory) as a result of an incision greater than 2 mm in depth
- Injury to a high-lying jugular bulb, dislocation of the incudostapedial joint, or injury to the facial nerve (rare)
- Atrophic scar at the site of the incision
- Possible permanent damage to or loss of hearing (rare)

A   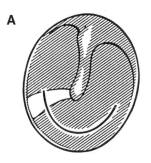   B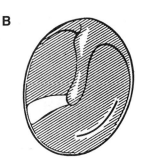

FIG. 30-2.
Myringotomy incisions. **A,** Wide incision through the drumhead might be used in a patient with refractory purulent otitis media or in which prolonged drainage of pus is necessary. **B,** A more limited incision is used for the same purpose or for inspection of the middle ear. (From Miglets AW, Paparella MM, Saunders WH: *Atlas of ear surgery,* ed 4, St Louis, 1986, Mosby. Used with permission.)

CPT/BILLING CODE

69420   Myringotomy or tympanocentesis

BIBLIOGRAPHY

Adams GL, Boies L, Jr, Hilger PA: *Boies' fundamentals of otolaryngology,* Philadelphia, 1989, W.B. Saunders.

Bluestone CD, Stool SE: *Pediatric otolaryngology,* ed 2, vol 1, Philadelphia, 1990, W.B. Saunders.

DeWeese DD et al: *Otorhinolaryngology: head and neck surgery,* St Louis, 1988, Mosby.

Miglets AW, Paparella MM, Saunders WH: *Atlas of ear surgery,* St Louis, 1986, Mosby.

CHAPTER 31

Cerumen Impaction Removal

Gregory J. Forzley

Gary R. Newkirk

Cerumen is a naturally occurring lubricant and protectant of the external auditory canal. The predominate form is a wet, sticky, honey-colored wax that can darken, but a dry scaly form occurs in some patients. Accumulation of cerumen can result in hearing loss, tinnitus, a pressure sensation, vertigo, and infection. Patients often do a poor job of removing cerumen with cotton-tipped sticks or over-the-counter preparations, leaving the physician to complete the procedure. Occasionally, anesthesia may be desired or foreign bodies must be removed as well (see Chapter 34, Removal of Foreign Bodies from the Ear and Nose). Removal of cerumen under direct visualization or by irrigation, without contributing to injury, remains the overall goal.

INDICATIONS

- Obscured visualization of the eardrum
- Patient complaint of decreased hearing on the affected side
- Patient complaint of otalgia on the affected side
- External otitis associated with cerumen

CONTRAINDICATIONS

- Uncooperative patient or infant who cannot be adequately restrained
- Operator lacks familiarity with the anatomy of the external auditory canal
- Patient with distorted anatomy (i.e., foreign body obstruction or injury obscuring normal anatomy)
- Previous ear surgery with resultant scarring and increased risk of perforation
- Known or suspected cholesteatoma
- The affected ear is the only hearing ear (Referral should be considered.)
- For irrigation, known or suspected perforation of the tympanic membrane

EQUIPMENT

- Ear curette
    Metal: *rigid,* Buck, Shapleigh, or Yankauer; *flexible,* Billeau flexible ear-loop
    Plastic: Flex-loop ear curette or infant ear scoop, both produced by Bionix Corporation, 757 Warehouse Rd, Toledo, OH 43615
- Ear syringe (large stainless steel syringe with irrigant deflector), **or** a commercially available oral jet irrigator (on "ENT table units," or a Water-Pik), **or** a 22-gauge butterfly intravenous catheter tubing (with needle and butterfly removed) and a 20 to 50 cc syringe
- Operating-head otoscope, or ear speculum and light source
- Towels or plastic drape
- Ear forceps
- Cotton strip
- *Optional:* various auditory suction catheters with suction source (Fig. 31-1)
- Emesis or ear basin to collect irrigant
- Cerumen softening agent such as mineral oil, triethanolamine (Cerumenex), carbamide peroxide (Debrox) or cresyl acetate (Cresylate)

PREPROCEDURE PATIENT EDUCATION

- For curette removal, discuss the chance of perforation and minor trauma to the ear canal associated with pain.
- For irrigation removal, discuss the risk of perforation and potential dizziness with the irrigation. Local discomfort may also be experienced, especially when the ear syringe is used.
- Stress the necessity of immobilization during the procedure.

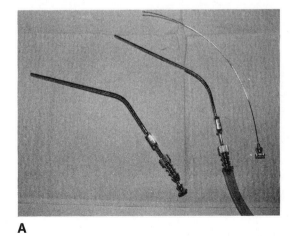
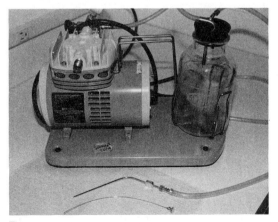

A   **B**

FIG. 31-1.
Suction catheters (**A**) and basic suction pump (**B**) can assist in managing ear canal obstruction.

TECHNIQUE

Curette Technique

This technique may be preferred for small amounts of easily visible and reachable wax. Irrigation will be required for dense or circumferential impactions.

1. Seat the patient on the examination table. Children often tolerate the procedure better supine with the parent or assistant stabilizing the head.
2. With the operating otoscope, visualize the cerumen in the canal using posterior traction on the helix as necessary.
3. Using the selected curette, gently remove the impacted cerumen, taking care to avoid trauma to the bony ear canal. Either work through the scope (Fig. 31-2, *A*), or, after identifying where the cerumen is, by direct vision (Fig. 31-2, *B*).
4. If hard wax is encountered, installation of mineral oil, 3% hydrogen peroxide or a commercially available preparation, such as Cerumenex or Debrox, for 5 to 10 minutes may facilitate removal. Cresylate may dissolve wax the fastest. For wax adherent to the tympanic membrane, irrigation or suction may be necessary.
5. Consider prescribing topical otic antibiotics if epithelium was disrupted.

Irrigation Technique (Figs. 31-3 and 31-4)

This technique takes longer than the curette technique and is often utilized when the curette technique has failed or caused pain. In only rare cases does it fail.

1. Fill the irrigator (syringe) with *body-temperature* tap water. This reduces the chance for stimulation of the vestibular reflex, causing nystagmus and nausea.
2. If the jet irrigator is used, adjust the pressure to the *lowest* setting to reduce the risk of perforation or acoustic trauma.

A

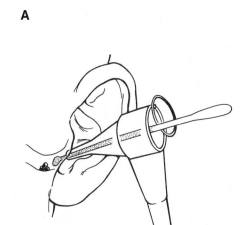

B

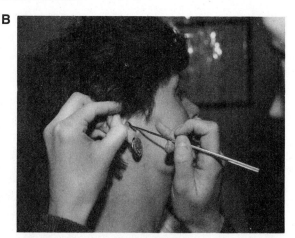

FIG. 31-2.
Often, foreign bodies or cerumen in the ear canal can be removed under direct vision once careful, magnified otoscopic examination is completed. Notice how the patient's head is supported and the physician's hand rests on the face.

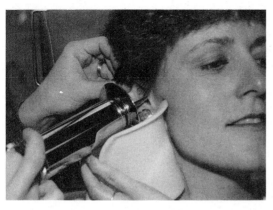

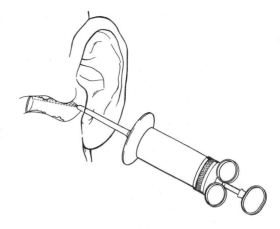

FIG. 31-3.
Typical commercial ear canal irrigation setup. The water should be at body temperature. The initial stream should be directed toward the superior canal. Patients often feel reassured when allowed to help hold the basin. Cover the upper torso with a splash bib.

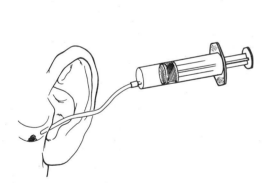

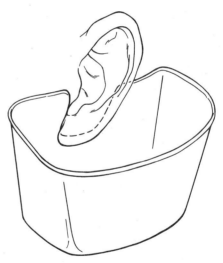

FIG. 31-4.
Alternative irrigation setup. Butterfly tubing with needle and butterfly removed.

FIG. 31-5.
Basin cup that fits under ear.

3. Protect the patient with a towel or plastic sheet to collect excess water.
4. Have the patient tilt the head to the side being irrigated while holding the ear basin (Fig. 31-5) below the earlobe.
5. Using the selected device, direct the water jet superiorly toward the occiput, allowing space for the return of the water and cerumen. The irrigation should *not* be directed onto the tympanic membrane. Fairly vigorous force is needed with the syringe techniques. Using large (25 to 50 cc) syringes will prevent excessive pressure.

6. Often the cerumen will wash out in one or two large pieces in a few seconds, at which point the canal is reexamined. If the canal is clear, stop the irrigation and dry the canal by inserting and removing a small length of cotton gauze.
7. Occasionally, the impacted cerumen will need to be prodded with an ear curette. If irrigation is still unsuccessful after a few moments, terminate the procedure and send the patient home to use a liquid ear wax softener and return in a few days for a repeat irrigation.
8. Consider prescribing topical otic antibiotics if the epithelium was disrupted to prophylax against external otitis.

POSTPROCEDURE PATIENT EDUCATION

- Instruct the patient to contact the physician's office if decreased hearing, vertigo, purulent drainage, or pain develop in the irrigated ear.
- Unless contraindicated, inform the patient to perform periodic ear cleansing using commercially available ear wax softeners, or mineral oil, and a squeeze bulb syringe. Otherwise, advise the patient to avoid self-instrumentation of the ear canal with cotton-tipped applicators.

COMPLICATIONS

- Tympanic membrane perforation and damage to ossicles with theoretical decreased or loss of hearing
- Otitis externa
- Vertigo, nausea and vomiting, or both
- Minor canal wall abrasions—some bleeding may occur if hard wax is adherent to the epithelium and causes desquamation with removal (If noted, antibiotic otic drops should be used for a few days.)
- Tinnitus

CPT/BILLING CODE

69210   Removal impacted cerumen (separate procedure), one or both ears

BIBLIOGRAPHY

Adams GL, Boies LR, Jr, Hilger PA: *Boies' fundamentals of otolaryngology,* Philadelphia, 1989, W.B. Saunders.
Dinsdale RC et al: Catastrophic otologic injury from oral jet irrigation of the external auditory canal, *Laryngoscopy* 101:75, January 1991.
Larsen G: Removing cerumen with a water pick, *Am J Nurs* 70:264, February 1976.

CHAPTER 32

Tympanometry

Gregory J. Forzley

Several methods are used to measure parameters of the middle ear and eardrum in an effort to determine whether there are dysfunctions that could ultimately affect the hearing ability of the patient or put him or her at risk for repeated infections. These modalities include pneumatic otoscopy, tympanometry, static immittance, and acoustic reflectometry. Tympanometry, routinely performed since the 1970s, is regarded as an objective technique for obtaining reproducible measurements of the compliance or mobility of the tympanic membrane and the pressure within the middle-ear system. These measurements aid in assessing eustachian tube function and in determining the continuity and mobility of the ossicular chain, even in a fairly uncooperative child.

The goal of tympanometry is the evaluation of the *immittance* of the tympanic membrane, which reflects the performance of the middle-ear transmission system. Immittance is the transfer of acoustic energy and is measured as the acoustic *admittance* (flow of energy into the middle-ear system), or as the reciprocal of the acoustic admittance—the acoustic *impedance* (opposition to the flow of energy into the middle ear).

A tympanometer contains an electroacoustic impedance bridge as a vital part of its instrumentation (Fig. 32-1). In addition, a small probe with three small openings is inserted into the patient's ear canal. One allows a controlled tone (220 Hz) to be delivered to the ear by a transducer. The second allows the microphone to measure the probe tone in the canal as the pressure varies. The third allows an air pump to vary the air pressure in the canal to create positive, negative, or atmospheric air pressure in the space between the probe tip and the tympanic membrane (Fig. 32-2). Measured parameters include compliance of the tympanic membrane and change in impedance as canal pressure varies. Devices that measure the acoustic admittance rather than the impedance obtain similar results but add the *tympanometric gradient* (curve width).

INDICATIONS

- To verify middle-ear abnormalities suspected by clinical otoscopy
- To check eustachian tube patency even when the tympanic membrane appears normal
- To evaluate hearing loss or ear pain, especially in the young

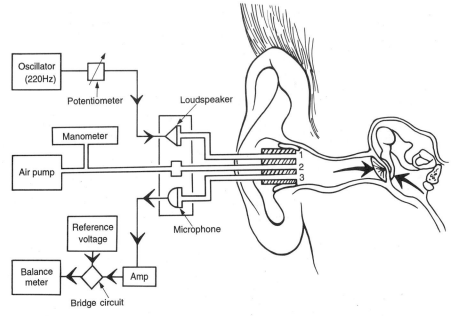

FIG. 32-1.
Electroacoustic impedance bridge. (Redrawn from Bordley J, Brookhauser P, Tucker G: *Ear, nose and throat disorders in children,* New York, 1986, Raven Press. Used with permission.)

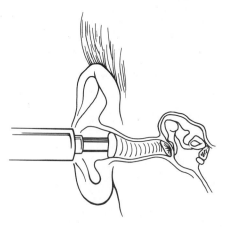

FIG. 32-2.
Tympanometric examination is performed with a probe inserted into the external ear canal. A 220-Hz tone is transmitted through the probe. Movement of the tympanic membrane in response to the tone is measured while the air pressure in the external canal is varied. The pressure at which peak movement (compliance) occurs is recorded.

- To detect tympanic membrane perforations
- To evaluate patency of pressure-equalization (PE) tubes
- To assist in evaluation of suspected fixation of the ossicular chain
- To help assess middle-ear function in a young child who cannot cooperate with audiometry
- To document or follow persistent middle-ear effusions

CONTRAINDICATIONS

- An ear canal totally occluded by cerumen
- Fulminant external otitis
- Age less than 7 months (because of the possibility of excessive canal-wall compliance, results may yield a misleading Type A or C curve)

EQUIPMENT AND SUPPLIERS

Tympanometry equipment is quite varied in size and features available. Some features to consider include the following:

- A 220-Hz probe tone is preferred; most supply 226-Hz probe tones.
- An air pressure range of −400 to +100 mm H_2O is preferable, however a range of −300 to +100 is acceptable. It should be noted that many instruments measure air pressure in decaPascals (daPa): 1.02 mm H_2O = 1.0 daPa.
- Results should be automatically obtained and easy to read.
- Results should be easily printable if desired.

Tympanometer manufacturers include the following:

Grason-Stadler, Inc.
537 Great Road, P.O. Box 1400
Littleton, MA 01460

Maico Hearing Instruments, Inc.
7375 Bush Lake Road
Minneapolis, MN 55435

American Electromedics Corporation
13 Sagamore Park Road
Hudson, NH 03051

Micro Audiometrics
3749-B, South Nova Road
Port Orange, FL 32019

Welch Allyn, Inc.
4341 State Street Road, P.O. Box 220
Skaneateles Falls, NY 13153-0220

PREPROCEDURE PATIENT EDUCATION

Explain the indications for the procedure and the necessity for the patient to remain immobile for a brief period after a seal has been obtained while taking measurements. Reassure the patient that this is a painless procedure.

TECHNIQUE

1. Check the ear canal for at least partial patency.
2. Have the patient sit, either independently or, in the case of a young child, in the parent's lap.
3. In the older child and adult, apply gentle traction to the helix in the posterior upward direction to straighten the auditory canal. In young children, posterior downward traction on the inferior helix is needed to straighten the canal.
4. Select the appropriate size of soft probe tip to occlude the ear canal adequately without entering it deeply.
5. Once a seal has been obtained, the tympanometer will automatically deliver the sound and air pressures and record the various parameters: the tympanic membrane compliance, the canal volume, and, in instruments so equipped, the acoustic reflex.

INTERPRETATION

The resultant tympanogram is a graph of the compliance of the middle-ear system on the vertical axis and the changes in ear pressure in the ear canal (in mm H_2O or daPa) on the horizontal axis. The graph may vary with the instrument, but the classically described types of tympanogram results are shown in Fig. 32-3. Since the maximum tympanic membrane compliance occurs when air pressure is equal on

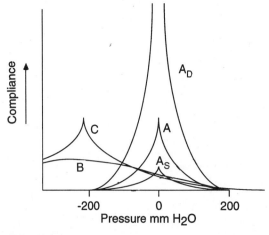

FIG. 32-3.
Tympanogram results. See text for details.

both sides of it, the peak of the normal tympanogram tracing (Type A in the figure) occurs at approximately 0 mm H_2O. With a shorter peak, but with maximum compliance still occurring at or near zero, the Type A_S indicates conditions such as ossicular fixation or stiffening, thickening of the tympanic membrane, or middle-ear effusion. The Type A_D tympanogram has a very high peak that exceeds the compliance scale and is obtained when there is ossicular disruption, a flaccid tympanic membrane, or a monomeric tympanic membrane (a single layer of membrane covering an old eardrum perforation). If the tympanogram is flat with no distinct peak, it represents Type B, and is typically considered to represent the presence of middle-ear fluid. Other conditions associated with a Type B tympanogram include cerumen impaction, perforation of the tympanic membrane, stenosis of the ear canal, a thickened eardrum, or an open functioning PE tube, but these can often be differentiated based on measuring the canal volume. Normal canal volume is 0.2 to 2.0 ml but varies widely according to the patient's age and bone structure. An excessive volume may indicate perforation or functioning PE tube, while decreased volume indicates obstruction or debris, such as cerumen. A Type C tympanogram is indicative of maximum compliance occurring with a negative pressure of more than -100 mm H_2O, and is associated with eustachian tube dysfunction with or without accompanying middle-ear fluid. Negative middle-ear pressures are generally considered clinically significant if they exceed -180 to -200 mm H_2O.

One precaution to be emphasized in interpreting tympanogram results is that a localized abnormality of the tympanic membrane can obscure measurements of the rest of the middle-ear system. For those devices equipped to measure auditory reflex, it may be useful for screening large populations, but has limited value in individual patients.

POSTPROCEDURE PATIENT EDUCATION

Discuss the management that the patient should follow and the possible need for further evaluation.

CPT/BILLING CODES

92567   Tympanometry (impedance testing)
92568   Tympanometry with acoustic reflex

BIBLIOGRAPHY

Adams GL, Boies LR, Hilger PA: *Boies' fundamentals of otolaryngology*, Philadelphia, 1989, W.B. Saunders.
Bluestone CD, Stool SD: *Pediatric otolaryngology*, Philadelphia, 1990, W.B. Saunders.
Bordley JE, Brookhouser PE, Tucker GF: *Ear, nose and throat disorders in children*, New York, 1986, Raven Press.
Bredfeldt RC: An introduction to tympanometry, *Am Fam Physician* 44:2113, 1991.
Holte L, Cavanaugh RM, Margolis RH: Ear canal wall mobility and tympanometric shape in young infants, *J Pediatr* 117(1):27, 1990.

CHAPTER 33

Ear Piercing

Gregory J. Forzley

Ear piercing is a procedure that the primary care physician may be asked to perform periodically. The mother of a young child may wish to maintain longitudinal, comprehensive care, and trusts the physician's ability to handle a particular child. Or a patient may trust that physicians use a more aseptic approach and have more knowledge of potential problems than others who pierce ears. At the very least, it is a procedure with which the primary care physician should have some familiarity.

INDICATIONS

- Either the patient or parent requests ear piercing

CONTRAINDICATIONS

- Local skin infection, severe eczema, a cyst, or any other significant skin disorder
- History of keloid formation
- Immunodeficiency
- Coagulation disorder

EQUIPMENT

- Commercial ear-piercing kit including gun, needles, and backing. Some models available include: Coren-PS disposable ear piercer (distributed by NEMSCO, Norwell, MA 02061); Debut Prestige ear-piercing kit (distributed by H & A Enterprises, Inc., 143-19 25th Ave, Box 489, Whitestone, NY 11357); and Grafco-Standard ear piercer (distributed by Goodrich-Universal, Inc., 500 Robert St., St. Paul, MN 55101)

- Surgical skin-marking pencil
- Cold-sterilizer basin and solution, such as cetyldimethylethylammonium bromide (Cetylcide)
- Sterile forceps
- Povidone-iodine (Betadine) wash or 70% isopropyl alcohol
- *Optional:* ice cubes for topical anesthesia

PREPROCEDURE PATIENT EDUCATION

Inform the patient or parent of the possible complications. The patient should also be informed that, in most cases, only mild discomfort will be felt.

TECHNIQUE

1. Cold-sterilize the gun, piercing needles, and backings for 20 minutes.
2. Have the patient or family member mark the anterior surface of the earlobe with the skin-marking pencil at the exact location desired for the earrings. It is recommended that the auricular cartilage be avoided to reduce the risk of complications.
3. Using the sterile forceps and sterile technique, load the ear piercer (proximally with the first needle, and distally with the backing in the stop plate of the piercing gun).
4. Generally, no anesthesia is required. If the patient desires some surface anesthesia, the earlobe may be held between two ice cubes for a minute or two, or the earlobe may be squeezed between the physician's thumb and index finger for 30 seconds.
5. Cleanse the earlobe with topical antiseptic, then pierce the earlobe at the marked site from anterior to posterior using the spring-loaded ear-piercer (Fig. 33-1). Follow universal blood and body fluid precautions.
6. If necessary, attach the backing more firmly to the piercing needle. Repeat the process for the other ear.

ALTERNATIVE TECHNIQUE

1. Using the patient's own earrings requires a modified technique. In place of the ear-piercing kit, the necessary equipment includes two 21-gauge and two 18-gauge, 1.5-inch needles (one of each for each ear), **or** two 20-gauge angiocaths and a pair of scissors. The patient's earrings (preferably 14-karat gold or stainless-steel posts to minimize the risk of contact dermatitis and infection) are used.
2. After following Steps 1, 2, and 4 (above), cleanse the earlobe with topical antiseptic, then pierce the earlobe from anterior to posterior at the marked site with either the 21-gauge needle or 20-gauge angiocath. Follow universal blood and body fluid precautions.

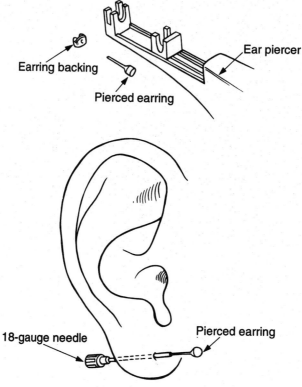

FIG. 33-1.
Ear-piercing technique.

3. If the needles are used, insert the 21-gauge needle from anterior to posterior at the marked site. This serves as a guide. The 18-gauge needle is then applied over the 21-gauge needle and inserted through the ear from posterior to anterior. Remove the 21-gauge needle from the lumen of the 18-gauge, and in its place, insert the earring post. Then withdraw the 18-gauge needle through the earlobe, pulling the earring post with it. Remove the 18-gauge needle and apply the backing to anchor the earring in place.
4. If the angiocath is used, insert it going anterior to posterior. Remove the needle introducer leaving the plastic cannula in the earlobe, and cut off the hub. Place the earring into the cut end of the cannula using the forceps. Then pull the cannula through the back of the earlobe, and discard it. Apply the backing to anchor the earring in place.
5. Repeat the procedure for the other ear, using the same technique.

POSTPROCEDURE PATIENT EDUCATION

Instruct the patient to do the following:

- Cleanse the earring post and backing daily with a cotton swab and 70% iso-propyl alcohol.
- Rotate the earring several times daily (to help prevent it from becoming embedded).
- Avoid exposure to strong soaps, hair spray, or cosmetics.
- Check the earlobe daily for redness or other signs of infection. If any is noted, apply moist, warm compresses to the lobe 4 times daily. If the problem has not cleared after 24 hours, call for further instructions.
- Leave the earring in place for six weeks, at which time it may be removed and another inserted. Again, stainless-steel or 14-karat gold posts minimize the chance of a local skin reaction.

COMPLICATIONS

- Local infection or sepsis
- Keloid formation
- Granuloma or cyst formation
- Bifid earlobe deformity if earring pulls through skin
- Auricular hematoma
- Nickel dermatitis
- Embedded earring stud or backing

CPT/BILLING CODE

69090   Ear piercing

BIBLIOGRAPHY

Driscoll CE: Procedures for your practice: ear piercing, *Patient Care:*194, August 1990.
Muntz HR et al: Embedded earrings: a complication of the ear-piercing gun, *Int J Pediatr Otorhinolaryngol* 19:73, 1990.
Zachowski DA: An IV cannula stent for ear piercing, *Plast Reconstr Surg* 80(5):751, 1987.

CHAPTER 34

Removal of Foreign Bodies from the Ear and Nose

John Harlan Haynes III

Gary R. Newkirk

The external auditory canal and nasal orifices occasionally collect small objects, such as beads, insects, peanuts, or beans. Foreign bodies in this area are especially common in pediatric patients and mentally impaired individuals. Simple attempts at removal should be pursued before instrumentation. In the external ear canal, pulsating irrigation through an 18-gauge catheter with saline directed posteriorly may dislodge the impacted object. In the nose, after using vasoconstrictive nasal solution (e.g., Neo-Synephrine) to reduce mucosal edema, have the patient blow forcefully. This may cause the object to dislodge. With infants, one may try briskly forcing air through the oropharynx (as in mouth-to-mouth resuscitation). Flushing or manual removal of the object is necessary if these methods are unsuccessful.

In determining whether to remove an object manually or by more aggressive flushing, one must consider several factors. If tympanic membrane perforation is suspected, irrigation is contraindicated. Knowledge of the type of the foreign body and how long it has been lodged in the orifice is very helpful. Some objects, such as plant materials, beans, or other seeds, can swell if left in place more than several hours or if saline is used to flush them out. When accompanied by a local response to the irritation, they may become further lodged in place as the canal swells and reactive debris accumulates. Manual removal or suction may be required to remove these objects. When the nasal passage is completely occluded by an expanding foreign body and is surrounded by marked edema and inflammation, local or general anesthesia may be necessary, along with a referral to an ear, nose, and throat specialist. The ultimate goal when removing a foreign body is to avoid pushing it further toward the tympanic membrane, middle ear, or posterior nasal passage. Attempts should be made to remove foreign bodies under direct visualization, if at all possible.

INDICATIONS

- Known foreign body

Note: A general rule of thumb for the ear is that if the object is in the outer two thirds of the canal and is easily accessible, it can generally be removed.

CONTRAINDICATIONS

- Lack of knowledge of normal anatomy of external ear canal or nasal passage
- Trauma-induced obscuration of the normal anatomy of the external ear canal or nasal passage
- An uncooperative patient who cannot be sedated (see Chapter 24, Pediatric Sedation)
- For the ear, see Chapter 31, Cerumen Impaction Removal

EQUIPMENT

- Traditional foreign-body extraction tools such as suction tips, alligator forceps, ear curettes, or wire loop curettes (Fig. 34-1)
- Ear speculum or nasal speculum (Select the largest that will fit the canal or nasal orifice.)
- Bright light that can be directed or focused
- Topical anesthetic (see Chapter 22, Topical Anesthesia)
- Irrigant such as saline
- For ear, irrigation materials as noted in Chapter 31, Cerumen Impaction Removal

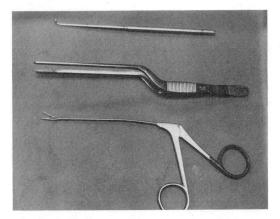

FIG. 34-1.
Traditional instruments used for foreign-body extraction. *From top to bottom:* ear curette, nasal forceps, and alligator forceps.

PREPROCEDURE PATIENT EDUCATION

- For curette removal, discuss the chance of perforation and minor trauma, which may be associated with pain.
- For irrigation, discuss risk of perforation, dizziness (for ear canal irrigation), and local discomfort.
- Stress the importance of remaining immobile during the procedure.

TECHNIQUE

1. Instill a topical anesthetic. After several minutes, suction pus, topical anesthetics, or blood as necessary to visualize the object. Small children may need to

A

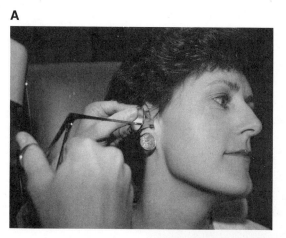

B

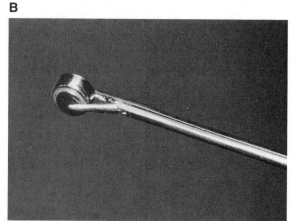

C

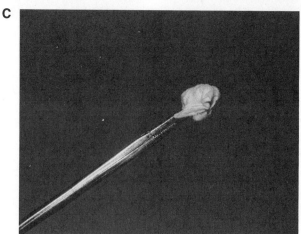

FIG. 34-2.
Alligator forceps (**A**) for retrieving small batteries (**B**) and paper balls (**C**) from auditory canal.

be sedated. (See Chapter 24, Pediatric Sedation.) With adults, visualization of the external ear is aided by pulling the auricle upward and backward to straighten the canal. In small children, the auricle is pulled downward. Extending the head and applying pressure on the nose in a superior and posterior direction helps to visualize the nasal canal.

2. The depth and surface qualities of the object to be removed often suggest the best tool. Grasp fibrous objects (cotton, plant matter) with the alligator forceps (Fig 34-2). Smooth objects, such as beans, seeds, or popcorn kernels, that are not completely blocking the canal might be dragged out by passing a wire loop beyond the object and gently withdrawing. Smooth, hard items, such as small batteries and BBs, may be teased out with a fine, 1 mm right-angle hook (Fig. 34-3). Occasionally, iron-containing items such as a BB can be removed with a small magnet probe fashioned from a nail that has been blunted. Such a nail can be magnetized by drawing across any strong permanent magnet, such as those available in hardware stores or found in the rear of stereo speaker cones.

   Note: Removal of small batteries, such as those for hearing aids, is a high priority because permanent damage to the ear can result if they are allowed to remain for more than a short time.

3. Irrigation may be useful in certain instances, such as when small fragments or debris remains.

4. Insects in the auditory canal should be drowned or smothered by instilling oil, lidocaine, or benzocaine solutions. Use alligator forceps to grasp and remove the insect.

5. In all cases, instruments introduced into the auditory canal or nasal passage require a steady hand resting on the patient's head in case of sudden movements, which can be involuntary if pain is elicited.

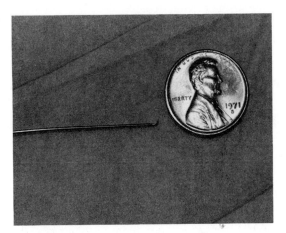

FIG. 34-3.
A precise right-angle hook made from bending a 1.5-inch, 21-gauge needle tip at a right angle is an excellent tool for removing smooth objects, such as beans and corn kernels.

6. Light, general (such as intramuscular or intravenous) anesthesia is mandatory to remove foreign bodies in individuals who cannot tolerate instrumentation with or without local agents.

ALTERNATIVE TECHNIQUE

This technique is a safe, reliable, and nontraumatic method of removing spherical foreign bodies from the ear and nasal cavity.

Equipment

- 30-inch plastic intravenous extension tubing or 10 Fr. suction catheter
- Heat source (burner, alcohol lamp, or lighter)
- Blunt end of metal ear curette handle or atomizer tip
- Wall or portable suction unit
- Hemostat

Technique

1. Cut off the tip of the tubing or suction catheter (Fig. 34-4, *A*). Heat the end of the curette handle or metal atomizer tip (Fig. 34-4, *B*). Flange the cut tube end with the preheated handle or tip so that it molds to the blunt rounded metal (Fig. 34-4, *C* and *D*).
2. Clamp the tubing and attach the opposite end to the suction unit.
3. Gently insert the flanged end into the orifice containing the foreign body under direct visualization and advance it to the object (Fig. 34-4, *E*).
4. When the flange is in contact with the object, quickly unclamp the suction catheter tubing (Fig. 34-4, *F*) and apply full suction immediately through the suction cup onto the foreign object.
5. While continuing suction, gently extract the tubing and suction-attached foreign body (Fig. 34-4, *G*).

ANESTHESIA FOR AUDITORY CANAL FOREIGN-BODY REMOVAL

- For local anesthesia, instill 5 drops of sterile 4% lidocaine or 20% benzocaine into the canal and allow it to remain for 10 minutes. Suction to remove fluid and canal debris before injecting local anesthetic (if needed) under direct visualization. If tympanic membrane rupture is suspected, ear drops and irrigation are contraindicated.
- For anesthesia of the external half of the auditory canal, inject small amounts (usually less than 2 cc) of 1% lidocaine with epinephrine at three or four sites equally spaced along the exterior verge of the canal. For deeper canal anesthesia (much more sensitive area), subcutaneous injections (0.5 to 1 cc total) of plain 1% lidocaine within the canal just external to the junction of the cartilaginous and bony canal (approximately half way into the canal) are useful.

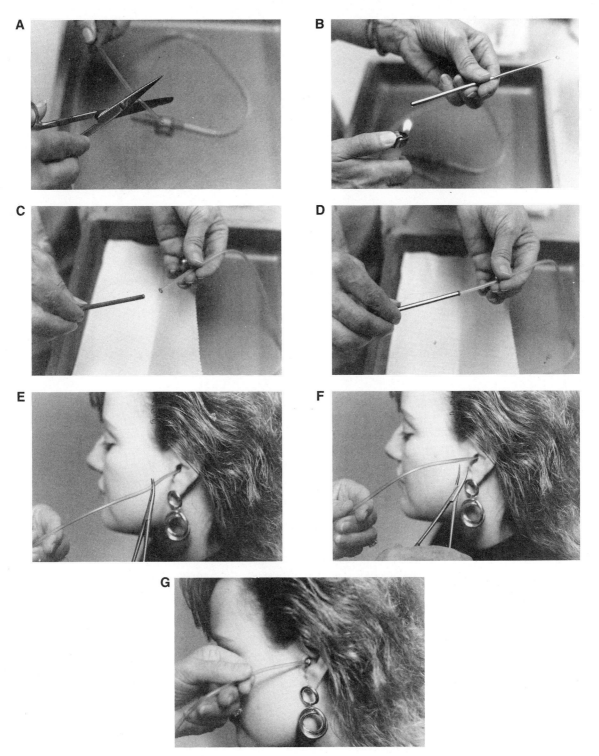

FIG. 34-4.
Technique for removing spherical foreign bodies from the ear. See text for details.

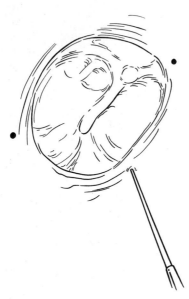

FIG. 34-5.
Local anesthetic block of the ear canal.

Beginning at the posterior and superior aspect of the canal, use a 27-gauge 1.5-inch needle to slowly infiltrate lidocaine (Fig. 34-5). Repeat this at two or three spots equally spaced around the canal. Allow the lidocaine to dissect down, "blanching" the ear canal and drum, if visible, during the injection. Topical lidocaine or benzocaine applied to the auditory canal before injections is often useful. Allow 5 to 10 minutes to elapse before resuming instrumentation.

POSTPROCEDURE PATIENT EDUCATION

Inform the patient to watch for signs of infection (see Chapter 31, Cerumen Impaction Removal). The patient should follow up with the physician in one to two days. Following removal of nasal foreign bodies, the patient should use saline irrigations 2 to 3 times a day for 2 or 3 days.

COMPLICATIONS

- Trauma to mucous membranes with the possibility of trauma-related infection or bleeding
- Injury to the canal, tympanic membrane, middle ear, or nasal passages
- Deeper progression of the object, resulting in inability to extract
- With foreign bodies of the ear, acute otitis externa is common and may result from injury caused by the foreign body itself or injury caused by its removal
- With the ear, the patient may experience nausea or vomiting (or both)

CPT/BILLING CODES

30300	Removal intranasal foreign body; without general anesthesia
30305	Removal intranasal foreign body; with general anesthesia
69200	Removal foreign body from external auditory canal; without general anesthesia
69205	Removal foreign body from external auditory canal; with general anesthesia

BIBLIOGRAPHY

D'Cruz O, Lakshman R: A solution for the foreign body in nose problem, *Pediatrics* 81:174, 1988.

DeWeese DD et al: *Otolaryngology: head and neck surgery,* ed 7, St Louis, 1988, Mosby.

Donlon JV: Anesthesia for eye, ear, nose and throat surgery. In Miller R, editor: *Anesthesia,* New York, 1986, Churchill Livingstone.

Jensen JH: Technique for removing a spherical foreign body from the nose or ear, *Ear Nose Throat J* 55:46, August 1976.

Simon R, Brenner B: *Emergency procedures and techniques,* Baltimore, 1987, Williams & Wilkins.

CHAPTER 35

Chalazion and Hordeolum Therapy

Lewis E. Mehl

A chalazion is an inflammation of the meibomian glands, which lie deep in the tarsal plate. Chalazia are often found in patients with marginal blepharitis, and probably originate when the gland orifices are blocked by infection. A hordeolum is an infection of a lash follicle and usually "points" or localizes on the lid border. Hot, moist compresses applied 10 minutes four times daily will cure about half the patients with hordeoli or acute chalazia of less than one week's duration. Topical antibiotics are not useful in the treatment of chalazia or hordeoli, except in a prophylactic sense to cure obvious external infection and prevent new lesions from developing. Systemic antibiotics, hot bathing, and analgesics may resolve acute chalazia when bacterial infection is prominent. When the inflammation and pain have subsided, a persistent mass, or chronic chalazion, may remain for many months and require removal by incision and curettage. For more detailed histological information, see Easty and Smolin.

CHALAZION

The chalazion lesion is usually identified with an area of a faint bluish discoloration under the palpebral conjunctiva. Exuberant lesions can sometimes break through to the skin surface or erode the conjunctiva, producing a pyogenic granuloma and resembling granulation tissue.

A chronic chalazion consists of a cystic swelling and a hard lump. In the chronic form, the swelling is relatively painless, and although vision may be disturbed by distortion of the cornea, the unsightly swelling is the major concern to the patient. A longstanding chalazion can induce an astigmatism, which will persist as long as the nodule remains.

Small chalazia are often absorbed spontaneously, but for larger ones removal may be desired.* Multiple and recurrent chalazia usually indicate an underlying

---

*All excised material should be submitted for pathological examination since meibomian gland carcinoma will often masquerade as a chalazion.

chronic abnormality such as chronic meibomianitis, blepharitis, or rosacea. As many as 50% of adults with chalazia may have rosacea. An underlying, low-grade staphylococcal infection is also often present.

Chronic chalazia have been treated effectively with injection of soluble steroids, but this carries a small but confirmed risk of central retinal artery obstruction, evidently the result of retrograde arterial infusion. It can also induce focal depigmentation in blacks. The presence of multiple, acute chalazionlike lesions along with preauricular adenopathy can be the presenting manifestations of tularemia.

EQUIPMENT (FIG. 35-1)

- Topical ophthalmic anesthetic
- 2% procaine or 1% to 2% lidocaine
- 25-gauge needle and 3 to 5 cc syringe
- Chalazion clamp
- Chalazion curettes
- Irrigator
- Delicate tissue forceps
- Suture scissors
- Needle holder
- Scalpel (small blade) for chalazion or No. 11 blade for hordeolum

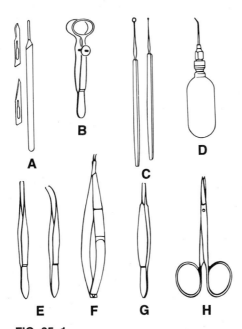

FIG. 35-1.
Instrument tray for acute chalazion removal. **A,** Knife; **B,** Chalazion forceps; **C,** Chalazion curette; **D,** Irrigator; **E,** Delicate tissue forceps; **F,** Needle holder; **G,** Suturing forceps; **H,** Suture scissors.

- Suture: nylon or chromic (5-0 or 6-0)
- Stevens scissors
- Graefe muscle hook
- Topical ophthalmic antibiotic ointment
- Eye patch
- Cotton-tipped applicator
- Lacrimal probe
- 1% silver nitrate stick

ACUTE CHALAZION REMOVAL

Preprocedure Patient Education

Obtain informed consent. Discuss the potential (but uncommon) risks of infection, damage to the eyelid, damage to the lacrimal duct, cosmetic scarring, and excessive bleeding with the patient.

Technique

1. Instill a topical anesthetic into the eye.
2. Inject local anesthetic through the palpebral conjunctiva into the retrotarsal fold with sufficient volume to cause it to balloon out. Also inject the anesthetic externally and subcutaneously around the swelling (Fig. 35-2, *A*).
3. Apply a chalazion clamp of sufficient size to hold the chalazion completely within it (Fig. 35-2, *B*).
4. Evert the eyelid.
5. Make a vertical incision with the scalpel into the chalazion, extending the incision slightly beyond it on both sides (Fig. 35-2, *C*).
6. Using the chalazion curette, thoroughly scrape the walls of the chalazion to remove all material (Fig. 35-2, *D*).
7. Release the clamp.
8. Apply antibiotic ointment and a firm patch to the eye.
9. The patch may be removed after several hours.

CHRONIC CHALAZION REMOVAL

Technique

The same procedures are followed for a chronic chalazion removal as for an acute chalazion until exposure of the mass has been accomplished. At that time, the following modifications to the above technique are followed:

1. Hold the mass with a small, curved hook and dissect it completely free with blunt Stevens scissors (Fig. 35-3).
2. Carefully curette the sac.

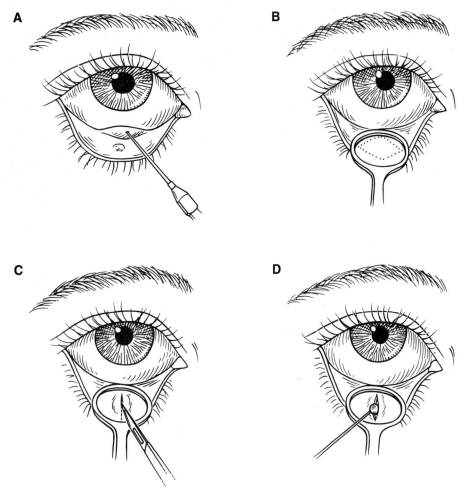

FIG. 35-2.
Removal of acute chalazion. See text for details.

3. Optionally, some physicians destroy the walls of the sac with chemical cautery. To accomplish this, a tightly wound cotton applicator is dipped in 1% silver nitrate and applied to the walls of the sac.
4. The conjunctival incision is left open.*

Alternatively, if the chalazion is very close to the skin, it can be approached externally and cutaneously through a horizontal skin incision. The previous procedures are followed, and the skin is closed by nylon or chromic sutures.

---

*Patients with chalazia large enough to require suture closure for subconjunctival removal should be referred to an ophthamologist.

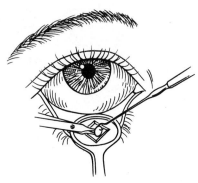

FIG. 35-3.
Excision of chronic chalazion. See text for details.

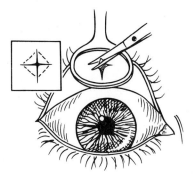

FIG. 35-4.
Excision of conjunctiva for adherent chalazion.

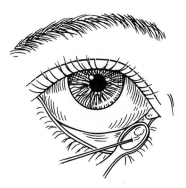

FIG. 35-5.
Protection of the canaliculus.

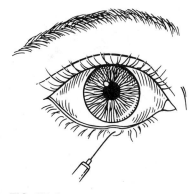

FIG. 35-6.
Diathermy.

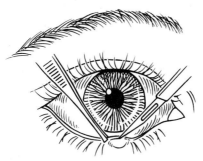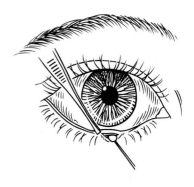

FIG. 35-7.
Marginal chalazion.

Special Situations

- If the conjunctiva is adherent to the chalazion, perform the removal in the same way as for an acute chalazion, except make a second incision at right angles at the midpoint of the first vertical incision. After the sac is curretted, excise the four tips of the incision with scissors (Fig. 35-4).
- A chalazion located near the tear duct must be carefully removed to prevent damage to the duct. Place a lacrimal probe in the duct for identification so that it can be protected during dissection (Fig. 35-5).
- A chalazion in the eyelid margin is difficult to treat surgically. It may be destroyed by surface diathermy (Fig. 35-6), curettage, or an incision in the gray line (Fig. 35-7). Excision of a **V**-shaped area of tissue that includes the chalazion may also be effective but requires a suture to close the lid edges.
- A chronic perforated chalazion can result in the formation of granulation tissue on the conjunctiva, which should be removed by excision or cautery.

HORDEOLUM

Hordeoli usually form on the lid border (Fig. 35-8) and open and drain spontaneously within 2 to 3 days. If the lesion points without draining, the patient may experience relief with a superficial horizontal stab from a No. 11 blade (Fig. 35-9). Localized cellulitis should be treated with systemic antibiotics.

CPT/BILLING CODES

67800	Excision of chalazion; single
67801	Excision of chalazion; multiple, same lid
67805	Excision of chalazion; multiple, different lids
67700	Blepharotomy, drainage of abscess, eyelid

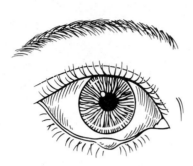

FIG. 35-8.
Hordeoli on the eyelid border.

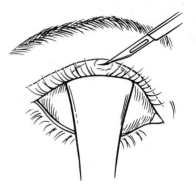

FIG. 35-9.
Hordeolum incised.

BIBLIOGRAPHY

Berens C, King JH: *An atlas of ophthalmic surgery,* Philadelphia, 1982, J.B. Lippincott.

Clayman HM, editor: *Atlas of contemporary ophthalmic surgery,* St Louis, 1990, Mosby.

Easty DL, Smolin G: *External eye disease,* Stoneham, Mass, 1988, Butterworth.

Griffith DG, Salasche SJ, Clemons DE: *Cutaneous abnormalities of the eyelid and face: an atlas with histopathology,* New York, 1987, McGraw-Hill.

King JH, Wadsworth JAC: *An atlas of ophthalmic surgery,* ed 2, Philadelphia, 1988, J.B. Lippincott.

CHAPTER 36

Corneal Abrasions and Removal of Corneal or Conjunctival Foreign Bodies

Grant C. Fowler

Corneal abrasions and corneal or conjunctival foreign bodies are common problems in both the primary care physician's office and the emergency department. In most cases, the management is uncomplicated and can be completed in the physician's office, but there are important guidelines for preventing impaired vision or blindness.

FLUORESCEIN EXAMINATION OF THE CORNEA AND CONJUNCTIVA

Indications

- Unilateral foreign body sensation, hypersensitivity to light, excess tearing, or pain—especially upon opening or closing the eye
- Red eye
- Eye trauma
- Unilateral eye irritation in contact lens wearers
- History of exposure to ultraviolet light from such sources as welding torches, sunlight, or tanning beds (UV light can penetrate the cornea even when the patient's eyes are closed if protective lenses are not being worn.)
- Mild chemical exposure to eye
- Neonates or infants with persistent crying, unilateral tearing, hypersensitivity to light, or conjunctival inflammation

Contraindications

Patients with the following should be referred to an ophthalmologist after immediate management:

- Suspected high-velocity injury to the eye (e.g., patients exposed to metal hammering or heavy machinery): high-speed metallic or nonmetallic fragments may penetrate the globe with unnoticable damage to the cornea and produce minimal symptoms. However, significant internal damage can result. A hyphema, lens opacification, an abnormal anterior chamber examination, or an irregularity of the pupil may suggest that the globe has been penetrated. Orbital X-ray films may confirm a metal foreign body.

  Note: A pressure patch is contraindicated in a penetration injury of the globe. For complex lid lacerations, a nonpressure protective eye shield should be applied before referral.

- Exposure to caustic or acidic media: immediate management includes copious irrigation, which should continue for at least 15 minutes (It can begin at home with tap water from a shower or hose.)
- Mild chemical exposure if the physician is not knowledgeable about the management of the specific chemical after contacting a Poison Control Center
- Ruptured globe
- An uncooperative patient (Infants may have to be sedated. See Chapter 24, Pediatric Sedation.)

Equipment

- Snellen's chart at 6 meters (20 feet), or an equivalent visual acuity chart (If a chart is unavailable, ask the patient to read a magazine at arm's length. If the patient cannot do so, measure and record the distance at which the patient can count fingers.)
- Topical ophthalmic anesthetic such as 0.5% proparacaine (Alcaine) or 0.4% benoxinate (Dorsicaine) unless contraindicated (e.g., ruptured globe, or, for benoxinate, allergy to ester local anesthetics)
- Fluor-I-Strip, sterile fluorescein sodium strips (Since fluoroscein is incompatible with preservatives effective against *Pseudomonas,* which can cause blindness, multidose dropper bottles of fluoroscein solution should not be used.)
- Bright white light source (A single point source such as a penlight is preferable.)
- Cobalt-blue light source (A Wood's lamp is adequate.)
- 8- to 10-power magnification (loupes, a magnifying glass, a colposcope, or an ophthalmoscope on the +20 to +40 diopter setting)
- Sterile cotton-tipped applicators
- Isotonic ophthalmic irrigant (sterile saline, Dacriose)

Preprocedure Patient Education

Emphasize the need for physician follow-up daily until completely healed; this will detect early complications such as infection. Instruct the patient to call the doctor if persistent or recurrent symptoms occur. Soft contact lenses should be removed before the eye is stained. Before instilling the topical anesthetic, tell the patient that it may cause a burning sensation until the eye becomes numb.

Technique

1. Check and document visual acuity in both eyes before instilling topical anesthetic. Initial anesthetic discomfort may later be wrongly suspected as the cause of impaired vision. If the patient normally uses corrective lenses for refractive error, check visual acuity with refraction. After the acuity check, the patient will probably be most comfortable in the supine position for the remainder of the examination.

    If the patient's corrective lenses are not available, pinhole myopia correctors can be used. These are commercially available, and they are easy to make. To make your own, use an 18-gauge needle to punch 8 to 10 holes within a 5 cm (2-inch) circle on an index card. Have the patient select the hole that provides the best vision for viewing the Snellen chart. This effectively corrects the patient's vision.

2. Instill 1 to 2 drops of topical anesthetic. (This is not mandatory but will facilitate patient cooperation and comfort.)

3. Inspect the affected eye with a bright white light source and compare it with the opposite eye. The sclera should be intact. The anterior chamber should be free of pus or blood. The iris should be normal in size and shape. The pupil should be normal in size, shape, and reactivity, and it should be symmetric with the other pupil unless there is already a history of asymmetry. *If all these conditions are not met, the patient should be referred.* (In the follow-up examination the next day, pupil dilation from the cycloplegic may persist. In this case, uneven pupil size should correlate with the half-life of the cycloplegic agent.)

4. Eversion of the upper lid is usually necessary to examine the entire conjunctiva (Fig. 36-1). Inspect the entire bulbar and palpebral conjunctiva for

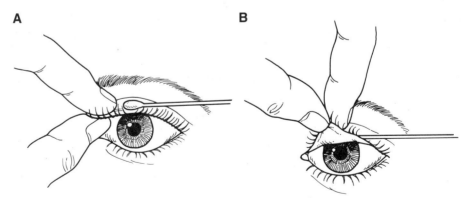

A   **B**

FIG. 36-1.
A, Grasp the upper eyelashes between the thumb and index finger and, with the tip of the other index finger or a cotton-tipped applicator, press gently on the skin at the upper lateral border of the tarsal plate. **B,** Pull outward on the lashes and rotate the tarsal plate upward until it forms a right angle with the eyeball. A gentle tug upward should flip the plate into eversion, clearly exposing the conjunctival surface of the upper lid.

trauma, foreign bodies, or other sources of symptoms, such as a hordeolum or inverted eyelash. For a foreign body, refer to the section later in this chapter, Corneal or Conjunctival Foreign Body Removal.

5. Instill fluorescein dye by moistening a fluorescein strip with one or two drops of sterile saline or topical anesthetic and gently touching the lower conjunctival sac for 3 to 5 seconds. When wetting the strip, use a minimal amount of solution so that only the defect is stained, not the entire eye.

6. Inspect the cornea with magnification under a cobalt-blue light source. If the entire cornea is stained, irrigate the eye and reexamine. Abraded areas of the cornea should remain highlighted with fluorescein. Make a drawing of the cornea for later reference, showing the areas of abnormality. If no source of symptoms is found or if vertical streaking is found on the cornea, suspect an embedded conjunctival foreign body in the eyelid and examine the entire conjunctiva under cobalt-blue light. Keep in mind that on the conjunctiva, fluorescein is taken up by mucus; therefore, dye uptake in conjunctival injuries is less specific than corneal injuries. At this time, if no source of symptoms can be found, the eye should be examined under a slit lamp. For deep, dendritic or central ulcerations or for ulcerations in which infection is suspected (i.e., if there is clouding of the cornea or a purulent discharge), the patient should be referred (Fig. 36-2).

TREATMENT OF UNCOMPLICATED CORNEAL ABRASIONS

Considerations

Some emergency department physicians send all patients to ophthalmologists for follow-up. Risk factors for permanent visual impairment include the abrasion's

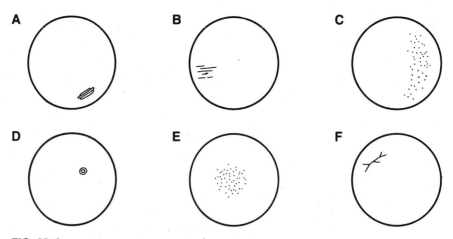

FIG. 36-2.
Corneal defect staining patterns for specific injuries. **A,** Typical abrasion; **B,** Abrasion around a corneal foreign body; **C,** Abrasion from a conjunctival foreign body under the upper lid; **D,** Abrasion from excessive wearing of a contact lens; **E,** Ultraviolet exposure (resulting from sunlamp exposure, welding, or snow blindness) and **F,** Herpetic dendritic keratitis.

depth, size, location, and susceptibility to infection. With minimal magnification, the depth of the abrasion is often difficult to assess, and referral should be considered for suspected deep or large lesions or those centrally located in the line of vision. One way to assess a borderline case is to wait until the follow-up examination the next day. The corneal epithelium is one of the fastest-healing areas of the body, and if considerable progress toward healing has not been made the next day or there are signs of infection, refer immediately.

Equipment

- Topical ophthalmic anesthetic
- Isotonic irrigant (sterile saline or Dacriose)
- Sterile eye patches and 1-inch (preferably nonallergenic) paper tape
- Ophthalmic antibiotics: tobramycin (3 mg per g ointment) or sulfacetamide (10% ointment)
- Cycloplegic drops such as 1% to 2% cyclopentolate HCl (Cyclogyl) are useful for pain control. Their duration of action ranges from hours to a day. For a longer duration of cycloplegia, especially in patients with darkly pigmented irises that absorb cyclopentolate and shorten its duration, 0.25% scopolamine HBr (Isopto Hyoscine) can be considered.

Technique

1. Irrigate copiously with ophthalmic irrigant, with the patient's head turned laterally toward the affected side.
2. Instill 1 to 2 additional drops of local anesthetic.
3. For significant pain, consider a cycloplegic. Trauma often results in spasm of the iris with subsequent discomfort.
4. Apply an antibiotic ointment. Even under the best of conditions, infection is a possibility because of the avascular nature of the cornea. Prophylaxis with antibiotics is important.
5. For all but very minor abrasions, use a double patch, with the first patch folded and the fold placed immediately under the brow (this adds padding and prevents opening of the eye). This patch is covered with the second patch.
6. With three to five strips of paper tape, secure the patches by placing the paper tape from the middle of the forehead to the ear (Fig. 36-3).
7. Do not use eye patches on young children. There is the theoretical chance of permanently affecting the use of one eye or of making amblyopia worse. Very young children will remove the patch anyway.
8. Pain medication should be prescribed in an amount appropriate to the symptoms. However, additional local anesthetic should not be prescribed, because it may retard corneal healing and result in corneal scarring.
9. Reexamine in 24 hours using fluorescein and magnification. If the abrasion has healed, antibiotic drops should be used for an additional 3 days. If the

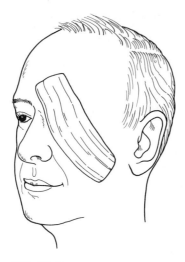

FIG. 36-3.
Pressure eye patch.

defect is smaller, instill a cycloplegic and the antibiotic ointment, repatch, and examine again in 24 hours. If at any time during the follow-up a cloudiness of the cornea or suppuration is seen, refer the patient to an ophthalmologist.

10. The visual acuity test should be repeated and documented just before the patient is discharged.

11. Tetanus immunity should be verified or provided.

Note: If infection is suspected, an eye patch is contraindicated. Abrasions resulting from fingernails or plant matter are notoriously slow to heal, but their progress should be followed as described previously, observing for any signs of early infection.

Postprocedure Patient Education

Instruct the patient not to rub the eyes, especially on awakening. Rubbing may disrupt the new layers of epithelializing cornea. Reepithelialization can take weeks to complete. Inform the patient that the local anesthetic will wear off in a few minutes to hours, and additional pain medication may be necessary. Moist compresses may be applied for some relief of discomfort if the patient's eye has not been patched. Instruct the patient to return to the office daily until healed and if persistent or recurrent symptoms develop. If cycloplegics were used, inform the patient; he or she should in turn tell the physician if seen in another center or if referred. Instruct the patient not to overuse the unpatched eye, such as by watching television or reading for prolonged periods. This is especially true for children or anyone with a history of amblyopia. It is important to document the degree of healing seen during the discharge examination. Safety goggles should be emphasized if the abrasion was an occupational injury.

Complications

- Infection
- Scarring (The highest morbidity occurs when the abrasion is near the central line of vision.)
- Permanent visual impairment

CORNEAL OR CONJUNCTIVAL FOREIGN BODY REMOVAL

Indications

- Noninfected, small, recent corneal or conjunctival foreign bodies

Contraindications

Same as contraindications for examination outlined in Fluorescein Examination of the Cornea and Conjuctiva as well as the following:

- Signs or symptoms that suggest infection, such as edema and clouding of the area of the cornea surrounding the foreign body, ulceration exceeding the size of the foreign body, or purulent discharge (If infection is suspected, patching is contraindicated and referral is necessary.)
- Large metal foreign bodies or those with potential to cause a large rust ring (i.e., those that have been embedded in the cornea for longer than 24 hours)
- Apparently deeply or centrally embedded foreign bodies
- Uncooperative patient

Equipment

- Topical ophthalmic anesthetic
- Sterile fluorescein sodium strips
- Sterile cotton-tipped applicators
- Bright white light source and cobalt-blue light source
- Magnification as previously listed (It may be necessary to have an assistant hold the magnifier to allow the operator the use of both hands.)
- Isotonic ophthalmic irrigant, such as sterile saline or Dacriose
- Snellen chart or equivalent visual acuity chart
- Sterile 18-gauge needle with small syringe
- *Optional:* Instead of an 18-gauge needle, a tuberculin syringe with a 26-gauge needle, a sterile eye spud, or a small, sterile chalazion curette may be substituted depending on user experience
- *Optional:* Sterile dental burr or cornea drill

Preprocedure Patient Education

Instruct the patient that it will be important to fix his or her gaze on a distant object, maintain that focus, and hold the head motionless, regardless of what is seen or experienced. Inform the patient that the eye will be numb from the local anesthetic, but that pressure may be sensed during the procedure.

Advise the patient of possible complications, and that referral may be necessary regardless of outcome. Some clinicians obtain signed informed consent.

Technique

Controversy exists about using a swab or spud to remove a corneal foreign body and whether more damage is caused in this manner. Only experienced users should consider a swab or spud for small corneal foreign bodies. The swab is more successful with recent, superficial foreign bodies. Irrigation alone is not usually successful unless the foreign object consists of carbon or is water soluble, since the patient's tears would have washed it away already.

1. Record the patient's visual acuity.
2. With the patient supine, hold the eyelids apart with your thumb and index finger, and position the patient's head so that the foreign object is at the highest point on the eyeball. The patient should fix his or her gaze. For conjunctival foreign bodies, the head should be positioned for maximal access.
3. Make an attempt to dislodge the object. Noting the controversy regarding swab or spud use, try to lift the object by lightly touching with a cotton swab moistened with local anesthetic. This occasionally dislodges the particle. Never use any force to rub the cornea, as this will dislodge the epithelium and cause a larger abrasion. The same maneuver can be attempted for a conjunctival foreign body.
4. To use a sterile needle, approach the object from a direction tangential to the eyeball, with the needle bevel upwards and the syringe held with a pencil grip (Fig. 36-4). Rest your hand on the patient's zygoma so that it moves with the patient. Use the needle tip to lift the object gently from its bed. Several attempts may have to be made, but referral for removal under slit lamp should

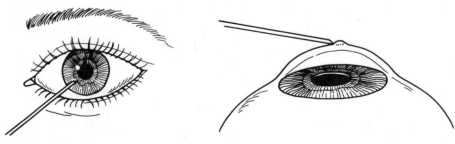

FIG. 36-4.
Removal of a superficial corneal foreign body. Side view illustrates the thickness of the cornea relative to the beveled needle edge. The needle or eye spud should be tangential to the cornea, and the object should be gently scraped off the cornea.

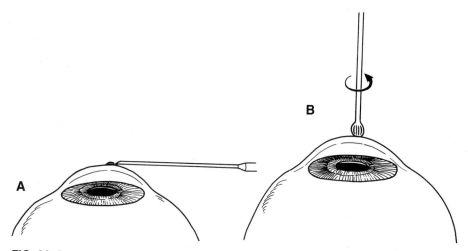

FIG. 36-5.
A, Disposable needle steadied with syringe. Note horizontal approach. **B,** Dental burr rotated once. Note vertical approach.

be considered if further corneal damage is anticipated. If several attempts with a needle are unsuccessful, (noting the controversy discussed) a spud or chalazion curette may be considered. For conjunctival foreign bodies, the technique is the same: attempt to lift them from their bed with the same instruments. More vigorous force, if controlled, may be used on the conjunctiva.

5. If a residual corneal rust ring is found under magnification, it can occasionally be removed with the sterile needle alone. A cornea drill may also be considered. It should have a pressure-sensitive automatic shutoff to minimize corneal damage. Another published technique involves the use of a sterile dental burr held between the thumb and forefinger to approach the rust ring vertically (Fig. 36-5). After the burr has made one gentle rotation, reexamine the eye under magnification to verify complete removal. Rust is toxic to corneal epithelium and prevents healing; it may also result in nighttime visual defects. If attempts to remove the rust ring are unsuccessful or they will result in further damage to corneal epithelium, referral should be made for management under slit lamp magnification.

6. Retest and record the patient's visual acuity.

Postprocedure Patient Education

Follow the guidelines for patching after an uncomplicated corneal abrasion. If the object cannot be removed, the resultant rust ring is too large, or the patient is referred to an ophthalmologist for any other reason, the ophthalmologist should provide further patient education.

Complications

- Same as complications associated with treatment of routine corneal abrasion, except the risk of corneal scarring is greater
- Perforation of the cornea or globe
- Incomplete removal of a foreign body
- Failure to heal due to a retained rust ring or other causes

CPT/BILLING CODES

65205	Removal of foreign body, external eye; conjunctival superficial
65210	Removal of foreign body, external eye; conjunctival embedded
65220	Removal of foreign body, external eye; corneal without slit lamp
99070	Eye tray: supplies and materials provided by physician over and above those that are usually included with the office visit

BIBLIOGRAPHY

Aquavella JV, Eiferman RA, Sher NA: Treating superficial corneal injuries, *Patient Care* 19:27, 1985.

May HL, editor: *Emergency medicine,* New York, 1984, Wiley Med Pub.

Reich JA: Removal of corneal foreign bodies, *Austr Fam Physician* 19:710, 1990.

Roberts JR, Hedges JR, editors: *Clinical procedures in emergency medicine,* Philadelphia, 1985, W.B. Saunders.

CHAPTER 37

Visual Function Evaluation

Fred D. Catrett

Malcolm L. Mazow

Vision evaluation encompasses testing for acuity, visual field defects, strabismus, and color vision. Deficits in any of these areas can have important ramifications, but usually they can be detected with relatively simple equipment.

Visual acuity loss may be insidious, slow, and painless, but it needs to be detected early, because it could be caused by diabetic or hypertensive retinopathy, as well as by numerous other treatable conditions, including senile cataract, chronic glaucoma, pituitary adenoma, choroiditis, creeping inferior retinal detachment, and choroidal melanoma. A reduction in the visual field can also be insidious and can indicate glaucoma, retinitis pigmentosa, intracerebral tumors, and detached retina (or hysteria if the size of the field loss is independent of distance).

Strabismus is misalignment of the eyes. It is called *comitant* if the misalignment of the eyes is about the same in all directions of gaze. Comitant strabismus is usually not caused by serious neurologic disease. Strabismus is called *noncomitant* when the amount of misalignment varies with the direction of gaze. Most noncomitant strabismus is paralytic and, if acquired, may indicate neurologic or orbital disease. Acquired strabismus, like other visual defects, may also occur with systemic diseases, such as hyperthyroidism, myasthenia gravis, cranial artery aneurysm, and multiple sclerosis.

In young children, strabismus should also suggest the possibility of amblyopia or asymmetric decreased visual acuity. Early recognition and correction of amblyopia might prevent blindness, especially if the patient is treated before five years of age. Therefore, newly diagnosed amblyopia or strabismus should be referred promptly to an opthalmologist.

INDICATIONS

- All newborns
- All infants
- All children as soon after the third birthday as possible, to detect asymmetry in visual acuity (using the Snellen chart)

- All school-age children
- Patients being evaluated for visual complaints
- Patients with ocular trauma
- All patients at screening physical examinations, to detect painless loss of vision
- Commercial aircraft pilots and people who operate heavy equipment (Color vision should be tested.)
- Patients with retinal or optic nerve disorders
- Patients at risk of glaucoma (Visual evaluation should be performed on a periodic basis.) (See Chapter 38, Tonometry.)

EQUIPMENT

- Very bright penlight for testing response to light and eliciting corneal light reflex (infants and children)
- Snellen and *Illiterate E* charts (Fig. 37-1): The latter, also called *Tumbling E,* consists of the letter *E* in various sizes and positions. A well-lit, 20-foot hallway is usually necessary to administer the test unless otherwise specified. (Reverse Snellen charts are available for use with mirrors if a 20-foot hallway is not available.)
- Pinhole cards for those with severely impaired vision
- Ishihara or Hardy-Rand-Rittler pseudoisochromatic plates for color-vision testing (These are a series of numbers or figures presented against a background of colored dots, arranged in such a way as to present a confusing and thus unreadable pattern to the person who has abnormal color discrimination.)
- Standard near vision chart for adults (Rosenbaum Pocket Visual Screener)

TECHNIQUE

Infants and Newborns

1. Test eye fixation on an object, and tracking of a moving object (opticokinetic testing) to demonstrate an intact visual pathway to the visual cerebral cortex.
   Step 1. Hold the infant upright and slowly move your face in front of the infant's face. The normal response is for the eyes to follow your facial movement briefly. If the test is abnormal, ask the parent to perform the same maneuver.
   Step 2. Hold three of your fingers together, palm toward you, in front of one of the patient's eyes, thus blocking the vision from it. Simultaneously test the uncovered eye as in Step 1. Repeat for the opposite eye. (The standard visual occluder is not necessary, and is more likely to be rejected by children.)
   Step 3. If any one of these tests is abnormal in patients aged 3 to 4 months, refer the patient to an ophthalmologist.
2. Next, test for intact third cranial nerves by looking for the expected positive reflex of pupillary constriction to light.
3. Visual field testing is performed by shining the light at the periphery of vision; expect the infant to turn its head in that direction.

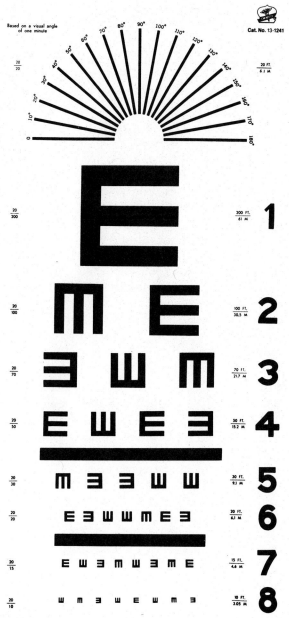

FIG. 37-1.
Illiterate E chart.

Distractions need to be minimized for these three tests, and the nursery lights need to be dimmed for the latter two.

Note: Gross retinal examination should be performed on all newborns by eliciting the *red reflex,* a symmetrical orange-red colored light reflected by both fundi. Hold the ophthalmoscope 1 to 2 feet from the eye and observe the color in the pupil. Asymmetry in color might indicate toxoplasmosis or a retino blastoma and should be evaluated further.

Young Children

1. Confirm that there is vision in each eye and screen for visual field deficits with an object such as a favorite toy to attract the patient's attention.
   Step 1. Cover one eye and pass the object successively from the periphery into each of the visual fields. Obvious facial brightening or verbal acknowledgment confirms detection of the object.
   Step 2. Repeat Step 1 with the other eye. If one eye is abnormal, the child may indicate that by crying when the normal eye is covered.
2. Test for strabismus. Shine a penlight or similar point light source towards the eyes, while having the patient gaze at a distant object. The reflection of light from each cornea should be symmetrically located. If symmetric, it is usually centered over the pupils. (Momentary eye wandering in infancy is common up to 3 or 4 months of age.)

Older Children

1. Test visual acuity. By the time they are 3 to 4 years of age, children should be tested for standard acuity using an Illiterate E chart (Fig. 37-1).
   Step 1. Show the child the chart at a distance from which it can be seen easily. Explain that he or she is to point with his or her fingers in the direction that the "legs" of the "E" point. Demonstrate how to do this. Allow the child to practice reading the letters, to help overcome confusion and anxiety.
   Step 2. With the child 20 feet from the chart, test from the largest to the smallest readable letters with one eye covered (use a patch if necessary). Record the lowest line on which the patient can correctly identify at least half the total number of letters. Repeat for the other eye, and then for both simultaneously.
   Step 3. If the child can read no line at 20 feet, walk him or her toward the chart, and record as the numerator the distance at which he or she can read the top line. (For example, if the child can read the top line, which normally can be read at 200 feet, at a maximum of 10 feet, record as 10/200 vision.)
   Step 4. If the patient is unable to see the top line at 3 feet, have him or her count fingers at maximal distance. Record as "CF/[insert the maximum distance]."
   Step 5. If the patient is unable to count fingers at 1 foot, have him or her determine the direction of hand motion. Record as "HM/[the maximum distance]."
   Step 6. Analogously, for progressively poorer vision, have the patient attempt to determine the position of a light ("LP with projection"), the presence of

light without being able to determine its position ("LP/no projection"), or no light perception ("NLP").

Step 7. Test any person who scores less than 20/20 vision by having him or her look through a pinhole. If the vision is improved, this suggests that corrective lenses will improve the vision.

Step 8. A difference in acuity between the two eyes of two or more levels is suggestive of amblyopia. Refer such patients to an ophthalmologist, who can assist in evaluating for additional disease, and in instituting appropriate corrective measures—such as temporary occlusion of vision in the stronger eye to strengthen the weaker one.

2. Test visual fields. Elicit cooperation from the older child in actively reporting when he or she detects an object in each successive visual field.
3. Test for strabismus.

Step 1. Observe for obvious deviation of one eye. A permanent nasal or inward deviation is designated *esotropia;* a temporal or lateral deviation is *exotropia.* Primary strabismus in children is most often esotropia. Exotropia is often secondary to another cause. Both should be evaluated further if persistent. If there is a misalignment, have the child look up, down, right and left to determine if the deviation is the same in all fields (comitant) or is significantly varied (neurologically significant paralytic stabismus).

Step 2. If Step 1 was negative, observe the corneal light reflection in each eye, looking for a more subtle degree of deviation.

Step 3. If still unable to detect strabismus, perform the maximally sensitive "cover/uncover" and "alternate cover" tests (Fig. 37-2): Have the child stare at a light source approximately 33 cm (12 inches) away; occlude the vision from the right eye with one hand; observe for any movement (which indicates abnormality) of the left eye (abnormal response).

Step 4. Watch for movement of the until-now occluded right eye as the cover is moved to the opposite eye. Any right eye movement, especially if there was none from the left eye in Steps 1 through 3, suggests that the right eye requires a constant visual stimulus to remain fixated. This indicates that there is a latent deviation, or phoria.

Step 5. Repeat Steps 3 and 4, covering and uncovering the left eye.

Step 6. Refer to an ophthalmologist if you diagnose previously unevaluated strabismus.

Adults

1. Test for distant acuity with the standard Snellen chart. With encouragement, patients will often read one line smaller to provide a more accurate assessment.

   Step 1. The Snellen chart is used in a fashion similar to the Illiterate E. Test adults as described for older children.
2. Test for near vision with standard near vision cards. If not available, use printed text and record size. Near vision should be checked if distant vision is difficult or if the patient has a complaint.
3. Test visual fields as for older children.

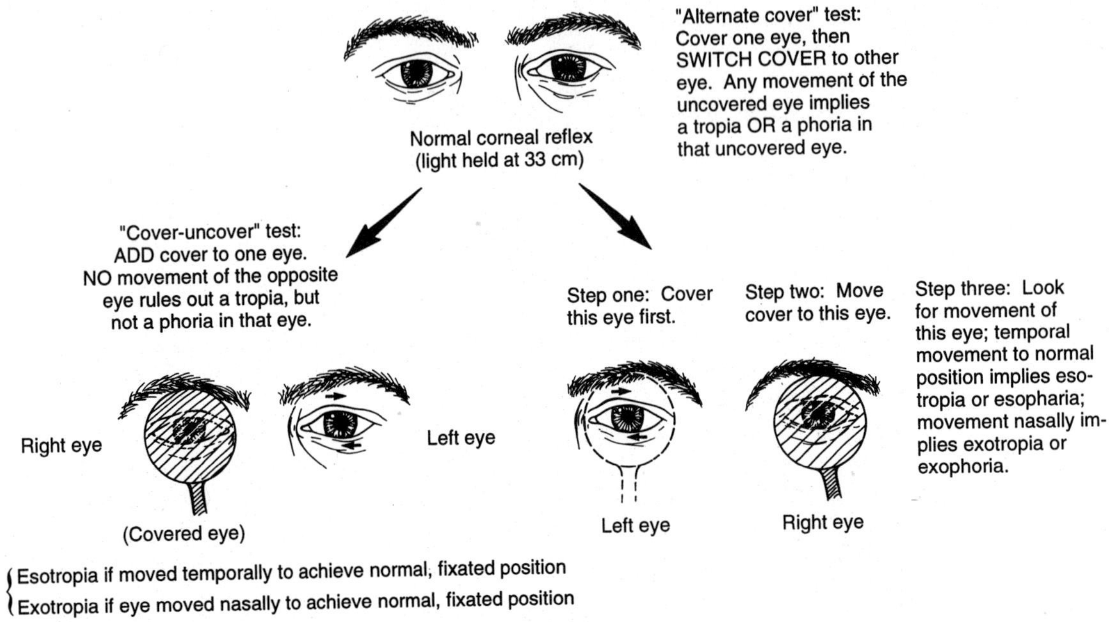

FIG. 37-2.
Tropia and phoria determination.

4. Test for strabismus as for older children.
5. Test for color vision, if indicated, using appropriate charts such as the Ishihara or Hardy-Rand-Rittler set. Ensure good illumination, and have the patient wear corrective lenses if they are normally used for near vision. Record the numbers of the charts that cannot be read. Refer to the specific instruction set for the chosen charts to interpret the specific type of color vision defect, if any.

CPT/BILLING CODES

Visual function evaluation cannot be billed separately; rather, it is to be considered within the context of the level of complexity and detail of the office examination.

BIBLIOGRAPHY

Helveston EM, Ellis FD: *Pediatric ophthalmology practice*, ed 2, St Louis, 1984, Mosby.
Leitman MW: *Manual for eye examination and diagnosis*, Oradell, N.J., 1981, Medical Economics.
Nelson LB et al: *Pediatric ophthalmology*, ed 3, Philadelphia, 1991, W.B. Saunders.
Scanlon JW et al: *A system of newborn physical examination*, Baltimore, 1979, University Park Press.

CHAPTER 38

Tonometry

John M. Boltri

Schiotz tonometry is used to detect increased intraocular pressure. Glaucoma is a leading cause of preventable blindness, the incidence of which increases with age. About 1.5 million persons in the United States have some degree of blindness caused by glaucoma. Although persons with intraocular pressure in the "normal" range can develop glaucoma, most patients at risk have increased intraocular pressure.

When used in combination with funduscopic examination and visual field testing, Schiotz tonometry can detect many patients at risk for developing glaucoma, making early treatment and prevention of blindness possible.

INDICATIONS

The risk factors for glaucoma include

- Age over 40 years
- Family history of glaucoma
- Black race
- Diabetes mellitus
- Ocular pain
- History of visual field loss
- Some medications: Corticosteroids, mydriatics, phenothiazines, and sympathomimetics can precipitate glaucoma.

Patients at risk for glaucoma should also be screened for visual fields defects, disc pallor, and increased cup-disc ratio.

CONTRAINDICATIONS

- Presence of eye infection
- History of recent eye trauma
- Patients who cannot keep their eyes still

EQUIPMENT AND SUPPLIER

- Schiotz tonometer kit (Each kit comes with the tonometer, three plunger weights, concave test block, conversion table, pipe cleaner, and instructions for care.)

  R.O. Gulden & Co.
  225 Cadwalader Ave, P.O. Box 7154
  Elkins Park, PA 19117
  215-884-8105

- Topical ophthalmic anesthetic, such as proparacaine hydrochloride 0.5%

PREPROCEDURE PATIENT EDUCATION

Explain the reason for measuring the intraocular pressure with the tonometer (presence of risk factors or positive physical findings). Briefly explain the procedure. Also tell the patient that this is a screening test that can detect increased intraocular pressure and lead to treatment to prevent the development of blindness. However, if the test is normal, it does not rule out glaucoma.

TECHNIQUE

1. Check and record the patient's visual acuity. Immediately following the funduscopic exam, place two drops of anesthetic into each eye. (The anesthetic will take effect while you prepare the tonometer.)
2. Assemble the tonometer with the 5.5 gm weight in place and test for accuracy on the convex metal test block (Fig. 38-1). The Schiotz tonometer is precalibrated by the manufacturer and must be returned for repair if it does not read "0" when resting on the test block.
3. Have the patient lie in the supine position on the table.
4. Ask the patient to relax and fix a gaze on a spot on the ceiling, with the line of vision perpendicular to the table. Retract the lids of the eye against the bony margin of the orbit with one hand and hold the tonometer by its handles with the thumb and middle finger of the other hand (Fig. 38-2). Center the foot plate of the tonometer over the cornea and gently lower the tonometer until it is resting on the cornea. The indicator will come to rest at a position to the right of 0. The tonometer should be perpendicular to the cornea in a vertical position.

   Note: Ask the patient to extend his or her arm straight upward and look at the thumbnail to help fix his or her gaze.

5. Record the scale reading. If it is less than 4, repeat the reading, because this indicates an elevated intraocular pressure. Perform another reading after add-

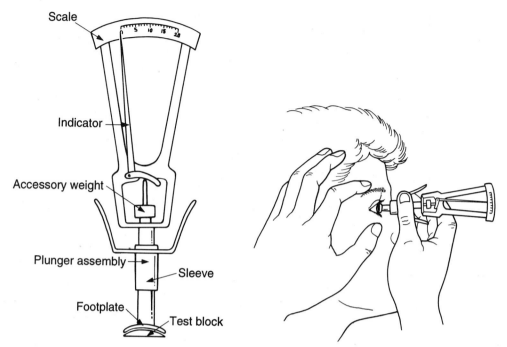

FIG. 38-1.
Tonometer.

FIG. 38-2.
Examination with the tonometer.

ing the 7.5 or 10 gm weight, as necessary, to obtain a scale reading between 4 and 8. Convert the scale reading to mm Hg using the calibration scale included with the kit (Table 38-1). Record this in the chart. Recommend a consultation with an ophthalmologist if the pressure in either eye is greater than 20 mm Hg.

6. Carefully clean the tonometer after each use to prevent transmission of disease. Alternatively, set the tonometer in an ultraviolet sterilizer stand, or cover the portion of the tonometer that contacts the eye with a disposable sheath (Tonofilm). The tonometer should be disassembled at the end of each day, and a pipe cleaner should be run through the barrel to remove dried secretions, which interfere with the motion of the plunger. The tonometer should not be oiled.

POSTPROCEDURE PATIENT EDUCATION

Although routine prophylactic topical antibiotics are unnecessary, warn the patient about the hazards of anesthetized eyes and to avoid rubbing or touching the eyes for 60 minutes. In addition, if symptoms of corneal abrasion subsequently occur, the patient should immediately contact the physician.

TABLE 38-1.

Sample Calibration Scale for Schiotz Tonometer

Scale reading	Plunger load (gm)			
	5.5	7.5	10.0	15.0
0	41	59	82	127
0.5	38	54	75	118
1.0	35	50	70	109
1.5	32	46	64	101
2.0	29	42	59	94
2.5	27	39	55	88
3.0	24	36	51	82
3.5	22	33	47	76
4.0	21	30	43	71
4.5	19	28	40	66
5.0	17	26	37	62
5.5	16	24	34	58
6.0	15	22	32	54
6.5	13	20	29	50
7.0	12	19	27	46
7.5	11	17	25	43
8.0	10	16	23	40
8.5	9	14	21	38
9.0	9	13	20	35
9.5	8	12	18	32
10.0	7	11	16	30
10.5	6	10	15	27
11.0	6	9	14	25
11.5	5	8	13	23
12.0		8	11	21
12.5		7	10	20
13.0		6	10	18
13.5		6	9	17
14.0		5	8	15
14.5			7	14
15.0			6	13
15.5			6	11
16.0			5	10
16.5				9
17.0				8
17.5				8
18.0				7

(From Schiotz Tonometer Kit. Courtesy of R.O. Gulden & Co., 225 Cadwalader Ave., P.O. Box 7154, Elkins Park, PA 19117.)

COMPLICATIONS

- Trauma to the cornea during Schiotz tonometry is uncommon; however, corneal abrasion can occur after the procedure while the cornea is still anesthetized.
- Infection is a complication that usually can be avoided with proper cleaning of the tonometer.

LIMITATIONS

Falsely elevated intraocular pressure readings can be a normal variant or can arise from pressure placed on the globe during the procedure, from a scarred cornea, or from an inflamed cornea. Falsely high readings can also occur with a thick or steeply curved cornea. Falsely low measurements can result from high-grade myopia or rapidly repeated measurements, or they may be a normal variant.

CPT/BILLING CODES

Ophthalmological services constitute integrated services. Itemization of tonometry is not applicable.

92002   Ophthalmological services: medical examination and evaluation with initiation of diagnostic and treatment program; intermediate, new patient

92012   Ophthalmological services: medical examination and evaluation with initiation of diagnostic and treatment program; intermediate, established patient

BIBLIOGRAPHY

Berson FG, editor: *Ophthalmology study guide,* San Francisco, 1987, American Academy of Ophthalmology.

Morse RM, Heffron WA: Preventive health care in family practice. In Rakel RE, editor: *Textbook of family practice,* Philadelphia, 1990, W.B. Saunders.

Moses RA: Tonometry. In Cairns JE, editor: *Glaucoma,* New York, 1986, Grune & Stratton.

Schottenstein EM: Intraocular pressure. In Ritch R, Shields MB, Krupin T, editors: *The glaucomas,* Philadelphia, 1989, Mosby.

CHAPTER 39

Management of Epistaxis

Nancy V. Schantz

Identification of the bleeding site is the key to appropriate management in epistaxis, a very common problem in primary care. Over 90% of nosebleeds are anterior, usually involving Kiesselbach's plexus of the nasal septum (Fig. 39-1). A brief history will help determine the bleeding site. Recent trauma, upper-respiratory infection, or age under 40 years should lead the physician to suspect an anterior nosebleed. In a patient over 40 years old, bleeds are often posteriorly located and associated with local or systemic disease. Possible causes include cancers of the nose or sinus, infections, hypertension, and coagulopathies.

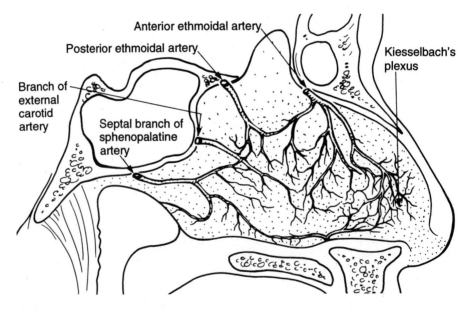

FIG. 39-1.
Anatomy of the septal blood supply.

Anterior epistaxis often can be stopped by digital pressure or simple cautery. Posterior bleeding can be life threatening, and requires posterior nasal packing with subsequent hospitalization.

INDICATIONS

- Epistaxis that persists despite continous external pressure for at least 10 minutes

RELATIVE CONTRAINDICATIONS

- Clotting abnormalities (Aggressive nasal packing, especially posterior packs, may cause further bleeding. Attempts should be made to normalize clotting mechanisms, especially before removing nasal packs.)
- Chronic obstructive pulmonary disease (Posterior packing in patients with chronic obstructive pulmonary disease may result in a significant drop in their oxygen partial pressure [P_{O_2}]. These patients should be given supplemental oxygen and closely monitored.)
- Known or suspected cerebrospinal fluid leak
- Trauma

EQUIPMENT

Anterior Pack

- Gowns for patient and physician
- Emesis basin
- Gloves
- Head lamp (or head mirror and light source)
- Nasal speculum (insulated, if electric cautery is to be used)
- Bayonet forceps
- Suction with No. 5 Fraser tip
- Cotton pledgets and applicator sticks (Q-Tips)
- 4% topical lidocaine mixed 1:1 with 1:1000 ephedrine (or topical 4% to 10% cocaine solution)
- Silver nitrate sticks or electric cautery
- Neosporin or bacitracin ointment
- Suture scissors
- Petrolatum (Vaseline) gauze packing in two sizes: ½ × 72 inch (anterior) and 3 × 36 inch (posterior)

Posterior Pack

- Benzocaine spray anesthetic (Cetacaine)
- Straight soft-rubber catheter (12 to 14 Fr.)

- Dental rolls and cotton gauze (2 × 2 inch or 4 × 2 inch and 4 × 4 inch)
- Umbilical tape (Heavy silk or nonabsorbable suture are alternatives.)
- *Optional:* Umbilical clamp
- *Optional:* Foley catheter 12 to 14 Fr., with 30 cc balloon
- *Optional:* 20 cc syringe
- Tongue depressor
- Goggles

PREPROCEDURE PATIENT EDUCATION

Allergy to local anesthetics should be determined (see Chapter 21, Local Anesthesia). Describe the risks to the patient as listed under Complications. Anterior packing and especially posterior packing are painful, and a mild sedative or narcotic may be helpful if the patient is stable. Warn the patient about the discomfort and ask him or her to attempt to hold as still as possible.

TECHNIQUE

1. Have the patient sit upright and face you. Give the patient an emesis basin to use as needed for bleeding. The patient should wear a gown to protect clothing. Ask the patient to blow his or her nose to evacuate all old clotted blood.
2. Using the nasal speculum and light source, examine both sides of the nose; use the suction tip to clear clots as needed.
3. Identify and examine the septum and middle and lower turbinates, paying close attention to Kiesselbach's area.
4. If the bleeding site appears to be anterior, insert cotton pledgets soaked in lidocaine/ephedrine mixture (or cocaine solution) into the nostril, using bayonet forceps. Have the patient apply pressure by pinching the nose for 10 minutes to stop the bleeding (Fig. 39-2).

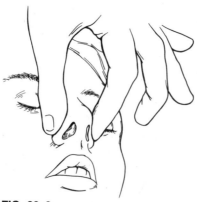

FIG. 39-2.
Apply pressure by pinching the nose to stop the bleeding.

5. Remove the pledgets and, with the nasal speculum, locate the bleeding site. If it is not readily seen, brush the area lightly with a cotton-tipped applicator. If it still cannot be located because of bleeding, suction gently with the Fraser tip while gradually proceeding posteriorly until posterior to the bleeding site (no blood return through the suction tip).

6. After locating the site, cauterize it with a silver nitrate stick or electrocautery. If silver nitrate is used, carefully dry the area with a cotton applicator stick to prevent the silver nitrate from spreading. If bleeding was limited, you may apply antibiotic ointment to keep the mucosa lubricated. You may choose to stop at this step and let the patient return home, with caution not to blow or pick the nose for the following week.

7. For a heavily bleeding anterior site, place an anterior pack. Coat petrolatum gauze (½ × 72 inch) with antibiotic ointment and fold in half. Insert the doubled end first to prevent the free end from entering the pharynx (Fig. 39-3). Fold layers into the nose from turbinates to floor (Fig. 39-4). The pack should be left in place for 48 hours.

8. If a posterior bleeding site is identified (i.e., if patient's chief complaint is blood in the throat, or if an anterior pack does not stop the bleeding), place a posterior nasal pack.

9. A standard posterior pack is made of 3 × 36 inch petrolatum gauze rolled into a tight cylindrical pack, 3 inches long (Fig. 39-5). The pack should be impregnated with antibiotic ointment.

10. Tie two 18-inch umbilical tapes around the middle of the pack.

11. Spray the posterior pharynx with benzocaine (Cetacaine) spray.

12. Insert the soft rubber catheter through the bleeding nostril. Through the patient's open mouth, visualize the catheter tip. Pull the tip from the pharynx and out the mouth with forceps.

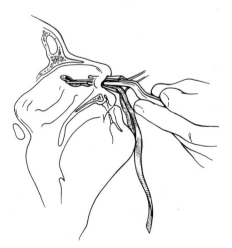

FIG. 39-3.
Insert anterior pack with folded end inserted first.

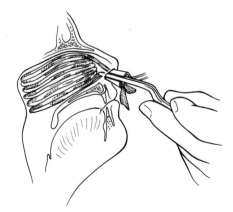

FIG. 39-4.
Fold gauze pack in layers.

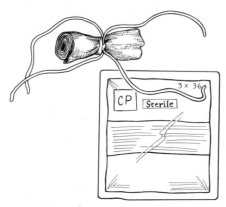

FIG. 39-5.
Prepare posterior pack.

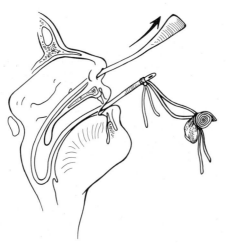

FIG. 39-6.
Tie or suture pack to catheter.

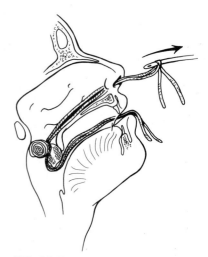

FIG. 39-7.
Pull pack into position.

13. Tie both ends of one piece of umbilical tape around the catheter (Fig. 39-6). Pull the catheter back through the nose, leaving the second piece of umbilical tape hanging from the mouth for pack removal (Fig. 39-7). Pull the pack into the posterior nose, pushing it around the soft palate with your finger.
14. Insert an anterior pack (Fig. 39-8).
15. Secure the posterior pack by tying the umbilical tapes to rolled 4 × 4 inch gauze pads held flush but not too firmly against the nares.

ALTERNATIVE TECHNIQUE FOR POSTERIOR PACK PLACEMENT

1. Remove and discard the tip of the Foley catheter that is distal to the balloon. Lubricate the catheter with antibiotic ointment.

2. Introduce the catheter into the bleeding nostril past the choana.
3. With the syringe, instill 5 cc of saline into the balloon and, using gentle traction, pull the balloon into contact with the choana. Once in place, fill the balloon with 10 to 15 cc of saline (Fig. 39-9).
4. Insert an anterior pack while maintaining traction on the catheter.
5. Fix the catheter with an umbilical clamp using padding between the clamp and the nose.
6. When bleeding ceases, deflate the balloon, but leave the catheter in place for 12 hours, in case of rebleeding.

POSTERIOR PACK CARE

- Hospitalize the patient and place on telemetry.
- Provide low-flow oxygen by mask.
- Order laboratory tests, including serial blood counts and coagulation studies.
- Monitor respiratory status carefully with frequent checks of vital signs and pulse oximetry.
- Begin broad-spectrum antibiotic therapy to cover pathogenic bacteria of the sinus while the pack is in place. The patient is at risk for stasis sinusitis.
- Remove the packs in 3 days. First remove the anterior pack. Cut the umbilical tapes around the gauze roll at the nares. Extract the pack through the mouth

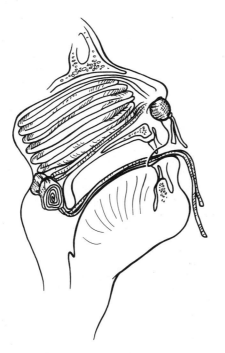

FIG. 39-8.
Secure posterior pack after placing anterior pack.

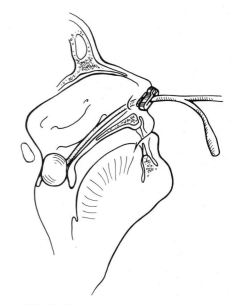

FIG. 39-9.
Foley catheter as alternate posterior pack.

by gently withdrawing the umbilical tapes. If a Foley catheter was used, deflate the balloon and, after appropriate observation period for rebleeding, gently remove it.

- If bleeding recurs, obtain an otolaryngology consultation.

POSTPROCEDURE PATIENT EDUCATION

If an anterior pack is placed, tell the patient that the pack will be left in place for 48 hours and that he or she may go home. Prophylactic antibiotics, such as a cephalosporin or amoxicillin/clavulanic acid, with good coverage of nasal pathogens should be initiated while the pack is in place. Ask the patient to report any recurrent bleeding or fever, and to return for removal in two days.

The patient with a posterior pack will require hospitalization for observation while the pack is in place. Risks include those outlined in Complications. If a posterior pack fails to stop the bleeding, consultation with an otolaryngologist may be required.

After either an anterior or posterior pack is removed, caution the patient to notify you if fever, facial or ear pain, or recurrent bleeding develop. Instruct the patient to return to the office in one week for reexamination.

COMPLICATIONS

- Rhinitis
- Otitis media
- Sinusitis
- Hemotympanum
- Bacteremia
- Respiratory distress
- Cardiac arrhythmias
- Pressure necrosis of nasal ala or mucous membranes
- Rupture of balloon with aspiration of saline (if Foley catheter was used for the posterior pack)
- Allergic reaction to local anesthetic

BIBLIOGRAPHY

McGill J, Kulig K: Epistaxis. In *Emergency medicine: concepts and clinical practice*, St Louis, 1988, Mosby.

Randall DA, Freeman SB: Management of anterior and posterior epistaxis, *Am Fam Physician* 43:2007, 1991.

VanderSalm TJ, Gacek RR: Control of epistaxis. In Vander Salm TJ, editor: *Atlas of Bedside Procedures* 1:207, 1979.

CHAPTER 40

Flexible Fiberoptic Rhinolaryngoscopy

Grant C. Fowler

In 1982, it was reported that fewer than 30% of practicing primary care physicians in Ohio were able to visualize a larynx, and that fewer than 4% included inspection of the larynx as part of their complete physical examination. Primary care physicians in Ohio are probably representative of those elsewhere, and a few commented anonymously that they had never visualized a larynx! Although the prevalence of carcinoma of the head and neck has not decreased for the last three decades, with early diagnosis, the cure rate is improving. This statistic, combined with the fact that the number of nasopharyngeal complaints continues to increase, has led primary care physicians to seek more satisfying techniques by which to visualize the upper airway. Fiberoptic rhinolaryngoscopy was first utilized in 1968; the ease of learning the technique, its low risk (especially for physicians already performing endoscopic procedures), the rapidity of the procedure (most procedures are completed in 5 to 10 minutes), and the relatively low cost of equipment ($3,500 to $5,000, exclusive of the light source) has led increasing numbers of primary care physicians to learn this technique.

INDICATIONS

Certain chronic upper-respiratory complaints encompass the primary indications for rhinolaryngoscopy, especially in smokers or those with unilateral conditions. As more studies become available, it may have applications for the management of common conditions such as sinusitis, a very common acute problem and the most common chronic disease in the United States. (One recent study found rhinolaryngoscopy almost as sensitive and more cost effective than radiography for diagnosing acute maxillary sinusitis.)

- Chronic hoarseness for more than 3 weeks
- Chronic sinusitis or sinus discomfort, especially unilateral
- Chronic serous otitis media in an adult, especially unilateral
- Recurrent otalgia

- Suspected neoplasia
- Chronic cough
- Chronic nasal obstruction or postnasal drip
- Chronic rhinorrhea
- Halitosis
- History of previous head and neck cancer
- Head or neck masses or adenopathy
- Recurrent epistaxis
- Dysphagia
- Chronic foreign-body sensation in pharynx
- Evaluation of snoring
- To further assure absence of disease in any chronic upper-respiratory condition

ACUTE CONDITIONS THAT MAY WARRANT RHINOLARYNGOSCOPY

- Hemoptysis
- Acute sinusitis
- Acute epistaxis
- Suspected nasal foreign body
- Suspected laryngeal foreign body
- Acute onset of hoarseness after straining voice

CONTRAINDICATIONS

- Acute epiglottitis (may precipitate complete airway obstruction)
- Acute epistaxis (The source of bleeding may be difficult to visualize with profuse hemorrhage.)

Note: Fiberoptic rhinolaryngoscopy is considered a very safe procedure. It is the only endoscopic procedure that does not require an informed consent statement in the state of Colorado.

EQUIPMENT AND SUPPLIERS

- Flexible fiberoptic rhinolaryngoscope with light source (Newer scopes are completely immersible, which simplifies cleaning and disinfection. Frequently, light sources used for other endoscopic procedures in the office may be compatible.)

Fujinon Corporation
Wayne, New Jersey
800-872-0196

Olympus Corporation
Lake Success, New York
800-645-8160

Pentax Precision Instruments Corporation
Orangeburg, New York
800-431-5880

Welch Allyn Corporation
Skaneateles Falls, New York
800-535-6663

Disposable Sheath Nasopharyngoscope
Vision Sciences
Natwick, Massachusetts
800-874-9975

- Nasal speculum
- Sterilizing solution, such as glutaraldehyde (Cidex)
- Decongestant
    Phenylephrine (0.25% to 2%) spray (Neo-synephrine)* or epinephrine
    1:50,000 (Adrenalin)
- Anesthetic
    Lidocaine (2% to 4%) spray (Xylocaine)†
    Benzocaine spray (14%) (Cetacaine)†
- Optional supplies include cotton balls or pledgets soaked in either deconges-
    tant or anesthetic. Three ear, nose, and throat spuds with soaked cotton appli-
    cators are another option. Cocaine solution (4% to 10%) can be used for both
    decongestion and anesthesia. At this strength, it does not produce a euphoric
    effect; however, many physicians choose not to stock cocaine because of the
    mandatory record keeping and the risk of burglary. With increased on-the-job
    drug screening, when cocaine is chosen as the anesthetic, the possibility that
    traces of cocaine metabolites might be found in the patient's urine should be
    explained to the patient.

PREPROCEDURE PATIENT EDUCATION AND EVALUATION

After a thorough head and neck history and examination, as well as the remainder
of a complete history and physical examination, explain the procedure to the

---

*Should be used with caution in those who are severely hypertensive or have a history of sensi-
tivity to the agent.
†Should be used with caution in those who have a history of an allergy or sensitivity to the
agent.

patient and schedule an appointment. When the patient returns for the procedure, obtain the interval history, examine the head and neck, and explain the procedure again. The procedure is brief enough that it can usually be done on initial visit.

Inform the patient that upon insertion of the scope, an intense tickling sensation may be experienced. Warning the patient beforehand can minimize his or her responses. The objectives of the procedure should be carefully described. Explain to the patient that he or she may talk to you during the procedure, and that he or she should tell you of any significant discomfort other than pressure. Tell the patient that he or she will be asked to say certain words or sounds, and may be asked either to swallow or to avoid swallowing at different stages.

Although rhinolaryngoscopy can be performed without anesthesia, visualization and patient tolerance is generally improved by utilizing a combination of decongestant followed by anesthetic, especially with inexperienced operators or anxious patients.

Ask the patient to gently blow the nose to clear the nasal passage. With the patient sitting up, apply decongestant with a generous spray of atomized solution to both nostrils. One spray should be directed superiorly and a second posteriorly. After the spraying, have the patient tilt the head back to allow the liquid to drain as far back as possible, and swallow any residual. Unless both nares are to be intubated, the nostril least obstructed by visual inspection after decongestion should be anesthetized for scope insertion.

After waiting 5 to 10 minutes for the decongestant to take effect, anesthetize the nostril(s) chosen for scope insertion. Spray liberal amounts of lidocaine or benzocaine aerosol spray; direct the spray superiorly and then posteriorly for about 1 second with the patient tilting the head back and again swallowing any residual. (Swallowing the anesthetic assists with suppression of the gag reflex.) For patients with a hyperactive gag reflex, gargles with lidocaine solution or generous spraying of the pharynx with benzocaine may also be helpful.

To use soaked cotton balls or pledgets, insert them through the nasal speculum with bayonet or offset forceps. One of each, either cotton ball or pledget, should be inserted superiorly, in the middle meatus, and posteriorly. They should remain for 5 to 10 minutes and be removed before insertion of the scope. Three ENT spuds with cotton applicators can be utilized in the same manner.

TECHNIQUE

1. Before insertion and while awaiting anesthesia, become reacquainted with the scope (for those who do not regularly perform endoscopic procedures) by deflecting the tip both ways to observe how far it moves for a given movement of the deflector. With the focal length on most scopes about 5 mm or greater, view an external object through the scope for a sense of proportion. In general, as it is advanced, the tip of the scope moves toward whatever structure is in the center of the field of view. A slight deflection of the tip can result in a marked change in direction of the scope.

2. Place the patient in either an erect sitting or supine position. Both examiner and patient should be in a position that they can maintain comfortably for 20 minutes. A small child may want to sit in his or her parent's lap. The patient is protected from injury caused by their own sudden movements or by their jumping away from the scope during the procedure if they are in the supine position, if a high, firm headrest is available for patients who are sitting, or if the parent maintains a firm hold on a child.

3. Rest the hand used for guiding the endoscope on the patient's cheek. Your middle, ring, and little fingers should form a tripod to support the index finger and thumb while handling and guiding the tip of the scope. As you gain more experience, you may wish to rest this tripod on the patient's forehead to sense for tensing of the frontalis muscle, which is often the first indication that the patient is experiencing significant discomfort. Turn on the light source. Tell the patient to close the eyes and expect a bright light. Insert the tip through the least-obstructed nostril, past the nasal hairs at the vestibule, and rest it against the nasal septum to warm it. Warming the scope usually defogs it.

4. The floor of the nasal cavity, which is within the inferior meatus, usually offers the most open channel and the best passage for intubations (Fig. 40-1). The meatus is the space below each tuberinate. Advance the scope only toward visualized objects and avoid advancing the scope blindly or against significant resistance. As with other endoscopic procedures, if only white is visible (a "whiteout"), the scope is probably resting against nasal mucosa and should be withdrawn until the structure is visualized. A deviated septum or large maxillary ridge may impede advancement of the endoscope along the floor. In this situation, make an attempt to pass the scope through the middle

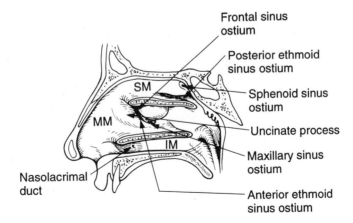

FIG. 40-1.

A sagittal section of the head with the turbinates removed to demonstrate ostia of the paranasal sinuses and nasolacrimal duct. *IM*, inferior meatus; *MM*, middle meatus; *SM*, superior meatus.

meatus, keeping in mind that the patient usually experiences more discomfort whenever the scope is directed or advanced superiorly. If this is unsuccessful, withdraw the scope and intubate the other nostril.

5. As the scope is advanced along the floor, the feet of the medial crura (of the lower lateral septal cartilages) can frequently be seen protruding from the medial aspect of the nasal passage. The inferior turbinate is visualized about 1 cm into the passage. Note the texture and size of the inferior turbinate, as well as any polypoid degeneration or swelling of the covering mucosal membranes. Flexion of the scope slightly upward often illuminates the middle turbinate in the distance and its meatus. The nasolacrimal duct drains into the inferior meatus and is usually not seen, but draining purulent fluid may be seen. Surgical antral windows into the maxillary sinus are frequently located in the inferior meatus and occasionally can be entered with a scope (Fig. 40-2). Again, note the condition of the mucosa.

6. Next, pass the scope posteriorly about 4 to 5 cm until the choana comes into view. The choana is the junction between the nasal fossa and the nasopharynx, and it looks just like a posterior "nostril" forming a halo in front of adenoid tissue. Adenoid tissue should be seen at this point. If desired, move the scope laterally and superiorly to allow entry into the middle meatus. However, since superior reflection of the scope may result in discomfort to the patient, you may elect to examine the middle meatus on the way out after visualizing the larynx. If the nasal floor is obstructed, there may be no choice but to attempt passage of the scope through the middle meatus.

7. Upon entering the choana, the adenoid pad appears on the posterior wall of the pharynx. Star-shaped scarring may be the residual of an adenoidectomy. Advance the endoscope into the nasopharynx, and when the posterior margin of the septum is passed (when it is no longer seen), slightly flex the tip of the endoscope and rotate 90 degrees laterally to observe the torus

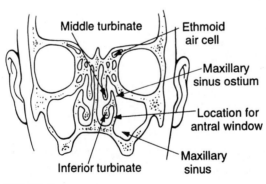

Middle turbinate Ethmoid air cell

Maxillary sinus ostium

Location for antral window

Maxillary sinus

Inferior turbinate

FIG. 40-2.
A frontal section of the head. In this section, eight ethmoid air cells (four on each side) are shown in their location medial to the orbit. A rather large maxillary sinus ostium is demonstrated, as well as the location in the inferior meatus for surgical placement of antral windows.

tubarius, or valve at the opening of the eustachian tube (Fig. 40-3). Ask the patient to say "key, key, key" while you observe tube function. The eustachian tube should open and close slightly. Adenoid or lymphoid hyperplasia may be noted in this area or anywhere throughout the procedure, and may block the torus tubarius. By advancing the scope slightly and rotating 180 degrees while making sure to avoid the septum, the opposite torus is illuminated. Its function should be observed. Posterior to both tori and anterior to the adenoid pad lie the clefts of Rosenmüller, each of which should be carefully inspected since most nasopharyngeal malignancies are found in this area.

8. Next, advance the scope inferiorly and toward the posterior wall of the oropharynx (Fig. 40-4). Instruct the patient to breathe through the nose to keep the soft palate from obstructing the view. As the patient swallows, or

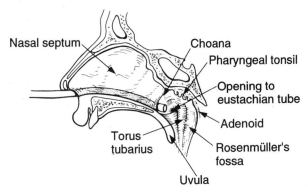

FIG. 40-3.
Anatomy of nasopharynx and oropharynx.

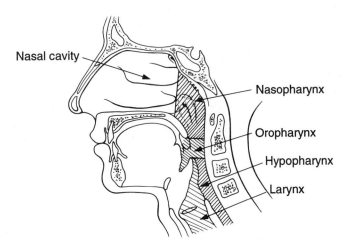

FIG. 40-4.
The anatomic divisions of the upper airway. All five divisions may be inspected with a fiberoptic endoscope.

talks, the normal movement of the soft palate can be seen. Flexion and slight rotation of the scope as it nears the posterior wall will allow for inspection of the uvula, the soft palate, and the lateral and posterior walls of the pharynx. The epiglottis should be seen in the distance. Note the presence of any masses, scarring, inflammation, exudate, mucosal irregularities, or pulsations. In some cases, dysphagia may be explained by lymphoid hyperplasia in this area, especially if associated with enlarged palatine tonsils and exudate.

9. When the scope has passed the soft palate, it enters the oropharynx. For the remainder of the procedure, keep the scope as close as possible to the posterior pharynx without touching it. Touching the pharynx may elicit the gag reflex. If the scope becomes fogged, tell the patient to swallow; often this clears the scope. With slight flexion and rotation, examine the posterior tongue, lingual tonsils, palatine tonsils, epiglottis, medial and lateral glossoepiglottic folds, and valleculae from above (Figs. 40-5 and 40-6). Ask the patient to stick out his or her tongue to improve visualization of the valleculae.

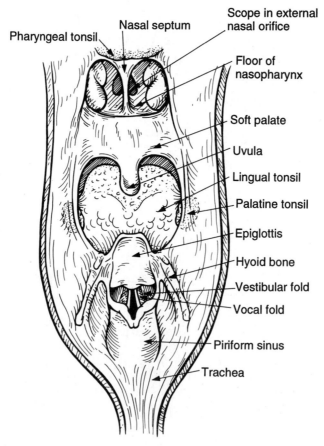

FIG. 40-5.
Oropharyngeal and laryngeal areas, viewed from posterior.

10. When the scope has passed the epiglottis, enter the hypopharynx (Fig. 40-4), and ask the patient to refrain from swallowing. At this level, swallowing can induce an unusual foreign-body sensation or provoke coughing. Assure the patient that if swallowing is unavoidable, it may seem as if he or she is trying to swallow the scope. If this sensation becomes too strong, the scope may be withdrawn until the sensation passes. At this level, the arytenoid cartilages, the corniculate and cuneiform cartilages, and the aryepiglottic folds can be visualized. The piriform sinuses posterior to the cords should be at least partially inspected. Closely examine the false and true vocal cords and the ventricles during quiet respiration (Fig. 40-6). Tell the patient to hold a prolonged high "eee" while you watch for symmetry of cord mobility, and edema, hemorrhages, erythema, nodules, or masses of the cords or surrounding structures. Note any mucosal or structural abnormalities. The scope should not touch or pass below the cords, even during accidental swallowing, because laryngospasm can result with subsequent patient asphyxia.

11. Withdraw the scope to a position just anterior to the choana and direct it very superiorly, almost inverted on itself (Fig. 40-7). With the tip in this position, carefully advance the scope anteriorly (withdraw), and the sphenoid bone should appear. (The sphenoid bone will appear in what was previously an anterior position in scope orientation before inversion.) The superior turbinate may be seen as well as an anatomical variant, the supreme turbinate. Medial to the superior turbinate, the ostia of the sphenoid sinus should be visible. The sphenoid sinus, which can be thought of as a large posterior ethmoid air cell (Fig. 40-8), is usually the only sinus in the posterior ethmoid group in which the ostia can be seen (Fig. 40-1). Superior direction of the scope into an area where anesthesia is frequently not complete may cause the patient some slight discomfort.

12. Straighten the scope and withdraw to the level where the complete choana comes into view. Move the scope in a superior and lateral direction to allow

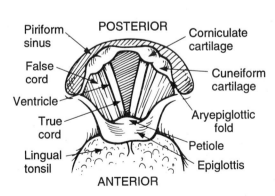

FIG. 40-6.
The larynx viewed from above and oriented as it would be seen with a fiberoptic endoscope.

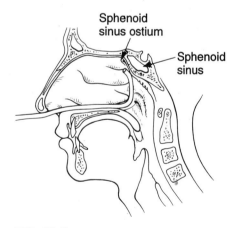

FIG. 40-7.
The endoscope is withdrawn to a position just anterior to the choana and retroflexed.

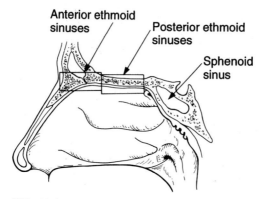

FIG. 40-8.
A parasagittal section of the head showing the relationship of the anterior and posterior ethmoid sinuses. The bone in this area is eggshell thin.

examination of the middle meatus. In most cases, it is easier to examine the middle meatus from posterior to anterior. The frontal sinus, anterior ethmoid cells, and maxillary sinus ostia are located in the middle meatus, with the maxillary sinus ostia most likely to be visualized. Note any drainage from ostia, any purulent fluid, inflammation, or polyps protruding from or occluding the ostia. The majority of polyps are seen in the middle meatus, originating from the anterior ethmoid cells. Typical polyps are slightly yellow, translucent, and relatively avascular. They can originate from nasal mucosa (most common) or they can be a polypoid degeneration of a turbinate; they can be mucous or fluid filled. Frequently they have a *stalk,* or extension of mucosa, that can be traced back to their sinus of origin. Through air drying and subsequent keratinization, polyps can develop benign squamous metaplasia and become more opacified and whiter/grayer in appearance. Upon completion of the examination, withdraw the scope and explore the opposite nasal cavity, if indicated.

13. As with any endoscopic procedure, the natural tendency during rhinolaryngoscopy is for an examiner to move toward whatever is visualized, resulting in a tight loop outside the patient's nose. To prevent this tendency, you should remember to relax and maintain the same distance from the patient throughout the procedure. If you straighten the scope at the end of the procedure before removing it from the patient's nose, the patient is usually most grateful.

CARE OF EQUIPMENT AND CLEANING

Although rhinolaryngoscopes are fairly indestructible, they are composed of fibers and lenses that can both be broken; hence you should avoid bending the scope into tight angles or traumatizing the tip. Clean the lens with lens cleaner and paper. Clean the scope thoroughly with soap and water followed by a 10-minute soak in glutaraldehyde between procedures.

COMPLICATIONS

- Adverse reaction to anesthetic or decongestant (most common)
- Sneezing and gagging severe enough to prevent completion of the examination
- Laryngospasm with possible asphyxia—prevented by remaining above the level of the vocal cords
- Blood pressure elevation (very rare and usually related to adverse drug reaction)
- Vasovagal reaction (rare)
- Epistaxis (It is possible to dislodge eschar or traumatize tumor.)
- Vomiting with possible aspiration

CPT/BILLING CODES

31575	Nasolaryngoscopy
92511	Diagnostic nasopharyngoscopy with endoscope
99070	Tray/room charge (supplies and disinfection charge)

BIBLIOGRAPHY

Corey GA, Hocutt JE, Rodney WM: Preliminary study of rhinolaryngoscopy by family physicians, *Fam Med* 20(4):262, 1988.

Fiberoptic examination of the pharynx and larynx, Lake Success, NY, Olympus Corp. (Videotape).

Hocutt JE, Corey GA, Rodney WM: Nasolaryngoscopy for family physicians, *Am Fam Physician* 42(5):1257, 1990.

Nasolaryngoscopy: the inside view, Lake Success, NY, Olympus Corp. (Videotape).

Patton D, DeWitt DE: Flexible nasolaryngoscopy: a procedure for primary care, *Primary Care & Cancer* 12(5):13, 1992.

Selner JC et al: *Rhinolaryngoscopy,* ed 2, 1989, Allergy Respiratory Institute of Colorado.

CHAPTER 41

Indirect Laryngoscopy

Grant C. Fowler

Despite readily available fiberoptic procedures enabling direct visualization of the upper respiratory tract, indirect laryngoscopy remains very useful. It is a rapid method of examining the upper tracheal rings, vocal cords, epiglottis, larynx, and hypopharynx. In certain instances, indirect laryngoscopy, combined with an adequate history, will complete the diagnosis. Performed by those comfortable with the procedure, it requires very little preparation, few instruments, and little time and care of equipment. This is especially true when compared to a procedure such as flexible rhinolaryngoscopy. Indirect laryngoscopy may also be useful when rhinolaryngoscopy is not available, for patients with low malignancy risk, and during follow-up for a known lesion after complete rhinolaryngoscopy has excluded other lesions. It may also be useful as a preliminary examination before rhinolaryngoscopy. However, the required coordination of instruments makes it difficult, if not impossible, to examine patients by indirect laryngoscopy—even by expert laryngologists—when not used on a regular basis.

INDICATIONS

- Chronic hoarseness for more than 3 weeks
- Suspected or previous neoplasia
- Chronic cough
- Halitosis
- Head or neck masses
- Dysphagia
- Chronic foreign-body sensation in pharynx
- Hemoptysis
- Suspected laryngeal foreign body
- Acute onset of hoarseness after straining voice
- Stridor, particularly inspiratory stridor
- Persistent earache or unilateral serous otitis

- Any clinical situation in which visualization of the hypopharynx and larynx will aid in diagnosis or therapy

CONTRAINDICATIONS

- Acute epiglottitis, since laryngoscopy may precipitate complete airway obstruction
- Acute inflammation or infection of the throat (*relative contraindication*)

EQUIPMENT

- Bright headlight or head mirror with external light source
- No. 4 and No. 5 laryngeal mirrors; smaller sizes for children
- 4 × 4 inch gauze sponges
- Local anesthetic: lidocaine* spray (2% to 4%) or benzocaine* spray (14%)
- Goggles
- *Optional:* alcohol lamp or bowl of hot water to warm mirrors

PREPROCEDURE PATIENT EDUCATION AND EVALUATION

After a thorough head and neck history and examination, as well as the remainder of a complete history and physical examination are performed, explain the procedure. Inform the patient that it is important to relax; that the mirror will be placed in the top of the back of the mouth, avoiding the throat; and that in most cases, if performed properly or if anesthetic is used, this procedure should not stimulate the gag reflex. Dentures should be removed.

TECHNIQUE

1. The patient should sit upright with the body straight, preferably in a high-backed chair with a headrest. Tell the patient to lean slightly forward. The head and jaw should jut forward in a "sniffing" position (Fig. 41-1).
2. Sit slightly to the side of the patient. Position the light source or mirror so that light is directed parallel to your visual axis and focused on the patient's posterior pharynx.
3. Spray the patient's pharynx with anesthetic and have him or her gargle and spit it out.
4. Select the largest mirror that will comfortably fit in the back of the throat and warm over the alcohol lamp, in the warm water, or inside the patient's

---

*Should be used with caution in those who have a history of an allergy or sensitivity to the agent (see Chapter 21, Local Anesthesia).

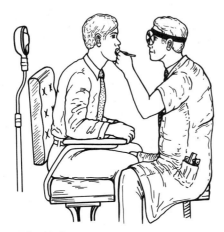

FIG. 41-1.
Proper positioning of the patient is essential for successful visualization of the larynx.

cheek. If it is externally warmed, check its temperature on the back of your hand before inserting it.

5. Cover the patient's protruded tongue with gauze and grasp it firmly between your thumb and middle finger. Do not pull hard enough to cause discomfort. Use your index finger to retract the upper lip.

6. Ask the patient to breathe in and out through the mouth or to "pant like a puppy." This opens the space between the soft palate and the tongue.

7. Apply the posterior aspect of the mirror to the uvula and lift it out of the way. Avoid the posterior pharyngeal wall and base of the tongue; touching these areas might stimulate the gag reflex (Fig. 41-2).

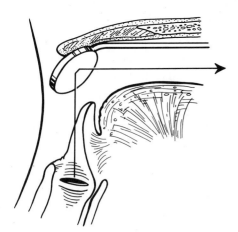

FIG. 41-2.
Laryngeal mirror is inserted into the pharynx, lifting the uvula but avoiding contact with the posterior pharyngeal wall.

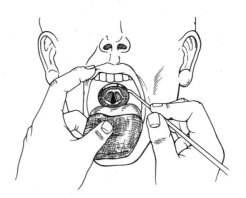

FIG. 41-3.
The tongue is pulled forward with gauze, and the mirror is tilted in various directions to visualize the larynx, the hypopharynx, and the anterior oropharynx.

8. In this position, tilt the mirror in various directions to visualize the larynx, the hypopharynx, and the anterior oropharynx including the base of the tongue. Move your head toward and away from the mirror to focus the light source maximally on visualized objects (Fig. 41-3).

9. As the larynx is visualized, observe vocal cord activity during quiet respiration. Next, observe cord activity while the patient holds a prolonged high "eee." Observe for symmetry of cord mobility; and edema, hemorrhages, erythema, nodules, or masses of the cords or surrounding structures. Note any other mucosal or structural abnormalities (see Fig. 40-6, Chapter 40, Flexible Fiberoptic Rhinolaryngoscopy).

Note: All structures viewed will be seen in mirror image (upside-down and backwards).

10. For those patients whose pharynx is not suitably visualized by this technique or for those in which a closer evaluation of an abnormality is indicated, flexible fiberoptic rhinolaryngoscopy should be performed or referral to an otolaryngologist considered.

COMPLICATIONS

- Possible laceration of the undersurface of the tongue from stretching the tongue firmly over the teeth
- Possible adverse reaction to anesthetic
- Vomiting—possible with aspiration
- Failure to diagnose an abnormality because of inadequate visualization

CPT/BILLING CODE

No separate code is available for this procedure.

BIBLIOGRAPHY

Passy V: Hoarseness, *Prim Care* 9(2): 1982.

Saunders WH: Indirect mirror larynogoscopy: the larynx, *Clin Symp* 16:67, 1964.

CHAPTER 42

Nasogastric Tube and Salem Sump Insertion

Julie Graves Moy

Most conditions that require nasogastric tube insertion will occur in the inpatient setting, the outpatient surgery setting, or the emergency room, but occasionally a patient will require nasogastric tube insertion in the office. For some patients, insertion is an irritating procedure that causes tearing, gagging, and sometimes emesis. More comfortable and less irritating insertion depends on adequate topical anesthesia and smooth, rapid insertion by the physician.

INDICATIONS

- To aspirate stomach contents for diagnostic or therapeutic reasons (such as assessment of gastrointestinal bleeding; determination of gastric acid content; treatment of paralytic ileus, intestinal obstruction, trauma, or overdose)
- To provide a route for feedings or administration of medications

CONTRAINDICATIONS

Blind nasogastric tube insertion should not be performed in patients with

- Facial fractures or basilar skull fracture with suspected cribriform plate injury
- Esophageal stricture
- History of caustic ingestions or esophageal burn
- Comatose patients with unprotected airway
- Penetrating cervical wounds
- Choanal atresia
- Recent oropharyngeal, nasal, or gastric surgery
- Zenker's diverticulum

EQUIPMENT

- Towel for covering patient's clothing
- Paper tissues
- Emesis basin
- 14 or 16 Fr. nasogastric tube (Much larger sizes are available for pill-fragment aspiration. Use 10 Fr. for children.)
- Cup of water with drinking straw
- Water-soluble lubricant jelly or lidocaine gel and cotton-tipped applicator (Benzocaine [Cetacaine] spray may be useful.)
- Goggles
- Latex gloves
- Stethoscope
- Hypoallergenic tape
- Catheter-tip syringe
- Vasoconstrictor nasal spray
- Magill forceps
- Suction device (wall suction, intermittent wall suction, or portable intermittent suction)
- *Optional*: soft nasal trumpet airway

There are three types of nasogastric tubes: firm straight suction tubes, sump suction tubes (Fig. 42-1) with two lumens, and soft feeding tubes. Sump tubes are less likely to be sucked against the stomach wall and become obstructed, but with the second air-inlet port, the suction lumen is smaller than that of the straight suction tubes. Soft tubes that minimize local trauma are available for prolonged feeding (Table 42-1).

PREPROCEDURE PATIENT EDUCATION

Explain the procedure to the patient and let the patient know that there are certain times that he or she will need to help. Explain the possible complications and the alternative treatments, if available. In most states, this procedure does not require

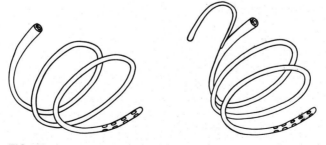

FIG. 42-1.
Firm straight and sump suction nasogastric tubes.

TABLE 42-1.

Enteral Alimentation Tubes

Trade name	Material	Circumference (French)	Length (inches/cm)	Feeding	Duration of use
Keofed	Silicone	5, 7.3, 9.6	43/107.5	Gastric or intestinal	Up to 6 weeks
Dobbhoff	Polyurethane	8	43/107.5	Gastric or intestinal	Up to 6 weeks
Duo-Tube	Silicone	5, 6, 8	40/100	Gastric or intestinal	Up to 6 weeks
Entriflex	Polyurethane	8	36, 43/90, 107.5	Gastric or intestinal	Up to 6 weeks

written informed consent, but either a narrative of the patient's agreement for the procedure in the medical record or a signed consent form is recommended.

TECHNIQUE

1. Position the patient in a sitting or a semi-sitting position with support for the back. Place a towel over the patient's chest and an emesis basin in the patient's lap. For unconscious patients, place them in the left lateral position with head turned to the downward side to prevent aspiration.
2. Select the more open naris while observing the patient inhale through the nose. Apply topical anesthetic to both nares and the pharynx: either spray the pharynx with benzocaine (Cetacaine) and place lidocaine gel 2% in the nares with a cotton-tipped applicator, or lubricate a soft nasal airway (10 Fr.) with 2% lidocaine gel and allow the patient to insert the lubricated airway into the nares. After 10 minutes, the nares and pharynx should be anesthetized since the patient swallows the gel running down the posterior nasopharynx.

   Note: In emergencies, anesthesia may not be an option, and patients do well with adequate lubrication alone.

3. Select the largest tube possible for that patient's nostril size; 16 Fr. is desirable for an adult. To determine the length of insertion, place the tip at the patient's nose, then loop the tube over the ear lobe and down to the xiphoid; mark this spot with tape before insertion. Another method to determine length of tubing needed is to measure the distance between the ear and the umbilicus.
4. Curve the end of the tube by coiling the first 6 inches. If significant nasal congestion is noted and the patient does not have hypertension or coronary artery disease, apply a spray of topical vasoconstrictor, such as ephedrine or phenylephrine hydrochloride.
5. Have the patient hold the water and straw to the mouth. Supporting the patient's head with your hand to prevent the patient from pulling away, insert the tube along the floor of the nose, directing the tube toward the floor of the nose, not toward the bridge. This will be at a 60-degree to 90-degree angle to the plane of the face (Fig. 42-2). Have the patient sniff and advance the tube straight back until resistance is felt (which means the tube has reached the nasopharynx). Ask the patient to swallow some water and flex the head

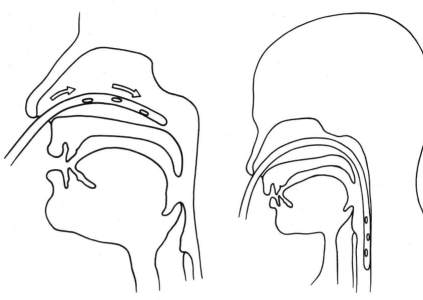

FIG. 42-2.
Nasogastric tube insertion.

FIG. 42-3.
Have the patient flex the head and gently
advance the tube, then ask the patient to swallow.

slightly (Fig. 42-3). When the patient swallows, advance the tube into the esophagus quickly. Once the tube is in the esophagus, it can easily be advanced into the stomach. The patient should be able to speak. If the patient is unable to speak, the tube is in the trachea and should be withdrawn. Violent coughing or gagging may also indicate trachael intubation. Patients with an altered mental status may not cough with tracheal intubation.

6. Advance the tube to the premarked distance; alternatively, advance to the first mark on a Salem sump tube. (This is at 45 cm, and the gastroesophageal junction is at about 40 cm.) If the stomach is full, an immediate return of fluid may occur; use the emesis basin to collect this. If there is no immediate return of fluid, confirm that the tube is not curled in the mouth or pharynx. Connect an air-filled, 60 cc catheter-tip syringe to the lumen and, while listening with a stethoscope over the left upper quadrant of the abdomen, push the air into tube. If a "whoosh" sound is heard immediately, the tube is probably in the stomach. If the "whoosh" is delayed, the tube could be in the esophagus. Reposition the tube if necessary, then reconfirm using the air-filled syringe. It may be necessary in some cases to confirm placement with X-ray, occasionally using liquid contrast media. Secure the tube (Fig. 42-4) after confirming proper placement. Feeding tubes should reach the proximal duodenum.

POSTPROCEDURE PATIENT EDUCATION

If the tube is removed before discharge, instruct the patient to avoid eating or drinking for 1 to 2 hours (to allow function of swallowing to recover from local

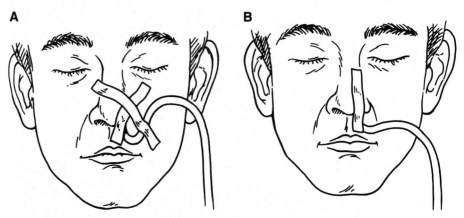

FIG. 42-4.
Secure the tube to the nose with tape in butterfly style (**A**) or vertically (**B**).

anesthetics, thus avoiding aspiration), and to eat only soft foods for the next 12 to 24 hours. If the patient is to go home with the tube (such as a feeding tube), provide explicit instructions about tube care and how to avoid pressure necrosis of the nose.

Family members should be aware of the risks of aspiration from feeding tubes for individuals with dementia or an altered mental status, and alternatives that are available, such as gastrostomy or jejunostomy tubes.

COMPLICATIONS

- Unnecessary patient discomfort and epistaxis can occur if the tube is forced.
- With nasogastric tubes for nutritional supplementation, the most dreaded complication is aspiration of feedings. Pneumonia may occur as a result. Risk of aspiration can be minimized by carefully checking placement before commencing feeding. Feeding tubes with radiopaque tips (Fig. 42-5) to enable plain X-ray verification of location are preferred. For patients who are uncooperative or attempt to pull the tube out, repeated verification of location is important. Checking for residuals after feedings may also minimize the risk of aspiration, especially in unresponsive patients.
- Placement of the nasogastric tube in the trachea or a bronchus may also cause a pneumothorax.
- Intracranial placement of a nasogastric tube has occurred in patients following pituitary surgery or severe head trauma.
- Hydrothorax, empyema, and hematemesis due to erosion of the right subclavian artery have been described.
- Forcing the tube can perforate the esophagus and lead to creation of a false passage.
- Necrosis of the nasal mucosa or erosion of the esophagus or stomach are possibilities if the tube remains in place for too long. Softer tubes should minimize the risk for long-term placement.

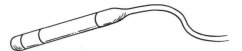

FIG. 42-5.
Feeding tube with radiopaque tip.

- Prolonged nasogastric suction can lead to significant fluid or electrolyte imbalance; fluid and electrolyte balance should be monitored daily.

CPT/BILLING CODES

89130	Gastric intubation and aspiration, diagnostic, each specimen, for clinical analyses or cytopathology
91100	Intestinal feeding tube, passage, positioning, and monitoring
91105	Gastric intubation, and aspiration or lavage for treatment (ingested poisons)

BIBLIOGRAPHY

Glauser JM: Nasogastric intubation. In Roberts JR, Hedges JR, editors: *Clinical procedures in emergency medicine,* Philadelphia, 1985, W.B. Saunders.

Knoarzewski WH, Richards GDH, Thomson SJ: Letter to editor, *Anaesthesia* 41(6):678, 1986.

Mills J et al, editors: *Current emergency diagnosis and treatment,* Los Altos, Calif, 1985, Lange Medical Publications.

Siegel IB, Kahn RC: Insertion of difficult nasogastric tubes through a nasoesophageally placed endotracheal tube, *Crit Care Med* 15(9):876, 1987.

CHAPTER 43

Emergency Cricothyroidotomy and Tracheostomy

Nancy V. Schantz

Cricothyroidotomy is an emergency procedure for securing an airway that is performed when other methods have failed. The advantage of this procedure is the speed with which it can be performed. The trachea is most superficial at the cricothyroid membrane, and landmarks are easily identified. Serious bleeding and perforation of other structures can usually be avoided.

Standard tracheostomy should be performed under controlled circumstances in the operating room. The complete procedure usually takes too long to be useful in emergency airway management and can be difficult to perform for the unskilled physician.

EMERGENCY CRICOTHYROIDOTOMY

Indications

- Airway obstruction (when endotracheal or nasotracheal intubation has failed, is contraindicated, or is unavailable)

Contraindications

- When a less radical means of airway management can be utilized
- Patient aged less than 12 years; needle cricothyroidotomy is the preferred procedure for this age group

Note: An 11-gauge needle inserted in the same area (needle cricothyroidotomy) may allow a patient to maintain spontaneous respirations for a few minutes. High-pressure oxygen ventilation is necessary if a 14- or 16-gauge needle is used, and the patient must be monitored for carbon dioxide retention. This is a very temporary airway that may be used to prevent respiratory arrest when no other equipment is available. However, it should be rapidly converted to tracheostomy or cricothyroidotomy since carbon dioxide will rapidly accumulate.

Equipment

- Povidone-iodine (Betadine) solution
- Sterile 4 × 4 inch gauze sponges
- Sterile fenestrated drape
- Sterile gloves
- Mask, cap, gown, goggles
- Lidocaine 1% with epinephrine in 10 cc syringe with 22-gauge ⅝-inch needle
- No. 11 scalpel blade with handle
- Size 4 to 6 endotracheal tubes or size 4 to 6 cuffed tracheostomy tubes
- Mosquito clamps (2)
- Kelly clamps (2)
- 10 cc syringe
- Adhesive tape
- Self-refilling bag-valve-mask unit (Ambu-bag), with tubing and oxygen source
- Suction and suction catheters
- Tracheal dilator (Delaborde) if available with curved scissors (Dilators are usually available in tracheostomy sets.)

Preprocedure Patient Education

No patient education is needed in the emergency setting. Risks include intraoperative bleeding, aspiration, infection, and subsequent tracheal stenosis at the cuff site. Documentation should be made in the patient's chart that an explanation of the procedure was given, if time allowed it.

Technique

1. Position the patient in the supine position with a towel between the shoulders and with the neck slightly hyperextended.
2. Clean the neck with povidone-iodine (if time allows).
3. Observe sterile technique (cap, gloves, mask, and drapes) if time allows, and universal blood and body fluid precautions.
4. Identify the cricothyroid membrane, which is located between the thyroid and cricoid cartilages (Fig. 43-1). It is the first indentation inferior to the hard thyroid cartilage, and it should be easily palpable even in obese individuals.
5. If the patient is awake, infiltrate lidocaine in a line across the membrane using the 10 cc syringe with the 22-gauge needle.
6. Immobilize the thyroid cartilage, and hold the skin taut over the cricothyroid membrane. Using the No. 11 blade, puncture the skin and cricothyroid membrane transversely to enter the trachea (Fig. 43-2). The posterior aspect of the cricoid cartilage should be avoided, but if the knife goes too deep, the cricoid cartilage should stop the progression of the knife.

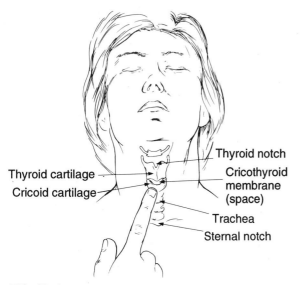

FIG. 43-1.
Identify cricothyroid membrane.

Thyroid notch
Cricothyroid membrane (space)
Thyroid cartilage
Cricoid cartilage
Trachea
Sternal notch

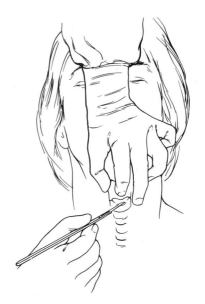

FIG. 43-2.
Open cricothyroid membrane.

7. Extend the incision laterally (a tracheal dilator can also be used in conjunction with spreading curved scissors for blunt extension) for approximately 1 cm on each side of the midline.
8. Insert a mosquito or Kelly clamp with the points downward into the incision and spread. A rush of air indicates patency of the airway.
9. Insert the endotracheal or tracheostomy tube through the incision (Fig. 43-3).
10. Connect the bag-valve unit to the tube and ventilate with 100% oxygen. Check for bilateral breath sounds to assure that the tube is properly placed and above the carina.
11. Inflate the cuff with enough air to stop any audible air leaks.

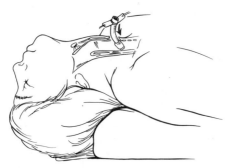

FIG. 43-3.
Insert tube into the incision.

12. Secure the tube and then apply a dressing. If an endotracheal tube is being used, secure the tube in place using tape. If a tracheostomy tube is being used, secure the tube with umbilical tape around the patient's neck.
13. Suction the trachea.
14. Obtain laboratory tests for arterial blood gases and a chest X-ray immediately.

Postprocedure Patient Education

If prolonged airway management is needed, convert the cricothyroidotomy to a tracheostomy and provide the appropriate patient education.

Complications

- Intraoperative and postoperative bleeding (Direct pressure will usually stop bleeding after the airway is established.)
- Hoarseness
- Misplaced tube placement with asphyxia
- Perforated esophagus
- Development of subglottic stenosis

TRACHEOSTOMY

Indications

- Laryngeal obstruction with or without temporary airway established by needle or surgical cricothyroidotomy
- Anticipated prolonged endotracheal intubation (more than 48 to 72 hours)
- Facial trauma
- Tracheal trauma
- Fractured larynx

Contraindications

- Lack of familiarity with the procedure
- Known preexisting laryngeal pathology
- Uncontrolled coagulopathy

Equipment

- Povidone-iodine (Betadine) solution
- Alcohol swabs
- 4 × 4 inch sterile gauze sponges
- Sterile gown, gloves, mask, goggles
- Sterile fenestrated drape
- 10 cc and 50 cc syringes

- 22- and 25-gauge ⅝-inch needle
- No. 15 scalpel blade with handle
- Mosquito hemostats (4)
- Trousseau dilator
- Allis clamps (2)
- Subcutaneous retractor
- Tracheal hook
- Tracheostomy tubes (various sizes)
- Needle holder
- Umbilical tape
- Suction apparatus and tubing
- Ventilation equipment: bag-valve-mask unit (Ambu-bag), with tubing and 100% oxygen available
- 3-0 Dexon or chromic absorbable suture on a cutting needle

Note: A very small, permanent indwelling transtracheal catheter is now available for continuous oxygen therapy. It is inserted under elective conditions below the crycothyroid membrane. (Scoop Transtracheal Catheters, Greenwood Village, Colorado: 800-527-2667)

Preprocedure Patient Education

Education of the patient and/or family should include the indication for tracheostomy and possible complications.

Technique

1. Position the patient in the supine position with a roll under the shoulders and with the neck extended (Fig. 43-4). (This position may be contraindicated in patients with epiglottitis or croup.) Placement of an endotracheal tube before elective tracheostomy or leaving an existing tube allows for better airway control and minimizes complications, especially in children. However, general anesthesia must be used for alert patients.
2. Prep the neck with povidone-iodine and apply the fenestrated drape.

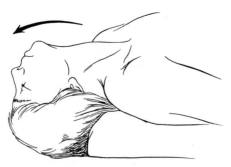

FIG. 43-4.
Position the patient.

3. Check the tracheostomy tube cuff for leaks. A second tube should be tested and available, if possible.
4. Palpate landmarks—the sternal notch, cricoid cartilage, and inferior border of the thyroid cartilage.
5. For conscious patients, inject lidocaine subcutaneously in the midline from the larynx to the fourth tracheal ring. Lidocaine can be injected down to the anterior tracheal wall.
6. Using the scalpel, make a vertical incision through skin and subcutaneous tissue to the strap muscles (pink color) approximately 4 to 6 cm superior to the sternal notch (Fig. 43-5).
7. Clamp the subcutaneous tissue with Allis clamps and retract laterally. Incise the fascia between the strap muscles in the midline and down to the pretracheal fascia (Fig. 43-6).

Note: Often the strap muscles are fused in the midline and can be covered by a network of troublesome veins. Attempts should be made to separate these veins. Occasionally they will have to be ligated.

8. Place retractor beneath the strap muscles and apply traction laterally. Incise the pretracheal fascia to expose the thyroid isthmus and tracheal ring (Fig. 43-7).
9. Retract the thyroid isthmus superiorly, if visible. If exposure is inadequate, extend the incision toward the sternal notch. If this is not possible, it may be necessary to divide the thyroid isthmus with clamps and suture the ligated edges (Fig. 43-8).

Note: It is important to remain in the midline with this procedure to minimize complications, especially in children.

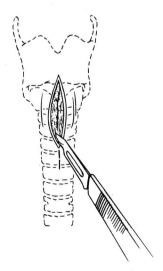

FIG. 43-5.
Make a vertical incision through the skin.

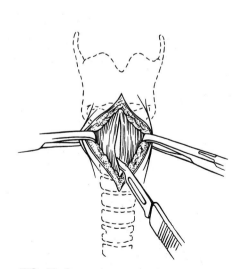

FIG. 43-6.
Clamp subcutaneous tissues and retract. Incise the fascia.

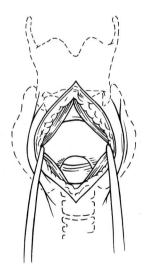

FIG. 43-7.
Place the retractor beneath the strap muscles.

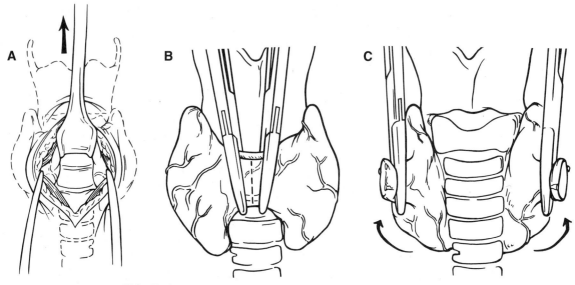

FIG. 43-8.
Retract the thyroid isthmus (**A**). If not possible, clamp (**B**) and divide (**C**).

10. If you are unsure that the object visualized is the trachea, you may wish to aspirate for air with a small-bore needle for confirmation before proceeding. After confirmation, place a tracheal hook into the first tracheal ring and elevate it anteriorly.
11. Make a transverse incision between the second and third ring (Fig. 43-9). Be prepared for a spurt of blood, air, or sputum and have suction ready.

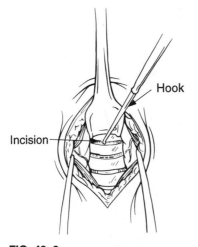

FIG. 43-9.
Place the tracheal hook in the first tracheal ring and elevate anteriorly. Make the incision between the second and third ring.

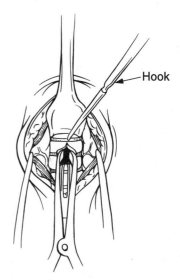

FIG. 43-10.
Insert the dilator into the trachea.

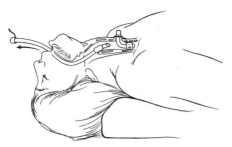

FIG. 43-11.
Remove the endotracheal tube and insert the tracheostomy tube.

12. Insert a Trousseau dilator into the trachea and dilate (Fig. 43-10).
13. Remove the endotracheal tube (if one is in place) and insert the tracheostomy tube through the dilator. Remove the dilator (Fig. 43-11).
14. Attach the tube to the Ambu-bag device and check for bilateral breath sounds with ventilation.
15. Secure tracheostomy tube around the neck with umbilical tape or with suture.
16. Apply a sterile dressing to the tube.
17. A chest X-ray should be taken immediately to assess placement and ventilation.

Postprocedure Patient Education

The patient will initially be cared for in the hospital and no postprocedure education will be necessary. If the patient is discharged with a tracheostomy, the patient will need someone trained to care for him or her.

Complications

In some studies of tracheostomy in children, mortality has been very high from the complications listed below, as well as from such complications as torn carotid arteries and completely severed tracheas.

- Bleeding
- Subcutaneous emphysema
- Pneumomediastinum
- Pneumothorax
- Tracheoesophageal fistula
- Recurrent laryngeal nerve damage
- Aspiration
- Malpositioned tube
- Tracheal stenosis
- Dysphagia
- Sepsis

Note: Placement of tracheostomies can be technically difficult, especially in children, obese patients, and patients with deformed or fixed cervical spines. They should be avoided, if possible, in emergency situations and performed at a later date under more controlled circumstances for these individuals.

CPT/BILLING CODES

31600	Tracheostomy, planned (separate procedure)
31603	Tracheostomy, emergency procedure; transtracheal
31605	Tracheostomy, cricothyroid membrane

BIBLIOGRAPHY

Cutler BS: Cricothyroidotomy for emergency airway, *Atlas of Bedside Procedures* 1(1):169, 1979.

Piotrowski JJ, Moore EE: Emergency department tracheostomy, *Emerg Med Clin North Am* 6:737, 1988.

Steinkraus L: Emergency cricothyroidotomy, *Patient Care* 21(9):147, 1987.

Subcommittee on Advanced Trauma Life Support: *ATLS student manual,* Chicago, 1993, American College of Surgeons Committee on Trauma.

CHAPTER 44

Reduction of Dislocated Temporomandibular Joint

Richard J. Bakeman

Grant C. Fowler

With trauma to the face and jaws, the temporomandibular joint (TMJ) is often affected. A blow to the chin while the mouth is slightly open is capable of causing an acute dislocation, which can be unilateral or bilateral. In addition, laughing excessively, stretching the mouth to its maximum open position, or yawning may cause a luxation of the TMJ. Dislocation occurs when the muscles and ligaments supporting the mandible are relaxed enough to allow the condyle to jump anteriorly or posteriorly over the articular eminence of the fossa. The luxation of the joint is exhibited by an open mouth that cannot be closed. Also, swallowing and talking are difficult. Unilateral dislocation causes a deviation away from the affected side. Once the dislocation occurs, trismus and muscle spasm prevent the joint from returning to its natural position.

INDICATIONS

- Unilateral or bilateral temporomandibular joint dislocation(s) without fractures (The dislocation should be confirmed with radiographs to rule out the possibility of a fracture.)

CONTRAINDICATIONS

- Fractured condyles (Patient should be referred to a maxillofacial surgeon.)

EQUIPMENT

- Gloves
- Parenteral muscle relaxation may be helpful (e.g., diazepam [Valium])
- Examination chair with firm neck rest
- *Optional:* 5 cc of 2% lidocaine in a 10 cc syringe with a 25-gauge needle
- *Optional:* povidone-iodine (Betadine) solution

PREPROCEDURE PATIENT EDUCATION

Inform patients that they may experience a feeling of considerable pressure on the molars as the joint is reduced. They may also experience some referred pain to the neck, face, or ear, as well as mild, aching TMJ arthralgia after the reduction. Stress the importance of relaxation and immobility during the reduction.

TECHNIQUE

Muscle spasms may be severe enough to inhibit simple reduction of the dislocated TMJ. Administering appropriate titrating doses of a muscle-relaxing drug, such as diazepam IV, is one possible approach to the problem. Often, if the muscle relaxant is titrated, the reduction of the joint occurs spontaneously.

Alternatively, after preparing the site with povidone-iodine, an injection of 3 to 5 cc of lidocaine into the TMJ may allow for spontaneous reduction (Fig. 44-1). One theory suggests that the dislocation is maintained by muscle spasm caused by painful stimuli arising from the capsule. A few minutes after localized unilateral injection, even with bilateral dislocation, the patient might be able to close the

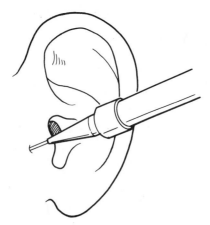

FIG. 44-1.
Injection of lidocaine into the joint.

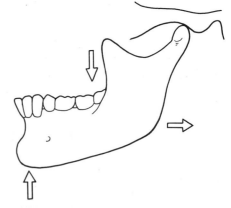

FIG. 44-2.
Direction and magnitude of force.

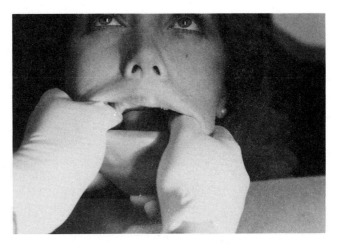

FIG. 44-3.
Reduction of a dislocated mandible from a position in front of the patient.

mouth and retract the mandible into its normal position. If passive reduction by muscle relaxation is not successful, active reduction may be necessary.

While standing in front of the patient, place the thumbs on the occlusal surfaces of the posterior lower teeth. Support the base of the mandible with the fingertips. Exert downward force on the molars (Fig. 44-2), and the condyles should clear the articular eminence. At the same time, apply very light pressure in a posterior direction and elevate the chin, sliding the mandible into its normal closed position (Fig. 44-3). Take care to protect your thumbs, since the mandible may snap sharply back into place. Gauze can be wrapped over the thumbs for protection. Should these procedures fail, use general anesthesia.

RECURRENT DISLOCATIONS

Search for possible causes:

• Occlusional disharmony resulting in muscle spasm
• Phenothiazine-induced trismus

POSTPROCEDURE PATIENT EDUCATION

In some instances, immobilization of the jaw is needed after reduction. For immobilization, refer the patient to a dentist. Some immobilize up to 2 weeks to allow the stretched muscles and ligaments an opportunity to heal and the edema to subside. If this precaution is not followed, the dislocation may recur. If the dislocation was not traumatic, inform the patient that reproducing the action that caused the dislocation will again result in dislocation. This is particularly true during the following 4 to 6 weeks while the ligaments heal. Warn the patient that recurrent dislocation may lead to permanent TMJ arthritis. In recurrent TMJ dislocation, the jaw should remain immobilized for 4 to 6 weeks, and the patient referred.

COMPLICATIONS (ALL RARE)

- Posterior dislocation of TMJ from reduction of anterior dislocation
- Anesthesia complications (e.g., allergic reaction to lidocaine)
- Permanent temporomandibular joint arthritis related to improperly managed, undiagnosed condylar fracture extending into the articular surface or from prolonged disarticulation (several days) or recurrent disarticulation

CPT/BILLING CODES

21480   Uncomplicated treatment of temporomandibular dislocation, initial or subsequent

21485   Complicated treatment of temporomandibular dislocation, initial or subsequent

BIBLIOGRAPHY

Henny A: The temporomandibular joint. In Kruger BS, editor: *Textbook of oral and maxillofacial surgery,* St Louis, 1979, Mosby.

Rowe NL, Williams JL: *Maxillofacial injuries,* vol I, New York, 1985, Churchill Livingstone.

Thoma KH: *Oral surgery,* vol I, St Louis, 1969, Mosby.

CHAPTER 45

Reimplantation of an Avulsed Tooth

Richard J. Bakeman

Grant C. Fowler

Traumatic damage to a tooth, ranging from a slight enamel chip to avulsion, is one of the most common injuries to the face. The primary care physician, in many instances, will be the first person to evaluate such injuries. Therefore, it is of great importance that physicians know the proper management.

Teeth are held in place by surrounding periodontal membrane fibers (Fig. 45-1). With trauma, these fibers may be concussed (Fig. 45-2), or an entire tooth may be avulsed (Fig. 45-3). In the event of avulsion, the blood supply must be restored by rapid reimplantation for the tooth to remain vital.

In addition, the proper storage and the duration of displacement of avulsed teeth are crucial factors in the success of reimplantation. Prognosis deteriorates rapidly as the tooth dries out, causing pulpal and periodontal damage.

Storage media available to prevent drying include physiologic (normal) saline, blood, milk, and saliva. These fluids have an osmotic pressure similar to those of the pulp and periodontal tissues and may help to preserve a tooth until it is reimplanted.

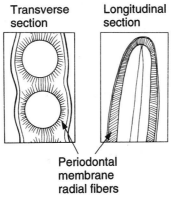

Transverse section

Longitudinal section

Periodontal membrane radial fibers

FIG. 45-1.
Arrangement of periodontal fibers.

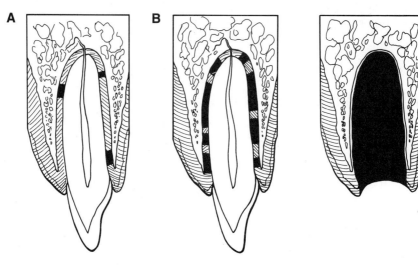

FIG. 45-2.
Slightly (**A**) and moderately (**B**) concussed tooth.

FIG. 45-3.
Avulsed tooth.

INDICATIONS

- Avulsed permanent tooth with minimal pulpal and periodontal damage, especially a tooth from the front of the mouth
- Tooth out of its socket for only a brief period of time
- Tooth stored in the proper physiologic medium

  Note: Saliva is a physiologic medium; therefore, the tooth can be stored in the patient's mouth (under the tongue), or in the mouth of a relative if the patient is unconscious, until reimplantation. Universal blood and body fluid precautions should be observed.

CONTRAINDICATIONS

- Deciduous (milk or temporary) teeth should not be reimplanted
- Gross caries or fractures in an avulsed tooth
- Significant loss of periodontal support before traumatic incident (periodontitis)
- Nonvital periodontal ligament (tooth has dried for one hour or more)

EQUIPMENT

- Sterile normal saline
- Irrigation syringe
- Local anesthetic and syringe
- Cotton gauze or tooth forceps
- Dental radiograph equipment and supplies

- Penicillin VK 500 mg tablets (18 to 26 tablets) or parenteral antobiotics for those at risk (See Chapter 133, Antibiotic Prophylaxis for Bacterial Endocarditis.)

PREPROCEDURE PATIENT EDUCATION

Explain the possible complications and the need for follow-up to the patient.

TECHNIQUE

1. Place the avulsed tooth in normal saline as soon as possible.
2. If the patient is at risk for bacteremia, administer parenteral antibiotics.
3. Conduct a systemic evaluation of traumatized individual (medical history).
   - Where, how, and when did the trauma occur? Are there fractures?
   - Is there any neurologic damage? Unconsciousness? Amnesia? Headache? Nausea?
   - Are there any underlying medical conditions? Immunocompromise? Diabetes? Prostheses or severe mitral valve prolapse? Heart murmurs?
4. Administer local anesthetic to the area if necessary.
5. Clinical examination:
   - Are there any other intraoral lacerations or disturbances?
   - Is the bite disturbed by other displaced teeth?
6. Take an X-ray of the area, if possible.
7. Examine the tooth socket and flush with normal saline. Remove all clot material.
8. Rinse the root and apex of the tooth with normal saline, being careful not to handle the root surface.
9. Hold the tooth with gauze or tooth forceps and replant the tooth as close as possible to its normal position using finger pressure. *Do not touch the root.*
10. Refer to a dentist for semirigid splinting and follow-up.
11. Administer penicillin VK 1 gram immediately (for those not already given parenteral dose), then 500 milligrams 4 times a day for 4 to 6 days (for those not allergic to penicillin).
12. Administer tetanus toxoid if the patient has not had a booster within 5 years.

POSTPROCEDURE PATIENT EDUCATION

Inform the patient that the prognosis depends on the length of time the tooth was out of the socket and the medium in which the avulsed tooth was stored. Fortunately, a tooth has two sources of blood supply (Fig. 45-4). However, pulpal revascularization of the pulpal arterioles is almost nonexistent in teeth after complete root development. It is unusual even with immature root development. Periodontal ligament preservation is also infrequent and dependent on the length of drying time to which the tooth was exposed. Fortunately, the periodontal ligament has a more diffuse blood supply and revascularizes more readily.

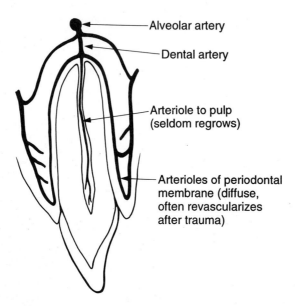

Alveolar artery

Dental artery

Arteriole to pulp
(seldom regrows)

Arterioles of periodontal
membrane (diffuse,
often revascularizes
after trauma)

FIG. 45-4.
Blood supply to tooth.

However, stress the importance of consulting a dentist for the appropriate follow-up care, especially for splinting to the next tooth.

COMPLICATIONS

- Necrosis of the pulp or periodontal ligament or complete loss of the tooth may occur. (Necrotic pulp tissue necessitates subsequent endodontic therapy.)
- With a nonvital periodontal ligament, ankylosis or osteoclastic root resorption may occur. This result requires an immediate root canal with calcium hydroxide root canal dressing.
- Bacteremia infection is a remote possibility.

CPT/BILLING CODE

D7270   Tooth reimplantation and/or stabilization of accidentally avulsed or displaced tooth and/or alveolus (HCPCS Code)

BIBLIOGRAPHY

Andreasen JO, Andreasen FM: *Essentials of traumatic injuries to the teeth*, Copenhagen, 1990, Munksgaard.

Ingle JI et al: Diagnosis and treatment of traumatic injuries and their sequelae. In Ingle JI, Beveridge EE, editors: *Endodontics*, Philadelphia, 1976, Lea and Febiger.

Rowe NL, Williams JL: *Maxillofacial injuries*, New York, 1985, Churchill Livingstone.

CHAPTER 46

Tongue-Tie Snipping (Frenotomy) for Ankyloglossia

Gary R. Newkirk

"Tongue-tie," or ankyloglossia, can be maxillary or mandibular. Maxillary ankyloglossia occurs when the tongue is ankylosed to the hard palate, the alveolar ridge, or the lower septal edge if cleft palate coexists. Mandibular ankyloglossia results from underdevelopment of the lingual frenulum, with the frenulum attaching in the midline near the tip of the tongue, along the floor of the mouth to the gingiva.

Infants and children differ substantially in the degree to which the frenulum attaches to the tongue. Most cases of tongue-tie are thought to resolve spontaneously by adulthood with little likelihood of feeding or speech-development problems. Usually, parents are the first to notice tongue-tie in their infant or child and bring this to the clinician's attention (Fig. 46-1). The condition can easily be

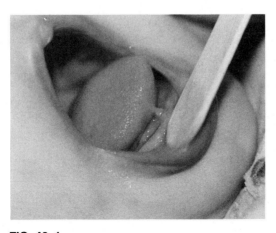

FIG. 46-1.
An 8-week-old infant with ankyloglossia (tongue-tie) noticed by the parents. This finding was not identified at the time of the newborn examination.

overlooked during the newborn examination, since infants typically retract their tongue when the mouth is opened, covering the short frenulum. Furthermore, newborn infants rarely stick their tongue out, which further obscures the limited tongue protrusion that accompanies this finding.

Since tongue-tie is a rare condition that lacks a precise definition, there have been no formal outcome studies comparing infants who have and who have not undergone frenotomy. However, problems with sucking, breastfeeding, chewing, swallowing, dentofacial growth and development, gingival hygiene, and speech have all been attributed to tongue-tie. Some researchers feel that the parents, not the child, have the problem. Others feel that simple frenotomy (referred to as snipping) remains a quick, easy, and safe procedure with benefits—even if only cosmetic—that in some instances outweigh the family anxiety generated by this condition.

The best method and timing for reducing partial ankyloglossia remains debatable as well. When ankyloglossia *severely* interferes with lingual function (e.g., "frozen tongue") few would argue the need for reduction; but in this case, Z-plasty is necessary, and the patient should be referred to a surgeon, since this procedure requires general anesthesia. Some clinicians feel if partial ankyloglossia contributes to poor infant sucking and other breastfeeding problems such as insufficient infant weight gain, or sore nipples or recurrent mastitis in the mother, frenotomy should be attempted. Simple frenotomy for infants and small children who have partial ankyloglossia can be performed readily in the outpatient setting.

INDICATIONS

- Clinical evidence of short lingual frenulum inhibiting tongue protrusion, feeding, swallowing, or speech

CONTRAINDICATIONS

- Lack of clinical evidence or suspicion that ankyloglossia is problematic to the infant or child
- Unstable medical conditions, such as bleeding disorders or diabetes mellitus
- Severe ankyloglossia, which requires frenectomy under general anesthesia (Usually this procedure involves Z-plasty or similar plastics reduction.)

EQUIPMENT

- Tongue retractor
- Small Metzenbaum scissors
- Small mosquito clip or hemostat
- Topical benzocaine 20% (e.g., Hurricane syrup)
- Lidocaine 1% with epinephrine
- Cotton-tipped swabs

PREPROCEDURE PATIENT EDUCATION

Describe the risks, including possible medication reaction (if used), injury, infection, and bleeding.

TECHNIQUE

1. Parents may help position and hold small infants or children if willing. *Note:* Crying often improves exposure of the frenulum.
2. Identify the frenulum and the degree of surgical lysis necessary. A limited "snipping" of the lucent, membranous portions of the distal frenulum is usually all that is required.
3. Dip a cotton-tipped swab in Hurricaine syrup to provide excellent local anesthesia. (Many clinicians clip membranous distal frenulums without topical agents.)
4. Retract the tongue (a small spoon or wooden tongue blade with a slit fashioned in the end works well).
5. With the tip of the mosquito clamp, grab and crush the frenulum to a depth and at the position where the scissor snip is to be made (Fig. 46-2, *A*).
6. Snip the crushed portion of the frenulum (Fig. 46-2, *B*).
7. Use a dry cotton-tipped swab, or one soaked in 1% lidocaine with epinephrine, to control oozing.

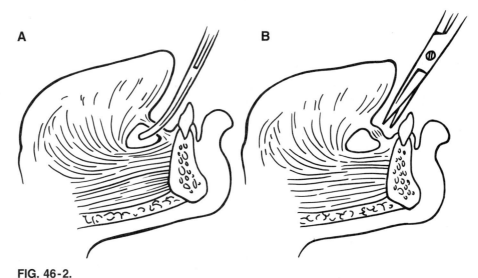

FIG. 46-2.
Tongue-tie snipping technique. **A,** Crush the frenulum where the snip is to be made. **B,** Cut through the crushed area.

POSTPROCEDURE PATIENT EDUCATION

- Ask the patient (or parent) to report significant bleeding or signs of infection.
- Instruct parent(s) to allow infants and children to resume normal feeding habits immediately.
- Ask the patient (or parent) to report any feeding difficulties, or significant swelling.
- Inform the patient to return for follow-up in 2 weeks, or sooner if complications arise.

COMPLICATIONS

- Bleeding
- Infection
- Injury to tongue or sublingual mucosa or tissue

CPT/BILLING CODE

41010   Incision of lingual frenulum (frenotomy)

BIBLIOGRAPHY

Berstein L: Congenital defects of the oral cavity. In Paparella MM, Shumrick DA, editors: *Otolaryngology, vol 3, head and neck,* Philadelphia, 1973, W.B. Saunders.

Conway A: Ankyloglossia—to snip or not to snip; is that the question? (editorial) *J Hum Lact* 6(3):101, 1990.

Marmet C, Shell E, Marmet R: Neonatal frenotomy may be necessary to correct breastfeeding problems, *J Hum Lact* 6(3):117, 1990.

Paradise JL: Evaluation and treatment for ankyloglossia, *JAMA* 263:2371, 1990.

Ward N: Ankyloglossia; a case study in which clipping was not necessary, *J Hum Lact* 6(3):126, 1990.

PART FOUR

Cardiovascular and Respiratory

CHAPTER 47

Percutaneous Arterial Line Placement

Grant C. Fowler

Intraarterial procedures have become common, with arterial dye studies and angioplasty joining arterial cannulation as invasive procedures that involve the arteries. Support staff and facilities must be properly trained and prepared to deal with the potential complications arising from procedures like percutaneous arterial line placement, which are more invasive—and much more prone to result in the development of complications—than simple intravenous cannulation or arterial puncture. The site (radial, brachial, or femoral) should be chosen according to the risks and priorities established in Chapter 51, Arterial Puncture.

INDICATIONS

- When continuous monitoring of arterial blood pressure is desired, especially in patients in shock, patients with resultant increased systemic vascular resistance, and during major surgery or administration of parenteral vasopressor or dilator medications
- When continuous access to arterial blood is desired to avoid repeated arterial punctures
- To measure cardiac output by dye dilution method
- Labile or accelerated hypertension and evidence of progressive vascular damage (Mean arterial pressure is a much more consistent blood pressure monitoring parameter for accelerated hypertension than the systolic or diastolic pressure alone.)

CONTRAINDICATIONS

- Inadequate collateral blood flow to a distant site, i.e., positive Allen test (see Chapter 51, Arterial Puncture)
- Severe atherosclerotic or vasospastic arterial disease
- Hypercoagulable states

- Anticoagulation from bleeding disorders, anticoagulant therapy, or potential future thrombolytic therapy
- Local skin compromise, such as with infection or a burn

EQUIPMENT

- Sterile gloves, drapes, and 4 × 4 inch gauze sponges
- Antiseptic skin preparation, such as povidone-iodine
- *Optional:* 1% lidocaine without epinephrine and a 3 cc syringe with 25-gauge 5/8-inch (1.6 cm) needle (in the alert patient)
- Short arm board for radial and brachial artery cannulation; and a gauze roll, about 3 inches in diameter, for radial artery cannulation
- For radial or brachial artery cannulation, an 18- to 20-gauge, 1.25- to 2-inch (3.2 to 5.1 cm) Teflon catheter-over-needle with a nontapered shaft (Deseret Angiocath, Becton-Dickinson IV Cath, etc.)
- For femoral artery cannulation, a 16 cm cannula
- For the Seldinger technique, a flexible guide wire small enough to pass through the catheter and needle
- Fluid-filled connector tubing attached to transducer (A stiff, low-capacitance tubing minimizes artifact, and a minimal length should be used.)
- Antibiotic ointment, such as povidone-iodine
- Silk or nylon 4-0 suture, preferably on a skin needle
- Hypoallergenic adhesive tape
- Suture scissors
- Sterile threeway stopcock and bag of sterile dextrose water (D_5W) intravenous fluid mixed with heparin to make a 1U/ml solution for flushing (This should be in-line with the connector tubing.)
- Razor for femoral insertion
- *Optional:* handheld Doppler

PREPROCEDURE PATIENT EDUCATION

Explain the indications, complications, and necessity of the procedure to the patient. Discuss the importance of immobilization while the procedure is being performed, and warn the patient of the discomfort that will be felt with the insertion.

Inform the patient that this catheter is more dangerous than an intravenous catheter and that care must be taken with the catheter after insertion. Obtain written consent for the procedure.

TECHNIQUE

1. The physician and patient should be in a comfortable position that can be maintained as long as necessary. When using nonclosed systems, observe universal blood and body fluid precautions.

2. Palpate the artery selected and immobilize it with two or three fingers along its course.
3. Prep the skin in an aseptic manner. For femoral cannulation, also shave the groin.
4. Local anesthetic (lidocaine) can be injected for a particularly anxious patient. Use minimal amounts to prevent anatomical distortion with resultant increased difficulty when palpating the pulse.
5. Drape the area with sterile towels.
6. Wearing sterile gloves, hold the catheter needle hub like a pencil with the needle bevel up.
7a. *For radial artery cannulation:* On the nondominant hand, slightly extend and immobilize the wrist by taping a gauze roll between the supinated extended wrist and the dorsally applied arm board. Apply tape over the proximal interphalangeal joints (excluding the thumb) and around the armboard. Also apply tape more proximally, securing the forearm to the armboard. Insert the needle one-half inch to one inch proximal to the wrist crease at about a 30-degree angle, and direct it slowly toward the pulsation (Fig. 47-1).
7b. *For brachial artery cannulation:* This location should be reserved for use only when radial artery catherization is impossible. Extend, supinate, and immobilize the nondominant arm with tape and an arm board, preventing flexion at the elbow. Insert the needle at about a 30-degree angle and direct it toward the pulsation in the medial aspect of the antecubital fossa slightly above the elbow crease (see Chapter 51, Fig. 51-5).
7c. *For femoral artery cannulation:* With the patient in a supine position and legs straight, insert the needle at a 45-degree angle and direct it toward the femoral artery pulsation 2 to 5 cm distal to the inguinal ligament at the inguinal crease. After the flash of blood, the angle can be lowered to 20 or 30 degrees relative to the leg. Large hematomas are not uncommon because of the soft tissue surrounding the area. Femoral artery cannulation carries the risk of more serious complications. A puncture proximal to the inguinal ligament could produce a retroperitoneal hematoma. The location near the groin may increase the risk of infection. This location is also less popular for cannulation if the patient is awake and mobile (see Chapter 51, Fig. 51-6).

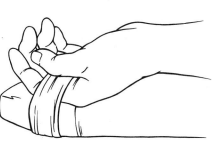
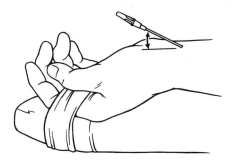

FIG. 47-1.
Position for radial artery cannulation.

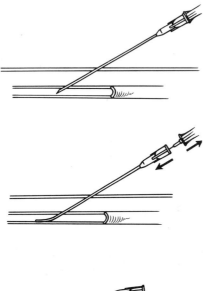

FIG. 47-2.

Insert the angiocatheter through the skin and cannulate the artery.

8. Puncture is detected when blood appears in the needle hub. For radial and brachial artery cannulation, while holding the needle fixed, advance the catheter-over-needle into the artery (Fig. 47-2). For femoral artery cannulation, do the same unless the Seldinger technique is desired. With the Seldinger technique, insert the wire through the needle into the artery, remove the needle, insert the catheter over the wire, and remove the wire. A modified Seldinger technique can be used for radial artery cannulation.

9. If the artery cannot be cannulated after the flash of blood has appeared, the posterior artery wall has probably been penetrated. Remove the needle entirely, slowly withdraw the catheter until blood flows into it, and readvance the catheter.

10. For the Seldinger technique, make sure the wire passes without *any* resistance at all to minimize the chance of intramural insertion or dissection.

11. If after three attempts, the artery has not been entered, discontinue the procedure on that side and attempt on the other side or at another site; a cutdown might also be considered. Pressure should be applied to the unsuccessful site for at least 10 minutes, followed by a pressure dressing.

12. After insertion, advance the catheter until the hub is in contact with the skin, and attach it to the connector tubing. Flush the catheter and observe the arterial tracing. It should be sharp and clean. If not, reposition the catheter. Otherwise, securely stitch it into position, apply antibiotic ointment, and

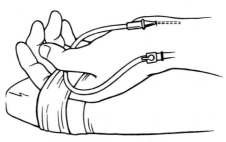

FIG. 47-3.
Attach to the catheter and fix in position.

cover with a sterile dressing (Fig. 47-3). For radial artery cannulation, remove the gauze roll.

13. While catheterized, the alert patient should be instructed to inform the staff
of any extremity pain, numbness, swelling or discoloration. The staff should
check the extremity every 4 hours for perfusion, and the site for signs of
hematoma, hemorrhage, or early cellulitis. The dressing should be changed
daily along with regular flushing of the line. Following catheter removal, observe the patient for bleeding, extremity pain, numbness, swelling or discoloration.

Note: The "liquid stylet" method may be useful in the non-Seldinger technique
cannulations. In those cases where a flash of blood is seen in the hub and the artery
cannot be cannulated, fill a 10 cc syringe with 5 cc of sterile normal saline. Attach the
syringe to the catheter hub, and aspirate 1 to 2 cc of blood to verify intraluminal
position. The blood should be very easy to aspirate. Slowly inject the fluid from the
syringe and advance the catheter behind the fluid wave.

Alternative Method for Radial Artery Cannulation: Doppler Ultrasound–Guided (Fig. 47-4)

1. Position the wrist in a slightly extended position and prep as previously described.
2. Using antiseptic ointment (such as povidone-iodine) as transmission gel, have
an assistant align the handheld Doppler with the radial artery and pass it back
and forth medial to lateral over the artery to determine the point of maximal
flow. The assistant should hold the Doppler in place at the point of maximal
volume.
3. Insert and advance the catheter slowly and with constant pressure at a 45-
degree angle to the skin directed toward the point of maximal flow.
4. Contact with the artery is discerned by a slight decrease in arterial flow sound.
5. As the needle compresses the artery before puncture, the flow sound may
transiently cease.
6. The characteristic sound of arterial blood flow should resume as the artery is
punctured and a flash of bright red blood is seen in the needle hub.
7. Advance the cannula and secure as described previously.

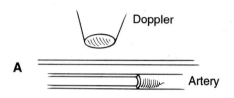

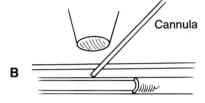

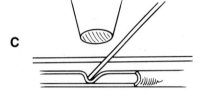

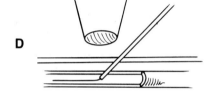

FIG. 47-4.
Radial artery cannulation is being guided by Doppler ultrasound. **A** and **B,** The Doppler locates the artery and helps in guiding the cannula. **C** and **D,** The catheter occludes the artery temporarily and then punctures the arterial wall and is placed intraluminally.

COMPLICATIONS

- Arterial thrombosis (risk minimized by reducing the duration of cannulation, by using larger arteries, and by flushing properly)
- Embolism
- Ischemia or necrosis distal to the site of arterial thrombosis or embolism
- Hemorrhage or local hematoma
- Aneurysm
- Infection
- Arteriovenous fistula
- Neurologic complications
- Vasovagal reactions
- Permanent radial artery stenosis or occlusion

Note: A vascular surgeon should be consulted immediately if arterial flow is compromised in any way.

CPT/BILLING CODE

36620   Arterial catheterization or cannulation for sampling, monitoring, or transfusion (separate procedure); percutaneous

BIBLIOGRAPHY

American Heart Association: *Textbook of advanced cardiac life support,* Dallas, 1988, The Association.

Maher JJ, Dougherty JM: Radial artery cannulation guided by Doppler ultrasound, *Am J Emerg Med* 7:260, May 1989.

May HL, editor: *Emergency medicine,* New York, 1984, John Wiley & Sons.

Roberts JR, Hedges JR, editors: *Clinical procedures in emergency medicine,* Philadelphia, 1985, W.B. Saunders.

CHAPTER 48

Central Venous Catheter Insertion

John F. Donnelly

John M. Passmore, Jr.

Over the past 25 years, the clinical use of central vein catheters has increased with other medical and technological advances, especially in emergency resuscitation protocols, sophisticated monitoring techniques, total parenteral nutrition, and transvenous pacemaker insertion.

Expeditious placement of large-bore central intravenous catheters presents a challenge to the physician, especially when dealing with the hypovolemic or critically ill patient. Fortunately, large veins (such as the subclavian vein and internal jugular vein) have constant, predictable relationships to easily identifiable anatomic landmarks.

Although peripheral veins can be used for many of the indications of central venous pressure (CVP) lines, they often require long catheters carefully guided into the superior or inferior vena cava. In other instances, peripheral veins may be collapsed, thrombosed, or otherwise difficult to locate or cannulate, and CVP lines remain the only option.

INDICATIONS

- Large-volume parenteral fluid administration (The fluid flow rate is directly proportional to the radius and length of the intravenous catheter. Therefore, if they are available and time allows, large-bore catheters are preferred for volume expansion. If access is available, a large-bore peripheral catheter is superior to a small-bore central catheter for large volume infusion.)
- Monitoring of central venous pressure
- Emergency venous access
- Administration of some medications (e.g., chemotherapy)
- Administration of hyperosmolar or irritating solutions, such as some parenteral

nutrition formulas (solutions associated with thrombophlebitis when given through small peripheral veins, and those that can cause soft-tissue necrosis if extravasation occurs)
- Alternative for repetitive venous cannulations of chronically ill patients or patients with small, thrombosed, or difficult-to-find veins (Burn patients with burns on all extremities may require central access.)
- Placement of Swan-Ganz catheter
- Placement of temporary transvenous pacemaker
- Performance of cardiac catheterization and pulmonary angiography
- Performance of hemodialysis or plasmapheresis

CONTRAINDICATIONS

- Distortion of local anatomy or landmarks (may result from surgery, trauma, or irradiation to the area)
- For subclavian insertion, chest wall deformities (moderate to severe with distortion in local anatomy or landmarks)
- Suspected injury to the superior vena cava (e.g., superior vena cava syndrome in which venous access below the diaphragm is preferable)
- Bleeding diathesis or anticoagulation therapy
- Full-thickness burn, cellulitis, or other infection over the anticipated insertion site
- Pneumothorax or hemothorax on the contralateral side, or inability to tolerate pneumothorax on ipsilateral side
- Uncooperative or combative patients, and patients unable to tolerate Trendelenburg position
- Prior injection of a sclerosing agent in the intended vein

RELATIVE CONTRAINDICATIONS

- Suspected prior injury to the vein (The vein on the contralateral side should be utilized if no associated pneumothorax or hemothorax is present.)
- Morbid or marked obesity
- Marked cachexia
- Vasculitis that predisposes to sclerosis or thrombosis of the veins
- Previous long-term central catheterization or recently discontinued subclavian catheter in the same area
- Mastectomy proposed on the side of subclavian insertion
- Patients receiving ventilatory support that have high end expiratory pressures (If possible, ventilation should be briefly interrupted while the catheter-introducing needle is being employed to locate the vein.)
- Patients undergoing cardiopulmonary resuscitation (Interference with chest compressions and chest wall motion makes infraclavicular subclavian vein puncture more difficult and more risky. However, internal jugular and supra-

clavicular subclavian vein puncture only requires a relatively motionless neck rather than chest, and can usually be performed without interruption of cardiopulmonary resuscitation.)

- Children less than 2 years old (The risk of complications is higher. For central access, the internal jugular vein is the best route for central access.)
- Severe hypovolemia, if peripheral access can be obtained with a large-bore catheter (16-gauge or larger)

Additional contraindications specific to *internal jugular vein* cannulation include significant carotid artery disease; distorted cervical anatomy; and recent, unsuccessful contralateral cannulation (to prevent bilateral neck hematomas, which could compromise the patient's airway).

EQUIPMENT

- Sterile prep solution (povidone-iodine, or hexachlorophene if the patient is iodine-allergic)
- Sterile swabs
- Prep razor
- Sterile gloves
- Sterile drapes
- Lidocaine 1%
- Small anesthetizing needle (25-gauge)
- A 3 to 5 cc syringe for anesthetic
- A 10 cc syringe
- Intravenous solution and connector tubing
- Central venous catheter and insertion set (Many products are commercially available, and they usually consist of an introducing needle and a radiopaque catheter, which is typically 30.5 cm long.)
- Bath towel
- 4 × 4 inch sterile gauze pads
- Needle holder
- Silk or nylon sutures (3-0, or 4-0) on a cutting needle
- Suture scissors
- Topical antimicrobial ointment
- Tincture of benzoin
- Adhesive or cloth tape, precut lengths
- Completed chest radiograph request form
- Goggles

Many authorities recommend the Seldinger guide wire technique of central vein access. This method is also indicated for the insertion of Swan-Ganz catheters and temporary transvenous pacemakers. With the Seldinger technique, a needle that is much smaller than the infusion catheter is used to cannulate the vessel. A guide wire is subsequently threaded through the needle; the needle is removed while the guide wire is left in place in the vessel, and a catheter is advanced over the guide wire into the lumen of the vessel. To prevent dissecting the vein, the wire must be withdrawn slowly while the catheter is advanced. The major advantage of this technique is the expeditious placement of a large catheter into the central circulation using a small-gauge needle, with minimal trauma to a vessel that may be collapsed or hidden.

In addition to the equipment listed above, materials for the Seldinger technique include the following:

- Introducing needle
- Guide wire or J-wire (flexible wire 35 cm long, 0.089 cm in diameter with a 3 mm radius of curvature)
- Catheter or sheath introducer
- No. 11 blade and scalpel

It is recommended to utilize one brand of central vein catheter routinely and ensure that all personnel are familiar with its use.

PREPROCEDURE PATIENT EDUCATION

Obtain informed consent for this procedure. Inform the patient of the possibilities of major complications and their management, which could require chest tube placement, surgery, or cardioversion. To minimize patient anxiety during the procedure, explain the major steps of the procedure, the necessity of remaining in the Trendelenburg position possibly for some time, and the near impossibility of complete anesthesia.

TECHNIQUE

Subclavian Venipuncture

Anatomy

The subclavian vein begins as a continuation of the axillary vein at the lateral border of the first rib, and it joins the internal jugular vein to form the innominate vein (Fig. 48-1). As it crosses behind the first rib, the subclavian vein lies posterior to the medial third of the clavicle; it is only in this region that an intimate anatomic relationship exists between the subclavian vein and the clavicle. The subclavian vein is valveless and has a diameter of 1 to 2 cm. The costoclavicular ligament lies anterior and inferior to the subclavian vein. The subclavian artery is superior and posterior to the vein; the anterior scalene muscle separates the subclavian vein from the artery. Contiguous structures of significance include the phrenic nerve; the thoracic duct (on the left side); and the lymphatic duct (on the right side), which enters the subclavian vein near its juncture with the internal jugular; and the dome of the pleura of the lung, which may extend above the first rib on the left side, but rarely extends this far cephalad on the right.

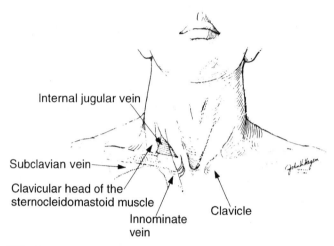

Internal jugular vein

Subclavian vein

Clavicular head of the
sternocleidomastoid muscle

Innominate
vein

Clavicle

FIG. 48-1.
Anatomic relationships of the subclavian vein. (From Schwartz RS et al: Cardiac catheterization and angiography. In Giuliani ER et al: *Cardiology: fundamentals and practice,* ed 2, St Louis, 1991, Mosby. © Mayo Foundation.)

Patient Position

Proper positioning of the patient is crucial for successful cannulation and for minimizing potential complications.

1. Place the patient in the Trendelenburg position at an angle of 15 to 30 degrees (or as much as the patient can tolerate). This position decreases the risk of air embolism by creating positive pressure inside the vein. The Trendelenburg position may also cause distension of the subclavian and internal jugular veins, which will make access easier. Raise the bed to a comfortable level for the operator.
2. Turn the patient's head to the opposite side. This may decrease the risk of contamination of the insertion site and minimize the patient's anxiety during the procedure. Turning the head to the opposite side has not been proven to influence vessel diameter or the relationship of the subclavian vein to the clavicle.
3. Consider placing a rolled bath towel between the patient's scapulae to allow the shoulders to fall backwards, making the clavicle more prominent. (Some physicians believe that the space between the clavicle and first rib narrows as the shoulders fall posteriorly, thereby making access to the subclavian vein more difficult.)
4. Both arms should be at the patient's sides, restrained if necessary, to prevent interference with the procedure.

Overview of the Procedure

1. You should obtain central access via the route with which you are most comfortable and most experienced. Inexperienced physicians should be supervised during the procedure. Sufficient knowledge of the regional anatomy is

important for successful cannulation of the central circulation and for minimal complications; however, you should keep in mind that each case is different, and always maintain a healthy respect for the possible complications of this procedure. It may help to outline the anatomy with a marking pen.

2. Strict adherence to sterile technique protocols is necessary to prevent infectious complications. Since optimal observation of aseptic technique is difficult during CPR, replace central lines placed during resuscitative efforts at the earliest opportunity.

Authors' note: We often administer one dose of prophylactic intravenous antibiotic therapy with cefazolin 1 g or vancomycin 500 mg to decrease the possibility of infection with skin pathogens if the CPR is successful.

3. Excluding intrinsic thoracic disease or other contraindications, the *right* subclavian vein is preferred over the left, because the dome of the pleura of the right lung is usually lower than the left, and because the large thoracic duct is not exposed to possible inadvertent laceration. If attempted catheterization is unsuccessful, try the ipsilateral internal jugular or supraclavicular approach before trying the contralateral subclavian; this reduces the risk of bilateral iatrogenic complications.

4. The desired final position of the catheter places the tip in the superior vena cava near the right atrium. Therefore, thread the catheter until it is approximately 2 to 3 cm below the manubrial-sternal junction. You can estimate this distance by placing the catheter parallel to the chest wall before insertion, and measuring the catheter with surface markers (Fig. 48-2).

Infraclavicular Approach
Procedure

1. Position the patient in the Trendelenburg position, with the head turned to the opposite side, as described.

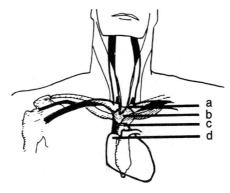

FIG. 48-2.
Surface markers on chest wall to determine length of catheter placement. *a,* Sternoclavicular joint, subclavian vein; *b,* Midmanubrial area, brachiocephalic vein; *c,* Manubrial-sternal junction, superior vena cava; *d,* 5 cm below manubrial-sternal junction, right atrium. (From *Textbook of advanced cardiac life support,* ed 2, Dallas, 1987, American Heart Association. Used with permission.)

2. Observe sterile technique and use sterile gloves. Some experts recommend use of a face mask, cap, and gown as well.

3. Scrub, shave, and prepare a wide area over the insertion site in sterile fashion. In sterile fashion, drape the infraclavicular and supraclavicular areas.

4. Assemble the introducing needle and 3 cc syringe, with the bevel of the needle aligned with the markings of the syringe. This alignment enhances awareness of the bevel direction after the skin is punctured.

5. Note important anatomic landmarks. Palpate the region that is inferior to the clavicle to locate the costoclavicular ligament connecting the first rib to the clavicle. This ligament lies at the junction of the medial third and middle third of the clavicle at the point where the clavicle bends posteriorly. Place your thumb over the costoclavicular ligament and your index finger in the suprasternal notch (Fig. 48-3). The subclavian vein traverses the imaginary line connecting these two points.

6. In the alert, conscious patient, anesthetize the skin at the puncture site with several milliliters of 1% lidocaine, using the 10 cc syringe and 25-gauge needle. Universal blood and body fluid precautions should be followed throughout the procedure. Anesthetize the subcutaneous tissue and periosteum of the clavicle along the anticipated route of cannulation. When anesthetizing, make sure that the needle is not in the vein before injecting lidocaine by aspirating as the needle is advanced.

7. Make sure that the bevel of the assembled introduction needle is aligned with the markings on the 3 cc syringe. It is helpful to fill the syringe with several milliliters of local anesthetic, so that during insertion, the subcutane-

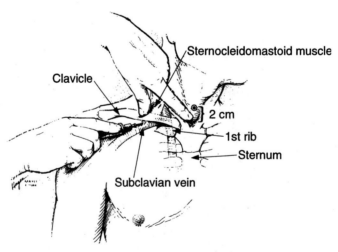

FIG. 48-3.

Technique of subclavian vein catheterization. With the index finger in the suprasternal notch and the thumb marking the costoclavicular ligament, insert the needle just medial to the thumb. (From Schwartz RS et al: Cardiac catheterization and angiography. In Giuliani ER et al: *Cardiology: fundamentals and practice,* ed 2, St Louis, 1991, Mosby. © Mayo Foundation.)

ous tissue can be further anesthetized as needed and so that the needle can be flushed of any skin plugs.

8. With your thumb over the costoclavicular ligament and index finger in the suprasternal notch, insert the needle caudad to the clavicle just medial to the thumb, and aim slightly cephalad and posterior to the index finger in the suprasternal notch.

9. If the patient is being ventilated with positive pressure, it is advisable to temporarily stop the ventilator or decrease the tidal volume as the needle punctures the chest wall. Ventilation should not be interrupted longer than 30 seconds. A respiratory therapist should be available to assist if necessary.

10. Advance the needle (while aspirating to detect puncture of a large vessel) at a 5- to 10-degree angle relative to the patient's chest wall until the needle contacts the patient's clavicle. At this point, decrease the angle of the needle so that it is parallel to the patient's chest wall, and carefully advance it under the clavicle while still directing it slightly cephalad to your finger in the suprasternal notch. Continue to aspirate, and advance the needle slowly while keeping the needle shaft parallel to the patient's chest wall (Fig. 48-4). Entry of the vein is indicated by a flash of dark venous blood, which usually occurs at a depth of 3 to 4 cm; blood return should flow freely if the needle is truly intraluminal and not lodged against the vessel wall.

Note: Some authorities recommend locating the vein first with a smaller needle, such as a 22-gauge needle attached to a 3 cc syringe. When the vein is located, the smaller needle is removed and the introductory needle assembly is directed at the same angle in the same direction.

11. A flash of pulsatile, bright red blood indicates inadvertent subclavian arterial puncture. In an elective situation, withdraw the needle and apply firm pres-

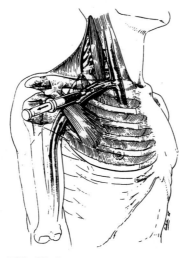

FIG. 48-4.
Proper needle advancement. See text for details. (From Phillips SJ: *Surg Gynecol Obstet* 127:1080, 1968. Used with permission.)

sure for 10 minutes over the puncture site. In an emergency situation, withdraw the needle and immediately repeat the process to attempt to cannulate the vein. The position of the artery should be noted to avoid puncturing it again.

12. If no flash of blood is observed, slowly withdraw the needle while maintaining negative pressure on the syringe. A flash will sometimes be encountered during needle withdrawal.

13. If the first attempt is unsuccessful, completely withdraw the needle and flush it with air to remove any tissue; otherwise, obstruction of the needle may result in failure of subsequent attempts. Repeat the process as previously described, but direct the needle approximately 5 degrees cephalad to the finger in the suprasternal notch and slightly more posteriorly.

Authors' note: We recommend changing the direction of the needle only after totally withdrawing it, to minimize the risk of puncturing neighboring structures. Seek assistance after three to four attempts, or consider cannulating the ipsilateral internal jugular vein or contralateral subclavian vein (after chest X-ray to rule out pneumothorax).

14. When the vein has been successfully entered, rotate the needle so that the bevel (which is still aligned with the syringe markings) faces caudally. Verify that blood flows freely with aspiration: rotating the needle may place its tip against the vessel wall. If blood does not flow freely, carefully withdraw or advance the needle 1 to 2 mm while aspirating slightly.

15. When the needle is positioned properly, stabilize it by grasping it with your thumb and index finger, and by firmly pressing it against the chest, while detaching the syringe. Immediately occlude the needle hub with your thumb to prevent air embolus. During this step, ask the alert patient to perform a Valsalva maneuver or to exhale, to raise intrathoracic pressure. If the syringe is firmly affixed to the needle, hemostats may be useful to grasp and anchor the needle during removal of the syringe; this may minimize the risk of needle displacement from the vessel lumen. Do not draw blood specimens until the catheter is securely threaded into the vessel. Drawing blood through the needle increases the chance of displacing the needle tip from the vessel lumen.

16. **Catheter-through-the-needle devices.**

    a. Quickly thread the catheter through the needle while stabilizing the needle with the other hand (Fig. 48-5). The catheter should advance without resistance. If resistance occurs, *do not force* the catheter; rather, recheck for blood return by aspirating before advancing the catheter again. Gently twisting and advancing the catheter may free a catheter trapped against the opposite vessel wall or one advanced past the junction of the subclavian vein and internal jugular veins. It may also help to unwind a kinked catheter. If the catheter cannot be advanced despite these measures, withdraw the catheter and needle as a unit. *Do not withdraw the catheter alone through the needle, since this may transect the catheter and result in a catheter fragment embolus.*

    b. When the catheter threads smoothly, advance it fully into the needle hub toward its desired final position in the super vena cava. If the patient is

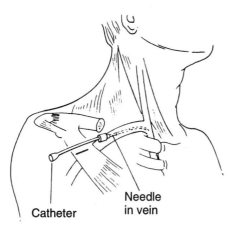

FIG. 48-5.
Catheter threading. After removal of the syringe, thread the catheter fully into the needle. (Used with permission of W.B. Saunders.)

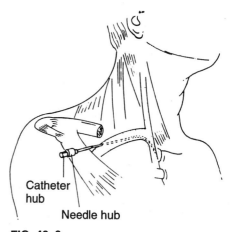

FIG. 48-6.
Withdrawal of the needle leaves only the catheter beneath the skin and in the vein. (From James P, Myers R: *Ann Surg* 175:695, 1972. Used with permission.)

cardiac monitored, the operator or assistant should observe the monitor for dysrhythmias while the catheter is advanced.

c. Withdraw the needle from the vein over the catheter until it is just outside the skin (Fig. 48-6).

d. Immediately attach the guard over the needle (Fig. 48-7).

e. Attach the syringe to the catheter hub and attempt to aspirate blood. Free blood return is presumptive, but not definitive, evidence of intravascular position of the catheter. (Blood return may also occur with hematoma or hemothorax if the catheter is not positioned within the vessel lumen.)

f. If blood return is obtained, remove the syringe and connect the intravenous tubing to the catheter hub. Before infusing intravenous fluids, lower the intravenous solution bag beside the bed to a level below the patient, and observe for backflow of blood. This further confirms intravascular catheter position.

g. Secure the catheter at the insertion site by placing a 3-0 or 4-0 silk suture through the skin, tying it, looping it around the catheter three to four times, and tying the suture again (Fig. 48-8). Ensure that the catheter lumen is not constricted by the suture. Alternatively, the needle guard may be affixed to the chest wall at two points parallel and caudad to the clavicle by placing silk suture through the skin and the two holes of the needle guard.

h. Apply antimicrobial ointment to the insertion site and cover it with a sterile 4 × 4 inch gauze sponge with a transparent cover to facilitate routine inspection. Tape the dressing in place. It is advisable to incorporate the catheter hub within the tape to minimize the risk of accidental disconnection (Fig. 48-8).

i. Ensure again that the catheter is neither kinked nor sharply angulated, check the integrity and patency of all connections, and tape all connections.

j. Remove the patient from the Trendelenburg position.

k. Confirm breath sounds bilaterally by auscultation to exclude the possibility of pneumothorax.

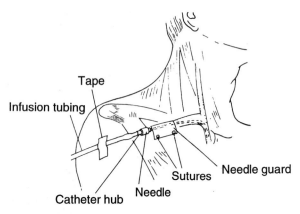

FIG. 48-7.
Place the guard and suture beneath the clavicle. (From Vander Salm TJ et al: *Atlas of bedside procedures,* Boston, 1979, Little, Brown & Co. Used with permission.)

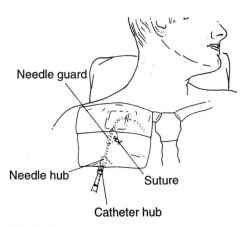

FIG. 48-8.
Alternative method of securing the subclavian catheter to allow free use of the arm. (From Vander Salm TJ et al: *Atlas of bedside procedures,* Boston, 1979, Little, Brown & Co. Used with permission.)

l. Order an immediate chest X-ray (preferably with the patient in the erect or semierect position) to verify catheter position and to check for possible pneumothorax or hemothorax. Reposition inadequately placed catheters. Obtain chest X-rays after unsuccessful attempts as well.

Catheter-over-needle-devices.

Advance the needle as described in Step 10 until venous backflow is observed. At this point, the needle tip, but not necessarily the catheter, is in the vessel lumen. Advance the needle 1 to 2 mm, then advance the catheter over the needle into the vessel lumen. Once the catheter is successfully threaded, withdraw the needle and syringe. Immediately place your thumb over the catheter hub to prevent air embolus, and connect the intravenous tubing after flushing it with fluids. *Again, never withdraw the catheter by itself, since this may result in a catheter fragment embolus.* Demonstrate backflow of blood by lowering the IV bag below the patient, secure and dress the catheter, and obtain an immediate chest X-ray.

Seldinger technique.

a. Advance an introducing needle large enough to accommodate the guide wire as described in Step 10 until venous backflow is noted.

b. Remove the syringe; occlude the needle hub with your thumb (Fig. 48-9, *A*), and thread the flexible end of the guide wire through the needle (Fig. 48-9, *B*). The guide wire should advance smoothly. If resistance occurs, gently rotate the needle and guide wire. If this maneuver is unsuccessful, withdraw the guide wire, reattach the syringe, and aspirate to determine if the needle is still positioned within the vessel lumen. Thread the guide wire until at least one fourth of its length is within the vessel lumen. If the patient is undergoing cardiac monitoring, watch the cardiac monitor for dysrhythmias that may result as the guide wire is advanced.

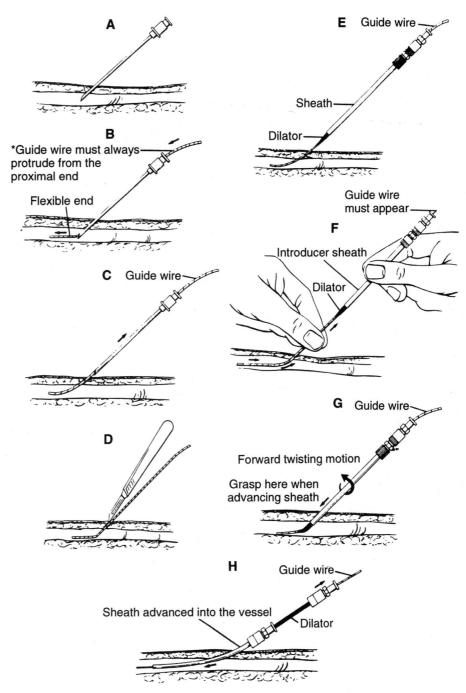

A

B

*Guide wire must always
protrude from the
proximal end

Flexible end

C   Guide wire

D

E   Guide wire

Sheath

Dilator

Guide wire
must appear

F

Introducer sheath

Dilator

G   Guide wire

Forward twisting motion

Grasp here when
advancing sheath

H   Guide wire

Sheath advanced into the vessel

Dilator

FIG. 48-9.
Placement of Seldinger-type guide wire and catheter. See text for details. (From Roberts JR, Hedges JR, editors: *Clinical procedures in emergency medicine,* Philadelphia, 1985, W.B. Saunders. Used with permission.)

b. Remove the needle so that only the guide wire remains in the vessel (Fig. 48-9, *C*).

c. Using a No. 11 mounted scalpel blade, make a small skin incision approximately the diameter of the catheter at the site of entry of the guide wire (Fig. 48-9, *D*).

d. Thread the catheter sheath and dilator over the guide wire to a point 1 to 2 cm from the skin surface (Fig. 48-9, *E*). It is critical to ensure that the guide wire is protruding through the proximal end of the sheath dilator unit enough to be grasped; otherwise, the guide wire may be lost in the vessel. If the guide wire is not visible, carefully withdraw the guide wire through the introducer unit until it is visible (Fig. 48-9, *F*).

e. Grasp the guide wire and advance the sheath-dilator introducer unit over the guide wire. Advance the dilator alone for several centimeters down to the vessel, then withdraw it to advance the sheath with the dilator to its full length in the vessel. As described above, the sheath should advance without resistance. Never force the sheath against resistance; rather, gently twist and push the sheath to advance (Fig. 48-9, *G*). Remove the dilator and guide wire together, leaving the sheath in the selected vessel (Fig. 48-9, *H*).

f. Confirm that the catheter is positioned within the vein, connect the flushed intravenous tubing, confirm blood return by lowering the IV bag below the level of the patient, secure and dress the sheath, and obtain an immediate chest X-ray.

Supraclavicular Approach

With the supraclavicular approach, the intent is to enter the subclavian vein in the superior aspect near its junction with the internal jugular vein. Advantages of the supraclavicular approach include the ability to cannulate the subclavian vein without interrupting chest compressions during CPR, little interference with airway management, and a relatively low complication rate. Again, the right side is preferred for the same reasons cited for the infraclavicular approach.

Procedure

1. Position, prepare, and drape the patient as previously described for the infraclavicular approach.

2. Anesthetize with 1% lidocaine at a point 1 cm lateral to the clavicular head of the sternocleidomastoid muscle and 1 cm cephalad to the clavicle. The needle may also be used to locate the vein (see Fig. 48-1).

3. While aspirating with a 3 cc syringe attached to a 14-gauge needle, advance the needle through the anesthetized site. Direct the needle toward the contralateral nipple in the male patient or the fifth intercostal space in the midclavicular line for a female. The needle shaft should be approximately 10 to 15 degrees above the patient's chest wall. Successful venipuncture is evidenced by freely flowing venous blood return, which usually occurs at a depth of 2 to 3 cm (Fig. 48-10).

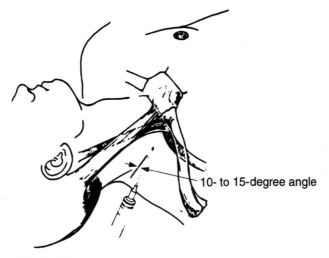

10- to 15-degree angle

FIG. 48-10.
Inserting needle in supraclavicular approach. (From Roberts JR, Hedges JR, editors: *Clinical procedures in emergency medicine,* Philadelphia, 1985, W.B. Saunders. Used with permission.)

4. The methods of inserting, securing, dressing, and evaluating the catheter position are identical to those described for the infraclavicular subclavian approach.

Internal Jugular Vein Catheterization

Advantages of the internal jugular technique include the ability to cannulate the vessel without interrupting chest compressions during CPR and a relatively low complication rate. Additionally, bleeding complications from attempted cannulation are more easily detected and compression can be more readily applied. As a result, the internal jugular approach is preferred over the subclavian approach for patients with coagulopathies. However, antecubital cutdown is probably the optimal approach for serious bleeding disorders in nonemergent situations. Disadvantages of the internal jugular approach include limited neck motion after insertion (especially troublesome for the conscious patient), interference with airway management, and increased neurologic complications (the recurrent laryngeal nerve, phrenic nerve, and brachial plexus may be injured in the procedure).

Anatomy
Like the subclavian vein, the internal jugular vein has relatively constant, predictable anatomical relationships. The internal jugular vein drains the intracranial region, and then travels with the carotid artery and vagus nerve in the carotid sheath. The internal jugular veins lie anterolateral to the carotid arteries throughout their course; therefore, palpation of the carotid pulse may be helpful when attempting to locate the internal jugular vein. The internal jugular vein travels under the apex of the triangle formed by the sternal and clavicular heads of the

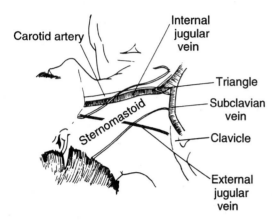

FIG. 48-11.
Anatomy of the internal jugular vein. (From *Textbook of advanced cardiac life support,* ed 2, Dallas, 1987, American Heart Association. Used with permission.)

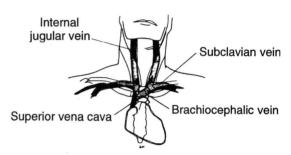

FIG. 48-12.
Anatomy of the subclavian vein.

sternocleidomastoid muscle and the clavicle (Fig. 48-11), and it courses inferomedially until it joins the subclavian vein cephalad to the clavicle (Fig. 48-12).

Patient Position
Proper positioning of the patient is crucial for successful catheterization of the internal jugular vein and is similar to that described for subclavian vein cannulation. It is not necessary to place a towel between the patient's scapula. The Trendelenburg position distends the internal jugular vein and creates positive pressure within the vein. The internal jugular vein may also be distended by asking the conscious patient to perform a Valsalva maneuver or by having an assistant compress the patient's epigastrium.

Overview of the Procedure
The same principles described for the subclavian route of access apply to the internal jugular approach.

Central Approach
Procedure.   Prepare the patient and equipment in a sterile fashion as described in subclavian catheterization via the infraclavicular approach, Steps 1 to 4.

1. Note important anatomic landmarks. Identify and palpate with the left index finger the triangle formed by the clavicle and the two heads of the sternocleidomastoid muscle (Fig. 48-13). Briefly palpate the carotid artery, which runs posteromedially to the jugular vein. Prolonged palpation of the carotid artery may decrease the caliber of the jugular vein and, therefore, should be avoided.
2. In the alert patient, use 1% lidocaine to anesthetize the skin at the catheter puncture site just caudad to the apex of the triangle formed by the two heads of the sternocleidomastoid muscle. Anesthetize the subcutaneous tis-

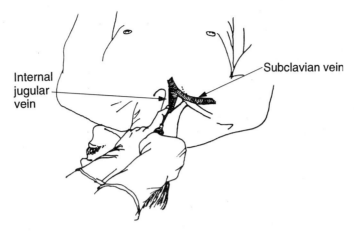

FIG. 48-13.
Central approach for internal jugular venipuncture. (From *Textbook of advanced cardiac life support,* ed 2, Dallas, 1987, American Heart Association. Used with permission.)

sue, directing the needle toward the ipsilateral nipple and the junction of the medial third and middle thirds of the clavicle. This direction courses parallel to the carotid artery. The angle of the needle shaft should be approximately 30 to 45 degrees above to the horizontal plane of the patient. Aspirate before injecting and check for absence of blood in the syringe to prevent injecting lidocaine intravenously.

3. Some clinicians initially attempt to cannulate with the catheter device, while others recommend using a smaller needle (i.e., 22-gauge) to locate the vein, thereby minimizing injury to neighboring structures.

4. Puncture the skin at the anesthesized site with the catheter device, and direct the needle caudally toward the ipsilateral nipple, as noted in Step 2. Palpate the carotid artery pulsation with your free hand. Some physicians recommend retracting the carotid artery medially and away from the internal jugular vein, but others feel that prolonged palpation of the carotid artery decreases the diameter of the internal jugular vein.

5. While aspirating with the syringe, slowly advance the needle while observing for dark venous blood return. Cannulation of the vein usually occurs at a depth of 1 to 3 cm. If the attempt is unsuccessful, withdraw the needle completely and reinsert it, angling 5 to 10 degrees lateral to the initial landmarks.

6. Return of bright red or pulsatile blood signifies inadvertent carotid artery penetration. In an elective situation, withdraw the needle and apply firm pressure for 10 to 20 minutes. In an emergency situation, withdraw the needle and immediately again attempt to cannulate, remembering, however, that a soft tissue hematoma may compromise an unprotected airway.

7. When blood returns, rotate the needle 360 degrees to ascertain that the bevel is completely within the vein. If blood flow is interrupted during this maneuver, slowly advance or withdraw the needle to bring the needle tip away from the vessel wall.

8. When the needle tip is properly positioned in the vessel lumen, disconnect the syringe in the same fashion as described for the subclavian approach and immediately occlude the needle hub with your thumb to prevent air embolus. If the patient is cooperative, ask him or her to exhale or to perform a Valsalva maneuver to increase pressure in the vein during this portion of the procedure.

9. Pass the catheter through the introducing needle; advance the catheter over the needle, or pass a guide wire through the needle, depending upon the catheter device being employed, as outlined beginning in Step 16 for subclavian venipuncture. Use the same precautions as discussed in the subclavian approach for each of these methods.

10. Confirm intravascular position of the catheter as previously described for the subclavian approach in Step 16.

11. Secure the catheter as described in Step 16(g) by placing a 3-0 or 4-0 silk suture through the skin, tying three square knots, looping the suture around the catheter three to four times, and again tying the suture. Check the catheter to make sure that the lumen is not constricted. Apply an antimicrobial ointment in a sterile dressing as outlined above in Step 16(h and i). Loop the catheter around the ipsilateral ear to reduce the risk of catheter kinking (Fig. 48-14).

12. Take the patient out of the Trendelenburg position.

13. Order an immediate chest X-ray to confirm the catheter position and to detect possible pneumothorax or hemothorax. Reposition inadequately placed catheters.

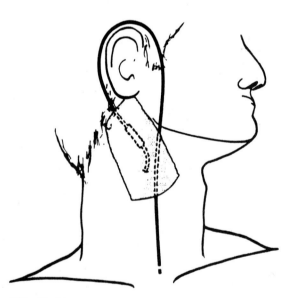

FIG. 48-14.
Internal jugular line secured by looping the catheter around the ipsilateral ear. (From *Can Anaesth Soc J* 23:609, 1976. Used with permission.)

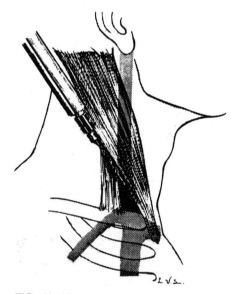

FIG. 48-15.
Posterior approach for internal jugular vein catheterization. (From Dunphy JE, Way LW, editors: *Current surgical diagnosis and treatment,* ed 5, New York, 1981, Appleton & Lange. Used with permission.)

Posterior Approach
Procedure

1. Insert the needle under the sternocleidomastoid muscle near the junction of the middle and caudal thirds of the lateral muscle border (Fig. 48-15). At this point, the external jugular vein crosses beneath the sternocleidomastoid muscle.
2. While aspirating with the syringe, direct the needle under the sternocleido-mastoid muscle toward the suprasternal notch at an angle of 45 degrees above the horizontal plane.
3. The vein is usually entered at a depth of 4 to 6 cm.
4. Follow the steps previously outlined for the central approach.

POSTPROCEDURE PATIENT EDUCATION

Instruct the patient with an indwelling catheter to report symptoms or signs of local or systemic infection, and explain the risks of hemorrhage. The patient should undergo formal training for management of the catheter, unless another trained individual is to manage care. When a central catheter is removed, the patient should be informed to notify a nurse or doctor if pain, swelling, or signs of infection occur at the insertion site. The patient should also notify the proper individuals for any related chest symptoms, such as chest pain (pleuritic or other), dyspnea, or hemoptysis.

COMPLICATIONS

- Hemorrhage, hematoma, or thrombosis
- Local and systemic infection
- Hydrothorax (results from infusion of intravenous fluids into the pleural space), pneumothorax, hemothorax, and chylothorax
- Perforation of the trachea
- Perforation of an endotracheal tube cuff
- Air embolus: detected when "squishy" heart sounds are heard and a sharp fall in blood pressure occurs (The patient should be immediately placed in a steep, head-down position with the right side elevated.)
- Catheter fragment embolus (especially with catheter-through-the-needle devices)
- Laceration of the subclavian or carotid artery
- With subclavian placement, laceration of the thoracic duct (on the left side) or lymphatic duct (on the right side)
- Arteriovenous fistula
- Superior vena cava obstruction
- Pericardial tamponade
- Injury to neighboring nerves (phrenic, recurrent laryngeal, brachial plexus)

- Cardiac dysrhythmias
- Catheter kinking
- Catheter malposition
- Soft tissue hematomas in the neck, which may compromise the airway

Complications may be minimized by proper patient selection, by thorough knowledge of the anatomy, by adherence to sterile technique, by having an experienced or supervised operator perform the technique, and by changing lines that were inserted under less than sterile conditions during CPR or are suspected of causing infection as soon as feasible.

CPT/BILLING CODES

36010	Introduction of catheter, superior or inferior vena cava
36011	Selective catheter placement, venous system; first-order branch (e.g., renal vein, jugular vein)

BIBLIOGRAPHY

American Heart Association: *Textbook of advanced cardiac life support,* Dallas, 1988, The Association.

Ho MT, Saunders CE, editors: *Current emergency diagnosis and treatment,* ed 3, Norwalk, Conn, 1990, Appleton & Lange.

Road II et al: The relationship between the thrombotic and infectious complications of central venous catheters, *JAMA* 271:1014, 1994.

Roberts JR, Hedges JR, editors: *Clinical procedures in emergency medicine,* Philadelphia, 1985, W.B. Saunders.

Schug CB, Culhone DE, Knopp RK: Subclavian vein catheterization in the emergency department: a comparison of guide wire and nonguide wire techniques, *Ann Emerg Med* 15:769, July 1986.

CHAPTER 49

Swan-Ganz Catheterization

Len Scarpinato

The utilization of the balloon-flotation, flow-directed pulmonary artery thermodilution Swan-Ganz catheter perhaps best symbolizes modern care of the critically ill patient. Yet, in the 32 years since its introduction, no large, randomized, double-blind sham-controlled study has ever shown that Swan-Ganz catheter placement is associated with reductions in morbidity or mortality. However, it is now such an important part of medical treatment of critically ill patients that such a study would probably never pass an institutional review board.

Partly because of the lack of such a study, the catheter has been maligned in the literature and abused in practice. Yet there are particular times during the care of critically ill patients that its utility is unquestioned. Urine output, blood pressure, central venous pressure (CVP), and other aspects of the physical examination are all very useful for monitoring critically ill patients; however, many physicians have voted: One million Swan-Ganz catheters are placed each year.

This chapter was written for the primary care physician preparing to insert a Swan-Ganz catheter, and thus it deals only with those applications that are not controversial. Almost all new Swans are cardiac-output capable (an option on older versions). None of the "add-on Swans," such as those that can also monitor continuous mixed venous oxygen saturation ($S_{\bar{v}}O_2$) (oximetric Swan), pacing (Paceport), 4-lumen position monitoring, and right ventricular ejection fraction or volume calculation are discussed here.

Although many physicians are proficient in similar procedures and may have cross-over skills, beginners should first observe Swan-Ganz catheter placement several times. Attempts at placement of the first few Swans should only be conducted under the guidance of a trained and skilled physician. Further study and use of the catheter will increase one's interest and knowledge. Courses devoted to the technology should facilitate proficiency, especially with the subtleties of the possible applications.

INDICATIONS

Diagnostic

- Suspected right ventricular dysfunction or infarction
- Evaluation of valvular lesions
- Evaluation of chronic congestive heart failure (CHF)
- Evaluation of left or right ventricular function
- Suspected pulmonary arterial hypertension
- Suspected pulmonary embolism
- Oxygen transport assessment

   Note: Contrary to the beliefs of many housestaff members and medical students, hypotension alone is not an indication for Swan-Ganz catheter placement; however, hypotension with no response to an adequate fluid bolus is an indication. This exemplifies the primary use of the Swan-Ganz catheter: to obtain more data to help make decisions about the medical care when we do not know exactly what is going on with the patient.

Differential Diagnosis

- Pulmonary edema (cardiogenic vs. noncardiogenic)
- Shock (cardiogenic vs. noncardiogenic)
- Low cardiac output syndrome
- Ventricular septal defect vs. pericardial tamponade vs. acute mitral regurgitation
- Electromechanical dissociation

Monitoring

- Titration of drug and other interventions in highly unstable patients (vasodilators, inotropes, pacemakers, and parenteral fluids)
- Congestive heart failure or cardiac ischemia
- Hemodynamically unstable patients unresponsive to conventional therapy
- Postinfarction angina
- Cardiac tamponade
- Cor pulmonale or chronic obstructive pulmonary disease (COPD) in a patient with both cardiac and pulmonary disorders
- Sepsis
- Myocardial infarction
- Perioperatively to enable optimization of the patient's status
- Overdose
- Continuous mixed venous oxygen saturation monitoring
- Right-sided heart failure due to severe obstructive lung disease, adult respiratory distress syndrome (ARDS), or pulmonary embolism

Therapeutic

- Pacing
- Aspiration of air emboli during seated neurosurgery

- Guidance of complex fluid management in certain difficult situations; e.g., shock, postoperative state, adult respiratory distress syndrome (ARDS), acute renal failure

RELATIVE CONTRAINDICATIONS

- Same as those for central venous catheterization (see Chapter 48, Central Venous Catheter Insertion)
- Prosthetic right heart valve patients
- Cardiac-paced patients (either permanent or pacer-dependent temporary)*
- Severely hypotensive patients or patients with known pulmonary hypertension
- Highly unstable arrythmias (especially ventricular)
- Highly unstable respiratory status
- Lack of nursing staff trained in use of Swan-Ganz catheters
- Lack of a compatible pressure-monitoring apparatus

If the underlying relative contraindication can be beneficially altered, catheterizaton is worth the risk.

EQUIPMENT

- Central venous access (see Chapter 48, Central Venous Catheter Insertion)
- Balloon flotation, flow-directed, thermistor-tipped pulmonary artery thermodilution catheter (see Fig. 49-1) with syringe for balloon inflation: 7 Fr. or larger for adults, or 5 Fr. for pediatric use
- Pressure transducer
- High-pressure tubing, connectors, and stopcocks (Fig. 49-2)
- Bedside monitor
- Heparinized saline flush system
- Sterile gowns, drapes, gloves, masks, and goggles
- Guide wire
- Suture
- Fully stocked code cart nearby

Many of these essentials are available in the manufacturer's kits.

---

*Left bundle branch block (LBBB) was previously a contraindication because of the high incidence of naturally occuring concomitant or induced right bundle branch block (RBBB) with an indwelling Swan (RBBB + LBBB = complete heart block). Recent evidence indicates that the risk of complete bundle branch block is lower than expected.

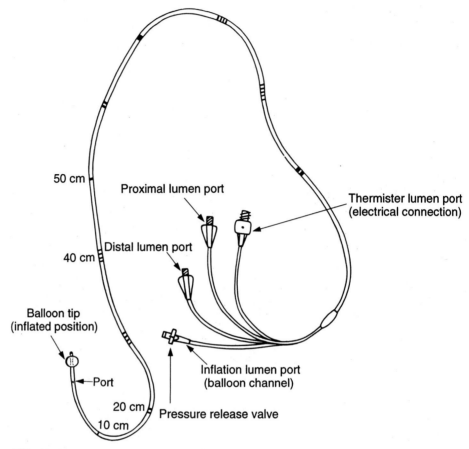

FIG. 49-1.
Balloon-tipped thermodilution catheter.

PREPROCEDURE PATIENT EDUCATION

Since Swan-Ganz catheterization is usually an emergency procedure, written informed consent cannot always be obtained. However, explain the indications, risks, and benefits of the procedure to the patient and the family, if possible. The implied consent should be documented with the potential complications (of both having and not having the catheter placed). Have the patient sign a standard informed consent form if he or she is able.

TECHNIQUE

Venous access is established by the procedure outlined in Chapter 48, Central Venous Catheter Insertion. As delineated in Chapter 60, Temporary Pacing, cath-

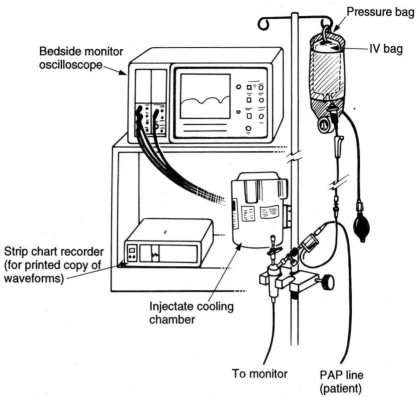

FIG. 49-2.
Pressure tubing, connectors, and stopcocks.

eterization of the right internal jugular vein provides the most direct access to the right atrium and ventricle, but subclavian catheterization is adequate. The broad curve of the left subclavian may make it more difficult to negotiate than the right. The most common central access used for Swan-Ganz catheterization is the right subclavian, which is the approach utilized for the purposes of this chapter.

Procedure Guidelines

- Observe strict sterile technique. Scrub after donning hair cover, goggles, mask, and gown; wear sterile gloves; and maintain sterile technique throughout the procedure. Follow universal blood and body fluid precautions.
- Whenever the heart undergoes invasive monitoring or an area of the heart is traversed, record an ECG tracing for future reference.
- To prevent the loss of a guide wire in a patient, do not let go of a guide wire while it is in a patient during catheter manipulation.
- Since this procedure may induce arrhythmias, an additional, separate intravenous access should be in place.

Conversion to a Sheath or an Introducer of Sufficient Size

If the venous catheter in place is not large enough to accept the Swan-Ganz catheter, it must be converted. You should use an 8 Fr. sheath for 7 Fr. Swan-Ganz catheter, or an 8.5 Fr. sheath for a 7.5 Fr. catheter.

1. Insert a guide wire of sufficient length through the existing venous access line.
2. Leaving the guide wire in place, remove the catheter over the guide wire.
3. Use the dilator in the kit to enlarge the lumen over the guide wire.
4. Leaving the guide wire in place, remove the dilator.
5. Place the obturator in the sheath and pass them over the guide wire and into the patient's central circulation.
6. Remove the guide wire and the obturator, and cap the sheath with the special cap that allows for Swan-Ganz catheter placement.

Insertion of the Swan-Ganz Catheter

1. Have an assistant set up, calibrate, and level the transducer.
2. Remove the Swan-Ganz catheter from its sterile packaging. Place the protective shield over the distal end of the catheter, making sure the docking mechanism is facing in the correct direction to attach it to the sheath that was inserted in the patient earlier. Flush the catheter by injecting sterile heparinized saline into the 3 or 4 ports of the catheter. Make sure the ports are patent. Saline is used because it conducts pressure gradations better than air.
3. Attach the smaller syringe to the balloon port. Fill the balloon with air. Usually a built-in safety mechanism prevents overdistention if the balloon is filled once. Place the balloon under sterile water or saline and check for bubbles, indicating a leak. A leaking catheter should be replaced. If possible, test the thermister by connecting the catheter connector cable to the cardiac output computer. It should read "ambient temperature." Deflate the balloon of the catheter.
4. Hand the proximal end of the catheter (proximal to the operator or the end that will stay outside the body) to the assistant so that the ECG can be monitored continuously during the procedure. The assistant should monitor the waveforms produced by the distal port. Have the assistant connect the catheter to the pressure tubing, which will allow for internal flushing with sterile saline.
5. Mark the patient's lateral mid-chest with an indelible ink spot so that the equipment can be lined up horizontally; this spot is considered the zero point. Record the height of the bed mattress from the floor. The strict recording of heights is necessary, because a change in height of 1 inch corresponds to a 1.8 mm Hg change in monitored pressure.

   Note: Passage of the catheter through the pulmonary artery can take as little as 10 to 20 seconds. If it takes too long to pass the catheter, it may soften (as it is supposed to do when exposed to body heat) and make it more difficult to advance. A good rule of thumb is that the catheter should pass from the right atrium to the wedge position in 20 to 30 seconds. There are no prizes for the most rapid passage, and more than likely, it will take longer than 20 seconds, especially with abnormal blood flow. Abnormal blood

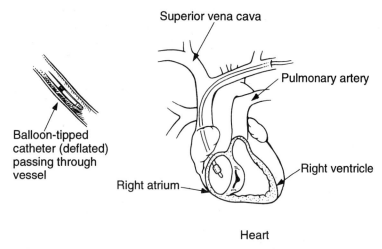

FIG. 49-3.
Balloon-tipped catheter passing through vessel to the 10 to 15 cm mark.

flow may be caused by valve abnormalities (tricuspid or pulmonic stenosis or insufficiency), cardiac dysfunction, and pulmonic disease with increased right ventricular pressure.

6. Pass the deflated balloon-tipped catheter through the sheath to the 10 or 15 cm mark; it is marked in 10 cm increments (Fig. 49-3).
7. Watch the waveform monitor for a characteristic central venous tracing or a right atrial tracing, the normal range of pressure from 0 to 10 mm Hg; they should show respiratory variation. Record these pressures. Three positive deflections can be seen if the scale is enlarged enough on the monitor: the *a, c,* and *v* waves (Fig. 49-4).
8. Verify that the appropriate scale was picked on the monitor.
9. Using the syringe provided with the kit, inflate the balloon with air to the recommended full volume as indicated on the package or the syringe (0.8 to 1.5 cc of air). Never advance the catheter beyond this point without an inflated balloon, unless using fluoroscopy to avoid vessel damage.

Author's note: I use 1.5 cc for patients with intracardiac shunts. In this case, carbon dioxide should be used to prevent left-sided air emboli.

The provided syringe has a hole that is set up in such a way that the entry of undesired air is prevented. As long as they are not overdistended, certain balloons provide a buffer around the distal hard tip of the catheter. Avoid overfilling the balloon, for it can burst with dire consequences, especially if already inserted, or if bursting goes unrecognized. Air should never be forced into a pulmonary artery catheter (Fig. 49-5).

10. Pass the catheter to the 30 or 40 cm mark in a quick but not too rapid fashion, while watching the pressure monitor for the characteristic right ventricular tracing. This tracing looks like a large square root sign without a dicrotic notch. A dramatic rise in the systolic pressure should occur during this manipulation, but there should be no change in the diastolic pressure (Fig. 49-4, *A*).

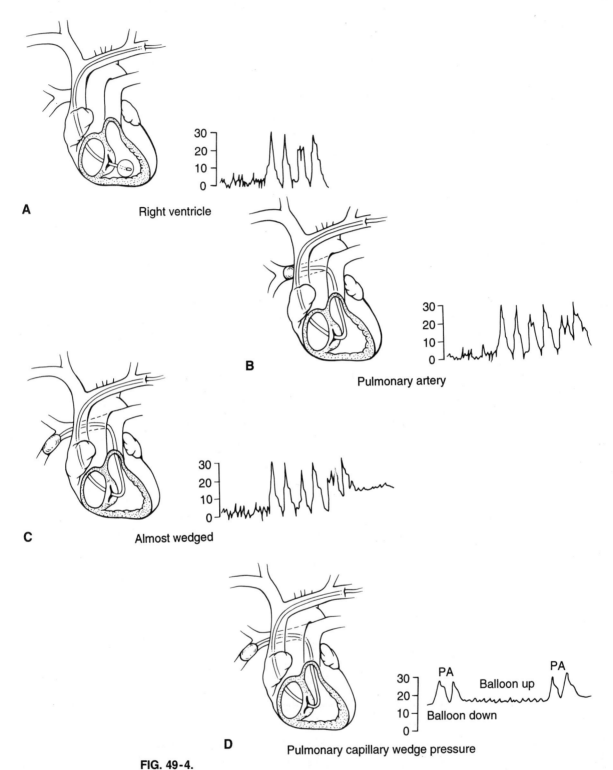

A   Right ventricle

B   Pulmonary artery

C   Almost wedged

PA   Balloon up   PA

Balloon down

D   Pulmonary capillary wedge pressure

FIG. 49-4.
Tracings recorded through the catheter as it traverses the right atrium, right ventricle, pulmonary artery, and finally the wedged position.

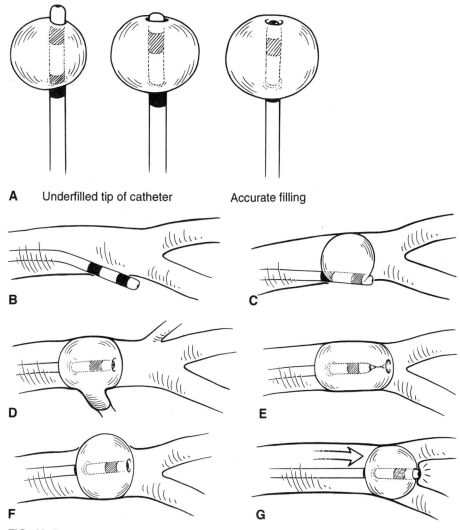

A   Underfilled tip of catheter   Accurate filling

FIG. 49-5.
Correct filling of the balloon and possible complications. **A,** Underfilled and accurate filling. **B,** Tip perforates wall of vessel when balloon is not inflated. **C,** Eccentric balloon (inaccurate wedge) and risk of wall rupture. **D,** Balloon inadvertently distending down side of vessel. **E,** Inaccurate and overdistention of balloon can cause catheter tip occlusion. **F,** Over wedge (see Troubleshooting). **G,** Underinflated catheter with protruding tip.

Record the right ventricular pressures. You should also watch the ECG tracing for any ectopy at this stage.

11. Once in the right ventricle, without delay pass the catheter rapidly to the 40 to 50 cm mark and into the pulmonary artery. The pulmonary artery gives a peculiarly shaped tracing, like a triangle with a dicrotic notch on the downhill distal side of the triangle (Fig. 49-4, *B*). Record the pressures. Normal pulmonary artery pressures are 15 to 25 mm Hg systolic, 8 to 16 mm Hg diastolic, with a mean of 10 to 20 mm Hg.

12. Once in the pulmonary artery, it is safe to continue passing the catheter at a much slower pace, watching for the characteristic pulmonary capillary wedge pressure (PCWP) tracing at about the 50 cm mark on the catheter. With PCWP tracings, one loses the characteristic pulmonary artery pattern, and the mean pressure decreases. This is the somewhat magical place where the vessel traversed has become occluded and the catheter starts reading the "back pressure" from the other side of the heart. The catheter no longer reads pulmonary artery pressures; rather, it reads pressure reflected back from the left atrium (LA) through the capillaries (Fig. 49-4, *C*). If the mitral valve is not obstructed and open during ventricular diastole, the PCWP approximates the left ventricular diastolic pressure. In the absence of elevated end expiratory pressures or obstruction of the pulmonary veins, PCWP approximates left atrial mean pressure within ± 2 mm Hg.

13. Once the balloon is wedged, allow it to passively deflate, and watch for the phasic pulmonary artery tracing. Do not aspirate to deflate the balloon; active deflation may cause rupture (Fig 49-4, *D*).

14. Inflate and deflate the balloon to observe the two different tracings. If the syringe and balloon were designed to hold 1.5 cc, this is the amount required to wedge the catheter safely. If any less accomplishes it, then the catheter's location is too distal; withdraw it until 1.5 cc wedges it. If 1.5 cc does not wedge the Swan, then it should be inflated and passed further. Even though the PCWP is called an occlusion pressure, the inflated balloon actually floats distally and *then* occludes the vessel. The vessel is not occluded from inflation at a fixed location.

15. Extend the catheter protective shield and attach it to the sheath with the docking mechanism.

16. Secure the entire assembly with suture and adequate tape. Apply sterile dressing.

17. Order a chest X-ray (portable anteroposterior and a cross-table lateral) and auscultate the patient's chest bilaterally to exclude a pneumothorax.

18. Begin infusion of necessary medications.

19. If the patient was moved, ask the assistant to rezero the equipment.

20. Document the procedure in the chart, including the tracings, and record end expiratory values. Additional documented values should include the pulmonary artery pressure, the pulmonary capillary wedge pressure, and the cardiac output (performed by the assistant and not detailed here).

TROUBLESHOOTING

- If salvos of premature ventricular contractions occur during catheter advancement, deflate the balloon and withdraw the catheter into the right atrium. (It may be coiled in the right ventricle.) If further attempts to pass it are unsuccessful, administer an intravenous bolus of 2% lidocaine (75 to 100 mg) and attempt passage under fluoroscopy.

- If a pulmonary artery or PCWP tracing cannot be obtained, keep the balloon deflated, pull the catheter back to 12 cm, and try again. Consider inserting the catheter using a clockwise twisting action. If that fails, try counterclockwise reinsertion. Having the patient take deep breaths may help pass the catheter.

- Some physicians recommend injecting cold, sterile saline solution to enhance passage; this may stiffen the catheter, which may have softened with the warmth of the body. Occasionally a guide wire and fluoroscope are necessary to advance the catheter. Repositioning the patient may help. In patients with a very low ejection fraction, an inotrope may have to be administered to facilitate passage.

- For a normal-sized adult, from the subclavian or internal jugular site, insertion beyond 50 cm (or 15 cm after entering the right ventricle) predisposes the catheter to coiling, which can lead to knotting.

- When a catheter's location is too distal in the vessel, a tracing called an overwedge may be seen. This is likely to occur when the balloon is not filled with enough air. After deflating the balloon, withdraw the catheter and attempt a wedge, this time with the balloon full to its correct volume (Fig. 49-5).

- Persistent underinflation of the balloon can damage pulmonary vessels or the endocardium, and may result in arrythmias, if the catheter tip is exposed (Fig. 49-5, *A* and *G*).

- There are several mechanisms that are proposed to cause rupture of the pulmonary artery, an unlikely but possible consequence related to either over- or underinflation of the balloon (Fig. 49-5, *F* and *G*).

- Damping can occur, which has an effect opposite to overwedging. When air is present in the catheter, it can damp the transmission of waveforms. It characteristically appears like a regular tracing but the variations are damped. Try to remove air bubbles from connecting tubes by aspirating and flushing the catheter. If blood cannot be aspirated, yet the catheter flushes easily, suspect a ballvalve thrombus at the catheter tip. Inject 5000 units of heparin into the lumen; allow 15 to 30 minutes for it to take effect. Initiate a continuous drip of heparin (not to exceed 20,000 units for 24 hours). If still unsuccessful, withdraw the catheter gradually 5 cm at a time, watching for waveforms.

- Lesions obstructing the mitral valve, such as mitral stenosis, can interfere with the ability of the PCWP to approximate left ventricular diastolic pressure. In these cases, PCWP may not be the best estimate of left ventricular end-diastolic pressure.

- Respirations can also cause significant variations in the pressure readings for the Swan-Ganz catheter. Make calibrated strip-chart recordings for all measurements derived from the catheter and then measure again at end expiration (Fig. 49-6). Patients on a ventilator requiring positive end expiratory pressure (PEEP) may not have the PCWPs that reflect left atrial pressures.

CATHETER CARE

- Inflate the balloon only when measuring the PCWP, and leave it inflated for a *maximum* of 60 seconds to prevent pulmonary infarction. To exclude the possibility of catheter obstruction before inflation, flush the catheter each time before inflating the balloon.

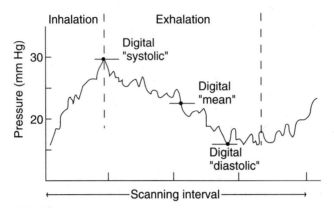

FIG. 49-6.
Respiratory variation of the pulmonary artery catheter tracing. (From Wiedemann HP, Matthay MA, Matthay RA: *Chest* 85:537, 1984. Used with permission.)

- Flush the catheter with heparinized saline every 30 minutes.
- Adjust the position of the catheter as necessary. The catheter may soften and migrate to a more distal site, predisposing to distal pulmonary artery or branch-vessel occlusion. If the pulmonary artery pressure tracing shows a loss in phasicity and begins to resemble the PCWP tracing (without balloon inflation), withdraw the catheter until the typical phasic pulmonary artery tracing reappears. Always deflate when withdrawing to avoid damage to intracardiac structures.
- Remove, inspect, and replace the sterile dressing daily.
- Obtain daily chest X-rays to check for catheter migration and exclude pulmonary infarction.

COMPLICATIONS

With Central Venous Catheterization (CVP)

- Same as complications for central venous catheterization (see Chapter 48, Central Venous Catheter Insertion)

With Swan-Ganz Catheter Placement

- Atrial and ventricular ectopy or conduction changes
- Knotting of the catheter, inside or outside of the heart (more likely with smaller-bore catheters, e.g., 5 Fr.)
- Malposition (including catheter puncture and insertion into many organs, such as the trachea, the subclavian artery, or even the endotracheal tube)
- Pulmonary infarction
- Destruction of vascular integrity
- Cardiac perforation and tamponade

With Continued Presence of the Swan-Ganz Catheter in the Central Circulation

- Same as complications for indwelling central venous catheters (see Chapter 48, Central Venous Catheter Insertion)
- Pulmonary hemorrhage
- Embolism (air or thrombotic)
- Pulmonary artery rupture
- Mural (or elsewhere) thrombus formation
- Pseudoaneurysm
- Balloon rupture or catheter fracture
- Valve or intracardiac structural damage
- Endocarditis
- Inaccurate diagnosis because of malfunctioning catheter
- Hemoptysis caused by flushing catheter when it is in the wedged position

CPT/BILLING CODE

93503   Insertion and placement of flow-directed catheter (e.g., Swan-Ganz), for monitoring purposes

BIBLIOGRAPHY

Ermakov S, Hoyt JW: Pulmonary artery catheterization, *Crit Care Clinics* 8(4):1992.

Amin DK, Shah PK, Swan HJC: The Swan-Ganz catheter, *Crit Illness* 1(4):24, 1986, and 1(5):40, 1986.

Kaye WE, Dubin HG: Vascular cannulation. In Civetta JM, Taylor RW, Kirby RR, editors: *Critical Care,* Philadelphia, 1988, J.B. Lippincott.

CHAPTER 50

Venous Cutdown

Grant C. Fowler

When percutaneous venous access is not available, venous cutdown (venesection) is a reliable and safe technique for administering large volumes of fluids, including blood. Very large-bore lines can be employed in this procedure, often allowing more rapid infusion of fluids than central lines.

INDICATIONS

- Hypotensive patient in whom major injury is suspected (Cutdown should occur simultaneously with attempts at large-bore antecubital vein cannulation.)
- Patient requiring emergency venous access or multiple intravenous lines in which antecubital or other veins cannot be visualized, palpated, or cannulated percutaneously

    Note: There is wide variation in opinion regarding how to prioritize locations for venous cutdown. The three most common locations, each with inherent advantages and disadvantages, are the distal saphenous vein at the ankle, the proximal saphenous vein at the groin, and the basilic vein in the antecubital fossa. Other peripheral locations are also available; however, before attempting to recall further anatomy of the venous system in an urgent situation, consider attaining central access instead.

CONTRAINDICATIONS

Venesection is contraindicated only when less invasive alternatives exist (routine venous catheterization) or when excessive delay would be required for the procedure to be performed. Evidence of severe venous obstructive disease should be considered when choosing the site. Choice of site should also take into account local arterial supply, and sites with local infection should be avoided.

EQUIPMENT

- Tourniquet
- Antiseptic skin preparation, such as isopropyl alcohol or povidone-iodine
- Sterile gloves and drapes
- 4 × 4 inch gauze sponges
- 1% lidocaine *without* epinephrine
- A 3 cc syringe with 25-gauge 5/8-inch (1.6 cm) needle
- Silk ligatures (4-0)
- Nonabsorbable skin suture (4-0)
- Fine forceps, with and without teeth
- Tissue dissection and suture scissors
- Curved hemostats and a mosquito hemostat
- No. 15 and No. 11 scalpel blades with handles
- Needle holder
- Intravenous fluids and setup
- Antibiotic ointment
- Adhesive tape
- Sterile cannula (Anything from a 2-, 3-, or 4-Fr. silastic catheter to a section of IV connector tubing can be used, based on the size of the vein to be cannulated.)
- Goggles

TECHNIQUE

1. If the patient is alert, explain the need for intravenous access and the procedure.
2. In an antecubital or distal saphenous cutdown, have an assistant apply a tourniquet proximal to the incision site and control it. This will enable you to more easily visualize the vein. A tourniquet applied high on the thigh may help with locating the proximal saphenous vein. To minimize bleeding, tourniquets should be released at the time of venipuncture.
3. Cleanse the area around the vein and incision site thoroughly with either 70% isopropyl alcohol or povidone-iodine.
4. Extend a wide sterile field 8 to 10 cm proximally and distally to provide you ample space.
5. For conscious patients, administer a local anesthetic to the area of incision.
6. Regardless of which cutdown site is chosen, incisions can all be made horizontally (laterally). All of these veins are in superficial fat layers; therefore, with an antecubital or proximal saphenous cutdown, if the excision exposes muscle fascia, it is too deep.
7. The vein should appear pulseless and thin-walled, and it should blanch when distal traction is applied. If a vein is not readily identified, have an assistant tighten the tourniquet, which may make it more apparent.
8. With all cutdowns, the vein should be dissected free and isolated for 4 cm along its axis.

CUTDOWN

Distal Saphenous Vein (Fig. 50-1)

Advantages

- Location does not disrupt other resuscitative measures, such as obtaining blood gases at the femoral artery or chest compressions during cardiopulmonary resuscitation (CPR).
- It provides IV access on both sides of the diaphragm if additional central access is obtained.
- It involves minimal training as well as minimal risk of complications compared with those of central access. Only the minor saphenous nerve is in the vicinity of the incision.

Disadvantages

- Phlebitis is more common in veins of lower extremity.
- Infection is more common in the presence of phlebitis.
- It offers a poor administration route for cardiac drugs during CPR.
- Hypertonic solutions should be avoided.
- The saphenous vein cannot be used if it has been used for a previous surgical procedure, such as coronary artery bypass grafting.

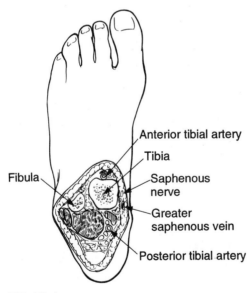

FIG. 50-1.
The greater saphenous vein may be isolated easily and safely at the ankle since no important structures lie nearby.

Specific Technique

1. Just above the medial malleolus, make an incision (only through skin) commencing at the anterior border (proximal) of the tibia or anterior shin and extending posteriorly to the posterior border of the tibia (Fig. 50-2).
2. Using a curved, closed hemostat with the point adjacent to the tibia, advance the instrument in the line of the incision from anterior to posterior just above the tibia and pick up all superficial tissue. Allow the tissue to slide over the back of the hemostat (Fig. 50-3).
3. Rotate the point of the hemostat upward while holding this tissue, and spread to reveal the distal saphenous vein, nerve, and tissue on the background of the hemostat.
4. Proceed to cannulation.

Proximal or Greater Saphenous Vein at the Groin

Advantages

- It provides IV access on both sides of the diaphragm if additional central access is obtained.
- It involves minimal training as well as minimal risk of complications compared with those of central access.
- This is a large vein that is easier to cannulate and that enables infusion of larger volumes to patients in profound hypovolemia.

Disadvantages

- Phlebitis is more common.
- Infection is more common in presence of phlebitis.
- It offers a poor administration route for cardiac drugs during CPR.
- Hypertonic solutions must be avoided.
- There is a possibility of damage to nearby structures if dissection is too deep.

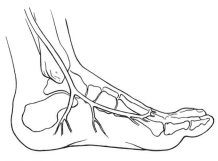

FIG. 50-2.
Anatomic relationships of the saphenous vein.

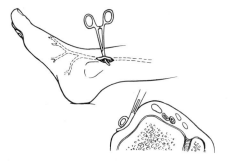

FIG. 50-3.
Insert the curved mosquito clamp into the anterior angle of the skin incision. Advance the mosquito clamp under the saphenous vein by sweeping it posteriorly. Lift the clamp and vein upward.

Specific Technique

1. With the patient supine, start a horizontal (lateral) incision (skin only) at the point where the scrotal fold (or labial fold) meets the medial thigh and extend it laterally to a point just past where an imaginary vertical (longitudinal) line would cross extended downward from the pubic tubercle, or the outer portion of the mons (Fig. 50-4). If muscle fascia is visible, the incision is too deep.
2. The proximal saphenous vein is located most frequently in an imaginary line running from the lateral aspect of the pubic tubercle downward where it crosses this incision. It is in the superficial fat layer.
3. Proceed to cannulation.

Basilic Vein

Advantages

- The basilic vein is located closer to the heart than the saphenous vein; hence, it affords a superior route of drug administration during CPR, although not as effective as central access.
- It has less risk of infection than the saphenous vein.
- It involves minimal training and minimal risk of complications compared with those of central access.

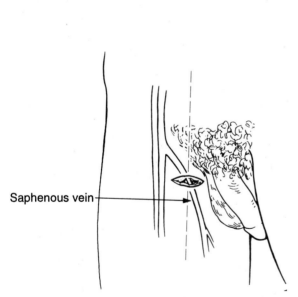

Saphenous vein

FIG. 50-4.
Cutdown location for greater saphenous vein at the groin.

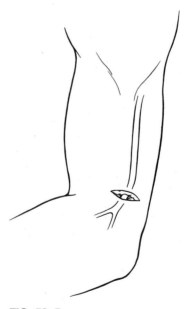

FIG. 50-5.
An incision is made between the biceps and triceps for basilic vein cutdown (right arm).

Disadvantages

- In CPR situations, ongoing attempts at percutaneous cannulation and/or chest compressions frequently make this a difficult site.
- Smaller diameter theoretically limits infusion volumes from what can be accomodated by the proximal saphenous vein, although frequently the cannulasused in both of these locations are the same size.
- There is a possibility of damage to nearby structures if dissection is too deep.

Specific Technique

1. The basilic vein lies in the groove of the medial arm between the triceps and the biceps muscles. It follows a course slightly anterior and superficial to the brachial artery. Divide the distance between the tip of the olecranon and the acromion into thirds and find the biceps/triceps groove in the middle of the distal third segment.
2. Make a horizontal, superficial incision at this level from the biceps across the groove to the triceps (Fig. 50-5).
3. The basilic vein is found with dissection of the superficial fat layer. If muscle fascia and the radial artery are observed, the dissection is too deep.
4. Proceed to cannulation.

CANNULATION

1. Dissect aside any loose adipose or adventitial tissue and isolate the chosen vein for a distance of 4 cm along its course.
2. Pass silk ties proximally and distally. If the distal vein is to be sacrificed, the distal ligature should be tied and left long to help control and manipulate the vein.
3. Place traction on the proximal ligature to minimize later bleeding; it should not be tied at this point.

A

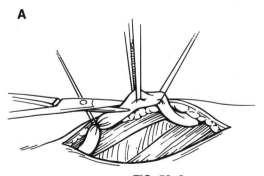

B

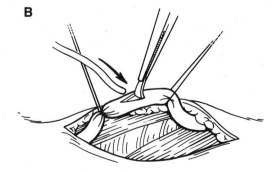

FIG. 50-6.
A, An angled wedge cut is made in the anterior wall of the vein. Maintain traction on the vein with proximal and distal ligatures. **B,** Introduce the cannula through the vein incision.

4. Loosen the tourniquet.

5. Incise approximately one third of the diameter of the vein with a scalpel or fine scissors in a distal-to-proximal direction and at a 45-degree angle to the axis (Fig. 50-6, *A*). Next, expand the diameter of the lumen with the mosquito hemostat while maintaining proximal traction on the ligature.

6. Once the skin has been entered through a separate stab wound, introduce the cannula through the vein incision following the 45-degree angle of the incision (Fig. 50-6, *B*). Threading the catheter into the vein is usually the most difficult portion of the procedure and requires patience and foresight. Relax slightly on the proximal ligature (Fig. 50-7). If the catheter cannot be threaded, the posterior wall of the vein may have been punctured or a false lumen may have been created. A catheter that is too large is another possible source of difficulty. If cannulation has not succeeded after multiple attempts, dilation of the vein with the mosquito hemostat followed by enlargement of the vein incision, as a last effort, may be considered.

   Caution: In greater saphenous vein cannulations, care must be taken to cannulate only the saphenous vein and to avoid blocking the lumen of the femoral vein, which would block all venous return from the lower extremities.

7. Next, aspirate air from the cannula by withdrawing blood and tie the proximal ligature around the vein wall and the cannula. Cut both ligatures and close the wound with skin suture (Fig. 50-8).

8. Completely remove the tourniquet and observe the incision for leakage of fluid or blood.

9. Secure the catheter to the skin with an additional stitch, and apply antibiotic ointment and a dressing (Fig. 50-9).

COMPLICATIONS

- Local hematoma and infection
- Phlebitis

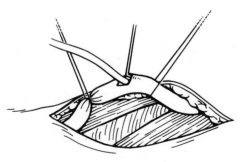

FIG. 50-7.
Catheter is threaded into the vein.

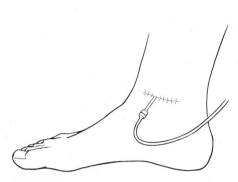

FIG. 50-8.
Incision closed and catheter sutured in place.

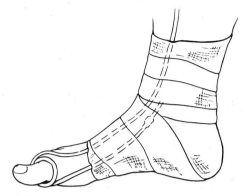

FIG. 50-9.
Dressing of the wound to prevent decannulation.

- Embolism
- Bacteremia and sepsis
- Injury to nearby structures in the cutdown process

The previously discussed locations are chosen to minimize the risks of these complications. If the cutdown is left in place less than 48 hours, the risk of infection is minimized. Closing the incision after initial cannulation also reduces the risk of infection.

CPT/BILLING CODES

36415	Routine venipuncture for collection of specimen(s)
36425	Venipuncture, cutdown; age one or over

BIBLIOGRAPHY

Kirkham J: Infusion into the internal saphenous vein at the ankle, *Lancet* 2:815, 1945.

May HL, editor: *Emergency medicine*, New York, 1984, John Wiley & Sons.

Roberts JR, Hedges JR, editors: *Clinical procedures in emergency medicine*, Philadelphia, 1985, W.B. Saunders.

Simon RR: Modified new approaches for rapid intravenous access, *Ann Emerg Med* 16:44, 1987.

CHAPTER 51

Arterial Puncture

Grant C. Fowler

Arterial punctures are used in urgent, acute, and some chronic conditions whenever arterial blood samples are needed. If frequent sampling will be required or intraarterial blood pressure monitoring is also necessary, consideration should be made for intraarterial line placement. With proper technique and equipment, an arterial puncture is a safe and simple procedure. However, advancements in technology of noninvasive monitoring may eventually make this procedure obsolete.

INDICATIONS

- To confirm a clinically suspected acute problem with carbon dioxide or oxygen exchange, or acid-base balance, such as those seen in patients with severe asthma, pulmonary thromboembolism, and refractory cardiac dysrhythmias, and in patients who are newly comatose
- To monitor a clinical intervention, such as oxygen supplementation, hyperventilation, or cardiopulmonary resuscitation
- To detect a change in clinical status in a patient with a chronic condition that affects gas exchange or acid-base balance, such as chronic obstructive pulmonary disease
- To confirm the need for home oxygen therapy
- To obtain blood for certain lab tests requiring arterial samples, such as serum ammonia, carbon monoxide, or lactate levels
- To obtain a blood sample in emergent situations when phlebotomy cannot be performed or when venous sites are inaccessible

CONTRAINDICATIONS

- Inability to palpate arterial pulsation
- Known or suspected severe arterial disease of aneurysmal, atherosclerotic, inflammatory, or vasospastic nature

- Bleeding dyscrasias, anticoagulant therapy, or possible later thrombolytic therapy
- Poor perfusion from the ulnar artery when the radial artery is the intended puncture site

EQUIPMENT

- 3 to 5 cc sterile plastic or glass syringe with a freely movable plunger (Kits are made in which the plunger should not be moved.)
- 25-gauge 5/8-inch (1.6 cm) needle for radial, brachial, and femoral puncture; in obese patients, a 22-gauge 1.5-inch (3.8 cm) needle
- Heparin 1000 units/cc
- Sterile gloves
- Antiseptic skin preparation, such as povidone-iodine (Betadine)
- 1% lidocaine *without* epinephrine
- 3 cc syringe with 25-gauge 5/8-inch (1.6 cm) needle for lidocaine
- Plug for sample syringe or rubber stopper for end of needle
- Sterile 4 × 4 inch gauze pads
- Container of crushed ice for transport (plastic bag or cup)
- Goggles

ARTERIAL SITE SELECTION

Each site for arterial puncture has its risks and its benefits. Because of its proximity to the skin surface, the radial artery is the preferred site for arterial sampling, especially on the nondominant hand, if there is adequate ulnar artery collateral circulation (see following section) and the clinical situation is stable. In severely hypotensive patients or during cardiopulmonary resuscitation, the femoral artery is usually the artery that is most readily palpable and most conveniently located, in spite of its association with a higher risk of complications. Alternative sites in decreasing order of preference include the brachial, superficial temporal, and dorsalis pedis arteries. The brachial artery should be reserved for use when radial artery puncture cannot be performed or is contraindicated. Operator experience should also be considered with choice of site. Avoid an artery where the overlying cutaneous defenses are not intact, such as sites in which there is infection, burn, or other skin damage.

ASSESSMENT OF ULNAR COLLATERAL CIRCULATION

Radial artery puncture or cannulation can result in thrombosis of the distal radial artery. Considering that up to 12% of hands have either poor collateral flow or an incomplete palmar arch with no collateral circulation, the collateral flow should be evaluated before the procedure so that the risk of ischemic damage to the hand can be minimized (Fig. 51-1).

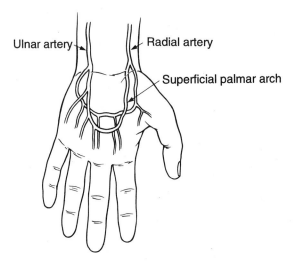

FIG. 51-1.
Anatomy of radial and ulnar arteries at wrist and superficial palmar arch.

The Allen test, used to evaluate ulnar collateral flow, was first described in 1929. It has since been modified to minimize falsely abnormal results. Emphasis should be placed on using the nondominant hand if possible. The modified Allen test is performed as follows:

1. Have the patient hold the arm above heart level, open and close the hand several times to exsanguinate it, and then clench the fist tightly. Compress the radial and ulnar arteries (Fig. 51-2, *A*). About a minute should be allowed for blood to drain from the hand. In a comatose or anesthetized patient, the hand can be clenched passively by the operator. The hand should be at least at room temperature (more than 70° F).

2. Next, the fist should be unclenched below the level of the heart (Fig. 51-2, *B*) and pressure released on the ulnar artery (Fig. 51-2, *C*). Care should be taken to avoid hyperextension of the wrist or fingers, which can result in a falsely abnormal test. When the pressure on the ulnar artery is released, the cadaveric color of the palm should return to normal color within 6 seconds, and color throughout the entire hand in less than 15 seconds (Fig. 51-2, *D*). If any area of the hand does not rapidly return to normal color, this is a positive test for abnormal ulnar collateral flow, and further tests or another location should be considered before performing the arterial procedure. The thumb, index finger, and thenar eminence are the most frequent areas involved in a positive test because of their frequent dependence on radial artery perfusion.

In the event of an abnormal or equivocal modified Allen test result, various types of noninvasive studies can be used to further evaluate collateral flow, including handheld or formal Dopplers.

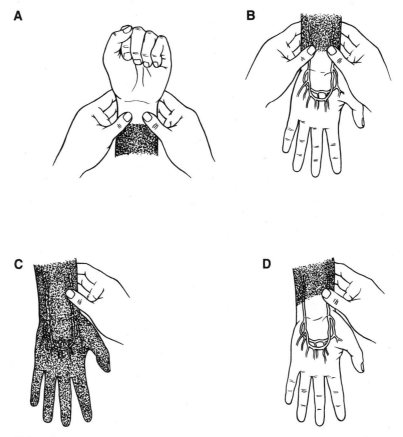

FIG. 51-2.
The modified Allen test. **A,** Hand is elevated and fist clenched while radial and ulnar arteries are occluded for one minute. **B,** Hand is lowered and fist is unclenched. Hand is cadaveric. **C,** Ulnar artery compression is released while radial artery compression is continued. The entire hand should regain color in less than 15 seconds. **D,** Positive test. In the presence of ulnar artery occlusion, the hand remains cadaveric while radial artery compression is maintained. A positive test demonstrates inadequate distal perfusion and another site should be considered.

To Perform Doppler Evaluation

1. After placing the probe between the heads of the third and fourth metacarpals on the palm, angulate the probe and advance it proximally until maximal auditory signal is obtained (Fig. 51-3).
2. With the palmar arch identified and maximal signal obtained, compression of the radial artery should result in no change of the signal, or it will result in an increase if the palmar arch is complete and supplied by collateral ulnar circulation. A decrease in signal indicates poor collateral flow. This is a much more sensitive and specific test than the Allen test.

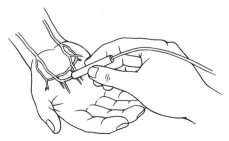

FIG. 51-3.
Assessment of the superficial palmar arch with Doppler instrument.

TECHNIQUE

1. The operator and patient should be in a comfortable position that can be maintained for quite a while if necessary. Explain the procedure and its necessity to the alert patient. The patient should be prepared to expect some discomfort. In nonclosed systems, you should observe universal blood and body fluid precautions.
2. Load the syringe for drawing the specimen with a small amount of heparin and then empty it. If a glass syringe is used, fill the barrel with heparin and attempt to eject it all. The main objective is to coat the syringe with heparin. The only remaining heparin should also fill the dead space of the needle and syringe. Certain kits contain syringes that are already heparinized and the plunger should not be moved.
3. Palpate the selected artery with the balls of two fingers, and immobilize it with two or three fingers along its course.
4. Prep the skin in an aseptic manner.
5. Local anesthetic (lidocaine) can be injected for a particularly anxious patient to minimize hyperventilation artifact. Use minimal amounts to prevent anatomical distortion and difficulty in palpating the pulse.
6. Wearing sterile gloves, hold the barrel of the syringe like a pencil, with the needle bevel up.
7a. *For radial artery puncture.* Extend and slightly rotate the wrist of (preferably) the nondominant hand. It should be supported by a firm surface. Insert the needle where the pulse is most prominent, one-half to one inch proximal to the wrist crease, at a 45- to 60-degree angle, and direct it slowly toward the pulsation (Fig. 51-4).
7b. *For brachial artery puncture.* Extend and supinate the arm and insert the needle at about a 45- to 60-degree angle toward the pulsation in the median aspect of the antecubital fossa, slightly above the elbow crease (Fig. 51-5).
7c. *For femoral artery puncture.* (Fig. 51-6). With the patient in a supine position and legs straight, insert the needle 2 to 3 cm distal to the inguinal ligament (inguinal crease) at a 60- to 90-degree angle toward the pulsation (Fig. 51-7).

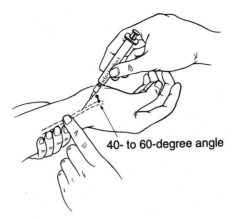

FIG. 51-4.
Palpate the patient's radial pulse with your left hand. While you are holding the heparinized syringe with your right hand (reverse hands in these directions if you are left-handed), puncture the skin at approximately a 60-degree angle, directing the needle toward the radial pulsation.

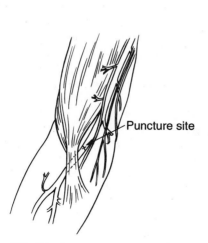

FIG. 51-5.
The right brachial artery, its branches, and the anatomic site for brachial artery puncture.

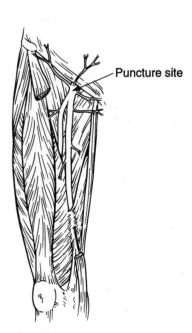

FIG. 51-6.
The right femoral artery and branches.

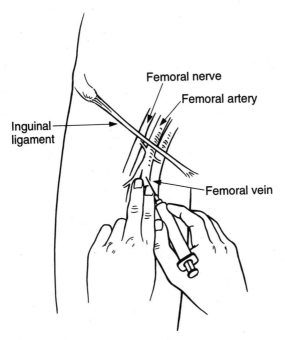

FIG. 51-7.
Technique of femoral artery puncture. The first two fingers of the free hand are used to palpate the femoral artery.

8. Puncture is detected when blood enters the syringe. It should enter the syringe spontaneously without withdrawing the plunger if the syringe is specifically designed for arterial punctures. With plastic syringes or in severely hypotensive patients, slight aspiration is sometimes necessary. Otherwise, avoid aspiration, if possible, to minimize the chance of obtaining venous blood. If blood is not obtained during the insertion, slowly withdraw the needle and stop when blood appears. If no blood appears, withdraw the needle to just beneath the skin and then advance again without changing the angle of approach but with the needle directed 1 mm to either side of the site of the previous attempt.

9. Collect 3 cc of blood and remove the needle from the artery with a smooth swift motion while applying pressure to the site. Steady pressure should be maintained for at least 5 to 10 minutes—longer in hypertensive patients and patients on anticoagulant therapy.

10. While applying pressure at the site with one hand, use the other hand to hold the syringe with the needle tip upright and expel any air bubbles. Tapping the syringe may help expel bubbles clinging to the sides.

11. Securely impale the needle tip in a rubber stopper or remove the needle and securely cap the syringe.

12. Roll the syringe between the palms of the hands 4 or 5 times to mix the blood uniformly with the heparin.

13. Label the syringe appropriately with the patient's name and number and place the syringe on ice. Immediately transport the syringe to the laboratory.
14. Return in 15 minutes and check the puncture site for hematoma formation and for adequate distal perfusion. Instruct the patient to inform you if the extremity becomes numb, painful, cold, or blue.

COMPLICATIONS

Repeated punctures at a site increase the chances of all complications.

- Hemorrhage or hematoma, the most common complication, can be minimized by prompt, continuous pressure application following the procedure, and by using a small-gauge needle.
- Thrombosis is a possible complication of any arterial puncture. It more commonly results from puncture of the radial artery and those arteries with occlusive disease. Prompt vascular surgical consultation should be considered. Ischemia and resulting gangrene are possible with this complication.
- Nerve damage directly from the needle insertion or from resultant hematoma pressure can occur.
- Infection is a possible complication.
- Spurious lab results are most often a result of mixing venous blood with the arterial sample, but they can also be due to an excessive quantity of heparin, which has a very low pH. Delay in analyzing the specimen or improper chilling can allow enough time for the blood to metabolize oxygen, or for oxygen to dissociate from hemoglobin. Air in the syringe may alter the P_{CO_2} or P_{O_2}. Vacutainers should not be used, because they contain measurable amounts of oxygen.

CPT/BILLING CODE

36600   Arterial puncture; withdrawal of blood for diagnosis

BIBLIOGRAPHY

Allen EV: Thromboangiitis obliterans: methods of diagnosis of chronic occlusive arterial lesions distal to the wrist with illustrative cases, *Am J Med Sci* 178:237, 1929.

American Heart Association: *Textbook of advanced cardiac life support,* Dallas, 1988, The Association.

Ho MT, Saunders CE, editors: *Current emergency diagnosis and treatment,* Norwalk, Conn, 1990, Appleton and Lange.

Kamienski RW, Barnes RW: Critique of the Allen test for continuity of the palmar arch assessed by Doppler ultrasound, *Surg Gynecol Obstet* 142:861, 1976.

May HL, editor: *Emergency medicine,* New York, 1984, Wiley Med Pub.

CHAPTER 52

Noninvasive Venous and Arterial Studies of the Lower Extremities

Grant C. Fowler

The accuracy of noninvasive vascular studies is *very* dependent on the skills of the operator and interpreter, and somewhat on the quality of the equipment. With state-of-the-art equipment and clinician confidence, some vascular surgeons will perform arterial surgery without arteriography, and physicians may initiate anticoagulation therapy on the basis of unequivocal venous studies alone.

NONINVASIVE VENOUS STUDIES

The incidence of deep venous thrombosis (DVT) increases with age and is more common in women than men. One third to one half of patients over 40 years of age experiencing an acute myocardial infarction, hip fracture, major surgery (especially orthopedic, pelvic, or urologic), or stroke will develop venous thrombi. Deep venous thrombosis can be found in about 80% of patients with a pulmonary embolus. As a result of previous DVT, the prevalence of postphlebitic sequelae in the adult population has been estimated at 5%. *Early* diagnosis of DVT is important to minimize long-term complications, such as venous stasis ulceration from chronic venous insufficiency. *Accurate* diagnosis is also crucial for minimization of the risk of anticoagulation therapy.

Clinical diagnosis of acute DVT has been notoriously inaccurate, with a rate of only about 50%. *Contrast venography* is regarded as the "gold standard" to verify the diagnosis; however, it is not without its risks—including allergic reactions and postvenography syndrome (10% to 20% of patients experience transient discomfort in the calf for 24 to 48 hours after contrast venography; most cases resolve without treatment, but some may progress to actual DVT). Venography is not easily repeated; it is usually only performed in one limb; it may be impossible to perform in those patients with poor venous access; and it may be difficult to perform in urgent situations without proper support staff.

Other diagnostic techniques are available:

Electrical impedance plethysmography (IPG) is the most extensively studied and commonly used noninvasive technique. Electrical impedance plethysmography provides a functional evaluation of the venous system for outflow obstruction. High false-positive rates are found with obesity, congestive heart failure, external venous compression (including that during pregnancy), and chronic DVT. It is also inaccurate in the diagnosis of thrombi in calf veins, although the clinical significance of thrombi in this area is debatable.

Ultrasound imaging (hi-frequency, B-mode, real-time) may also have limitations with obese patients. Ultrasound's other limitation is an inability to visualize the venous system above the inguinal ligament (the iliac veins) or distal to the popliteal vein. Using this technique on accessible vessels, the veins, valves, and the thrombus may be actually visualized. Compressibility of the vein, normal valve motion, and absence of visualized thrombi may help exclude the possibility of DVT.

Duplex scanning is the combination of velocity measurements by Doppler technique and ultrasound imaging. Current studies indicate that color enhancement of the Doppler velocities may improve accuracy, especially in smaller vessels. Duplex scanning may be necessary in special cases where impedance plethysmography has limitations. Impedance plethysmography, combined with duplex studies, yields results essentially as accurate as venography.

Doppler (handheld or with recorded velocities) may add information to IPG studies, such as information about the calf veins. Handheld Doppler studies were included in the protocol of many of the original noninvasive venous studies.

Risk Factors for Deep Venous Thrombosis

- Previous DVT or pulmonary embolism
- Persons who are more than 50 years old
- Venous stasis
- Persons with paralysis or otherwise immobilized
- Local injury to veins
- Hypercoagulant states
- Oral contraceptive therapy
- Pregnancy or postcesarean section
- Trauma
- Fractures, especially long bone fractures or multiple fractures
- Postoperative state from major surgeries
- Heart disease, especially congestive heart failure
- Ulcerative colitis and Behçet's syndrome
- Malignancies
- Blood type (Persons with type A may be at higher risk than those with type O.)

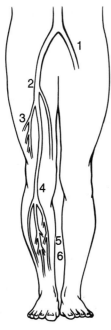

FIG. 52-1.
Six most common sites of deep venous thrombosis in the lower body. *1,* Left iliac vein; *2,* Common femoral vein; *3,* Termination of deep femoral vein; *4,* Popliteal vein at adductor canal; *5,* Posterior tibial vein; *6,* Intramuscular veins of calf.

Venous thrombi arise at bifurcations and in valve cusps (Fig. 52-1). The aging thrombus adheres to the vein wall, and nearby valves can be damaged or destroyed. The two most important valves for controlling venous hydrostatic pressure are the valve of the proximal superficial femoral vein and the valve of the distal popliteal vein. Destruction of those valves is more likely to lead to sequelae.

INDICATIONS

Nongravid

- Verification of clinically suspected acute deep venous thrombosis (This may require serial studies if calf thrombosis is suspected, and if IPG or ultrasound imaging are the diagnostic studies employed. Neither of these techniques is highly sensitive for calf thrombosis, and serial studies are recommended to monitor for more proximal progression of a thrombus.)
- Diagnosis of recurrent deep venous thrombosis
- Evaluation before discontinuing anticoagulation for deep venous thrombosis (The IPG should be repeated every 4 to 6 weeks after discharge from the hospital until the results return to normal.)
- Venous evaluation of patient with pulmonary embolism
- Preoperative study before saphenous vein stripping

- Preoperative study before venous sclerotherapy
- Venous insufficiency

Gravid

- Superficial venous thrombosis in the gravid patient should be thoroughly evaluated since about 17% of patients will also have deep venous thrombosis, which places the patient at high risk of pulmonary thromboembolism (One review of maternal deaths revealed that pulmonary embolism was the second leading cause of death.)

CONSIDERATIONS

- Unilateral or unexplained edema of the lower extremity
- Screening of certain groups of high-risk patients (e.g., postoperative)

Electrical Impedance Plethysmography (IPG)

Various plethysmography techniques are used to study a change in physical function with a change in volume. Electrical impedance plethysmography (IPG) is used to study the impedance of the lower extremity as the blood volume varies. When venous return is restricted in the lower extremity by a cuff, venous volume in the lower extremity increases. Conductivity in the lower extremity also increases (i.e., resistance or impedance decreases), since blood is a good conductor of electricity. This is measured by administering a weak electrical current that is imperceptible to the patient and measuring the current's strength after it passes through the area. When the cuff is released, conductivity should rapidly decrease if the deep venous system is patent. The rate of change of electrical conductivity is reduced in patients with thrombosis of the popliteal vein or more proximal veins. IPG has been proven to be safe, painless, reliable, and cost effective. With proper patient selection in certain large centers, accuracy approaches 98% for detecting proximal DVT, and treatment decisions can be based on unequivocal IPG studies alone. Drawbacks include expense and nonportability of equipment.

Relative Contraindications

- Significant pain or the inability to relax (may result in false-positive results)
- Patients with any potential risk of false-positive test results, i.e., patients with congestive heart failure, external vein occlusion (including that resulting from pregnancy), obesity, or chronic DVT (The risk of a false-positive result should be weighed against the risks and the availability of other venous studies.)
- Patients who are unable to remain supine, such as those with severe orthopnea

Personnel and Equipment

- A physician or technician trained to perform and record IPG
- A physician trained to interpret IPG

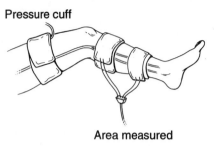

Pressure cuff

Area measured

FIG. 52-2.
For impedance plethysmography testing, elevate the leg 25 to 35 degrees. Apply electrodes around the calf, and place a pressure cuff around the thigh.

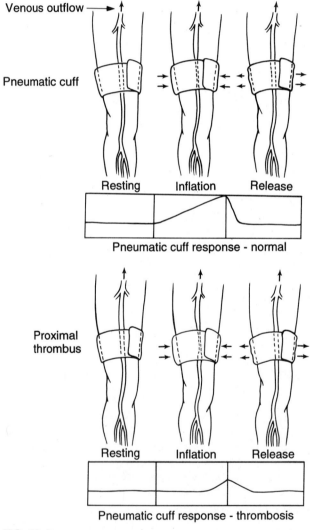

Venous outflow

Pneumatic cuff

Resting   Inflation   Release

Pneumatic cuff response - normal

Proximal thrombus

Resting   Inflation   Release

Pneumatic cuff response - thrombosis

FIG. 52-3.
Normal and abnormal impedance plethysmography tracings.

- IPG recorder
- Appropriate cuffs and electrodes

Technique

1. Place the patient in the supine position with legs elevated 25 to 30 degrees (Fig. 52-2). All tight garments should be removed and the leg well exposed.
2. Place a pneumatic cuff around the thigh, and place electrodes circumferentially around the calf.
3. Inflate the cuff to 50 mm Hg to block the venous outflow but not impair arterial inflow.
4. After the cuff has been inflated for 2 minutes, suddenly release the pressure in the compression cuff.
5. The total rise of the IPG tracing during cuff occlusion and the fall during the first 3 seconds of deflation will be plotted on a two-way graph (see Fig. 52-3 for normal and abnormal IPG tracings and Fig. 52-4 for plotting).

Interpretation and Sources of Error

Overall, the major shortcoming of IPG is that it is associated with a false-positive rate of approximately 5%. Sensitivity increases in the symptomatic patient and is

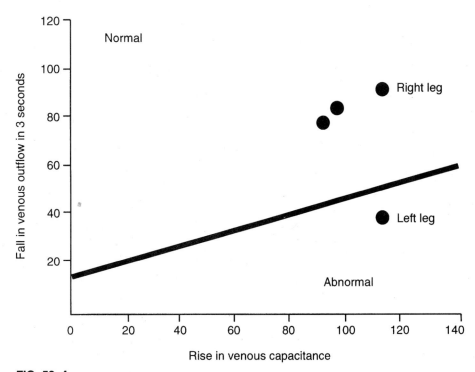

FIG. 52-4.
Typical result of impedance plethysmography. This reading suggests deep venous obstruction in the left leg, with normal venous function in the right leg.

slightly reduced when evaluating for silent proximal thrombosis, such as with postoperative screening. The error rate can be minimized by a physician with experience who takes into consideration the following factors:

- If the first result falls below the discriminant line, it is not necessarily abnormal. With repeated testing, the values may fall above the discriminant line, where they are considered normal. In the presence of *true* outflow obstruction, the result remains fixed.
- The closer the result falls to the discriminant line on either side, the more likely that it is abnormal. Such test results (close to line) should be confirmed with either venography or duplex scanning.
- Some references suggest that if abnormal results are found with both lower extremities, they are likely false-positive results, and therefore, the patient should be further evaluated with another technique.
- Excessive tightness of the cuff, particularly in obese patients, may cause tension on the skin during cuff occlusion and a false-positive result.
- Patients who are unable to relax (such as those who are apprehensive or in pain) may impede venous return with involuntary muscle restriction, which may result in a false-positive test.
- A full bladder, particularly in the elderly patient, may cause muscle tension.

Ultrasound Imaging

Real-time, B-mode sonography in the higher frequency ranges (5 to 10 MHz) allows direct "visualization" (imaging) of the venous system, and it allows the technician to search for thrombus. Sound waves are best transmitted in fluid; therefore, large veins and arteries are easily visualized with the proper probe and adequate acoustic gel interface. Arteries are differentiated from veins by their thicker walls and pulsatile nature. They also are not as easily compressible when pressure is applied on the leg with the probe. Arteries do not engorge with a Valsalva maneuver or vary with respiration.

In some situations, such as after hours in the emergency department, ultrasound may be the only diagnostic modality available. Studies of such situations have indicated that accuracy of diagnosis of DVT by ultrasound approaches the accuracy of venography.

Personnel and Equipment

- A physician or technician familiar with venous anatomy (Fig. 52-5) as well as ultrasound technology
- 5 to 10 MHz probe (transducer) and scanner
- Acoustic gel

Technique

1. Place the patient in the supine position with the lower extremities lowered at about 20 degrees and moderately externally rotated. This position increases the fluid volume in the veins and facilitates scanning.

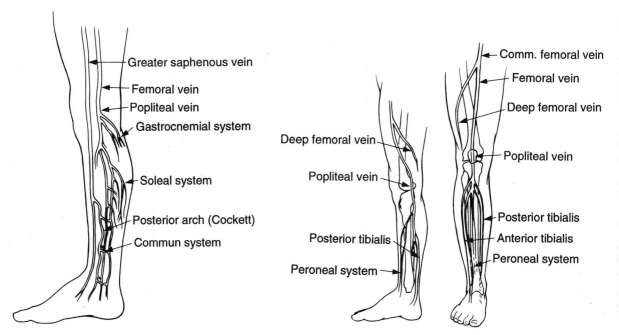

FIG. 52-5.
Venous system of the lower extremity.

2. Apply ample acoustic gel. With the probe perpendicular to the vessel, scan the common femoral and superficial femoral veins in the longitudinal and transverse dimensions. *Echogenic* matter (which appears white) within the vessels should be carefully studied to exclude a possible thrombus. Presence or absence of thrombus should be recorded. Partially obstructing thrombi occur and may be confused with scarred thickened venous walls, making it important to comment about or record wall thickness.

3. If no thrombus is visualized, apply gentle pressure with the probe to compress the vessel walls. If the vessel walls are not compressible, an early thrombus may be preventing compression, but it may not be organized or dense enough to be echogenic. Compressibility of the vessel walls should be recorded.

4. Proceed distally and continue scanning vessels in the longitudinal and transverse dimensions to the medial thigh. Fascial planes at the adductor hiatus may obscure visualization of the superficial femoral vein at that level.

5. Scan the popliteal vein either with the patient in this position or by rotating the patient to a prone position with the knees flexed 20 or 30 degrees.

6. In about 30% of patients, infrapopliteal vessels can be scanned, with the anterior and posterior tibial veins more likely than peroneal veins to be visualized.

7. Valve thickness and motion should be recorded when observed.

8. Vein response to Valsalva maneuver and deep inspiration should be recorded at the level of the common femoral, superficial femoral, and popliteal veins.

Interpretation

- Visualization of an intraluminal thrombus is *diagnostic*. This is further confirmed when the Valsalva maneuver produces minimal changes in vein diameter and when the vessel wall is incompressible. Early studies indicate that these diagnostic criteria are superior to all other techniques except venography. In a symptomatic patient, treatment (anticoagulation) can be initiated with the visualization of a thrombus alone. Ultrasonography is also a superior diagnostic technique for screening for silent DVT, which is occasionally seen in the postoperative patient. Again, absence of a visible thrombus does not completely rule out the presence of a *new* (acute) thrombus, which may have the same density as flowing blood. Other indirect signs or Doppler studies should be utilized in suspicious cases where a thrombus is not visualized, before withholding treatment.
- A *possible positive* study is one in which the veins are incompressible or do not distend with Valsalva. Consider duplex scanning for confirmation if a thrombus is not visualized by ultrasonography. The accuracy and outcomes of duplex scanning have been extensively studied, producing diagnostic results similar to venography in cases where a thrombus is not visualized.
- Differentiation of an acute thrombus from a chronic thrombus can occasionally be obtained. Acute thrombi have a homogenous texture, can be free floating, and are somewhat compressible. They often result in distal dilation of the vein. Chronic thrombi are usually not compressible, have heterogeneous echogenicity, and are firmly attached to the walls with a normal-sized or slightly contracted distal vessel.
- Increased wall thickness can be due to either previous or chronic DVT or to a partially obstructing thrombus. All of these possibilities should be strongly considered in a symptomatic patient, since all of these scenarios also place the patient at risk for DVT.
- At least one published study indicates safety in withholding treatment with a completely negative ultrasound study. This result should be weighed against the availability of duplex scanning.

Duplex Scanning

Duplex scanning provides an additional measurement of venous blood flow velocity to a routine ultrasound study using Doppler technology incorporated within the probe of the ultrasound scanner. Duplex scanning is accurate and reproducible. Compared with those of venography, the sensitivity for DVT and specificity in most series are more than 90%. Both the positive and negative predictive values, or the ability to predict the presence or absence of DVT, are in the 90% to 95% range. The drawbacks to duplex scanning include its cost to the patient (averaging $250 to $300 per study), the cost and nonportability of equipment, the time required for a complete examination, and the experience required for the technician and physician to perform and interpret the study. As with ultrasound, the ability to study the venous system above the inguinal ligament, and occasionally the superficial femoral and tibial veins at the adductor hiatus, is poor compared to IPG capabilities.

Normal venous physiology provides *spontaneous* blood return to the heart, which can be heard in the area of the vein with a handheld auditory Doppler or recorded with a Doppler velocity instrument. This spontaneous flow should be *phasic* with respirations and decrease with a Valsalva maneuver. Compression of the limb distal to probe placement should augment this flow as well.

Duplex scanning has special advantages over routine ultrasound in areas where compressibility of the vein cannot be determined because of physical restrictions, such as with smaller vessels (infrapopliteal) or with a suspected thrombus. With duplex scanning, other measurable or demonstrable parameters of venous physiologic function can be evaluated if a suspected thrombus is not clearly visualized with routine sonography. Even with a thrombus that is clearly visualized, confirmation by these four factors can be comforting data before anticoagulation therapy is initiated.

Technique

The technique of duplex scanning is the same as for ultrasound, except that there are three additional criteria for a positive result: (1) the absence of phasicity during quiet respiration, (2) the absence of spontaneous blood flow, and (3) the absence of augmentation of flow when the limb is compressed distal to the site of probe placement. The effect of the Valsalva manuever should also be observed. Valve function can be assessed by compressing the limb proximal to the site of probe placement. Functional valves should not allow augmentation of reverse flow with proximal compression. The extent of valve function at the following locations should be routinely recorded: at the level of the common femoral, femoral, and popliteal veins. They should also be evaluated and recorded as far distally as possible.

Interpretation

Treatment decisions in most large centers are based on duplex scan results alone. Occasionally, venogram and duplex results will differ. Clearly abnormal findings on a duplex scan with normal findings on venography may be due to the presence of duplicate veins in up to 20% of patients. Also, thrombosis of a superficial femoral or popliteal vein can be missed by a venogram. For a patient with a normal venogram, significant symptoms, and a clearly abnormal duplex scan, treatment is not out of the question.

Venous Dopplers

Doppler studies, including those with handheld Dopplers, have been used by themselves to qualitatively assess the venous system. The probe utilizes Doppler ultrasound technology to translate the velocity of venous blood into an audible signal or chart recording while the patient undergoes various maneuvers. This technology has not been studied as extensively as IPG or duplex scanning. One advantage is that Doppler ultrasound equipment is inexpensive and, in most cases, much more portable than IPG equipment. The safety of withholding anticoagulant treatment in patients with normal Doppler results has never been formally evaluated. For anyone performing noninvasive venous studies, a working knowledge of this technique is important for understanding basic venous physiology.

Indications
Practical indications are slightly different than for those previously discussed; for example, Dopplers may be used alone when other diagnostic methods are unavailable for confirming proximal DVT in a symptomatic patient, and they may be used to diagnose postphlebitic syndrome. This technique can also be utilized for screening those patients for whom duplex scanning or IPG may be indicated, if those studies are not readily available. If the screening test is positive, the additional cost or effort of obtaining a duplex or IPG study may be warranted. A Doppler is more reliable than IPG for the diagnosis of DVT in patients with severe arterial insufficiency or with a leg in traction. Used alone, a Doppler provides mainly qualitative evidence of venous function.

Relative Contraindications
Obese patients and patients with massive leg swelling may be difficult to study.

Personnel and Equipment

- A physician or technician familiar with venous anatomy and Doppler ultrasound technology (Since the vein cannot be visualized with this technique, a better knowledge of anatomy may be required than when using ultrasound technology [see Fig. 52-5]. Experience increases the accuracy of this examination significantly.)
- 5 to 10 MHz probe (transducer)
- Acoustic gel

Technique

1. Prepare the room and patient. The room temperature should be warmer than 70° F to prevent vasoconstriction. Place the patient in the supine position with the head slightly elevated. All tight garments should be removed and the leg well exposed. (Tight-fitting garments may interfere with venous return.) The leg should be slightly abducted, externally rotated, and slightly flexed at the knee. It should also be relaxed to prevent compression of the deep veins. Support the knee with a pillow for better muscle relaxation.
2. Locate the common femoral vein by first finding the artery and then moving the probe medially until the characteristic venous flow or tone is found. The best tone is usually obtained with the probe angled toward the heart (in the direction of venous flow). Use minimal probe pressure to keep from compressing the vein. Arterial flow is characterized by a high-pitched, usually abrupt tone. Venous flow is usually lower-pitched and more continuous.
3. Examine the patient from the level of the common femoral vein distally to the superficial femoral, popliteal, and posterior tibial veins (Fig. 52-6). When you reach the level of the popliteal vein, the patient may be turned to a prone position with knees slightly flexed and feet resting on two pillows.
4. Compare the sound or tracing from one leg to that of the other leg at each level of the examination and record the results.

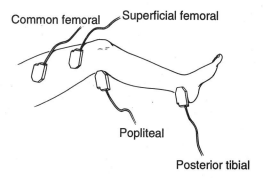

Common femoral   Superficial femoral

Popliteal

Posterior tibial

FIG. 52-6.
Doppler sonographic examination. The patient is supine with the head slightly elevated. Examine the common femoral, superficial femoral, popliteal, and posterior tibial veins sequentially.

Interpretation

Four characteristics describe normal venous flow: It is *patent* if flow is heard at the anatomic level of the vein. It is *spontaneous* if it can be heard at all levels of the vein. It varies with respiration, or is *phasic*. It is *augmented* by distal compression of the limb or by release of proximal compression.

Patent.   Rarely does the flow completely disappear with DVT, because some flow is usually preserved around a thrombus or through collateral vessels. Differences between one side and the other may be more important, and DVT is frequently associated with a continuous, high-pitched signal. A pulsatile tone that varies with the cardiac cycle is not normal and indicates increased venous pressure.

Augmented.   Firm, gentle compression of the limb for a few seconds distal to the vein should result in augmentation of the flow. Proximal compression followed by release should also result in augmentation. Deep venous thrombosis results in a more abrupt and shorter augmentation compared to that of a normal leg—if augmentation remains present at all. Augmentation produced by proximal compression before release, or distal compression after release, indicates valvular incompetence. Presence of augmentation provides support that the vein is patent.

Spontaneous.   DVT results in loss of spontaneous flow. Other causes of loss of spontaneity include anything causing vasoconstriction. As previously stated, low ambient room temperature can cause patient anxiety or vasoconstriction. The posterior tibial vein may not have a spontaneous signal in normal individuals. Presence of spontaneity is usually found when venous flow is phasic.

Phasic.   This characteristic variation with respiration may be lost with DVT. A Valsalva maneuver should decrease the signal and a deep breath should augment the signal with normal venous physiology.

False-negative results may occur in patients with incomplete venous obstruction by thrombi, and false-positive results may be caused by extrinsic venous compression.

When making treatment decisions, the physician must weigh the fact that no good outcome studies of treatment decisions based on the results of Doppler alone are available—against the availability of duplex, IPG, or contrast studies. Abnormal Doppler results are frequently confirmed with another technique. Available portable equipment, such as plethysmography, may provide additional types of quantitative data, which may be helpful to the physician in determining those patients who need further evaluation.

ARTERIAL STUDIES

Peripheral artery disease (PAD) affects 12% to 15% of the population who are more than 50 years old. Although only a small proportion of individuals with PAD and intermittent claudication develop skin breakdown or limb loss, the associated pain and disability often restrict ambulation and the overall quality of life. Men are affected nine times more frequently than women. Diabetics also develop this disease more frequently and at an earlier age; and unlike that in nondiabetics, the prognosis is grave since the disease almost always progresses. Diabetics also have a greater incidence of vessel involvement between knee and ankle than nondiabetics. Diabetic PAD is responsible for about one half of all amputations.

A history of intermittent claudication or absent/diminished peripheral pulses are unreliable indications for PAD. Peripheral artery disease most frequently involves the superficial femoral artery, with the aortoiliac and popliteal arteries next in frequency. The absence of a posterior tibial pulse is a more useful finding on examination than the absence of a dorsalis pedis pulse: 10% to 15% of the population has congenitally absent dorsalis pedis pulses. However, neither finding is very accurate.

Multiple noninvasive techniques are available for *diagnosing* lower-extremity PAD. A comprehensive history and physical examination, and a combination of at least two noninvasive tests should be employed to confirm both the diagnosis and the location of the lesion. If the location of a hemodynamically significant lesion is known, the risks associated with tests involving contrast dye can be minimized; and this knowledge can also guide the radiologist's approach for optimal contrast visualization. Different information, or sometimes more useful information, can be gained from noninvasive studies than from contrast studies; as a result, some surgeons operate without subjecting the patient to contrast studies. Contrast studies may also be avoided if noninvasive studies fail to demonstrate a hemodynamically significant lesion consistent with the patient's symptoms.

Note: The physician must always consider the possibility of cardiac disease in patients with PAD. Intermittent claudication is often the first symptom of generalized arteriosclerotic vascular disease, and these patients most frequently succumb to myocardial infarctions or cerebrovascular accidents.

Regarding *screening,* although noninvasive studies are more accurate than physical examination, there has been little literature that reveals any benefits to early detection of PAD. Additional data are needed before noninvasive testing should be considered for routine screening.

Risk Factors for Peripheral Artery Disease

- Diabetes
- Hypertension
- Cigarette smoking
- Family history
- Hyperlipidemia

INDICATIONS (ESPECIALLY IN DIABETICS)

- Intermittent claudication
- Nonhealing foot ulcer

CONSIDERATIONS

- To screen before surgery on the lower extremity of a diabetic patient
- To screen patients with a neuropathy who may have ischemia without symptoms due to the underlying neuropathy
- To follow a patient after reconstructive arterial surgery or for whom nonoperative therapy is selected

It has been said that an experienced physician can establish the presence of PAD in most patients by utilizing history and examination alone. However, many physicians who are inexperienced in management of vascular disease examine patients with extremity pain, and noninvasive studies allow for an objective diagnosis.

Segmental Pressure Measurement

The segmental pressure study is the most generally accepted and widely applied noninvasive test. Segmental pressures are often the initial study for arterial abnormalities.

Personnel and Equipment

- A physician or technician familiar with arterial anatomy of the foot and Doppler ultrasound technology
- 5 to 10 MHz probe (transducer) with audio
- Acoustic gel
- Aneroid (gauge) manometer
- Four cuffs for each leg (They can be of the same diameter. If eight are available, study time is considerably reduced.)

With arterial stenosis and especially with collateral flow, arterial resistance is significantly increased. This increased resistance results in a large or asymmetric drop in arterial blood pressure, compared to the other leg, over the particular arterial segment with obstruction. The brachial pressure can be used as a reference to compare the pressures of the lower extremity. At a minimum, brachial pressure should always be recorded along with its ratio to the pressure at the ankle (ankle-arm pressure index [API]).

Since an aneroid manometer is more mobile, faster, and more convenient than a mercury manometer, it is used by most technicians for studying segmental blood pressure measurements. Artifact is not a concern if the same gauge is used throughout the study, since ratios and gradients are the values obtained as opposed to absolute blood pressure measurements.

Likewise, the same cuff widths can be used throughout the lower extremities without concern for cuff artifact. Interpretation has taken into account cuff artifact. In most cases, this technique produces a high-thigh systolic pressure greater than brachial artery pressure, which is acceptable for calculating ratios.

Technique

1. With the patient in the supine position, measure both arm systolic pressures with the aneroid manometer and record.
2. Apply four lower-limb segmental cuffs (Fig. 52-7). The systolic values recorded refer to the cuff level rather than the artery studied.
3. Using the Doppler, evaluate each of the three major arteries of the foot (dorsalis pedis, posterior tibial, and peroneal) for the strongest signal. Use the artery that has the strongest signal throughout the study. When determining

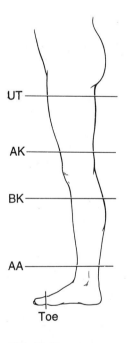
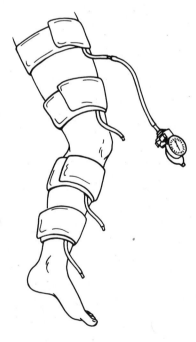

FIG. 52-7.
Segmental arterial pressure measurement. Cuff positions: *UT* = upper thigh; *AK* = above knee; *BK* = below knee; *AA* = above ankle.

pressures, hold the Doppler probe consistently over the artery in the direction and at the angle that produces the strongest signal.

4. Use the same aneroid manometer throughout. Attach it to a cuff, and inflate the cuff until the Doppler signal in the foot disappears.
5. Deflate the cuff slowly until the first signal is audible in the foot, and record this systolic value for that cuff level.
6. Sequentially inflate and deflate and record the systolic values for each cuff level throughout both lower extremities.
7. Calculate the ankle-arm pressure index (API) for both ankles, which is the ankle systolic pressure divided by the brachial systolic pressure.

Sources of Error

Most errors arise when the examiner moves the probe off the artery while inflating the cuff. One limitation with this technique is that although it is fairly sensitive for diagnosing PAD, it is not extremely satisfactory for localizing lesions.

Vessel calcification, such as that found in patients with diabetes and chronic renal failure, may result in an arterial segment that is only compressible at very high pressures and produce unusual results. Segmental pressures appear to follow a so-called reverse gradient.

With an API less than 1.0, always consider the possibility of an obstructed aorta or bilateral iliac arteries as well. Due to cuff artifact, high-thigh pressures may be greater than brachial pressures and mask aortic or iliac obstruction.

With an abnormal study, consider comparing the systolic pressure in all the arteries of the foot. This prevents the artifact that might be produced in event of localized obstruction of just one pedal artery.

Interpretation

The single best method of quantitative screening for peripheral artery disease is the ratio of the resting arm blood pressure to ankle blood pressure as determined by Doppler ultrasound. Normally, the ankle pressure is equal to or slightly greater than the arm pressure. Any API less than 1.0 is abnormal. Typically, patients with rest claudication or gangrene have APIs less than 0.5. Patients with intermittent claudication usually have APIs between 0.5 and 0.9.

A high-thigh pressure less than the arm pressure, or any pressure drop of 30 mm Hg or more from one segment to the next or a difference of 30 mm Hg or more between extremities at the same segmental level, signifies an obstruction in that segment. Some asymmetry of results in the lower extremities is normal. Remember that pressure drops may represent the sum of more than one lesion.

Waveform Analysis

Velocity or *pulse volume* waveform analysis is indicated whenever there is an abnormal API or segmental pressure study. Each of these can confirm the above studies and assist in localization of obstruction.

Velocity Waveform Analysis

Personnel and Equipment

- A physician or technician familiar with arterial anatomy of the lower extremity and Doppler ultrasound technology
- 5 to 10 MHz probe (transducer) with audio and chart recorder
- Acoustic gel

(This same equipment can be used for venous Doppler studies.)

Technique

1. Prepare the room and patient. The room temperature should be greater than 70° F to prevent vasoconstriction. The patient should rest in the supine position for at least 10 minutes. The leg should be well exposed, slightly abducted, externally rotated, and slightly flexed at the knee. Support of the knee with a pillow may provide increased patient comfort.
2. Beginning at the common femoral artery, apply acoustic gel and auscultate with the probe for maximal tone and amplitude on the recorder. The best tone is usually obtained with the probe pointed away from the heart in the direction of arterial flow. Arterial flow is characterized by a high-pitched, usually abrupt tone. This should be differentiated from the sound of venous flow, which is usually lower-pitched and more continuous.
3. Obtain tracings from common femoral, popliteal, and posterior tibial arteries. For the popliteal arteries, the patient may be turned to a prone position with knees slightly flexed and feet resting on two pillows if this position is more comfortable.
4. Compare the sound or tracing from one leg to the other leg at each level of the examination and record.

Sources of Error

- Dense objects or tissue, such as local excess fat, hematoma, scar tissue, or plaque on the anterior wall of the vessel, may significantly interfere with ultrasound transmission, making it more difficult to obtain a tracing.
- Prosthetic vessels are almost impossible to study.
- In severe disease, tracings may be unobtainable in spite of being able to hear a tone, especially in distal extremities.
- With incorrect probe angle, the multiphasic components of a tracing can be missed or lost.

Interpretation

The normal arterial velocity signal is multiphasic. It should be characterized by one systolic and one or more diastolic components. With a directional Doppler study, the diastolic component may at first be briefly negative followed by a positively directed diastolic flow component (Fig. 52-8). The diastolic component may be decreased in a vasodilated individual and increased in a vasoconstricted individual.

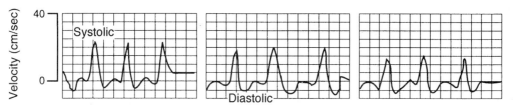

FIG. 52-8.
Normal arterial Doppler velocity tracings.

Pre-occlusion

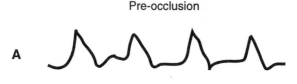

Over-stenotic

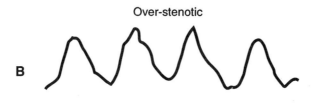

Post-stenotic

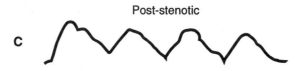

FIG. 52-9.
Examples of pre-stenotic (**A**), over-stenotic (**B**), and post-stenotic (**C**) tracings.

The arterial velocity signal produced *just proximal* to an occlusion is characteristically of short duration and low amplitude (Fig. 52-9, *A*). The arterial velocity signal produced *over* a stenotic segment is characteristically high-pitched with less prominent diastolic components (Fig. 52-9, *B*). The arterial velocity signal produced *distal* to a stenotic segment is characterized by a dampened systolic signal and absent diastolic signal. It is not as high-pitched as the stenotic signal (Fig. 52-9, *C*). The arterial signal *far distal* to a stenotic segment is like the poststenotic segment but is likely to have an even lower amplitude. *Collateral* signals are high-pitched and almost continuous.

To differentiate the contour of normal arterial signals from the contour of obstructed arterial signals, physicians describe them as "tepees" and "igloos." "Tepees" refer to the rapid upstroke with resultant high amplitude signal of a normal artery. The sluggish upstroke and minimal amplitude signal of a postobstructed artery might well be described as an "igloo."

A rule of thumb is that presence of a *multiphasic* Doppler signal in a distal vessel, such as that of the foot, strongly suggests that the proximal artery is normal.

Pulse Volume Waveform Analysis

Pulse volume recordings (PVRs) are less operator dependent, are not limited by calcification of the vessel walls, and are readily and rapidly obtained using the same cuffs that are already in place for segmental pressure measurements. This is a quantitative measurement that allows reasonably accurate localization of a lesion or lesions.

Equipment

- Pulse volume recorder
- Four cuffs for each leg (They can be of the same diameter. If eight are available, the study time is much reduced.)

Technique

1. Place the patient in the supine position. Cuffs are placed in the same locations as for segmental pressure determinations and are inflated to 65 mm Hg.
2. Record the PVR at each level.

Interpretation

Changes in waveforms with progression of PAD are seen in Fig. 52-10, *A*. To simplify the description as a progression, first noted is the loss of the reflected diastolic wave. Next, with more progressive disease, a decrease in the rate of fall of the catacrotic limb, or the downsloping portion, of the wave is seen. Last, a further delay in the rise of the anacrotic limb, or the upsloping initial portion, of the wave is noted. With moderate to severe disease, an "igloo" is the predominant feature.

Source of Error

With severe proximal disease, it is occasionally difficult to assess the degree of distal disease since the PVRs in the entire extremity are flat.

Other Studies

For the patient with intermittent claudication or a history compatible with claudication for whom all of the previous evaluations are normal, various other studies are available. Vascular stress testing is probably the most common, but it is limited in its application outside of a vascular laboratory because of the equipment cost.

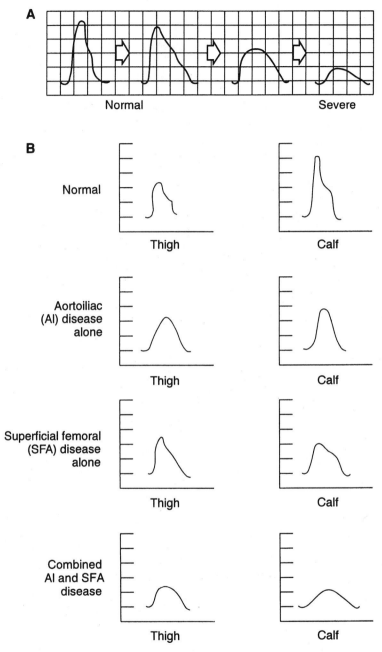

FIG. 52-10.
A, Alterations seen in pulse volume waveform as arterial occlusive disease progresses from mild to moderate to severe. **B,** Various thigh and calf waveform patterns characteristic of aorto-iliac and superficial femoral arterial occlusive disease. In the normal example, notice the contour of both the thigh and calf waveforms as well as the characteristic increase in amplitude of the calf pulse volume recordings.

CPT/BILLING CODES

93922	Noninvasive physiologic studies of upper- or lower-extremity arteries, single level, bilateral
93965	Noninvasive physiologic studies of extremity veins, complete bilateral study
93970	Duplex scan of extremity veins including responses to compression and other maneuvers; complete bilateral study
93971	Follow-up or limited study

BIBLIOGRAPHY

Barnes RW, Russell HE, Wilson MR: *Doppler ultrasonic evaluation of venous disease: a programmed audiovisual instruction*, Iowa City, 1975, University of Iowa Press.

Barnes RW, Russell HE, Wilson MR: *Doppler ultrasonic evaluation of peripheral arterial disease: a programmed audiovisual instruction*, Iowa City, 1976, University of Iowa Press.

Chance JF et al: Real-time ultrasound for the detection of deep venous thrombosis, *Ann Emerg Med* 20(5):494, 1991.

Darling RC et al: Quantitative segmental pulse volume recorder: a clinical tool, *Surgery* 79:21, 1972.

Fronek A: *Noninvasive diagnostics in vascular disease*, New York, 1989, McGraw-Hill.

Hobson RW et al: Current status of duplex ultrasonography in the diagnosis of acute deep venous thrombosis. In Bergan JJ, Yao JST, editors: *Venous disorders*, Philadelphia, 1991, W.B. Saunders.

Kempczinski RF: *The ischemic leg*, Chicago, 1985, Year Book Medical Publishers.

Leclerc JR, Illescas F, Jarzem P: Diagnosis of deep vein thrombosis. In Leclerc JR, editor: *Venous thromboembolic disorders*, Philadelphia, 1991, Lea & Febiger.

Report of the ultrasonography task force: Doppler sonographic imaging of the vascular system, *JAMA* 265(18):2382, 1991.

Satiani B et al: Noninvasive diagnosis of deep venous thrombosis, *Am Fam Physician* 44(2):569, 1991.

CHAPTER 53

Ambulatory Blood Pressure Monitoring

Peter Hanson

Diane Lillis

The diagnosis and treatment of hypertension have traditionally been based on clinical blood pressure measurements. However, these sporadic measurements are subject to a variety of physiological and psychological factors that may acutely affect the actual blood pressure. For example, the physician-induced pressor response, known as white-coat hypertension, results in higher values obtained in the office than those obtained by the patient at home.

Because of the potential variability of clinical blood pressure measurements, it is helpful to obtain more frequent measurements over a 24-hour period, during which the patient performs the usual activities of daily living, at work, and during sleep. Ambulatory blood pressure monitoring (ABPM) provides a record of average blood pressure and the variations associated with daily activities. Both of these parameters are better predictors of hypertension-related target-organ damage (e.g., left ventricular hypertrophy) and morbidity than are blood pressure measurements obtained in the clinic.

For patients who demonstrate variable clinic blood pressures, ABPM is successful for determining the presence of sustained hypertension. It is also useful for documenting the efficacy of antihypertensive drug therapy, especially since the patient can be monitored at the work site and under similar conditions where activity and psychological stress are high.

INDICATIONS

- Monitor patient with multiple blood pressure variations over 24 hours (labile hypertension)
- Monitor nonpharmacologic, or single/serial antihypertensive drug therapy for mild or borderline hypertension
- Monitor efficacy of multiple drug therapy for moderate to severe hypertension
- Documentation of breakthrough hypertension

- Determination of diurnal variability in patients with diabetes or autonomic insufficiency
- To evaluate the discrepancy between home and office blood pressure measurements

LIMITATIONS

- Noise, aberrant recordings that occur during exercise and sleep
- Patient characteristics may impair recording quality and accuracy
- Calibration is required before each recording period
- Lack of normal reference data
- Cost (varies with geographic region)

EQUIPMENT

Ambulatory blood pressure monitoring utilizes a microprocessor-controlled pump to inflate a standard blood pressure cuff at preset time intervals of 15 to 30 minutes (or on demand). Either a piezoelectric microphone that detects Korotkoff sounds is placed over the brachial artery, thereby measuring the blood pressure; or another method is used measuring the oscillometric patterns of cuff pressure.

Serial measurements are stored in the microchip's memory and are subsequently transferred to a microcomputer for analysis and graphic display. Most ABPM units report the mean blood pressure for each 1-hour interval during 24 hours, the mean daytime blood pressure, the mean nighttime blood pressure, and the percent of readings that are higher than 140/90. New units weigh less than 1 kg and are approximately the size of a Holter monitor recorder; their characteristics are summarized in Table 53-1.

TECHNIQUE

1. Carefully place the microphone over the brachial artery on the inside of the upper arm, just above the elbow. Use the nondominant arm (Fig. 53-1).
2. Choose an appropriately sized blood pressure cuff so that valid readings will be obtained. The manufacturer should provide standard-sized cuffs (obese, pediatric, adult).
3. If electrocardiogram gating is used, the electrode sites should be free of body hair and should be prepped using alcohol and light sandpaper. Be sure to use an ECG lead (usually II) with a large positive R wave.
4. Explain to the patient that the accuracy of the measurements depends on the cuff arm being quiet and free of extraneous noise during measurement.
5. It is crucial that the monitor be calibrated for each patient, both in the sitting position and the standing position.

TABLE 53-1.

Types of Noninvasive Ambulatory Blood Pressure Units

Method	Design Features	Advantages	Disadvantages	Company
Auscultatory	1. Transducer over brachial artery detects Korotkoff (K) sounds	1. R-wave gating diminishes interference from extraneous noise and muscle movement	1. Microphone is affected by ambient noise, may detect K sounds not audible to human ear, and, therefore, may result in higher systolic and lower diastolic blood pressure readings	Suntech Accutracker II Delmar Avionics Pressurometer IV
	2. K sounds are recorded following the R wave of ECG (R-wave gating)		2. ECG electrodes may decrease patient compliance or comfort	Colin Model ABPM 630 (both auscultatory and oscillometric)
Oscillometric	1. Oscillations (pressure waveform changes) transmitted from brachial artery to cuff permit discrimination of systolic and mean blood pressure	1. Increased patient comfort and ease of application	1. Accuracy is affected by muscle movement artifacts and vibrations under the cuff	Spacelabs Model 90207
	2. Diastolic blood pressure is calculated from systolic and mean blood pressure algorithm		2. Pulse pressure is influenced by cardiac output; algorithm may not be appropriate for all patients	
Indirect Continuous	1. Cuff around finger transmits arterial oscillations via a light-emitting diode that detects change in arterial size	1. Beat-by-beat continuous blood pressure analysis	1. New technology (may not be universally available)	Finapres (Portapres)
	2. The measurement of systolic and diastolic blood pressure is estimated using a special algorithm	2. Light, very compact	1. Systolic and diastolic blood pressure may be underestimated compared to brachial artery pressures	

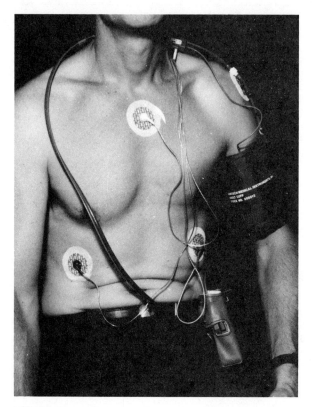

FIG. 53-1.
Subject wearing ambulatory blood pressure monitoring Accutracker unit.

Authors' note: In our laboratory, three consecutive seated and standing blood pressure measurements must be within 5 mm Hg of each other for the instrument to be considered calibrated.

The ideal calibration method is to measure simultaneously with a mercury sphygmomanometer attached to the monitor with a T-tube device.

6. Explain the necessity of writing a 24-hour diary. The patient should write down the time of work activities and home activities, medications taken, and driving, eating, sleeping, and waking times. Activities to avoid during monitoring are those that require predominant isometric arm movements, such as lawn mowing, golfing, running, and racquet sports.

INTERPRETATION

Normal subjects exhibit a characteristic diurnal variation in blood pressure (Fig. 53-2). During the first hours after awakening, the blood pressure is usually increased for several hours because of the activation of baroreflexes and neurohu-

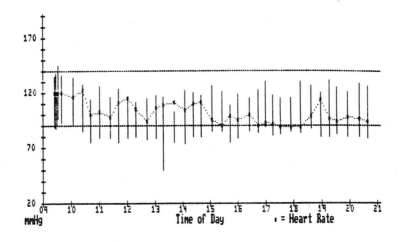

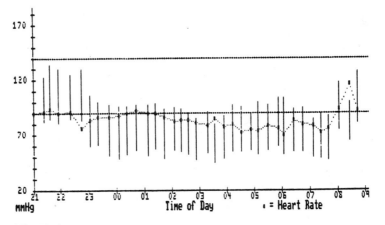

FIG. 53-2.

Normal 24-hour ambulatory blood pressure monitoring graph. Vertical lines indicate mean systolic and diastolic blood pressure. Dotted line connects heart rate. Note blood pressure and heart rate values are slightly higher in early morning and fluctuate within normal range during daytime activities. Nighttime blood pressure and heart rate show a prominent decline during sleep.

moral mechanisms that were attenuated during sleep. During daytime activities, blood pressure generally coincides with physical activity and is proportionally higher during work or exercise. Emotional stress also increases blood pressure, independent of activity. Office meetings, driving, smoking, and public speaking are examples of stressful events that frequently elicit increased blood pressure in ABPM studies. During sleep, systolic blood pressure shows a normal decline of 10 to 20 mm Hg, and diastolic, 5 to 10 mm Hg. Heart rate also decreases by 10 to 15 beats per minute. The reference values for 24-hour, daytime, and nighttime blood pressure are summarized in Table 53-2.

Cardiac dysrhythmias, such as atrial fibrillation or frequent ventricular ectopic beats, will greatly decrease the accuracy of measurement.

TABLE 53-2.

Reference Values for Ambulatory Blood Pressure.

	24-hour	Day	Night
Normal	118/72	123/76	106/64
Hypotension	97/57	101/61	86/48
Probably hypertension	139/87	146/91	127/79
Definite hypertension	149/94	157/99	137/87

Adapted from meta-analysis of 23 ABPM studies reported by Staessen et al. "Hypotension" and "Probably hypertension" are "Normal" ± 2 SD. "Definite hypertension" is "Normal" + 3 SD.
From Staessen IA et al: *Am J Cardiol* 67:723, 1991. Used with permission.

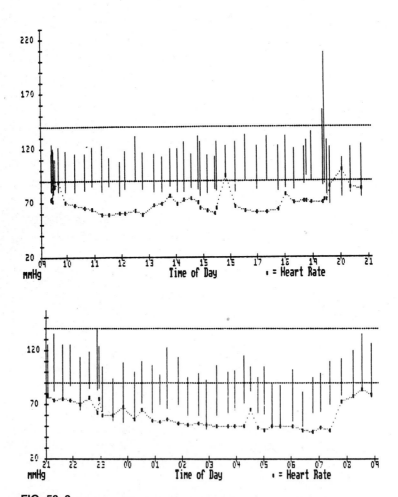

FIG. 53-3.
Clinical hypertension. Note hypertensive readings only during calibration with otherwise normotensive readings throughout the subsequent ambulatory blood pressure monitoring study.

Clinical hypertension may be suspected during the calibration phase of ABPM studies. Fig. 53-3 illustrates this pattern of apparent hypertensive values only during the three calibration readings. Pressures thereafter normalize and remain so throughout the day.

Hypertensive subjects, like normotensive subjects, show a pattern of diurnal variation, but increased systolic and diastolic blood pressure are maintained throughout daytime and sleep (Figs. 53-4 and 53-5). Some hypertensive patients exhibit a more pronounced increase during initial daytime readings after awakening. In addition, stress-related increases may be more pronounced than those of normal subjects. Older patients frequently show predominant systolic hypertension with minimal elevation of diastolic blood pressure. Nighttime blood pressures usually decline in hypertensive patients, but remain higher than those in normal

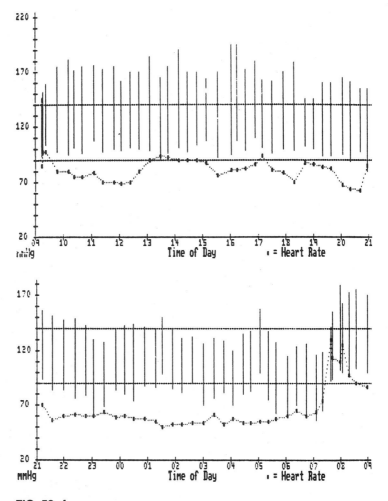

FIG. 53-4.

Untreated hypertension. Note predominant hypertensive values throughout daytime ambulatory blood pressure monitoring, continuing mild hypertension during sleep and hypertensive rise in blood pressure in early morning.

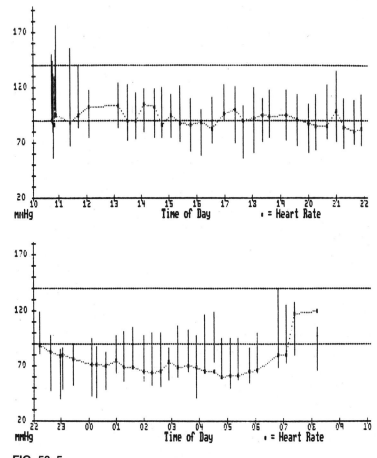

FIG. 53-5.
Treated hypertension. The same patient (Fig. 53-4) treated with transcutaneous clonidine (TTS-2), which normalizes blood pressure throughout day and night ambulatory blood pressure monitoring.

subjects. Reference values for probable hypertension and definite hypertension are also summarized in Table 53-2.

CPT/BILLING CODES

93784	Ambulatory blood pressure monitoring, utilizing a system such as magnetic tape and/or computer disk, for 24 hours; including recording, scanning analysis, interpretation, and report
93786	Recording only
93788	Scanning analysis with report
93790	Physician review with interpretation and report

Third-party coverage varies with geographical area and specific insurance carrier. Most third-party insurers reimburse for ABPM.

BIBLIOGRAPHY

Health and Public Policy Committee, American College of Physicians, Philadelphia: Automated ambulatory blood pressure monitoring, *Ann Intern Med* 104:275, 1986.

Hornsby JL, Mongan PF, Taylor AT: Ambulatory blood pressure monitoring in hypertension, *Am Fam Physician* 43(5):1631, 1991.

Meyer-Sabellek, Schultel KL, Gotzen R: Noninvasive ambulatory blood pressure monitoring: technical possibilities and problems, *J Hypertens* 8(Suppl 6):S3, 1990.

National High Blood Pressure Education Program Working Group Report on Ambulatory Blood Pressure Monitoring, *Arch Intern Med* 150:2270, 1990.

O'Brien E, O'Malley K: Twenty-four-hour ambulatory blood pressure monitoring: a review of validation data, *J Hypertens* 8(Suppl 6): S11, 1990.

The Scientific Committee: Consensus document on noninvasive ambulatory blood pressure monitoring, *J Hypertens* 8(Suppl 6):135, 1990.

Staessen IA et al: Mean and range of the ambulatory pressure in normotensive subjects from a meta-analysis of 23 studies, *Am J Cardiol* 67:723, 1991.

CHAPTER 54

Holter Monitoring

Ken Grauer

Norman Holter developed ambulatory electrocardiography, or Holter monitoring, in the early 1960s. The first device weighed about 85 pounds. Although in the past, Holter recordings were almost exclusively the domain of cardiologists and internists, the procedure is becoming increasingly popular among all primary care physicians. Primary care physicians are further encouraged to utilize Holters by their ability to acquire ambulatory monitoring systems for their practice at a reasonable cost, and by their increasing competence in interpreting the results.

Family physicians consider the procedure attractive because it is a time-efficient, income-generating test that provides useful information allowing more complete (and often definitive) management for many patients. Another benefit of Holter monitoring: the results usually enable a more appropriate referral, if referral is necessary.

Acquiring an office Holter monitoring system is not a decision to be taken lightly. The physician must first clearly have an interest in cardiac arrhythmias and be willing to invest the time needed to learn the system. The physician must also make the commitment to promptly interpret the results of all tests performed. Realistically, with training and a modicum of practice, most physicians can interpret and dictate the results of most Holter reports within 5 to 15 minutes. The ability to conduct office Holter monitoring may be an invaluable clinical resource with potential benefits that more than justify the effort expended.

Holter monitoring should not be considered a routine procedure, because it is expensive and time consuming. It should be reserved for specific indications. It is relatively easy to interpret the results; it is considerably more difficult to apply them clinically.

COMPARISON OF AVAILABLE ARRHYTHMIA MONITORING METHODS

Physical Examination and Cardiac Auscultation

- Unreliable for distinguishing between premature supraventricular and ventricular beats (PVCs), and for diagnosing rhythm abnormalities

12-Lead ECG and Rhythm Strip

- Only monitors cardiac rhythm for short period of time

24-Hour Holter Monitor

- Gold standard for arrhythmia monitoring
- Subject's diary enables the correlation of symptoms to timing of arrhythmias
- Expensive ($200 to $350 in most institutions)
- May not identify subjects with infrequent but potentially lethal arrhythmias
- Interpreter must be aware of the tremendous spontaneous variability in ectopic frequency
- May identify subjects with silent ischemia and quantify amount

Transtelephonic Monitoring

- Helpful in documenting arrhythmias that occur infrequently
- Subject must be aware of arrhythmias when they occur, and must maintain consciousness long enough to transmit the arrhythmia over the telephone

Patient History

- Unreliable in subjects who are unaware of arrhythmia or ectopic beats
- Potentially valuable for subjects who can accurately sense the occurrence of arrhythmias (i.e., "poor person's Holter monitor")

Stress (Exercise) Testing

- Demonstrates the effect of activity on ventricular arrhythmias
- May detect some forms of complex ventricular ectopy not detected by Holter monitoring
- Good screening test for the presence of underlying ischemia or coronary artery disease
- ST-segment depression in the absence of chest pain may alert physician to silent ischemia
- Not nearly as sensitive as Holter monitoring for detection of premature ventricular contractions (PVCs)

BENEFITS AND DRAWBACKS OF AVAILABLE MONITORING METHODS

Physical examination and cardiac auscultation are unreliable for distinguishing supraventricular from ventricular premature beats. The cheapest reliable method to document these arrhythmias is to obtain a standard 12-lead ECG with a short rhythm strip. Unfortunately, the cardiac rhythm is monitored only for a short period of time. Considering that the commonly accepted definition of "frequent" ventricular ectopy is more than 10 to 30 PVCs as infrequently as every few minutes, it becomes easy to see how even "frequent" PVCs can be overlooked by this method. On the other hand, if any PVCs are noted at all on a short rhythm strip, it is likely that both frequent and complex ventricular ectopy are present, and would be detected during a longer period of monitoring.

In the past, Holter recordings of only a few hours' duration were used for arrhythmia detection. Although practical and economical, such recordings do not accurately reflect the severity of cardiac arrhythmias in many individuals. This is because of the tremendous spontaneous variability in the frequency of ectopic beats that exists between one Holter recording and the next. For example, in a study by Winkle et al. of 57 patients who had three consecutive 24-hour Holter recordings performed during the late phase of acute myocardial infarction, ventricular tachycardia was detected in 12 of the 57 patients. In those patients who were found to have ventricular tachycardia, this arrhythmia occurred very sporadically during the 72-hour monitoring period. Ventricular tachycardia was seen on all three 24-hour recordings of only one of the 12 patients, and was not detected at all on 2 of the 3 days of monitoring in 9 of the 12 patients.

Marked variability in PVC frequency also occurs in ambulatory patients with chronic ventricular arrhythmias. As demonstrated by Morganroth, PVC frequency varies greatly from one day to the next, between successive 8-hour monitoring periods, and even from hour to hour within a single day. Certain individuals exhibit PVCs primarily during the day; others have them manifest principally at night. As might be expected, PVC frequency often varies with physical activity and emotional state. However, in many individuals, marked spontaneous variability in PVC frequency persists even when monitoring conditions are kept absolutely constant.

Because of such fluctuations in PVC frequency, a monitoring period of at least 24 hours is usually recommended for adequate characterization of an arrhythmia. For most individuals, 24-hour monitoring permits recognition of diurnal variations in arrhythmia frequency and allows detection of the maximal grade of ectopy.

Appreciation of the phenomenon of spontaneous variability in PVC frequency is essential if one is to interpret Holter recordings accurately and evaluate the effectiveness of antiarrhythmic therapy in a clinically relevant manner.

Although a reduction in PVC frequency from 5000 to 2500 PVCs per day following institution of an antiarrhythmic agent would seem to suggest drug efficacy, one cannot statistically exclude spontaneous variation by this response. To do so, a reduction in PVC frequency of at least 80% between Holter recordings is required. In this case, the number of PVCs would have to be decreased from 5000 to less than 1000 before one could confidently conclude that the reduction was truly a response to the medication and not simply due to chance.

Assessment of drug efficacy by follow-up Holter monitoring is made even more difficult by the fact that antiarrhythmic agents themselves have a proarrhythmic effect. Five to ten percent of all antiarrhythmic drugs paradoxically worsen the very arrhythmia that the clinician is trying to treat.

Proarrhythmic effects are most commonly seen in patients with impaired left ventricular function who have malignant ventricular arrhythmias and who are treated with antiarrhythmic agents that reduce conduction velocity, such as class I.a. or I.c. drugs and moricizine, or agents that prolong refractoriness, such as amiodarone or sotalol. However, they may also occur in patients who have simple ventricular ectopy without couplets, salvos, or longer runs of PVCs; who do not have underlying heart disease; and who are treated with beta blockers or class I.b. antiarrhythmic agents. Spontaneous variability in PVC frequency and the possibility of proarrhythmia can make it very difficult to determine whether a particular drug is making the patient better or worse.

In general, subjects with frequent ventricular ectopy almost always develop complex forms. However, the converse does not necessarily hold true. Certain individuals with potentially lethal ventricular arrhythmias only have infrequent ventricular ectopy between periods of ventricular tachycardia. Malignant ventricular arrhythmias may thus pass undetected if they do not happen to occur on the day of monitoring.

As an example, consider the case of a man with coronary artery disease who has fewer than 100 PVCs during the course of a day, but who develops an asymptomatic 20-beat run of ventricular tachycardia. This patient's arrhythmia definitely places him at increased risk of sudden cardiac death, and many clinicians would consider placing him on antiarrhythmic therapy. Although this would not be inappropriate, it may be problematic for a number of reasons. First, antiarrhythmic treatment of *asymptomatic* nonsustained ventricular tachycardia has never been shown to improve prognosis. On the contrary, empiric antiarrhythmic treatment of such patients could be potentially deleterious. Furthermore, short of invasive electrophysiologic testing, there is no reliable way to monitor the success of treatment. Even a follow-up Holter that fails to detect ventricular tachycardia cannot be taken as assurance that this infrequent but potentially lethal arrhythmia is no longer occurring!

A key caveat of Holter monitoring is that no conclusions can be reached about the existence of a symptomatic arrhythmia unless symptoms occur on the day of monitoring. As noted previously, patients may even have malignant ventricular arrhythmias that occur only intermittently, sometimes as infrequently as every few weeks. To exclude this possibility, one would either have to extend the period of Holter monitoring, or consider another method for arrhythmia detection. Performing Holters for two or more consecutive days until symptoms occur is both cumbersome to the patient and extremely expensive. A far more effective method for documenting the occurrence of sporadic ventricular arrhythmias is to employ transtelephonic monitoring. The patient is issued a set of electrode leads and a device that transmits the patient's signals over the telephone. This equipment remains with the patient for a few days or weeks. When symptoms occur, the patient simply puts on the electrode leads and a rhythm strip may be transmitted via telephone to the central monitoring station. The principal drawback of this method is that the patient must be aware of arrhythmias when they occur, and be able to maintain consciousness long enough to transmit the rhythm.

One suggested practice is to always obtain a standard 24-hour Holter as the first study. However, only in a rare situation is it necessary to order transtelephonic monitoring. Nevertheless, it occasionally is invaluable for documentating the occurrence of an infrequent arrhythmia that was not picked up by the standard Holter.

An often-ignored adjunct for monitoring is the patient's history (perception) of arrhythmia occurrence. Although many individuals are totally unaware of their arrhythmias, others are able to sense each and every ectopic beat. In selected individuals with non-life-threatening arrhythmias who have this awareness—and in whom electrocardiography has confirmed a temporal relation between symptoms and the occurrence of their arrhythmias—the *patient's account of symptoms* may serve as a fairly reliable and cost-effective adjunct for long-term monitoring. As such (the "poor person's Holter monitor"), it may greatly reduce the need for (and expense of) repeated Holter recordings for judging the effect of treatment.

Consider the case of a patient who is markedly symptomatic from extremely frequent ventricular ectopy. Baseline Holter monitoring reveals several thousand PVCs during the day of monitoring, but no runs of ventricular tachycardia. Correlation of notations on the patient's diary with the Holter confirms a definite relation between symptoms and periods of greatest ectopy. Treatment with an antiarrhythmic agent is well tolerated and results in complete resolution of symptoms. Need you repeat the Holter?

Practically speaking, the key question for the physician to ask is whether repeating the Holter would be likely to reveal anything that might alter treatment. Or, is the patient's account of symptoms (that is, the "poor person's Holter") adequate for guiding management? In many instances, such as this particular case, it is adequate.

INDICATIONS

- **Evaluation of patients with symptoms of suspected cardiac origin**
  Not all patients with symptoms such as palpitations, dizziness, and syncope need Holter monitoring. Symptom duration and severity, the likelihood of underlying cardiac disease, the existence and effect of potentially reversible extracardiac factors (e.g., caffeine, alcohol, electrolyte abnormalities, and nonessential medications), the patient's or physician's "need to know," and cost concerns should all be considered. Therefore, on a patient's first visit, do *not* routinely order Holter monitoring for patients that lack underlying heart disease or risk factors, especially if symptoms are of recent onset and are not particularly bothersome to the patient. On the other hand, you *should* order a Holter for a patient with activity-limiting symptoms, especially when the symptoms are persistent, and especially when the patient has underlying heart disease.
- **Evaluation of heart disease in which the presence of symptomatic (or asymptomatic) arrhythmias is felt to be of prognostic significance**
  The dilemma in using Holter monitoring to evaluate patients with ventricular arrhythmias is the lack of evidence that treatment of PVCs *per se* improves prognosis.

  One of the most common indications for Holter monitoring in the elderly is to diagnose and evaluate patients with sick sinus syndrome; however, pacemaker implantation in asymptomatic individuals has not been shown to prolong life.

- **Evaluation of antiarrhythmic drug therapy**

  Although it makes intuitive sense to evaluate the efficacy of antiarrhythmic treatment with follow-up Holter monitoring, doing so is not only expensive, but also problematic. Thus, drug-induced phenomena such as proarrhythmia effects or spontaneous variability in baseline PVC frequency often make it exceedingly difficult to assess the degree of efficacy (if any) of a particular drug. Moreover, even when antiarrhythmic therapy results in near-total abolition of arrhythmic events, prognosis is not necessarily improved because the precipitating cause of the arrhythmia, heart disease, remains. Surprisingly, monitoring *after* discontinuing antiarrhythmic medications is sometimes more useful.

- **Evaluation of patients for silent ischemia**

  This is the newest and most controversial indication for Holter monitoring. Although it may have great potential, using the Holter monitor to analyze ST-segment changes and their clinical implications (possible ischemia) in an unselected population is often even more problematic than using the procedure to evaluate and manage patients with ventricular arrhythmias. Practically speaking, in patients without known coronary disease, and who have Holter monitoring for evaluation of possible cardiac arrhythmias, most ST-segment shifts are *not* the result of silent ischemia.

STRESS TESTING VS. HOLTER MONITORING

The final method for evaluating PVCs is stress testing. This modality demonstrates the effect that exercise has on the arrhythmia. In general, PVCs that diminish with progressively increasing degrees of activity are less worrisome and tend to be associated with a better prognosis than those that are brought on by low levels of exercise. Although not nearly as accurate as Holter monitoring for quantitative or qualitative assessment of PVCs, complex ventricular arrhythmias (including ventricular tachycardia) and symptoms are sometimes elicited only by vigorous exercise. In addition, stress testing serves as a convenient, noninvasive screening tool for detecting the presence and the likely severity of underlying coronary artery disease. Holter monitoring and exercise testing are thus complementary procedures that provide different information, and both tests should be considered for the complete evaluation of patients with ventricular arrhythmias.

Detection of PVCs per se on exercise testing is not indicative of an ischemic response. However, PVCs become cause for much more concern when they occur in association with ST-segment depression in patients who are likely to have coronary artery disease. Thus, it is not advisable to allow a middle-aged individual who has coronary risk factors to exercise in an unsupervised manner if stress testing produces PVCs and ST-segment depression. Instead, further evaluation, including cardiac catheterization, is warranted.

On the other hand, many physicians are much more comfortable allowing healthy young adults who have frequent, asymptomatic ventricular ectopy to exercise vigorously if stress testing does not produce ST-segment depression and if PVCs resolve with exercise. This is because when these younger, asymptomatic, and otherwise healthy adults go out and exercise, their PVCs will probably resolve with activity in a similar manner as they did on the treadmill. Moreover, such individuals are much less likely to have underlying heart disease.

SILENT MYOCARDIAL ISCHEMIA

In recent years, increasing importance has been attached to the finding of silent myocardial ischemia (SMI). Diagnosis of this entity is made by objective documentation of transient myocardial ischemia in the absence of chest pain or anginal equivalents.

Silent myocardial ischemia is felt to be much more prevalent than is generally appreciated, occurring in asymptomatic individuals as well as those with known coronary artery disease. Among the latter group, it is thought that silent ischemic episodes are actually far more common than painful ischemic episodes. Clinical implications are obvious. Because episodes of SMI are not alarming to the patient, they frequently go undetected and are left untreated. This predisposes the individual to a significant increased risk of morbidity from coronary artery disease.

The two modalities most commonly used for diagnosing SMI are Holter monitoring and exercise testing. At the present state of technology, detection by Holter monitoring is still problematic, especially when transient ST-segment depression is noted in otherwise asymptomatic individuals without cardiac risk factors. It appears that in most cases, these abnormalities reflect false-positive results. In contrast, when episodes of transient ST-segment depression are detected on Holter monitoring or during exercise testing of individuals with multiple risk factors and/or known coronary artery disease, such findings are much more likely to represent true disease.

The reason that detection of SMI is important in patients with ventricular ectopy is that ischemia may be the underlying or exacerbating cause of the arrhythmia. In such cases, treatment with nitroglycerin (NTG) or calcium channel blockers may be far more appropriate than antiarrhythmic therapy. Among the antiarrhythmic agents, beta blockers offer the advantage of potentially benefiting both ischemia and the arrhythmia.

Reservations about using Holter monitoring for detection and evaluation of SMI include the following:

- Right-sided monitoring leads (such as lead V_1) that are commonly used for detection of cardiac arrhythmias only rarely demonstrate ST-segment depression.
- Special attention must be directed at ensuring optimal lead placement to rule out position-induced ST-segment deviations.
- A relatively long period of monitoring (48 to 72 hours) may be needed to adequately assess the true frequency and duration of ischemic episodes in many patients.
- Follow-up of patients identified as having SMI is both expensive and problematic.

Intuitively, it would seem logical that patients with coronary artery disease who are identified as having significant SMI should be treated with nitroglycerin, beta blockers, and calcium channel blockers, and that follow-up Holter monitoring should be done to demonstrate the efficacy of such treatment (that is, to document that the number and duration of silent ischemia episodes is less with treatment). Unfortunately, spontaneous variability of both the frequency and duration of silent ischemia episodes detected on Holter monitoring among patients with chronic stable coronary artery disease is even greater than the spontaneous variability in PVC frequency. Nabel et al. have shown that in order to statistically exclude spontaneous variability, one must virtually eliminate *all* episodes of silent ischemia on the follow-up Holter. Needless to say, this is an almost impossible task.

TECHNIQUE

- The patient's report form should be completed with relevant patient information such as cardiac risk factors, medications, activity level, and other medical problems that may assist in interpretation.
- Monitoring parameters on the equipment should be set.

Equipment Settings

Most Holter systems allow the operator some flexibility in selecting the parameters for the abnormalities that will be scanned. Some routine settings are shown in Box 54-1.

Thus, the computer should record a full-size rhythm strip for those tachycardias that are faster than 120 beats/minute (automatic high rate); for bradycardias slower than 40 beats/minute (automatic low rate); and for pauses longer than 2.00 seconds (automatic pause). Since automatic abnormal is set at 3, the machine should record the first three incidents of tachycardia that occur during any given hour, to a maximum of 5 strips per hour for any reason—which may still yield a total of 60 pages of rhythm strips to wade through (up to 5 strips per hour × 24 hours = 120 strips ÷ 2, since two rhythm strips are displayed per page).

Since periodic storage is set at 2 hours, the computer should record at least one rhythm strip every 2 hours, even if no abnormalities occur. This guarantees that the interpreter will have at least 12 rhythm strips to look at, even if the Holter is completely normal.

BOX 54-1. EQUIPMENT SETTINGS

Automatic high rate	120 beats/min	Periodic storage	2 hour
Automatic low rate	40 beats/min	Strips per hour	5
Automatic pause	2.00 sec	Report full revision	10.00
Automatic SVE	25%		
Automatic ST level	2 mm		
Automatic abnormal	3/hour		

Author's note: I generally have not felt comfortable accepting the computer's reading of "normal" unless a certain minimal number of normal full-size rhythm strips are displayed.

One reason for favoring 120 beats/minute as the upper rate limit is that lower numbers (i.e., 100 or 110 beats/minute) are more likely to produce an excessive number of benign sinus tachycardia strips, while higher numbers (i.e., 130 or 140 beats/minute) might prevent the detection of potentially significant tachycardias with relatively slow rates, such as ventricular tachycardia at 125 beats/minute.

Note: Selecting equipment settings always involves a compromise, and the setting of 120 beats/minute may occasionally yield a monotonous deluge of sinus tachycardia strips at 120 to 125 beats/minute.

For similar reasons, a lower rate limit of 40 beats/minute is favored. For example, selecting a lower rate limit of 50 beats/minute might result in a deluge of benign sinus bradycardia strips if the Holter was performed on an otherwise healthy individual who happened to have a slow pulse.

Pauses of up to 2.00 seconds are common, especially in the elderly, and are usually benign. Longer pauses, especially those accompanied by frequent episodes of bradycardia with rates less than 40 beats/minute, suggest the possibility of sick sinus syndrome.

The automatic SVE setting of 25% should record rhythm strips demonstrating a greater than 25% variation in R-R interval. This is how supraventricular ectopies (SVEs) such as premature atrial contractions (PACs) are picked up. Setting the SVE lower (i.e., at 10%) would detect many more PACs, but would also pick up sinus arrhythmia. Higher settings might miss too many PACs. But even with a setting of 25%, imagine the number of strips that would result when the underlying rhythm is atrial fibrillation!

The most controversial parameter is the automatic ST level, which is usually set at 2 mm, unless the reason for performing the Holter is to "seek and search" for silent ischemia. Resolution of ST-segment images may be less than ideal, and in an otherwise unselected population, a majority of individuals with episodes of ST-segment depression between 1 and 2 mm will be false positives; that is, they will not have true silent ischemia. Setting the ST-segment parameter at 2 mm greatly increases the specificity of this finding for true silent ischemia. The tradeoff is that some patients with coronary artery disease may have frequent episodes of silent ischemia with lesser degrees of ST-segment depression. Although the ST-segment trend analysis (see Fig. 54-4) should reflect this, it is important to document the phenomenon by recording at least a few full-size strips that demonstrate definite ST-segment depression. This is one benefit of lowering the ST-segment parameter to 1 mm when the principal reason for performing the Holter is to evaluate the patient for silent ischemia.

PREPROCEDURE PATIENT EDUCATION AND PREPARATION

- Explain to the patient why Holter monitoring is necessary.
- Attach the ECG electrodes in the same locations as in an office ECG (see Chapter 55, Office Electrocardiograms), except place the limb leads more cen-

trally, toward the chest (see operating instructions of the particular model of Holter).
- Explain to the patient the need to keep an event diary.

An essential part of the Holter recording is the patient event diary. Considering how commonly supraventricular and ventricular ectopy are found in the general population (and how frequently patients come to a physician with symptoms suggestive of cardiac arrhythmias), the importance of establishing a cause-and-effect relationship between the two becomes evident. For example, if symptoms are noted at 10 AM, 2 PM, 5 PM, and 11 PM, but no cardiac arrhythmias are seen at these times, it is likely that the symptoms are not cardiac-related. Much useful information may therefore be obtained from Holter recordings even if no arrhythmias occur—provided that the diary is carefully filled out.

In symptomatic individuals who actually demonstrate cardiac arrhythmias on Holter monitoring, one can infer whether or not the arrhythmias are likely to be the cause of symptoms by their temporal relation to events noted on the diary. For example, if long runs of ventricular bigeminy occur while the patient is relaxed and totally unaware of the arrhythmia—and palpitations or chest discomfort are noted only during periods of sinus rhythm—ventricular bigeminy is probably not related to the patient's symptoms.

Unfortunately, in clinical practice, completion of the diary is all too often neglected. As a result, consider the following:

- Emphasize the importance of filling out the diary to your patient.
- Be sure that the patient can read and write before providing the diary. If the patient is unable to do so, see if there is someone who can help the patient fill out the diary.
- For hospitalized patients, consider actively involving the nursing staff to ensure accurate completion of the patient diary.

EQUIPMENT

- Holter monitor with desired capabilities (Check for cracked or broken wires, dead batteries, or damage to the carrying case.)
- Printer paper, ink, extra cassettes (for the report to be printed out for interpretation)
- Razor
- Rubbing alcohol
- Electrodes
- Electrode cream, if disposable electrodes are not used
- Lead attachment kit

Most of the time, hospitals and commercial Holter laboratories employ trained technicians to scan Holter recordings for the interpreting physician. This is a tremendous time-saving feature because the technician can highlight the principal findings, thus sparing the physician the need to meticulously scan each of the full-disclosure printouts.

On the other hand, the luxury of having a trained technician scan full-disclosure tracings is not available to many physicians in private practice who have purchased their own Holter monitoring system. Options include:

- Having the hard copy of the Holter recording processed and scanned by a commercial laboratory—a costly option!
- Hiring or training a technician to scan may be the most cost-effective solution for the busy practitioner who has a nurse or technician with interest and expertise in arrhythmia interpretation.
- Not printing 24-hour full disclosure. Depending on your area's third-party payment regulations, you may not receive full reimbursement unless 24-hour full disclosure is printed out.
- Printing but ignoring 24-hour full disclosure, or looking only at those portions of the printout that seem relevant to the clinical problem (i.e., looking at full disclosure only at times when symptoms are noted on the diary, or at times of densest ectopy as suggested on the hourly summary). This will save time, but if something was missed, it will be documented.
- Printing 24-hour full disclosure and scanning the printout yourself. Although this takes a greater amount of time to accomplish, it may be time well spent.
- Purchasing a Holter system that does not provide full disclosure. If reimbursement for this modality in your area is comparable to that for full-disclosure systems, this alternative may be cost- and time-effective if you do not have great interest or expertise in arrhythmia interpretation. Realize however, that such systems are more likely to yield equivocal findings, and that they may overlook potentially important arrhythmias. Your interpretation of Holters recorded on such systems is only as good as the system's computer software in the system.

Author's note: I feel full 24-hour disclosure is indispensable for optimal Holter interpretation. In my experience, I feel it is essential that someone scan all full-disclosure tracings, even when trend analyses, hourly summaries, and selected rhythm strips are normal. At the very least, the first 10 to 20 Holters performed on the system in your office should be meticulously scanned, as a quality control measure; that is, when the Holter printout says "no runs of tachycardia," you can be confident of its accuracy. I have been "burned" more than once for not manually scanning the 24 hours of full disclosure.

INTERPRETATION

Appreciation of the wide range of normal is essential for meaningful interpretation of ambulatory ECG recordings. Premature supraventricular and ventricular contractions, as well as cardiac arrhythmias, are commonly found in otherwise healthy, asymptomatic individuals who are not in need of costly evaluation or treatment (which can be associated with unpleasant side effects or is even harmful).

Although detailed description of all of the variants of "normal" is beyond the scope of this review, a brief discussion of the prevalence of ventricular arrhythmias may be helpful.

Prevalence of PVCs in the General Population

Premature ventricular contractions are common. They are found in up to 50% of otherwise healthy, asymptomatic young adults. Their frequency increases with age; thus, most adults over 60 have some ventricular ectopy during a 24-hour period of monitoring. Less well appreciated is the fact that in the absence of underlying heart disease, complex forms of ventricular ectopy (e.g., multiform PVCs, ventricular couplets, salvos, or longer runs of ventricular tachycardia) are not commonly seen in most individuals. In contrast, both frequent and complex ventricular ectopy are common when underlying heart disease is present.

The term *frequent* when used to quantify ventricular ectopy is subject to interpretation. In a population of middle-aged individuals with underlying heart disease, frequent ventricular ectopy is most often defined as an average of more than 10 to 30 PVCs per hour over 24 hours of monitoring (i.e., at least 240 PVCs/day). In contrast, among otherwise healthy, asymptomatic young adults, a much lower definition of "frequent" should probably be used. As noted above, although up to half of these individuals have some PVCs during 24 hours of monitoring, it is unusual for them to have as many as 100 PVCs in a day.

A notable exception to these generalities is in the small subset of patients with primary electrical disease. These individuals have extremely frequent and complex ventricular ectopy despite an apparent absence of underlying heart disease. Seventy-three such subjects (with a mean age of 46) have been studied by Kennedy et al., and followed for a period of up to 10 years. Holter monitoring initially demonstrated a mean frequency of 566 PVCs/hour (range 78 to 1994 PVCs/hour) for the group. Multiform PVCs were present in 63%, ventricular couplets in 60%, and ventricular tachycardia in 26%. Extensive noninvasive cardiologic examination failed to reveal underlying heart disease in these asymptomatic individuals, although subsequent cardiac catheterization did disclose coronary artery disease in a small percentage of them. Survival data for the group showed a significantly lower mortality rate than would be expected for age-matched controls. Thus, even individuals with exceedingly frequent and complex ventricular ectopy will often have a relatively benign course when overt evidence of underlying heart disease is absent.

Clinical Significance of PVCs

The significance of ventricular ectopy depends on the clinical setting in which it occurs. Patients with PVCs who do not have underlying heart disease tend to have a benign prognosis. Even among individuals with primary electrical disease who may have alarmingly frequent and complex PVCs (as noted above), treatment is probably not indicated in the absence of symptoms when there is no underlying heart disease. In contrast, in the setting of acute ischemia with angina, any ventricular ectopy at all must be viewed as potentially significant and as a potential trigger of ventricular fibrillation.

Although left ventricular function is the most important predictive factor of mortality during the year following acute myocardial infarction, PVCs are also an independent risk factor. Mortality in this year is related to the frequency of ventricular ectopy detected by Holter monitoring prior to discharge from the hospital. Patients with less than one PVC per hour tend to have a low (less than 10%) mortality. The figure rises sharply as a function of PVC frequency. About half of this PVC-associated mortality increase is achieved at frequencies of three PVCs per hour, with a mortality plateau (20% to 30% for the ensuing year) being reached above PVC frequencies of 10 per hour. Thus, a predischarge Holter monitor recording obtained on a myocardial infarction patient needs to be interpreted in a different light from one obtained on a patient with chronic ventricular ectopy, and the definition of "frequent" ventricular ectopy should probably be adjusted downward in such individuals.

The frequency of ventricular arrhythmias detected in the postinfarction period is time-dependent. Premature ventricular contractions are minimal 3 to 5 days following infarction. They tend to increase over the next 6 to 12 weeks, and finally level off. Despite this tendency of PVCs to increase after discharge from the hospital, it may be more practical to obtain a baseline Holter monitor in selected patients before they are sent home.

Repetitive forms of ventricular ectopy (for example, ventricular couplets, and especially salvos and longer runs of ventricular tachycardia) are additional cause for concern. Their presence more than doubles the first-year mortality risk over that of patients who do not demonstrate repetitive forms. In contrast to what was previously thought, the prognostic significance of multiform PVCs and R-on-T complexes is much less than that of repetitive forms.

Much less can be said about the clinical benefit derived from drug treatment of postinfarction patients with PVCs. In the absence of extremely frequent and complex forms, many physicians consider beta blocker therapy first because beta blockers are generally well tolerated, have a low incidence of proarrhythmia, and may lower postinfarction mortality *and* reduce ventricular ectopy.

Despite acknowledgment of the increased risk that postinfarction ventricular arrhythmias confer, data showing benefit from treating such arrhythmias is still lacking. On the contrary, the CAST study demonstrated a twofold to threefold *increase* in mortality when postinfarction patients with ventricular arrhythmias were routinely treated with flecainide or encainide. Treatment of such patients with a class I.a. or I.b. antiarrhythmic agent when beta blockers are contraindicated remains controversial. Because of the drugs' potential for producing a proarrhythmic effect and for increasing the risk of mortality, the decision to initiate empiric antiarrhythmic therapy should never be taken lightly.

SAMPLE HOLTER MONITOR

There are many types of Holter monitor systems on the market. Each has its own advantages and disadvantages. The field continues to evolve at an amazingly rapid pace, so that today's drawbacks of a particular system may be corrected by tomorrow. Therefore, it behooves the interested physician to become familiar at least in general terms with the pros and cons of several types of Holter systems so as to be better prepared to select those operative features that are likely to be most applicable for a particular practice setting.

On the following pages, the information provided by one type of full-disclosure Holter system is illustrated. Although resolution quality of P-wave and ST-segment morphology is admittedly less than optimal with this particular system, it should still be adequate for office monitoring in most cases.

CASE STUDY

A 60-year-old man has dyspnea on exertion, which has been progressively increasing for one month. He had a myocardial infarction in the distant past, but had been active for years and was doing well without the need for cardiac medications until recently. He did not complain of chest pain or palpitations, but instead described frequent episodes of intense dyspnea associated with weakness and dizziness that most often occurred with activity. Physical examination was unremarkable, and a resting ECG revealed normal sinus rhythm without any acute changes. Because of the frequent occurrence of symptoms with activities of daily living, it was decided to obtain a Holter prior to stress testing.

Patient Diary

It is very important that the patient keep a diary to aid in interpreting the results of a Holter monitoring. This is because symptoms of potential cardiac etiology and arrhythmias are very common in the general population. The only way to prove that symptoms are cardiac-related is to document a temporal correlation between their occurrence and the occurrence of arrhythmias on a Holter.

Unfortunately, the sad reality of clinical practice is that most patient diaries simply do not get filled out. All too often this is because the physician failed to take the extra moment needed to explain to the patient the vital importance of completing the diary. It is impossible to correlate the occurrence of symptoms and arrhythmias if the diary is blank.

As emphasized earlier, completion of a diary may provide the physician with much useful information, even if the Holter is entirely normal. Thus, if multiple symptoms are noted on the day of monitoring and no arrhythmias are detected on the Holter, the patient can be reassured that symptoms are unlikely to be cardiac-related. The patient diary is especially helpful in this case (Fig. 54-1) because it indicates eight symptomatic episodes (of weakness, dizziness, and/or shortness of breath).

12-Lead ECG

Many physicians obtain a baseline 12-lead ECG on all patients scheduled for Holter monitoring. Doing so will largely eliminate the occasional problem of interpreting a

Time	Activity	Symptoms
1PM	Lunch, relax	
2PM	Rake leaves	Weak, dizziness
4PM	Sitting, resting	Weak, dizziness
6PM	Resting	Weak
7PM	Watching TV	Dizziness
9PM	Went to bed	Dizziness
7AM	Breakfast	Short of breath
8AM	Resting	Short of breath, dizzy
9AM	Drove to doctor's office	Weak, dizziness

FIG. 54-1.
Patient diary for Holter monitoring.

patient's underlying rhythm in the presence of so much artifact on the Holter recording that it precludes accurate assessment of P-wave morphology. Despite the fact that P-wave amplitude is small on this patient's 12-lead ECG (Fig. 54-2), the underlying rhythm can be clearly identified as sinus (since the P wave is upright in lead II). Sinus rhythm is harder to identify with certainty on many of the selected rhythm strips provided on this Holter.

Additional advantages found with having a baseline 12-lead ECG include accurate determination of intervals (PR, QRS, and QT), and a much better appreciation of the baseline ST segment. As a result, determination of ST-segment shifts (i.e., silent ischemia) is greatly facilitated. In this case, all intervals are normal. There is some nonspecific ST-T wave flattening in the inferolateral leads, but no frank ST-segment depression and no acute changes.

Narrative Summary

Most Holters include a narrative summary (Box 54-2) that consolidates the principal findings detected by the computer. Practically speaking, the main task of the interpreter is to verify that this computerized summary of pertinent findings is accurate.

The narrative summary in this particular case indicates a number of abnormal findings. The interpreter will certainly want to see representative examples of

- episodes of tachycardia (with a heart rate of up to 160 beats/minutes)
- episodes of bradycardia (with a heart rate between 36 to 39 beats/minute)
- pauses (between 2.14 and 3.29 seconds in duration)

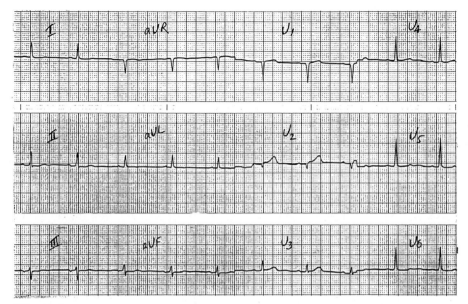

FIG. 54-2.
Baseline 12-lead ECG.

BOX 54-2. NARRATIVE SUMMARY OF HOLTER RECORDING

The patient was monitored for a period of 23:36 hours and minutes.

During this period the average heart rate was 75 BPM with a maximum heart rate of 160 BPM at 16:45 and a minimum heart rate of 36 BPM at 03:38.

There were 29 tachy episodes detected during the monitoring period.

These episodes ranged from 120 BPM to 160 BPM.

There were 7 brady episodes detected during the monitoring period.

These episodes ranged from 36 BPM to 39 BPM.

There were 57 pause episodes detected during the monitoring period.

These episodes ranged from 2.14 sec to 3.29 sec.

There were 25 SVE episodes detected during the monitoring period.

The patient pressed the event button 2 times during the monitoring period.

There were no ST episodes detected during the monitoring period.

During the monitoring period there were 1151 abnormal beats detected.

There were 2 successive abnormal episodes detected during the monitoring period.

- rhythm strips at the time the patient activated the event button (which occurred on two occasions)
- "abnormal beats" (which were recorded as occurring 1151 times), including the two episodes of "successive abnormalities"

As the interpreter, you do not need to pick out each of the 1151 abnormal beats. Moreover, there is really no need to do so. Nevertheless, you should verify that the beats are truly abnormal and not artifact; whether the "abnormal" beats are truly PVCs; and whether these PVCs seem to be occurring frequently enough to explain the computer count. Practically speaking, it matters little if there are 1151 abnormal beats or 1100 abnormal beats—or 800 or 500, for that matter—since the difference between 1151 and 800, or 500, is still well within the range for spontaneous variability. Clinically, it is unlikely that treatment decisions would differ for a patient who has 1151 PVCs or 500 PVCs, and it is probably sufficient to say that there are "frequent" PVCs.

Remember: To evaluate any intervention, a reduction of at least 80% in PVC frequency from one Holter to the next must first be demonstrated to statistically rule out the possibility of spontaneous variation. Therefore, in this particular case, the number of PVCs would have to be reduced from 1151 to *less than* 230 to eliminate this possibility.

Finally, this particular Holter system does not indicate whether PVCs are uniform or multiform; it simply gives the sum of all "abnormal" beats. Once again, practically speaking, this really does not matter in view of the following facts:

- The prognostic implications of multiformity is not nearly as ominous as was thought in the past. Much more important than multiform PVCs is the occurrence of *repetitive* PVCs (for example, couplets, salvos, and longer runs of ventricular tachycardia).
- Almost all individuals with frequent ventricular ectopy over a 24-hour period will also demonstrate at least some degree of multiformity.

Trend Analysis of Abnormal Beats

The trend analysis of abnormal beats allows us to see at a glance when PVCs occur most frequently during the day. The trend analysis of abnormal beats in this particular case demonstrates minimal ventricular ectopy at night and maximal ectopy during the daytime and evening hours (that is, between noon to midnight) when the patient is active (Fig. 54-3).

Author's note: In my experience, PVCs are most often distributed throughout the 24-hour period of monitoring. However, some patients manifest a distinct diurnal variation, in which ventricular ectopy is minimal at night and peaks in the early morning hours (at about 6 to 7 AM)—at or shortly before awakening. A second, less well-defined peak is sometimes seen in the early evening hours.

Identifiable periods of peak ventricular ectopic activity may suggest a specific approach to treatment. For example, patients who manifest diurnal variation or

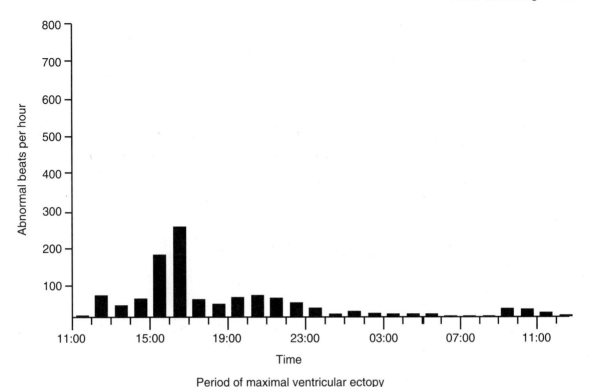

Period of maximal ventricular ectopy

FIG. 54-3.
Trend analysis of abnormal beats during 24-hour Holter monitoring.

increased ectopic activity during the hours of maximal daily activity often have an increase in sympathetic tone as part of the etiology of their arrhythmia. Therefore, these patients are optimal candidates for beta blocker therapy. Patients on antiarrhythmic therapy who demonstrate a peak in ectopic activity 6 to 10 hours after the last dose of their medication may benefit from increasing the dosing frequency or by using a sustained-release product.

Trend Analysis of Heart Rate and ST-Segment Level Trend

The heart rate trend analysis demonstrates at a glance heart rate variations during the day. For example, in this case it is easy to see that a tachycardia of approximately 150 beats/minute was sustained for most of the period between 16:00 and 17:00 (Fig. 54-4). The ST-level trend analysis shows that 1 mm of ST-segment depression was sustained throughout most of this same period (*arrow*), suggesting that the ST-segment depression is likely to be at least partially rate-related.

The ST-level trend analysis may facilitate quantitative assessment of the type and duration of ST-segment depression in patients with silent ischemia.

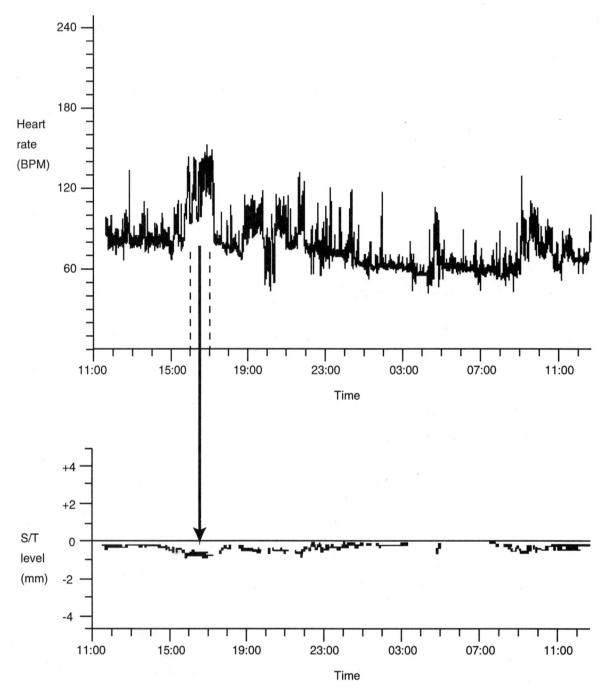

FIG. 54-4.
Heart rate and ST trend analysis during Holter monitoring.

Hourly Summary

Most Holter systems include some type of tabular hourly summary. Although it usually takes some time and practice to become familiar with this format, doing so tremendously facilitates interpretation. The hourly summary shows exactly where to look on the full-disclosure tracings to verify abnormal findings.

The hourly summary in this case (Fig. 54-5) indicates the following:

- The lowest heart rate (36 beats/minute) was recorded between 03:00 and 04:00.
- The fastest heart rate (160 beats/minute) was recorded between 16:00 and 17:00.
- The greatest hourly frequency of PVCs, or "isolated abnormalities," (235) occurred between 16:00 and 17:00.
- The event button was activated twice (once between 15:00 and 16:00, and once between 09:00 and 10:00).
- The 57 pause episodes (38 + 19) all occurred between 19:00 and 21:00.

TIME	HEART RATE AVG	MAX	MIN	S/T LEV	SLP	TACHY EPS	BRADY EPS	PAUSE EPS	SVE	ISO ABN	COUP.	SUCC. ABN	PAT. EVENT
11:00	87	105	70	-0.4	-02	0	0	0	0	5	0	0	0
12:00	82	105	62	-0.4	-02	0	0	0	0	64	0	0	0
13:00	80	139	63	-0.4	-01	0	0	0	1	40	0	0	0
14:00	81	114	68	-0.4	-02	0	0	0	0	67	0	0	0
15:00	94	153	63	-0.8	-09	3	0	0	2	176	0	0	1
16:00	129	160	89	-1.0	-17	8	0	0	10	235	0	0	0
17:00	83	159	67	-0.4	-04	4	0	0	3	71	0	0	0
18:00	82	136	63	-0.2	-01	2	0	0	0	57	0	0	0
19:00	85	141	37	-0.4	-01	4	3	38	1	79	0	0	0
20:00	87	129	44	-0.4	-02	4	0	19	0	86	0	0	0
21:00	84	144	50	-0.4	-06	4	0	0	1	62	0	0	0
22:00	73	126	51	-0.2	-03	0	0	0	1	51	0	0	0
23:00	73	124	56	-0.2	-03	0	0	0	0	32	0	0	0
00:00	62	94	43	0.0	-04	0	0	0	0	9	0	0	0
01:00	61	122	53	0.0	-05	0	0	0	0	16	0	0	0
02:00	58	81	39	0.0	-04	0	1	0	2	9	0	0	0
03:00	58	110	36	0.0	-05	0	1	0	0	6	0	1	0
04:00	63	105	42	0.0	-03	0	0	0	0	7	0	1	0
05:00	58	91	50	0.0	-03	0	0	0	1	4	0	0	0
06:00	56	91	39	0.0	-03	0	1	0	0	3	0	0	0
07:00	56	99	38	0.0	-03	0	1	0	1	4	0	0	0
08:00	87	137	53	-0.4	-01	0	0	0	1	23	0	0	0
09:00	72	101	55	-0.2	-01	0	0	0	0	20	0	0	1
10:00	70	93	48	-0.2	-01	0	0	0	1	13	0	0	0
11:00	70	105	55	-0.2	-03	0	0	0	0	5	0	0	0
AVG	75			-0.2	-04	1	0	2	1	48	0	0	0
TOTAL						29	7	57	25	1144	0	2	2

FIG. 54-5.
Hourly summary for 24-hour Holter study.

Automatic,   13:03:20

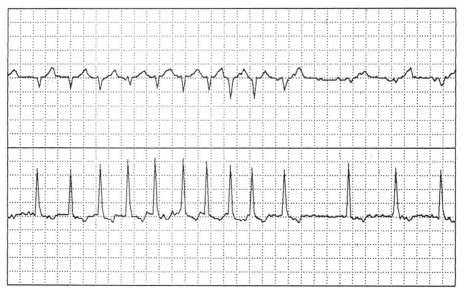

FIG. 54-6.
Selected rhythm strip at 13:03:20.

Periodic,   15:03:20

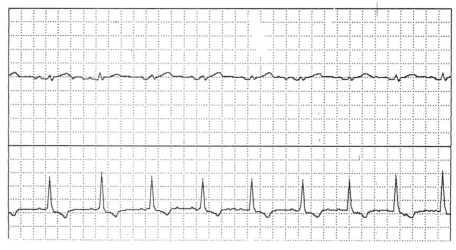

FIG. 54-7.
Selected rhythm strip at 15:03:20.

Selected (Full-Size) Rhythm Strips

Inspection of selected representative full-size rhythm strips is essential for verifying pertinent computer findings. Thus, it can be seen that this patient had a 10-beat run of paroxysmal atrial fibrillation at 13:03:20 (Fig. 54-6). He was in a regular, presumably sinus rhythm at 80 beats/minute at 15:03:20 (Fig. 54-7). An ever-so-slightly irregular supraventricular tachycardia (rapid atrial fibrillation) is evident at 15:51:09 (Fig. 54-8). This strip was "patient activated," which means that the patient was symptomatic at this time and activated the event button to record the strip.

Another rhythm strip was automatically recorded at 15:55:53 (Fig. 54-9), presumably because of the rapid, irregular rhythm and associated ectopic activity. Finally, a rhythm strip is shown at 21:56:13 (Fig. 54-10). Although it is possible that the computer may have mistakenly interpreted this tracing as showing ventricular ectopic beats, inspection of this strip strongly suggests that the baseline irregularity is due to artifact.

Full-Disclosure Strips

Many states now require full (that is, 24-hour) disclosure as a prerequisite for maximal financial compensation. The obvious advantage of having this miniaturized recording of the entire 24 hours of monitoring is that it enables the interpreter to review all events of the day and to print out a full-size rhythm strip of any abnormalities not initially recognized by the computer. Interpretation of full disclosure tracings will probably seem like an overwhelming task to the uninitiated. This need not be the case.

Patient Activated,   15:51:09

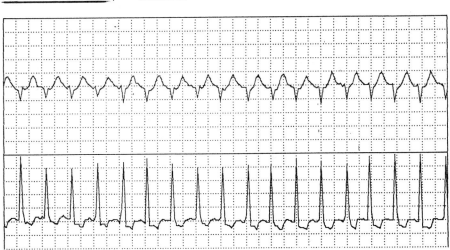

FIG. 54-8.
Selected rhythm strip at 15:51:09.

<u>Automatic,</u>   15:55:53

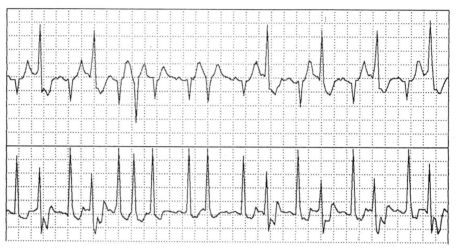

FIG. 54-9.
Selected rhythm strip at 15:55:53.

<u>Automatic,</u>   21:56:13

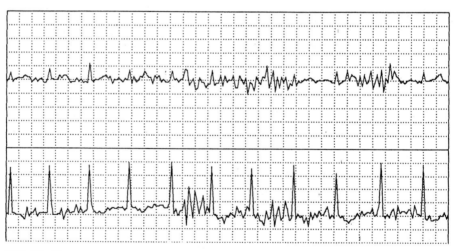

FIG. 54-10.
Selected rhythm strip at 21:56:13.

To orient you to the use of full-disclosure tracings for Holter interpretation, we will use portions of three pages from the Holter monitoring session of the patient in our case study. Normally, each page contains a miniaturized account of a full hour of the Holter recording from a single monitoring lead, and one minute of recording is represented by each of the 60 lines on the page. Because of space constraints, only half of a page (30 minutes) is shown for the selected hours. Thus, the period from 13:00 to 13:29 is shown on Fig. 54-11; from 15:30 to 15:59 on Fig. 54-12; and from 16:00 to 16:29 on Fig. 54-13.

Scan the first few lines of Fig. 54-11. Note how deceptively easy it is to identify the short run of supraventricular tachycardia that occurs between 13:03:10 and 13:03:20. (See Fig. 54-6, which showed the full-size recording of this short burst of tachycardia.) Note also how easy it is for your eye to fall upon the different looking (i.e., "abnormal") beats, which are PVCs, and for you to see that the baseline undulation on the 13:06 and 13:12 lines is likely due to artifact.

With practice, self-discipline, and diligent concentration, you should be able to rapidly scan each page (i.e., each hour of recording) in less than 10 seconds, and still be able to identify most major abnormalities on the page.

Now look at Fig. 54-12. The selected full-size rhythm strips previously reviewed demonstrated rapid atrial fibrillation at 15:51:09 (Fig. 54-8) and rapid atrial fibrillation with frequent ventricular ectopy at 15:55:53 (Fig. 54-9). Find these arrhythmias on the full disclosure tracing.

Once you see how a particular abnormality looks on the miniaturized full-disclosure tracing, it becomes relatively easy to pick up other episodes of that abnormality. Thus, we can see other short runs of frequent ventricular ectopy on lines 15:52, 15:53, 15:54, and 15:56.

Finally, turn to Fig. 54-13. Note how the patient has sustained tachycardia for a subtantial portion of this monitoring period. Actual-size rhythm strips reveal persistent of rapid atrial fibrillation during much of the hour.

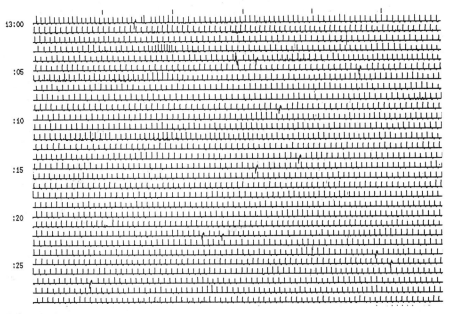

FIG. 54-11.
Full disclosure strip between 13:00 and 13:29.

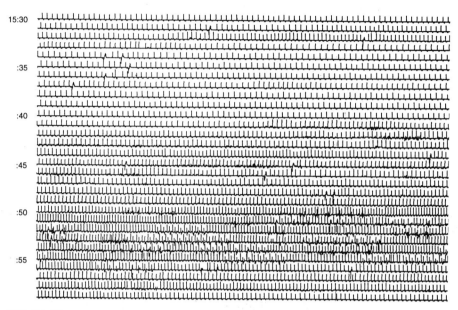

FIG. 54-12.
Full disclosure strip between 15:30 and 15:59.

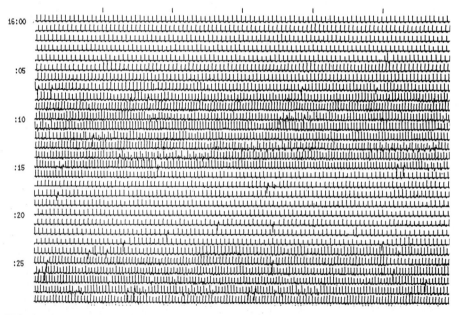

FIG. 54-13.
Full disclosure strip between 16:00 and 16:29.

INTERPRETATION OF CASE STUDY

This case study is an excellent example of how Holter monitoring can assist the physician in determining the cause of a patient's symptoms. In this particular case, the patient's symptoms were not well defined; they included increasing dyspnea, weakness, and dizziness over the previous month. There were no palpitations, and apart from some nonspecific ST-T wave changes, the patient's baseline ECG was unremarkable. Although a cardiac arrhythmia would certainly be included in the differential diagnosis, other entities would merit equal attention. In conjunction with the diary, the Holter monitor in this case is diagnostic.

Final Interpretation

- Sinus rhythm with periods of sinus bradycardia down to 36 to 40 beats/minute
- Several episodes of rapid, paroxysmal atrial fibrillation lasting minutes, with heart rates up to 160 beats/minute
- Normal intervals
- No significant ST-segment shifts
- Frequent PVCs (1151 recorded), especially during the waking hours—but virtually no repetitive forms
- Diary indicating eight symptomatic episodes of weakness, dizziness, and dyspnea that correlate well with episodes of rapid, paroxysmal atrial fibrillation—suggesting that this patient's symptoms are cardiac related (and should be treated)

Despite notation on the narrative summary of 57 pause episodes of up to 3.29 seconds, close inspection of full-disclosure tracings did not reveal any sustained pauses, which suggests that this count may reflect computer error.

Standard Interpretation Form

Use of a standardized form greatly facilitates the task of Holter interpretation. The two-sided form that we have developed (Fig. 54-14) organizes the key components of an ambulatory ECG study. In so doing, it not only saves time, but also ensures consistency in interpretation, provides clear documentation of findings, and facilitates the reporting of information in an easily understood, clinically relevant manner.

Several components of this form deserve special mention. Because artifact is often misread by the computer as ventricular ectopy, a boxed commentary (under Arrhythmias) is included on the form to reflect the interpreter's assessment of the computer's PVC count (indicating whether the count is likely to be accurate or a distortion produced by artifact). Rather than exclusively focusing on the number of ectopic beats, greater emphasis is placed on whether the occurrence of premature atrial, junctional, and ventricular contractions (including couplets and runs of ventricular tachycardia) are "common," "occasional," or "rare/absent."

HOLTER Interpretation Form

Name of patient_____ Name of physician_____ Date _____

Baseline ECG Interpretation_____

_____

PR interval _____ QRS duration _____ QTc: Normal ☐ Borderline ☐ Long ☐

Trend Analysis:
The heart rate varies from _____ to _____ , with an average rate of _____/min .

- **ST Segment Shifts ?** Yes ☐ *No significant ST segment shifts* ☐
ST elevation? ☐ ST depression? ☐ with Sx? ☐ without Sx? ☐
Estimated *duration* of ST segment depression over 24 hours_____ .

Rhythm:
Selected strips show the rhythm to be _____ .

Arrhythmias:

Number of **PVCs** *counted* by computer_____ .

Probable *accuracy* of computer **PVC count:**

```
|----------|----------|----------|----------|----------|
          Poor              Moderate            Excellent
     (PVCs are rare;                        (Computer count
   much artifact present)                  is probably accurate)
```

- *True* **PVCs appear to be:** Common ☐ Occ ☐ Rare/Absent ☐ Multiform? ☐
  - Number of ventricular couplets_____ . Couplets are: Common ☐ Occ ☐ Rare/Absent ☐
  - Number of runs of VT (≥ 3PVCs) _____ . VT runs are: Common ☐ Occ ☐ Rare/Absent ☐

- Number of **PACs/PJCs** counted by computer_____ .
  PACs/PJCs are: Common ☐ Occ ☐ Rare/Absent ☐

- Longest tachyarrhythmia (type) _____ . *No significant tachyarrhythmias* ☐
  Duration of run _____ Time _____ with Sx? ☐ without Sx? ☐

- Longest bradyarrhythmia (type) _____ . *No significant bradyarrhythmias* ☐
  Duration of run _____ Time _____ with Sx? ☐ without Sx? ☐

- Longest pause (type)_____ . *No significant pauses* ☐
  - Number of pauses >2.0 sec_____ at _____ . with Sx? ☐ without Sx? ☐

FIG. 54-14.
Standardized interpretation form. (From Grauer K and Leytem B: *Am Fam Physician* 45:1641, 1992. Used with permission.)

Diary:

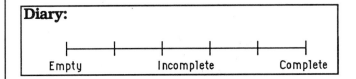

Empty   Incomplete   Complete

- *Activities* during the day:

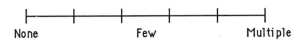

None   Few   Multiple

- **Symptoms** during the day:

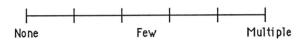

None   Few   Multiple

- Apparent *correlation* on Diary
      between **symptoms** and **arrhythmias**:

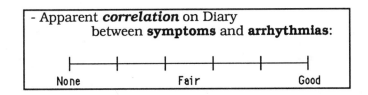

None   Fair   Good

Summary of Findings:

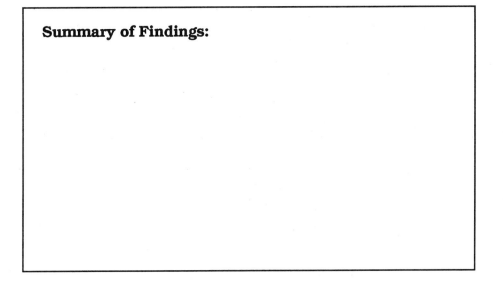

_____   _____
Interpreting Physician   Date

Finally, it is often difficult to convey the clinical relevance of a patient's diary in relation to the ambulatory ECG recording. The relative scales on the back of the interpretation form helps resolve this problem by clarifying the interpreter's assessment of the validity of the patient's diary and the correlation (if any) between patient symptoms and the arrhythmias that are noted.

CPT/BILLING CODES

93224	Continuous original ECG waveform recording and storage, with visual superimposition scanning; includes recording, scanning, analysis with report, physician review and interpretation
93230	Continuous original ECG waveform recording and storage, without superimposition scanning utilizing a device capable of producing a full miniaturized printout; includes recording, microprocessor-based analysis with report, physician review and interpretation
93235	Continuous computerized monitoring and noncontinuous recording, and real-time data analysis utilizing a device capable of producing intermittent full-size waveform tracings, possibly patient activated; includes monitoring and real-time data analysis with report, physician review and interpretation

BIBLIOGRAPHY

Bigger JT, Coromilas J: Identification of patients at risk for arrhythmic death: role of Holter ECG recording, *Cardiovasc Clin* 15:131, 1985.

Brodsky M et al: Arrhythmias documented by 24-hour continuous electrocardiographic monitoring in 50 male medical students without apparent heart disease, *Am J Cardiol* 39:390, 1977.

The Cardiac Arrhythmia Suppression Trial (CAST) Investigators: Increased mortality due to encainide or flecainide in a randomized trial of arrhythmia suppression after myocardial infarction, *N Engl J Med* 321:406, 1989.

Grauer K: Silent myocardial ischemia: dilemma or blessing? *Am Fam Physician* 42 (suppl):13S, 1990.

Grauer K, Cavallaro D: *ACLS: certification preparation,* vol I, ed 3, St Louis, 1993, Mosby.

Grauer K, Gums J: Ventricular arrhythmias:
  Part I: Prevalence, significance, and indications for treatment, *JABFP* 1:135, 1988.
  Part II: Special concerns in evaluation, *JABFP* 1:201, 1988.
  Part III: Benefits and risks of antiarrhythmic therapy, *JABFP* 1:255, 1988.
  Part IV: New agents, additional treatment modalities, and overall approach to the problem, *JABFP* 1:267, 1988

Grauer K, Leytem B: A systematic approach to Holter monitor interpretation, *Am Fam Physician* 45:1641, 1992.

Hatch R, Grauer K, Gums J: Cardiac arrhythmias. In Taylor RB, editor: *Family medicine: principles and practice,* ed 4, New York, 1993, Springer-Verlag.

Kennedy HL et al: Long-term follow-up of asymptomatic healthy subjects with frequent and complex ventricular ectopy, *N Engl J Med* 312:193, 1985.

Morganroth J et al: Limitations of routine long-term electrocardiographic monitoring to assess ventricular ectopic frequency, *Circulation* 58:404, 1978.

Nabel EG et al: Variability of transient myocardial ischemia in ambulatory patients with coronary artery disease, *Circulation* 78:60, 1988.

Skluth H, Grauer K, Gums J: Ventricular arrhythmias: an assessment of newer therapeutic agents, *Postgrad Med* 85:137, 1989.

Winkle RA, Peters F, Hall R: Characterization of ventricular tachyarrhythmias on ambulatory ECG recordings in post-myocardial infarction patients: arrhythmia detection and duration of recording, relationship between arrhythmia frequency and complexity, and day-to-day reproducibility, *Am Heart J* 102:162, 1981.

CHAPTER 55

Office Electrocardiograms

Mark E. Clasen

Grant C. Fowler

The office electrocardiogram (ECG) is a relatively simple procedure. With the availability of software that facilitates ECG interpretation, it has become an even more reassuring and commonplace procedure. The physician must be familiar with the proper use of the machine and electrode placement; however, patient comfort, alignment, and warmth are very important for good results.

INDICATIONS

- Chest pain of suspected cardiac origin
- History suspicious of recent or remote myocardial infarction
- Dysrhythmia recognition and management (see Chapter 54, Holter Monitoring)
- As an integral addition to the data preceding further cardiovascular investigation
- Baseline data before an exercise prescription
- Baseline or longitudinal data for patients with hypertension, screening particularly for left ventricular hypertrophy
- Inclusion in the baseline data when certain risk factors for cardiovascular disease are detected and/or patients reach certain age criteria
- Preoperative screen to exclude recent infarction for patients at high risk for or with known coronary artery disease

Note: Due to lack of data on the effectiveness of the screening ECG for detection of coronary artery disease, the optimal interval for such testing is uncertain. Prospective studies in asymptomatic individuals suggest that Q-waves, ST-segment depression, T-wave inversion, left ventricular hypertrophy, and ventricular arrhythmias are associated with increased risk for coronary events and sudden death. However, there are important limitations to the sensitivity and specificity of electrocardiography when used in this manner, and a normal ECG does not exclude coronary artery disease.

The American College of Cardiology recommends that all adults receive a baseline 12-lead ECG at an unspecified age, followed by periodic ECG testing every five years, or annually in high-risk persons. The American Heart Association recommends a baseline ECG at age 20, followed by repeat tracings at age 40 and 60 in normotensive persons. The Institute of Medicine has recommended obtaining a baseline ECG at age 40 or 45. A number of reviewers and the Canadian Task Force have recommended against routine ECG. Considering optimal ECG interpretation requires clinical correlation (patient signs, symptoms, data) and availability of a prior tracing for comparison (especially in symptomatic individuals).

CONTRAINDICATIONS

- Patient phobia, refusal, or inability to remain in one position
- Emergent need for airway maintenance, or management of breathing, or circulation (These needs should be met before an electrocardiogram is performed.)

EQUIPMENT

- Electrogel, or conduction pads
- Electrocardiogram machine with identifiable leads, and paper correctly loaded (Computerized ECG machines may require the clinician to type in certain data, such as patient identifiers [vital signs, age, sex, height, weight, blood pressure, drugs], time, and so forth. If a modem is used for remote computer interpretation, the number for its access and use is another requisite.) (See Chapter 56, Stress Testing, for a list of manufacturers.)

PREPROCEDURE PATIENT EDUCATION

- Explain the procedure to the patient, and discuss why the patient needs to remain as immobile as possible, to maintain normal respiration, and to not talk during the procedure. Occasionally, there is a need to assure the patient that the procedure is safe and will not cause an electrical shock.
- Inform the patient that a normal ECG does not eliminate the possibility of coronary artery disease or significant heart disease. Moreover, abnormal ECGs do not always indicate significant disease.
- Inform the patient that further cardiac workup may be necessary regardless of the outcome of the ECG.

TECHNIQUE

Review the operator's manual regarding standardization, which should be consistent. One should standardize the machine when it is tracing at 25 mm/second by briefly depressing the standardization button. One millivolt (mV) should deflect exactly 10 mm, and full standardization should be used if possible. If this varies, evaluation of serial tracings is less accurate.

Perform the ECG in a quiet, pleasant room, away from powerful electrical equipment (electric motors, X-ray equipment, etc.), if possible.

1. Place the patient in the supine position on the table with the head elevated enough for respiratory comfort. The patient should be relaxed physically and mentally, if possible. Arms should rest at the sides of the torso. Legs should be flat, apart, and not touching each other. Make certain the patient is not experiencing orthopnea from lying too flat. (If necessary, the office ECG may be performed with the patient seated in an upright position. If the patient is in a position other than lying flat, the heart's electrical axis is altered, making serial tracings difficult to compare. Whenever this is the case, a note should be made on the ECG strip. Also note the position on the ECG.) While the patient's chest and distal extremities are exposed, keep the rest of the body covered. This should prevent shivering and possible compromise of the quality of the electrocardiogram.

2. Bring the ECG machine next to the table, and turn it on. Some equipment requires a minimum of two minutes to warm up. Usual settings include sensitivity at 1N (can be verified when standardizing) and paper speed at 25 mm/ second.

3. If the skin is covered with dirt, ointment, or lotion, clean it. Place small dabs of electrogel on the distal third of the lower legs on the anterior medial surfaces. Similarly, place small dabs of electrogel on the volar surfaces of the distal third of the forearms bilaterally, and rub in briskly to mildly abrade the skin.

   Note: Electrogel contains electrolytes and an abrasive intended to break down the waterproof horny layer of the skin. Brisk rubbing enables the gel electrolytes and body electrolytes to form a continuous conductive matrix and produce the best results.

4. Place the limb electrodes: The red electrode is for the left leg, and is so labeled. The electrode for the right leg is universally green, and is labeled "right leg." The electrode for the right arm is often banded in white and labeled "RA." The electrode for the left arm is banded in black and labeled "LA." (Display the color coding for your machine so it is readily visible; colors listed here are often used.)

5. Place electrogel on the six locations of the anterior chest leads (Fig. 55-1) and rub in briskly. Place the chest electrodes:

   V_1: Fourth intercostal space at right sternal border—red
   V_2: Fourth intercostal space at left sternal border—yellow
   V_3: Halfway between V_2 and V_4—green
   V_4: Fifth intercostal space at the midclavicular line—blue
   V_5: Anterior axillary line directly lateral to V_4—tan
   V_6: Midaxillary line directly lateral to V_5—violet

The nipples are in the midclavicular line, and on men they usually overlie the fourth intercostal space. Location of the nipple varies in women. For consistent

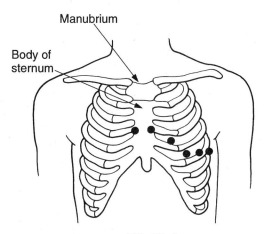

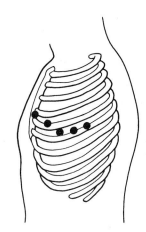

FIG. 55-1.
Location of unipolar precordial leads.

placement, utilize only bony landmarks for precordial electrodes. The sternal angle, usually palpated between the manubrium and body of the sternum, is immediately above the second intercostal space. V_4 through V_6 are placed in the same horizontal plane as V_4 (directly lateral).

6. Perform the electrocardiogram. Once the electrodes are in their proper locations and attached to the patient over the electrogel, set the machine in the run mode. Often the clinician becomes adept at "eyeballing" a good tracing devoid of artifact. Sometimes it is time-efficient to have the person ordering the test evaluate the tracing for adequacy before removing the electrodes from the leads. An extended rhythm strip or another attempt at a 12-lead ECG may be indicated for improved technical quality to further recognize and evaluate dysrhythmias.

7. Remove the electrodes from the patient, and cleanse the electrogel from the patient and from the electrodes so that the machine will be ready for immediate use.

8. For monitoring purposes, any lead can be used; however, most coronary care units use a modified bipolar chest lead. The negative electrode is near the left shoulder and the positive is the traditional V_1. A third is placed at a more remote area of the chest and serves as a ground. For rhythm evaluation, the ground electrode is optimal. To monitor for ischemia with ST-segment changes, V_4 or V_5 may be advisable.

For heat-sensitive paper, if the baseline is too light or thin, the stylus is not hot enough. If the baseline is too thick, the stylus is too hot (refer to the operating manual). Improper stylus pressure is detected by using the standardization pulse. With proper pressure, the standardization pulse should produce a tracing with sharp corners. Rounded or exaggerated angles indicate improper pressure.

For a wandering baseline, the machine has been inadequately warmed up or has a poor electrode connection (loose or dirty or not enough gel), or the patient is slowly moving or breathing deeply.

A jagged baseline is from alternating wall current (AC) interference, a broken wire, improper grounding, or a blown fuse.

POSTPROCEDURE PATIENT EDUCATION

- For persistent symptoms, the patient should schedule a follow-up visit with his or her physician, regardless of the ECG result.
- The patient should be given the results of the ECG, as well as instructions for medications, follow-up, or further workup, as necessary.

Note: If a normal baseline ECG is found, the physician may wish to give the patient a copy of the ECG, or ECG interpretation, for his or her personal records.

COMPLICATIONS

- Local skin irritation or allergic reaction to electrode placement or adhesive
- Unexpected deterioration of clinical status while undergoing ECG
- Patient distress over abnormal ECG
- Incorrect interpretation due to improper lead placement or ECG performance
- Unnecessary diagnostic workup due to no prior ECG tracing with which to compare, an inadequate clinical correlation, or a normal ECG variant

CPT/BILLING CODES

93000	Electrocardiogram, routine, with at least 12 leads; with interpretation and report
93005	Tracing only, without interpretation and report
93010	Interpretation and report only

BIBLIOGRAPHY

Grauer K: *A practical guide to ECG interpretation,* St Louis, 1992, Mosby.

U.S. Preventive Service Task Force: *Guide to clinical preventive services,* Baltimore, 1989, Williams & Wilkins.

CHAPTER 56

Stress Testing

Terrence L. Meece

Stress testing, or graded exercise testing, is a low risk, cost-effective method to diagnose and detect asymptomatic coronary artery disease (CAD) and to evaluate low-risk patients with atypical chest pain. It is also used for functional assessment to determine prognosis in patients with known heart disease and for monitoring patients during their ongoing cardiac rehabilitation. More recently, the stress test has been employed in health promotion programs to determine participants' aerobic fitness level and to motivate those involved in an exercise program by providing feedback of their progress.

PHYSIOLOGY OF EXERCISE AS APPLIED TO STRESS TESTING

The physiologic response to exercise is increased demand or *total* oxygen consumption, with increases in ventilation, cardiac output, and oxygen extraction by tissues. Despite increased stroke volume being a more efficient method of increasing cardiac output (requiring less oxygen to meet this demand), cardiac output usually increases in a less efficient manner by increasing the heart rate. The *myocardial* oxygen demand during exercise is met primarily through increases in coronary artery flow rather than improvement in oxygen extraction. Significant blockage in coronary arteries will produce a threshold at which the heart cannot obtain adequate oxygen. In normal persons, there is a linear relationship between oxygen uptake and heart rate. The heart rate increases with exercise intensity to a maximum that can be crudely estimated based upon age. (Graphic estimates based upon age are the best when determining maximum heart rate, but calculated estimates are possible.)

As exercise begins, oxygen uptake increases rapidly until the end of the second minute of constant exercise. Thereafter, oxygen uptake remains stable. Large muscles such as leg muscles (treadmill or bicycle) rapidly increase oxygen demand with increased exertion. Maximum oxygen uptake ($V_{O_2 \, max}$) is the greatest amount (volume) of oxygen that a person can extract from inspired air while performing dynamic exercise such as aerobic exercise. $V_{O_2 \, max}$ varies with body weight, heredity, gender, and exercise habits; and it often decreases progressively with age. Regular aerobic exercise can maintain or increase the $V_{O_2\ max}$. There is a nearly linear relationship between $V_{O_2\ max}$ and the maximum cardiac output; therefore, the $V_{O_2\ max}$ is a noninvasive measurement of the functional capacity of the cardiovascular system. It can be measured with inspired/expired gas analysis or more readily determined indirectly from a graded maximal exercise test.

The $V_{O_2\ max}$ is often represented as multiples of the basal oxygen consumption, which is 3.5 ml/kg/minute, or 1 metabolic equivalent (MET). (3.5 ml/kg/minute = 1 MET.) For instance, moderately active young males usually have a $V_{O_2\ max}$ of at least 42 ml/kg/minute, or 12 METs. Walking 2 mph on a level ground is approximately equal to 2 METs. 4 mph on level ground is approximately 4 METs.

Normal clinical responses to exercise testing include

- A gradual increase in pulse to maximum rate achievable for that patient (To estimate maximum heart rate, use the equation 220 − age.)
- A rise in systolic blood pressure to approximately twice the resting value (A drop in systolic blood pressure may indicate CAD.)
- A return of systolic blood pressure to its resting value by approximately 6 minutes postexercise
- A minimal change or decrease in diastolic blood pressure during exercise

INDICATIONS*

Class I: Conditions for which there is general agreement that exercise testing is justified

- To assist in the diagnosis of coronary artery disease (CAD) in male patients with symptoms that are atypical for myocardial ischemia (When evaluating atypical chest pain, risk factors should be weighed. Consider referring high-risk patients to a cardiologist. Unstable angina can occasionally present as atypical chest pain.)
- To assess functional capacity and to aid in assessing the prognosis of patients with known CAD (This is a higher-risk situation; physician should have experience in stress testing.)
- To evaluate the prognosis and functional capacity of patients with CAD soon after an uncomplicated myocardial infarction, before discharge or soon after discharge (Results are more difficult to interpret.)
- To evaluate patients after coronary artery revascularization by surgery or by coronary angioplasty (This is a higher-risk situation; physician should have experience in stress testing.)

---

*Adapted from Schlant RC, Friesinger GC, Leonard JJ: Clinical competence in exercise testing: a statement for physicians, from the ACP/ACC/AHA/ Task Force on Clinical Privileges in Cardiology, *Circulation* 82(5): November 1990. Used with permission.

- To evaluate patients with symptoms suggestive of recurrent exercise-induced arrhythmias (see Chapter 54, Holter Monitoring)
- To evaluate the functional capacity of selected patients with congenital heart disease
- To evaluate patients with rate-responsive pacemakers

Class II: Conditions for which exercise testing is frequently performed, but for which there is a divergence of opinion about its value and appropriateness

- To evaluate asymptomatic male patients over the age of 40 with special occupations (pilots, air traffic controllers, fire fighters, police officers, critical-process operators, bus or truck drivers, and railroad engineers)
- To evaluate asymptomatic males over the age of 40 with two or more risk factors for CAD
- To evaluate sedentary male patients over the age of 40 who plan to enter a vigorous exercise program (Vigorous is defined as more than 60% of maximal capacity.)
- To assist in the diagnosis of CAD in women with a history of typical or atypical angina pectoris
- To assist in the diagnosis of CAD in patients who are taking digitalis or who have complete right bundle-branch block (Results are more difficult to interpret.)
- To evaluate the functional capacity of patients with CAD or heart failure, and their response to medical therapy
- To evaluate patients with variant angina
- To perform serial evaluations (at intervals of 1 year or longer) in patients with known CAD (This is a higher-risk situation; physician should have experience in stress testing.)
- To evaluate patients with a Class I indication who have baseline ECG changes or coexisting medical problems that limit the value of the test (In some of these patients, exercise testing may still yield clinically useful information such as duration of exercise, blood pressure response, and production of chest discomfort. The results of testing may be more difficult to interpret.)
- To evaluate patients who have sustained a complicated myocardial infarction but who have subsequently "stabilized" before discharge or soon after discharge (This is higher-risk situation; physician should have experience in stress testing.)
- To evaluate on a routine, yearly basis patients who remain asymptomatic after a revascularization procedure (This is a higher-risk situation; physician should have experience in stress testing.)
- To evaluate the functional capacity of selected patients with valvular heart disease
- To evaluate the blood pressure response of patients being treated for systemic arterial hypertension who wish to engage in vigorous dynamic or static exercise
- To evaluate selected children and adolescents with valvular or congenital heart disease

CONTRAINDICATIONS*

- Very recent acute myocardial infarction (generally less than 6 days)
- Angina pectoris at rest, or unstable angina
- Severe symptomatic left ventricular dysfunction
- Potentially life-threatening cardiac dysrhythmia
- Acute pericarditis, myocarditis, or endocarditis
- Severe aortic stenosis, or suspected dissecting aneurysm
- Severe arterial hypertension (resting greater than 200 mm Hg systolic or 120 mm Hg diastolic)
- Acute pulmonary edema, embolus, or infarction
- Acute thrombophlebitis or deep vein thrombosis
- Acute or serious general illness
- Neuromuscular, musculoskeletal, or arthritic condition that precludes exercise
- Uncontrolled metabolic disease such as diabetes, thyrotoxicosis, or myxedema (Medication intoxication should be avoided [digoxin, diuretics, sedatives, psychotropic agents].)
- Inability or lack of desire or motivation to perform the test
- Nonavailability of advanced cardiac life support (ACLS) equipment or of an individual certified to perform ACLS

Some of these are relative contraindications. In selected cases, testing may be performed by a skilled cardiologist, generally in a referral center. All are contraindications to testing in the office. Most of these conditions result in a difficult-to-interpret or worthless study anyway.

EQUIPMENT AND PERSONNEL

Exercise equipment for office stress testing

- Treadmill with adjustable speed and grade is by far the most common method used (Fig. 56-1). Advantages include its comfort and its ability to test under actual physiologic conditions during exercise of most patients, since walking is the norm. In addition, a variation in patient motivation during the treadmill test causes less variation in results as compared with the bicycle method. However, the treadmill may be difficult for some patients because of its elevation. It may also be a problem for patients with lower-extremity or lower-back orthopedic problems, or for patients who are very obese.
- Bicycle ergometer with adjustable resistance and pedal frequency (Fig. 56-2). With the bicycle ergometer, the test can be terminated instantly. Many patients feel more secure on the bicycle. This method is associated with less artifact, and blood pressure measurements are easier to obtain. Unfortunately, leg

*Adapted from Schlant RC, Friesinger GC, Leonard JJ: Clinical competence in exercise testing: a statement for physicians, from the ACP/ACC/AHA/ Task Force on Clinical Privileges in Cardiology, *Circulation* 82(5): 1990. Used with permission.

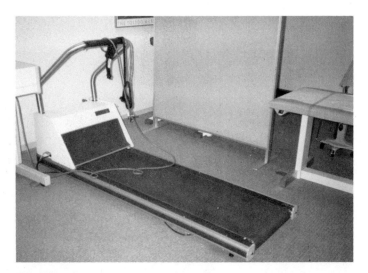

FIG. 56-1.
Treadmill.

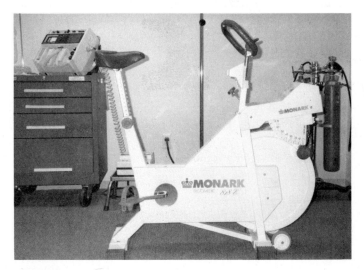

FIG. 56-2.
Bicycle ergometer.

fatigue is common because many patients do not bike. In fact, the $V_{O_2 \, max}$ often is not obtained because of fatigue. This test is dependent on motivation throughout its duration.

- Arm ergometer (Fig. 56-3). The arm ergometer enables patients with orthopedic problems to be tested. However, muscle fatigue often occurs before the maximum heart rate is achieved.

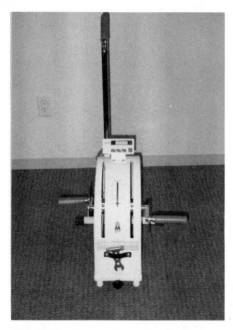

FIG. 56-3.
Arm ergometer.

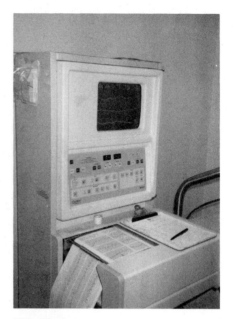

FIG. 56-4.
ECG monitor.

ECG

- Twelve-lead ECG recorder and monitor (oscilloscope) (Fig. 56-4); three-channel model is desirable; continuous tracing with screen-freeze option is desirable
- Electrodes and cables

Sphygmomanometer, including various cuff sizes
Stethoscope

Supplies

- Electric razor
- Rubbing alcohol
- Electrodes: Silver plate or silver chloride crystal pellets improve recordability; disposable electrodes are more convenient, but also more expensive
- Electrode cream if not using disposable electrodes

Emergency equipment (Fig. 56-5)

- Defibrillator
- Oxygen
- Airways, intubation, and suction equipment
- Emergency drug kit, including intravenous fluids and tubing (Available drugs should enable ACLS protocols to be followed.)

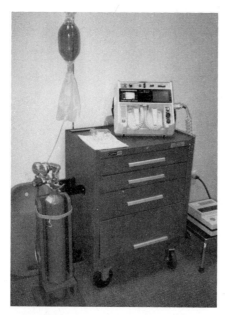

FIG. 56-5.
Emergency equipment. See text for details.

It is helpful to have a trained test technician (Fig. 56-6). Technician certification for stress testing is available through the American College of Sports Medicine. In many centers, the technician prepares the patient; monitors the ECG, the patient's response to exercise, the heart rate, and the blood pressure; and prepares the report of results for interpretation. The physician should watch the oscilloscope screen when the technician is taking blood pressure readings.

WRITTEN PROTOCOLS

- Informed consent procedure (Box 56-1)
- Medical history and physical examination form review (Fig. 56-7)
- Criteria for stopping exercise test (see Technique)
- Emergency response plan (This should be designed for every office and kept on file in event of a complication from stress testing.)
- Quality assurance plan, including calibration and testing of equipment: The emergency equipment should be checked daily and medications should be checked weekly to monthly, depending on utilization. The stress-testing equipment should be inspected and calibrated periodically based on manufacturer recommendations. ACLS cards should be kept on file along with the above records.

TABLE 56-1.

Stress Testing Systems and Manufacturers

Manufacturer	Product	Cost (approximate list price)
Marquette Electronics, Inc. 8200 W. Tower Ave. Milwaukee, WI 53223 Telephone: 414-355-5000 or 800-558-5120	Max 1 (and monitor) 1900 (treadmill)	$12,000 $6,000

Burdick, Inc.
15 Plumb St.
Milton, WI 53563
Telephone: 800-777-1777
	E350 ST (noninterpretive
	  recorder, includes treadmill)
	E550 (interpretive recorder,
	  includes treadmill)
		$14,700
		
		$16,250

Quinton Instrument Co. 2121 Terry Ave. Seattle, WA 98121 Telephone: 800-426-0337	Q4000 (monitor and recorder) Q50 (treadmill)	$11,000 $5,400
Marquette, Burdick, and others	Office defibrillators Electrically braked ergometer Manually braked ergometer	$2,000 to $3,000 $3,500 $1,200

Other Manufacturers

Health Watch Technology, Inc.   Mortara Instrument, Inc.
3400 Industrial Lane, Suite A   7865 N. 86th St.
Broomfield, CO 80020   Milwaukee, WI 53224
Telephone: 800-892-0012   Telephone: 414-354-1600

From Evans CH, Karunaratne HB: *Am Fam Physician* 45:121, 1992. Used with permission.

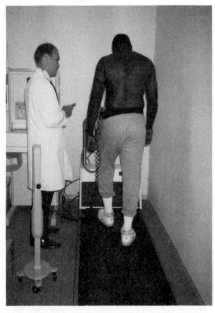

FIG. 56-6.
Trained technician monitoring patient.

BOX 56-1. CONSENT FORM
STRESS TESTING

Your physician has decided that an exercise stress test will be helpful in the diagnosis and evaluation of your medical condition. Stress testing is designed to evaluate the function of your heart, lungs, and blood vessels, especially the coronary (heart) arteries. Before the stress test, you will be screened by a physician experienced in stress testing, and a resting electrocardiogram will be recorded. You will then be asked to walk faster and faster on a treadmill (or pedal a bicycle or exercise on some other device) until the amounts of fatigue, breathlessness, chest pain, and/or other symptoms are too much for you, and you feel you should stop. If you feel you should stop the test, notify the medical personnel in the room with you.

Your blood pressure, pulse, and electrocardiogram will be monitored during the test. In some instances, blood may be drawn for testing.

Risks of stress testing include occasional changes in the rhythm of the heart beats and the possibility of very high changes in blood pressure. There is a rare chance of fainting and an even rarer chance of a heart attack (about 1 in 10,000).

Benefits of testing include learning how much exercise you can safely do and determining if there are any problems with your heart. The knowledge gained from the stress test allows a better diagnosis of your medical condition and makes more accurate treatment and prognosis possible.

Consent

Your signature on the line provided below indicates that (1) you have read, understood, and agreed to all of the above statements; (2) you have had an opportunity to ask questions about the stress test; (3) the test has been adequately explained to you, and you have sufficient information regarding the test, its risks and benefits; and (4) your consent to take the stress test is given voluntarily, as you have the right not to take the test if you so choose.

I hereby consent to undergo the performance of the stress test under the supervision of

_____

Doctor's name

_____   _____

Date   Patient's name

_____   _____

Time   Patient's signature

                                                               _____

                                                               Witness' signature

Exercise Stress Testing

Exercise stress test results

Patient's name ______________________

Date ______________
Protocol ______________
Age ______ Wt ______

Heart rate (beats per minute)

200, 190, 180, 170, 160, 150, 140, 130, 120, 110, 100, 90, 80, 70, 60

Blood pressure

Speed																
Grade	%	%	%	%	%	%	%	%	%	%	%	%	%	%	%	%
METS	1.6	2	3	4	5	6	7	8	9	10	11	12	13	14	15	
Functional class (AHA)	IV		III		II		I									

PMHR ______
(100%) (85%)
Rate attained ____% ______
METS ____ Double prod ____
Endpoint ______________

Medications ____

Angina began ______________ Angina subsided ______________ Arrhythmias ______________

Interpretation:

Physician ______________________ M.D.

FIG. 56-7.
Exercise stress test results form. (From Evans CH, Karunaratne HB: *Am Fam Physician* 45:121, 1992. Used with permission.)

PREPROCEDURE PATIENT EDUCATION

Before arrival:

- Instruct the patient not to eat for 2 hours before the test.
- If the indication for the test is disease screening or diagnosis instead of determination of pharmacologic efficacy, instruct the patient to discontinue any cardiac or hypertension medications the day of the test. (Digoxin can cause artifact even at therapeutic doses. If possible, digoxin should not be taken for 2 weeks, the amount of time necessary for its elimination.) Beta blockers, long-acting nitrates, and calcium channel blockers can suppress the development of ischemia or "prolong a positive." Patients who discontinue beta blockers should be watched closely to avoid "rebound" symptoms, and if they develop symptoms, they should restart their beta blockers. Angiotensin-converting-enzyme inhibitors have little or no effect on performance of a stress test. Sublingual nitrates can be used on an as-needed basis if other antiangina medications are discontinued, since sublingual nitrates have a much shorter duration of action.
- Instruct the patient to bring shoes and clothing that are comfortable for walking and possible jogging.

After arrival:

- Explain the reasons for the test.
- Explain the procedure: how work load will be increased, how blood pressure measurements will be taken.
- Assure the patient of close monitoring.
- Discuss symptoms the patient should report during test.
- Explain to the patient how he or she can terminate the procedure.
- Obtain informed consent.

TECHNIQUE

1. Review the patient's medical history and physical examination.
2. Select the mode (treadmill, bicycle ergometer, or arm ergometer) based on the individual's condition.
3. Select the protocol. There are many excellent protocols in use; therefore, the choice is often dependent on patient demographics and on physician preference.
   - Choose a protocol that starts at a low level (2 to 3 METs).
   - A protocol with stage durations of at least 3 minutes allows more physiologic adaptation to the work load of each stage.
   - Work load increases that are no greater than 1 to 3 METs at each stage also allows more physiologic adaptation.
   - Choose a protocol that allows completion of the study in less than 20 minutes, beyond which fatigue and overheating may independently affect results.

In the United States, the Bruce protocol is the most common, and has been the most extensively studied and validated. It is especially useful in active patients and takes less time than other protocols because it involves rapid increases in work load. It does have its disadvantages: By the fourth or fifth stage, the patient must run, which increases artifact. In addition, the patient often experiences difficulty in accommodating to increases in both slope and speed with each stage. In general, most "modified" protocols (such as the modified Bruce or modified Balke protocol) have a reduced progression of workload and are more easily tolerated by elderly or debilitated patients. Gradual but continuously increasing workload (RAMP) protocols are being studied in several large centers and show promise.

4. Obtain the resting blood pressure.
5. Prepare the patient for the ECG machine to be used in the test (Fig. 56-8).
   a. Locate sites on chest for electrodes, which are the same locations as for office ECG (see Chapter 55, Office Electrocardiograms), except that the arm electrodes are placed in the infraclavicular fossae and the leg electrodes are placed on the upper abdominal quadrants just above the beltline.
   b. Shave any hair off sites.
   c. Cleanse the skin at these sites with gauze soaked in alcohol and let dry thoroughly.
   d. Apply electrodes to these sites.
   e. Attach the exercise ECG *octopus* on a belt around the patient's waist. (An ECG octopus is the set of leads usually provided by the equipment

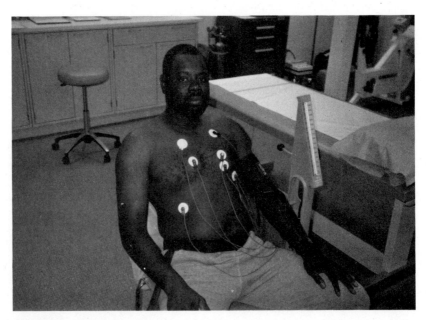

FIG. 56-8.
Patient with electrodes attached.

manufacturer to accompany its ECG machine.) The octopus can be bundled and affixed to the patient with extra expansion loops to allow a variation of distance from ECG machine and to minimize motion artifact. More recent equipment utilizes filters that minimize motion artifact.

    f. Attach lead wires from the octopus to the appropriate electrodes.

    g. For female patients, a gown or loose-fitting shirt should be worn over the lead wires.

6. Obtain the supine resting ECG.
7. Have the patient sit, and obtain the resting ECG.
8. Have the patient hyperventilate for 20 seconds, and repeat the ECG.

    Occasionally ST-segment depression occurs with hyperventilation. This makes it very difficult to interpret the actual test, because if ST-segment depression occurs during exercise, it could be either a normal result of hyperventilation or a pathologic state.

> *Note:* Some authorities no longer have every patient hyperventilate before each procedure. If the patient has a positive result, attempts should be made to evaluate the possibility of hyperventilation artifact *after* the recovery period. This trend is especially useful in the office setting where few positives should be seen; hence, this saves a lot of individuals from unnecessary hyperventilation.

9. Begin the exercise test using preselected protocol. If using the treadmill for determining a fitness level or for prognosis, do not allow the patient to hold on, as this will falsely elevate the fitness level.
10. Monitor the patient's symptoms and pulse rate at all times. Instruct the patient to give adequate warning before he or she wants the test stopped. Encourage the patient to go as far as he or she can.
11. Record a 12-lead ECG at the end of each stage, any time an abnormality is noted on the oscilloscope, immediately on stopping, and every minute for 8 minutes postexercise.
12. Termination of exercise test:
    - Keep patient exercising for 3 to 4 minutes during recovery to prevent venous pooling.
    - Monitor blood pressure, symptoms, and oscilloscope during recovery. Observe the patient in recovery until symptoms or ECG changes have resolved completely, or for at least 8 minutes.
13. Test termination criteria:

Absolute Indications

- Systolic blood pressure (SBP) drops below resting value, despite an increase in work load
- Worsening anginal chest pain (severe enough that the patient desires to stop)
- Central nervous system symptoms
- Signs of poor perfusion (cyanosis, pallor) or severe ventricular dysfunction (dyspnea)

- Serious arrhythmias
- Technical problems with ECG or SBP monitoring
- Patient request to stop
- Marked ECG changes (greater than 3 mm of horizontal, downsloping ST-segment depression, or greater than 2 mm of ST-segment elevation)

Relative Indications

- Worrisome ST or QRS changes such as excessive junctional depression or marked axis shift
- Increasing chest pain
- Fatigue, shortness of breath, wheezing, leg cramps, or intermittent claudication
- Worrisome appearance
- Hypertensive response (SBP greater than 240 mm Hg, diastolic blood pressure [DBP] greater than 115 mm Hg)
- Less serious dysrhythmia, including supraventricular tachycardia
- Development of bundle-branch block that cannot be distinguished from ventricular tachycardia

DIAGNOSTIC INTERPRETATION OF STRESS TEST

Normal ECG responses to exercise (Fig. 56-9):

- P-wave amplitude increases.
- PR interval decreases.
- Below a heart rate of 150, the R-wave amplitude is unchanged or increased; above 150 or near maximal exercise, the R wave in a healthy heart usually decreases in amplitude (the so-called Brody effect).
- *J-point,* or the junction between the S wave and ST segment, is depressed in the lateral leads at maximum exercise and gradually returns to normal during recovery.
- The ST-segment slope is usually upsloping so that at 0.04 to 0.06 seconds after the J-point, the ST segment has returned to a baseline level.

Abnormal ECG responses to exercise:

- ST-segment depression is the most widely held indicator of an abnormal stress test. Flat and downsloping depression are more likely a true positive result than a rapid upsloping ST-segment. For a true positive result, ST-segment depression must be seen in at least two leads for at least three consecutive complexes.
- There is varying opinion on the amount and type of ST-segment depression that indicates an abnormality.
- Interpretation for patients with abnormal baseline ECGs can be problematic. Table 56-2 lists the recommended criteria for significant ST-segment depression as described by Ellestad for both normal and abnormal baseline ECGs.
- ST-segment elevation may also be an indication of ischemia or of a dyskinetic area from a previous myocardial infarction. If ischemia is suspected, the test should be terminated.

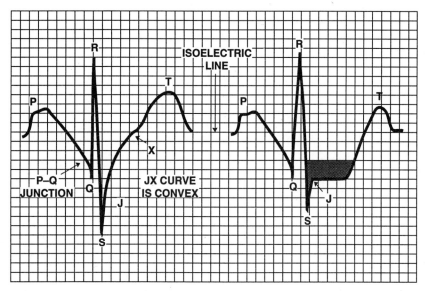

FIG. 56-9.

Left, The normal exercise ECG complex. Note that the P-Q segment is deflected below the isoelectric line. This point is considered to be a baseline for determining S-T segment abnormalities. *Right,* A horizontal S-T segment depression of 2.0 mm as measured from the P-Q segment. (From Ellestad MH: *Stress testing principles and practice,* Philadelphia, 1987, F.A. Davis. Used with permission.)

TABLE 56-2.

Recommended Criteria for Significant ST-Segment Depression with Maximal Exercise

Resting ST-T Configuration	Exercise or Postexercise ST Configuration	ST Depression and Point of Measurement
Normal	Horizontal	1.0 mm at 60 ms from J-point
	Upsloping	1.5 mm at 80 ms from J-point
	Downsloping	1.0 mm more depressed than at rest
Flat or sagging ST and T	Horizontal	1.0 mm more depressed than at rest
	Upsloping	1.5 mm more depressed than at rest at 80 ms from J-point
	Downsloping	1.0 mm more depressed than at rest
Inverted T	Horizontal	1.5 mm at 60 ms from J-point
	Upsloping	1.5 mm at 80 ms from J-point
	Downsloping	1.5 mm at 20 ms from J-point

Note that these current criteria are slightly different depending on the configuration of the resting ST segment and T wave.
From Ellestad, MH: Horizontal and downsloping ST segments. In *Stress testing: principles and practice,* ed 3, Philadelphia, 1987, F.A. Davis, p. 236. Used with permission.

- Ventricular tachycardia as well as multifocal and frequent PVCs (> 30% of contractions) may be indicators of underlying coronary artery disease. Occasional PVCs are seen in normal patients, especially at high work loads, or in elderly patients.
- Transient atrial fibrillation or flutter during exercise may be an indicator of heart disease or other conditions.
- Exercise-induced second- or third-degree heart block is significant.

Other physiologic changes of clinical significance:

- A drop in systolic pressure or a systolic blood pressure that does not rise with exercise intensity may indicate underlying heart disease. In most cases, the earlier the drop during the procedure, the more severe is the disease.

GENERAL INTERPRETATION OF EXERCISE TEST

- The test should not be labeled simply as normal or abnormal, but rather the specific responses found to be abnormal should be identified.
- Age and risk factors for heart disease should be taken into account when interpreting results.
- Many conditions and circumstances can cause a false-positive or a false-negative test (Box 56-2).
- The lateral leads are the most important to watch (V_4, V_5, V_6). They are directly over the left ventricle and are most likely to show ischemic ST changes.
- Prognosis of patients attaining 10 METs is as good with medical therapy as with coronary artery bypass surgery, regardless of ST-segment response.

RULES*

Methodology

1. ST-segment elevation is measured from the ST level before the test (the baseline level):

   - If it occurs over or adjacent to diagnostic Q waves, it can be due to a ventricular aneurysm or a wall motion abnormality.
   - If it occurs with a normal ECG or absence of previous infarction, it indicates transmural ischemia, and the test should be stopped. This type of ischemia is extremely arrhythmogenic.

2. Another source measures ST-segment depression is measured at the J-point (ST zero, also known as the beginning of the ST segment, or end of the QRS complex) and is considered abnormal only if the slope over the following 60 ms is horizontal or downsloping.

---

*Adapted from Froelicher VF, Marcondes GD: *Manual of exercise testing,* Chicago, 1989, Year Book Medical Publishing. Used with permission.

BOX 56-2. CAUSES OF FALSE-POSITIVE TESTS

1. A preexisting abnormal resting ECG (for example, ST-T abnormalities)
2. Cardiac hypertrophy
3. Wolff-Parkinson-White syndrome and other conduction defects
4. Hypertension
5. Drugs (e.g., digitalis)
6. Cardiomyopathy
7. Hypokalemia
8. Vasoregulatory abnormalities
9. Sudden intense exercise
10. Mitral valve prolapse syndrome
11. Pericardial disorders
12. Pectus excavatum
13. Technical or observer error

CAUSES OF FALSE-NEGATIVE TESTS

1. Failure to reach an adequate exercise work load
2. Insufficient number of leads to detect ECG changes
3. Failure to use other information (systolic blood pressure drop, symptoms, dysrhythmia, heart rate response) in test interpretation
4. Single vessel disease
5. Good collateral circulation
6. Musculoskeletal limitations before cardiac abnormalities occur
7. Technical or observer error
8. Medications: Long-acting nitrates, beta blockers, and calcium-channel blockers have antianginal effects, and may prolong the time of study until it becomes positive.

From Blair SN et al: False positive and false negative tests. In *Guidelines for exercise testing and prescription,* ed 3, Philadelphia, 1986, Lea & Febiger, p 28. Used with permission.

3. ST depression should be measured depending upon the baseline ST segment:

- If the ST segment is isoelectric or elevated before exercise (that is, J-point ≥ 0), the amount of ST depression due to exercise is measured from the PR isoelectric line.
- If the ST segment is depressed before exercise (that is, J-point < 0), the amount of ST depression is measured from the preexercise level.

ST Analysis Interpretation

- If left bundle-branch block (LBBB) or Wolff-Parkinson-White (WPW) is present, ST-segment depression does not necessarily indicate ischemia.

- If right bundle-branch block is present, ST-segments can only be analyzed in V4, V5, or V6.
- If coronary artery bypass surgery has been performed, exercise-induced ST-segment depression has less prognostic value.
- If anterior and/or lateral Q waves are present, exercise-induced ST-segment depression does not have prognostic value.
- If a patient recovering from a myocardial infarction has LBBB, prognosis is guarded.
- If ST depression occurs only in II, III and/or AVF or any combination of the three and not in the lateral leads as well, it is usually a false positive response due to atrial repolarization. These patients will frequently have a short PR interval as well. (The artrial repolarization wave, which is negative, "pulls down" the ST-segment when superimposed.)
- ST-segment depression does not localize ischemia. Ischemia is a global subendocardial phenomena.

THE GRADING SYSTEM*

Normal electrocardiographic response (negative test):

- Absence of any change in the ST segment at maximal or near maximal heart rate
- Junctional depression with rapidly rising ST-segment slope (This should disappear within 1 minute into recovery phase.)
- Development of isolated T-wave inversion without ST-segment displacement
- Ventricular ectopic beats occurring infrequently, especially those occurring at heart rates exceeding 130 beats/minute
- Appearance of atrial arrhythmias
- Development of right bundle-branch block

Uninterpretable exercise test responses:

- Failure to attain at least 85% of the age-predicted maximum heart rate, with absence of ischemic changes in a well-motivated patient (unless taking B-blocker)
- Presence of baseline ECG abnormality known either to predispose to false-positive results should ST abnormalities occur during exercise, or to mask possible ST changes (These include ECG evidence of left ventricular hypertrophy; left bundle-branch block [fixed or rate-dependent]; accessory atrioventricular conduction of the Wolff-Parkinson-White type; mitral valve prolapse with rest-

---

*Adapted from Selzer A, Cohn K, Goldschalager N: On the interpretation of the exercise test, *Circulation* 58(2):194, 1978. Used with permission.

ing or hyperventilation-induced ST-T changes; ST segment and/or T wave abnormalities that occur with standing or develop in the preexercise hyperventilatory period; and digitalis therapy.)

Note: In most of these instances, a radionuclide study combined with the stages test may offer additional information and sensitivity as well as accuracy.

Mildly positive electrocardiographic response (-):

- Horizontal ST-segment depression between 1 and 1.5 mm (0.1 to 0.15 mV)
- Junctional depression with slowly rising ST slope that remains depressed 1.5 mm or more, 80 ms after the J-point

Moderately positive electrocardiographic response:

- Horizontal ST depression of between 1.5 and 2.5 mm (0.15 to 0.25 mV)
- Slowly upsloping ST-segment depression with the ST segment being depressed in excess of 2.5 mm, 80 ms after the J-point
- Downsloping ST depression with the J-point depressed 1 to 2 mm
- Frequent ventricular ectopic activity (15% to 20% of QRS complexes over a period of time), especially when appearing during exercise at low heart rates (under 130 beats/minute) and when associated with ischemic ST-segment abnormalities

Strongly positive electrocardiographic response:

- Downsloping ST-segment depression, J-point depression of 2 mm or greater
- Downsloping or flat ST-segment depression in excess of 2.5 mm*
- Horizontal or downsloping ST-segment depression appearing during the first stage of exercise and/or persisting beyond 8 minutes in the recovery phase*
- Complex ventricular ectopic activity, including multiform ventricular ectopic beats, salvos, or runs of ventricular tachycardia; or occurrence of ventricular fibrillation

Note: For uninterpretable tests through mildly positive tests, additional studies may be desired versus following serial MSETs. This should be determined on an individual basis with cardiology consultation.

Most authorities denote a maximal stress exercise test (MSET) as one achieving a heart rate of greater than 85% of the predicted maximal heart rate for that patient's age (roughly 220 − age) or to the point of symptoms. Since predicted maximal heart rate is not patient specific and frequently is in error, most cardiologists exercise patients to maximal effort (to the point of symptoms). This also gives the physician knowledge about patients' cardiac response at a level of exercise that they are not likely to reproduce on their own and is certainly reassuring to the physician as he or she gives an exercise prescription.

---

*This criterion holds only if exercise is terminated within 1 to 2 minutes after ischemic ST changes appear. Marked ischemic changes will appear in many patients with mild coronary disease if they are exercised beyond their ischemic threshold.

CONTROVERSIES IN USING EXERCISE TESTING FOR DIAGNOSING CORONARY ARTERY DISEASE

- The task force on Assessment of Cardiovascular Procedures of the American College of Cardiology and the American Heart Association called exercise testing in asymptomatic men with risk factors a Class II indication—a condition in which exercise testing is frequently used, but in which there is a divergence of opinion about its value. The divergence of opinion is largely due to the higher likelihood of a false-positive result in this population. However, in this population, there is no noninvasive method of screening without false-positives.
- Current guidelines for periodic screening (such as the Report of the U.S. Preventive Services Task Force) do not recommend routine exercise test screening for the general population.
- The major reasons for controversy about performing additional exercise testing for screening include the lack of consensus about absolute criteria for determining a positive test, and the unknown natural course of asymptomatic coronary artery disease.
- Performing exercise testing on selected individuals with known cardiac risk factors may increase the likelihood that a positive test is due to coronary artery disease.
- The majority (more than 50%) of CAD cases are currently diagnosed *after* an individual's first myocardial infarction or sudden cardiac death. Therefore, we as physicians are not performing enough screening.

COMPLICATIONS OF EXERCISE TESTING

- Hypotension
- Congestive heart failure
- Severe cardiac arrhythmia
- Cardiac arrest
- Acute myocardial infarction
- Acute central nervous system event, such as syncope or stroke
- Death

SAFETY OF STRESS TESTING

- Mortality is approximately 1 out of 10,000.
- Hospital admission related to arrhythmia, prolonged chest pain, or myocardial infarction is approximately 4 out of 10,000.

EXERCISE TESTING FOR FITNESS EVALUATION AND EXERCISE PRESCRIPTION

General principles:

- A graded exercise test can be used to actually determine an individual's maximum heart rate.
- A maximum heart rate is necessary to calculate a training heart rate range, which can be used as a guideline for aerobic training.
- An exercise test can also estimate an individual's $V_{O_2 \, max}$, which is helpful in determining a current level of aerobic conditioning.

$V_{O_2 \, max}$ and aerobic fitness levels:

- The $V_{O_2 \, max}$ can be determined for various exercise protocols using standard formulas (see Blair SN et al: *Guidelines for exercise testing and prescription*).
- Tables 56-3 and 56-4 show $V_{O_2 \, max}$ determined for individuals according to the length of time they are able to continue exercise on a treadmill with a Bruce protocol.
- Using estimated $V_{O_2 \, max}$, an individual's approximate level of aerobic conditioning can be determined using age/sex matched tables.

Note: For most patients, their perceived exertion (see Box 56-3) is reproducible at a given level of exercise and correlates fairly well with their heart rate. Ask patients to indicate on a scale of 0 to 10 how hard they feel they are working with each stage. Most feel they increase 2 to 3 on the exertion scale. People who highly underestimate their effort must be taught to measure their pulse before receiving an exercise prescription. Individuals with good exertion perception may not have to measure their pulse as frequently.

BOX 56-3. PERCEIVED EXERTION SCALE

```
   0 Nothing at all
 0.5 Very, very weak
   1 Very weak
   2 Weak
   3 Moderate
   4 Somewhat strong
   5 Strong
   6
   7 Very strong
   8
   9
  10 Very, very strong
```

TABLE 56-3.

$V_{O_2\ max}$ from Bruce Protocol Using Treadmill Time, Female

$2.95 \times$ (min.) $+ 3.74 =$ ml/kg/min					
TM	VO_2	TM	VO_2	TM	VO_2
3.0	12.59	7.1	24.68	11.2	36.78
3.1	12.88	7.2	24.98	11.3	37.07
3.2	13.18	7.3	25.27	11.4	37.37
3.3	13.47	7.4	25.57	11.5	37.66
3.4	13.77	7.5	25.86	11.6	37.96
3.5	14.06	7.6	26.16	11.7	38.25
3.6	14.36	7.7	26.45	11.8	38.55
3.7	14.65	7.8	26.75	11.9	38.84
3.8	14.95	7.9	27.04	12.0	39.14
3.9	15.24	8.0	27.34	12.1	39.43
4.0	15.54	8.1	27.63	12.2	39.73
4.1	15.83	8.2	27.93	12.3	40.02
4.2	16.13	8.3	28.22	12.4	40.32
4.3	16.42	8.4	28.52	12.5	40.61
4.4	16.72	8.5	28.81	12.6	40.91
4.5	17.01	8.6	29.11	12.7	41.20
4.6	17.31	8.7	29.40	12.8	41.50
4.7	17.60	8.8	29.70	12.9	41.79
4.8	17.90	8.9	29.99	13.0	42.09
4.9	18.19	9.0	30.29	13.1	42.38
5.0	18.49	9.1	30.58	13.2	42.68
5.1	18.78	9.2	30.88	13.3	42.97
5.2	19.08	9.3	31.17	13.4	43.27
5.3	19.37	9.4	31.47	13.5	43.56
5.4	19.67	9.5	31.76	13.6	43.86
5.5	19.96	9.6	32.06	13.7	44.15
5.6	20.26	9.7	32.35	13.8	44.45
5.7	20.55	9.8	32.65	13.9	44.74
5.8	20.85	9.9	32.94	14.0	45.04
5.9	21.14	10.0	33.24	14.1	45.34
6.0	21.44	10.1	33.53	14.2	45.63
6.1	21.73	10.2	33.83	14.3	45.93
6.2	22.03	10.3	34.12	14.4	46.22
6.3	22.32	10.4	34.42	14.5	46.52
6.4	22.62	10.5	34.71	14.6	46.81
6.5	22.91	10.6	35.01	14.7	47.11
6.6	23.21	10.7	35.30	14.8	47.40
6.7	23.50	10.8	35.60	14.9	47.70
6.8	23.80	10.9	35.89	15.0	47.99
6.9	24.09	11.0	36.19	15.1	48.29
7.0	24.39	11.1	36.48	15.2	48.58

From Health Services Center, Kimberly-Clark Corporation, Neenah, Wisconsin.
Note: 1 MET = 3.5 ml/kg/min

TABLE 56-4.

$V_{O_2\ max}$ from Bruce Protocol Using Treadmill Time, Male

$2.94 \times (min.) + 7.65 = ml/kg/min$					
TM	VO$_2$	TM	VO$_2$	TM	VO$_2$
3.0	16.47	7.4	29.40	11.8	42.34
3.1	16.76	7.5	29.70	11.9	42.63
3.2	17.06	7.6	29.99	12.0	42.93
3.3	17.35	7.7	30.28	12.1	43.22
3.4	17.64	7.8	30.58	12.2	43.51
3.5	17.94	7.9	30.87	12.3	43.81
3.6	18.18	8.0	31.17	12.4	44.10
3.7	18.52	8.1	31.46	12.5	44.40
3.8	18.82	8.2	31.75	12.6	44.69
3.9	19.11	8.3	32.05	12.7	44.98
4.0	19.41	8.4	32.34	12.8	45.28
4.1	19.70	8.5	32.64	12.9	45.57
4.2	19.99	8.6	32.93	13.0	45.87
4.3	20.29	8.7	33.22	13.1	46.16
4.4	20.58	8.8	33.52	13.2	46.45
4.5	20.88	8.9	33.81	13.3	46.75
4.6	21.17	9.0	34.11	13.4	47.04
4.7	21.46	9.1	34.40	13.5	47.34
4.8	21.76	9.2	34.69	13.6	47.63
4.9	22.05	9.3	34.99	13.7	47.92
5.0	22.35	9.4	35.28	13.8	48.22
5.1	22.64	9.5	35.58	13.9	48.51
5.2	22.93	9.6	35.87	14.0	48.81
5.3	23.23	9.7	36.16	14.1	49.10
5.4	23.52	9.8	36.46	14.2	49.40
5.5	23.82	9.9	36.75	14.3	49.69
5.6	24.11	10.0	37.05	14.4	49.98
5.7	24.40	10.1	37.34	14.5	50.28
5.8	24.70	10.2	37.63	14.6	50.57
5.9	24.99	10.3	37.93	14.7	50.87
6.0	25.29	10.4	38.22	14.8	51.16
6.1	25.58	10.5	38.52	14.9	51.46
6.2	25.87	10.6	38.81	15.0	51.75
6.3	26.17	10.7	39.10	15.1	52.05
6.4	26.46	10.8	39.40	15.2	52.34
6.5	26.76	10.9	39.69	15.3	52.63
6.6	27.05	11.0	39.99	15.4	52.93
6.7	27.34	11.1	40.28	15.5	53.22
6.8	27.64	11.2	40.57	15.6	53.52
6.9	27.93	11.3	40.87	15.7	53.81
7.0	28.23	11.4	41.16	15.8	54.10
7.1	28.52	11.5	41.46	15.9	54.40
7.2	28.81	11.6	41.75	16.0	54.69
7.3	29.11	11.7	42.04	16.1	54.98

From Health Services Center, Kimberly-Clark Corporation, Neenah, Wisconsin.
Note: 1 MET = 3.5 ml/kg/min

Giving an aerobic exercise prescription:

- Cardiorespiratory endurance is enhanced by regular (3 episodes per week) aerobic exercise.
- Aerobic exercise involves raising the heart rate to a specified point and maintaining that level of exercise for 15 to 45 minutes per session.
- A safe training range is at a heart rate of 60% to 80% of maximum heart rate. This range is called the *target heart rate* (perceived exertion scale of 5 to 7).
- A repeat exercise test after an aerobic exercise program has been implemented can help determine levels of improvement.
- An exercise prescription should include a target heart range, duration of exercise sessions, frequency of sessions, and types of exercises that can be used to achieve the goals of cardiovascular conditioning. The American Heart Association recommends that a prescription include a minimum three sessions of exercise per week for 30 minutes per session.
- Competitive athletes want to use their training program to raise their anaerobic threshold (level of exercise at which they can no longer oxygenate all tissues).
- Anaerobic thresholds are now best determined by expired gas analysis combined with exercise stress testing. (This equipment is very expensive, and the technique is beyond the scope of this text.)

CPT/BILLING CODES

93000	Electrocardiogram routine ECG with at least 12 leads; with interpretation and report
93015	Cardiovascular stress testing with continuous electrocardiographic monitoring and interpretation

BIBLIOGRAPHY

Blair SN et al: False positive and false negative tests. In *Guidelines for exercise testing and prescription,* ed 3, Philadelphia, 1986, Lea & Febiger.

Ellestad MH: The normal exercise electrocardiogram. In *Stress testing, principles and practice,* ed 3, Philadelphia, 1987, F. A. Davis.

Evans CH, Karunaratne HB: Exercise stress testing for the family physician: Parts I & III, *Am Fam Physician* 45(1 & 2):121; 679, 1992.

Froelicher VF, Marcondes GD: *Manual of exercise testing,* Chicago, 1989, Year Book Medical Publishers.

Mead WF, Hartwig R: Fitness evaluation and exercise prescription: Procedures in family practice, *JFP* 13(7):1044, 1981.

Schlant RC, Friesinger GC II, Lenoard JJ: *Clinical competence in exercise testing:* a statement for physicians from the ACP/ACC/AHA task force on clinical privileges in cardiology, *Circulation* 82(5): 1990.

Selzer A, Cohn K, Goldschlager N: On the interpretation of the exercise test, *Circulation* 58(2):194, 1978.

CHAPTER 57

Cardioversion

Thomas J. Zuber

John L. Pfenninger

Transthoracic direct-current electrical shock, or cardioversion, is a safe and effective procedure for terminating most sustained tachyarrhythmias. Cardioversion is useful for converting arrhythmias that are causing acute deterioration of the patient's condition, and chronic tachyarrhythmias that are unresponsive to drug therapy. Cardiac arrhythmias often can be converted to sinus rhythm with medications, but the term *cardioversion* refers to the application of direct electrical current. Defibrillation is a similar procedure in which nonsynchronized electrical current is applied to convert chaotic fibrillation or other rhythms that result in unstable clinical conditions. This chapter focuses on the indications for and technique of synchronized cardioversion.

In synchronized cardioversion, cardiac cells are depolarized at a specific time to restore a stable heart rhythm. An electrical impulse is delivered immediately after a QRS complex. External paddles are used to apply the electrical current, which causes total depolarization of the atria and ventricles. This depolarization frequently results in the instantaneous conversion of a tachyarrhythmia to sinus rhythm.

ELECTRODES AND PLACEMENT

Either handheld paddle electrodes or self-adherent pad electrodes 8 to 12 cm in diameter will deliver adequate energy for cardioversion. To maximize the current flow to the heart, correct paddle or electrode placement is crucial. One electrode should be placed below the right clavicle just to the right of the upper sternum, and the second electrode to the left of the left nipple with the center of the electrode in the midaxillary line. This is the standard positioning; however, a front-back placement can also be used. In this alternative approach, one electrode is placed anteriorly over the left precordium, and the other electrode is placed behind the heart below the left scapula. The anteroposterior position may reduce energy requirements for cardioversion by up to 50%.

Paddles or electrodes must be positioned far enough apart so that electricity travels to the heart. Avoid paste or gel smeared on the skin between electrodes, which might allow the current to travel along the chest wall. Electrodes should also be placed far enough away from a pacemaker generator to prevent damage to its electrical components.

SYNCHRONIZATION

Synchronization refers to the delivery of electrical current to the myocardium during a nonrefractory period. Shocking the myocardium during the relative refractory period (the T wave) can induce the more ominous rhythm of ventricular fibrillation. In synchronized mode, the energy is delivered a few milliseconds after the R wave, or the peak of the QRS complex. Synchronized administration reduces the energy requirements and complication rates of electroshock therapy.

Most defibrillators highlight the QRS peak when active synchronization is selected. Very rapid tachycardias may prevent a defibrillator in a synchronized mode from discriminating between the peak of the QRS complex and the peak of a T wave. Therefore, machines may fail to discharge when attempting to synchronize a very rapid heart rate. Physicians should switch off the synchronization switch if the machine cannot adequately detect the QRS complexes.

Any attempted cardioversion that results in ventricular fibrillation should be nonsynchronously defibrillated immediately with 200 joules (J) of energy. On some defibrillators, the synchronization must be manually shut off to administer a nonsynchronized shock, i.e., for defibrillation.

ENERGY SELECTION

Cardioversion is accomplished by passing an electrical current of sufficient magnitude (with energy expressed in joules and flow expressed in amperes) through the heart to depolarize the tissues. Current flow is determined by the energy flow in joules and the resistance of the thoracic wall tissues. The transthoracic resistance in an average adult is 70 to 80 ohms. If the transthoracic resistance is too high, the energy may fail to accomplish cardiac depolarization.

Some supraventricular arrhythmias are very sensitive to electrical current. Low energy settings may depolarize the myocardium in atrial flutter and allow the heart to assume a sinus rhythm. Recommended initial energy settings for cardioversion of various arrhythmias are listed in Table 57-1.

Cardioversion energy for ventricular tachycardia (VT) depends on the rate and morphologic features of the electrical activity. Monomorphic VT presents with a regular ECG form and rate, and is generally responsive to cardioversion beginning at energies of 100 J. Polymorphic VT has an irregular form and rate, and is less responsive to electroshock therapy. Polymorphic VT behaves like ventricular fibrillation, and the initial shock energy should be 200 J.

TABLE 57-1.

Recommended Initial Energy Settings for Cardioversion

Atrial flutter	50 J
Paroxysmal supraventricular tachycardia (PSVT)	50 J
Atrial fibrillation	100 J
Monomorphic ventricular tachycardia	100 J
Polymorphic ventricular tachycardia	200 J
Children	0.55 J/kg
Defibrillator of ventricular tachycardia*	200 J

* Not a true cardioversion, but often referred as such.

If the first shock fails to cardiovert any arrhythmia, repeated attempts should be undertaken with stepwise energy increases. The standard sequence for synchronized cardioversion is 100 J, 200 J, 300 J, and 360 J; the energies used are dependent on the initial energy selected. For example, the second attempt to convert polymorphic VT should be with an energy of 300 J.

Note: Some sources start as low as 25 J for initial elective cardioversion (or 5 to 10 J for patients taking digitalis) and double the energy for each successive discharge. Patients with large thoraces, chest wall deformities, or large amounts of adipose tissue may require larger initial settings.

INDICATIONS (SYNCHRONIZED CARDIOVERSION)

- Hemodynamically stable ventricular tachycardia unresponsive to pharmacologic therapy
- Hemodynamically unstable supraventricular arrhythmias
- Certain supraventricular arrhythmias unresponsive to pharmacologic therapy
- Supraventricular tachycardia
- Atrial fibrillation
- Atrial flutter
- *Urgent:* Serious signs and symptoms (Box 57-1) usually with heart rate above 150 beats per minute
- *Elective:* Hemodynamically stable, sustained tachyarrhythmias

---

BOX 57-1. SERIOUS SIGNS AND SYMPTOMS INDICATING URGENT CARDIOVERSION

Chest pain
Dyspnea
Decreased level of consciousness
Hypotension
Shock
Pulmonary edema
Congestive heart failure
Acute myocardial infarction

CONTRAINDICATIONS (SYNCHRONOUS CARDIOVERSION)

Urgent Cardioversion

- Absent pulse
- No QRS complex on ECG rhythm
- Severely unstable patients

   Note: Defibrillation or nonsynchronized cardioversion may be indicated.

- Ventricular tachycardia (*relative contraindication*)
- Unstable ventricular tachycardia (The American Heart Association recommends using nonsynchronized shocks to avoid the delay associated with attempts to synchronize.)

Elective Cardioversion

- Severe electrolyte disturbances
- Digitalis toxicity
- A left atrial diameter greater than 4.5 cm (because of the low likelihood of maintaining sinus rhythm) (*relative contraindication*)
- Patients with sick sinus syndrome or sinoatrial node block (should not undergo cardioversion until a pacemaker has been placed)
- Patients with a history of minimal hemodynamic or symptomatic improvement with sinus rhythm (may not need cardioversion)
- Multifocal atrial tachycardia and sinus tachycardia (do not normally respond to cardioversion)

EQUIPMENT

See Chapter 56, Stress Testing, for suppliers of defibrillators/cardioversion equipment.

- Handheld paddle electrodes, **or** 8 to 12 cm diameter self-adherent pad electrodes
- Advanced cardiac life support (ACLS) equipment:

   Oxygen
   Airways and intubation equipment
   Suction equipment
   Emergency drug kit, including IVs
   Medication to follow ACLS protocols

- ECG monitoring capabilities
- Direct current defibrillator/cardioversion unit, preferably with synchronization capabilities and "quick look" paddles
- Sedatives for elective cardioversion

PREPROCEDURE PATIENT EDUCATION

Urgent Cardioversion

If the patient is alert, briefly explain the procedure while connecting the equipment. Informed consent is not necessary for a life-threatening situation. Document the indications and risk to patient without cardioversion.

Elective Cardioversion

Instruct the patient to fast for 4 to 6 hours before the procedure. Explain the indications for the procedure and the risk of complications to the patient. Obtain informed consent. Explain that sedation will be used, but the patient may experience a mild shock as well as some achiness in the arms and chest following the procedure. Remove any dentures before beginning the procedure.

TECHNIQUE

Scheduled or elective cardioversion should be performed in a prepared environment, generally in a cardiac care unit. The procedure steps include:

1. Administer anticoagulant (if indicated) until satisfactory clotting times are obtained.
2. Confirm that electrolyte balance and serum digoxin level is within normal range.

   Note: Some experts recommend for any patients taking digitalis a prophylactic dose of lidocaine 1 mg/kg intravenously.

3. Keep the patient NPO after midnight.
4. Obtain informed consent.
5. Premedicate the patient with a sedative.
6. Set up equipment so that the patient's cardiac, oxygenation, and blood pressure status can be monitored. The patient should be lying on a flat, dry surface.
7. Initiate intravenous access. Apply supplemental oxygen.
8. Have suction, resuscitation equipment, and support staff immediately available.
9. Apply conductive material and electrodes.
10. Select the appropriate energy level.
11. Turn on the defibrillator.
12. Turn on the synchronizer circuit.
13. Charge the capacitors.
14. Assure proper paddle or electrode placement.
15. Make sure that no personnel are in physical contact with the patient or the bed.
16. Call "all clear."
17. Deliver countershock by depressing discharge buttons.

18. Assess the cardiac rhythm.
19. Assess the patient.
20. If necessary, repeat cardioversion process (at higher setting).
21. If necessary, resynchronize the defibrillator before each use.

Many experts recommend anesthesia standby if this service is available. Administration of a sedative (such as diazepam, midazolam) or a barbiturate can be combined with an analgesic (such as meperidine or fentanyl) to improve patient comfort. At the time of cardioversion, consider 5 mg of diazepam intravenously, followed by 2.5 mg in increments every 2 to 3 minutes until adequate sedation is achieved.

Several studies have confirmed the benefit of treating atrial fibrillation with direct-current countershock. Patients with atrial fibrillation of more than several days' duration may develop intraatrial thrombi. The risk of embolic events following cardioversion is increased in patients with left atrial dimensions greater than 4.0 cm. The incidence of emboli may be up to 5% for the first 2 weeks after cardioversion. Many experts recommend anticoagulation with warfarin prior to attempted cardioversion of a patient with chronic atrial fibrillation. The international normalized ratio (INR) for anticoagulation should be maintained between 2.0 and 3.0 (or the protime 1.3 to 1.5 times the control using North American thromboplastin) for 3 weeks before and 4 weeks after the procedure.

Some physicians advocate a trial of an antiarrhythmic medication, such as quinidine sulfate, for 48 hours prior to cardioversion, and continuation of drug therapy if the cardioversion is successful.

Patients should be monitored carefully for several hours after cardioversion, with a longer period of monitoring indicated if antiarrhythmic drug therapy is continued.

Urgent cardioversion should precede antiarrhythmia therapy in a rapidly deteriorating patient. Antiarrhythmic medications can be administered as soon as possible after the procedure. Urgent cardioversion generally precludes administration of sedatives unless they are immediately available.

POSTPROCEDURE CARE

Inform the patient that the original dysrhythmia may recur. Monitor the patient in a critical care setting while he or she is stabilizing and undergoing complete diagnostic and therapeutic interventions.

COMPLICATIONS

Complications following cardioversion are uncommon in the absence of digitalis toxicity, or hypokalemia, and with properly delivered shock.

- Bradycardia is sometimes noted immediately after cardioversion in patients with a prior history of inferior myocardial infarction.

- Transient mild arrhythmias or creatine kinase elevations may be noted, but they are generally insignificant.
- Atrial and ventricular ectopy is not uncommon in the first 15 to 30 minutes following cardioversion. Intravenous lidocaine may be used.
- Skin burns can be minimized by using adequate amounts of electrode paste.
- Electrical shock is a possibility for anyone in contact with the patient or the patient's bed. Any attached electrical equipment can be damaged.
- Systemic emboli may develop if the patient is not adequately anticoagulated.
- Original arrhythmia may recur.

Note: With any cardioversion, especially with repeated or nonsynchronized, there is a risk of producing a worse rhythm, such as ventricular tachycardia or fibrillation. High-energy or repeated shocks may also damage the myocardium.

CPT/BILLING CODES

92950	Cardiopulmonary resuscitation
92960	Cardioversion, elective; electrical conversion of arrrhythmia, external

BIBLIOGRAPHY

American Heart Association: *Textbook of advanced cardiac life support,* ed 2, Dallas, 1987, The Association.

Clark A, Cotter L: Practical procedures: DC cardioversion, *Br J Hosp Med* 46:114, 1991.

de Silva RA et al: Cardioversion and defibrillation, *Am Heart J* 100:881, 1980.

Dunn M et al: Antithrombotic therapy in atrial fibrillation, *Chest* 89:68s, 1986.

Emergency Cardiac Care Committee and Subcommittees, American Heart Association: Guidelines for cardiopulmonary resuscitation and emergency cardiac care, III: advanced cardiac life support, *JAMA* 268:2199, 1992.

Mann DL et al: Absence of cardioversion-induced ventricular arrhythmias in patients with therapeutic digoxin levels, *J Am Coll Cardiol* 5:882, 1985.

Reiffel JA et al: Direct current cardioversion: effect on creatine kinase, lactic dehydrogenase and myocardial isoenzymes, *JAMA* 239:122, 1978.

CHAPTER 58

Chest Tube Insertion

Nelly A. Otero

Chest tube placement is a very common therapeutic procedure, frequently performed in the emergency department. The first known chest tube placement with sealed drainage took place in 1875, as developed by Bulan. The objective for this procedure is to provide an appropriate evacuation of an abnormal collection of air or fluid from the pleural space.

INDICATIONS

- Pneumothorax: iatrogenic, spontaneous, tension, or traumatic
- Hemothorax
- Chylothorax
- Empyema
- Drainage of recurrent pleural effusion
- Following thoracotomy

CONTRAINDICATIONS

Relative contraindications include the following:

- Systemic anticoagulation therapy or bleeding dyscrasia
- Small, stable pneumothorax (may resolve spontaneously)
- Empyema caused by acid-fast organisms
- Loculated hydrothorax or pneumothorax
- Previous chest tube insertion, thoracic surgery, or pleurodesis may cause pleura to become stuck together (preventing chest tube insertion)

EQUIPMENT

- Sterile gloves and gown
- Surgical mask, cap, and goggles

- Antiseptic solution (povidone-iodine [Betadine])
- White petrolatum-impregnated gauze
- Adhesive tape (hypoallergenic)
- Chest tubes
    22 to 36 Fr. for adults (32 Fr. is average)
    16, 20, 24 Fr. for children
- Appropriate suction-drainage system (a three-bottle system or a commercial model such as the Pleur-Evac or Thoradrain [Fig. 58-1])
- Rubber clear plastic tubing (6-foot length, ½-inch diameter)
- Thoracostomy tray (Box 58-1)
- Sterile towels or paper drapes (if not included in the thoracostomy tray)
- Sterile Y-connector

PREPROCEDURE PATIENT EDUCATION AND EVALUATION

- Explain the procedure and its indications to the patient and obtain written informed consent if possible.
- Sedate the patient if he or she is not in severe respiratory distress. This procedure is rather painful.
- If possible, obtain prothrombin time, partial thromboplastin time, and platelet count (or simply a bleeding time).

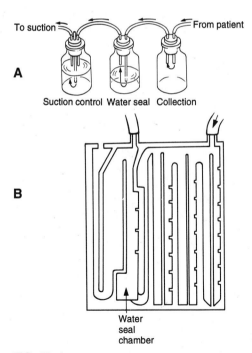

FIG. 58-1.
A, Three bottle suction. **B,** Disposable suction unit.

BOX 58-1. THORACOSTOMY TRAY

Lidocaine 1%, with 10 cc syringe and 25- and 22-gauge needles
Sterile towels (4)
Basin for antiseptic solution
Sterile 4 × 4 inch gauze pads
Towel clips (optional)
Large straight scissors
Large curved (Mayo) scissors
Large clamps (Kelly) (2)
Medium clamps (2 to 4)
Needle holder
No. 1-0 or 2-0 nonabsorbable sutures on large cutting needles (2)
No. 10 or No. 11 mounted scalpel blades
Forceps

TECHNIQUE

Sterile technique should be followed, including usage of face mask and sterile gown.

1. Prepare all the necessary equipment. Be sure everything is sterile, and wear the proper gown and face mask. Follow universal precautions for blood and body fluids.
2. Select the proper chest tube. For a pure pneumothorax, an 18- to 20-Fr. catheter should be large enough. For fluid accumulation or hemothorax, a 32- to 36-Fr. catheter is suggested. Some physicians suggest using a 38- to 40-Fr. catheter in trauma patients.
3. Assemble the suction-drain system according to manufacturer's recommendations.
4. Connect the suction system to a wall suction outlet. Adjust the suction as needed until a steady stream of bubbles is produced in the water column.
5. Position the patient. For axillary line insertion, elevate the head of the bed 30 to 60 degrees, and place the arm on the affected side over the patient's head. It is advisable to restrain the patient's arm in this position.
6. Determine the insertion site and mark it with a fingernail indentation or skin marker. The most common site is the lateral thorax at the anterior axillary line, lateral to the nipple in males, or lateral and about two finger breadths above the sternoxiphoid junction in females. At this site, the tube will be in the fourth or fifth intercostal space, above the diaphragm.

   Warning: The liver or spleen can be lacerated if the patient is not properly positioned or the tube is inserted below this level. The diaphragm and liver/spleen may shift superiorly with certain chest abnormalities.

7. Observing sterile technique, and with sterile gloves, open the thoracostomy tray, arrange the instruments, and verify the tray's inventory.

8. Sterilize the skin with antiseptic solution, covering a wide area.

9. Proper application of local anesthesia will minimize discomfort. At the rib chosen for the pleural *insertion* site, anesthetize the skin over the mid- to superior aspect of the rib with 1% lidocaine using the 10 cc syringe and 25-gauge needle. Through the skin wheal at the *incision* area (the rib below the rib chosen for pleural insertion), infiltrate the subcutaneous tissue, the muscle, the periosteum, and the parietal pleura with the 22-gauge needle (Fig. 58-2). Be careful to remain near the superior border of rib. With the anesthetic needle and syringe, aspirate the pleural cavity and check for the presence of fluid or air. If none is obtained, repeat the procedure or change the insertion site.

10. Anesthetize the skin at the incision area and make a 2 to 4 cm transverse incision through the skin and the tissues overlying the rib. Direct the incision toward the intercostal space above (Fig. 58-3). Using a Kelly clamp, extend the incision by blunt dissection down to the fascia overlying the intercostal muscle. Bluntly dissecting between planes, continue tunneling toward the superior aspect of the rib above (Fig. 58-4, *A*).

11. Once the previously anesthetized superior border of the rib above is reached, close and turn the Kelly clamp and push it through the parietal pleura with steady, firm, and even pressure (Fig. 58-4, *B*).

12. Once inside the pleural cavity, open the clamps widely and withdraw. Either air or fluid will rush out when the pleura is opened. Insert a gloved index finger.

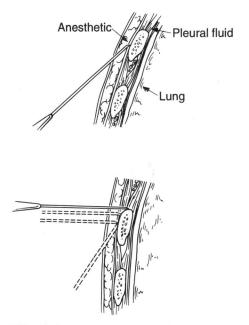

FIG. 58-2.
Infiltration of skin and pleura with local anesthetic.

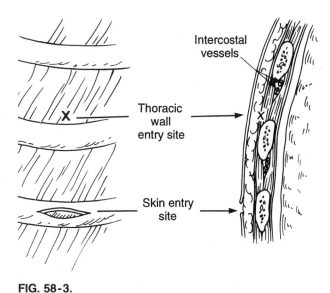

FIG. 58-3.
Incision is made one intercostal space below the space through which the tube will pass.

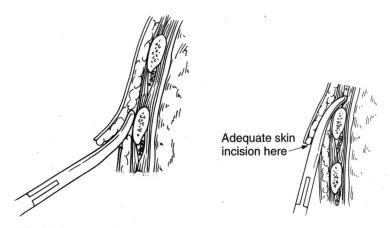

FIG. 58-4.
Location of the intercostal neurovascular bundle and tunnel procedure diagram. See text for details.

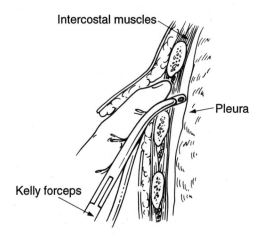

FIG. 58-5.
Using the finger as a guide, place the tip into the pleural cavity.

13. *Important:* Use your finger to verify that the pleural space has been entered and not the potential space between the pleura and chest wall, and that there are no pleural adhesions. Also check for unanticipated findings, such as the diaphragm.

14. Now grasp the chest tube with a curved clamp so that the tip of the tube protrudes beyond the jaws of the clamp. Clamp the free end of the tube with a separate clamp, and cut the beveled distal end so that it is square and will fit the suction connector better. Place the tube into the pleural space using your finger (which should still be inside the pleural space) as a guide (Fig. 58-5). Direct the tip of the tube superiorly, medially, and *posteriorly* for fluid drainage. Smaller tubes may be directed *anteriorly* and superiorly for

pneumothorax evacuation. Regardless of direction, all the ventilation holes in the chest tube must finally rest within the pleural space.

Note: Chest tubes that are equipped with an intraluminal trocar are not recommended, because they are associated with a higher incidence of intrathoracic complications.

15. Attach the tube to the previously assembled suction-drainage system. If no underwater seal is available, attaching a Penrose drain in line with the tube temporarily can act as a one-way valve, allowing air to exit through the Penrose but not to enter the chest. When the underwater seal is available, release the distal clamp. Ask the patient to cough and observe if bubbles form at the water seal level. This will check the system patency. (There are several types of suction-drainage systems, so be sure you understand the mechanics and the proper use of the particular system before doing this procedure.)

16. If the tube has not been properly inserted in the pleural space, no fluid will drain and the level in the water column will not vary with respiration.

17. To suture the tube in place, use 1-0 or 2-0 silk or nonabsorbable suture material. Place the first suture next to the tube and tie firmly (Fig. 58-6). Leave the ends long. Wind both suture ends around the tube, starting at the bottom and working toward the top. Tie the ends of the suture very tightly around the tube and cut the ends. With a second suture, place a horizontal mattress stitch or purse-string stitch around the tube at the skin incision site (Fig. 58-7); this will be used to close the incision when the tube is removed. Pull both ends of this suture together, and close the skin tight around the tube with a surgeon's knot. Wind the loose ends tightly around the chest tube, and make a bow for the final knot. This bow will identify the suture that will be used to close the skin when the tube is removed.

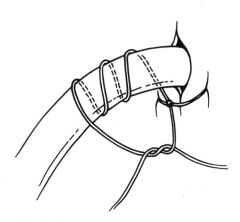

FIG. 58-6.
Chest tube is fastened by a stay suture.

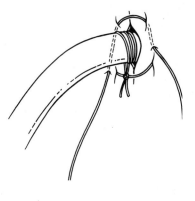

FIG. 58-7.
A purse-string suture is placed to ensure a seal when the chest tube is withdrawn.

18. Wrap the petrolatum-impregnated gauze around the tube where it enters the skin. Cover the tube with two or more 4 × 4 inch sterile gauze pads into which you have made Y-shape cuts so that they fit around the tube. Tape the gauze and tube in place. Tape together the connection between the chest tube and the suction tube, and tape the chest tube to the patient's side.
19. Obtain an erect posteroanterior (PA) and lateral chest X-ray to confirm tube placement, and document the degree of resolution of initial condition for which the chest tube was inserted.
20. Chest tubes are generally removed when there has been no fluid or air drainage for more than 24 hours.

CHEST TUBE REMOVAL

1. Place the patient in the same position in which the tube was inserted.
2. Using sterile technique, prep the area. Remove the suture holding the tube, loosen the purse-string stitch, and prepare this stitch for tying.
3. Clamp the chest tube and disconnect the suction system.
4. If awake, ask the patient to hold his or her breath, and remove the tube with a swift motion. If the patient is receiving ventilator support, pause the ventilator.
5. Tie the purse-string suture.
6. Apply an occlusive dressing (gauze impregnated with petrolatum or antibiotic ointment) and tape securely.
7. Observe for any new symptom or complication after chest tube removal, repeat the chest X-ray, and after 48 hours, remove the dressing and follow routine wound care.

COMPLICATIONS

- Injury to heart and great vessels or lung
- Subdiaphragmatic placement of tube
- Open pneumothorax
- Tension pneumothorax
- Dislodgment of the tube
- Subcutaneous emphysema
- Unexplained or persistent air leakage
- Hemorrhage from an injured intercostal artery
- Local or more generalized infection

CPT/BILLING CODE

32020   Tube thoracostomy with or without water seal (e.g., for abscess, hemothorax, empyema)

BIBLIOGRAPHY

Condon E, Nyhus LM, editors: *Manual of surgical procedures*, Boston, 1985, Little, Brown & Co.

Graber RF, Garvin JM: Chest tube insertion, *Patient Care:*159, September 1988.

Ho MT, Saunders CE, editors: *Current emergency diagnosis and treatment*, Norwalk, Conn, 1990, Appleton & Lange.

May HL, editor: *Emergency*, New York, 1984, Wiley & Sons.

Roberts JR, Hedges JR, editors: *Clinical procedures in emergency medicine*, Philadelphia, 1985, W.B. Saunders.

CHAPTER 59

Endotracheal Intubation

Len Scarpinato

In an emergency, primary care physicians may be called upon to perform an endotracheal intubation—a life-saving procedure. Endotracheal intubation can be accomplished by primary care physicians in large university hospital intensive care units when no specialist is available, or in small rural hospitals where they are the best and sometimes the only caregivers capable of performing this procedure.

Endotracheal tubes may be inserted in many different ways: through the mouth or nose, with direct visualization or blindly, with the patient awake or unconscious, through a cricothyrotomy, or with the assistance of bronchoscopy.

The method described in this chapter is used primarily for emergent direct oral intubation in the unconscious patient. This method causes minimal nasal bleeding and sinusitus, results in easier suctioning, and can be learned relatively quickly.

During this procedure, consider concomitant medical problems. Arrythmias, congestive heart failure, and many other diseases may be affected by this procedure.

A respiratory therapist and a trained assistant should be present throughout the procedure.

Note: Reading this chapter alone is not sufficient to master this skill. Manikins are available for practice and should be utilized. They are often owned by hospitals for use in advanced cardiac life support (ACLS) classes. Reading some of the references at the end of this chapter and reviewing pertinent anatomy can be instructional, as well as taking a course in ACLS. Observing trained anesthesiologists in the operating room under controlled circumstances can add to the practitioner's experience. Observing in a code situation can truly make one appreciate that conditions are not always optimal for intubation. While learning this skill, utilize a mentor. Initial attempts should be supervised by trained personnel. Universal blood and body fluid precautions should be followed.

INDICATIONS

- Respiratory failure: Hypoxia (consider when $P_{A_{O_2}} < 60$ with $F_{I_{O_2}} > 0.5$), hypercapnia, tachypnea, or apnea from causes including adult respiratory distress syndrome (ARDS), pulmonary edema, and infection

- Maintenance or protection of an intact airway: To assist the collection and removal of bronchopulmonary secretions, to prevent aspiration of gastric contents, or to bypass oropharyngeal trauma or obstruction

CONTRAINDICATIONS

- A patient not able to extend the head, with severe degenerative cervical spine disorders, or with severe rheumatoid arthritis involving the cervical spine
- Moderate to severe trauma to the cervical spine or anterior neck (Patients with gunshot wounds to this area are candidates for cricothyroidotomy.)
- Infection in the epiglottal area
- Mandibular fracture
- Mild hypoxia (*relative contraindication*: Administer 100% oxygen through a bag-mask assembly first, then redraw arterial blood to determine if the P_{O_2} has risen to a normal level.)
- Intact tracheostomy (*relative contraindication*: Endotracheal intubation can be done if a tracheostomy tube falls out; however, obviously the best action is to replace the tube.)

EQUIPMENT (FIG. 59-1)

- Laryngoscope
- Blades, curved (MacIntosh) *and* straight (Miller) (Inexperienced physicians will find the curved blades easier to use.)
- Endotracheal tubes of various sizes (for neonates and full-term infants, Nos. 0 and 1; for adults, 6.5 to 7.5 mm tube for women, 7.5 to 8.5 mm for men; suppliers include Mallincrot, Portex, and Rusch)
- Lubricant (sterile and water-soluble)
- 10 cc syringe (to inflate endotracheal tube cuff)
- Adhesive tape ½-inch and ¾-inch rolls
- Tincture of benzoin
- Oxygen (100%) supply and tubing
- Manual resuscitation bag with mask (anesthesia or bag valve mask)
- Pulse oximeter (if available)
- Ventilator
- Suction and suction catheter (Yankauer, 10 to 12 Fr.)
- Cardiac monitor
- Defibrillator
- Clock or watch with a second hand
- Stethoscope
- Local anesthetic (benzocaine spray, cocaine, lidocaine); intravenous skeletal muscle relaxant (succinylcholine); benzodiazepine (midazolam); or narcotic
- Sterile gloves

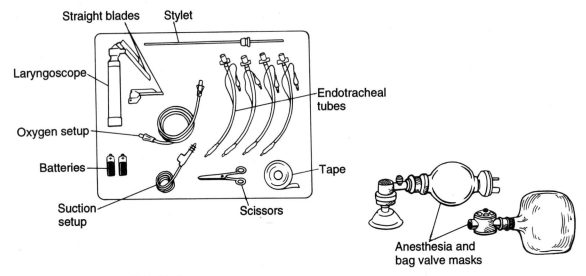

FIG. 59-1.
Intubation equipment.

Optional

- Suction tube trap to catch the first intubated specimen for Gram stain and culture
- Malleable stylet
- Magill forceps (for nasal intubation)
- Scissors
- Bite block
- Bed with removable headboard and lockable wheels

PREPROCEDURE PATIENT EDUCATION

Endotracheal intubation is often an emergency procedure, and there is usually no time for written informed consent. Talk to the patient and family, explain the situation, and document an *implied* consent. Complications of the procedure should be mentioned, as well as what might happen to the patient if the procedure is not performed.

TECHNIQUE

1. Obtain informed consent, if possible.
2. Decide whether to use a local anesthetic, or a combination of a skeletal muscle relaxant, a benzodiazepine, and sodium pentothal. In most emergent

situations, muscle relaxants and general anesthetics are not necessary. If needed, consider using intravenous midazolam (or diazepam), a short-acting barbiturate (sodium pentothal), and a skeletal muscle relaxant (vecuronium, atarcuronium, or succinylcholine). Remember that once the patient is paralyzed, you must be prepared to take over all respirations. If you cannot intubate, a tracheostomy is indicated.

3. Position the patient supine. Use a chin lift or jaw thrust (Fig. 59-2) to allow the patient to continue spontaneous respiration during the procedure. Place towels under the occipit, and arrange the patient's head and body so that the mouth, pharynx, and trachea are all in a line (Figs. 59-3 and 59-4). Remove full or partial dentures, or any foreign bodies in the mouth.

    Stand behind the patient's head. Remove the headboard if possible, and raise the bed to a comfortable working height.

4. Arrange and check that all equipment and personnel are present and working. Arrange the equipment in order of need. Attach the pulse oximeter to the patient and turn it on.

5. Select and attach the appropriate blade. The curved blade is easy to use; the straight blade, however, is the anesthesiologist's favorite (Fig. 59-5).

6. Verify that the light on the laryngoscope is working.

7. Check the cuff by filling the syringe with air and inject it into the cuff; if the cuff loses air, it leaks! Change the endotracheal tube. After checking for leaks, deflate the cuff.

8. Check the length of the endotracheal tube by placing it next to patient's neck. The tube should extend from the mouth to beyond the sternal notch.

9. Using sterile gloves, remove the endotracheal tube from its package, lubricate the outside, and insert the stylet inside. Do not allow the stylet to extend beyond the last 1 to 1.5 cm of the endotracheal tube.

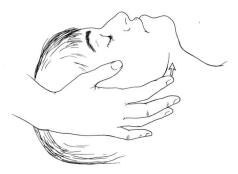

FIG. 59-2.
Jaw thrust. Rotate mandible forward by using index fingers. Arrow indicates motion to bring soft tissues foward to relieve airway obstruction.

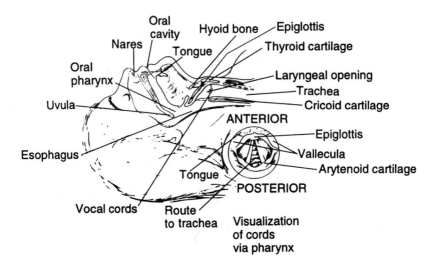

Cutaway side view of head and neck

FIG. 59-3.
Anatomic landmarks of the head and neck.

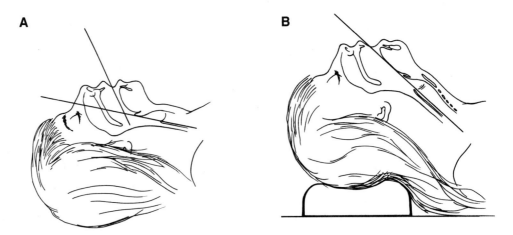

FIG. 59-4.
Proper head position is important for successful orotracheal intubation. Axes of the mouth, pharynx, and larynx need to be aligned. **A,** Divergent axes; **B,** Axes in line, "sniffing position."

10. Administer 100% oxygen via mask for 1 minute.
11. Begin a 20-second count. Intubation must be accomplished in 20 seconds or else oxygen should be reapplied.
12. Remove the patient's mask and open the patient's mouth. Recheck for dentures and other possible obstructions; remove if found.

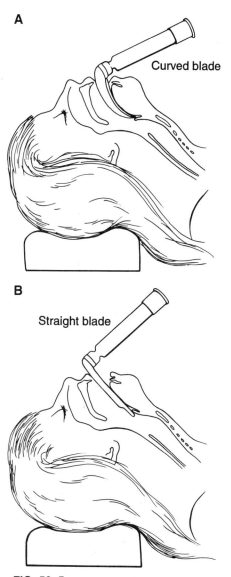

FIG. 59-5.
Blade placements. **A,** Curved blade (Macintosh) may be less traumatic and less reflex stimulating because it avoids the larynx (tip of blade is in vallecula). **B,** Laryngoscopic technique with straight blade (Miller). This is mechanically easier if patient has no large central incisors.

13. Regardless of your "handedness," pick up the laryngoscope with your left hand, and turn it on by flipping the blade. Place the suction catheter in your right hand, and place the scope in the patient's mouth. If you are using a straight blade, insert the scope on the right side and push the tongue to the left side. If you are using a curved blade, insert the scope in the center of the mouth and pass it up into the vallecula (Fig. 59-5).

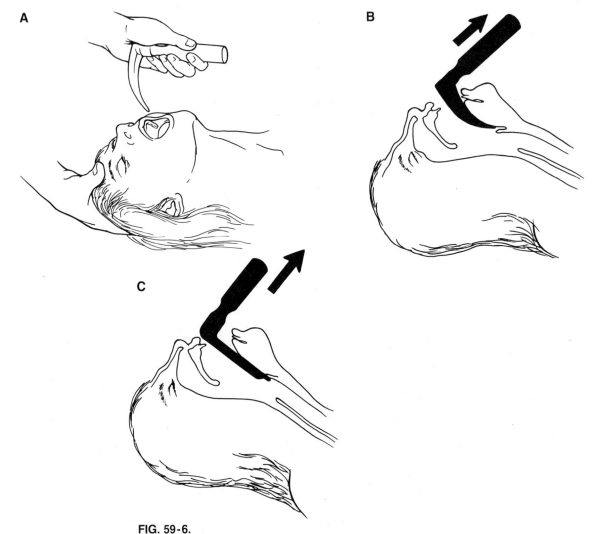

FIG. 59-6.
A, Insertion of laryngoscope. **B,** Correct nonfulcrum movement of curved laryngoscope blade.
C, Straight blade.

14. Push the blade posteriorly to the correct position (in which no part of the tongue can be visualized distally).

15. Use suction to remove secretions and fluids that are in the posterior pharynx. Always keep suction nearby. (If the patient still exhibits a gag reflex, reconsider using topical lidocaine or Cetacaine spray. Intravenous general anesthetics or benzodiazepines might also be appropriate.)

16. Lift the whole blade assembly and laryngoscope toward the ceiling. Avoid fulcrum movement, which you can feel in your biceps (Fig. 59-6).

17. Watch for the vocal cords (Fig. 59-7). If they are not visible, have an assistant gently press the cricoid cartilage using the Sellick maneuver (Fig. 59-7),

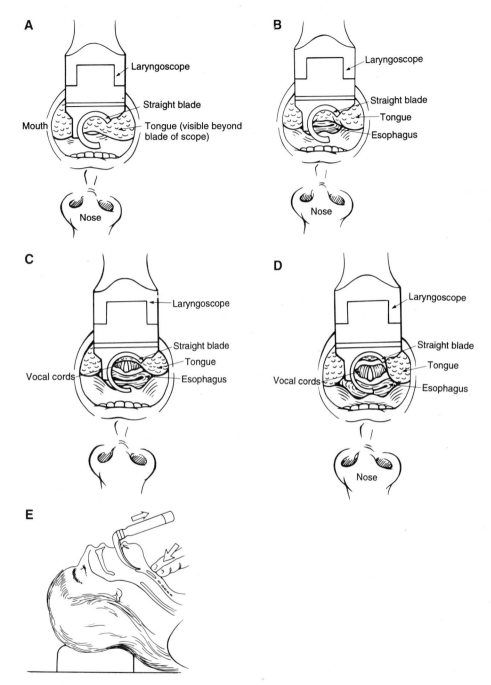

FIG. 59-7.

Different views with correct and incorrect placement of laryngoscope. **A,** Blade is not inserted far enough, only the tongue is visible. Push blade in further. **B,** Blade is in too far; the esophagus is visible, but no vocal cords are visible. Pull the blade out. **C,** Correct position with partial view of vocal cords. Lift the blade in a nonfulcrum movement (see Fig. 59-6). **D,** Correct view for intubation. **E,** Sellick maneuver (some suggest utilizing early with every attempt to prevent aspiration).

which also helps prevent aspiration of gastric contents. This is especially important when the timing of the last meal is unknown. If cords still cannot be seen, modify the patient's position. If more than 20 seconds have elapsed, stop the attempt, administer 100% oxygen via bag ventilation for 1 minute, and then retry intubation.

Note: Some authorities recommend the Sellick manuever throughout the procedure to prevent aspiration.

18. Once the vocal cords have been visualized, pick up the endotracheal tube in your right hand *without looking away from the scope* (Fig. 59-8). Place the

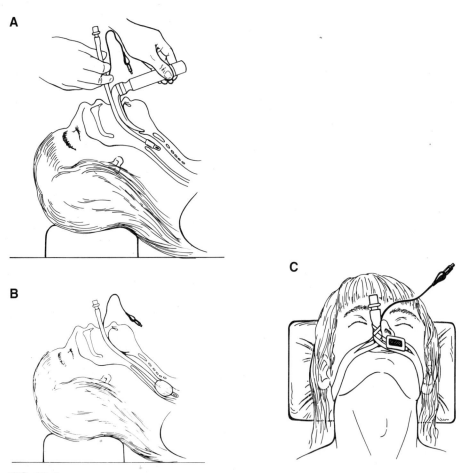

FIG. 59-8.
Insertion of endotracheal tube with laryngoscope in place. **A,** Insert the tube just lateral to the path of the laryngoscope so a clear view can be maintained at all times. Watch the tube pass through cords. **B,** The tube is correctly positioned when the proximal end of the tube cuff is just below the vocal cords. When the tube is in place, remove the laryngoscope and carefully withdraw the stylet. **C,** Secure the tube to minimize patient discomfort while maintaining correct positioning.

distal end of the tube in the patient's mouth, into the posterior pharynx, and *through* the vocal cords. Visualization of the tube going through the cords is crucial for proper tracheal intubation—otherwise, the tube may enter the esophagus. Insert the tube just far enough for the cuff to rest slightly below the vocal cords. This correlates to about where the 23 cm mark on the tube would rest in the corner of the mouth in men, and 21 cm in women (distal tip will be 2 cm above the carina).

19. Keep holding the endotracheal tube in your right hand and stabilize it against the patient's face. Remove the laryngoscope.

20. Remove the stylet from the endotracheal tube with your left hand while continuing to stabilize the tube with your right hand.

21. Ventilate oxygen via bag. Auscultate over the lungs for air flow to check for symmetry, and over the stomach, to be sure there are no air sounds (Fig. 59-9). If lung sounds are asymmetric (the right side is usually the louder side), the endotracheal tube is too deep and the right lung has been intubated since it has a straighter path. Mark the tube and pull it back 1 to 2 cm. Auscultate again. Air excursion should be symmetric and effective. The tube needs to rest just above the carina.

22. Attach oxygen source (bag valve mask or ventilator).

23. Apply tincture of benzoin to the skin, place the bite block on the endotracheal tube, and tape the tube. If desired, obtain a specimen for Gram stain and culture.

24. Using the syringe, inflate the endotracheal tube cuff with air until it is full. (Fullness is indicated by a senescent bag; do not overinflate or it will feel *hard* to compress.)

25. Obtain a chest X-ray to verify tube location and check for complications.

26. Insert a nasogastric, or feeding, tube (to deflate the stomach and act as a reminder to supplement nutrition early).

27. Order the ventilatory parameters for respiratory therapy: rate (usually 14 to 18 inhalations per minute), tidal volume (usually 8 to 10 cc/kg), and $F_{I_{O_2}}$. When in doubt, start with 100% oxygen and rapidly reduce the percentage, depending on the readings from a pulse oximeter and results of judiciously timed arterial blood gases.

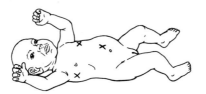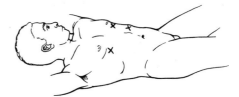

FIG. 59-9.
Auscultation points of right and left chest for respiratory movement and over stomach for lack of sound.

Remember:

- If intubation requires more than 20 seconds, abort the attempt, ventilate the patient with 100% oxygen (bag valve mask or mouth-to-mask), and then try again. Consider continuous positive airway pressure (CPAP) using a tight-fitting mask. It can improve oxygenation if a routine mask is not sufficient while awaiting intubation.
- Check tube position and reposition as needed.
- Suction excess debris.
- The stylet can be bent against the hard palate while in the mouth, if needed.
- Prior placement of a nasogastric tube will show you where *not* to go.

Further questions and considerations: Does the patient have an anteriorly displaced larynx? Need the Sellick maneuver? Is pharyngeal anatomy such that you need more extension? Flexion? Do you need to make a blind passage through arytenoids (not desirable, but sometimes necessary)?

POSTPROCEDURE CARE

- Order daily chest X-rays to verify tube placement.
- The Respiratory Services department of the hospital usually supplies the ventilator, tape, etc., and provides care; however, the physician is ultimately responsible.
- Check the patient and the respiratory setup frequently.

COMPLICATIONS

- Short-term laryngeal edema: sore throat occurs in almost 100% of patients following extubation (Repeated attempts at intubation by unskilled personnel may result in enough edema to preclude intubation by highly skilled clinicians.)
- Trauma:
  - Broken teeth
  - Avulsion of arytenoid cartilage
  - Oral lacerations or ulcerations (lip, tongue, esophagus, and even trachea)

- Hypoxia, due to the following:
  - Long duration of procedure
  - Esophageal intubation (most commonly results from not visualizing the vocal cords)
  - Pneumothorax
  - Aspiration of vomited material, especially in conscious or semiconscious patient

- Laryngospasm with resultant noncardiogenic edema
- Hypertension/hypotension

- Bradycardia
- Tachycardia with or without arrhythmias
- Sequelae (of long-term endotracheal tube placement)
- Nosocomial infection
- Pneumothorax
- Corneal abrasions
- Epistaxis
- Sinusitus
- Vocal cord paralysis (left cord more frequently involved than right)
- Tracheomalacia and stenosis (occurs more frequently in males; more common with older tubes that use higher cuff pressures)
- Tracheoesophogeal fistula
- Innominate artery erosion by endotracheal cuff

CPT/BILLING CODE

31500   Intubation, endotracheal; emergency procedure

BIBLIOGRAPHY

Gallagher TJ: Endotracheal intubation, *Crit Care Clinics* 8(4):665, 1992.

Gammage GW: Airway management. In Civetta et al, editors: *Critical Care,* Philadelphia 1988, J.B. Lippincott.

Hines D, Bone RC: The technique of E-T intubation, *J Crit Illness* 1(9):59, 1981.

Kaur S, Heard SO, Welch GW: Airway management and endotracheal intubation. In Rippe JM et al, editors: *Intensive care medicine,* ed 2, Boston, 1991, Little, Brown & Co.

CHAPTER 60

Temporary Pacing

Len Scarpinato

In rural or underserved health care settings, or if first on the scene, primary care physicians may be required to perform temporary cardiac pacing. As an integral part of the algorithms for advanced cardiac life support, pacing can be a life-saving procedure, especially when the problem is resistant to drug therapy and the tertiary care provider cannot get to the patient in time.

This chapter is merely an introduction toward gaining competence with this procedure. One should practice on the equipment and observe the procedure performed by trained individuals to gain additional proficiency. When this procedure is first attempted, a trained and competent individual must be present for supervision.

Various options are available for temporary pacing. This chapter will deal primarily with the intravenous route of emergency ventricular pacing. External pacing will also be covered briefly.

EXTERNAL (TRANSCUTANEOUS) PACING

Most defibrillator units available on crash carts are now "external-pacing capable." Modern units represent a major improvement on the older, crude machines that inflicted significant chest and back muscle stimulation and discomfort and even burns to the skin. At least one suicide has been recorded of a pacer-dependent patient who removed the leads from one of the older units to end the pain.

Even with today's somewhat more sophisticated external pacing equipment, it is rare for patients not to complain of some pectoral muscle stimulation. Therefore, always remember to add analgesics, narcotics, and/or sedatives when using the external pacer.

The high voltages required for external pacing produce significant muscle twitching, and conventional ECG recordings are useless since they display these impulses and their aftermath. Fortunately, most external pacer units have a monitor capable of filtering these spikes, allowing one to perform an ECG.

About one fifth of the patients who have an external pacer applied will not have effective pacing. There are several reasons for difficult or ineffective external

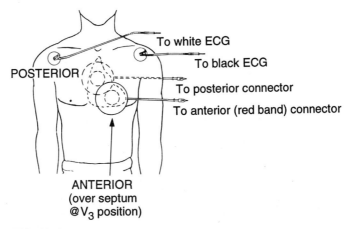

To white ECG

To black ECG

POSTERIOR

To posterior connector

To anterior (red band) connector

ANTERIOR
(over septum
@V$_3$ position)

FIG. 60-1.
External (transcutaneous) pacing. Large electrode patches are attached to the anterior and posterior chest walls, and the output is adjusted upward to obtain ventricular capture. (From Dahlberg ST, Benotti JR: Temporary cardiac pacing. In Rippe JM et al, editors: *Intensive care medicine,* ed 2, Boston, 1991, Little, Brown.)

pacing, including increased intrathoracic air (such as barrel chests or chronic obstructive pulmonary disease), pericardial effusion or tamponade, or patient size or electrode placement.

To perform external pacing, first affix the exposed adhesive surfaces of two large electrode patches to the anterior and posterior chest walls (Fig. 60-1). Set the heart rate and stimulation, pacing, and sensing thresholds in a manner similar to that used for internal pacing; however, remember that larger outputs are necessary. Keep in mind that for demand pacing, external units often do not have sensing thresholds. Pacing is usually set at 1.25 times the initial capture threshold. Patients with conditions that cause difficult or ineffective pacing may require higher outputs for capture. At these higher outputs, the resultant muscle twitches may preclude external pacer use.

The use of the external pacer probably has reduced the number of prophylactic internal pacers placed; however, external pacers have a 20% failure rate. To minimize the possibility of a "code" situation, prophylactic intravenous access via the right internal jugular vein may be helpful. Should external pacing fail, an internal wire can be passed for transvenous pacing. Keep in mind that external pacing is always a temporary measure that is used until an internal (probably transvenous as described below) pacer can be placed in nontransient situations where pacing is absolutely indicated.

INTERNAL (TRANSVENOUS) PACING

Access Route

The most direct route for internal pacemaker insertion is through the right internal jugular. The right subclavian vein can be used, especially for relatively long-term

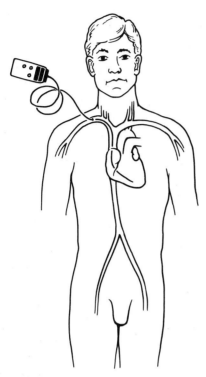

FIG. 60-2.
Temporary pacer in right subclavian vein.

use, but the insertion may be more difficult due to the turns the electrode has to negotiate with this route of access (Fig. 60-2).

INDICATIONS

Note: The indications for temporary transvenous cardiac pacing can be divided into therapeutic, prophylactic, and diagnostic categories. For the purposes of this chapter, only the first two categories will be covered. In addition, "medicinal" pacing can be attempted following ACLS guidelines (atropine, isoproterenol, etc.). Overdrive pacing to terminate arrhythmias is useful but beyond the scope of this chapter, as is atrioventricular sequential pacing and transthoracic cardiac electrode placement.

- Symptomatic or life-threatening bradyarrhythmias, including sick sinus syndrome
- Asystole
- Sinus or junctional bradycardia that is unresponsive to atropine and that results in hemodynamic compromise
- Variants

1. Atrioventricular (AV) block (Pacing is indicated whenever rate-dependent hypotension is present.)
   a. High-degree block, either complete or Möbitz type II
   b. Möbitz type I block with slow sinus rate and low AV conduction rate (Pacing is rarely indicated with Möbitz type I.)
   c. Inferior myocardial infarction (MI) with complete heart block
   d. Idioventricular rhythm (usually with slow rate)
2. New bifascicular block
   a. Right bundle branch block (RBBB) with left anterior hemiblock or left posterior hemiblock
   b. Left bundle branch block (LBBB) alone following acute anterior MI (controversial)
   c. Alternating RBBB and LBBB in acute MI
   d. Old bifascicular block with new PR-interval prolongation (especially indicated to prevent complete AV block in anterior MI)

- Bradycardia-dependent ventricular tachycardia
- *Torsades de pointes* (polymorphic ventricular tachycardia with prolongation of QT intervals)
- Medically unresponsive, recurrent ventricular tachycardia that requires multiple direct-current cardioversions
- Atrial flutter with hemodynamic compromise
- Intra-AV-nodal tachycardias with hemodynamic compromise
- Extra-AV-nodal tachycardias (e.g., Wolfe-Parkinson-White syndrome) with hemodynamic compromise

CONTRAINDICATIONS

(Same general contraindications as in Chapter 48, Central Venous Catheter Insertion)

- Bleeding diatheses of a significant nature including, but not limited to, elevated prothrombic time, partial thromboplast time, or low platelets
- Patient undergoing anticoagulant or thrombolytic drug therapy
- Presence of a prosthetic tricuspid valve
- Atrial fibrillation (not indicated for atrial pacing)
- Depending on access site, neck or clavicle surgical procedures or fracture history

EQUIPMENT

- Bipolar transvenous pacing electrodes, 4 to 6 Fr. catheter (Fig. 60-3)—may be elastic, stiff, semifloating, or composed of flexible Dacron (A flow-directed, flexible balloon-tipped catheter; a pacer-equipped pulmonary artery catheter; or a Swan-Ganz catheter with pacemaker lumen may be used.)

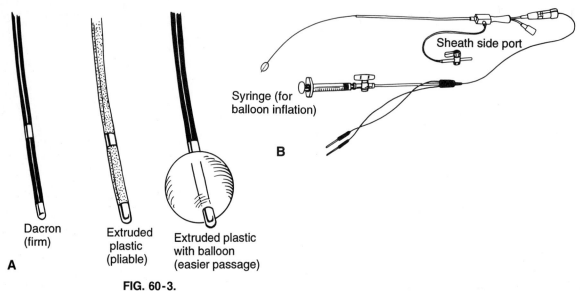

Dacron
(firm)

Extruded
plastic
(pliable)

Extruded plastic
with balloon
(easier passage)

A

FIG. 60-3.
A, Distal tips of transvenous pacers. **B,** Transvenous balloon-tipped temporary pacer.

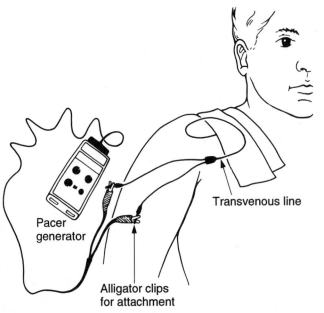

FIG. 60-4.
Transvenous line in place.

- Pacer, pulse generator (Fig. 60-4)
- ECG monitoring capability during insertion (Availability of fluoroscopy is ideal.)
- Venous insertion site (The right internal jugular vein is the preferred route for placement of temporary pacers.)

PREPROCEDURE PATIENT EDUCATION

This is an emergency procedure, and usually written informed consent cannot be obtained. However, the situation, risks, and benefits should be explained to the patient and family, and *implied* consent should be documented. Always outline the complications of both performing the procedure and withholding the procedure.

TECHNIQUE

All steps should be performed using aseptic technique and following universal blood and body fluid precautions. Venous access is established by the procedure outlined in Chapter 48, Central Venous Catheter Insertion.

Catheter Conversion

If necessary, insert a larger catheter into the established venous access site.

1. Place a guide wire down the central venous access line.
2. Remove the catheter.
3. Use an obturator over the wire to enlarge the lumen.
4. Pass an introducer with catheter assembly over the guide wire.
5. Remove the introducer.
6. Check for venous return.

Pacer Placement

Fluoroscopy technique.
By far, the best method of temporary pacer placement involves fluoroscopic guidance of the balloon-tipped bipolar pacing leads. Many intensive care units and some emergency rooms have beds that will accommodate C-arms for fluoroscopy. If C-arms cannot be accommodated, and if time and clinical conditions permit, the patient might also be moved to the radiology suite.

1. Pass the balloon-tipped catheter to the 10 to 12 cm mark (10 cm graduations are marked on the catheter).
2. Blow up the balloon and advance the catheter; it should move easily into the right atrium (RA).
3. Pass the tip across the tricuspid valve and advance it to the apex of the right ventricle (RV). Ask the patient to take deep breaths or to cough; this will facilitate passage across the valve. Deflate the balloon once the radiopague tip is at

the apex, the last 2 to 3 cm of the lead should show minimal or no longitudinal motion with further advancement under fluoroscopy; the rest of the catheter will have horizontal and longitudinal motion (Fig. 60-5).

4. Hook up the pacer electrodes to the pacer unit.

Nonfluoroscopy technique.

The flexible balloon-tipped catheter can be advanced and positioned much like the Swan-Ganz (see Chapter 49, Swan-Ganz Catheterization), except that the distal negative electrode catheter is attached to an ECG machine (usually the V lead, a unipolar lead), and the change in the recorded QRS complex allows one to approximate the tip location (Fig. 60-6). The passage route is the same: into the right atrium, across the tricuspid valve, and to the apex of the right ventricle. While the lead is in the atrium, the P wave will appear quite large, and then as it passes the tricuspid valve, the QRS amplitude increases. Once the catheter is correctly placed, a large elevated ST segment can be seen.

Emergency technique.

Unfortunately, emergency situations frequently dictate that a temporary pacer be placed during the most extreme and urgent conditions, such as during a code with the patient lying in a hospital bed. The catheter may be inserted blindly to about 12 cm, attached to the pacemaker, and turned on, with the rate set higher than the patient's highest heart rate the amperage (ventricular output current) set at the highest setting, and the mode set at asynchronous (sensitivity off). The surface or conventional ECG or rhythm strip should be running while the catheter is being passed. Multiple attempts at passage may be necessary until capture is noted by an

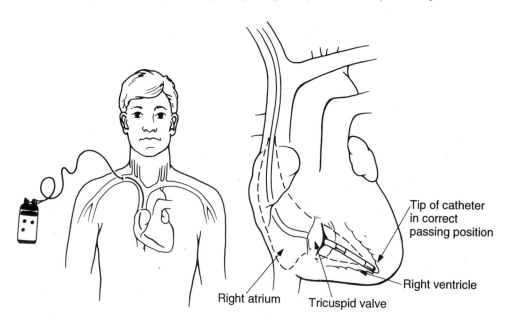

FIG. 60-5.
Correct positioning of pacer catheter. When the tip reaches the apex, it quits moving under fluoroscopy.

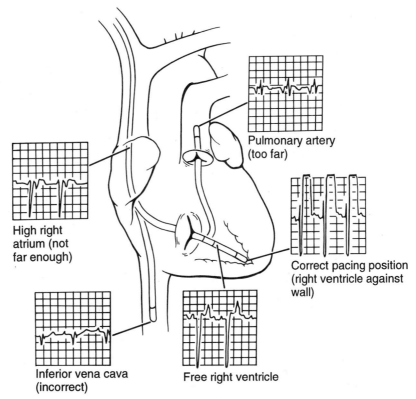

FIG. 60-6.
Pattern of recorded ECG from intracardiac pacemaker electrodes at various locations in the venous circulation.

obviously paced rhythm seen on the surface ECG. Unfortunately, even experienced clinicians occasionally fail after multiple attempts, which underscores the benefits of fluoroscopic guidance.

Parameter Settings

Determine the parameters and record each when it is set. Once the pacer guide wire is in place, the pacer should be attached positive terminal to positive lead and negative to negative, much like a car battery.

Rate.
If the patient shows no intrinsic heart rate, set the pacing rate at 70 to 80 beats per minute to simulate the normal beating heart. If the patient is bradycardic, the same range can be used to raise the blood pressure and heart rate. Record the rate chosen after setting the machine.

Ventricular output.
The ventricular output signal is the current generated by the pacer, adjustable from 0.1 to 20 milliamperes (mA). Most situations discussed in this chapter require the

maximum output at initiation of pacing, with gradual reduction afterward. After reaching the level of output necessary to capture the ventricle, large spikes followed by bundle branch block (BBB) pattern complexes (wide QRS complexes, ST-segment depression, and T-wave inversion depending on the lead) are seen. A pulse should also be palpable and should generate a blood pressure. The ventricular output setting can then be gradually reduced, and capture should be maintained at a setting less than 2 mA (optimally less than 1 mA). For the final operating output setting, the stimulation or pacing threshold must be determined. If spikes are seen but no capture occurs, catheter manipulation is indicated. If spikes and BBB pattern are seen with no pulse, the possibility of pulseless electrical activity must be considered, as should the proper ACLS management protocol (electromechanical dissociation [EMD]).

Stimulation or pacing threshold.
To determine the actual stimulation or pacing threshold, set the rate at 10 to 15 beats above the patient's intrinsic rate (not below 60), set the sensitivity between 1.5 and 3 millivolts (mV), and use a ventricular output of about 5 mA. With the pacer turned on, the ECG should show capture (Fig. 60-7). Decrease the mA until the capture of the heart is lost and the patient's heart reverts to its intrinsic rhythm. The amperage of the ventricular output signal at the time that capture is lost is the *stimulation* or *pacing threshold*. Optimally, this should be less than 1 mA, which indicates that the electrode is in adequate contact with the endocardium. In actual use, the output is maintained well above this setting (usually about 2 times, and some physicians suggest 3 to 5 times this threshold level). If levels of 5 to 6 mA or greater are required (which is common in fibrosis, but is usually a result of poor electrode positioning), repositioning should be attempted.

Demand Pacing

If the patient's intrinsic rhythm is inadequate, a sensing threshold must be determined. Occasionally a sensing threshold cannot be determined when the patient has a significantly slow rhythm.

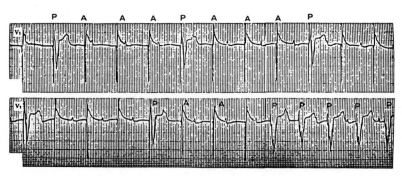

FIG. 60-7.
Pacing with intermittent capture. "P" indicates paced beats. "A" indicates pacer artifact without capture. (From Dahlberg ST, Benotti JR: Temporary cardiac pacing. In Rippe JM et al, editors: *Intensive care medicine,* ed 2, Boston, 1991, Little, Brown.)

Sensitivity is the control on the pacer that detects the amplitude of the patient's intrinsic R wave. The most sensitive setting is 1 mV, corresponding to full clockwise rotation of the knob. This is opposed to the least sensitive setting, called *asynchronous pacing,* where the pacer does not care if there is a rhythm and functions oblivious to the intrinsic rate. The asynchronous setting should be avoided when there is an intrinsic rhythm because the additional electric spikes generated by the pacer can set up an arrhythmia.

To determine sensing threshold, first set the rate about 10 beats per minute below the patient's intrinsic rate. Gradually adjust the sensitivity control toward the highest sensitivity or entirely clockwise (to detect even the lowest amplitude waves), which is known as the *full demand* setting. Pacer pulses should no longer be seen because all deflections are sensed and interpreted as QRS complexes, and every intrinsic or artifactual QRS complex should generate a flash of the sense indicator on the pacer. At this level, the pacer senses almost all electrical activity, and its firing is thus prevented. In fact, T waves, sometimes P waves (if your catheter is close to the atrium), chest muscle contractions, or even artifact may prevent the pacer from firing. This is called the *oversensing point.* This full demand setting is obviously too high for the pacer to function. The sensitivity control should then be turned counterclockwise, changing or decreasing the sensitivity toward higher numbers until ECG pacer spikes are seen that correspond to the patient's intrinsic rhythm, regardless of their capture. This level is the *sensing threshold* of the pacer. The pace indicator light (if the machine has one) should also flash. For *demand pacing,* the sensing should be set at a level halfway between the oversensing point and the sensing threshold. This level should be recorded.

Keep in mind that pacers can fail to sense when the sensitivity setting on the pacer is too low, when the lead is malpositioned, or when the intrinsic signal is of poor quality.

Once pacing effectively, the length of wire that has been inserted transvenously should be recorded. Secure the electrode catheter to the skin with two sutures at two sites.

Confirmation of Lead Placement

1. A cross-table lateral and anterioposterior chest radiograph should be ordered. The tip of the catheter should be at the distal right ventricle in the apex, with no loops, kinks, or doublings (no redundancies). On the lateral view, the pacer should be to the left of the spine and slightly inferior and anterior (retrosternally).
2. A 12-lead ECG should demonstrate the expected LBBB pattern due to the origination of electrical current in the right ventricle (Fig. 60-8).

While a temporary pacer is in place, a hardwire or telemetry rhythm strip should be recorded and monitored. Patients should be restricted to bedrest for at least 24 hours. Aseptic technique must be maintained when handling the catheter, and appropriate skin care should be ordered. Sterile bandage changes should follow the intensive care unit's central venous line protocol. Unnecessary catheter manipula-

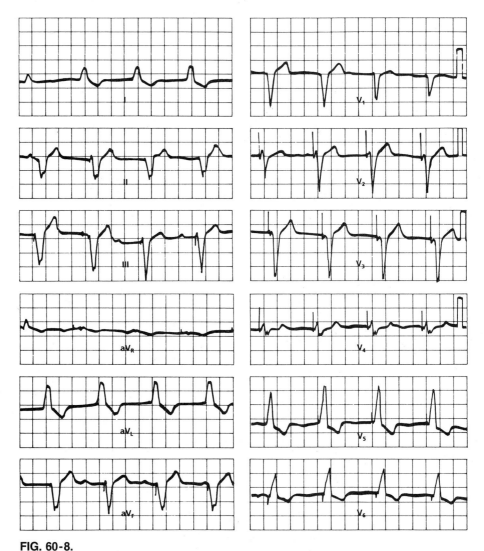

FIG. 60-8.
Finished product: 12-lead ECG with pacer in place. (From Morelli RL, Goldschlager N: *J Crit Ill* 2(3):71, 1987. Used with permission.)

tions should be avoided. Pacemaker function should be checked daily with a 12-lead ECG, and pacing threshold determinations documented. Daily physical examination for friction rubs (a clue to perforation) or clicking noises (muscle stimulation) must be documented.

Troubleshooting—Failure to Pace

Failure to pace can occur from a variety of reasons including—but not limited to—a faulty battery, dislodged or malpositioned leads, a loose connection, a damaged or fractured wire, electronic interference, or a faulty pacer. Some cardiac conditions cause very high pacing thresholds or preclude intrinsic pacing: myocardial fibrosis or ischemia, drug toxicity from cardiac agents, myocardial perforation, ventricular refractoriness from a low-grade unsensed intrinsic QRS complex.

If the pacer fails to work after it had been previously functioning, several questions should be considered: Has the catheter dislodged? Are the wires loose or disconnected? Are the pacemaker settings correct? Has the battery failed? Is there electrical interference? Has the ventricle been perforated as a result of synchronous diaphragmatic or intracostal muscle contractions?

In an emergency situation, consider increasing the stimulation or pacing threshold to regain capture. Occasionally the area in the heart near the electrode can become fibrotic and require a higher stimulation. Also, the catheter tip could have become partially dislodged. If the problem is oversensing, that threshold should be reset.

If all else fails, another emergency maneuver is to switch the polarity of the lead connections to the pacer. Occasionally this will regain pacing, although this has not been well documented in the medical literature.

COMPLICATIONS

(Same as those for central venous line insertion; see Chapter 48, Central Venous Catheter Insertion.) These are seen more frequently in emergency situations:

- Loss of pacing (failure of pacer, lead dislodgement, fracture of pacer wire)
- Pericardial friction rub, myocardial damage or infarction
- Arrhythmia
- Interventricular septum or right ventricular perforation, with or without cardiac tamponade
- Infection, including bacteremia
- Arterial or venous injury, including phlebitis and thrombosis (incidence is higher than expected)
- Diaphragmatic stimulation, chest wall stimulation
- Pulmonary embolism
- Air embolism
- Endocardial structural damage
- Electrical hazards (Any extraneous currents, even micro currents, can cause ventricular fibrillation if applied to a pacemaker catheter.)

CPT/BILLING CODES

36489	Placement of central venous catheter, over age 2
92953	Temporary transcutaneous pacing

BIBLIOGRAPHY

American Heart Association: *Advanced cardiac life support,* ed 2, Dallas, 1987, The Association.

Dahlberg ST, Benotti JR: *Temporary cardiac pacing in intensive care medicine,* ed 2, Boston, 1991, Little, Brown & Co.

Higgins JR: Temporary cardiac pacemakers. In Civetta JM, Taylor RW, Kirby RR, editors: *Critical care,* Philadelphia, 1988, J.B. Lippincott.

Jafri SM, Kruse JA: Temporary transvenous pacing in critical care clinics, *Procedures in the ICU* 8(4):713, 1992.

Morelli RL, Goldschlager N: Temporary transvenous pacing, *J Crit Ill* 2(3):71, 1987; and 2(4):73, 1987.

CHAPTER 61

Thoracentesis

Terry S. Ruhl

The pleural "space" is normally a potential space between the visceral pleura, which is adherent to the lung, and the parietal pleura, which is adherent to the chest wall. Normally, it contains only a thin film of lubricating fluid. Any time this space becomes filled with air or extra fluid, the work of breathing increases. Many diseases produce pleural effusions, and sampling this fluid often helps in determining the diagnosis. Other patients may gain relief of symptoms by removal of air or fluid by thoracentesis.

INDICATIONS

- Any pleural effusion of unknown etiology (Effusions with an easily explained cause, such as congestive heart failure, may be observed for response to therapy.)
- Large symptomatic effusion
- Stable spontaneous pneumothorax

CONTRAINDICATIONS

- Patient refuses the procedure
- Chest wall pyoderma or local skin compromise (cellulitis, burn, etc.)
- Herpes zoster on chest wall
- When tube thoracostomy is more appropriate
- Ruptured diaphragm

CONDITIONS ASSOCIATED WITH INCREASED RISK

- Coagulopathy or patient undergoing anticoagulant therapy
- Inability of patient to cooperate
- Very small effusions (less than 10 mm thick on a decubitus film)

- Removal of large amounts of fluid (greater than 1 liter)
- Unstable medical condition
- Patients with positive ventilatory pressures
- Pleural adhesions (due to previous tuberculosis infection, hemopneumothorax, or empyema)

EQUIPMENT

Commercial trays such as Pharmaseal (American Hospital Supply Corporation, Valencia, CA 91355) are available, or the following equipment can be assembled:

Preparation

- Sterile tray
- Sterile 4 × 4 inch gauze pads
- Povidone-iodine solution
- Sterile gloves
- Mask
- Fenestrated drape or sterile towels
- Oxygen by nasal cannula

Anesthesia

- 10 cc Luer-Lok syringe
- 25-gauge or smaller needle
- 1.5- to 2-inch 22-gauge needle
- 10 cc lidocaine 1% with epinephrine

Insertion

- 50 cc Luer-Lok syringe
- 2-inch 18-gauge needle (for air)
- 2-inch 15-gauge needle (for fluid)
- 3-way stopcock
- 2 curved clamps
- Specimen tubes: 1 red top, 1 lavender top, culture tubes (aerobic and anaerobic), 10 to 50 cc red top for cytology; possibly 1 green top

Optional

- Sterile plastic tubing
- 1-inch 15-gauge needle
- 500 or 1000 cc vacuum bottles

Dressing

- Sterile gauze pads
- Adhesive tape

PREPROCEDURE PATIENT EDUCATION

Explain the procedure and its attendant risks to the patient. Provide a patient education handout (Box 61-1), detailing the procedure. Obtain informed consent (Box 61-2).

BOX 61-1. PATIENT EDUCATION HANDOUT
THORACENTESIS

What Is Thoracentesis?
Thoracentesis is the removal of air or fluid from the area around the lung.

Why Is a Thoracentesis Performed?
It is not normal to have fluid or air in the area around your lung. Sometimes the only way to figure out why someone has this fluid is to take a sample. Sometimes fluid or air around the lung can make it hard to breathe. Removing it may make you feel better.

How Is a Thoracentesis Performed?
An area on your chest or back will be washed off and numbing medicine will be injected. Then a needle will be inserted between your ribs, and the air or fluid pulled out.

Does It Hurt?
Yes, but most people say it is not much worse than having blood drawn.

What Sort of Things Can Go Wrong?
The most common problem that occurs from thoracentesis is for more air to get into the area around the lung, causing the lung to "collapse." This happens 5% to 20% of the time. Most often the collapsed lung gets better on its own, but sometimes a tube has to be put in to get the air out. This tube would stay in for several days. You would have to remain in the hospital.

You may feel short of breath immediately after the procedure, but this should get better. Very rarely, the needle goes through an organ, causing bleeding. Sometimes the needle can cause an infection. The goal of thoracentesis is to gain important information and to make you feel better, but there is always the chance it will make you worse.

What Can I Do to Make Things Go Smoothly?
The most important thing is to lie or sit still. Let the doctor know if you are having any chest pain or shortness of breath. After the procedure, you will probably have to lie quietly and breathe oxygen for a while. You can take off the bandage 24 hours after the procedure and wash the area. Inform the physician if you have a hard time breathing, or develop a new fever or chills, or redness at the puncture site.

```
┌─────────────────────────────────────────────────────────────────────┐
│              BOX 61-2. DOCUMENTATION OF INFORMED CONSENT              │
│                                                                       │
│      I, _____ authorize Dr. _____ · ____ or │
│   an assistant to perform a thoracentesis. I have read this handout and have had the │
│   procedure explained to me. All my questions have been answered. I understand │
│   that every procedure has associated risks and that not all of the risks associated │
│   with thoracentesis may be listed here. I understand that I have choices other than │
│   the thoracentesis, but I choose freely to go ahead with the thoracentesis. │
│                                                                       │
│         Signed: _____ Date: _____ │
│         Witnessed: _____ Date: _____ │
└─────────────────────────────────────────────────────────────────────┘
```

TECHNIQUE

Insertion Site and Patient Position

1. Position the patient comfortably (Fig. 61-1). *For removal of fluid,* have the patient sit and lean forward with arms supported on a table. *For air removal,* the patient should be lying supine, with the head of the bed elevated at a 30- to 45-degree angle.
2. Confirm the location and extent of fluid or air by percussion, auscultation, and study of posteroanterior and lateral chest radiographs.

   Note: If available in the office or emergency department, ultrasound may also be helpful for completing this step. See Chapter 144, Emergency Department Ultrasound.

3. Select the needle insertion site. *For air removal,* use the second or third intercostal space, in the midclavicular line or more lateral. *For fluid removal,* use an area one or two interspaces below the fluid level and 5 to 10 cm lateral to the spine. Do not use an area below the eighth intercostal space. *For high-risk patients or for small effusions,* consider using ultrasound to guide the insertion. Perform the thoracentesis at the time of the ultrasound or in exactly the same location as fluid was shown on ultrasound.
4. Mark the insertion site with a marker or by applying pressure from the hub of a needle.

Preparation and Anesthesia

1. Prepare the skin with povidone-iodine. Use sterile technique and universal blood and body fluid precautions. Wear a mask, and drape with sterile towels.
2. Raise a skin wheal with lidocaine with epinephrine solution, using a 25-gauge or smaller needle attached to a 10 cc syringe.
3. To infiltrate the anesthetic, change to a 1½-inch 22-gauge needle. Angle the needle slightly downward, and insert it through the skin wheal, so that it

A

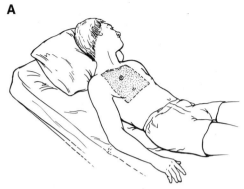

B

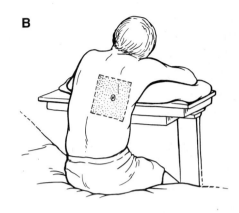

FIG. 61-1.
Position for air (**A**) and fluid (**B**) removal.

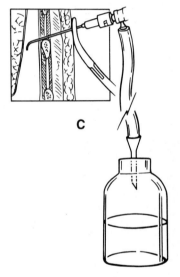

A

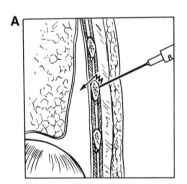

B

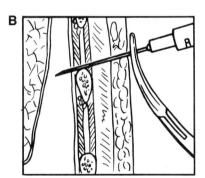

C

FIG. 61-2.
Anesthetizing the intercostal muscle layers. **A,** Needle is "walked" over the rib. **B,** Clamp is placed to mark depth of effusion. **C,** Needle in pleural space. Fluid draining into evacuated bottle.

touches the superior border of a rib, aspirating and injecting as you advance. "Walk" the needle over the superior margin of the rib and deeper into the interspace, anesthetizing the intercostal muscle layers.

Note: Do not remove the needle before Step 4 (see Fig. 61-2, *A*).

4. Confirm the presence of fluid or air with the small anesthesia needle. Continue advancing the needle, and continue aspirating and injecting until the parietal pleura has been penetrated. (A pop will be felt, or fluid or air will

be aspirated.) Warn the patient that there may be a twinge of pain as you go through the pleura. Place a clamp on the needle at skin level to mark the depth (Fig. 61-2, *B*). Withdraw the needle. If no fluid is obtained, try the next higher intercostal space. If air is unexpectedly obtained, try a lower intercostal space.

Needle-Only Insertion Technique

1. Prepare the equipment. Attach a 15-gauge needle (for fluid) or an 18-gauge needle (for air) to a 50 cc syringe with a 3-way stopcock. Mark the previously measured depth on this needle with a clamp. Test the equipment to be sure you are well acquainted with the use of the stopcock. Open the stopcock to the syringe.
2. Insert the thoracentesis needle in the same tract as the anesthesia needle, and advance it to the level of the clamp. Aspirate to confirm placement. Keep the clamp attached to prevent penetrating too far.

Catheter-Through-Needle Insertion Technique

(Use a commercially prepared thoracentesis needle, such as that made by Pharmaseal.)

1. Prepare the equipment. Place the syringe and stopcock on the Y sidearm. Advance and then retract the catheter to break the seal. Mark the measured depth on this needle with a clamp.
2. Insert the thoracentesis needle in the same tract as the anesthesia needle, and advance it to the level of the clamp. Aspirate to confirm placement. Keep the clamp attached to prevent penetrating too deeply.
3. Next, insert the catheter. While holding the hub, advance the Y sidearm until it engages the hub. Remove the split tube. Withdraw the needle, leaving the catheter in the pleural space.

Completing the Procedure

1. *For stopcock and open container:* Pull the fluid into the syringe. Turn the stopcock off to the needle, being careful not to open the needle to the environment. Push the fluid out of the syringe into the containers. Alternate aspiration into the syringe with deposition of the syringe contents into the container by rotating the stopcock.
   For stopcock and evacuated container: Attach one end of the tube to the stopcock and the other end to a needle. Place the needle in an evacuated container and open the stopcock to the thoracentesis needle (Fig. 61-2, *C*).
2. After withdrawal of necessary fluid, remove the needle while the patient is exhaling.

Caution: It may not be safe to withdraw more than 1000 cc of fluid.

3. Dress the site with a sterile dry dressing.
4. Send the fluid for study. See the following section for details. In most cases, a volume of 100 cc is sufficient for diagnostic tests.
5. Check expiratory chest radiograph for pneumothorax.

PLEURAL FLUID ANALYSIS

There are many tests that can be performed on pleural fluid, and, therefore, much money can be wasted. Numerous strategies have been suggested to reach a diagnosis in a cost-effective way. Specific tests depend on the clinical situation, and many times the fluid will not yield a definitive answer. Measurement of total protein and lactate dehydogenase (LDH) in pleural fluid and serum is usually sufficient to determine if the fluid is a transudate or an exudate. Additional studies on transudate fluid are unlikely to give useful information. One approach is to send some of the fluid for protein and LDH measurement, while storing the remaining fluid for the other tests if they are needed. See Table 61-1 for potentially useful tests and their significance, and see the bibliography for references on pleural fluid analysis.

COMPLICATIONS

- Pneumothorax may result if air is introduced through the needle or catheter, or if the visceral pleura is punctured. Five to twenty percent of procedures are associated with resulting pneumothorax, which requires treatment with a chest

TABLE 61-1.

Potentially Useful Tests in the Evaluation of Pleural Effusions

Test	Abnormal Values	Frequently Associated Condition
Protein (PF/S*)	>0.5	Exudate
LDH (PF/S)	>0.6	Exudate
LDH (IU†)	>200	Exudate
Red blood cells (per mm³)	100,000	Malignancy, trauma, pulmonary embolism
White blood cells (per mm³)	10,000	Pyogenic infection
neutrophils (%)	>50	Acute pleuritis
lymphocytes (%)	>90	Tuberculosis, malignancy
eosinophilia (%)	>10	Asbestos effusion, pneumothorax, resolving infection
mesothelial cells	Absent	Tuberculosis
Glucose (mg/dl)	<60	Empyema, tuberculosis, malignancy, rheumatoid arthritis
pH	<7.20	Esophageal rupture, empyema, tuberculosis, malignancy, rheumatoid arthritis
Amylase (PF/S)	>1	Pancreatitis
Bacteria	Positive	Etiology of infection
Cytology	Positive	Diagnostic of malignancy

*PF/S = pleural fluid to serum ratio.
† IU = concentration in international units.

From Kinasewitz GT, Fishman AP: Pleural dynamic and effusions. In Fishman AP, editor: *Pulmonary diseases and disorders*, vol 3, New York, 1988, McGraw-Hill. Used with permission.

tube about 20% of the time. Pneumothorax incidence may be reduced by using ultrasound-guided thoracentesis. Insert the needle only as far as needed to obtain fluid. Be comfortable with the equipment, especially the stopcock, before insertion. Smaller needles, short bevels, and removal of less fluid may also decrease the risk of pneumothorax.

• Hemothorax may result from laceration of intercostal vessels or internal mammary vessels. To reduce the risk of hemothorax, insert the needle just above the rib. The neurovascular bundle runs below each rib; this area should be avoided. Never puncture within the area medial to the midclavicular line.

• The spleen, liver, or diaphragm may be lacerated. To avoid lacerations to these organs, do not allow the needle to penetrate lower than the eighth intercostal space posteriorly. Mark the intended depth of penetration each time with a clamp.

• Hypoxia is very common and is caused by ventilation-perfusion mismatch in the newly expanded lung. To prevent hypoxia, administer oxygen for several hours after the procedure, and evaluate oxygenation with pulse oximetry or by obtaining arterial blood gases.

• Reexpansion pulmonary edema can be minimized by removing no more than one liter of fluid at a time. Remove fluid slowly and stop if the patient develops a cough, dyspnea, or chest pain.

• A catheter fragment may be left in the pleural space. To avoid this possibility, *never* withdraw the catheter through the needle.

• Failure to obtain fluid can occur. For better success, pay close attention to landmarks obtained by auscultation, percussion, and X-ray. Consider ultrasound guidance.

• Infection can occur. To minimize this possibility, use sterile technique and avoid inserting through infected skin.

• Hypovolemia can occur. To reduce the incidence of hypovolemia, remove less than one liter of fluid at a time.

• Pain is associated with thoracentesis. Use adequate local anesthesia.

• Hypoproteinemia is a possibility. To reduce this problem, avoid repeated thoracenteses.

CPT/BILLING CODE

32000   Thoracentesis, puncture of pleural cavity for aspiration, initial or subsequent

BIBLIOGRAPHY

American College of Physicians: Diagnostic thoracentesis and pleural biopsy in pleural effusions, *Ann Intern Med* 103:799, 1985.

American Thoracic Society: Guidelines for thoracentesis and needle biopsy of the pleura, *Am Rev Respir Dis* 140:257, 1989.

Jay SJ: Diagnostic procedures for pleural disease, *Clin Chest Med* 6:33, 1985.

Peterman TA, Speicher CE: Evaluating pleural effusions: a two-stage laboratory approach, *JAMA* 252:1051, 1984.

CHAPTER 62

Pulmonary Function Testing

Edward A. Jackson

Pulmonary function studies are helpful in the diagnosis and management of many medical conditions. Conditions such as asthma, bronchitis, and chronic obstructive pulmonary disease (COPD) can be evaluated, quantified, and documented with pulmonary function testing (PFT). Having PFTs available in the office setting allows longitudinal tracking of pulmonary function, early detection of occupational disease, or early intervention with deterioration of a medical condition. In fact, for screening, PFTs have become so generally used that they are often part of the complete physical examination. However, it should be kept in mind that PFTs support or exclude a diagnosis, but are not definitive in making a diagnosis.

Common clinical measurements of airflow include the volume of air in the lungs after a maximal inspiration (total lung capacity [TLC]), the residual after a maximal expiration (residual volume [RV]), and the volume of gas exhaled when going from TLC to RV (vital capacity [VC]). Using very simple principles and these measurements, pulmonary function testing is most useful when it produces at least a printed and graphic representation of flow and volume versus time with a forced expiration.

INDICATIONS

- For early detection of respiratory defects in asymptomatic individuals: industrial screening and environmental exposures; smokers; patients with a strong family history of pulmonary disease; patients taking medications with possible toxic pulmonary effects (bleomycin, amiodarone)
- For screening of patients with systemic diseases that can involve the lungs, such as rheumatoid arthritis, systemic lupus erythematosus (SLE), or sarcoidosis
- For preoperative evaluation of patients undergoing any major surgery or intervention who have underlying pulmonary disease; or of patients undergoing surgery involving or affecting pulmonary functions, such as major thoracoabdominal surgery, chest radiation therapy, or chemotherapy

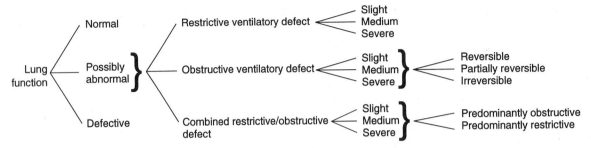

FIG. 62-1.

Differential assessment of airways obstruction and restriction. (From Garbe BR, Chapman TT: *The simple measurement of lung ventilation,* Lenexa, Kan, 1986, Vitalograph. Used with permission.)

- For evaluation of symptomatic adults with persistent cough, wheezes, shortness of breath, chest tightness
- For evaluation of pediatric patients with history of wheezes, chronic cough, cough after exertion/exercise, scoliosis, asthmalike symptoms
- To evaluate or monitor therapy and intervention strategies, such as response to bronchodilators, challenge testing (formal testing with methacholine should be performed in a lab), or response to corticosteroids (check 10 to 14 days after initiation)
- To exclude or support an intrapulmonary versus extrapulmonary diagnosis (Fig. 62-1)
- To monitor patients with known COPD (perhaps annually)
- To assess for disability or impairment

CONTRAINDICATIONS

- Severe debilitation and excessive tiring (patients who cannot expend the required effort for testing)
- Extreme or moderately severe respiratory distress
- Patients not motivated or willing to cooperate

EQUIPMENT

- Pulmonary function testing machine/spirometer
- Comfortable chair and area of office to allow private testing (avoids patient embarrassment)
- Nose clips
- Various inhalants for testing response to bronchodilators

Note: Peak flowmeters are advantageous for patients to use at home but do not provide the documentation needed in office. The PFT machine should meet the American Thoracic Society Standards (Box 62-1). In addition, a helpful checklist is also suggested (Box 62-2).

BOX 62-1. RECOMMENDED SPECIFICATIONS FOR PULMONARY FUNCTION EQUIPMENT

Flow
Accuracy: ±5% or ± 0.1 L/s (whichever is greater)
Response: ±5% to 8 Hz

Volume
Accuracy: ±3% of reading or 30 mL (whichever is greater)
Sensitivity: 20 to 40 mm of chart = 1 L
Response: ±5% to 5 Hz

Time
Discrimination 0.05 s/mm
Timer threshold 50 mL/s

Dynamic calibration
Low inertia
Amplitude response ±5% to 15 Hz

Other considerations
Closed circuit or pneumotachygraph to assess adequacy of inspiratory effort
(Should produce or print the curve)

BOX 62-2. CHECKLIST FOR THE CORRECT CHOICE OF SPIROMETER

1. Simplicity—in operation and maintenance
2. Accuracy—ease of checking and adjusting calibration
3. Test visualization—ideally while the test is in progress
4. Permanent record—of spirometric tracings
5. Robust—and easily transported
6. Hygenic—designed for prevention of cross-contamination
7. Electrical safety—preferable to meet recognized standards
8. Tolerance—of climatic changes

SUPPLIERS

Puritan Bennett
Boston Division
265 Ballardvale St.
Wilmington, MA 01887

Vitalograph
8347 Quivira Rd.
Lenexa, KS 66215

Medical Systems Corp.
One Plaze Rd.
Greenvale, NY 11548

PREPROCEDURE PATIENT EDUCATION

Before performing a PFT, review the patient's respiratory history, including any medications taken for respiratory problems. A clear explanation of the test and what is to be expected is essential to the patient's performance. The PFT has both effort-dependent and effort-independent portions. The best overall result is from a maximal effort. Patients not previously experienced in performing a PFT should take two to three practice attempts until a maximal effort is obtained. Usually the patient should be seated in an upright position to perform the test. An average of three test attempts is usually standard, with reproducibility to within 3% considered to be valid.

A demonstration of the test may be helpful. A few practice maneuvers by the patient may also be helpful. Explain that this test helps to measure lung function and that best results are obtained when the patient takes a deep breath and then blows out as hard and as fast as possible for as long as possible.

Note: Smokers should try to abstain from smoking for 1 hour before testing.

TECHNIQUE

Since the forced vital capacity (FVC) is among the most common of spirometric measurements, the technique of this test is described here.

1. Prepare the equipment. Machine calibration and parameter set-up vary with the spirometer. See the individual instructions pertaining to the particular instrument for this portion of the procedure.
2. The patient should be seated; nose clips are recommended.
3. Have the patient breathe in and out several times with the nose clips in place to become comfortable.
4. Ask the patient to take as deep a breath as possible to completely fill the lungs.
5. Have the patient place the mouthpiece *into* the mouth (rather than "trying to play a flute or trumpet").
6. Have the patient blow out as hard and as fast as possible, for as long as possible (try for at least 6 seconds) (Fig. 62-2). Enthusiastically coach the patient

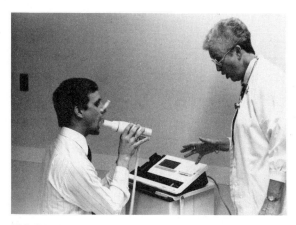

FIG. 62-2.
Patient takes a deep breath, inserts the mouthpiece, and blows out as fast and as hard as possible.

to breathe out "fast, fast, faster" or "breathe, breathe, breathe" until the forced vital curve flattens out (usually 5 to 6 seconds).

7. When the lungs are completely emptied, have the patient breathe in as deeply as possible to obtain the inspiratory parameter and complete the evaluation.

8. Repeat the test three times.

   Note: An FVC is invalid if the patient exhales for less than 6 seconds, if the patient coughs during inspiration or exhalation, or if the patient performs a Valsalva maneuver.

9. If a pre- and postbronchodilator segment of the examination are being performed, after the previous three tests of the prebronchodilator segment, administer a beta-agonist with a bronchodilator via a handheld inhaler.

10. Wait about 20 minutes and then repeat the FVC maneuver as in Steps 1 through 8.

INTERPRETATION

Definitions

1. FVC: Forced vital capacity
2. FEV_1: Forced expiratory volume in the first second
3. $FEV_1\%$: (FEV_1/FVC × 100)
4. FEF_{25-75}: Forced midexpiratory flow or average of forced expiratory flow during the middle half of the FVC (This is the slope of a line drawn from the 25% to 75% point of FCV. Most spirometers calculate this slope automatically and include this value in their printout [Fig. 62-3].)

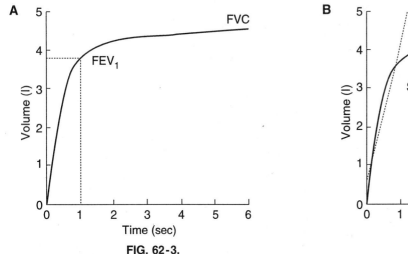 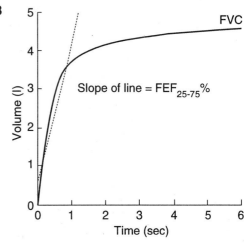

FIG. 62-3.
Volume-time spirometer printouts. **A,** FEV, and FVC measured. **B,** A straight line drawn between the 25% point and the 75% point of the forced expiratory curve. Slope of the line is the FEV_{25-75}.

FLOW-VOLUME LOOPS

- May be useful in conjunction with the volume-time spirogram.
- May help in determining whether an obstruction is in the larger or the smaller airways. Flow-volume loops may only be derived if the spirometer is accurate in displacement and time.
- Usually the most useful information obtained from flow-volume loops is in the expiratory portion of the flow loop (Fig. 62-4).

CRITERIA FOR INTERPRETATION OF PULMONARY FUNCTIONS

Vital Capacity (FVC)

FVC

80% to 120% of predicted value	Normal
70% to 79% of predicted value	Mild reduction
50% to 69% of predicted value	Moderate reduction
<50% of predicted value	Severe reduction

Restrictive lung disease is characterized by reduced vital capacity and relatively normal airflow rates. If obstruction is present (see Flow Rates), the reduction in vital capacity may only be reported as "probably secondary to obstruction" if the severity of the reduced vital capacity and that of the obstructive findings are approximately equal. In comparing vital capacities obtained at different times (including those obtained before and after bronchodilator administration) the importance of the expiratory time must be considered and the raw curves compared.

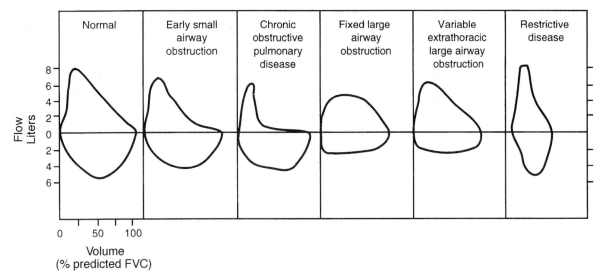

FIG. 62-4.
Characteristic flow-volume curves of restrictive disease and various types of obstructive diseases compared to normal.

Flow Rates

FEV_1 can be plotted as the percentage of vital capacity ($FEV_1/FVC \times 100$)

FEV_1

>75%	Normal
60% to 75%	Mild obstruction
50% to 59%	Moderate obstruction
<49%	Severe obstruction

Note: For patients less than 25 years old, add 5% to these figures; for those more than 60 years old, subtract 5%.

The FEF_{25-75} is currently thought to reflect small airway function. The terminology for the FEF_{25-75} as a percentage of *predicted* FEF_{25-75} will be as follows:

FEF_{25-75}

>79% of predicted value	Normal
60% to 79% of predicted value	Mild obstruction
40% to 59% of predicted value	Moderate obstruction
<40% of predicted value	Severe obstruction

In most cases of *obstructive* lung disease, the percentage of the predicted value of the FEF_{25-75} will be "worse" than the percentage of the predicted value of the FEV_1. However, the modifier used to describe the type of *obstruction* (as mild, moderate, or severe) should be that associated with the value of the FEV_1, not the FEF_{25-75}. The FEF_{25-75} may be separately referred to with such statements as "... particularly affecting small airways, as reflected in the FEF_{25-75}." Should the

FEF_{25-75} *alone* be abnormal, the diagnosis of obstructive lung disease should not be assumed; rather, the reduction should be interpreted as compatible with "early small airways disease." Again, for comparisons over time the raw curves should be examined to determine adequacy of effort.

Therefore, an $FEV_1\%$ less than 75% indicates some degree of loss of elastic recall (e.g., emphysema) or obstructive disease (e.g., asthma), whereas reduced FVC and FEV_1 (but $FEV_1\%$ greater than 75%) indicates restrictive disease, such as that caused by infiltrative parenchymal disease (e.g., sarcoidosis, interstitial fibrosis, silicosis), loss of lung volume (e.g., pneumothorax, pleural effusion), extrathoracic compression (e.g., obesity, ascites, pregnancy); or chest wall disease (e.g., kyphosis, neuromuscular disorders). Suspicion of restrictive disease warrants referral.

ERRORS IN PULMONARY FUNCTION TESTING

Some technical errors and their effects in pulmonary function testing include the following:

- Air leak due to poor fit of noseclip or mouthpiece can result in a wandering baseline, which can lead to underestimation of many spirometric measurements.
- Incomplete expiration may give a falsely low reading of FVC and a spurious increase in $FEF_{25-75\%}$.
- Poor initial expiratory effort may give a falsely low reading of the FEV_1 and $FEF_{25-75\%}$.

CPT/BILLING CODES

94010	Spirometry, including graphic record, total and timed vital capacity, expiratory flow rate measurements
94060	Bronchospasm evaluation; spirometry before and after bronchodilator
94160	Vital capacity screening test: total capacity with timed FEV (duration and peak flow rate must be stated)
94375	Respiratory flow-volume loop
94664	Aerosol or vapor inhalation for sputum mobilization, bronchodilation, or sputum induction for diagnostic purposes; initial demonstration and/or evaluation

BIBLIOGRAPHY

Enright P, Hyatt R: *Office spirometry,* Philadelphia, 1987, Lea & Febiger.

Morris AH et al: *Clinical pulmonary function testing: a manual of uniform laboratory procedures,* ed 2, Salt Lake City, 1984, Intermountain Thoracic Society.

Petty T: Diagnostic procedures for the primary care office: spirometry, *Prim Care Cancer* 13:8, 1993.

Pinkowish MD: Spirometry: who? when? how? *Patient Care:*59, February 1991.

Polagar G, Promadhat V: *Pulmonary function testing in children: techniques and standards,* Philadelphia, 1971, W. B. Saunders.

PART FIVE

Urinary and Male Reproductive

CHAPTER 63

Bladder Catheterization

Robert E. James

James R. Palleschi

Urethral catheterization may be performed for diagnostic or therapeutic indications. Familiarity with the anatomy of the urethra and with the catheters that are available will increase the ease and success of bladder catheterization.

In the male patient with a normal lower urinary tract, there are two points of potential obstruction when passing a urethral catheter: The first is at the point of acute upward angulation between the bulbous and the membranous urethra. The second is at the bladder neck, where a bladder neck stenosis or an enlarged median lobe of the prostate gland may be present (Fig. 63-1).

In the female patient, the angle between the urethra and the bladder neck increases with age. Consequently, in the older patient, the urethra is normally directed toward the sacrum, while in the younger patient it is angled toward the umbilicus. Keeping these urethral angles in mind will improve the physician's technique, thereby reducing the patient's discomfort and facilitating the passage of a urethral catheter.

Catheter size is noted in French (Fr.). As the number increases, the size increases (i.e., a 16 Fr. catheter is larger than a 12 Fr.). One "French unit" is approximately 0.33 mm.

INDICATIONS

- Acute or chronic urinary retention
- Measurement of the residual urine
- Collection of a urine specimen for culture and sensitivity
- Diagnostic studies of the lower urinary tract (voiding cystourethrogram and urodynamics)
- Urinary output monitoring

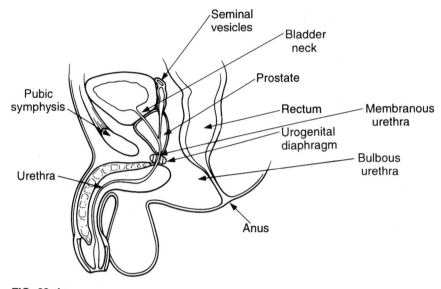

FIG. 63-1.
Urethral anatomy of the male.

CONTRAINDICATIONS

- Known urinary tract obstruction, such as urethral stricture
- Recent reconstructive surgery of the urethra or bladder neck
- A combative or uncooperative patient
- Known or suspected urethral disruption due to pelvic trauma
- Acute infection of the prostate and/or urethra

EQUIPMENT

- Urethral catheter

   Foley catheter. The Foley catheter is a straight urethral catheter with a single port that is used to inflate the retaining balloon (Fig. 63-2). A 16 Fr. to 18 Fr. Foley catheter may be used for adults who require either a temporary or chronic indwelling catheter.

   Coudé catheter. This catheter is similar to a Foley catheter with one exception: The terminal two inches are curved upward (Fig. 63-3). This is used in adult males for whom a Foley catheter cannot be inserted because of an enlarged

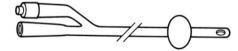

FIG. 63-2.
Foley catheter.

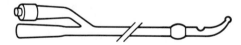

FIG. 63-3.
Coudé catheter.

median lobe of the prostate gland or an elevated bladder neck. Some physicians advocate using a Coudé catheter in all men more than 50 years old. A 16 Fr. to 18 Fr. catheter is normally used.

- Lubricant: Either a water-soluble lubricant (K-Y Jelly) or a lubricant with a local anesthetic (2% lidocaine jelly) may be employed. When available, the latter is preferred; 10 cc is sufficient for female patients and 10 to 20 cc for male patients.
- Sterile towels and gloves
- Antiseptic solution
- Closed urinary drainage system

PREPROCEDURE PATIENT EDUCATION

The specific indications for catheterization and the technique should be reviewed with the patient. Catheter care should be discussed with the patient if it is to remain in place.

TECHNIQUE

1. The female patient is placed in the lithotomy or the supine position with the legs abducted. The male patient is placed in the supine position; the legs may either be abducted slightly or straight.
2. Cleanse the urethral meatus and surrounding area with an antiseptic solution, and isolate the genitalia with sterile drapes or towels.
3. Inject the 2% lidocaine jelly into the urethra and leave it in place for approximately 5 to 10 minutes. Some manufacturers place the anesthetic jelly in a syringe with a smooth conical end that can be inserted into the urethra. Otherwise, draw the anesthetic jelly into a 10 cc syringe. Place the end of the syringe *(without a needle)* gently inside the urethral meatus and inject the lidocaine jelly into the urethra. The male patient should be asked to compress the midurethra between his index finger and thumb to prevent the jelly from leaving the urethra.
4. For an adult patient, select a 16 Fr. or 18 Fr. catheter. A Foley catheter is used for *female* patients. Following the anticipated course of the urethra, pass the catheter 3 inches into the bladder. Once urine is obtained, the balloon may be inflated with 5 cc of normal saline or water. Then gently pull the catheter outward until the balloon is resting against the bladder neck.

   A Foley catheter may be used for *male patients less than 50 years of age.* Pass the catheter into the bladder the full length until the junction of the Foley catheter and inflation port for the balloon is visible (Fig. 63-4).

   Caution: If this is not done, the balloon may be inflated within the urethra. The balloon is normally inflated with 5 cc of normal saline or water. If the balloon does not inflate easily, or if the patient experiences discomfort as the balloon is being inflated, you should

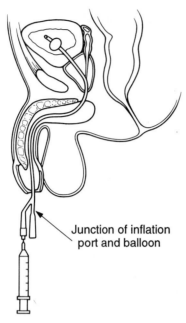

Junction of inflation
port and balloon

FIG. 63-4.
Foley catheter is passed into the bladder until the junction of the catheter and inflation port for the balloon is met.

suspect that the balloon is located within the urethra. In such a case, the balloon should be deflated, and the catheter reinserted.

Once the balloon has been inflated, pull it gently down against the bladder neck.

For male patients over the age of 50, select a Coudé catheter. The curve of the catheter should be directed at the 12 o'clock position. This will permit the catheter to glide over an enlarged median lobe of the prostate gland or an elevated bladder neck. If the catheter does not pass easily, it should be removed and the procedure should be repeated. Occasionally, the tip of the catheter will rotate as it is being inserted. If this occurs, the catheter will not pass through the prostatic urethra into the bladder. If you cannot pass a 16 Fr. Foley or Coudé catheter into the male urethra, there is usually a urethral stricture, bladder neck stenosis, or very large median lobe of the prostate gland. In such a case, you may consider using a 12 Fr. Foley or Coudé catheter. If the smaller catheter does not pass, a urology consultation is advised.

COMPLICATIONS

- Urinary tract infection
- Transient hematuria
- Creation of a false passage resulting from the use of a small catheter, excessive force, or the presence of a urethral stricture
- Urethral stricture

CPT/BILLING CODES

53670	Simple catheterization
53675	Complicated catheterization

BIBLIOGRAPHY

Cancio LC, Sabanegh ES, Thompson IM: Managing the Foley catheter, *Am Fam Physician* 48(5):829, 1993.

Hopkins TB: Urethral catheterization. In Vander Salem TJ, editor: *Atlas of bedside procedures,* Boston, 1979, Little, Brown & Co.

Thuroff JW: Retrograde instrumentation of the urinary tract. In Tanagho EA, Macanich JW, editors: *General urology,* East Norwalk, Conn, 1988, Lange Medical Publications.

CHAPTER 64

Suprapubic Catheter Insertion/Change

Robert E. James

James R. Palleschi

Suprapubic catheters are normally used to provide short-term urinary drainage. If the patient's age or comorbid conditions preclude corrective surgery, the temporary catheter may be left in place or, with the aid of an exchange wire and appropriate dilators, may be replaced with a permanent suprapubic catheter.

INDICATIONS

- Impassable urethral stricture, bladder neck contracture or obstruction
- Inability to pass a urethral catheter over an elevated bladder neck or enlarged median lobe of the prostate gland
- Urethral trauma
- Recent urethral or bladder neck reconstructive surgery
- Inability to tolerate a urethral catheter, and unwilling or unable to perform intermittent self-catheterization
- Bladder drainage required in the presence of a significant urethral or prostate infection

CONTRAINDICATIONS

- Uncooperative patient
- Bleeding disorder or the use of systemic anticoagulants

EQUIPMENT

- Local anesthetic: 10 cc lidocaine 1% to 2%
- 10 cc syringe, 1½-inch 22-gauge spinal needle
- Antiseptic skin preparation
- Sterile towels

- Mask and sterile gloves
- Mounted scalpel blade (No. 11 or No. 15)
- Suture scissors, needle holder, and 2-0 silk suture
- Closed urinary drainage system
- Suprapubic catheter set

  Note: There are many manufacturers of suprapubic catheters, including the following: Bonnano catheter (Becton-Dickinson Corp.), Stamey percutaneous suprapubic catheter set (Cook Urological), and the Simplastic suprapubic catheter (Franklin Medical).

  The principal components of each set are a metal obturator and the suprapubic catheter. The metal obturator is placed down through the suprapubic catheter and is subsequently removed when the catheter is appropriately positioned within the bladder. The end of the catheter may consist of a pigtail tip, malecot, winged-tip, or Foley catheter. These are equally effective in retaining the catheter within the bladder.

PREPROCEDURE PATIENT EDUCATION

Explain to the patient that mild to moderate suprapubic pain may be experienced for a few hours to days following this procedure. As long as the catheter is in place, intermittent hematuria and irritative voiding symptoms may be present. Review catheter care, including the use of a leg bag and overnight drainage bag. Tell the patient to contact the physician if increasing pain, excessive bleeding, temperature greater than 101° F, or a nonfunctioning catheter is noticed. Informed consent should be obtained.

TECHNIQUE

1. Place the patient in the supine position. If the bladder is not palpable, the procedure should be delayed until the bladder can be easily identified or it should be completed with ultrasound guidance.

   Note: If the patient has a bladder or pelvic anatomic abnormality from previous surgery, cancer, or trauma, the procedure should be completed with the aid of ultrasound guidance.

2. Prepare the suprapubic skin with an antiseptic solution, and drape with sterile towels. Inject the local anesthetic into the skin overlying the abdominal wall and dome of the bladder.
3. Make a half-inch lateral skin incision 2 inches above the symphysis pubis in the midline (in both the adult and pediatric patient). At this point, some physicians prefer to pass a 22-gauge spinal needle into the bladder. This will localize the bladder before the suprapubic catheter is inserted. If the bladder is distended, this procedure is not necessary.
4. Once the skin incision has been made, place the metal obturator into the lumen of the suprapubic catheter, with the sharp oblique end of the obturator extending beyond the tip of the catheter (Fig. 64-1). Advance them together through the skin incision at a 60-degree caudal angle toward the

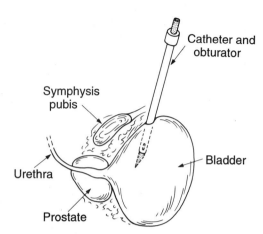

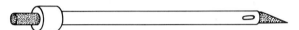

FIG. 64-1.
Suprapubic catheter with obturator in place.

FIG. 64-2.
Insertion and advancement of the catheter and obturator.

bladder neck (approximately the mid-perineal area) (Fig. 64-2). With momentary pressure, advance the catheter through the rectus sheath and muscle, and into the dome of the bladder. This requires inserting it a total of approximately 2 inches below the skin.

5. Advance the catheter and obturator an additional 2 inches to assure appropriate position. Remove the obturator; urine will be seen passing from the suprapubic catheter. After the obturator is removed, the wings of the malecot type of catheter (Stamey suprapubic catheter) will expand, or the pigtail tip of the Bonnano catheter will coil inside the bladder to prevent it from falling out.

6. If the catheter has a balloon tip, once it has been appropriately positioned within the bladder, inflate the balloon with sterile saline.

7. Pull back the catheter until the balloon, coil, or wings are resting against the dome of the bladder.

8. Secure the catheter in place with a silk suture.

9. Using sterile saline, irrigate the catheter to ensure appropriate drainage and position.

10. Connect a drainage bag to the catheter.

COMPLICATIONS

- Perivesicle bleeding
- Gross hematuria
- Intestinal perforation (more likely when the bladder is not distended, when the normal anatomy is distorted by previous surgery or trauma, or when the obturator and catheter are not introduced at the correct angle; normally, a small perforation will seal spontaneously without consequence)

SUPRAPUBIC CATHETER REPLACEMENT

If the catheter has been in place for several weeks and a mature tract is established, the existing catheter may be removed and replaced with a similar catheter. To replace a percutaneous suprapubic catheter, fill the bladder with sterile saline or water, and remove the catheter. The sterile water or saline will begin to pass through the suprapubic catheter site and, consequently, the catheter needs to be replaced promptly. Place an obturator in the new catheter, and advance it down the tract until the sterile water or saline begins to exit through or around the catheter. Usually a local anesthetic is not required.

If the catheter needs to be replaced before the tract is mature, the bladder should be filled with sterile saline or water before removing it. If the catheter is obstructed, it should be removed and another catheter inserted once a distended bladder can be palpated. At that time, a new catheter may be inserted in the same tract, employing the technique described previously. Ultrasound guidance should be used if the bladder cannot be positively identified or palpated.

If an open suprapubic cystotomy has been performed, a mature tract between the skin and the bladder usually is formed within 3 to 4 weeks. If the catheter must be replaced, select a similar-sized catheter. Normally, a catheter guide or obturator is not required. The new catheter should be introduced into the bladder immediately after removing the initial one. After inflating the balloon with 5 to 10 cc of sterile saline, irrigate the bladder to ensure that the catheter is draining properly. Usually, a suprapubic catheter is replaced every 8 to 12 weeks, or whenever it is not draining properly.

CPT/BILLING CODES

51010	Insertion of a percutaneous suprapubic catheter
51705	Changing a suprapubic catheter, simple

BIBLIOGRAPHY

Hagen IK: Instrumental examination of the urinary tract. In Smith DR, editor: *General urology,* East Norwalk, Conn, 1984, Lange Medical Publications.

Hopkins TB: Percutaneous suprapubic cystostomy. In Vander Salem TJ, editor: *Atlas of bedside procedures,* Boston, 1979, Little, Brown & Co.

CHAPTER 65

Suprapubic Taps or Aspirations

Robert E. James

James R. Palleschi

Suprapubic aspiration is a valuable diagnostic procedure, and occasionally, it may even be a valuable therapeutic tool. In most cases, suprapubic aspiration can be performed safely at the bedside or in the physician's office.

INDICATIONS

- Collection of a sterile urine specimen for analysis, culture, and sensitivity
- Temporary relief of acute urinary retention

CONTRAINDICATIONS

- Blood dyscrasia, coagulation disorder, or anticoagulant therapy
- An uncooperative patient

EQUIPMENT

- Local anesthetic: 10 cc lidocaine 1% to 2%
- Needles:
  Anesthetic needle: 1½-inch 25-gauge (The spinal needle can also be used without the stylet.)
  Localization needle: 4-inch 22-gauge spinal needle
  Aspiration needle: In most cases, the localization needle will be sufficiently large to obtain an adequate urine specimen. If not, an 18- or 20-gauge intravenous needle may be used.
- 10 cc syringe
- Microscope slide for direct examination, methylene blue, and Gram stain
- Sterile urine culture collection container

PREPROCEDURE PATIENT EDUCATION

Review the purpose of the procedure and the technique with the patient and family. Following this procedure, the patient may experience pain in the suprapubic area or mild hematuria for 24 to 48 hours. Obtain informed consent.

TECHNIQUE

1. Place the patient on the examination table in the supine position. Examine the suprapubic area by palpation and percussion to identify the distended bladder. If the distended bladder cannot be positively identified, the procedure should be delayed until the bladder can be identified, or the procedure may be performed with ultrasound guidance.
2. Cleanse the suprapubic area with an antiseptic solution and drape in a sterile fashion.
3. In the midline, anesthetize the skin approximately 2 inches above the symphysis pubis (in both the adult and the pediatric patient). Next, aspirate before injecting down to the fascia and bladder. In the adult, usually 10 cc is required to anesthetize the skin, abdominal wall, and abdominal bladder. In a child, the same can be accomplished with 5 to 10 cc of anesthetic.

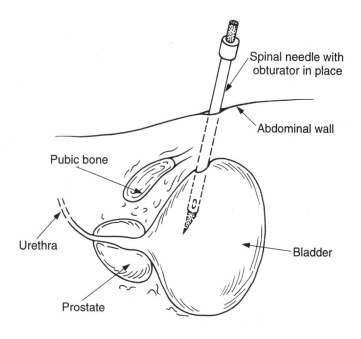

Spinal needle with obturator in place

Abdominal wall

Pubic bone

Urethra

Bladder

Prostate

Midsagital view

FIG. 65-1.
Insertion of the spinal needle with the obturator in place.

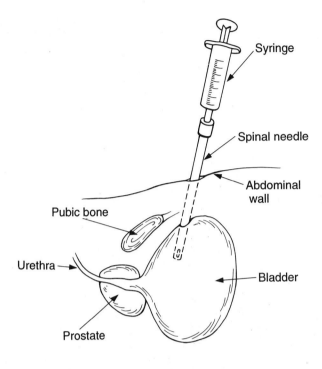

Midsagital view

FIG. 65-2.
Connect the syringe to aspirate urine from the bladder.

4. Direct the 22-gauge spinal needle with the obturator in place (Fig. 65-1) through the anesthetized skin at a 60-degree caudal angle directed toward the bladder neck. If the bladder is distended, after the needle has been advanced approximately 2 inches, it will enter the abdominal bladder.

5. Remove the obturator and connect a sterile syringe (Fig. 65-2) to aspirate urine from the bladder. If urine is not obtained, slowly advance the needle, applying continuous suction on the syringe. If, after advancing the needle an additional 2 inches, the specimen cannot be obtained, terminate the procedure and start once again as outlined above. If you are unsuccessful a second time, the procedure should be delayed until the bladder is further distended, or the procedure should be performed with ultrasound guidance. If continued difficulties are encountered, a urology consultation should be obtained.

COMPLICATIONS

- Transient hematuria
- Perivesicle hematoma
- Intestinal perforation (If this occurs with a 22-gauge needle, it should seal spontaneously and should not be a problem.)

CPT/BILLING CODE

51000   Suprapubic bladder aspiration

BIBLIOGRAPHY

Hagen IK: Instrumental examination of the urinary tract. In Smith DR, editor: *General urology,* East Norwalk, Conn, 1984, Lange Medical Publications.

Hopkins TB: Percutaneous suprapubic cystotomy. In Vander Salem TJ, editor: *Atlas of bedside procedures,* Boston, 1979, Little, Brown & Co.

CHAPTER 66

Basic Urodynamic Studies for Urinary Incontinence

J. Christopher Hough

Urinary incontinence is very common among the growing elderly population: As many as one third of patients over age 60 have experienced urinary incontinence to some degree. This disorder can severely affect the physical health, psychosocial well-being, and health care costs of patients and their caregivers. Unfortunately, the majority of afflicted patients do not seek help, even though about 80% of cases could be cured or greatly improved with proper therapy. This chapter provides primary care clinicians with a basic strategy for the initial assessment and management of urinary incontinence.

The first step in assessing an incontinent patient is to determine whether the incontinence is persistent or is of acute onset. In acute-onset incontinence, the onset has occurred within the last 2 weeks, and if this is the case, all the potentially reversible causes of acute incontinence should be explored and treated; these causes include urinary tract infection, atrophic vaginitis, adverse drug effects, urinary retention, stool impaction, and acute conditions that cause delirium or restricted mobility.

There are four basic types of persistent urinary incontinence: stress, urge, overflow, and functional. The diagnostic evaluation of persistent types of urinary incontinence generally includes a history, physical examination, urinalysis and culture, and a basic assessment of lower urinary tract function. A 1-week voiding diary may also help determine the daily volume and frequency of fluid consumed and voided, and the number of episodes of incontinence.

The assessment of lower urinary tract function may include a pad test to detect stress incontinence, a postvoid residual urine volume determination, and simple cystometry. The assessment can be carried out by a physician, a nurse practitioner, or a physician assistant, and it can be performed in a clinic office, at a patient's bedside in a nursing home or hospital, or even in the patient's own home. For a cooperative, reasonably mobile patient, these tests take 15 to 20 minutes. Although they can be carried out by a single examiner, it is usually helpful to have an assistant available. The procedures are generally well tolerated, and the incidence of symptomatic urinary tract infection following urodynamic testing is less than 5%.

INDICATIONS

- Persistent urinary incontinence of unsure etiology

CONTRAINDICATIONS

- Acute incontinence without therapeutic trial
- Uncooperative patient
- Patient for whom urinary catheterization is contraindicated

EQUIPMENT

- 12 or 14 Fr. straight catheter
- Sterile catheter tray
- 50 cc catheter-tipped syringe (without piston)
- 1 L of sterile water for irrigation
- Fracture pan (*females*) or urinal (*males*)
- Commode (either portable commode or commode adjacent to examination room)
- Small absorbent pads (for stress test)
- 32 oz. graduated cylinder; disposable (plastic)

PREPROCEDURE PATIENT EDUCATION

Explain the entire procedure to the patient. Then, during the procedure, explain each step before proceeding with it.

TECHNIQUE

The simplified tests of lower urinary tract function should be preceded by a focused history and physical examination.

1. *Stress Maneuver.* If possible, start the tests when the patient feels his or her bladder is full. Place a small pad over the urethral area. Ask the patient to cough forcefully three times in the standing position. Leakage of urine coincident with the stress maneuver confirms the diagnosis of stress incontinence. Prolonged loss of urine, leakage occurring 5 to 10 seconds after coughing, or urine loss with provocation indicate that stress incontinence is unlikely.

2. *Normal Voiding.* Prepare the patient for urine specimen collection with antiseptic solution and pads. Ask the patient to void (privately) in his or her usual

fashion into a commode that contains a measuring hat. Signs of voiding difficulty (hesitancy, straining, or intermittent stream) may indicate bladder obstruction or contractility problem. To help quantify volume and timing, an approximate flow rate can be calculated by dividing the amount of urine voided by the approximate time required to pass the urine (the normal rate is 15 to 20 cc/sec).

3. *Postvoid Residual Determination.* Using sterile technique, insert a 14 Fr. straight catheter into the bladder, within 5 to 10 minutes of the patient's voiding. If it is very difficult to pass the catheter, the bladder may be obstructed. If the residual volume is elevated after a normal void (more than 100 cc), bladder obstruction or a contractility problem may be present. For elevated postvoid residual volumes, repeat the test; the initial test result could be due to an isolated instance of nonpathologic urinary retention.

4. *Bladder Filling.* For females, position a fracture pan under the buttocks; for males, have a urinal available to measure any leakage during filling. Attach a 50 cc catheter-tipped syringe (without the piston) to the catheter, and use this as a funnel to fill the bladder. Fill the bladder with room-temperature, sterile water, allowing 50 cc at a time to flow in under the pressure of gravity. Hold the syringe so that it is approximately 15 cm above the pubic symphysis. Bladder pressure should not normally exceed 15 cm of water during filling. Continue until the patient feels the urge to void. Next, use 25 cc increments until the bladder capacity is reached (Fig. 66-1).

   Note: Do not fill the bladder beyond 500 cc.

   When the patient experiences an involuntary contraction or says "I would rush to the toilet now; I can't hold any more," remove the catheter.

   Involuntary contractions (detected by continuous upward movement of the column of fluid, sometimes accompanied by leaking around or expulsion of the catheter) or severe urgency at relatively low bladder volume (e.g., less than 250 to 300 cc) suggests urge incontinence, especially when urge incontinence is consistent with the patient's symptoms.

5. *Repeat Stress Maneuvers.* Ask the patient to cough forcefully three times in the supine position and three times in the standing position (see Step 1). Stress maneuvers with a full bladder are more sensitive for detecting stress incontinence.

6. *Bladder Emptying.* Ask the patient to empty his or her bladder into the commode with the measuring hat (see Step 2). The validity of the calculated postvoid residual may be greater if the patient did not feel full at the beginning of tests. The postvoid residual may be calculated by subtracting the amount voided from the amount instilled.

POSTPROCEDURE PATIENT EDUCATION

Instructions to the patient will be based on the clinical test results and be appropriate to the patient's diagnosis. Ask the patient to report any new dysuria, which may indicate an iatrogenic urinary tract infection.

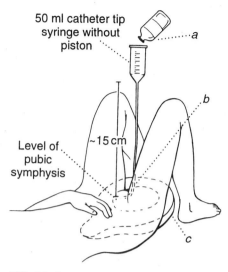

50 ml catheter tip
syringe without
piston

_a_

_b_

~15 cm

Level of
pubic
symphysis

_c_

FIG. 66-1.

Cystometry procedure: _a,_ Assistant pours sterile water in 50 cc increments and holds the syringe erect with the center 15 cm above the pubic symphysis; _b,_ Examiner holds 12 to 14 Fr. catheter in place and pinches the catheter while the water is poured to ensure accurate volume calculation; _c,_ Fracture pan (for females) in the event of involuntary bladder contraction (urinals for males). (Redrawn from Ouslander J, Leach G, Staskin D: Simplified tests of lower urinary tract function in the evaluation of geriatric urinary incontinence, _J Am Geriatr Soc_ 37(8):706, 1989. Used with permission.)

CRITERIA FOR REFERRAL

The history, physical examination, and simplified tests of lower urinary tract function must be used in conjunction with several criteria for referral to develop an appropriate initial management plan. The recommended criteria for referral are outlined in Box 66-1. Marked pelvic prolapse is depicted in Fig. 66-2 and defined

---

BOX 66-1. CRITERIA FOR REFERRAL OF ELDERLY INCONTINENT PATIENTS FOR UROLOGIC, GYNECOLOGIC, OR FORMAL/COMPLEX URODYNAMIC EVALUATION

- History of lower urinary tract or pelvic surgery or irradiation
- Relapse or rapid recurrence of symptomatic urinary tract infection
- Marked pelvic prolapse
- Stress incontinence that has not responded to nonsurgical treatment
- Marked prostatic enlargement or suspicion of prostate cancer
- Severe hesitancy, straining, low flow rate, or interrupted urinary stream
- Difficulty passing a 14 Fr. straight catheter
- Postvoid residual volume greater than 100 cc (test should be repeated before referral)
- Hematuria
- Uncertain diagnosis

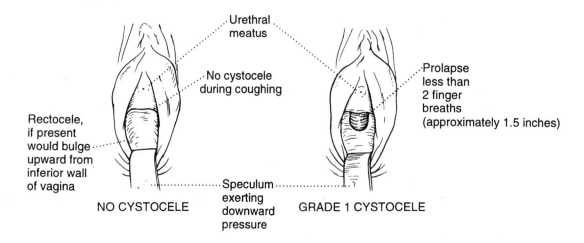

Urethral meatus

No cystocele during coughing

Rectocele, if present would bulge upward from inferior wall of vagina

Speculum exerting downward pressure

NO CYSTOCELE

Prolapse less than 2 finger breaths (approximately 1.5 inches)

GRADE 1 CYSTOCELE

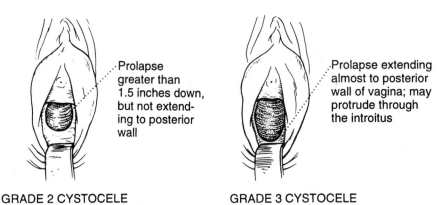

Prolapse greater than 1.5 inches down, but not extending to posterior wall

GRADE 2 CYSTOCELE

Prolapse extending almost to posterior wall of vagina; may protrude through the introitus

GRADE 3 CYSTOCELE

FIG. 66-2.

Example of clinical grading system for cystoceles. A Grade 2 cystocele extends beyond one third of the height of the vaginal introitus and is best detected by having the patient strain in the standing position. (Redrawn from Ouslander J, Leach G, Staskin D: Simplified tests of lower urinary tract function in the evaluation of geriatric urinary incontinence, *J Am Geriatr Soc* 37(8):706, 1989. Used with permission.)

as a Grade 3 cystocele. It should be recognized that Grade 1 and Grade 2 cystoceles are nonspecific findings in elderly women and may or may not be related to symptoms of incontinence. All women with stress incontinence warrant a trial of conservative therapy. For properly selected patients (with or without pelvic prolapse) who do not respond to conservative and/or medical therapy, surgical treatment of stress incontinence may be very effective. The decision about whether to undertake such surgery in an elderly woman must be individualized, and the patient's symptoms, physical findings, overall health, and personal preference must be taken into account.

The initial treatment of patients with urge, stress, and mixed incontinence generally involves behavioral and/or pharmacologic interventions. Detailed discussions of these therapeutic modalities can be found in other sources.

CPT/BILLING CODES

51725	Simple cystometrogram (CMG), e.g., spinal manometer or as discussed above with the use of a 50 cc syringe; this is to be differentiated from the complex cystometrogram using calibrated electronic equipment
51736	Simple uroflowmetry (UFR), e.g., stop-watch flow rate, mechanical uroflowmeter
51795	Voiding pressure studies (VP); bladder voiding pressure, and technique

When multiple procedures are performed in the same investigative session, either modifier −51 or code 09951 are employed. All procedure codes above imply that procedures were performed by or under the direct supervision of a physician and includes supplies.

BIBLIOGRAPHY

Burton JR et al: Behavioral training for urinary incontinence in elderly patients, *J Am Geriatr Soc* 36:693, 1988.

Ouslander JG: Geriatric urinary incontinence, *Clin Geriatr Med* 2:4, 1986.

Ouslander JG, Leach GE, Staskin DR: Simplified tests of lower urinary tract function in the evaluation of geriatric urinary incontinence, *J Am Geriatr Soc* 37:706, 1989.

Ouslander JG, Sier HC: Drug therapy for geriatric incontinence, *Clin Geriatr Med* 2:789, 1986.

Pfenninger JL, Fowler GC, James RE: Selected disorders of the genitourinary system. In Taylor RB, editor: *Family medicine: principles and practice,* ed 4, New York, 1994, Springer-Verlag.

CHAPTER 67

Androscopy

John L. Pfenninger

Androscopy is an office procedure that examines the male genitalia under magnification after acetic acid application to identify condyloma.

Recent literature documents the close association of the human papillomavirus (HPV) with cervical dysplasia and cervical cancer. Whether the virus *alone* leads to cancer is unknown. It is likely, however, that HPV is the necessary cause (if not the single sufficient cause) for cervical cancer. Human papillomavirus is very contagious, and it is most readily spread through sexual contact; it may be transmitted in yet unknown ways in a minority of cases.

The clinical significance of condyloma and HPV in men is uncertain, but men act as carriers and may transmit the disease to sexual partners.

There are over 70 types of HPV. Eight to ten of these characteristically infect the genital areas. Condyloma acuminata, the visible lesions that we commonly see, are caused by noncarcinogenic strains such as types 6 and 11. The subclinical types identified by magnification after acetic acid staining are more likely to cause neoplastic changes; frequently these are types 16 and 18.

There is no evidence that treatment of male partners of women who have dysplasia lessens the likelihood of persistence or recurrence in the female. Wearing a condom has little benefit since the virus is generally a regional disease. In men, it is present on the penis, scrotum, perineum, and perianal areas. In women, it is present on the cervix, the vagina, the vulva, and the perineal and perianal areas.

Some clinicians question the value of carrying out an androscopic examination. Identification and treatment of condyloma is not the only reason to perform androscopy. Patient education is a valuable aspect of this procedure. The male must be informed of the significance of his disease and the necessity of maintaining a single-partner committed relationship. It is no longer a matter of moral or religious persuasion, but rather a good health practice to be monogamous (as is exercising, not smoking, eating low-fat foods, and so forth).

Although it is rare, the human papillomavirus is associated with penile cancer. Differentiating mild, moderate, and severe dysplasia of the penis (penile intraepithelial neoplasia [PIN]) is nearly impossible without obtaining biopsy samples. It is known that anorectal cancer in homosexual men frequently contains the human papillomavirus.

INDICATIONS

- Visible condyloma on the penis, scrotum, or anus (Staining and examination with magnification will identify smaller lesions that are easier to treat. Early treatment may reduce recurrence of clinically obvious acuminate lesions, although there are no studies to document this.)
- Partner with recurrent or persistent condyloma acuminata or cervical dysplasia (There is some evidence that if the male presents a high viral load, the immune system response of the partner may be overwhelmed by the virus. High viral load exists if the male has visible acuminate lesions or a diffuse acetowhite staining of the penis.)
- Psychological reassurance
- Chronic perineal or perianal irritation
- Recurrent condyloma
- Medical/legal examinations in child abuse cases
- History of other sexually transmitted diseases
- Necessity for patient education (Doing the procedure is better received by the patient than "just talking." A biopsy-proven diagnosis speaks a thousand words of reinforcement.)

EQUIPMENT

- Spray bottle with 5% acetic acid (white vinegar); or 200 cc of 5% acetic acid and four 4 × 4 inch gauze pads (or a roll of 3-inch gauze)
- Colposcope (or possibly a high-quality handheld magnifying lens)
- High-quality fine-tissue scissors
- Pickups with teeth
- Formalin jars
- Monsel's solution
- 3 cc lidocaine 1% or 2% *without* epinephrine
- 30-gauge needle
- 1 to 5 cc syringe (depending on size and number of lesions)

PREPROCEDURE PATIENT EDUCATION

It is always best if the patient is well informed of the nature of the disease prior to the procedure. Provide the patient with an educational handout (Box 67-1). Encourage the patient to watch a 30-minute videotape that discusses the implications of HPV infection in men and women prior to the visit. (The videotape is available from Creative Health Communications, 809 Elm St., Essexville, MI 48732;

**BOX 67-1. PATIENT EDUCATION HANDOUT
ANDROSCOPY**

Androscopy is a procedure for examining the male genitals in a very detailed and thorough fashion, using a special microscope (the colposcope). Androscopy is done to identify *genital warts*. The medical term for these warts is *condyloma acuminata*. They are caused by the *human papillomavirus (HPV)*. These lesions are very contagious and are passed readily by sexual intercourse. There is an 80% chance of getting warts with just one sexual contact with an infected person. Genital warts may occasionally be spread without sex, but this is very rare. Warts may lay dormant or inactive for up to 20 years after infection before they become visible or cause a problem.

Long-term effects on males are not totally certain, but there is a possibility that genital warts may cause penile and rectal cancer. It has been proven that HPV infection is the primary cause of cervical cancer in females. If there is evidence of infection in the female, which is often picked up on a Pap smear, then the male sexual partner may need to be examined. Although it is not always necessary, *both* partners may need to be treated. It is almost impossible to totally "cure" a person of the infection. The cervix can be treated and cancer can be prevented 97% of the time, but it is difficult to completely eradicate the virus from the penis, vagina, and rectal areas. The goal of the procedure is to try to remove any visible warts and to make the virus go inactive.

Symptoms that indicate that treatment is necessary include visible warts (lesions), itching, or a large number of lesions seen on staining. Even with treatment, the warts frequently return and the infected male must assume he is contagious for the rest of his life.

Although many warty type lesions are visible to the naked eye, many others are too small to be seen and require examination with great magnification to identify or confirm their warty nature. Vinegar, sprayed on the penis, causes the warty tissues to turn whiter than the surrounding skin, making it easier to identify and examine. Men can have the virus and look totally normal before staining and examination.

Men who are infected are advised to be *monogamous* so as not to spread the disease further. *Condoms* make sex safer but not totally safe. Previous sexual partners should be advised to get their Pap smears regularly and possibly have a colposcopic examination since the *Pap smear is known to miss 25% of lesions.* You have the legal liability to tell any future partners that you have the warts.

Women who smoke have twice the risk of cervical cancer. EVEN IF YOU SMOKE your partner's risk for cervical cancer increases. It is recommended that you *stop smoking.*

Description of the Procedure

The procedure takes approximately 20 minutes. You will be asked to undress from the waist down and will be draped appropriately. You will lie on the examination table with your feet in stirrups. The penis and entire genital area will be soaked with vinegar for at least 5 minutes.

You will first be examined to detect any readily visible lesions, then the colposcope (a special microscope) will be used to confirm the nature of the lesions.

Once warty lesions have been identified, they may be biopsied to confirm their diagnosis. Larger lesions may be treated by excision, strong acid, cryocautery (freezing), or laser vaporization. All these methods are quite simple, and no time off work (other than for the office visit) is necessary. A cream called Efudex or a solution called Condylox can also be used to treat warts. You will receive a special handout if these are used.

You may need to have *follow-up* examinations to assure that there are no other recurrent or new lesions. Times for these re-checks will vary depending on the treatment used. Your physician will advise you.

Videotapes that discuss the above information in more detail are available for your viewing at home. Ask your physician for details. It often helps to review the tapes *before* your examination.

telephone 800-462-2492.) Viewing the videotape will help the patient focus on questions that he or his partner may have, and it will allow the practitioner to avoid repetitious explanations of the same counseling information. No preoperative medication is needed for the procedure, and the patient can be reassured that there will be minimal discomfort, even if biopsies are obtained.

TECHNIQUE

1. Place the patient on an examination table with stirrups, and position as a female is positioned for a Pap smear. Conduct a visual inspection and note any lesions.
2. Spray the entire perineal area with 5% acetic acid (white vinegar) and allow to soak for 5 minutes. Alternatively, the entire penis and scrotum can be wrapped with a 3-inch gauze or several 4 × 4s that are liberally soaked with acetic acid. Allow the solution to run freely over the perineum and anus.
3. Remove the gauze if used. Inspect the entire anogenital area under magnification. Generally a colposcope is used on low power (×3 to ×7). There is no study comparing good handheld magnification with colposcopic evaluation.
4. Grossly apparent warts that were previously seen will turn white with the acetic acid. Previously unseen "flat" or subclinical lesions will also now be identifiable on the penis, scrotum, perineum, or rectum. They will show up as white areas known as acetowhite changes.
5. Take a biopsy sample of any atypical lesions with an unusual vascular pattern (mosaicism or punctation; see Chapter 81, The Colposcopic Examination) or pigmentation. The pigmentation of worrisome lesions will look different from that of a freckle or nevus; it will be a nondiscrete, brownish discoloration. If no atypical lesions are seen, biopsy one or two of the acuminate lesions or the acetowhite areas to document the presence of HPV. It is very convincing to have the pathology report confirm your clinical diagnosis, which is thereby reinforced to the patient.
6. A penile biopsy specimen is easily obtained using sharp tissue scissors. If only one or two small lesions are to be sampled, simply tent up the skin by pinching it at its base. Looking through the colposcope, obtain a 1 to 2 mm sample with the sharp tissue scissors. No anesthetic is required, and this method is often less painful than an injection. Only a very superficial sampling is needed. If the lesions are larger, or more than two samples are to be obtained, it is best to premedicate with 1% to 2% lidocaine *without* epinephrine. Using a 30-gauge needle minimizes any discomfort.
7. If lesions are numerous, diffuse, or large, they may need to be removed with radiofrequency surgery, 85% trichloroacetic acid, cryosurgery, Efudex, or excisional therapy. A dorsal penile nerve block may facilitate this removal.
8. Monsel's solution may be needed as an astringent to limit postoperative bleeding.
9. Treatment of only punctate acetowhite changes on the penis, acetowhite changes of the scrotum, and mild perianal acetowhite changes is unnecessary and of little benefit, although biopsies will confirm HPV.

10. Unless the patient has had significant excision of his warts, he can return to full activity with no modification of his daily routine.

POSTPROCEDURE CARE

No definite recommendations can be made regarding treatment of dysplastic lesions on the penis since studies of long-term follow-up have not been conducted. Five to ten percent of the lesions biopsied will come back with a report of mild or moderate bowenoid dysplastic change. Rarely, a severe dysplasia will be found. (Unlike dysplastic cervical lesions in females, it is difficult to predict the degree of dysplastic change observed on examination with magnification in males.) In such situations, ask the patient to return for reexamination to confirm that the entire lesion was removed. The patient should report any unusual growths or ulcerations at once. Advise him to discuss his HPV history with the physician during future examinations. Sexual partners should be examined.

COMPLICATIONS

There are essentially no complications. There may be minimal scarring or bleeding. The penile skin is very thin, and the biopsy should be kept very superficial. Condyloma acuminata can be confused with other lesions such as condyloma lata, molluscum contagiosum (commonly seen), keratoses, bowenoid dysplasia, and other nondescript papular lesions.

CPT/BILLING CODE

There presently is no CPT code for androscopy. Use 55899, unlisted procedure, male genital system (documentation suggested).

54100   Biopsy, penis, cutaneous

BIBLIOGRAPHY

Barrasso R, DeBrux J, Croissant O: High prevalence of papilloma virus: associated penile intraepithelial neoplasia in sexual partners of women with cervical intraepithelial neoplasia, *N Engl J Med* 317:916, 1987.

Brinton LA et al: Risk factors of penile cancer: results from a case-control study in China, *Int J Cancer* 47:504, 1991.

Burmer GC, True LD, Krieger JN: Squamous cell carcinoma of the scrotum associated with human papillomavirus, *J Urol* 149:374, 1993.

Epperson WJ: Androscopy for anogenital HPV, *JFP* 332:143, 1991.

Krebs HB: Management of human papilloma virus: associated genital lesions in men, *Obstet Gynecol* 73:312, 1989.

Krebs HB, Helmkamp F: Does the treatment of genital condylomata in men decrease the treatment failure rate of cervical dysplasia in the female sexual partner? *Obstet Gynecol* 76:660, 1990.

Palefsky JM et al: Detection of human papillomavirus DNA in anal intraepithelial neoplasia and anal cancer, *Cancer Res* 51:1014, 1991.

Patton D, Rodney WM: Androscopy of unproven benefit, *JFP* 332:135, 1991.

Pfenninger JL: Androscopy: technique for examining men for condyloma, *JFP* 29(3):286, 1989.

Pfenninger JL: Letter to the editor, *JFP* 33(6):566, 1991.

Rando RF: Human papilloma virus: implications for clinical medicine, *Ann Int Med* 108:628, 1988.

Rosenberg SK: Sexually transmitted papilloma viral infections: IV, the white scrotum, *J Urol* 33(6):462, 1989.

Von Krogh G: Clinical relevance and evaluation of genitoanal papilloma virus infection in the male, *Seminars in Dermatology* 11(3):229, 1992.

Zabbo A, Stein BS: Penile intraepithelial neoplasia in patients examined for exposure to human papillomavirus, *J Urol* 41(1):24, 1993.

CHAPTER 68

Vasectomy

George C. Denniston

John L. Pfenninger

Vasectomy is a safe, inexpensive, permanent form of contraception. Unlike tubal ligation for females, vasectomy is usually performed in an office setting, is associated with fewer and less severe complications, and is considerably less expensive. There is no reported mortality from vasectomy, while in the United States, approximately 10 women die annually from complications of tubal ligation. Although both procedures have similar low failure rates, failure of vasectomy can be detected easily when men bring in their postprocedural semen specimens.

In the chain of events that leads to vasectomy, the key person is usually not the surgeon; rather it is the person who helps the man make the decision to have a vasectomy. Therefore, it is important that all doctors, nurses, and others who wish to help men come to a decision about vasectomy be knowledgeable and give factual statements about vasectomy (Box 68-1).

INDICATIONS

Vasectomy is appropriate for a man who does not wish to have children—or to have any more children—but who wishes to continue having sexual intercourse.

CONTRAINDICATIONS

- Local infection
- Coagulation disorders
- Inability to palpate and elevate both vasa
- Marked stress from a recent event, such as divorce or financial setback (*relative contraindication*)
- Lack of adequate informed consent

BOX 68-1. PATIENT EDUCATION HANDOUT
VASECTOMY

Every man has a basic right to a vasectomy, a valuable medical procedure. Before you actually have a vasectomy, you should think about it carefully, because a vasectomy is designed to be permanent. *Vasectomy is a small procedure, but a large decision.* When children are definitely not wanted in the future, vasectomy relieves the man and woman from fear of pregnancy. In today's world, it is important for men to have a responsible role in birth control.

Vasectomy simply blocks the travel of sperm to the penis. Vasectomy prevents the sperm from getting out of the man's body. It does not cause voice changes, hair loss, impotence, or loss of sexual desire. Male hormones are *not* affected by vasectomy, and they continue to circulate normally.

How is the procedure performed? Usually the doctor gives an injection of local anesthetic into the skin of the scrotum (the sac holding the testicles). This may feel like a brief pinch. The anesthetic numbs the area. The doctor then makes one or two small, half-inch openings, gently pulls up each tube (vas deferens), cuts it, and burns or ties it shut. The procedure takes about 30 minutes to complete.

What is the "no-scalpel" method of doing vasectomy? The *no-scalpel technique* is a method developed by Dr. Li, a Chinese physician. The doctor uses a special instrument instead of a scalpel to enter the scrotum. This instrument has a sharp point and spreads the skin instead of cutting it. This makes a smaller opening, and may cause less bleeding and less postprocedural pain.

When can I go back to work? You should have a day or two of rest after the vasectomy. You should avoid heavy lifting or other strenuous activity for at least one week.

Is there much pain after vasectomy? No. You may experience a few days of mild discomfort, like a pulling or aching feeling in the groin. This discomfort can usually be relieved with ibuprofen (Advil or Nuprin) and good support with tight underwear. Some bruising may occur, but this is perfectly normal. A very small number of men have more serious side effects, such as significant bleeding, infection, or painful sperm leakage (sperm granuloma).

Will my sex life be affected? That depends: If a couple has been worried about pregnancy, their sex life could improve, especially as they come to trust the vasectomy. The procedure does not change anything, except that there will no longer be sperm in the semen. Sex, orgasm, and ejaculation are not affected. However, if you do *not* want a vasectomy and are having one because you think you should, or because your partner wants you to, then you may note some resentment. If you have been worried about other facets of your sex life before the procedure, chances are that a vasectomy will not improve those other conditions.

When can I have sex again? You should wait one week until some healing has taken place. *Use another form of birth control until your semen has been examined and no sperm is present.*

When is the vasectomy effective? It is effective when the semen has been tested and has been found to be free of sperm. A sperm count is usually done 6 weeks after the procedure, and after at least 15 ejaculations.

What happens if my vasectomy is not successful? In the rare cases where the sperm can still get through, a repeat vasectomy may be required.

Continued.

BOX 68-1.—cont'd

When I have an orgasm, will I still ejaculate? Yes. The sperm are produced by the testicles, and they make up only 5% of the semen (the fluid that is produced with ejaculation). The other 95% of semen is produced by other glands that continue to function normally. Unless the semen is placed under a microscope, it is impossible to tell whether or not sperm are present.

What happens to sperm after a vasectomy? The sperm continue to be produced by the testicles, but their passage to the penis is blocked. Therefore, the sperm cells break down in the body and their component parts are recycled. This process is normal and it occurs in men who have not had a vasectomy.

What are the complications? In a few cases, a small blood vessel may continue to bleed inside the scrotum, causing *bruising* or even a larger accumulation of blood. *Infection* in the scrotum may also occur. *Pain* after a vasectomy is generally quite minimal; on a scale of 1 to 10, it is rated a 3. *Failure* rates vary between 1 per 200 and 1 per 1500 vasectomies. Recently there have been some concerns that having a vasectomy may increase the chances of getting *prostate cancer.* After careful review of all the data, several major organizations, including the American Cancer Society and the National Institute of Health, have concluded that there should be no change in vasectomy recommendations. Similarly, there do not appear to be any increased risks of any other diseases.

Is vasectomy reversible? Vasectomy should always be considered permanent, so do not undergo a vasectomy if you feel there is any chance you will change your mind. Forty to fifty percent of the reversal operations are unsuccessful.

What are the other options for contraception? There are many other temporary and reversible options for contraception: condoms, spermicides, diaphragm, IUD, Norplant, contraceptive sponge, and birth control pills.

Is vasectomy anything like castration? No. *Castration* means removal of the testicles. Vasectomy does not touch the testicles and does not reduce the production of male sex hormones.

Are there men who should not have vasectomies? Perhaps. Some examples are men who feel masculine only when they can cause a pregnancy; men or partners who change their minds a lot; men who may get divorced and then marry someone else who wants children; men who think they might want children later. We will consider performing a vasectomy for any man who has seriously thought about the implications of his decision and who feels quite sure he has had all the children he will ever want. This applies equally to men who are single, married, divorced, widowed, childless, or with families, regardless of age.

Why do you offer only local anesthetic? There are certain well-established health risks associated with general anesthesia. Because vasectomy is such a simple and quick procedure, we feel that it is unwise to subject our patients to these unnecessary risks. While some doctors use general anesthesia, the vast majority of vasectomies in the United States are performed using local anesthesia.

Do you need the consent of my partner? Only your written consent is required, although it is wise for you to discuss this decision with your partner. Her consent is not required by law. However, we prefer to have her present during counseling, if possible.

Continued.

BOX 68-1.—cont'd

What can I expect after vasectomy? After the procedure, you will need to remain in the office for a short time, and when you leave, you should take it easy for the rest of the day. It is a good idea to take another day or two off work. You may shower the next day. For adequate support, you should wear tight cotton briefs or an athletic supporter for the next two weeks. Some men get bruising that can be quite extensive. This is quite harmless and is caused by leakage of blood under the skin. It fades slowly. Some men ache about six hours after the procedure. Others may begin to ache about five days after the procedure. If swelling or pain persists, or if the incision looks infected, call your physician. If you can let the area heal for seven days before having an ejaculation, you are more likely to have a successful result.

What should I do to prepare for the day of surgery?

* Do not take any aspirin for 2 weeks before surgery. You may use acetaminophen (Tylenol).
* Clip the hair in front of the scrotum with a scissors. A razor can cut the skin and lead to infection.
* Shower before coming into the office. Wash well with soap and water.
* Take 3 or 4 ibuprofen 200 mg tablets (Advil or Nuprin) 2 hours before surgery.
* Bring in your jock strap or tight, snug-fitting underwear to the office with you.

PREPROCEDURE PATIENT EDUCATION

Fully informed consent can be obtained and confirmed by providing the patient with a vasectomy fact sheet (Box 68-1), and then by having him answer several true-false questions *in writing* (Box 68-2). Questions answered incorrectly should be discussed, and the patient should correct the answer and initial it. Finally, he should sign the questionnaire and the formal consent form (Box 68-3). This is an improvement over other methods of obtaining informed consent for vasectomy. It ensures adequate knowledge by the patient, and it offers better legal protection to the physician. It is wise to include the wife or partner, if any, in the consent process; however, a man has a right to vasectomy even in the absence of spousal consent.

Authors' note: The standard consent form has been changed to a request for vasectomy. Men are not consenting to vasectomy, they are *requesting* that it be done. This puts more of the decision-making responsibility on the patient.

Our policy has always been to operate on any man who is fully informed and is certain that he wants a vasectomy. We make it clear that it is his decision. This is almost always appreciated. It also makes it more difficult for him to say, "You should never have permitted me to have a vasectomy." If he is young and without children, these factors should be considered; however, these are not grounds to discriminate against him. Nevertheless, the doctor still retains responsibility to try to prevent him from making a decision for a procedure that he will later regret.

Boxes 68-1 to 68-4 review the material necessary to achieve fully informed consent. The preprocedure counseling visit can be documented using the encounter form in Box 68-5, which reviews the patient's pertinent history, physical and

Text continued on p. 528.

BOX 68-2. VASECTOMY QUESTIONNAIRE

After you have read the vasectomy fact sheet, please answer the following questions. It is simply to confirm that you understand the procedure. If you answer some of the questions incorrectly, the counselor or the doctor will discuss them with you.

Please circle the correct answer. Correct answers to these questions confirm that you understand the basic facts about vasectomy.

1. Vasectomy keeps the sperm from getting out.	F	T
2. Most vasectomies are done using local anesthetic.	F	T
3. After vasectomy, men are still fertile for some time.	F	T
4. After vasectomy, the amount of fluid ejaculated is about the same as before the procedure.	F	T
5. A complication can occasionally occur after a vasectomy.	F	T
6. Vasectomy is very different from castration.	F	T
7. Vasectomy should be considered permanent.	F	T

_____   _____
Signature   Date

[The correct answer to all questions is True.]

BOX 68-3. VASECTOMY REQUEST FORM

I, _____ , the undersigned, request Doctor _____ and the doctor's assistants to perform a vasectomy on me.

It has been explained to me that this operation is intended to result in sterility. I understand that a sterile person is not capable of becoming a parent. I also understand that the operation may not result in sterility and that no guarantee of sterility has been given to me.

I have been told that the operation has possible complications, the most common of which are infection, pain, hematoma (bleeding and bruising), sperm granuloma (a reaction to sperm in the scrotum), reuniting of the channels (failure), and reaction to the local anesthetic.

I voluntarily request the operation, and I understand that if it proves successful, the results will be permanent, and if they are, it will be impossible for me to father children.

I have been advised that, because of the supply of sperm in the reservoir beyond the vasectomy site, I will remain fertile after the procedure until this reservoir is empty. I have been advised to bring a semen sample after at least 15 ejaculations and that a sperm count will be performed on it; if necessary, repeat counts may be advised.

I have read this entire statement and agree to its terms and conditions. I understand the risks, the benefits, the procedure itself, and the alternatives to this operation. I have been given a chance to have all my questions answered.

_____   _____
Patient   Date

_____   _____
Wife, partner [optional]   Witness

BOX 68-4. PATIENT INSTRUCTIONS AFTER VASECTOMY

Keep the incision(s) dry until the next day; then you may shower. Keep clean gauze over the area for three days.

Some **bruising, drainage,** and **swelling** are not unusual. The scrotum and penis may turn "black and blue." The edges of the incision may pull apart, and may heal rather slowly. A **"knot" may be present** on each side for several months. This is part of the normal healing process.

Please return directly to your home, and **take it easy** for at least 12 hours. Put your feet up. An **ice bag** on the scrotum may help to prevent swelling. **The day after surgery,** you may walk and shower. You may increase your activity on the third day, but vigorous exercise (jogging, basketball, etc.) is not advised.

If you have discomfort, one or two acetaminophen (Tylenol) tablets taken every 4 to 6 hours, or up to three 200 mg ibuprofen tablets every 6 hours, usually will provide relief.

Wear **tight underwear or an athletic supporter** for increased support and comfort during the next week.

No heavy lifting or very strenuous activity for 10 days.

If there is **bleeding or severe pain,** or if you develop a **fever,** call us immediately.

It is recommended that you refrain from having sexual intercourse and ejaculation for one week. This is to permit the cut ends of the vas deferens to close before pressure is put on them.

Do not be surprised if your ejaculate contains some blood. It is usually old blood, and nothing to worry about.

You will not be sterile for some time after the operation because the reservoirs may still contain live sperm. **Continue to use another method of birth control** until you have had a sperm count, and have received a statement that sperm are no longer present in the semen.

At 6 weeks or 15 ejaculations (whichever is later), bring in a semen specimen to the doctor's office or to the lab as directed. Collect it in a clean, small jar, medicine vial, or in a container the doctor provides. To collect the semen, have intercourse and withdraw prior to ejaculation, or stimulate yourself. Take the specimen to the doctor's office within two hours of collection. A second specimen is often recommended three months after surgery.

If you have any concerns about any possible complications or any other questions, please call at once for advice.

Remember: Use another form of contraception until you have had your semen check(s) and your doctor gives the okay that you do not need to use other contraception.

BOX 68-5. VASECTOMY ENCOUNTER FORM

PATIENT TO FILL OUT

Date _____

Referring physician _____

Phone (H) _____ (W) _____

Name _____

Wife's name _____

Age _____

Age _____

Education _____

Education _____

Occupation _____

Occupation _____

Marriage: 1st, 2nd, 3rd

Marriage: 1st, 2nd, 3rd

    years _____

    years _____

What is the quality of your marriage? _____

Any marital problems? _____

How is sexual functioning? _____

Any sexual problems? _____

Children's ages and sex _____

Religion _____

Do you have religious conflict with vasectomy?   Yes No

Current contraceptive _____

Are you or your wife experiencing any problems with this? _____

Considered tubal? _____ Other temporary methods?_____

Why do you want a vasectomy? _____

How long have you been thinking about limiting your family size? _____

Patient's health?   Good   Poor
Wife's health?   Good   Poor

Is there any genetic disease in the family?   Yes   No

    If YES, please explain _____

Are you concerned about anything in particular in regards to the vasectomy? If so, describe: _____

_____

Continued.

BOX 68-5. VASECTOMY ENCOUNTER FORM—cont'd

How well do you tolerate pain?   Well   OK   Poorly

Do you have a tendency to faint?   Yes   No

Past medical history

Epididymitis?	Y	N	Do you have bleeding tendencies?	Y	N
Lumps in the testicles?	Y	N	Do you take aspirin?	Y	N
Hernia/surgery?	Y	N	Do you take any regular medications?	Y	N
Trauma in the groin?	Y	N	Have any major illness?	Y	N
VD, prostatitis, urine infection?	Y	N	Psychological counseling?	Y	N

Allergies to medications: _____

Have you read and understood the handouts explaining vasectomy?   Y   N

PHYSICIAN TO FILL OUT

Physical exam

Hernia?   _____ Yes   _____ No
Testicles?   _____ Normal   _____ Abnormal
Vas-palpable bilaterally? _____ Yes   _____ No
Urethral discharge?   _____ Yes   _____ No
Scrotal contents?   varicocele   R L   spermatocele R L
Skin

Counseling

Anatomy and physiology   Impression: _____
Technique   _____
Effect on patient
Complications   Plan: _____
Vasovasostomy/sperm banking   _____
Patient preparation
Permits
Cost
Follow-up regimen/postoperative care
Diagram handout given to patient _____ Yes _____ No   _____
                                                              Physician Signature

POST OP

Date surgery performed _____

	RESULT	DATE	INITIALS	PT. NOTIFIED
Semen check #1	_____	_____	_____	_____
Semen check #2	_____	_____	_____	_____

PROBLEMS (see dictated note)		DATE		
I.		_____	_____	_____
II.		_____	_____	_____
III.		_____	_____	_____

counseling points, and documents the follow-up semen specimen checks. Box 68-6 is a checklist of the counseling material reviewed with the patient. The original sheet is for the patient, and a copy is placed in the chart. For a more detailed description of the preprocedural counseling visit, see Pfenninger (1984).

Many legal authorities now recognize the educational value of patient education videotapes. The patient can review the material several times in the privacy of his home. A vasectomy counseling videotape by Thomas J. Zuber, M.D., is available from Creative Health Communications (517-892-7614 or 800-462-2492).

EQUIPMENT

- Electrocautery unit and handpiece, with a fine-needle electrode (The unit should be set at the lowest level that quickly cauterizes small "bleeders.")

  Authors' note: Based on Schmidt's findings, a disposable battery-powered cautery unit may be the instrument of choice for optimal sealing of the vas ends; however, it may not be the best choice for achieving hemostasis.

- 3 hemostats (small)
- Scalpel handle with a No. 15 blade or the no-scalpel dissecting vas forceps (Fig. 68-1, *A*)
- Adson tissue forceps (1 × 2 teeth)
- Tissue scissors
- Needle holder
- 4-0 chromic catgut suture on an atraumatic needle
- 10 cc syringe (1.5-inch 27-gauge or smaller bore needle)
- 1% lidocaine *without* epinephrine (10 cc)
- Sterile sodium bicarbonate solution for less pain during anesthetic infiltration. (Just before injection of the anesthetic, draw up 1 cc of sodium bicarbonate and then 10 cc of the lidocaine.)
- Vas clamps for isolating vas

  Authors' note: The Soonawala vasectomy forceps were developed by Dr. Soonawala of Bombay, India. If these are not available, they can easily be made by filing off both sides of a baby Allis forceps until only three teeth are left: one tooth on one side, and two teeth on the other (1 × 2 teeth). Otherwise use sharp or blunted towel clips as an alternative, or a 5 mm no-scalpel vasectomy clamp.

- 4 × 4 inch gauze (large pack)
- Povidone-iodine or Hibiclens prep
- Fenestrated sterile drape and nonfenestrated drape
- Sterile gloves and mask
- Single sterile glove (into which the cautery unit is placed)
- Pair of nonsterile gloves for prep
- Specimen jar

Alternative equipment includes the following:

- Small hemoclips with clip applicator for closing vas sheath

BOX 68-6. PATIENT EDUCATION WORKSHEET
VASECTOMY

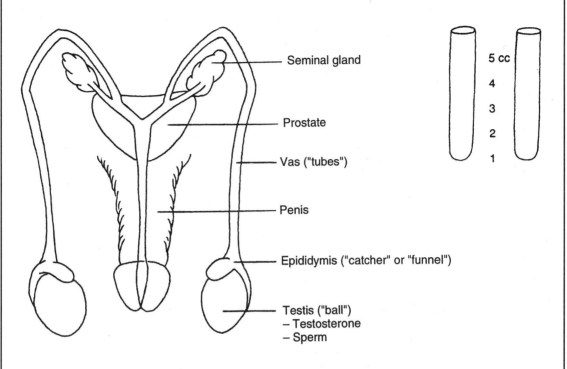

Seminal gland

Prostate

Vas ("tubes")

Penis

Epididymis ("catcher" or "funnel")

Testis ("ball")
– Testosterone
– Sperm

5 cc
4
3
2
1

1. **Anatomy and Procedure**
   - Lidocaine
   - Clamp around vas
   - Insert forceps
   - Remove 1/4 inch
   - Cauterize
   - Tissue wall separating ends

2. **Complications**
   - Pain
   - Bleeding
   - Infection
   - Granuloma
   - Long-term
   - Failure

3. **Prep-Day of Surgery**
   - No aspirin for 10 days
   - Clip hair
   - Shower after clip
   - Take 4 ibuprofen
   - Sign permit if not already done
   - Jock strap or bikini underwear

4. **After Surgery**
   - Day of: home, feet up, ice, jock
   - Day 2: walk, shower, jock
   - Day 3: whatever is comfortable

5. **Sex**
   - Week 1—1x at end of week
   - Week 2—2x
   - Thereafter, as desired

6. **Follow-up Specimens**
   - Six weeks (after 15 ejaculations) and three months
   - Call the office. Be sure I'm in.
   - No need for appointment, just drop off specimen.

7. **Costs**
   - Counseling
   - Procedure
   - Semen checks
   - Follow-up problems for 1 year

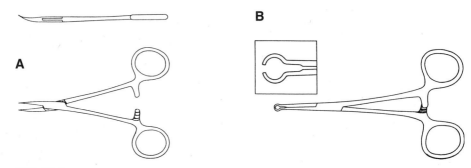

FIG. 68-1.
No-scalpel vasectomy instruments. **A,** The dissecting forceps; **B,** Percutaneous vas clamp. (From Li S et al: *J Urol* 145:341, 1991. © 1991 American Urological Association, Inc. Used with permission.)

- No-scalpel percutaneous vas clamp (5 mm) (Fig. 68-1, *B*) or sharp towel clips to isolate vas

TECHNIQUE

There are many techniques for performing vasectomy. Some use one incision in the midline, while others recommend two separate incisions. The no-scalpel technique from China is only a method of entering the scrotum and isolating the vas. Once that is accomplished, any number of occlusion techniques may be used. Some surgeons merely incise the vas and cauterize both ends. Others resect 1 to 2 cm of vas and cauterize. Ligation of the vas has been generally replaced by cautery of the ends or end and interposing a layer of fascia between the two ends. The fascia can be closed over with chromic suture or with hemoclips. The latter are quicker and avoid the bleeding one occasionally has when placing suture. (For a discussion of various techniques, see Lipschultz.)

The open-ended technique is described here, using electrocautery only on the prostatic end of the cut vas, and chromic catgut suture to close the fascia over that end. It differs from other techniques in that the testicular end of the vas is left open. The open-ended technique was first recommended and used more than 50 years ago. Recently, its merits have been documented by Errey and Edwards. It minimizes the problem of back pressure on the testicle and the associated long-term pain in the occasional patient (congestive epididymitis). Symptomatic sperm granulomas may be reduced. The incidence of vasectomy failure is not increased if the cauterized end is properly covered with surrounding fascia. Finally, dilation of the proximal vas (testicular end) does not occur, making surgical reanastomosis, if desired, easier. Some vasectomists prefer this technique for men less than 40 years old because they may be more likely to request reversal. Many surgeons still routinely cauterize both resected ends.

1. Have the patient lie down and cover his scrotum with a warm, hot water bottle wrapped in a plastic bag or with gauze that has soaked in warm water. After sufficient relaxation is obtained (the key to an easy vasectomy), clip any remaining excess scrotal hair that has not already been removed. Non-

sterile gloves are recommended for the prep. A warm disinfectant scrub is used to complete the prep. Cover the area with sterile surgical drapes.

2. Isolate the left vas between the fingers high in the scrotum, and bring to the surface. The vas has the diameter of a ballpoint pen refill. Roll it gently upwards until it is immediately beneath the skin. With sufficient relaxation, the vas and surrounding skin may be lifted above the scrotum, then held from beneath with two fingers, the vas forming an arc. Alternatively, use *three-point fixation* to secure the vas. Using the middle finger of the left hand (if right-handed), press up from beneath the scrotum. On top of the scrotum, hold the vas between the thumb and index finger (Fig. 68-2).

3. Anesthetize the skin and vas. Use 0.5 to 1 cc of lidocaine to infiltrate subcutaneously along the midline. The small volume will help prevent anesthetic distortion over the site of entry. Execute a bilateral high perivasal block (Fig. 68-3). Enter the skin from the midline and inject 3 to 5 cc around the vas on the left in several areas. Let the vas fall back, then grasp the right vas. Redirect the needle to the right vas and inject another 3 to 5 cc.

4. In the open-ended technique (Fig. 68-4), use one of the types of vas clamps suggested to anchor the vas (Fig. 68-4, *A*). Make a quarter-inch skin incision (Fig. 68-4, *B*). Enlarge the incision with a hemostat.

Authors' note: The more experienced vasectomist will generally make one midline entry and resect each vas through the same site. For those less experienced, it is easier to

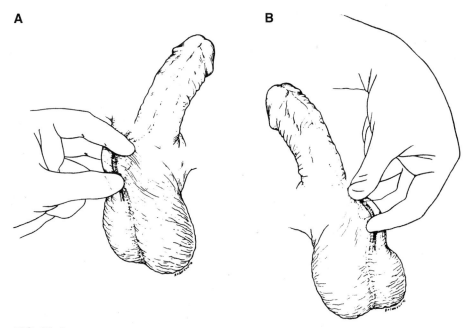

A   **B**

FIG. 68-2.
Three point fixation of the vas beneath the skin. **A,** Right side; **B,** Left side. Proper immobolization of the vas is a crucial factor in ease of performing a vasectomy. For single entry, isolate the vas beneath the midline raphe. (From Li S et al: *J Urol* 145:341, 1991. © 1991 American Urological Association, Inc. Used with permission.)

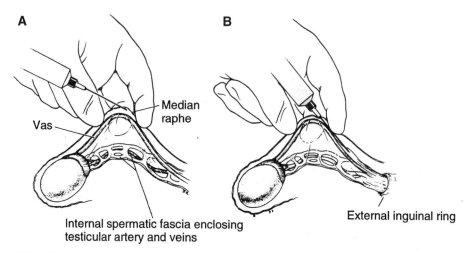

A

Vas

Median raphe

Internal spermatic fascia enclosing testicular artery and veins

B

External inguinal ring

FIG. 68-3.
Technique of perivas nerve block. **A,** Skin wheal with anesthetic is placed over the midline raphe. **B,** The 1½-inch needle tracks along the vas towards the inguinal area. Anesthetic is injected around the vas at the base of the scrotum. (From Li S et al: *J Urol* 145:341, 1991. © 1991 American Urological Association, Inc. Used with permission.)

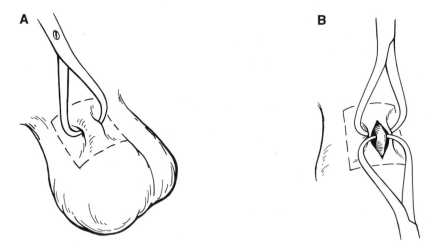

A

B

FIG. 68-4.
Sequence of vasectomy using the traditional technique. **A,** Isolate the vas with a clamp (sharp towel clip) and make an incision over the right vas (two incision technique). **B,** Grasp the vas through the incision with a second vas clamp. **C,** Insert hemostats beneath the vas and strip away the perivas fascia. **D,** Apply downward pressure to isolate the vas. **E,** Secure the vas with hemostats on the perivas fascia and make an incision. **F,** Partially transect the vas, then cauterize one or both ends. Complete the incision after cautery. If a partial excision of the vas is to be done, partially transect the vas in two areas 1 cm apart. Cauterize one or both ends. **G,** Complete the excision and place the vas section in formalin. **H,** Fascial interposition is carried out using 3-0 or 4-0 chromic suture and creating a "purse-string" effect similar to the technique of inverting an appendical stump. **I,** Alternatively, a hemoclip can be applied to close the fascial sheath.

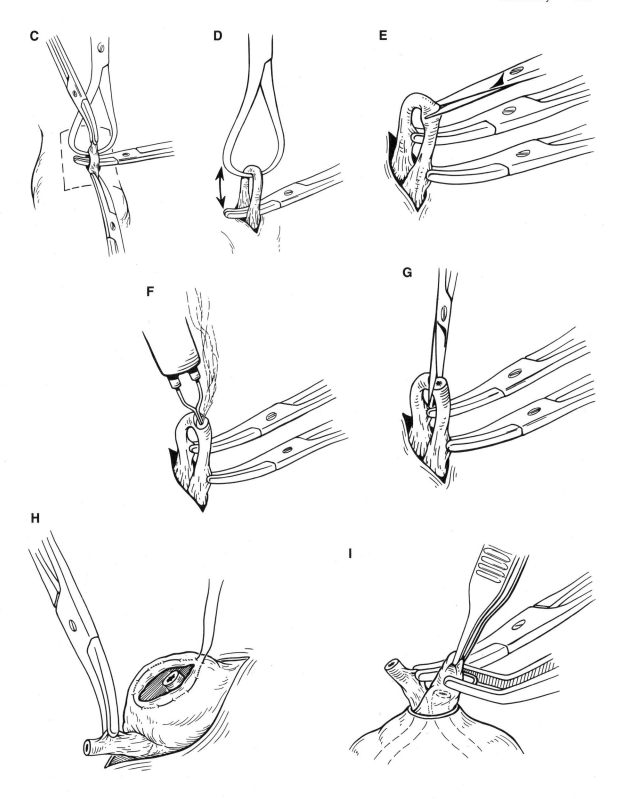

make two entries, over each isolated vas. In this case, additional lidocaine will be needed to anesthetize the skin over the entry sites.

Grasp the vas through the incision with a Soonawala forceps or towel clip. Make certain that the forceps surround the vas. Cut down through the peri-vas fascia with a scalpel to the vas and strip away any adherent fascia (Fig. 68-4, *C*). Use a hemostat to create a small loop of vas. Using a twisting motion, push a hemostat through the tissue in the loop and apply downward pressure to "strip" the tissue off the vas (Fig. 68-4, *D*). Apply hemostats to the fascial tissue of the isolated vas as a safety measure (Fig. 68-4, *E*). Incise the vas, leaving the prostatic end of the vas short (Fig. 68-4, *G*). (Small pieces of vas may be removed and preserved in formalin, but as soon as the physician can identify the vas in vivo with certainty, this may no longer be necessary.)

5. Cauterize the prostatic end(s) of the vas by inserting the cautery tip 5 mm into the lumen, activating the cautery unit, and then quickly withdrawing the tip (Fig. 68-4, *F*). The objective is to create a graduated burn, minimal at the upper portion, and maximal at the cut tip so that fibroblasts can close the vas somewhere in between. If too much burning is done, the entire tip may slough.

6. With 4-0 chromic, create a "purse-string closure" using three suture points in a triangle and draw the fascia over the prostatic end of the vas, being careful to prevent the open testicular end from falling back into the sheath (Fig. 68-4, *H*). After hemostasis is assured, drop the vas back into the scrotum.

7. Identify the *right vas*. (If a second incision is made, provide additional anesthesia of the skin.) Isolate the right vas. Confirm that it is the right vas by tugging gently to move the right testicle. The procedure carried out on the left side is now carried out on the right.

8. A single 4-0 chromic catgut or vicryl suture may be needed to close the skin; although generally, small incisions can be left open.

9. Place several 4 × 4 inch gauze pads over the incision to provide a compression dressing. This may be held in place with an athletic supporter or tight underwear.

10. Give the patient appropriate instructions for care, provide him with two containers for semen samples, and caution him to use alternative birth control until his semen checks are negative.

11. Discharge the patient after it is determined he understands the instructions on postprocedure care and follow-up.

The No-Scalpel Technique

The no-scalpel vasectomy technique is merely a method for delivering the vas from the scrotum. The specifics of occlusion are left up to the operator. Developed in China by Dr. Li Shun-Quiang, it has been used on more than 800,000 men. In trained hands, there are few complications, and the procedure is faster. The name of this technique desensitizes the patient and makes the procedure less psychologically adversive. In addition, studies suggest there is less pain, bleeding, and infection with the no-scalpel technique (Fig. 68-5).

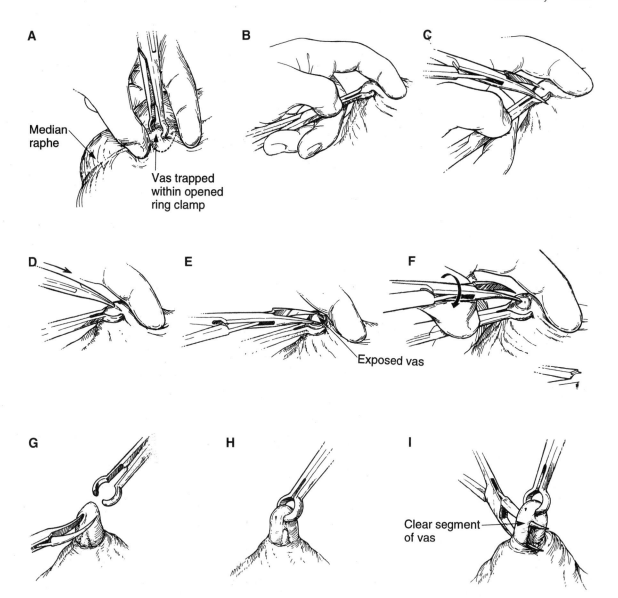

FIG. 68-5.

The no-scalpel vasectomy technique. **A,** Percutaneous isolation of the vas with a special vas clamp. If single incision technique is used, grasp the vas over the midline raphe. **B,** Stretch the skin to thin out the area over the vas. **C,** The vas dissecting forceps are opened and one jaw is pierced through the skin into the vas lumen. **D,** and **E,** Dissecting forceps are closed and inserted *down to the vas,* then opened to spread the perivas tissue. This frees the vas. It is essential to have all the perivas tissue freed up to facilitate the next step. **F,** Open the dissecting forceps again and paritally penetrate the vas as if on a skewer. Rotate the forceps 180 degrees, maintaining upward pressure. **G** and **H,** Release the vas clamp and reapply it, clamping directly through the vas. **I,** Strip away the perivas fascia for 1 to 1.5 cm, creating a free loop. At this point, proceed as with conventional vasectomy using any of a variety of occlusion techniques. (From Stockton MD, Davis LE, Bolton KM: *Am Fam Physician* 46(4):1153, 1992. Used with permission.)

After anesthetizing the area, grasp the vas through the skin with the special vas clamp, and tent it up. Use the dissecting forceps (similar to a hemostat sharpened to a point) to pierce the skin and deliver the vas. Once the vas is out, any of various means can be used to complete the vasectomy.

CAUTERY INSTRUMENT STERILITY

It is difficult to maintain sterility of the reusable cautery instrument. The method shown in Fig. 68-6 can be used for an electrical unit with handpiece or a battery unit.

COMPLICATIONS

- Swelling and discomfort are routinely prevented by using an ice pack and mild analgesic.
- Ecchymosis makes the scrotum look bad, but is harmless. Careful cautery of the skin margins of the incision usually prevents it.
- Hematoma, a major concern, may be prevented through good hemostasis.
- Infection is always a risk, but is prevented by careful sterile technique. Prophylactic antibiotics are generally not indicated.
- Sperm granuloma is only a problem if symptomatic; the risk of symptomatic sperm granuloma is not increased if the open-ended technique is used.
- Vasectomy failure is a rare occurence (less than 1%). Stress the importance of returning for semen specimen testing to the patient.
- Uncommon complications: _Neuroma_ is characterized by exquisite sensitivity at the vasectomy site and can be definitively treated by a single injection of procaine. _Congestive epididymitis_ may occur weeks to months after the procedure, and is associated with the occlusion of the testicular end of the vas. It may cause _chronic testicular pain_ in vasectomized men. Leaving the testicular end of the vas open decreases the incidence of this complication.
- Chronic diseases: In large, long-term studies of vasectomized men, no increase in incidence of chronic disease has been found, including, among other diseases studied, hypertension, diabetes, autoimmune diseases, and cardiovascular diseases. The possibility of a slight increase in prostate cancer has been proposed; however, the data suggest only a weak association, if any, and no change in current practices have been recommended by any of the major associations.

REVERSAL

Many men request vasectomy reversal because a new partner wishes to have children. With fully informed consent, the true regret rates are extremely low, and patient and partner satisfaction with the procedure are extremely high. Rosenfeld

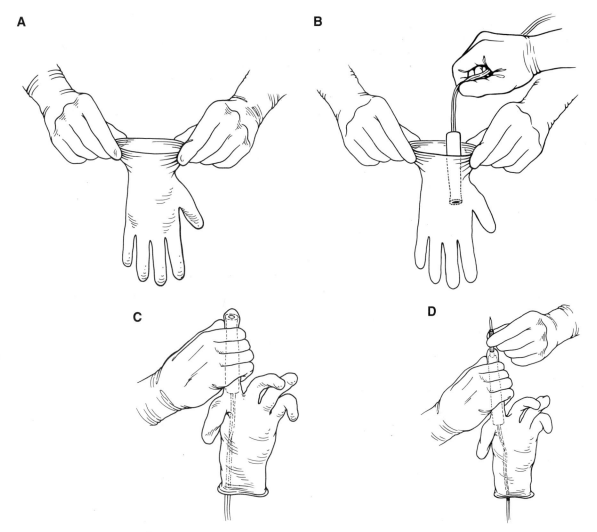

FIG. 68-6.
Maintaining sterile cautery instrument. **A,** Gloved physician holds the sterile glove. **B,** Assistant holds the cautery unit without the tip by wire and carefully drops into finger of glove. **C,** Gloved physician grasps finger that is protecting the cautery handle inside and keeping it sterile. **D,** Sterile tip is punctured through rubber glove. The unit can now be handled in a sterile fashion being careful not to contaminate the surgical field with the wire. (If it is a battery unit without wire, activate the unit and the tip will burn through the glove and be exposed for use.)

showed it is the only contraceptive method with which 100% of women are satisfied. With tubal ligation, the method with next highest acceptance rate, only 78% of women are satisfied.

POSTPROCEDURE CARE

No routine postprocedure examination is necessary. For the physician who is just beginning to perform vasectomy procedures, it may be advisable to see the patients in 1 to 2 weeks to gain an appreciation for the normal postprocedure changes.

It is customary to obtain two postprocedure semen checks: the first after 6 weeks (or 15 ejaculations, whichever is later) and the second in 3 months. This method will detect essentially all failures. If recanalization occurs, it generally takes place in the early postprocedure period. Some define a positive specimen as any visualized sperm under high power (unspun specimen). Others claim that only live sperm are significant. It may be prudent to document at least one completely sperm-free sample. The seminal vesicles are sperm repositories; therefore if the specimen is obtained too soon after vasectomy, sperm may be seen in the ejaculate even though the procedure was successful.

Edwards recently reported that testing can be done 4 weeks after vasectomy, regardless of the number of postvasectomy ejaculations. As long as the examination was done within 12 hours of collection, the specimen was read as negative if no motile sperm were seen. Repeat tests were recommended only if motile sperm were seen. Whether this study becomes the accepted standard is uncertain.

If a true surgical failure is suspected on the basis of semen analysis, it may be advisable to have the patient produce a specimen in the office before proceeding with repeat vasectomy.

RESOURCES

Videotapes for patient education:
Creative Health Communications, Inc.
809 Elm St.
Essexville, MI 48732
517-892-7614; 800-462-2492

Association for Voluntary Surgical Contraception
799 Madison Ave.
New York, NY 10016
212-561-8000

Written patient education handouts:
Association for Voluntary Surgical Contraception (see above)

Procter & Gamble Pharmaceuticals
Norwich, NY 13815-0231

Technique videotapes for physicians:
  Health Sciences Center for Educational Resources
  Contact: Dr. George Denniston
  University of Washington
  T252 Health Sciences Center
  Seattle, WA 98195

  Association for Voluntary Surgical Contraception (see above)

  Network for Continuing Medical Education (NCME)
  1111 Secaucus Road
  Secaucus, NJ 07094

No-scalpel instrument suppliers:
  Zinnanti Surgical Instruments
  21540-B Prairie St.
  Chatsworth, CA 91311
  800-223-4740

  Advanced Meditech International
  86-20 53rd Ave.
  Suite One
  Flushing, NY 11373
  718-672-7150; Fax: 718-672-8501

Hemoclips and clip applicators:
  Weck
  11311 Concept Blvd.
  Largo, FL 34643
  800-237-0169

  Ethicon, Inc.
  P.O. Box 151
  Somerville, NJ 08876-0151
  800-438-4426

Battery operated cautery:
  Ellman
  1135 Railroad Ave.
  Hewlett, NY 11537
  800-835-5355

BIBLIOGRAPHY

Alderman PM: Complications in a series of 1224 vasectomies, *JFP* 33:576, 1991.
Denniston GC: The effect of vasectomy on childless men, *J Reproductive Med* 21(3):151, 1978.

Denniston GC: Vasectomy by electrocautery: outcomes in a series of 2,500 patients, *JFP* 21(I):35, 1985.

Der Simonian R et al: Vasectomy and prostate cancer risk: methodological review of the evidence, *J Clin Epidemiol* 46(2):163, 1993.

Edwards IS: Early testing after vasectomy, based on the absence of motile sperm, *Fertil Steril* 59(2):431, 1993.

Errey BB, Edwards IS: Open-ended vasectomy: an assessment, *Fertil Steril* 45:843, 1986.

Giovannucci E et al: A long-term study of mortality in men who have undergone vasectomy, *N Engl J Med* 326(1):1392, 1992.

Giovannucci E et al: A prospective cohort study of vasectomy and prostate cancer in U.S. men, *JAMA* 269:873, 1993.

Giovannucci E et al: A retrospective cohort study of vasectomy and prostate cancer in U.S. men, *JAMA* 269:878, 1993.

Greenberg MJ: Vasectomy technique, *Am Fam Physician* 39(1):131, 1989.

Guess HA: Is vasectomy a risk factor for prostate cancer? *Eur J Cancer* 29A(7):1055, 1993.

Howards SS, Peterson HB: Vasectomy and prostate cancer—chance bias, or a casual relationship, *JAMA* 269:913, 1993.

Kendrick JS et al: Complications of vasectomy in the United States, *JFP* 25:245, 1987.

Li PS et al: External spermatic sheath injection for vasal nerve block, *J Urol* 39(2):173, 1992.

Li PS et al: The no-scalpel vasectomy, *J Urol* 145:341, 1991.

Lipshultz LI, Benson GS: Vasectomy 1980, *Urol Clin North Am* 7:89, 1980.

McKay W, Morris R, Mushlin P: Sodium bicarbonate attenuates pain on skin infiltration with lidocaine, with or without epinephrine, *Anesth Analg* 66:572, 1987.

Pfenninger JL: Complications of vasectomy, *Am Fam Physician* 30(5):111, 1984.

Pfenninger JL: Preparation for vasectomy, *Am Fam Physician* 30(4):177, 1984.

Raspa RF: Complications of vasectomy, *Am Fam Physician* 48(7):1264, 1993.

Rosenfeld JA et al: Women's satisfaction with birth control, *JFP* 36(2):169, 1993.

Schmidt SS: Prevention of failure in vasectomy, *J Urol* 109:296, 1973.

Schmidt SS: Vasectomy: principles and comments, *JFP* 33:571, 1991.

Schmidt SS: The vas after vasectomy: comparison of cauterization methods, *Urol* 40(5):468, 1992.

Stockton MD, Davis LE, Bolton KM: No-scalpel vasectomy: a technique for family physicians, *Am Fam Physician* 46(4):1153, 1992.

Vasectomy: procedures for your practice, *Patient Care:*116, October 1991.

CHAPTER 69

Prostate Massage

Robert E. James

James R. Palleschi

Prostate massage has been used therapeutically and diagnostically in the management of recurrent or chronic prostatitis and prostatodynia. At this time, its primary benefit is in establishing the diagnosis of chronic prostatitis.

INDICATIONS

- Diagnosis of chronic or subacute prostatitis
- In the management of prostatosis and prostatodynia *infrequently*

CONTRAINDICATIONS

- Acute prostatitis
- Prostatic abscess
- Significant difficulty voiding

EQUIPMENT

- Examination glove and water-soluble lubricant
- Microscope slide
- Sterile culture container

PREPROCEDURE PATIENT EDUCATION

Tell the patient that he may have an urge to urinate and may feel rectal pressure for 15 to 60 minutes after prostatic massage. Tell the patient to contact the physician or the nearest emergency room if he experiences chills, myalgia, rigors, or temperature above 101° F.

TECHNIQUE

1. Place the patient in a comfortable position for the prostate examination. A variety of positions may be employed: the knee/chest position, left lateral decubitus position, or bent over the examination table. (With this position, the patient should place his elbows on the examining table and spread his heels apart. The patient is thus immobilized, which facilitates the prostate examination and the subsequent massage.) In addition, the patient may assist you in collecting the expressed prostatic fluid by holding the microscope slide below the glans penis.

2. Apply a generous amount of lubricant to the anus and to your gloved index finger. The examination will be more comfortable for the patient if he performs a mild Valsalva maneuver as the finger passes through the anus. In patients with a high-riding prostate, a Valsalva maneuver may bring the gland down to the examining finger.

3. For the prostate massage, press the pad of your index finger into the substance of the prostate. Start on the superior and lateral aspect of the prostate. Move your index finger laterally to medially, from the base or superior aspect of the prostate gland to the inferior portion or apex (Fig. 69-1). This motion is carried out several times bilaterally. Last, massage the median furrow, or midaspect, of the prostate gland, from the base to the apex. The prostatic secretions will be massaged toward the prostatic urethra. These secretions will

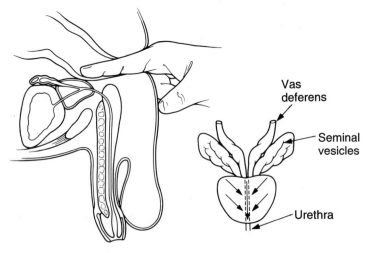

FIG. 69-1.
Technique of prostatic massage. The glandular substance is compressed from its lateral edges to the urethra, which lies in the center. (Drawing at right shows direction of pressure.) The seminal vesicles are then stripped from above downward.

then pass through the distal urethra, and can be collected for microscopic examination and culture and sensitivity if desired. Normally, you will need to repeat the prostatic massage for a period of 30 to 90 seconds before any secretions are obtained. The quantity collected may vary from a few drops to 2 to 3 cc. Some patients will not discharge any secretions (despite correct performance of the prostate massage as described) or may have discomfort sufficient to abort the procedure. Clinically, more than 15 white blood cells per high-power field would suggest an infectious process.

COMPLICATIONS

- Rarely, bacteremia or urosepsis may occur after a prostate massage. This can be avoided by not performing prostate massage on a patient suspected of having acute prostatitis or a prostate abscess.
- Occasionally, a patient with significant prostatism secondary to prostatic hypertrophy may develop sufficient prostate edema following a massage to produce temporary difficulty urinating or urinary retention.
- Hematuria and hematospermia occur infrequently after a prostate massage.

CPT/BILLING CODE

87205   Prostatic smear

There is no CPT code for prostate massage.

BIBLIOGRAPHY

Tanagho EA: Physical examinations of the genitourinary tract. In Tanagho EA, Macaninch JW, editors: *General urology,* East Norwalk, Conn, 1988, Lange Medical Publications.

CHAPTER 70

Adult Circumcision

Donald E. DeWitt

Adult circumcision is a procedure about which little is written, even in the urological literature. It is often performed for reasons that are not purely medical, yet it also has clearly defined medical indications. Some patients have their own nonmedical reasons.

General anesthesia may occasionally be necessary, but usually local anesthesia is sufficient in the outpatient setting, including the properly equipped office. Informed consent should be obtained after a thorough discussion with the patient (and partner, if appropriate), during which the indications, the procedure, the postprocedure care, and the potential complications are explained. This should be done for all patients, and it should always be documented. This serves as a record of the authenticity of the complaint of the *patient,* and is important because individual physicians may vary in their judgments of the need for surgery. The physician must make sure that the patient's reasons for requesting circumcision are medically sound and that his expectations of the results are realistic.

INDICATIONS

- Phimosis (tightness of the foreskin so that it cannot be drawn back from over the glans); possibly related to complaints of pain with erections and intercourse
- Paraphimosis (retraction of a narrow inflamed foreskin which cannot be replaced)
- Penile hygiene; recurrent balinitis (inflammation of the glans penis)
- Posthitis (inflammation of the prepuce) not relieved by medical treatment
- Preputial neoplasms
- Excessive foreskin redundancy
- Frenular tears

CONTRAINDICATIONS

- Active inflammation in the genital area
- Infection in the genital area

- Psychiatric disorder or history (*relative contraindication:* Carefully screen these patients.)
- Bleeding dyscrasias (handle appropriately)
- History of penile surgery, significant trauma, or unusual-appearing or ambiguous genitalia (Patient should be referred to a specialist.)

EQUIPMENT

- 10 cc syringe with a 1-inch 27-gauge needle and a half-inch 30-gauge needle
- Prep bowl with a dozen 4 × 4 inch gauze sponges
- Iodine solution or other antiseptic for scrub
- Ring forceps
- 4 sterile towels
- 1 fenestrated drape
- 6-inch segment of half-inch Penrose drain
- 6 straight mosquito forceps
- 1 large straight forceps
- 1 curved Mayo scissors
- 1 suture scissors
- 5-inch needle holder
- 1 Brown-Adson thumb forceps
- 1 medium-size straight Metzenbaum scissors
- 4-0 plain and 4-0 chromic gut suture on FS-2 needle
- Xeroform gauze
- 1-inch Kling bandage
- 1 malleable 4- to 6-inch silver probe

PATIENT PREPARATION

If the patient has preprocedural anxiety, a preprocedural dose of an oral, sublingual, intramuscular, or intravenous anxiolytic (such as diazepam) may be administered. If this is used, there must be someone who can drive the patient home after the procedure.

The patient should be supine and comfortable. Shave the area around the base of the penis, *preferably* with surgical clippers. Surgically prep the entire genitalia, scrotum, and pubic area with an appropriate antiseptic solution. Use a fenestrated drape.

ANESTHESIA

1. Using a 10 cc syringe filled with 1% lidocaine *without* epinephrine and a 1-inch 27-gauge needle, inject 0.5 to 1 cc subcutaneously over the dorsal vein so that the wheal is raised at the junction of the penis and the pubis (Fig. 70-1).

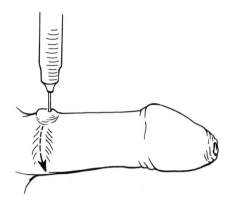

FIG. 70-1.
Site of initial injection over dorsal vein.

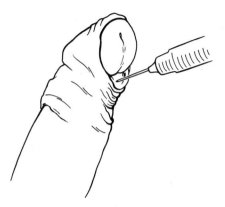

FIG. 70-2.
Additional anesthetic injected into the frenulum.

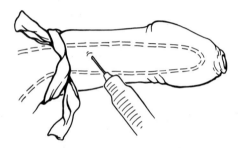

FIG. 70-3.
Use of tourniquet if additional anesthetic is needed.

2. Without withdrawing the needle, angle it toward both sides of the dorsal vein and inject additional lidocaine.

3. Extend the needle subcutaneously downward to the tunica albuginea, an area of firm resistance, and continue injecting circumferentially, staying close to the tunica albuginea. The penile skin is loose; therefore, complete circumferential deployment of the anesthetic agent can be accomplished, and the ventral surface can be reached from both sides. Inject approximately 4 cc in this manner on each side. Do not penetrate the fascia.

4. Wait a few minutes, and then inject 1 cc of the local anesthetic subcutaneously into the frenulum using a half-inch 30-gauge needle (Fig. 70-2).

5. Wait several more minutes and then test the depth of local anesthesia by cautiously grasping the edge of the foreskin with a mosquito hemostat. Should more anesthesia be required, use a Penrose drain as a tourniquet around the midportion of the penis. Tie the tourniquet tightly or hold the Penrose drain with a clamp to obstruct venous return. Inject an additional 2 cc lidocaine into both corpora cavernosa just distal to the tourniquet (Fig. 70-3).

6. After approximately 5 minutes, retest for anesthesia; if anesthesia is adequate, remove the tourniquet.

TECHNIQUE

An assistant is of considerable help in carrying out this procedure.

1. Using small straight hemostats, grasp the distal foreskin at the 11 o'clock, 1 o'clock, 5 o'clock, and 7 o'clock positions, and gently pull the foreskin over the glans (Fig. 70-4).
2. Use a maleable silver probe on the undersurface of the dorsal foreskin to determine a point 1 cm distal to the corona.
3. Place a large straight hemostat at the 12 o'clock position, close it firmly, and compress and crush the foreskin to the point that you previously determined with the silver probe.
4. Remove the forceps and use a straight Metzenbaum scissors to incise through the center of this crushed area (Fig. 70-5). Crushing the tissue reduces the bleeding from this incision.
5. Repeat this procedure at the 6 o'clock position, making an incision *up to the base of the frenulum* (Fig. 70-6).
6. Using a curved Mayo scissors, carefully excise these two lateral tissue flaps, maintaining a 1 cm margin from the corona (Fig. 70-7). Fulgurate all bleeders or tie with a 5-0 plain catgut.

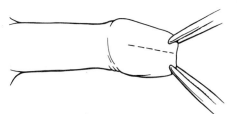

FIG. 70-4.
Straight hemostats applied at very distal tip of foreskin.

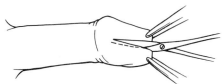

FIG. 70-5.
Dorsal slit through crushed tissue.

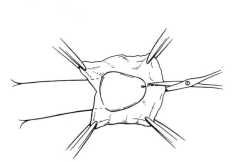

FIG. 70-6.
Ventral slit to base of frenulum.

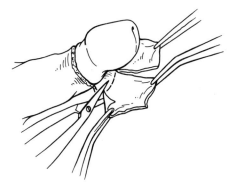

FIG. 70-7.
Excising foreskin.

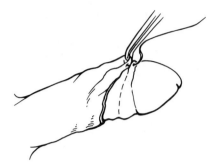

FIG. 70-8.
Suturing the skin to the shaft mucosa just proximal to corona.

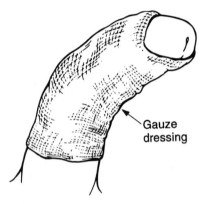

Gauze
dressing

FIG. 70-9.
Cover suture with gauze dressing.

7. If the large dorsal vein is cut, ligate with 3 or 4 1-0 plain catgut sutures.
8. After complete hemostasis, sew the outer layer of skin just proximal to the glans to the underlying muscosal layer (1 cm skin remnant of prepuce) with multiple 4-0 or 5-0 chromic sutures (Fig. 70-8).
9. Place two layers of Xeroform gauze dressing over the suture line around the entire circumference and overlay with a light layer of Kerlix or Kling (Fig. 70-9).

POSTPROCEDURE CARE

- Prescribe 5 days worth of adequate analgesics appropriate for the patient's pain tolerance. A combination product containing codeine, such as Tylenol #3, or a similar product is sufficient.
- Instruct the patient to soak in a tub of warm water 24 to 36 hours later, and to remove all of the dressing at that time.
- Give the patient instructions on how to replace the Xeroform gauze and Kling gauze, which should be done every day until the patient returns to the office for the follow-up visit in one week.

- Tell the patient to call if there is any undue pain or active bleeding.
- Instruct the patient to avoid sexual arousal and sexual intercourse for about 4 weeks.

COMPLICATIONS

- Late bleeding
- Hematoma
- Infection
- Pain with erection (prevented by leaving an adequate "cup" (1 cm margin) of coronal skin [see Step 6 under Technique])
- Stricture and scarring (rare)

CPT/BILLING CODE

54161   Circumcision, surgical excision other than clamp device, or dorsal slit, other than newborn

BIBLIOGRAPHY

An argument for circumcision: prevention of balanitis in the adult, *Arch Dermatol* 126(8): 1990.

Circumcision at the 121st Evacuation Hospital: report of a questionnaire with cross-culture observations, *Milit Med* 154: April 1989.

Dorsal penile nerve blocks, *Letter to J Am Bd FP:* October 1990.

Pories WJ, Thomas FT: *Office surgery for family physicians,* Stoneham, Mass, 1985, Butterworth.

CHAPTER 71

Self-Injection Therapy for the Treatment of Impotence

Robert E. James

James R. Palleschi

Significant advances have recently been made in the diagnosis and treatment of impotence. The self-injection of vasoactive agents into the corpora cavernosa (Fig. 71-1) now enables many patients to resume satisfactory sexual activities without surgery.

The currently available vasoactive agents include *papaverine hydrochloride,* a nonspecific smooth-muscle relaxant, which may be used with *phentolamine mesylate,* a smooth-muscle relaxant that enhances the effect of papaverine; and *prostaglandin E_1 (PGE$_1$),* a vasodilator and a smooth-muscle relaxant. For several years, these agents have been used extensively for impotence, although this remains an unlabeled indication.

These vasoactive agents induce an erection by increasing arterial blood flow, relaxing the sinusoidal spaces within the cavernosal tissue, and increasing venous resistance. An excellent erection that lasts for 30 to 90 minutes usually occurs in patients with mild to moderate arterial insufficiency, mild to moderate venous incompetence, psychogenic impotence, neurogenic impotence, and medication-induced impotence.

INDICATIONS

- Impotence due to arterial insufficiency
- Impotence due to mild to moderate venous incompetence
- Psychogenic impotence (Patients with performance anxiety may be treated with counseling and short-term intracavernosal agents. If this is ineffective, sexual therapy or psychotherapy should be advised.)
- Neurogenic impotence

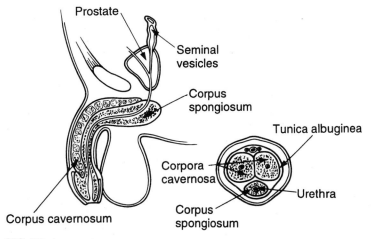

FIG. 71-1.
Side view of penis and scrotum (*left*) and cross-sectional view of penis (*right*).

- Medication-induced impotence, when drug therapy cannot be altered or terminated
- Diagnostic erection

CONTRAINDICATIONS

- Blood dyscrasia, coagulation disorder, or anticoagulation drug therapy
- Unstable cardiovascular disease
- Impaired manual dexterity or vision
- The presence of a prosthetic penile device
- Valvular heart disease
- Intolerance to the test dose of the vasoactive agent

EQUIPMENT

- 1 to 3 cc syringes with half-inch 27- and 30-gauge needles
- Alcohol swabs
- Vasoactive agents

  Papaverine HCl 30 mg/cc is available in 10 cc multidose vials.
  Papaverine and phentolamine solution: Inject 5 mg (or 10 mg) of phentolamine (Regitine) into a 10 cc vial of papaverine 30 mg/cc. The (approximate) concentrations will be papaverine 30 mg/cc and phentolamine 0.5 mg/cc (or 1 mg/cc).
  Prostaglandin E_1 (PGE_1, or alprostadil) is available in 1 cc ampules from Upjohn as Prostin VR Pediatric 500 mcg/cc. For the desired concentration,

inject 0.2 cc of this preparation into each of five 10 cc vials of bacterio-static normal saline for injection. Each vial will contain PGE_1 10 mcg/cc.

Open vials or compounded solutions should be refrigerated to maintain sterility and effectiveness. A 30-day expiration date is recommended; however, sufficient effectiveness has been reported for up to 3 months.

- Antidote
  Alpha-adrenergic agents will cause vasoconstriction and thus will usually result in prompt detumescence. Some of the available agents include ephedrine sulfate, epinephrine, and, for prolonged or painful erection, *phenylephrine hydrochloride* (Neo-Synephrine).

PATIENT EDUCATION

Discuss the self-injection program, alternatives, and potential complications with the patient and, when possible, his partner. Patients using this program may experience bruising at the injection site and local or systemic infection (less than 0.05% incidence). Chronic fibrosis at the injection site may occur with repeated injections, and this may result in pain or penile curvature. Papaverine may elevate the results of liver function tests. Consequently, patients should obtain pretreatment liver function tests, and should be retested every 3 months while using papaverine. If the liver function test values begin to rise, the medication should be discontinued. If the initial liver function tests are elevated, use PGE_1 instead of papaverine. Approximately 20% of patients using PGE_1 may experience an ache in the penis that may last for several hours and that may recur with each injection. Priapism, an erection lasting longer than 4 hours, may occur in up to 10% of patients receiving any of the vasoactive agents, but it is reported to occur less frequently with PGE_1. Systemic side effects, such as dizziness and orthostatic hypotension, occur in 2% of patients receiving these vasoactive agents and are believed to be secondary to penile venous incompetence.

Instruct the patient to contact the physician if he experiences a significant erection that persists for more than 4 hours. This will need to be treated promptly to prevent intracorporal fibrosis.

TECHNIQUE

1. Complete the patient's history and physical examination to provide a preliminary diagnosis.
2. Select the agent and the dose. If psychogenic or neurogenic impotence is suspected, use a smaller dose of the vasoactive agent. In psychogenic impotence, one fourth of the maximum dose should be used; and in neurogenic impotence, no more than one sixth of the maximum dose should initially be used. The maximum dose of papaverine is 60 mg, and of PGE_1, is 20 mcg. To reduce the risk of priapism and to prevent other untoward reactions, even when

vascular disease is suspected as the cause of impotence, the initial dose should not exceed 30 mg of papaverine or 10 mcg of PGE$_1$. If a satisfactory erection does not occur, the dose may be appropriately increased at the time of the next office appointment.

3. Once the desired dose of the vasoactive agent has been selected, extend the patient's penis and prepare the lateral surface with an alcohol swab. Locate the neurovascular bundle at the 12 o'clock position and the urethra at the 6 o'clock position (Fig. 71-2). Select as the injection site an area between these two structures in which there are no superficial veins. With the patient standing, gently direct the penis to the left or the right to expose its lateral surface. Introduce a 27- to 30-gauge needle perpendicular to the skin and tunica albuginea, and into the corpora cavernosum. Normally, the needle is advanced one-quarter to one-half inch. Inject the vasoactive agent into the corpora cavernosum. The medication will enter the opposite corpora caverno-sum through cross-circulation. If resistance is met as the medication is injected, withdraw the needle slowly as you continue to inject. The resistance normally occurs because the needle is against the opposite wall of the corpora caver-nosum. To prevent injection of the medication into the subcutaneous space, it is recommended that the needle be advanced the entire half-inch and then slowly withdrawn.

4. Once the injection is completed, have the patient apply pressure to the injec-tion site for 2 minutes. Concurrently, the patient should place the thumb and index finger of the other hand around the base of the penis to reduce sys-temic distribution of the medication. This pressure should be applied for 2 to 5 minutes.

5. Evaluate the condition of the patient periodically during the first 15 minutes following the injection. The quality of the erection should be evaluated, with the patient in the standing position, at 15-minute intervals during the first hour. To evaluate the quality of the erection the patient will experience with sexual stimulation, you may ask the patient to apply manual stimulation. Once the erection has started to subside, the patient may be discharged from the office. Instruct the patient to contact you if priapism occurs later. If the erec-tion does not begin to subside within one hour after the injection in your of-fice, you may wish to administer the antidote at that time.

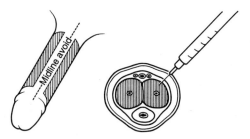

FIG. 71-2.
Intracavernous injection site. Grasp the glans. Pull firmly outward to tense penis. Do not rotate.

TREATMENT OF THE PERSISTENT ERECTION

If the patient does not have significant hypertension or unstable cardiac or cerebrovascular disease, an intracavernosal alpha adrenergic agonist is safe and very effective in the treatment of priapism. Before injecting the antidote, you should attempt to treat the priapism by first aspirating 20 to 30 cc of blood from the corpora cavernosum. Inject the skin over the aspiration site (shaft of the penis) with 0.5 to 1 cc of local anesthetic (1% to 2% lidocaine). Then aspirate, using aseptic technique, with a 30 cc syringe and a 16- to 18-gauge needle. Insert the needle one-half inch and withdraw the blood slowly.

The following agents may be considered for the treatment of priapism if aspiration of blood is unsuccessful:

* *Ephedrine sulfate.* A vial contains 50 mg (25 mg per cc). Initially inject 10 to 25 mg into the corpora cavernosum. If detumescence does not begin within 15 to 30 minutes, the dose may be repeated. A maximum of 50 mg may be given. Ephedrine is the drug of choice because of its efficacy, simplicity, and safety.
* *Epinephrine.* Inject 1 cc of dilute epinephrine (10 to 20 mcg/cc) slowly into the corpora cavernosum every 5 to 10 minutes. This may be repeated twice, and if satisfactory detumescence does not occur, a urology consultation should be obtained. (To prepare the proper dilution, use epinephrine 1: 10,000 solution. For 10 mcg per cc, dilute 0.1 cc of epinephrine with 0.9 cc of normal saline. For 20 mcg per cc, dilute 0.2 cc of epinephrine with 0.8 cc of normal saline.)
* *Phenylephrine hydrochloride* (Neo-Synephrine) 1%. Inject 1 cc slowly into the corpora cavernosum every 5 to 10 minutes. If satisfactory detumescence does not occur after the second dose, a urology consultation should be obtained. (To prepare the proper dilution, use phenylephrine 0.1 cc diluted with 0.9 cc of normal saline for 100 mcg/cc. Use phenylephrine 0.2 cc diluted with 0.8 cc of normal saline for 200 mcg/cc.)

These medications should be given individually and never in combination. Monitor the blood pressure and pulse closely in all patients. Cardiac arrhythmias and significant hypertension may occur.

If these measures are ineffective, obtain a urology consultation. Surgical intervention may be required at this time.

COMPLICATIONS

* Priapism
* Infection
* Subcutaneous ecchymosis or hematoma
* Fibrosis to the corpora cavernosum with repeated injections
* Curvature of the penis occurring after repeated injections
* Painful erections

- Dizziness or postural hypotension
- Myocardial infarction and/or stroke in patients with unstable cardiac or cerebrovascular disease

CPT/BILLING CODE

54325   Injection of corpora cavernosum

BIBLIOGRAPHY

Bernard F, Lue TF: The roles of the urologist in patient auto-injection therapy for erectile dysfunction, *Contemp Urol J:*21, 1990.

Broderick GA, Lue TF: Treatment of priapism. In Rafer J, editor: *Common problems in infertility and impotence,* St Louis, 1990, Yearbook Medical Publishers.

Zorgniotti AW: Pharmacologic erection therapy. In Rafer J, editor: *Common problems in infertility and impotence,* St Louis, 1990, Yearbook Medical Publishers.

PART SIX

Gynecology and Female Reproductive

CHAPTER 72

Diagnostic Hysteroscopy

Barbara S. Apgar

The hysteroscope has emerged as a valuable tool for viewing the endocervical canal and uterine cavity. Diagnostic hysteroscopy is not intended to replace tissue diagnosis, but rather to make current sampling techniques more precise. The hysteroscopist has three goals: (1) to transform the uterine cleft into a cavity by the use of distending agents, (2) to illuminate the uterine cavity by a light source and light transmission, and (3) to transmit the image by an optical system. Hysteroscopes are designed to apply optical physics to a small dark space (the endometrial cavity) through a narrow aperture (the cervical canal). With the smaller-diameter scopes, diagnostic hysteroscopy can be performed in the office setting without the need for cervical dilatation or local anesthesia. Controlled-rate carbon dioxide insufflators allow safe distention of the uterine cavity with minimal side effects.

Hysteroscopy is best performed in the early follicular phase when the endometrium is the thinnest.

INDICATIONS

- Suspicion of endometrial polyps or submucous uterine myomas
- Evaluation of abnormal uterine bleeding in a premenopausal or postmenopausal patient
- Localization of lost intrauterine devices
- Diagnosis of uterine or cervical carcinomas
- Infertility evaluations (with hysterosalpingography), including recurrent miscarriage
- Evaluation of postpartum bleeding

CONTRAINDICATIONS

- Acute pelvic infections
- Acute uterine bleeding (if using carbon dioxide insufflation)

- Pregnancy
- Recent uterine perforation
- Known uterine or cervical carcinoma

EQUIPMENT

- Flexible or rigid (0-degree or 30-degree viewing angle) panoramic hysteroscope, 3.6 mm to 5 mm in diameter (suppliers include Olympus, Cabot Medical, Storz, Cooper Surgical, Circon ACMI, Fujinon)
- Carbon dioxide insufflator (constant flow/variable pressure)
- Halogen or xenon lamp light source
- Vaginal speculum (unhinged on one side)
- Antiseptic solution
- *Optional:* lidocaine 1% *without* epinephrine
- *Optional:* 10 cc syringe, 4-inch needle extender, 27-gauge needles
- Tenaculum
- Uterine sound

PREPROCEDURE PATIENT PREPARATION

Explain the procedure to the patient and obtain informed consent. Be sure that full resuscitative equipment is available. For patients of reproductive age who are not using reliable birth control, obtain a pregnancy test. In patients at high risk for pelvic infection, obtain cervical or uterine cultures before performing hysteroscopy.

TECHNIQUE

1. Place the patient in the dorsal lithotomy position. Perform a bimanual pelvic examination to determine uterine position and size.
2. Place a sterile vaginal speculum (unhinged on one side), and cleanse the cervix with antiseptic solution.
3. Most patients will tolerate insertion of the diagnostic scope without anesthesia, but a pudendal block may be necessary in some patients. A pudendal block is accomplished by administering 5 cc of 1% lidocaine *without* epinephrine into each uterosacral ligament at the 4 and 8 o'clock positions. A small amount (0.5 cc) of 1% lidocaine can be placed intracervically on the anterior or posterior lip where the tenaculum is placed.
4. Grasp the anterior cervix with a tenaculum. Sound the uterus to determine the depth and direction of the central axis.
5. Engage the hysteroscope at the external os, and begin carbon dioxide insufflation through the instillation port on the scope at an initial rate of 30 cc/minute. As the hysteroscope traverses the endocervical canal, the carbon dioxide will create a visual space ahead of the scope. Advance the scope only

if the view is clear. After increasing the carbon dioxide insufflation rate to 40 to 50 cc/minute, examine the uterine cavity systematically.

6. *The flexible hysteroscope* has ultrathin glass fibers with a view that is ground glass–appearing. The scope is rotated by a movement of the hand; the distal end has a maximum up-and-down deflection of approximately 100 to 120 degrees. Deflection of the distal tip is accomplished by the thumb, which moves the deflection control lever on the handle of the scope. The distal tip can be maneuvered around lesions so that structures obscured by masses (such as polyps) can be visualized.

   The rigid hysteroscope consists of a telescope with a 0-degree or 30-degree viewing angle and a sheath measuring 3 to 5 mm in diameter. The telescope consists of an eyepiece, a barrel, and a terminal lens. The sheath that fits over the telescope has a port for carbon dioxide installation. The 0-degree scope provides a straight-on view. The 30-degree scope provides a view that is 30 degrees off the horizontal. The 0-degree scope approximates normal vision. The 30-degree scope allows dexterous examination of the cornual area.

7. The average time required to perform diagnostic hysteroscopy is 5 to 10 minutes. The carbon dioxide insufflation must be critically controlled during the procedure. If the gas is instilled too quickly, obstructive bubbles of carbon dioxide will form. Intrauterine pressure should not exceed 100 mm Hg.

8. After the uterus is inspected, withdraw the hysteroscope.

9. Clean the scope with a disinfectant solution.

10. Complete the written report and record all abnormal findings in detail.

POSTPROCEDURE INSTRUCTIONS

1. Place the patient in the Trendelenburg position if she experiences shoulder pain secondary to the carbon dioxide instillation.
2. Administer analgesics to control mild uterine cramping.
3. If infection develops following the procedure, initiate therapy with broad-spectrum antibiotics effective against anerobes.

COMPLICATIONS

- Uterine perforation can occur if the hysteroscope is forcibly advanced without a panoramic, unobstructed view.
- Infection is rare if strict protocols are followed in screening for pelvic infections in high-risk patients.
- Complications related to carbon dioxide insufflation are rare with use of a constant-flow insufflator. Acidosis and hypercarbia are rare events.
- Shoulder pain can be experienced by patients after carbon dioxide insufflation.

CPT/BILLING CODES

56350	Hysteroscopy, diagnostic (separate procedure)
56351	Hysteroscopy, surgical; with sampling (biopsy) of endometrium and/or polypectomy; with or without D & C
56355	Hysteroscopy, surgical; with removal of impacted foreign body

BIBLIOGRAPHY

Apgar B, DeWitt D: Diagnostic hysteroscopy, *Am Fam Physician* 46(5):19S, 1992.

Frey DL: Should you be doing hysteroscopy? *Fam Pract Management:* 63, April 1994.

Gimbleson RJ, Rappold HO: A comparative study between panoramic hysteroscopy with directed biopsies and dilatation and curettage, *Am J Obstet Gynecol* 158(3):489, 1988.

Heury LA: A buyer's guide to hysteroscopes, *Fam Pract Management:* 68, April 1994.

March CM: Hysteroscopy, *J Reprod Med* 37(4):293, 1992.

Mencaglia L, Perino A, Hamou J: Hysteroscopy in premenopausal and postmenopausal women with abnormal uterine bleeding, *J Reprod Med* 32(8):577, 1987.

Shapiro BS: Instrumentation in hysteroscopy, *Obstet Gynecol Clin N Am* 15(1):13, 1988.

Taylor PJ: Hysteroscopy: where have we been, where are we going? *J Rep Med* 38(10):757, 1993.

Valle RF: Hysteroscopy in the evaluation of female infertility, *Am J Obstet Gynecol* 137(4): 425, 1980.

Wheeler JM, DeCherney AH: Office hysteroscopy, *Obstet Gynecol Clin N Am* 15(1):29, 1988.

CHAPTER 73

Endometrial Biopsy

Barbara S. Apgar

Endometrial biopsy is a safe, relatively painless, and cost-effective diagnostic means of evaluating the endometrium for abnormal uterine bleeding, infertility, and malignancy.*

INDICATIONS

- Determination of the causes of abnormal uterine bleeding: ovulation/anovulation, hormone-replacement therapy adjustment, malignancy/hyperplasia, and postmenopausal bleeding
- Infertility evaluation, short luteal phase determination, ovulation/anovulation
- Prior to hormone replacement in women at higher risk of uterine cancer (obesity, onset of menopause in women more than 52 years old, pelvic irradiation, strong family history, polycystic ovarian disease, infertility, diabetes, liver disease, chronic oligomenorrhea, other cancers)
- Follow-up to previous diagnosis of adenomatous hyperplasia or atypia
- Evaluation of enlarged uterus (in conjunction with ultrasound examination)
- Monitoring adjuvant hormonal therapy (tamoxifen citrate)

CONTRAINDICATIONS

- Pelvic inflammatory disease/cervicitis
- Pregnancy
- Cervical stenosis
- Coagulation disorders, anticoagulant drug therapy

---

*The *ACOG Technical Bulletin* (1991) concludes that the accuracy of office endometrial biopsy under optimal conditions approaches that of dilation and curettage.

PREPROCEDURE PATIENT PREPARATION

1. Explain the procedure to the patient and obtain informed consent (Box 73-1).
2. Offer the patient a nonnarcotic oral analgesic 1 hour prior to the procedure (e.g., ibuprofen 600 to 800 mg).

BOX 73-1. PATIENT CONSENT FORM
ENDOMETRIAL BIOPSY

_____   _____   _____
           Patient Name   ID #   Birthdate

_____has explained the procedure and anesthesia necessary
         Clinician
to diagnose or treat (circle one): a. my condition
                              b. my dependent's condition
I understand the nature of the procedure summarized below. I request and authorize the performance of these procedures:

   Endometrial biopsy (taking a small tissue sample from the lining of my uterus)

I have been informed and understand that the following are risks associated with this procedure:

   Perforation of uterus, which may require hospitalization
   Infection (rare)
   Pain during procedure and cramping afterwards for 1 to 2 days
   Bleeding (slight or severe) which may be controlled with outpatient treatment
     or may require hospitalization
   A D & C in the hospital, if tissue is not diagnostic
   A missed abnormality by biopsy (rare)

I have been informed of the following benefits of this procedure:
   It helps to plan future therapy.
   Having tissue from inside the uterus will help make a diagnosis of my condition.
   It may detect cancer or early precancerous changes.

I have been informed of the alternative(s) to diagnose or treat my condition (state "none," if none).

I have been given an explanation of the procedures, read and understand this information, and have had all questions answered to my satisfaction.

_____   _____
        Patient Signature   Witness

_____   _____
           Date   Date

3. Antibiotic prophylaxis is indicated in those patients with prosthetic heart valves. It is not needed in those patients with murmurs or mitral valve prolapse.

EQUIPMENT

There are various instruments used to obtain endometrial tissue (Fig. 73-1). Three of the more popular ones are described for comparison.

Novak Curette (reusable)

- Vaginal speculum (preferably large Graves)
- Antiseptic solution (povidone-iodine)
- Novak/Randall curette
- Tenaculum
- Uterine sound
- 20 cc syringe
- Formalin sample bottle with labels

Tis-u-Trap Endometrial Curette and Vabra Aspirator (disposable)

- Vaginal speculum (preferably large Graves)
- Antiseptic solution (povidone-iodine)
- Tis-u-Trap sampler device (Milex Products, Inc., 5915 Northwest Hwy., Chicago IL 60631; telephone 1-800-621-1278 [Fig. 73-2, *A*]) or Vabra Aspirator (Berkeley Medevices, Inc., 907 Camelia St., Berkeley, CA 94710; telephone 415-526-4046)—requires external suction pump
- Tenaculum
- Uterine sound
- Formalin sample bottle with labels

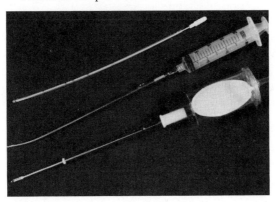

FIG. 73-1.
Three common instruments used to obtain an endometrial sample. *Upper:* the pipelle; *middle:* the Novak curette; *lower:* the Tis-u-Trap.

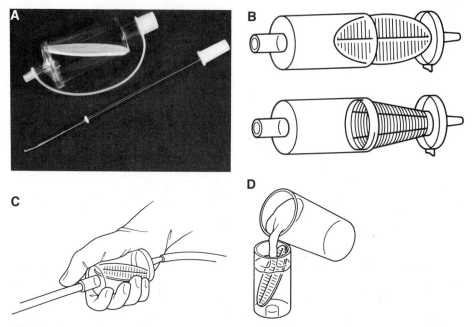

FIG. 73-2.
A, Tis-u-Trap sampler device. **B,** The plastic grid onto which the tissue will rest. **C,** Initiate suction by covering the suction hole on the curette. **D,** Remove the curette from the tissue trap and cap the opening. Pour formalin into the container to cover the plastic grid, then seal with cover.

Pipelle Endometrial Aspirator (disposable)

- Vaginal speculum (preferably large Graves)
- Antiseptic solution (povidone-iodine)
- Pipelle Endometrial Suction Curette or similar device (Unimar, 475 Danbury Rd, Wilton CT 06897; telephone 800-243-6608. Similar devices can be purchased from Milex; ZSI, 21540-B Prairie St., Chatsworth, CA 91311; telephone 800-223-4704; and Wallach, 291 Pepe's Farm Rd., Milford, CT 06460; telephone 203-783-1818)
- *Optional:* tenaculum
- Scissors
- Formalin sample bottle with labels

TECHNIQUE

When using endometrial biopsy (instead of dilation and curettage) to rule out neoplasm, endocervical curettage generally precedes endometrial sampling. Introduce a Kevorkian endocervical curette into the external os, and up to the internal os.

Curettage the entire endocervical canal 360 degrees—twice—from the internal os to the external os (see Chapter 81, The Colposcopic Examination). Follow the endocervical curettage with the endometrial biopsy.

The Novak Curette, the Tis-u-Trap Endometrial Curette, and the Vabra Aspirator may be used to obtain a microcurettage consisting of one to four strips of endometrium. The latter two instruments use suction curettage to obtain the sample; they require an external electric pump.

The Pipelle Endometrial Suction Curette may be used to obtain an endometrial sample without external suction. It also may be more successful for the patient with a stenotic os. The Pipelle consists of an outer plastic sheath with a circular curette opening that is proximal to the closed distal tip, and an internal piston that creates negative pressure within the instrument sheath. This unit is inexpensive, requires little office setup, and is associated with diagnostic accuracy at least equal to that of dilation and curettage (except for endometrial polyps) (Fig. 73-3).

With all techniques, cleanse the cervix with antiseptic solution, and insert the sterile sampling device through the cervical os without touching the vulva or vaginal walls. Do not touch the part of the sampler that is placed into the uterus. Sterile gloves and speculum are not necessary if a "no touch" technique is used. Drapes are not necessary if the procedure is followed. A Kevorkian endocervical curette will usually be necessary to perform an endocervical curettage before the endometrial biopsy specimen is obtained.

The Novak Curette

1. Perform a bimanual examination to determine the position of the uterus.
2. Insert a vaginal speculum, and visualize the cervix.
3. Cleanse the cervix with antiseptic solution.
4. Apply a tenaculum to the anterior or posterior lip.
5. Insert a uterine sound to the top of the fundus, and measure the length of the uterine cavity (up to 8 cm is normal).
6. Apply gentle traction with the tenaculum as you insert the curette into the fundus.
7. Attach a 20 cc syringe to the curette hub. Create suction by pulling the syringe plunger back.
8. Perform one to four single-strip curettages: apply pressure against the side walls of the uterus and sample straight out from the fundus to the lower uterine segment. One sample from each quadrant is advised.
9. Withdraw the curette from the uterus and express the sample by pushing the plunger toward the curette.
10. Discharge the specimen into the formalin sample bottle, then label and cap the bottle.
11. Remove the speculum from the vagina.

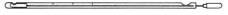

FIG. 73-3.
Pipelle endometrial suction curette.

Tis-u-Trap or Vabra Aspirator

1. Perform a bimanual examination to determine the position of the uterus.
2. Insert a vaginal speculum, and visualize the cervix.
3. Cleanse the cervix with antiseptic solution.
4. Apply a tenaculum to the anterior or posterior lip.
5. Insert a uterine sound to the top of the fundus, and measure the length of the uterine cavity (up to 8 cm is normal).
6. Hook up the device to the suction pump, and activate the pump.
7. Insert the curette through the os and into the fundus, and initiate the suction by covering the suction hole.
8. Perform a curettage of the entire endometrium. The tissue will travel through the curette and into the trap, where it will collect on the grid.
9. When sufficient tissue is in the trap, release the suction and remove the curette from the uterus.
10. Turn off the suction pump and remove the curette from the trap.
11. Add formalin to the trap, ensuring that all the tissue is exposed to the solution. Cap and label the trap, preparing it for transport to pathology (see Fig. 73-2).
12. Remove the speculum from the vagina.

The Pipelle Endometrial Suction Curette, or Similar Instrument

1. Perform a bimanual examination to determine the position of the uterus.
2. Insert a vaginal speculum, and visualize the cervix.
3. Cleanse the cervix with antiseptic solution.
4. Introduce the device (with the piston fully inserted to the distal tip of the sheath) through the cervical canal, into the uterine cavity, and up to the fundus. A tenaculum may be placed on the cervix, but usually this is not necessary (Fig. 73-4, *A*).
5. Document the depth of the uterus.
6. Stabilize the sheath with one hand, and draw the piston completely back in one continuous motion to create negative pressure within the lumen (Fig. 73-4, *B*).
7. Rotate the sheath between the thumb and index finger, and move it in and out between the fundus and the internal os three or four times. These combined actions pass the curette opening through a helical arc against the walls of the uterus. During this passage, the negative pressure within the sheath draws the endometrial tissue into the curette opening, where it is sheared away and carried into the sheath lumen. Fill the lumen with tissue as completely as possible (Fig. 73-4, *C*).
8. Withdraw the device.
9. Cut off the distal tip (Fig. 73-4, *D*) with the scissors, and expel the sample into the formalin by advancing the piston into the sheath (Fig. 75-4, *E*).
10. Remove the speculum from the vagina.

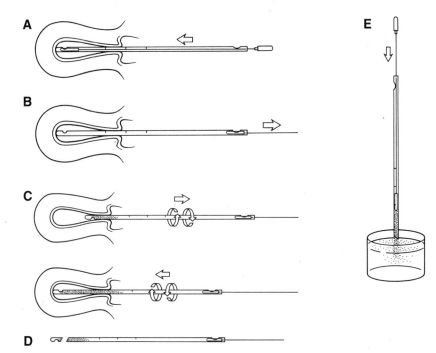

FIG. 73-4.
A, With the piston fully advanced within the sheath, insert the Pipelle through the cervical canal into the uterine cavity. **B,** While holding the outer sheath, pull the piston back completely without interruption to the proximal piston stop creating maximum negative pressure within sheath. **C,** Simultaneously roll the sheath between your fingers while moving the sheath laterally and back and forth between the fundus and internal os 3 or 4 times to obtain the sample. **D,** Remove the Pipelle from the uterus and cut off the distal tip just proximal to the curette opening. **E,** Advance the piston rod to expel the sample into the transport medium.

POSTPROCEDURE CARE

1. Ask the patient to remain supine for a few moments following the endometrial biopsy. Assess for vasovagal reaction.
2. Painful uterine cramps (if present) usually subside rapidly or are relieved by nonsteroidal antiinflammatory agents.
3. If heavy bleeding is not observed and the vasovagal reaction (if it has occurred) has resolved, discharge the patient.
4. The patient may resume sexual relations in 2 to 3 days, or after bleeding has stopped.
5. Instruct the patient to report any fever, cramping after 48 hours, or bleeding for 24 to 48 hours that is heavier than a normal menses.

COMPLICATIONS

- Bacteremia, septicemia, and endocarditis have been reported following endometrial biopsy, although they are very rare.
- Reports indicate a 0.1% to 1.3% risk for uterine perforation. Patients in whom perforation is suspected should be observed closely for bleeding complications and infection.
- Excessive uterine bleeding may occur following endometrial biopsy, especially in patients with undiagnosed coagulation disorders or perforation.
- Less than 10% of patients have been reported to have some degree of vasovagal reaction after the procedure.

CPT/BILLING CODE

58110   Endometrial and/or endocervical sampling without cervical dilator

BIBLIOGRAPHY

Baugham DM: Office endometrial aspiration biopsy, *Fam Pract Recert* 15(5):45, 1993.

Carcinoma of the endometrium, *ACOG Technical Bulletin* 162:1, 1991.

Check JH et al: Clinical evaluation of the Pipelle endometrial suction curette for timed endometrial biopsies, *J Reprod Med* 34(3):218, 1989.

Grimes DA: Diagnostic dilation and curettage: a reappraisal, *Am J Obstet Gynecol* 142(1):1, 1982.

Jaber R: Detection of and screening for endometrial cancer, *JFP* 26(1):67, 1988.

Kaunitz AM et al: Comparison of endometrial biopsy with the endometrial Pipelle and vabra aspirator, *J Reprod Med* 33(5):429, 1988.

Koonings PP, Grimes DA: Endometrial sampling techniques for the office, *Am Fam Physician* 40(4):207, 1989.

Koonings PP, Moyer DL, Grimes DA: A randomized clinical trial comparing Pipelle and Tis-u-Trap for endometrial biopsy, *Obstet Gynecol* 75(2):293, 1990.

Perkins RL, Hernandez E, Berenberg JL: Septicemia in a postmenopausal woman after endometrial biopsy, *Am J Gynecol Health* 4(2):20, 1990.

Schneider L: Causes of abnormal vaginal bleeding in a family practice center, *JFP* 16(2):281, 1983.

Silver MM, Miles P, Rosa C: Comparison of Novak and Pipelle endometrial biopsy instruments, *Obstet Gynecol* 78:828, 1991.

Stovall TG, Photopulos GJ, Poston WM: Pipelle endometrial sampling in patients with known endometrial carcinoma, *Obstet Gynecol* 77:954, 1991.

CHAPTER 74

Hysterosalpingography

Steven Fettinger

Hysterosalpingography (HSG) is a radiologic examination of the female genital tract. It allows for the evaluation of the cervical canal, endometrial cavity, tubal lumen, and the periadnexal area. Some physicians feel that it has been superseded by laparoscopy with hysteroscopy, but others feel that it remains an integral part of many diagnostic workups. Hysterosalpingography is a relatively easy procedure, requires no anesthesia, and has a low complication risk. Its employment as a therapeutic procedure for enhancing fertility is promoted by some and doubted by others. The radiation exposure is usually minimal, in the 50 to 500 mrem range.

INDICATIONS

- Infertility (uterine)
    Endometrial adhesions (Asherman's syndrome)
    Polyps; endometrial, pedunculated leiomyomata
    Uterine anomalies
    Diethylstilbestrol (DES); T-shaped uterus
- Infertility (tubal)
    Assessment of tube patency
    Salpingitis isthmica nodosa
    Periadnexal adhesive disease
- Habitual abortions
    Asherman's syndrome
    Uterine anomaly
    Diethylstilbesterol (DES) changes
    Leiomyomata
- Pre- and postoperative evaluation
    Tubal reanastomosis/reimplantation, tuboplasty
    Uterine septal resection, metroplasty
    Myomectomy

- Localization of lost intrauterine contraceptive device (IUD)
- Cervical incompetency (controversial indication)

CONTRAINDICATIONS

- Allergy to contrast medium
- Recent history of salpingitis
- Pregnancy
- Recent dilation and curettage
- Untreated sexually transmitted disease (STD)

GENERAL EQUIPMENT

Cannulas

Many types of HSG cannulation devices are available. Choice may depend on procedure rationale and physician preference. Three general types are in common use, with multiple modifications:

1. *Olive-tipped cannulas.* A small cannula traverses the cervical canal, and an olive- or cone-shaped seat is held against the cervix to seal it.
2. *Suction cannulas.* A small cannula is held in place and sealed by a suction cup on the cervix.
3. *Balloon cannulas.* One or two balloons are used to fix and seal the cervix. A primary intrauterine balloon is pulled down against the internal cervical os by a second balloon, a spring-loaded platform, or manual traction. The balloon catheters (including pediatric Foley catheters) obscure the lower uterine anatomy; however, the balloon can be deflated after the procedure, and additional contrast dye can be injected to evaluate this area.
4. Special selective cannulation catheterization sets are available from most vendors (see Suppliers). These catheters are used to selectively cannulate and evaluate a fallopian tube in special circumstances; i.e., unilateral or bilateral nonvisualization, salpingitis isthmica nodosa, or prior ectopic pregnancy.

TABLE 74-1.

Selection of Contrast Medium

Medium	Advantages	Disadvantages
Water-soluble	Rapidly absorbed Less need for delayed films Improved visualization of details Extravasation tolerated	No enhancement of fertility
Oil-based	Possible fertility enhancement	Delayed films may be needed Granuloma formation possible Pulmonary embolism if extravasated

Contrast Medium

Most centers are currently using water-soluble dye. There has been continued controversy regarding the use of water-soluble versus oil-based media (Table 74-1). The question of ionic or nonionic water-soluble dye depends on the preference of the radiologist. The majority of centers are using the cheaper ionic dyes, except in patients with a history of iodine allergy.

SPECIFIC EQUIPMENT

- Prep tray, including 4 × 4 inch gauze pads, ring forceps, povidone-iodine solution, medicine cups, lubricating jelly, and a plastic speculum
- Cannula (See Fig. 74-1)
    Jaco, or Kuhn (nondisposable)
    Hysterocath (Cook)
    HUI (Unimar)
    HUI Mini-Flex (Unimar)
    Bard Cervical Cannula (Bard)
    ZUMI 2.0/4.0/4.5 (Zinnanti)
    H/S Catheter Set (Ackrad)
    Pediatric Foley catheter
- Contrast medium
    Water-soluble
    Oil-based (Lipoidol or Ethiodol)
    Nonionic water-soluble

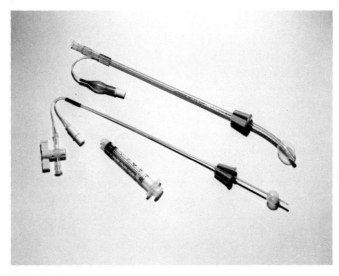

FIG. 74-1.
Examples of uterine catheters for injection of dye for hysterosalpinography. *Top:* Zinnanti ZUI 4.0. *Bottom:* Zinnanti ZUI 2.0.

- Vaginal speculum
  - One-armed Graves (removable after placement of cannula)
  - Plastic nonradiopaque
- Tenaculum (if needed to fixate cervix for cannula placement)
- Syringe, 10 or 20 cc

SUPPLIERS

Unimar
475 Danbury Rd.
Wilton, CT 06897
800-243-6608

Cook Ob/Gyn
110 W. Morgan St.
P.O. Box 271
Spencer, IN 47460
800-541-5591

C.R. Bard, Inc.
200 Ames Pond Dr.
Tewksbury, MA 01876
800-826-BARD

Ackrad Laboratories, Inc.
70 Jackson Dr.
P.O. Box 1085
Ranford, NJ 07016
908-276-6390

Zinnanti Surgical Instruments, Inc.
21540-B Prairie St.
Chatsworth, CA 91311
800-223-4740

PREPROCEDURE EVALUATION

Hysterosalpingography should be performed in the proliferative (preovulatory) phase of the menstrual cycle to avoid exposing an embryo to radiation; to decrease the risk of infection, which is higher if the procedure is performed during the secretory phase; and to avoid the possibility of dislodging a preimplantation conception and causing an ectopic pregnancy.

Patients with a history of salpingitis require negative cultures for sexually transmitted disease, normal sedimentation rate or C-reactive protein, and nontender preprocedure pelvic examination.

Patients with a history of pelvic inflammatory disease or prior tuboplasty should be treated with prophylactic antibiotics. Two options have been shown to be effective: doxycycline 200 mg the morning of the procedure and 100 mg twice a day for 5 days following the procedure; or metronidazole 200 mg three times a day for 5 days following the procedure. Antibiotic prophylaxis is controversial for patients without a history of pelvic inflammatory disease or prior tuboplasty. Currently, many physicians utilize prophylaxis with all patients undergoing HSG.

Preoperative medications may include a nonsteroidal antiinflammatory agent, such as ibuprofen 600 mg, given 1 to 2 hours preoperatively to decrease pain and cramping; diazepam 10 to 20 mg 1 to 2 hours preoperatively may be given for extreme apprehension.

PREPROCEDURE PATIENT EDUCATION

- Discuss the procedure, the typical findings, alternatives to, risks of, and possible complications of the procedure with the patient; obtain informed consent.
- Explain to the patient that mild discomfort will be experienced during the procedure, and that spotting for up to a few days after the procedure is expected.
- Educate the patient about the warning signs of complications: for example, increasing pain, heavy bleeding, and fever.

TECHNIQUE (FIG. 74-2)

1. Check all equipment to ensure that the setup is complete and in proper working condition.
2. Draw up the contrast material and preload the cannula (bubbles may obscure intrauterine disease).
3. Position the patient on a high-resolution image-intensifier fluoroscopy table in the dorsal lithotomy position. An adequate light should be available.
4. Perform a bimanual pelvic examination to assess the degree of flexion or retroflexion of the uterus and to exclude pelvic tenderness (the latter is a contraindication to HSG if associated with inflammation).
5. Insert the vaginal speculum.
6. Prepare the cervix and upper vagina with povidone-iodine.
7. If indicated by the cannula choice, grasp the anterior lip of the cervix with the tenaculum (slowly, to minimize pain).
8. Insert the cannula and seat it as indicated by the specific cannula:
   Inflate the upper balloon then the lower balloon (*Bard*).
   Inflate the upper balloon and set spring platform (*Unimar*).
   Inflate the balloon and pull down (*pediatric Foley* and *Zinnanti*).
   Insert the cannula and set spring to tenaculum (*Jaco*).
   Insert the cannula and seat suction cup onto the cervix; then apply suction to the cup.
9. Remove the speculum (nonradiopaque plastic speculums may be left in place).
10. Place the patient in the recumbent position for fluoroscopy.
11. Inject the contrast slowly: 1 to 3 cc may be sufficient to show intrauterine detail; greater volumes may obscure small polyps or adhesions. The injection should be viewed concurrently, and a single spot film taken. Upward or downward movement will often change the degree of flexion to obtain a better view.
12. Continue to inject dye until the tubes are very full. A spot film at this point may show tubal detail that will be obscured after spill.

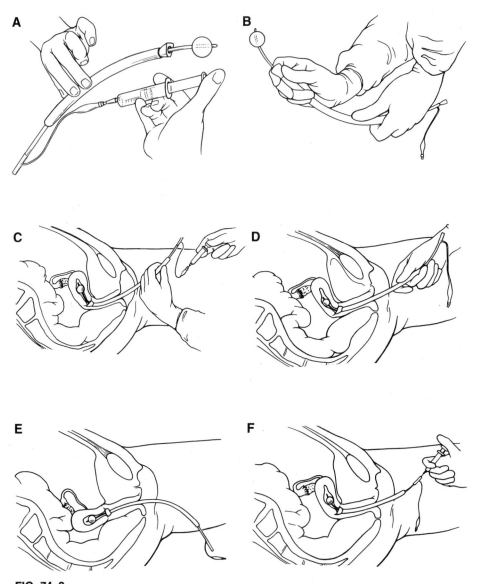

FIG. 74-2.
Technique of using the ZUMI 4.5 (Zinnanti) for HSG. **A,** Testing catheter cuff balloon. **B,** Adjusting catheter for uterine depth. **C,** Placement of catheter and inflation of cuff. **D,** Gentle downward traction to test placement and to seal against cervix. **E,** Placement for posteriorly flexed uteri. **F,** Injection of contrast media. For more detail, refer to the product package informatiion.

13. Continue to inject dye until a spill of dye is seen bilaterally. A spot film at this point will sometimes show peritubal detail. A delayed spot film may be needed to confirm location of dye in peritubal adhesions.
14. Rolling the patient from side to side during the procedure sometimes helps the clinician to visualize lesions.
15. If visualization of one tube cannot initially be accomplished, relax tubal spasm by relieving the pressure and waiting 1 to 2 minutes.
16. Remove the instruments.
17. Observe the patient for 30 minutes for allergic reactions and heavy bleeding.

INTERPRETATION

Interpretation is beyond the scope of this chapter, but a few points may be helpful.

- Correlation of HSG and laparoscopy may be as poor as 25% false-positive and false-negative. Absolute statements based on tubal patency should not be made.
- Uterine anomalies are classified according to the American Fertility Society, but may require laparoscopy to fully define the abnormality.
- Association of renal and uterine developmental anomalies may be as high as 20%; therefore, renal evaluation may be indicated.

COMPLICATIONS

- Infection rates may be as high as 3%. Antibiotic prophylaxis is indicated in select patients (as mentioned previously) to decrease this risk.
- Tenaculum site bleeding is rare, but may require suturing.
- Extravasation of dye into the intravascular space warrants discontinuation, especially if an oil-based dye is used (there is a risk of oil pulmonary embolus).
- Granuloma formation after oil-based dye is a rare late complication.
- Uterine perforation should prompt discontinuation.

CPT/BILLING CODE

58340   Hysterosalpingography

BIBLIOGRAPHY

Garcia CR: *Current therapy of infertility,* ed 3, Toronto, 1988, B. C. Decker.
Mishell DR Jr: *Infertility, contraception & reproductive endocrinology,* ed 3, Boston, 1991, Blackwell Scientific Publications.
Sciarra JJ: *Gynecology and obstetrics,* vol 5, Philadelphia, 1990, J. B. Lippincott.
Speroff Leon et al: *Clinical gynecology endocrinology and infertility,* ed 4, Baltimore, 1989, Williams & Wilkins.
Taymor ML: *Infertility,* New York, 1990, Plenum Publishing.

CHAPTER 75

IUD Insertion

John L. Pfenninger

The ParaGard T380A has been approved by the U.S. Food and Drug Administration (FDA), the American College of Obstetricians and Gynecologists (ACOG), and the World Health Organization (WHO) as an effective and safe contraceptive method for selected women. A recent editorial in *Ob-Gyn Clinical Alert* by Leon Speroff encouraged clinicians to increase the use of the ParaGard intrauterine contraceptive device (IUD) based on recent studies.

Although it was previously believed that the IUD acted mainly by preventing implantation, it is now felt that the primary mode of action may be the inhibition of conception: Thick cervical mucus inhibits sperm migration. Should this mode fail, the IUD may then have the back up effect of inhibiting implantation.

A progesterone-releasing IUD, Progestasert, is less frequently used because it must be replaced annually. The ParaGard T380A has been approved for 8 years of continuous use before replacement is needed. However, the Progestasert is less expensive and may be preferred by women seeking a shorter period of contraception.

INDICATIONS

To be considered a candidate for an IUD, the patient must be parous, in a stable mutually monogamous relationship, and have no history of pelvic inflammatory disease or ectopic pregnancy. The patient must also be willing to check for the presence of IUD strings on a monthly basis. The IUD is especially appropriate for women who have difficulty remembering to take oral contraceptives regularly, who desire reversible contraception, and who want to avoid hormonal contraception.

CONTRAINDICATIONS*

- Pregnancy
- Uterine cavity malformations

---

*Modified from Pfenninger JL: *Fam Pract Recert* 14:131, 1992. Used with permission.

- Acute sexually transmitted disease
- Present or past pelvic inflammatory disease (PID)
- Less than 8 weeks postpartum (If there was a postpartum endometritis or an infected abortion, there should be at least a 3-month interval and complete resolution of infection before insertion.)
- Uterine or cervical malignancy (including unresolved abnormal Pap smear)
- Excessively heavy periods or marked dysmenorrhea with periods (*relative contraindication*)
- Abnormal uterine bleeding, unresolved
- Marked cervicitis or vaginitis
- Wilson's disease (the ParaGard IUD contains copper)
- Allergy to copper
- History of ectopic pregnancy
- Multiple current partners (unstable relationships)
- Immunodeficiency states (leukemia, diabetes, AIDS, intravenous drug use, chronic corticosteroid therapy)
- Genital actinomycoses
- Previously inserted IUD that has not been removed, or marked intolerance to IUDs
- Small uterine cavity (*relative contraindication*)

EQUIPMENT

- The ParaGard T380A or the Progestasert (The ParaGard is a polyethylene "T" wrapped with copper. The Progestasert is polyethylene impregnated with progesterone. Monofilament threads attached to the vertical arm protrude through the cervix after insertion. The devices are radiopaque.)
- Speculum
- Basin with cotton balls moistened with antiseptic solution
- Cervical tenaculum
- Uterine sound
- Sterile gloves (for insertion)
- Nonsterile gloves (for bimanual examination prior to insertion)
- Sterile towel for tray top
- Long suture scissors

PREPROCEDURE PATIENT PREPARATION

Federal regulations require that the patient be given an IUD patient information brochure. These are provided by the manufacturer of the Paragard T380A (Gyno-Pharma Inc., 50 Division Street, Summerville, NJ 08876: 201-725-3100 or 1-800-322-Gyno) and the Progestasert (Alza Corp., 950 Page Mill Rd., P.O. Box 10950, Palo Alto, CA 94303-0802: 415-496-8073 or 1-800-634-8977). The brochures are excellent and also serve as consent forms, as the patient fills out a checklist and signs the entire handout. After the procedure, give the patient an extra handout to take home.

Generally, the patient is seen and counseled in a separate visit. This allows time for her to review the educational materials and to make a more informed decision about insertion. The procedure ideally should be scheduled for the last day or two of menstruation or within five days of the last day of menstruation.

Patients at risk for developing subacute bacterial endocarditis should receive prophylactic antibiotic therapy (doxycycline 200 mg 1 hour before the procedure; or erythromycin 500 mg 1 hour before IUD insertion and 500 mg 6 hours after the procedure). The risk of endometritis is greatest in the first month after insertion or with a new partner. Many physicians prefer to give all patients this prophylactic antibiotic therapy.

A nonsteroidal antiinflammatory drug taken an hour before IUD insertion may help alleviate cramping.

It is essential that a Pap smear be performed within 6 months of insertion and that it be normal. There should be no evidence of sexually transmitted diseases or pelvic inflammatory disease.

The clinician should stress the importance of a mutually monogamous relationship.

TECHNIQUE

1. Perform a pelvic examination to establish the position of the uterus.

   Note: Use sterile technique and wear sterile gloves from this point throughout the procedure.

2. Insert a warm vaginal (preferably large) speculum.
3. Cleanse the cervix with antiseptic solution.
4. Apply a single-tooth tenaculum to the anterior lip of the cervix. Apply slight traction to correct any angulation and to stabilize the cervix. Some clinicians prefer to use a small amount of 2% lidocaine with epinephrine to minimize discomfort. However, the discomfort from the tenaculum is brief and most clinicians do not use local anesthetics.
5. Sound the uterus. The depth should be between 6.5 and 8.5 cm. The incidence of complications is increased in women with uterine depth less than 6.5 mm; the incidence of expulsion is increased in women with uterine depth greater than 8.5 cm.
6. Open the IUD package and place the contents on a sterile towel. Insert the vertical arm of the IUD into the polyethylene inserter tube. Fold the horizontal arms down and place inside the tube (Fig. 75-1).
7. Insert the solid white inserter rod so that it just touches the tip of the vertical arm of the IUD (Fig. 75-2).
8. Adjust the blue flange on the inserter rod to the depth of the uterus as indicated from the uterine sounding. Be sure that the horizontal arms of the IUD are parallel to the horizontal orientation of the blue flange. This will ensure proper placement in the uterus (Fig. 75-3).

A

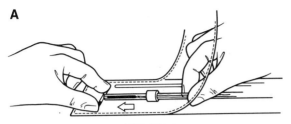

B

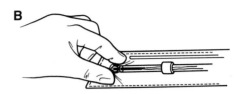

FIG. 75-1.
A, After the bimanual examination and antiseptic solution preparation and after the uterus has been sounded, insert the IUD into the inserter tube. **B,** Bend the arms and insert them just far enough to retain them in the tube. (Redrawn from Pfenninger JL: *Fam Pract Recert* 14:131, 1992. Used with permission.)

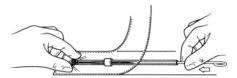

FIG. 75-2.
White inserter rod is placed into insertion tube so it just touches the bottom of the vertical arm of the IUD. (Redrawn from Pfenninger JL: *Fam Pract Recert* 14:131, 1992. Used with permission.)

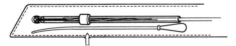

FIG. 75-3.
Set the blue flange so that the distance from the tip of the IUD to the flange is the same distance as indicated by the uterine sound. (Redrawn from Pfenninger JL: *Fam Pract Recert* 14:131, 1992. Used with permission.)

9. Grasp the single-tooth tenaculum to stabilize the cervix. Insert the IUD into the cervical canal up to the flange. Have an assistant hold the tenaculum at this juncture while you hold the solid white rod stationary with your right hand and *withdraw the clear plastic insertion tube* approximately 2 cm with your left hand. *The solid rod should not move.* Using this technique, the IUD "falls" into place (Fig. 75-4).
10. Gently push the tube inserter toward the fundus until resistance is felt. This helps reassure high placement of the IUD.
11. Withdraw the inserting device (Figs. 75-5 and 75-6).
12. Cut the threads to leave 3 to 5 cm protruding from the os. It is better if they are left slightly long since they can always be shortened at the follow-up visit. If cut too short, they can be irritating to a male partner.

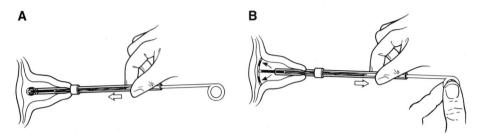

FIG. 75-4.
A, Insert the IUD into the cervical canal up to the flange. **B,** Withdraw the insertion tube approximately 2 cm, holding the solid inserting rod stable and "dropping" the IUD into place. (Redrawn from Pfenninger JL: *Fam Pract Recert* 14:131, 1992. Used with permission.)

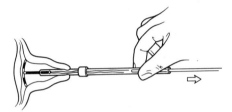

FIG. 75-5.
Withdraw the solid inserting rod. Gently advance the inserting tube to ensure high placement of IUD. (Redrawn from Pfenninger JL: *Fam Pract Recert* 14:131, 1992. Used with permission.)

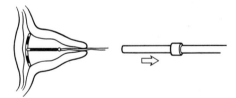

FIG. 75-6.
Withdraw the insertion tube ensuring that the threads are adequately long. (Redrawn from Pfenninger JL: *Fam Pract Recert* 14:131, 1992. Used with permission.)

COMPLICATIONS

In general, the use of the IUD is associated with less morbidity and mortality than pregnancy and delivery (see Table 75-1).

- Contraception failure (less than 1%) is possible. Should this occur, remove the IUD as soon as pregnancy is diagnosed. There is a risk of inducing an abortion, and, if the IUD is left in place, there is increased risk for premature labor and delivery, sepsis, and abortion. Consider ectopic pregnancy, since it is unlikely that there is an intrauterine pregnancy.
- There is an association of pelvic inflammatory disease (PID) with IUD use, but the incidence appears to be increased only during the first 30 days after

TABLE 75-1.

Annual Number of Birth-Related (B) or Method-Related (M) Deaths Associated with Control of Fertility per 100,000 Nonsterile Women by Fertility Control Method According to Age.

Method of control and outcome	Cause of death	Patient Age (years)					
		15-19	20-24	25-29	30-34	35-39	40-44
No fertility control	B	7.0	7.4	9.1	14.8	25.7	28.2
Oral contraceptives (nonsmokers)	M	0.3	0.5	0.9	1.9	13.8	31.6
Oral contraceptives (smokers)	M	2.2	3.4	6.6	13.5	51.1	117.2
IUD	M	0.8	0.8	1.0	1.0	1.4	1.4
Condom	B	1.1	1.6	0.7	0.2	0.3	0.4
Diaphragm/spermicide	B	1.9	1.2	1.2	1.3	2.2	2.8
Periodic abstinence	B	2.5	1.6	1.6	1.7	2.9	3.6

From Ory HW: Mortality associated fertility and fertility control, *Fam Plann Perspect* 15:57, 1983. Used with permission.

insertion or if there are new sexual partners. Should there be any question of PID, broad-spectrum antibiotics should be initiated and the IUD removed.

- The risk of perforation can be limited if the IUD is inserted only after the uterus has fully involuted after pregnancy or an abortion.
- Embedment of IUD into the endometrium can result in difficult removal.
- Some patients experience heavier periods and increased dysmenorrhea. Generally, this will subside within 2 to 3 months. If it does not, it may be necessary to remove the IUD. Patients can also expect to have some spotting for the first month or two after insertion.
- Copper can precipitate symptoms of Wilson's disease.
- Medical diathermy is contraindicated in women with copper-containing IUDs in place.
- In partial or complete expulsion, the patient may not realize that the IUD has passed spontaneously. Therefore, the patient must check for the presence of strings monthly. Occasionally, the IUD will partially expel and be caught in the endocervical canal. The patient may experience excessive uterine cramping, and if this occurs, she must be seen and evaluated. (If the IUD is spontaneously expelled or if it is removed for a complication and another IUD is to be inserted later, the company will replace the used IUD free of charge if the original is returned to them. Similarly, if the IUD is contaminated during the insertion process and subsequently cannot be used, it may be returned to the manufacturer for a refund.)
- Should the patient develop an abnormal Pap smear, doing the cervical biopsy and endocervical curettage during colposcopy, LEEP/LETZ/LOOP procedure, or cervical conization becomes difficult. Although there is no known association between cervical dysplasia and use of the IUD, it is essential that the Pap smear be normal prior to insertion.
- Since patients do not need to see their health care provider regularly as they do for prescription renewal of birth control pills, they potentially may not return for annual Pap smears. It should be emphasized to them that an annual

Pap smear is essential, and that even though they do not need to return for birth control pills, they must return for their annual Pap smear and pelvic examination. (It is a concern that with the long-acting contraceptives, for example, IUDs and the Norplant system, diagnosis of cervical malignancy might be delayed.)

POSTPROCEDURE PATIENT EDUCATION

Give the patient a copy of the handout provided by the company. It is important to reemphasize the major concerns:

- She must check for the threads of the IUD after each menstrual period. If they are not palpable, she should contact her physician immediately.
- Alert the patient to signs of partial or total expulsion—primarily cramping.
- Tell the patient to report any of the following: excessive pain, malodorous discharge, excessive bleeding (other than spotting for a few months), fever, prolonged pelvic discomfort, any type of genital lesions, suspicion of sexually transmitted disease, a missed period, any other concerns that she might have.

SUPPLIERS

ParaGard T380A: GynoPharma Inc.
                 50 Division St.
                 Summerville, NJ 08876
                 201-725-3100 or 1-800-322-Gyno
Progestasert: Alza Corporation
                 950 Page Mill Rd.
                 P.O. Box 10950
                 Palo Alto, CA 94303-0802
                 415-496-8073 or 1-800-634-8977

CONCLUSION

Recent research results indicate that the IUD should receive strong consideration as a long-term contraceptive method in those patients who have a monogamous relationship and who do not have a history of PID or ectopic pregnancy. Pregnancy rates are less than 1%, and 80% of patients will continue use of the IUD after one year. The IUD is intercourse independent, has very low complication rates, and is significantly cheaper than the cost of 8 years of oral contraceptives. Since the primary mode of action is prevention of conception (as opposed to prevention of implantation), it has now become more morally acceptable to patients and physicians alike.

CPT/BILLING CODES

58300	Insertion of intrauterine (IUD), not including device
58301	Removal of intrauterine device (IUD)
X4633	Charge for cost of copper IUD
X4634	Charge for cost of progesterone IUD

BIBLIOGRAPHY

Alvarez F, Brache V, Fernandez E: New insights on the mode of action of intrauterine contraceptive devices in women, *Fertil Steril* 49:768, 1988.

Attico NB: Contraception update: barrier methods, IUDs, and sterilization, *Fam Pract Recert* 14(1):45, 1992.

Farley TM et al: Intrauterine devices and pelvic inflammatory disease: an international perspective, *Lancet* 339:785, 1992.

FDA Pink Sheet. October 21, 1991.

Kronmal R, Whitney C, Mumford S: The intrauterine device and pelvic inflammatory disease: the Women's Health Study reanalyzed, *J Clin Epidemiol* 44:109, 1991.

Lee N, Rubin G, Boruchi R: The intrauterine device and pelvic inflammatory disease revisited: new results from the Women's Health Study, *Obstet Gynecol* 72:1, 1988.

Ory HW: Mortality associated fertility and fertility control, *Fam Plann Perspect* 15:57, 1983.

Pfenninger JL: Technique for inserting an IUD, *Fam Pract Recert* 14:131, 1992.

Speroff L: Levonorgestrel and copper IUDs are excellent contraceptive devices, *Obstet/Gynecol Clincial Alert* 10(12):89, 1994.

Speroff L: The IUD and PID, *Ob-Gyn Clinical Alert* 9:9, 1992 (editorial).

CHAPTER 76

IUD Removal

John L. Pfenninger

Generally, intrauterine contraceptive device (IUD) removal is a simple and uncomplicated procedure that takes only a few minutes. The rare case in which the IUD string is not visible presents a more challenging situation.

REMOVAL WITH IDENTIFIABLE STRINGS

The usual IUD removal is uncomplicated, and there is no need for sterile technique. Insert the speculum, and visualize the strings. Using ring forceps, grasp the IUD strings and then pull toward the introitus in a firm and deliberate motion until the IUD is delivered. The patient will experience momentary discomfort, which may be prevented somewhat by premedicating with 800 mg of ibuprofen. Remove the speculum and send the patient home. Some minor spotting may be expected for a few days.

WHEN THE IUD STRINGS ARE NOT VISIBLE

If the speculum is inserted and IUD strings cannot be visualized after a diligent search, one of several approaches may be used. The simplest procedure employs a long-handled, hemostatlike instrument such as uterine packing forceps. Insert this instrument into the os, with the instrument opened as much as the os will allow. Close the jaws in hopes that the strings are grasped. If the strings are indeed grasped, resistance will be felt when the instrument is removed. Carry out this maneuver four or five times in an attempt to grasp the strings. If unsuccessful, or if the os is too small, other methods will be needed to find the strings.

Some suggest using an endocervical speculum along with the colposcope. Frequently the end of the string is just within the os. Once visualized, it is much more easily grasped with forceps and removed.

Should these techniques fail, proceed with a more invasive technique. Perform a bimanual examination to identify the position of the uterus. Prepare the area with an antiseptic solution. Grasp the anterior lip with a cervical tenaculum and apply slight traction to straighten the uterus. A uterine sound may be used to dilate the internal os. Alternatively, one of the variety of IUD removers can be used to enter

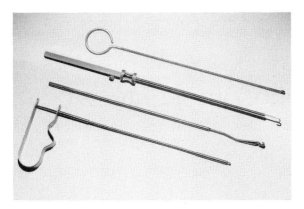

FIG. 76-1.
IUD removal instruments. *From top to bottom:* simple IUD hook, universal IUD hook, double IUD extractor, and flexible IUD hook.

the intrauterine cavity (Fig. 76-1). The double IUD extractor and flexible IUD hook are more commonly used. The double IUD extractor resembles a crochet hook and will frequently "hook" the IUD. Use a twisting motion to wrap the strings around the hook for removal. The flexible IUD hook is actually a forceps. Insert the stem into the uterus and compress the handle to open the jaws. When the handle is released, the jaws grasp the IUD as they close. Then withdraw the unit. If the string or the IUD is grasped, resistance will be felt. Using the larger-sized instrument will prevent or minimize perforation of the uterus.

If the IUD has been in place for a significant length of time, it may have become embedded in the endometrium, and significant force will be required to remove it. If the force seems to be extreme or there is any question whether or not the IUD is still in place, it may be best to defer removal. Although a flat plate of the abdomen will identify whether the IUD is present (IUDs are radiopaque), the X-ray will not indicate whether the IUD is intrauterine. A pelvic ultrasound examination, on the other hand, will confirm whether it is present *and* whether it is intrauterine. If it has moved to an extrauterine position, surgery will be required.

If an intrauterine IUD is confirmed by ultrasound, the patient must return for a subsequent visit when further, more aggressive attempts can be made to remove it. If all else fails, the patient may require a dilation and curettage procedure, with the IUD removed under anesthesia or hysteroscopy-guided removal.

SUPPLIERS

The various IUD removal instruments should be available from most medical supply firms. Those seen in Fig. 76-1 are from Zinnanti Surgical Instruments, 21540-B Prairie St., Chatsworth, CA 91311; 1-800-223-4740.

CPT/BILLING CODE

58301   IUD removal

CHAPTER 77

Culdocentesis (Colpocentesis)

Steven H. Eisinger

Culdocentesis is a procedure performed in female patients to detect and sample free intraperitoneal fluid. With this procedure, critical diagnostic information can be obtained for a variety of important gynecologic conditions, such as ectopic pregnancy and pelvic inflammatory disease. The implications of the results are usually clear-cut, but must always be considered in the context of the patient's total clinical picture.

INDICATIONS

Broadly speaking, any suspicion of free fluid within the peritoneal cavity of a woman may be an indication for culdocentesis.

Ectopic Pregnancy

The classic and most widely applied indication for culdocentesis is a suspected leaking or ruptured tubal ectopic pregnancy. Approximately one in a hundred pregnancies is ectopic. In a typical tubal ectopic pregnancy, intraperitoneal hemorrhage will eventually occur. Hemoperitoneum will cause pelvic peritonitis, which is manifested by rebound tenderness in the lower abdomen without guarding, and tenderness on cervical motion. Surprisingly, the signs of peritonitis may sometimes be very subtle or absent, even in the presence of relatively large amounts of free blood in the abdomen. Eventually, more generalized peritonitis will occur, causing abdominal pain and distension, ileus, shoulder pain, and a "doughy" feel to the abdomen. The cul de sac may bulge into the vagina on speculum examination. When these signs of pelvic peritonitis are combined with the classic signs of ectopic pregnancy—positive pregnancy test, amenorrhea followed by vaginal bleeding—emergency culdocentesis is indicated to determine whether intraperitoneal bleeding is occurring. While other more sophisticated methods exist to diagnose ectopic pregnancy (such as ultrasound, B-HCG determinations, and laparoscopy), in the emergency room setting, culdocentesis remains the fastest, easiest, and surest way to confirm the diagnosis. Indeed, a culdocentesis showing blood, along with a positive pregnancy test, is associated with ectopic pregnancy more than 99% of the time.

Acute Salpingitis

The second major indication for culdocentesis is acute salpingitis, also known as pelvic inflammatory disease (PID). Clinical signs and symptoms of acute salpingitis vary and are sometimes difficult to interpret. Classically, a woman will have progressive aching lower abdominal pain, often beginning during or after her menstrual period. On examination she will have fever, rebound tenderness, and exquisite tenderness on motion of the cervix or palpation of the adnexa, which may be enlarged. Again, pelvic peritonitis is the key finding, indicating irritating fluid (in this case, pus) free in the lower abdomen. Accurate diagnosis is important; however, false-negative and false-positive diagnoses of acute salpingitis are quite frequent. The fastest means of establishing the diagnosis is by obtaining pus through culdocentesis. Many authorities are now advocating that culdocentesis be considered in all cases of suspected acute salpingitis when laparoscopic diagnosis is not feasible.

Other Indications

A ruptured cyst may cause pain and pelvic peritonitis. Culdocentesis will demonstrate the cyst fluid free in the abdomen. Occasionally, a ruptured cyst will create a hemoperitoneum as dramatic and dangerous as that associated with a ruptured ectopic pregnancy.

Ascitic fluid may be obtained through culdocentesis either for diagnostic purposes—such as sampling for the cytology laboratory to assess for ovarian cancer—or for relief of the symptoms of excessive ascites.

CONTRAINDICATIONS

- A cul de sac mass is a contraindication for culdocentesis, because such a mass could be a benign or malignant neoplasm, an endometrioma, an abscess, or an unruptured ectopic pregnancy whose rupture would be harmful.
- If the uterus is in fixed retroversion, then the cul de sac will be obliterated and culdocentesis will be impossible.

EQUIPMENT

The equipment required for culdocentesis is simple and should be available in any well-equipped office or emergency room (Figs. 77-1 and 77-2).

- Speculum
- Single-tooth tenaculum or Allis forceps

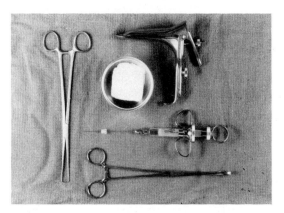

FIG. 77-1.
Equipment required to perform culdocentesis: single-tooth tenaculum, sponges, graves speculum, three-finger control syringe with 20-gauge spinal needle, and sponge forceps.

- 10 or 20 cc syringe
- 20-gauge spinal needle or a 3-inch needle extender
- 1½-inch 20-gauge needle
- Sterile swabs or sponges
- Forceps
- Antiseptic solution
- *Optional:* three-finger control syringe (helpful but not essential; it allows the clinician to aspirate with one hand)

The instruments should be sterile. Universal blood precautions should be followed, although technically face masks, drapes, and so forth are not necessary.

TECHNIQUE

1. Perform a standard pelvic examination prior to culdocentesis. During the speculum examination, vaginal cultures may be obtained or other tests performed. A bulging of the cul de sac into the posterior fornix of the vagina is a finding suggestive of the presence of intraperitoneal fluid.
2. During the bimanual examination, determine the size, position, and mobility of the uterus. If the uterus is fixed in retroversion, culdocentesis should not be performed. On the other hand, a mobile retroverted uterus may be manipulated and moved out of the way by lifting or pulling on the cervix with a tenaculum. An anterior uterus presents no problem. The cul de sac must be determined to be free of masses by examination. A fixed mass in the cul de sac is a contraindication to culdocentesis.
3. Position the patient. Allow the patient to walk or sit up for a short time before the procedure. Fluid will then collect in the cul de sac. To prevent a

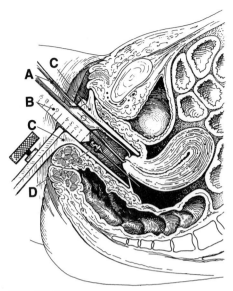

FIG. 77-2.
The instruments as they are used for culdocentesis: *A,* Allis forceps or tenaculum; *B,* syringe; *C,* speculum; *D,* 20-gauge spinal needle. (From *Stedman's Medical Dictionary,* ed 25, Baltimore, 1990, Williams & Wilkins. Used with permission.)

syncopal episode, observe caution in raising a patient with suspected intraperitoneal hemorrhage to an upright position.

The correct position for culdocentesis is the lithotomy position, with the head and shoulders raised slightly. The procedure may be performed in the office or emergency room setting on a regular examining table with stirrups.

4. Place the speculum. A medium Graves speculum is suitable for most patients. Open it as wide as the patient can tolerate. This will expose the posterior vaginal fornix and stretch the mucosa taut, making the procedure easier.
5. Cleanse the vagina with a suitable antiseptic solution.
6. Grasp the cervix with a tenaculum or Allis forceps (Fig. 77-3). The tenaculum may be placed vertically or horizontally on the anterior or posterior lip of the cervix, as the clinician desires. Grasping the cervix with a tenaculum causes discomfort for most women; therefore, a small amount of local anesthetic may be injected at the tenaculum site.
7. Choose the puncture site. Manipulate the cervix gently with the tenaculum either by pulling in and out or up and down. This maneuver is to identify the point of reflection of the vaginal mucosa below the cervix where the mucosa sweeps off the cervix and crosses or covers the cul de sac. Insert the needle about 1 cm below this reflection, in the midline. If the puncture site is too high, the needle will hit the substance of the cervix. If the needle is placed too low, it may enter the rectum or tunnel beneath the posterior peritoneum of the cul de sac.
8. Administer anesthesia, if desired. Culdocentesis is generally perceived by women as quite painful. Some clinicians recommend injecting a small

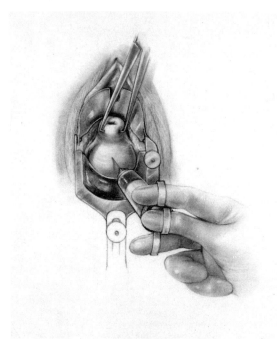

FIG. 77-3.
Operator's view of culdocentesis. Note the widely opened speculum, the tenaculum grasping the lower lip of the cervix and elevating it in the vagina, and the bulging posterior vaginal fornix. The puncture site is about a centimeter below the deflection of the mucosa from the cervix onto the posterior fornix. The needle is held approximately horizontally to seek the pool of fluid and to avoid puncturing the rectum. (From Eisinger SH: Procedure in family practice: culdocentesis, *JFP* 13:95, 1981. Used with permission.)

amount of local anesthetic into the puncture site. Others believe that the anesthetic injection is painful and that it may confuse the issue by causing some intraperitoneal bleeding. A calm and complete explanation of the procedure usually improves patient cooperation and minimizes anxiety. The patient may be reassured that although the pain is sharp, it is bearable and will only last for a few seconds. Judiciously selected intravenous narcotics or sedatives, such as 50 mg of meperidine (Demerol) or 3 to 5 mg of midazolam (Versed), can be very helpful.

9. Make the puncture. Elevate the cervix in the vagina to stretch the mucosa, and retract it outward to pull the uterus out of retroversion, if necessary. Two or three cubic centimeters of air may be placed in the syringe prior to puncture, although this step should be omitted if infection is suspected. Perform the puncture itself with a bold, smooth movement, inserting the needle 3 to 4 cm through mucosa. The needle should be approximately horizontal.

10. Inject the air in the syringe. If there is resistance to air injection, the needle tip is in a solid organ, such as the uterus, and should be repositioned;

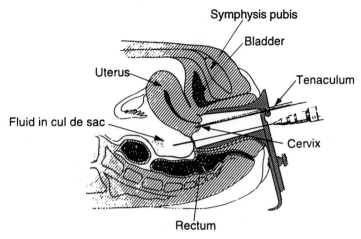

FIG. 77-4.
Midline sagittal view of pelvis during culdocentesis showing anatomic relationships and position of instruments. Note the depth of the needle puncture and the proximity of the tip to adjacent structures. (From Eisinger SH: Procedure in family practice: culdocentesis, *JFP* 13:95, 1981. Used with permission.)

usually, the air passes freely. Sometimes the air may be heard bubbling through free fluid.

11. Pull back on the syringe plunger, strongly aspirating while withdrawing the needle slowly. If fluid is obtained, the syringe should be filled and the needle withdrawn. If no fluid is obtained, a second or even third attempt may be made at a slightly different location or angle. A spray of bloody, frothy fluid is often seen just as the needle emerges from the mucosa. This is blood from the venus plexus of the vaginal mucosa and should not be interpreted as a bloody tap.

12. Terminate the procedure when fluid is obtained, or when three taps fail to yield any fluid. Remove all instruments from the vagina and allow the patient to rest. Bleeding from the puncture and tenaculum sites is usually slight and will abate in a few hours.

13. Examine the fluid from the cul de sac. Observe blood from the cul de sac for several minutes for clotting that would indicate a traumatic tap. Blood-tinged or frankly bloody fluid should be spun for a hematocrit. Turbid or clear fluid should be examined microscopically by means of a Gram stain, and cultures—both aerobic and anaerobic—should be obtained.

COMPLICATIONS

Culdocentesis is generally quite free of complications. Both the small and large bowel are probably pierced rather frequently with no observed ill effects. A serious potential complication is in puncturing or rupturing various pathologic pelvic structures listed under Contraindications.

Intrapelvic hemorrhage as a result of the procedure must be very rare inasmuch as the great vessels of the pelvis lie away from the midline and should not be approached by the needle tip. The most significant hazard of the procedure is a deceptive result, providing unwarranted reassurance or leading to unnecessary treatment.

INTERPRETING RESULTS

Blood obtained from the cul de sac should be tested in two ways: for clotting ability and hematocrit. Pooled blood within the peritoneal cavity is defibrinated and will not clot. However, in a ruptured ectopic pregnancy, bleeding is occasionally so brisk that the blood does not have time to become defibrinated.

It is surprising how low the hematocrit can be in fluid that appears quite bloody. As a rough rule, a hematocrit below 15% probably indicates either a minor amount of bleeding or a bloody tap. Frank blood is an indication for immediate surgery, but blood-tinged fluid can usually be managed with observation. In medical centers and well-equipped hospitals, laparoscopy is increasingly the procedure of choice for both definitive diagnosis and surgical treatment. There is still a place, however, for emergency laparotomy in the presence of hemoperitoneum, particularly if the patient shows any sign of hemodynamic instability.

Pus or turbid fluid should always be Gram stained and microscopically examined: white blood cells and bacteria are often identified. Cultures of specimens obtained from the cul de sac are the best means of assessing the bacteriology of a pelvic infection without performing surgery. However, cultures obtained from culdocentesis fluid do not always accurately reflect the bacteriology of the infection. Pus, particularly watery pus, indicates that acute salpingitis is the problem in most cases, and treatment should be medical. Appendicitis can also produce an exudate with white blood cells in it.

Clear fluid commonly is obtained in three situations: clear fluid may be the contents of a ruptured ovarian cyst; it may be ascites; or, in small amounts, it may be normal. In general, aspirated clear fluid is reassuring, and no active management is required. Dark brown, chocolate-like material is old blood. A ruptured endometrioma is the most likely cause, but any cyst that contains old blood, including the cyst of a chronic ectopic pregnancy, can contain chocolate-like fluid.

Somewhat less than half the time, no fluid at all can be obtained, even with repeated efforts. This phenomenon should be referred to as a dry tap, not a negative tap. *No diagnostic assumptions should be made on the basis of a dry tap.* The needle may simply not have found the pool of fluid. When a dry tap occurs, physicians must resort to ultrasound, laparoscopy, or other expensive and invasive techniques, or they must rely wholly on their clinical acumen to make the correct diagnosis.

CPT/BILLING CODE

57020   Colpocentesis

BIBLIOGRAPHY

Droegemueller W et al: *Comprehensive gynecology,* St Louis, 1987, Mosby.

Eisinger SH: Procedures in family practice: culdocentesis, *JFP* 13:1, 1981.

Hager WD et al: Criteria for diagnosis and grading of salpingitis, *Obstet Gynecol* 61(1):113, 1983.

Romero R et al: Value of culdocentesis in the diagnosis of ectopic pregnancy, *Obstet Gynecol* 65(4):519, 1985.

Schneider D et al: Outcome of continued pregnancies after first- and second-trimester cervical dilatation by laminaria tents, *Obstet Gynecol* 78(6): 1121, 1991.

Vermesh M, Graczykowski JW, Sauer MV: Reevaluation of the role of culdocentesis in the management of ectopic pregnancy, *Am J Obstet Gynecol* 162:411, 1990.

CHAPTER 78

Bartholin's Cyst/Abscess: Word Catheter Insertion

Barbara S. Apgar

Simple incision and drainage of a Bartholin duct cyst or abscess may give immediate and dramatic results, but the recurrence rate after such a procedure is unacceptably high. The glands are located at the vaginal opening at the crease between the hymen and labia minora (at approximately the 5 and 7 o'clock positions). Total excision of the gland and duct is rarely required. Total excision requires a hospital operating room, involves excessive cost, and is associated with increased morbidity. It is preferable to create an epithelialized tract from the vulvar vestibule to the cyst, which allows for continued functioning of the Bartholin's gland, proper drainage, and minimal recurrence. Use of a Word catheter creates a fistulous tract that preserves the gland and allows for adequate drainage. Recurrence using this technique is between 2% and 15%. The Word catheter has a short latex stem with an inflatable bulb at the distal end (Fig. 78-1).

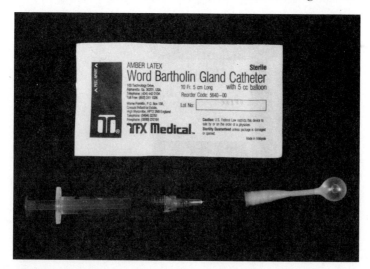

FIG. 78-1.
Word Bartholin gland catheter.

INDICATIONS

- Treatment of symptomatic Bartholin's gland cyst
- Treatment and culture of Bartholin's gland abscess (often gonococcal)

CONTRAINDICATIONS

Any condition that would preclude normal incision and drainage of a vulvar cyst or abcess would preclude use of the Word catheter. Small asymptomatic glands do not need to be drained.

PREPROCEDURE PATIENT EDUCATION AND PREPARATION

Explain the procedure to the patient and obtain informed consent. Administer a nonnarcotic oral analgesic to the patient prior to the procedure, if desired.

EQUIPMENT

- Word Bartholin's gland catheter (One source is FX Medical, 100 Technology Drive, Alpharetta, GA; telephone: 800-241-1926; however the catheter is available from most medical supply companies.)
- 3 cc syringe (for catheter inflation)
- 22-gauge 1-inch needle (for catheter inflation)
- 1% to 2% lidocaine for anesthesia
- 30-gauge 1-inch needle (for anesthesia)
- 3 cc syringe (for anesthesia)
- No. 11 blade
- Pickups with teeth
- 4 × 4 inch gauze pads
- Normal saline for irrigation
- Antiseptic solution (povidone-iodine)

TECHNIQUE

1. Prepare the vestibule with the antiseptic solution. Inject lidocaine just inside the hymen, if possible. If the incision is to be made external to the hymen, plan to insert the catheter approximately in the area of the original duct orifice, immediately adjacent to the hymenal ring.
2. Lance or incise the cyst or abcess with the scalpel blade. It is essential that the stab wound penetrate the cyst wall, which will be evidenced by the free flow of pus or mucus. Culture contents if indicated. The stab wound must be just

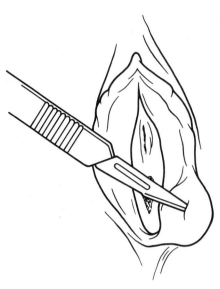

FIG. 78-2.
Incision should be just large enough to admit the uninflated Word catheter.

large enough for the catheter to be inserted, usually 3 to 4 mm (Fig. 78-2). It may be difficult to enter the cyst after the incision is made and the sac is compressed. To preserve the tract, grasp the cyst wall using pickups with teeth as the incision is made. One arm of the pickups slides down the side of the blade into the lumen while the other grasps externally. This enables stabilization of the tissue while the catheter is inserted. Grasping the cyst wall in this fashion also prevents the creation of false tracts outside the cyst itself.

3. Insert a small hemostat into the stab wound and break away any loculations. Instill 25 to 50 cc of normal saline into the cyst to wash out the cyst cavity.

4. Insert the sterile catheter into the incision and inflate the bulb by injecting 2 to 3 cc of saline through the sealed-stopper end. Use just that quantity of water necessary to ensure that the catheter will not fall out with normal activity. Do *not* use air to inflate the catheter. A common problem occurs when the clinician injects the fluid into the balloon, lets go of the syringe plunger, and checks the tightness of the balloon in the cavity. The increased pressure in the balloon will push the saline back up into the syringe; the balloon then deflates and the catheter may fall out. To prevent this, *maintain pressure* on the syringe plunger while checking the bulb (Fig. 78-3).

5. If the incision was made inside the hymen, tuck the catheter stem into the vagina, where it will rest perpendicular to the perineum. With the catheter in the vagina, the patient has freedom of movement and activity without the added awareness of protrusion of the catheter stem, which can occur if an external incision site is used. Most patients tolerate the catheter without discomfort.

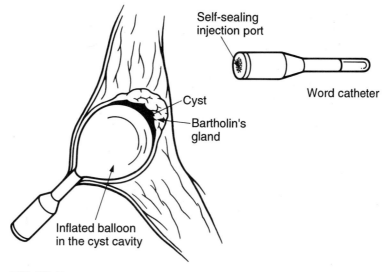

Self-sealing
injection port

Word catheter

Cyst

Bartholin's
gland

Inflated balloon
in the cyst cavity

FIG. 78-3.
A balloon is inflated within the cavity of the cyst so that it will not fall out through the stab wound.

POSTPROCEDURE CARE

- Tell the patient to expect a discharge, as the catheter will allow for drainage of the cyst or abcess.
- The catheter is left in place for 4 to 6 weeks until epithelization of the new tract is complete.
- Advise the patient that sexual activity may be resumed after 2 weeks, but it may cause expulsion of the catheter. If this happens, the catheter may need to be reinserted. If possible, it is best to defer sexual activity until the catheter is out.
- Encourage daily showers or tub baths.
- Schedule a return visit with the patient in 4 to 6 weeks. At that time, the catheter is removed by inserting a needle into the catheter sealed-stopper end and drawing out the saline. The catheter is then withdrawn from the incision.

COMPLICATIONS

- Continuous pain after insertion of the catheter may occur. The bulb may be too large for the cyst cavity, which may be corrected by withdrawing some of the fluid, thus reducing the size of the bulb.
- With an abscessed Bartholin's gland, there may be cellulitis around the vulvar opening of the duct. Simple incision and drainage may not correct the cellulitis, and antibiotics may need to be administered for 48 to 72 hours after insertion of the catheter.

- If the needle used to introduce the saline into the catheter punctures the stem, the catheter will gradually deflate and fall out before epithelization is complete.
- If the stab wound is too large, the catheter will fall out. It may be necessary to suture the stab wound around the catheter to keep it in place.

CPT/BILLING CODES

56405	Incision and drainage of vulvar or perianal abscess
56420	Incision and drainage of Bartholin's gland abscess
56440	Marsupialization of Bartholin's gland cyst
56740	Excision of Bartholin's gland or cyst

BIBLIOGRAPHY

Cohen SD et al: Management of the Bartholin's abscess, *Am J Gynecol Health* 4(3):42, 1990.

Goldberg JE: Simplified treatment for disease of Bartholin's gland, *Obstet Gynecol* 35:109, 1970.

Heah J: Methods of treatment for cysts and abscesses of Bartholin's gland, *Br J Obstet Gynecol* 95:321, 1988.

Oliphant MM, Anderson GV: Management of Bartholin's duct cysts and abscesses, *Obstet Gynecol* 16:476, 1960.

Word B: New instrument for office treatment of cyst and abscess of Bartholin's gland, *JAMA* 190:777, 1964.

CHAPTER 79

The Pap Smear: Screening for Cervical Cancer

Gary R. Newkirk

Despite the controversies surrounding Papanicolaou (Pap) smear testing, it remains an effective tool for cancer prevention and detection. Numerous studies have documented a statistically valid drop in the incidence and mortality rates of invasive cervical carcinomas since the introduction of the Pap smear. Unfortunately, cervical cancer screening has not eradicated this potentially preventable disease. The current cervical cancer detection system relies on a complex system of clinical and laboratory procedures that have potential for error at numerous places. Koss's landmark discussion summarizes major sources of error including (1) problems with the initial clinical examination, (2) inappropriate smear collection technique, (3) laboratory errors in sample preparation and interpretation, (4) errors in report interpretation, (5) failure of the clinician to understand or appropriately respond to Pap smear–generated data, and (6) failure of the patient to follow the clinician's recommendations.

Compelling arguments link cervical neoplasia with human papillomavirus (HPV) infection. Epidemiologic data further document the epidemic proportions of new genital HPV infections. There appears to be escalating pressure to rely on Pap smear screening methodology, yet recent reports documenting between 20% and 40% false-negative results alarm patients and clinicians alike. Clinicians can continue to make significant contributions to cancer prevention in women by refining their method of Pap smear sampling, by enhancing their understanding of Pap smear report interpretation, and by clarifying their recommendations for patient management. This chapter focuses on a contemporary approach to Pap smear screening; it is assumed that basic pelvic examination skills have been mastered. Table 79-1 offers a brief summary of the terminology used throughout this discussion.

It must be remembered that the Pap smear is a *screening test only;* it is *not diagnostic*. Thus, if an abnormality is seen or palpated at the time of the examination, it should be examined with a colposcope. The physician cannot rely on the Pap smear alone to be diagnostic for that particular lesion.

TABLE 79-1.

Terminology and Definitions (Also see Chapter 81, The Colposcopic Examination)

1. Ectocervix	Also called exocervix. The flat portion of the cervix that is readily visible. Cervical os is located centrally.
2. Exocervix	See *ectocervix.*
3. Squamous cells	Epithelial cells that line the ectocervix; nonkeratinized, stratified epithelium. These cells appear smooth and pink on the cervix.
4. Columnar epithelium	Sincle-layer, mucin-secreting epithelium that lines the endocervix.
5. Endocervical cells	Glandular, columnar-shaped cells obtained from the endocervical epithelium (endocervical canal).
6. Squamocolumnar junction	Area where the squamous epithelium of the ectocervix joins the mucus-secreting columnar epithelium of the endocervix.
7. Squamous metaplasia	A type of tissue present where columnar epithelium is being replaced (transformed) by squamous epithelium. This normal tissue occurs within the cervical transformation zone.
8. Transformation zone	Area of transformation or replacement of the endocervical columnar epithelium by squamous epithelium through a process called metaplastic change. Principal site of origin for precancerous and invasive squamous cell carcinomas of the cervix.
9. Koilocytotic	Equivalent terms include condylomatous atypia and HPV effect; these terms describe cells that have perinuclear halos or vacuoles that vary in shape and configuration, and that show a distinct zone of clearing between the nucleus and cytoplasmic membrane. The abnormal nuclei are characterized by wrinkling, variation in size and shape, binucleate forms, and hyperchromasia. Usually indicative of HPV infection.
10. Dysplasia CIN	Cervical intraepithelial neoplasia. An abnormality of cervical epithelium displaying proliferation of parabasal cells with disordered polarity, loss of cellular junctions, coarse nuclear chromatin clumping, abnormal nuclear cytoplasmic ratio, and high mitotic index. Reported as grades I (low grade) to III (high grade, including carcinoma in situ) dysplasia.
SIL	Squamous intraepithelial lesion. Reported as either low or high grade, corresponding to increasing severity of dysplasia (Bethesda terminology).
11. Carcinoma in situ	Synonomous with severe dysplasia, CIN III.
12. Microinvasive cervical cancer	Invasion 3 mm or less below the basement membrane.
13. Frankly invasive cervical cancer	Invasion greater than 3 mm below the basement membrane.

INDICATIONS

- Screening: All women by age 18 or with onset of sexual activity; annually thereafter. (Some clinicians will screen a subset of women with low risk factors every 3 years providing that there are three negative yearly Pap smears and the risk factors do not change. Box 79-1 summarizes these risk factors for cervical dysplasia. Most clinicians find this modified screening methodology impractical and clinically difficult to apply.)

BOX 79-1. RISK FACTORS FOR ABNORMAL PAP SMEARS

1. Early age of first intercourse (under age 18)
2. Multiple sexual partners (more than three) or history of sexual abuse
3. Tobacco smoking
4. Other sexually transmitted disease
5. Illicit drug use (intravenous or oral)
6. History of genital condylomata
7. History of abnormal Pap smear
8. Sexual partner with genital condylomata
9. A sexual partner with more than three sexual partners

- Diethylstilbestrol (DES)–exposed offspring: At least by age 14, onset of menstruation, or initial sexual activity; every 6 to 12 months thereafter if colposcopy and biopsy is performed and tissue is found to be benign. DES-exposed offspring require colposcopic evaluation (and repeat colposcopy with biopsy as necessary). The appropriate Pap smear follow-up usually requires modified routines determined by coordinated exchange of expert opinion between the clinician, pathologist, and, quite often, a gynecologist familiar with this small subgroup of women.
- Any visible or palpable lesion of the cervix. Follow precaution that Pap smear is *not* diagnostic and further assessment may be necessary.
- Any abnormal vaginal bleeding or discharge.
- Posthysterectomy (hysterectomy for benign disease): Every 3 years if patient's risk for cancer remains low.
- Posthysterectomy (hysterectomy for dysplasia, carcinoma): annually after three to four normal Pap smears at 4- to 6-month intervals.
- Posttreatment for cervical dysplasia, malignancy: Every 4 months for three visits; every 6 months for two visits; annually thereafter.
- Victims of rape, incest, abuse: As part of initial work-up. Repeat in 6 to 12 months.

There are numerous schemes for follow-up after treatment for cervical dysplasia and carcinoma. All involve increased frequency of Pap smear testing for a period of time. Repeat colposcopic examination is often performed with endocervical curettage or cervical biopsy, if necessary. All women with a history of cervical dysplasia remain at significant risk for disease recurrence and should undergo Pap smear testing at least annually for life.

CONTRAINDICATIONS

There are no absolute contraindications to obtaining a Pap smear. Relative contraindications include clinical circumstances where sample collection is difficult to obtain or difficult to interpret (e.g., active vaginitis or cervicitis, pelvic inflammatory disease [PID], or menses). The clinician must weigh the benefits versus the risk of obtaining the screening Pap smear under these circumstances. For instance, if a woman presents with abnormal vaginal bleeding, a Pap smear is advised, despite the presence of blood. This contrasts with a patient who comes in for a routine Pap smear screening and has begun to menstruate. In the later instance, the Pap smear can be deferred to a more favorable time.

EQUIPMENT AND SUPPLIERS

- Examination table appropriate for placing the patient in the lithotomy position
- A warm, well-lighted examination room
- Various-sized speculums: Graves (metal)—many suppliers, $14.00 to $20.00 each; Pederson (metal); plastic, disposable—25/box about $1.60 each (Welch-Allyn, Inc; Durr-Fillauer Medical, Inc.; Miltex Instrument Company)
- Water-soluble lubricant (e.g., K-Y Jelly)
- Nonsterile examination gloves for the clinician
- Large swabs for gently blotting excess discharge
- Method for warming the speculum (warm water or speculum drawer warmer [lightbulb])
- Cotton swabs (numerous sources)
- Wooden spatulas (Hardwood Products Co., Cervical Scraper No. 7, P.O. Box 149, Guilford, ME 04443) or plastic spatula (Cervical Scraper, 8.5″, Milex-Western, P.O. Box 46305, Los Angeles, CA 90046) for ectocervical sample
- Cytobrush Plus for endocervical sample (Mediscand USA Inc., P.O. Box 7733, Hollywood, FL 33081; telephone: 800-235-7697)
- As an alternative to taking two samples, a "broom" device can be used for ecto/endocervical sample (Cervexbrush, Unimar, 475 Danbury Road, Wilton, CT 06897; telephone: 203-762-9550; Papette, Wallach Surgical Devices, 291 Pepe's Farm Road, Milford, CT 06460; telephone: 203-783-1818)
- Microscope slides, fixative (common hairspray; consult with reference laboratory performing cytology)
- Appropriate patient identification, history forms to accompany Pap smear and other tests
- Culture or transport media and swabs as necessary for gonorrhea, chlamydia, herpes, fungal, and KOH/wet mount
- Cervical tenaculum or cervical hook (rarely needed)
- Ring forceps
- *Optional:* Lugol's solution (approximately $6.00/pint, local pharmacy)
- *Optional:* 5% acetic acid solution ($3.00/gal, white vinegar, local grocery store)

SAMPLING DEVICES

Concern over the frequency of false-negative results of the Pap smear has led to the development of newer Pap smear sampling techniques. Despite the higher costs for

AGE 12
(puberty)

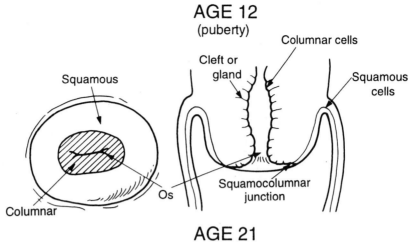

AGE 21
(sexually active)

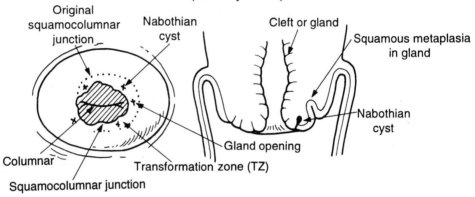

AGE 45
("perimenopausal")

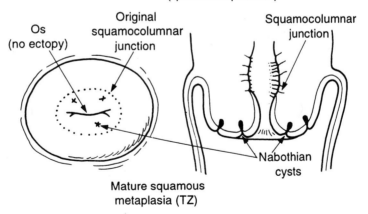

FIG. 79-1.

Appearance of cervix in various age groups. The area most at risk in all age groups is the transformation zone (TZ), including the squamocolumnar junction (SCJ). Note how location varies with age. The entire TZ must be sampled to maximize efficacy of the Pap smear. The SCJ migrates inward with aging.

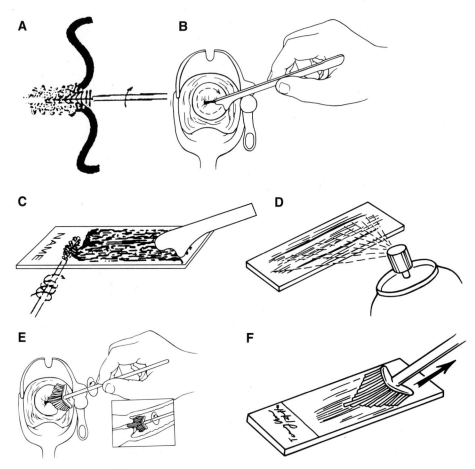

FIG. 79-2.
Obtaining the pap smear. **A,** Endocervical sample with cytobrush. **B,** Ectocervical sample obtained with a woooden or plastic spatula. **C,** A single-slide technique is preferred. First, the spatula sample is spread followed by "unrolling" the brush sample directly over the first sample. **D,** Immediate fixation of the slide with cytologic fixative. **E,** Alternatively, a single sampling device may be used. (Cervexbrush or "broom") to obtain both electrical and endocervical sample at the same time. **F,** Spreading the sample from broom device on to slide.

these sampling devices (nominally $0.40 to $0.60 each), the increased quality of smears, the improved detection rates, and, ultimately, the fewer patients who must return for "inadequate" repeat smears more than justify this added expense. The routine use of the Cytobrush, Cervexbrush, Papette, or similar devices is recommended by most authorities. Sampling of the endocervical canal should always be coupled with sampling of the entire transformation zone (Figs. 79-1 and 79-2).

The Pap smear test is considered exfoliative cytology; the transformation zone need not be dermabraded of its mucosa to obtain an adequate sample. Sharp, fine-edged plastic devices are advocated by some physicians; however, wood works fine. A bloody Pap smear sample decreases detection rate. Fig. 79-3 illustrates several of the common sampling devices that achieve satisfactory sampling. Clinicians should not be locked into using a single method of

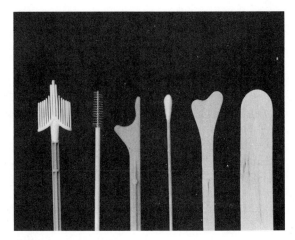

FIG. 79-3.
Papanicolaou sampling devices. *Left to right:* Cervexbrush, Cytobrush, Miltex plastic sampler, cotton swab, wooden ayre spatula, and tongue blade.

transformation zone sampling; they should choose a technique based on patient anatomy. The days of the "one size fits everybody" Pap smear sampling device should be over.

PREPROCEDURE PATIENT EDUCATION

Your patient should understand the reason for performing the Pap smear. The Pap smear is best performed during midcycle. The patient should avoid douching, vaginal medications, and intercourse for 24 hours prior to the procedure. Reschedule the examination if the patient is actively menstruating. The patient should void before unclothing for the examination. Inform the patient of the mechanisms you use to follow up on test results (Pap smear, cultures, etc.).

TECHNIQUE

1. Obtain history, review systems, and answer questions. Clarify the patient's risk factors for cervical dysplasia.
2. Proceed with the general medical and breast examination, leaving the pelvic examination for last.
3. Label the frosted end of the glass slide with the patient's name and other identifying data as necessary.
4. Place the patient in the lithotomy position, and begin the examination. Wear gloves. Inspect the vulva, and assess hair pattern, anatomy, estrogen effect, discharge, and any abnormal areas. Ask the patient if she has any concerns.
5. Place a small amount of water-soluble lubricant on the speculum and insert it. Carefully advance the speculum, applying gentle pressure posteriorly.

Consider using a vaginal stint in patients whose vaginal walls prolapse and obstruct view. This can be fashioned by cutting off both ends of a single finger of a latex rubber glove and placing it over the blades of the speculum (Fig. 79-4).

6. Adjust the speculum to obtain adequate visualization of the cervix, and tighten the screw or lock the speculum open.

7. Determine whether the vagina or cervix appears inflamed or infected. Avoid rubbing or otherwise traumatizing the cervix.

8. Identify cervical landmarks, including the transformation zone with its squamocolumnar junction. Note the nature of the cervical mucus. Excess mucus or discharge may be gently blotted, not rubbed, from view. Note any gross cervical lesions such as erosions, leukoplakia, nabothian cysts, or condylomata (see Table 79-1). Examine the vaginal fornices for obvious abnormalities.

9. Obtain the Pap smear by using an endocervical sampling device (Cytobrush, Papette, or Cervexbrush). If the two-sample method of obtaining cells is used, first insert the Cytobrush into the canal and rotate 90 to 180 degrees. Follow this by a gentle smear of the entire transformation zone with a spatula device, fitting the contour of the patient's remaining transformation zone. Broom devices (Papette, Cervexbrush) are inserted and rotated 360 degrees five times. They obtain both endo and ectocervical samples at the same time.

   Sampling the vaginal pool has little advantage during Pap smear screening unless the patient has had a hysterectomy. In this instance, be sure to sample the vaginal cuff. If vaginal abnormalities are seen, another Pap smear of these areas (using a spatula) may be submitted on a separate slide. Areas that appear abnormal on visualization will ultimately require colposcopy and biopsy.

10. If a one-slide smear technique is suggested by your reference lab (check with your pathologist), withhold smearing the endocervical Cytobrush

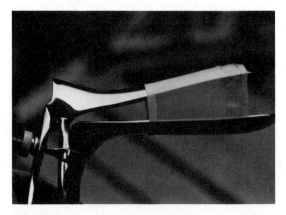

FIG. 79-4.
Vaginal speculum stint. To aid in the visualization of the cervix, a single finger of a latex examination glove can be cut off and placed over the blades of a standard vaginal speculum. This is helpful if there is redundant vaginal mucosa as seen with pregnancy, obesity, or multiparity.

sample on the slide until the spatula sample is smeared first. Follow this quickly by applying the Cytobrush sample (which is much less subject to drying artifact). If a two-slide technique is used, each preparation is evenly applied to its appropriate slide immediately after sampling, and then the slide is sprayed or dipped in preservative within 5 seconds.

11. Perform the appropriate cervical cultures after cytologic sampling, if indicated.

12. Some experienced colposcopists have recognized the benefit of routinely using acetic acid staining of the cervix following the Pap smear, especially in women who have significant risk factors for cervical dysplasia. Five percent acetic acid (white vinegar) applied to the cervix turns abnormalities white. Any observed cervical abnormality that cannot be readily explained by normal anatomic variants (e.g., nabothian cysts), either before or after acetic acid application, warrants colposcopic evaluation—even if the Pap smear report is normal.

13. Examine the vagina by slowly withdrawing the speculum, which is held slightly open allowing the vagina to collapse over the blades. Note abnormalities.

14. Lubricate the gloved hand as necessary and proceed with the bimanual examination. Pay particular attention to palpated abnormalities of the introitus, vagina, fornices, and cervix. Palpate the areas of the Skene's and Bartholin's glands. Ask your patient to bear down and observe for uterine or pelvic floor prolapse, and for leaking of urine. Having her cough facilitates assessment of pelvic support.

15. Complete the remainder of the bimanual examination, noting the size, contour, tenderness, and mobility of the uterus and adnexal structures.

16. Perform a rectal examination. Be sure to put on a new glove before the rectal examination to prevent the spread of HPV or other infectious agents to the anus.

17. Allow the patient to dress.

18. Make sure the Pap smear requisition form includes all pertinent data regarding your patient. Be sure to include clinical findings, patient risk factors, or your concerns as part of this "referral" (Bethesda recommendation).

COMPLICATIONS

The Pap smear is only a screening test. False-negative rates are high (10% to 40%, with an average of 25%), and significant disease can be missed or underestimated. More frequent Pap smear screening or colposcopy may be indicated, depending upon patient history and risks for having or developing genital malignancy.

"GOLDEN RULES"

• Identify cervical landmarks and gross abnormalities, and sample both the endocervical canal and the entire transformation zone. Choose a transformation zone sampler that fits your patient.

- All Pap smears reported as abnormal require some form of intervention. A report of dysplasia warrants colposcopy. Many clinicians recommend colposcopy for reports of atypia also, especially in patients with numerous risk factors.
- Clarify your patient's risk factors for having HPV infection and cervical dysplasia as part of the routine examination.
- An observed abnormality on the cervix that cannot be readily explained by normal variants (e.g., nabothian cysts) warrants colposcopic examination. A normal Pap smear report in the face of an observed abnormal cervix should not dissuade the clinician from performing colposcopy and biopsy.
- The presence of cervicovaginitis alters the *timing* for colposcopic examination, not the indication.
- Know your cytopathologist. Interpretive problems should be discussed directly with the pathologist, who can address your questions—including the option to review the cytology at issue.

TABLE 79-2.

Classification and Approximate Comparative Nomenclature of Cervical Smears

Papanicolaou Numerical	NCI Class	CIN System* Cytodescriptive	Bethesda
Class I normal smear; no abnormal cells	negative	normal	normal
Class II atypical cells; no neoplasia	atypical	reparative or atypical	atypia[†]
Class III smear contains abnormal cells consistent with dysplasia	suspicious	CIN I or II mild, moderate dysplasia	low-grade SIL (HPV changes and CIN I)
Class IV smear contains abnormal cells consistent with carcinoma in situ	positive	CIN III, CIS[‡]	high-grade SIL (CIN II, CIN III, CIS)
Class V smear contains abnormal cells consistent with carcinoma of squamous origin[§]	positive	carcinoma	invasive carcinoma

[*]CIN = cervical intraepithelial neoplasia.
[†]Discourages the use of the term *atypia*. Recommends using only when all other explanations have been exhausted. Excludes HPV changes.
[‡]CIS = carcinoma in situ.
[§]Further subcategorization of carcinoma is confirmed by histologic features demonstrated by biopsy. Microinvasion = < 3 mm penetration; frankly invasive > 3 mm (some argue 5 mm as depth of differentiation).

INTERPRETATION

Adequacy

The Pap smear report should indicate whether the smear was adequate. Unless the patient has had a hysterectomy, this should include cytologic evidence that the transformation zone was sampled. Ordinarily, the reporting of endocervical cells along with squamous cells implies adequate sampling. Many cytologists attribute "squamous metaplasia" the same significance as the reporting of "endocervical cells present." Either are considered objective evidence that the transformation zone was sampled, which implies an adequate sample.

Interpretation System

Table 79-2 summarizes the various Pap smear reporting systems. The Bethesda system attempts to address much of the confusion regarding Pap smear terminology. Regardless of the reporting system utilized, the following general principles should apply to all Pap reports:

- The Pap smear report should use terminology that is understood by the clinician.
- The clinician should be able to discuss the Pap report with the cytopathologist if questions arise.
- All abnormal Pap smears require some form of intervention in addition to the routine yearly screening interval.

Indications for Colposcopy (See Chapter 81, The Colposcopic Examination)

Pap Report

- Persistent squamous atypia
- Evidence of dysplasia of any degree (CIN I-III, low- and high-grade SIL)
- Evidence of malignant cells
- Evidence of HPV infection including: koilocytosis, hyperkeratosis, atypia, or inflammation that cannot be explained, especially if patient has significant risk factors for HPV infection
- Evidence of glandular (adenomatous) atypia

  Note: A report describing glandular or adenomatous atypia (to be differentiated from squamous atypia) warrants immediate colposcopy and evaluation of possible cervical adenocarcinoma (10% to 18% of cervical carcinomas). Furthermore, endometrial carcinoma may be suggested by abnormal cytology detected by a Pap smear. In such instances, formal endometrial sampling is indicated.

Pelvic Examination Findings

- Abnormal-appearing cervix
- Abnormal-feeling cervix or vagina
- Genital condylomata at any site

Other Indications

- A positive HPV-DNA screen
- DES offspring
- A partner with genital condylomata
- History of sexual abuse
- Other sexually transmissible disease

CPT/BILLING CODES

90070	Pap smear*
88150	Pap smear interpretation[†]
57500	Biopsy of cervix[‡]
57505	Endocervical curettage[‡]

BIBLIOGRAPHY

Baker RM: Improving the adequacy of Pap smears, *Am Fam Physician* 39(6):109, 1989.

Cervical cytology: evaluation and management of abnormalities, *ACOG Technical Bulletin* 183: August 1993.

Koss LG: The Papanicolaou test for cervical cancer detection: a triumph and a tragedy, *JAMA* 261:737, 1989.

Lundber GD: The 1988 Bethesda system for reporting cervical/vaginal cytological diagnoses, *JAMA* 262(7):931, 1989.

Nelson JH, Averette HE, Richart RM: Cervical intraepithelial neoplasia and early invasive cervical carcinoma, *Cancer Journal for Clinicians:*157, 1989.

Reissman SE: Comparison of two Papanicolaou smear techniques in a family practice setting, *JFP* 26(5):525, 1988.

Richart RM: Causes and management of cervical intraepithelial neoplasia, *Cancer* 60 (Suppl 8):1951, 1987.

The 1988 Bethesda system for reporting cervical/vaginal cytological diagnoses: National Cancer Institute workshop, *JAMA* 252(7):931, 1989.

---

*Many clinicians include the professional fee for performing the Pap smear as part of the female annual examination—in many cases, an "extended visit."

[†]A code used by the cytopathologist for billing. Very few clinicians (i.e., nonpathologists) interpret their patients' cytology.

[‡]The majority of cervical biopsies and endocervical curettage will be performed as part of the formal colposcopic examination. Please refer to the chapter on colposcopy for appropriate billing information.

CHAPTER 80

HPV-DNA Testing of the Cervix

Gary R. Newkirk

The presence of human papillomavirus-deoxyribonucleic acid (HPV-DNA) in the female genital system correlates with cervical dysplasia. Addressing the false-negative rate of traditional Pap smear testing has led to the development of tests with the ability to detect and confirm evidence of HPV infection, especially when equivocal, low-grade, or atypical Pap smear results are reported. Of the 62 or more subtypes of HPV, at least seven are known to infect almost exclusively the genital system. Each subtype has a number based on the order of discovery. Subtypes 6 and 11 correlate with typical exophytic condylomatous lesions and are thought to have low malignancy potential. Subtypes 16 and 18 produce typically flat condylomata that are harder to identify without magnification and acetic acid staining and that are highly correlated with advanced dysplasia. Subtypes 31, 33, and 35 have intermediate dysplastic potential. Several tests are now available for testing of HPV subtypes (e.g., ViraPap and ViraType, available from Digene Diagnostics). ViraPap checks for the presence of one or more of the seven most common genital infective subtypes (6, 11, 16, 18, 31, 33, 35). ViraType will further characterize the sample into one of three subtype groups: 6, 11; 16, 18; or 31, 33, 35. Neither test is intended as a screening method for the general population. The clinician is provided with a kit to obtain the samples from a Pap smear. DNA testing can be performed either on a smear or a tissue biopsy.

INDICATIONS

Although they are controversial, indications include the following:

- An adjunct to the Pap smear to identify individuals at risk for the development of cervical dysplasia
- A test for HPV as a sexually transmissible disease
- Patients with an equivocal Pap smear
- Women with numerous risk factors for HPV (A positive screen would then indicate the need for closer Pap and/or colposcopic monitoring.)

613

- Identifying individuals with more aggressive subtypes, such as 16 and 18
- Patients considering conservative treatment or no treatment
- Victims of possible sexual abuse

Note: At the present time, HPV-DNA testing is considered to have a sensitivity and specificity of 75% to 85%. Most authorities recommend that therapy be based not on HPV typing, but rather on colposcopic findings and biopsy diagnosis. As science progresses, recommendations may change.

TECHNIQUE

Material can be obtained via the Pap smear technique at any time, and sample collection is similar to the Pap smear procedure. Use the rayon swab enclosed in the kit to sample cervical mucus. Place the sample in a small test tube with transport and incubating media. The ViraPap report will be returned 4 to 21 days later, and the results are read as either positive or negative for the group of seven subtypes of HPV. If a ViraType study is ordered as well, the same swab submitted for the ViraPap can be used. The ViraType report will then indicate which of the three subtype groups are found in the specimen.

Alternatively, a tissue sample (at least 3 mm in size) can be submitted in formalin or on dry ice for HPV screening or typing. This method, in situ hybridization, allows for a tissue- and site-specific determination for the presence of the HPV-DNA of the screened subtypes.

Polymerase chain reaction (PCR) technology greatly enhances the sensitivity for detecting HPV-DNA. This technology can be applied to both smears and tissue samples. By means of amplifying HPV-DNA, as few as 10 viruses per 1 million cells can be detected. False-positive results can easily occur from contamination by sampling technique or within the laboratory during confirmatory testing. Many feel that although this technology holds great promise, it is currently best reserved for research protocols and not for routine clinical use.

HPV DETECTION TESTS

- Digene
- Enzo
- ONCOR
- ViraPap
- ViraType

This is only a partial listing of available HPV detection tests.

COST

- ViraPap: $45 to $80
- ViraType: $45 to $80

- Both: $90 to $150
- In situ hybridization (HPV-DNA testing on biopsy tissue): $100 to $150

CPT/BILLING CODE

There is no specific CPT code for physician obtaining the sample, other than routine procedure (i.e., Pap smear, cervical biopsy, etc.).

BIBLIOGRAPHY

Koutsky LA, Galloway DA, Holmes KK: Epidemiology of genital human papillomavirus infection, *Epidemiol Rev* 10:122, 1988.

Moscicki A et al: Variability of human papillomavirus-DNA testing in a longitudinal cohort of young women, *Obstet Gynecol* 82:578, 1993.

Reid R, Lorincz AT: Should family physicians test for human papillomavirus infection? *JFP* 32(2):183, 1991.

Richart RM et al: HPV-DNA: quicker ways to discern viral types, *Contemp Obstet Gynecol* 33(4):112, 1989.

CHAPTER 81

The Colposcopic Examination

Gary R. Newkirk

Addressing the widespread human papillomavirus (HPV) and genital epithelial dysplasia epidemic requires mastery of colposcopy, cervical biopsy, and endocervical curettage. The most frequent indications for these procedures include evaluating the abnormal Pap smear (see Chapter 79, The Pap Smear: Screening for Cervical Cancer), visible cervical abnormalities, or evidence of clinical HPV infection. Current evidence suggests that more than 90% of cases of cervical dysplasia can be managed entirely in the outpatient setting. Successful colposcopy requires *strict compliance with established protocol* and the support of the pathologist, urologist, and gynecologist. Mechanisms for excellent documentation and rigorous follow-up are mandatory. Physicians who assimilate colposcopy skills into their practices will benefit from responding to a major public health problem and will enhance their patients' access to care.

The colposcope is essentially a stereoscopic (4× to 40×), portable operating microscope with a focal distance long enough to examine the genitalia and cervix. The colposcopic examination serves to (1) identify normal landmarks, (2) identify abnormal areas in relation to these landmarks, (3) facilitate directed biopsy of abnormal areas for histologic diagnosis, and (4) rule out invasive cancer. Based on the findings, patients will be triaged for outpatient procedures (cryotherapy, loop electrical excision procedure [LEEP]), inpatient intervention such as cervical conization (laser or conventional), or definitive therapy for invasive carcinoma.

Colposcopic-directed biopsy will provide histologic clarification of abnormal Pap smears; this is mandatory before definitive therapy. Premalignant and malignant cervical conditions produce colposcopically identifiable epithelial changes that are often characteristic, and generally occur within the transformation zone, which can be carefully examined during the colposcopic examination. Ultimately, it is the pathologist who provides the histologic diagnoses for abnormalities identified during the colposcopic examination. Therefore, the major challenge for the colposcopist is, with assistance of staining (acetic acid, concentrated iodine solution) and magnification, to distinguish the normal from the abnormal, and to sample the most abnormal appearing changes for histologic confirmation. The endocervical curettage is always performed as part of the routine colposcopic examination (in nonpregnant patients) to confirm the absence of occult disease within the endocervical canal.

Colposcopy itself, without the benefit of histologic confirmation, is not considered a diagnostic tool. Even though colposcopically defined visual abnormalities correlate with cervical dysplasia or frank carcinoma, the ultimate diagnosis rests on the traditional histologic interpretation of submitted samples and not with the visual pattern recognition. Accordingly, diagnostic accuracy requires that the colposcopist perform *liberal* biopsy of the abnormal cervix.

In the past decade, major changes in our understanding of the epidemiology and science of cervical carcinoma have yielded efforts to develop a unified terminology to be used throughout the international scientific community. The International Federation of Cervical Pathology and Colposcopy (IFCPC) approved a basic colposcopic terminology at its Seventh World Congress in Rome in May 1990 (Box 81-1). These terms should be used to describe findings during the colposcopic examination.

COLPOSCOPIC FINDINGS

The prudent colposcopist must be completely familiar with the normal findings and the visual abnormalities that correlate with dysplasia and malignancy (Fig. 81-1; also see Fig. 79-1).

Normal Colposcopic Findings

- **Original squamous epithelium.** A featureless, smooth, pink epithelium. There are no features suggesting columnar epithelium such as gland openings or nabothian cysts. Epithelium was "always" squamous and was not transformed from columnar to squamous.
- **Columnar epithelium.** A single layer of mucus-producing, tall epithelium that extends between the endometrium and the squamous epithelium. Columnar epithelium appears irregular, with stromal papillae and clefts. With acetic acid application and magnification, columnar epithelium has a grapelike or "sea-anemone" appearance. It turns mildly acetowhite. Columnar epithelium is found in the endocervix, surrounding the cervical os and is generally visible in the reproductive age group.
- **Transformation zone.** The geographic area between the original squamous epithelium and the columnar epithelium that is occupied by metaplastic epithelium in varying degrees of maturity. The *active transformation zone* contains gland openings, nabothian cysts, and, typically, islands of columnar epithelium surrounded by metaplastic squamous epithelium. It is the area of most active metaplasia.
- **Squamous metaplasia.** The physiologic, normal process whereby columnar epithelium is thought to develop into mature squamous epithelium. Squamous metaplasia typically occupies the transformation zone. At the squamocolumnar junction, it appears as a "ghost white" film with the application of acetic acid.

BOX 81-1. COLPOSCOPIC TERMINOLOGY
(See text for definitions)

I. Normal colposcopic findings
   A. Original squamous epithelium
   B. Columnar epithelium
   C. Normal transformation zone
   D. Squamocolumnar junction (SCJ)
   E. Squamous metaplasia
II. Abnormal colposcopic findings
   A. Within the transformation zone
      1. Acetowhite epithelium (areas of white after application of vinegar)
         (a) Flat
         (b) Micropapillary or microconvoluted
      2. Punctation (red dots)
      3. Mosaicism (linear, tilelike patterns)
      4. Leukoplakia (white change *before* application of vinegar)
      5. Iodine-negative epithelium (tissue that is *not* deeply stained by iodine)
      6. Atypical vessels
   B. Outside the transformation zone (ectocervix, vagina)
      1. Acetowhite epithelium
         (a) Flat
         (b) Micropapillary or microconvoluted
      2. Punctation
      3. Mosaicism
      4. Leukoplakia
      5. Iodine-negative epithelium
      6. Atypical vessels
III. Colposcopically suspect invasive carcinoma
IV. Unsatisfactory colposcopy
   A. Squamocolumnar junction not visible
   B. Severe inflammation or severe atrophy
   C. Cervix not visible
   D. Entire lesion not seen (i.e., goes into canal)
   E. Most advanced lesion not biopsied
V. Miscellaneous findings
   A. Nonacetowhite micropapillary surface
   B. Exophytic condyloma
   C. Inflammation
   D. Atrophy
   E. Ulcer
   F. Other (polyp, hemorrhage, cysts, etc.)

Adapted from Adolf Stafl, GD Wilbanks: An international terminology of colposcopy: report of the nomenclature committee of the International Federation of Cervical Pathology and Colposcopy, *Obstet Gyn* 77(2):313, 1991. Used with permission.

- **Squamocolumnar junction (SCJ).** Generally, a clinically visible line seen on the ectocervix or within the distal canal (e.g., postcryotherapy or postmenopausal age group) that demarcates endocervical tissue from squamous tissue or from squamous metaplastic tissue (conceptually comparable to the vermillion border around the mouth where mucosa meets squamous epithelium).

Abnormal Colposcopic Findings

- **Atypical transformation zone.** A transformation zone with findings suggesting cervical dysplasia or neoplasia.

  1. *Acetowhite.* Epithelium that transiently whitens following the application of acetic acid. Areas of acetowhiteness correlate with higher nuclear density.
  2. *Punctation.* A stippled appearance of capillaries viewed end-on; often found within acetowhite areas, where they appear as fine-to-coarse red dots.
  3. *Mosaicism.* An abnormal change made up of small red blood vessels appearing in linear form suggesting a confluence of tile or chickenwire pattern. This is best seen after staining with acetic acid.
  4. *Leukoplakia (hyperkeratosis).* Typically an elevated, white plaque seen *before* the application of acetic acid.
  5. *Abnormal blood vessels.* Atypical, irregular true vessels with abrupt courses and patterns; often appear as commas, corkscrews, or spaghetti shapes. No definite pattern is recognized as with punctation or mosaicism.

- **Suspect invasive cancer.** A complex pattern consisting of roughened, irregular cervical epithelium, typically with abundant irregular vessel patterns and dense acetowhite change with a slight yellowish hue. It may also appear as ulcerated, friable, necrotic tissue.

Unsatisfactory Colposcopy

The entire squamocolumnar junction or the limits of all lesions cannot be completely visualized. Proper examination can also be hampered if an active inflammatory process is present or if the patient is not estrogen primed (e.g., postmenopausal without replacement therapy).

Other Colposcopic Findings

- Vaginocervicitis
- Traumatic erosion
- Atrophic epithelium
- Endocervical polyps
- Changes from DES
- Abnormal pigmentation
- Nabothian cysts

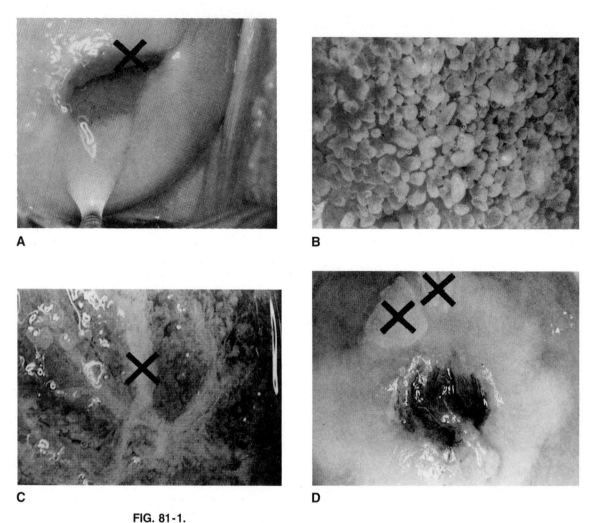

FIG. 81-1.
Colposcopic findings. *Normal:* Squamocolumnar junction (**A**); Endocervical tissue (**B**); Squamous metaplasia overlying endocervical tissue (**C**). *Abnormal:* Acetowhite areas from the 12 to 2 o'clock positions (**D**); Lugol's solution highlighting acetowhite area (**E**); Leukoplakia, abnormal white lesion before acetic acid (**F**); Punctation in lower left corner (**G**); Coarse punctation (**H**); Mosaicism (**I**); Abnormal blood vessels (**J**). The "X" indentifies findings noted. (From Cartier R, Cartier I: *Practical colposcopy,* Paris, 1993, Cartier Laboratoire. Used with permission.)

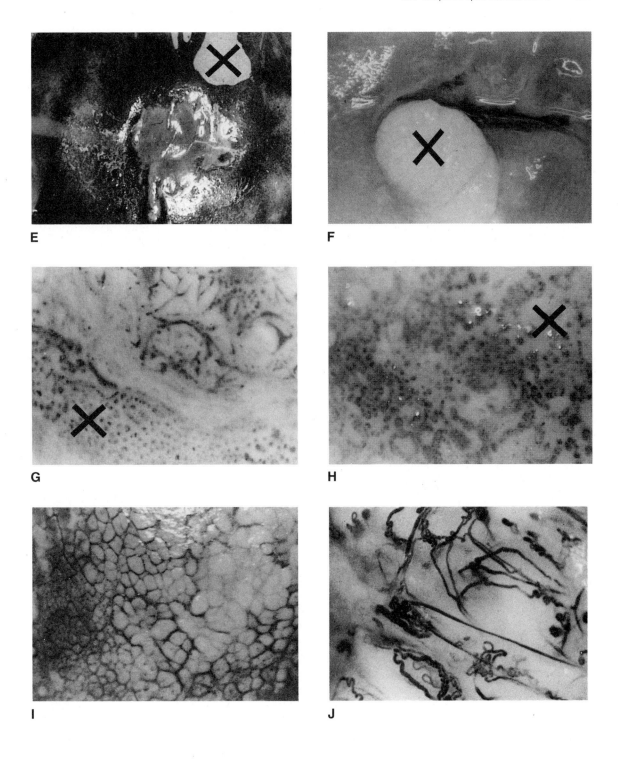

E

F

G

H

I

J

Guidelines regarding visual colposcopic findings help ensure sampling of the most advanced sites of cervical dysplasia. The classic hallmark of cervical dysplasia includes the change that dysplastic epithelium undergoes following the application of 3% to 5% acetic acid (vinegar) or Lugol's (concentrated iodine) solution. *Dysplastic epithelium* typically turns whiter than the surrounding normal epithelium following the application of acetic acid (*acetowhite epithelium*). More advanced dysplasia typically appears whiter, thicker, more sharply bordered; areas have straight edges, few or no satellite lesions, and more rough or thickened as the severity of dysplasia advances. Changes in the vasculature pattern also correlate with cervical dysplasia. These abnormal patterns, which often occur within an acetowhite or leukoplakia patch, include *punctation, mosaicism,* and frankly *abnormal vessel variations.* The more coarse the punctation or mosaicism, the more severe the dysplasia. Frankly abnormal vessel patterns imply severe dysplasia or potential invasive carcinoma. Typically, Lugol's solution will cause an immediate blackening (staining) of normal epithelium (iodine uptake is high in normal cells that are rich in cytologic glycogen); abnormal dysplastic tissue, whose cells contain much less intracellular glycogen, are not stained by iodine (*Lugol's negative epithelium*).

Squamous metaplasia, a normal finding, may appear slightly acetowhite and may take up Lugol's iodine incompletely; therefore, this tissue can cause some degree of confusion. Squamous metaplasia is the physiologically normal tissue in which the columnar epithelium is thought to develop into mature squamous epithelium. This occurs at the transformation zone—the same site where dysplasia generally occurs. Squamous metaplasia is especially prominent with certain conditions such as active cervicitis, where healing and reparative activities occur. *Questionable areas always warrant biopsy.* If squamous metaplasia without dysplasia is reported on biopsy, the prudent colposcopist must look elsewhere to explain the finding of dysplasia on the Pap smear. A report of squamous metaplasia among other biopsies revealing dysplasia reflects the difficulty encountered by the colposcopist in evaluating this normal variant of acetowhite change. (Indeed, not all appendixes removed for an acute abdomen are the source of the pain either!) The only other common areas that normally turn slightly white with acetic acid are the *endocervical (columnar) cells,* which are located within the cervical canal and variably extend to the exocervix. Endocervical tissue can generally be differentiated from abnormal areas by colposcopic examination. Biopsy is still warranted if there is any confusion.

This chapter focuses upon the evaluation of the abnormal Pap smear as it typically relates to cervical disease. *The complete examination also includes the colposcopic examination of the remainder of the genital system in women.* The colposcope can also be used to examine male genitalia (see Chapter 67, Androscopy). Ultimately, the patient's cytological, colposcopic, and histologic data are used in concert to direct appropriate management. A well-managed colposcopy program provides effective treatment for all patients with identified abnormalities of the cervix and genital tract.

Many colposcopists keep their scopes immediately available to augment the routine Pap and pelvic examination. Although complete formal colposcopic examination and biopsy can be performed when visual abnormalities are identified, many clinicians prefer to reschedule patients for full colposcopic examination at a later date. This allows more time for patient education and thorough evaluation.

INDICATIONS

- Pap smear consistent with dysplasia or cancer
- Pap smear with unexplained atypia
- Pap smear with evidence of HPV infection (koilocytosis)
- Suspicious visible lesion or palpable lesion of the cervix
- History of intrauterine diethylstilbestrol (DES) exposure
- Follow-up of previously treated patients or high-risk patients

STRONG CONSIDERATION FOR COLPOSCOPY

- Patient with visible genital condylomata or sexual partner with evidence of condylomata
- History of genital warts or sexual partner with history of genital warts
- Unexplained vaginal discharge, vulvodynia, cystitis
- Multiple sexual partners
- Early age of first coitus
- History of or current sexually transmitted disease
- Intravenous drug abuse
- Positive findings of HPV-DNA on cervical screening (see Chapter 80, HPV-DNA Testing of the Cervix)
- Patients with HIV infection (Pap smear is unreliable.)

CONTRAINDICATIONS

Most contraindications relate to temporary or treatable conditions that alter the timing of the colposcopic examination rather than absolutely preventing it from occurring. The adequate colposcopic examination requires excellent visualization with a compliant and cooperative patient.

- Active, inflammatory cervicitis
- Noncooperative patient
- Postmenopausal patient who is not estrogen-primed (intravaginal or oral estrogens)
- Heavy menses (may prevent adequate examination)

EQUIPMENT

The equipment and supplies used during routine colposcopy should be within reach in the colposcopy examination room (Figs. 81-2 to 81-5). Monsel's (ferric

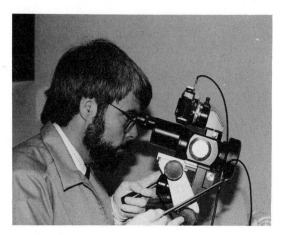

FIG. 81-2.
The colposcope and colposcopist in position for examination and biopsy.

subsulfate) solution should be thoroughly shaken in its original bottle and then allowed to evaporate until it is the consistency of a thick, greenish-brown paste; this renders it a potent astringent to control biopsy-induced bleeding.

- Colposcope—variable fixed power or zoom lens (3× to 7× low power to 15× to 40× high power)
- Biopsy forceps* (e.g., Tischler, baby Tischler, Kevorkian)
- Endocervical curette* (Kevorkian, no basket)
- Endocervical speculum[†] (Kogan, narrow and wide)
- Ring forceps*
- Tenaculum[†] (rarely used)
- Cervical hook[†] (rarely used)
- Pap smear materials[†]
- Vaginal speculums (e.g., metal Graves or disposable plastic speculum) in various sizes and lengths (use largest tolerated), or a clear, lighted, plastic speculum setup (e.g., Welch-Allyn) for selected cases
- Full-strength Lugol's iodine solution[†,‡] (30 cc)
- Monsel's solution[‡] (ferric subsulfate), 15 cc
- Acetic acid solution 3% to 5%, (white vinegar), (4 to 6 oz. or 120 to 180 cc)[§]
- Cotton- or rayon-tipped swabs (8 to 10)
- Jr. scopettes/OB-GYN applicators (6 to 10)
- 4 × 4 inch gauze
- Urine or sputum cups for vinegar
- Vaginal retractor[†]

---

[*]Included in "colpo pack." These must be sterilized before procedures. "No touch" technique is used on the ends of instruments touching the patient. Reusable instruments are sterilized, but colposcopy is not a "sterile" procedure.

[†]Available in colposcopy room but not used at every procedure.

[‡]Hospital pharmacy.

[§]Grocery store or mix to make 3% to 5% acetic acid.

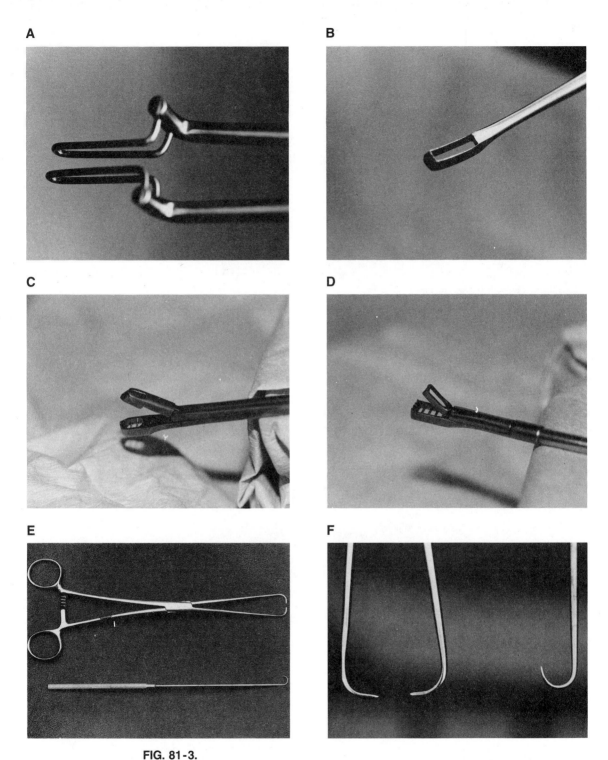

FIG. 81-3.
The key instruments required for the colposcopic examination with biopsy. **A,** Kogan endocervical speculum; **B,** Kevorkian endocervical curette without basket; **C,** Tischler cervical biopsy forceps; **D,** Kevorkian biopsy forceps; **E,** Cervical tanaculum and hook; **F,** Close-up of tenaculum and hook.

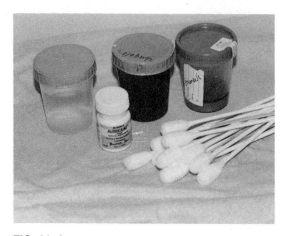

FIG. 81-4.
A typical colposcopy tray (Mayo stand) holding plastic cups (sputum cups) of acetic acid, Lugol's and Monsel's solution, specimen bottles, and cotton-tipped swabs.

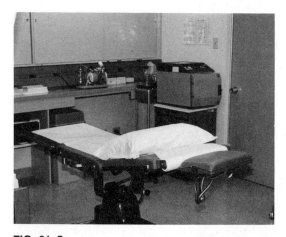

FIG. 81-5.
A typical Ritter table, which facilitates patient positioning during colposcopic examination.

- Underpads (17 × 24 inch)
- Cotton balls (15 to 20)
- Power-assisted patient examination table that can be raised or lowered

Optional items include: 2 oz 20% benzocaine topical gel (e.g., Hurricane), preprocedural dose of an oral nonsteroidal antiinflammatory agent, paracervical injection setup (rarely used), aromatic ammonium capsules ("smelling salts") for vasovagal responses, and a camera/video attachment.

PREPROCEDURE PATIENT EDUCATION

- Discuss the indications for colposcopy with the patient. The patient should acknowledge the importance of long-term follow-up. The patient should advise the physician's clinic of change of address or telephone number.
- Instruct the patient to continue contraceptive practices before and after the colposcopic examination until treatment or management decisions have been made.
- Explain to the patient that a pregnancy test will be performed on the day of the procedure if pregnancy is a possibility.
- Instruct the patient to consume a regular diet on the day of the procedure and not to skip a meal before the procedure. This lessens the possibility of a vasovagal episode.
- Warn against taking aspirin, or medications containing aspirin, for 7 days before the procedure. Aspirin consumption within the past week does not ordinarily contraindicate colposcopy with biopsy, but you should be aware of the potential for excessive bleeding. Normally, nonsteroidal antiinflammatory drugs, such as ibuprofen, do not significantly prolong bleeding; therefore, they may be taken before the procedure for pain control.
- Review the medical history with particular attention to in-utero exposure to DES; drug allergies; asthma; diabetes mellitus; the need for subacute bacterial endocarditis (SBE) prophylaxis; history of vagal sensitivity (frequent fainting); bleeding disorder; recent symptoms of cervicitis or pelvic inflammatory disease; symptoms suggesting pregnancy; symptomatology suggestive of an endometrial disorder that may require endometrial sampling; and history of prior cervical treatment, including conixation, laser therapy, or cryotherapy.
- Explain that the procedure will take about 20 to 30 minutes. Most clinics ask patients to arrive at least 15 minutes early, to allow for appropriate education, a pregnancy test, and questions.
- If pictures will be taken, inform the patient, and establish consent, before the actual procedure.
- Review the risks before the procedure: infection, bleeding, discharge, and missing disease (all very rare).
- Explain that colposcopy with biopsy ordinarily renders a diagnosis and is not a therapeutic procedure per se. Definitive therapy will be determined by correlation of historical, colposcopic, cytologic, and histologic data.
- Discuss treatment options. Ordinarily, cervical cryotherapy, if indicated, will be performed after the cervix has had time to heal from the biopsy and pathology reports are available. This typically can be performed as early as 2 weeks later or after the next menstrual cycle.
- If applicable, inform the patient that she may likely receive a separate bill for the interpretation of the pathology samples obtained during the biopsy procedure.

Many physicians mail patient education information to their patients before their colposcopy examination (see Box 81-2). This has been proven to decrease patient

BOX 81-2. PATIENT EDUCATION HANDOUT
COLPOSCOPY WITH BIOPSY

Your physician has recommended that you undergo colposcopy with biopsy. Colposcopy is an examination in which an instrument is used to magnify and examine carefully the surface of the external genitalia, vagina, and cervix. Colposcopy allows the physician to identify and sample any abnormal tissue. During the biopsy, a small pinch of tissue is removed and sent to a specialist for careful examination under the microscope. This tissue analysis allows your physician to determine whether or not a premalignant or cancerous condition of the birth canal exists, and whether specific treatment is needed.

When you come to the office, you will lie on the examination table with your feet in stirrups. Vinegar will be placed in the vagina; this helps to identify the abnormal tissue. Your physician will then look with the colposcope and obtain biopsies, if necessary. Next, the physician will scrape the cervix (birth canal). This causes a sensation similar to menstrual cramps and only lasts 30 to 60 seconds. Generally, this procedure causes little pain. Taking 3 or 4 ibuprofen 200 mg tablets an hour before the procedure will help to minimize the pain.

During the colposcopy and biopsy procedure, your physician may use the colposcope to photograph your cervix or vagina for medical documentation. These pictures are cataloged and used for future reference to help evaluate and treat your specific problem. Occasionally, these pictures may be used to help teach other physicians about the abnormal appearance of the birth canal.

The major risks of colposcopy and biopsy include the following:

Bleeding. Since a small piece of tissue is removed during a biopsy, there may be some bleeding. Normally this is controlled with a solution that is applied to the biopsy site during the procedure. Occasionally, a stitch may be required. Rarely, bleeding may show up as a late complication after you have gone home. If bleeding occurs and the flow is heavier than that of your usual period, you should call the physician's office to receive further treatment. You may also notice some spotting after intercourse.

Infection. Normally the cervix is fairly resistant to infection following biopsy. Occasionally infection does occur, and signs of infection may include unusual pain, discharge, bleeding, fever, or bad odor. If any of these signs appear, you should call the physician's office. If you develop an infection, you may have to take antibiotics.

Missing disease. The main purpose of using the colposcope to direct a biopsy of the birth canal is to help find the most diseased areas for sampling. Occasionally this area is not visualized well with the colposcope, and significant disease may be missed. In this circumstance, further biopsies and treatment may be necessary. It is *very important* that you follow up with all recommended treatment and testing. It is also important to realize that colposcopy with biopsy is not a "treatment" procedure, but a procedure to help clarify the type and extent of disease that you might have in your birth canal. Further treatment will be then recommended following the results of your biopsy.

Other precautions. If it is possible that you are pregnant, please tell your physician at the time of your colposcopy and biopsy. Special precautions can be taken during the procedure to help prevent complications with the pregnancy. A specialist referral may be necessary.

You should realize that the evaluation and treatment of abnormal tissue in the birth canal causing the abnormal Pap smear often requires you to make many visits to the doctor for treatment and further follow-up testing. This is generally a life-long process. The minimum requirement will be that you must have a Pap smear every year for the rest of your life. Failure to comply with recommended treatment could place you at risk for progressive disease of the birth canal and the possibility of developing a serious cancer or dying.

Please feel free to discuss any questions you may have regarding colposcopy and biopsy before undergoing testing.

anxiety and improve understanding of the disease process. Videotapes are available to further enhance patient education and informed consent (Creative Health Communications, see Suppliers list).

TECHNIQUE

Box 81-3 provides a summary protocol for the colposcopic examination and highlights the key patient management issues. Clinicians are also advised to either dictate or write their findings in the medical record to supplement the colposcopic examination form. See Box 81-1 for the suggested terminology to be used to describe findings.

With practice and skill, the colposcopic examination with appropriate tissue sampling can be effectively assimilated into the contemporary clinician's practice. In addition to the necessary technical skills, the successful colposcopy program requires close attention to data interpretation and careful patient follow-up. The patient who has an abnormal Pap smear and who ultimately has biopsy-confirmed cervical dysplasia remains at a lifetime risk for recurrence or reexpressions of genital malignancy.

1. Prepare the colposcopy room. Make sure the room is warm. Some patients benefit from quiet background music. Have all necessary solutions and equipment readily at hand. Make sure the appropriate culture media, KOH, and wet prep materials are in the room. Keep all sizes of speculums in your colposcopy room.

2. Prepare your patient. Mail information before the procedure. Answer her questions. Use a pelvic model or diagrams when you explain the procedure. Review medical history. Are there significant medical conditions such as diabetes or bleeding disorders? Is there a recent history of symptoms suggesting pregnancy, vaginosis, pelvic inflammatory disease? What are her drug allergies? Is she sensitive to iodine? Ibuprofen 800 mg may be offered 30 minutes before the procedure.

3. Obtain informed consent. Allow patient to review a written description of the procedure, its risks, and complications (see Box 81-2). Address questions and concerns. Obtain informed consent, which often includes a signed permit.

4. Obtain a pregnancy test as necessary. Endocervical curettage is contraindicated in pregnancy. Occult pregnancy at the time of colposcopy is common.

5. Perform a bimanual examination. Is the uterus enlarged or tender? What position is the cervix? Can the cervix be moved? How long is the vagina? Are there palpated abnormalities of the introitus, vagina, fornices, or cervix? Examine the vulva for obvious condylomata.

6. Warm the speculum. Colposcopy requires the widest speculum the patient can comfortably tolerate. The examination requires greater cervical and vaginal exposure than a screening Pap smear. Because of the relative duration of the colposcopic examination, the vaginal walls may migrate inward, which makes visualization more difficult. (A carefully inserted wide, large Graves speculum is far more comfortable in the long run than constant prodding

BOX 81-3. COLPOSCOPY

PATIENT INSTRUCTIONS: Please complete questions in this box

Date _____ Age _____ Referring Physician _____

Name _____ Reason for Colposcopy _____

Phone (home) _____ (work) _____

HISTORY

Previous abnormal paps?	Y N	Age _____	
History of previous cryocautery (freezing)?	Y N	Number of pregnancies _____ Children _____	
Personal history of cancer?	Y N	Date of last menstrual period _____	
Family history of cancer?	Y N	Type of contraception _____	
History of venereal diseases (circle)	Y N	Number of sexual partners (lifetime) _____	

• gonorrhea • aids • herpes • syphillis   Age at first sexual intercourse _____

Do you desire testing for   Do you smoke   Y   N
  any of these diseases?   Y   N   Partner(s) with warts?   Y   N
History of genital warts?   Y   N   History of sexual abuse?   Y   N
Visible warts now?   Y   N   Other PMH: Y   N
Previously treated?   Y   N
  If so, how? _____

PROCEDURE (Doctor will fill out)

Observation without staining: _____

Pap repeated?   Y   N   LK = Leukoplakia
SCJ seen?   Y   N   WE = White epithelium
  Endo spec needed?   Y   N   PN = Punctation
ECC done: Y   N   MO = Mosaicism
Entire lesion seen?   Y   N   ATZ = Abnormal Transformation Zone
                                        AV = Abnormal vessels
Vaginal vault: BE = Bulk effect
                                        AG = Atypical glands
Urethra: X = Biopsy sites

Labia:

Perineum:

Rectum:

IMPRESSION: _____

_____

RECOMMENDATIONS

Cryocautery   Y N
Referral to specialist   Y N
LETZ   Y N
Other:

PLAN:
  Discourage smoking
  Partner needs information
  Need at least annual Paps for the rest of life
    no matter what others say
  Handout on cryocautery - LETZ - Andro - Ellman
    vitamins - Ca prev. diet

cc: _____   _____
                                        Physician's Signature

and manipulating of the vagina to move it out of the field of view if an inappropriately narrow speculum is used.) If necessary, use a vaginal retractor. A thin layer of water-soluble vaginal lubricant can be applied on the speculum. This thin coating significantly facilitates the insertion of the speculum, will rarely interfere with Pap smear testing (if necessary), and does not interfere with biopsy interpretation. Use both thumbscrew dimensions of the speculum to gain maximum exposure. Ideally, the colposcopic examination is facilitated by having the cervix facing anteriorly and virtually "suspended" between the blades of the speculum.

7. Grossly examine the cervix and vaginal fornices. Does the cervix appear inflamed or infected? An active cervicitis confuses colposcopic detail. Characterize the vaginal and cervical discharge. It is permissible to gently blot (never rub) excess secretions away to view the cervix more clearly. Use magnification to quickly scan the cervix to identify landmarks, such as the transformation zone with its squamocolumnar junction. Are there areas of gross vessel atypia? It is important to scan the cervix for gross leukoplakia before applying acetic acid. Although acetic acid greatly enhances the elucidation of diseased areas, its mild vasoconstricting properties can render significant vessel detail less obvious.

8. Obtain specimens for cultures, KOH and wet preparations, HPV-DNA probe, and Pap smear, as necessary. Even a correctly performed Pap smear irritates the cervix, may cause bleeding, and may change fine colposcopic detail. The Pap smear may need to be repeated because the original Pap smear was performed at a different lab; because more than 3 months have elapsed since the last Pap smear; because the patient is pregnant (Pap smears are less reliable during pregnancy and colposcopy is more difficult; it is important to maximize clinical assessment); and because of the need to allay any concern or confusion regarding the adequacy or interpretation of the original Pap smear results.

9. Apply 5% acetic acid. One method is to use 4 × 4 inch gauze rolled up tightly and held longitudinally in a ring forceps. This saturates the cervix with vinegar quickly and without trauma. Cotton balls or large swabs also work well. Use large swabs or Jr. scopettes to repeat the application. Refer to acetic acid as "vinegar" or simply as "douche solution" when discussing it with the patient. Warn her of brief stinging and coldness. Repeat application every 5 minutes, because the acetowhite effect is only temporary.

10. Perform the colposcopic examination. Start with low power (typically 5×). Scan the entire cervix with white light. Use a vinegar-soaked cotton-tipped swab to help manipulate the cervix and transformation zone into view. It is almost never necessary to use the tenaculum to move the cervix. The cervical hook can be used; however, it is rarely necessary. The Kogan endocervical speculum greatly aids the examination of the distal endocervical canal. Use this instrument gingerly to prevent bleeding and pain. Use higher magnification to carefully document abnormal findings. The entire transformation zone, including the squamocolumnar junction, must be seen and evaluated. Abnormalities will turn white (acetowhite).

11. Use the green filter to enhance vascular detail. All abnormal areas demand biopsy. Lugol's solution aids with the identification of abnormal (dysplastic) areas, but is rarely used (it is unnecessary and messy). Dysplasia and reparative (metaplastic) tissue will incompletely stain with concentrated iodine because of low levels of cellular glycogen as compared with the staining of healthy, mature squamous epithelium. The sharply outlined borders afforded by Lugol's can be dramatic, and this can help clarify biopsy sites. Iodine staining does not interfere with histology. However, Lugol's may obscure the underlying vascular pattern. Lugol's solution should be used when further clarification of potential biopsy sites is necessary or when no lesion is seen with acetic acid. Applying Lugol's solution will also help delineate the squamocolumnar junction for the beginning colposcopist and is used for performing cervical loop diathermy procedures (LEEP, LLETZ) since its effects last longer than those of acetic acid.

12. Mentally map the cervix. The main goal of colposcopy is to identify areas for biopsy. The colposcopist must be able to differentiate normal tissues from abnormal. Acetowhite areas that have sharp geographic borders and that appear thick or raised are likely to be histologically more abnormal. The presence of coarse punctation or mosaic patterns, or of frankly abnormal vessels, is associated with a more severe degree of dysplasia. Ultimately, however, it is the histopathologist who makes the diagnosis from biopsy samples. Be prepared to draw a careful record of what is observed and where biopsy samples were taken. The colposcopic impression of severity of disease must be recorded to compare and correlate later findings. Coppleson et al. have proposed scoring indexes to help discern colposcopically identifiable lesions. Many physicians find these helpful when beginning colposcopy (see Reid, 1993).

13. Is the colposcopic examination satisfactory? The entire transformation zone, including all the squamocolumnar junction, must be visualized. The borders of all lesions must be entirely seen (lesions should not disappear into the canal, for example). Patients who are uncooperative or who have a severely flexed uterus with inadequate visualization are potential "real world" causes of inadequate colposcopy. An inadequate colposcopic examination with cytologic evidence of dysplasia may require obtaining a cervical cone biopsy sample for evaluation. In summary, the adequate colposcopic examination requires the following: (1) visualizing of the entire transformation zone including the squamocolumnar junction, (2) identifying the area of abnormality producing the abnormal Pap smear, (3) confirming that the limits of all abnormal areas are clearly seen, (4) obtaining a biopsy sample of all abnormal areas, and (5) verifying no colposcopic evidence of malignancy. If these conditions are met *and* no lesion extends greater than 5 mm into the canal; the ECC is negative; there is no colposcopic evidence of malignancy; any high grade lesion is only focal in size; and there is correlation between Pap, colposcopic impression, and histology (see Chapter 83, Crycone of the Cervix), then the patient is a candidate for ablative therapy.

14. Perform the endocervical curettage (ECC). Topical 20% benzocaine (Hurricaine) gel is an excellent topical anesthetic, although the FDA has not

approved labeling for this purpose. Generally, local anesthesia is not necessary. Use a Kevorkian curette without basket. Insert gently until the internal cervical os is reached, which is manifested by a slight puckering of the cervix with further advancement. In multiparous women, the internal os is not well defined; the curette should not be advanced farther than 2 cm. Scrape the entire lining of the canal (360 degrees) twice. The procedure may be done with or without colposcopic observation. The sample appears as a coagulum of mucus, blood, and small gray or tan tissue fragments. The scope can then be used to examine tissue and to further tease the sample from the canal. Sometimes a Cytobrush will retrieve the ECC sample, which may persistently remain stuck in the canal. Submit the ECC as a separate sample on a piece of paper towel, lens paper, or Telfa. Ordinarily, it is not necessary to place a sample pad in the posterior vaginal fornix as it is with formal dilation and curettage. Do *not* perform an ECC on pregnant patients or patients with evidence of active cervicitis or PID. All other patients must have a documented negative ECC prior to ablative therapy. Some physicians prefer to do the ECC after the cervical biopsy samples are obtained.

15. Obtain cervical biopsy samples. Sample the posterior areas first to prevent blood from dripping over future biopsy sites. The cervix can be manipulated with a cotton-tipped swab, a Jr. scopette, or a hook to provide an adequate angle for obtaining the biopsy sample. A 3 mm deep sample is all that is necessary. It is *not* necessary to include normal-appearing tissue with biopsy samples (that is, to include the margins of lesions in the sample). Beginning colposcopists can enhance their skills by placing samples from different biopsy sites in separate bottles and subsequently correlating them with colposcopic impression. After sufficient experience, biopsy samples that appear of similar severity can be placed together. If bleeding is profuse from a particular site and more samples are needed, hold a cotton-tipped swab to the area and proceed with obtaining the next sample. (To control persistent bleeding, see Complications). Do not apply Monsel's solution until all samples are obtained. Monsel's solution in a biopsy specimen ruins good histology. Some physicians prefer to obtain the cervical biopsy samples before the ECC.

16. Apply Monsel's solution to bleeding areas. To be most effective, the Monsel's should be as thick as toothpaste. This consistency can be achieved by allowing the Monsel's solution to evaporate down to paste consistency. Swab out the excess Monsel's and bloody debris, which appears as a black mass of coagulum which may alarm the patient and irritate the vulva. Observe the cervix until all evident bleeding ceases.

17. Remove the speculum and examine the vagina. Gently retract the speculum with a twisting motion and observe as the vaginal wall collapses around the receding blades. Are abnormal vaginal areas apparent? Be sure to colposcopically examine vaginal areas that were abnormal when palpated during the bimanual examination.

18. Examine the vulva and anus. Vulvar examination may be performed at this time. Acetic acid application will yield an acetowhite effect in most sites with condylomata. It is mandatory to do a careful vulvar colposcopic examination

with acetic acid in women at high risk for vulvar dysplasia including those with unexplained vulvar itching; smokers over age 40, especially those with vulvar symptoms; and those with abnormal-appearing areas of vulvar tissue.

The easiest way to examine the vulva is to begin superiorly. Use two hands to separate the vulva and slowly raise the power table with the foot pedal. Examine carefully from clitoris to anus. *The finding of perianal condylomata warrants anoscopy.* The clear plastic, disposable anoscopes are ideal. Acetic acid can be used in the anal canal, but is rarely necessary. Small anal canal condylomata can usually be palpated.

19. Allow the patient to recover. Have the patient rest supine for at least several minutes, then sit up slowly, and rest again.

20. Document your findings. Carefully draw a picture of lesions and biopsy sites. Photos of the cervix do not replace accurately drawn diagrams of the colposcopic cervical findings. Include whether or not you feel the colposcopic examination was adequate.

    Chart whether the colposcopic impression supports outpatient cervical cryotherapy and which cryotip should be used (size and shape). See Chapter 83, Crycone of the Cervix. This is not a decision based solely on colposcopic appearance. Only histologic reporting and correlation of cytologic, colposcopic, and histologic data together can define the appropriate therapeutic intervention. Factors such as lesion location, grade of severity, number, and size also dictate treatment options. For instance, large lesions (over 25 mm in diameter, more than 15 mm from the os, or involving more than two cervical quadrants), even if they are only mildly dysplastic, may be more appropriately treated with loop diathermy or laser therapy than would a small focal severe dysplasia, which may respond to ambulatory cryotherapy very well.

21. Discuss the findings, and give postprocedure instructions. After your patient has recovered and is dressed, review your impressions but withhold the specific diagnosis until the histology report and review of all the clinical data have been examined. Provide careful postprocedure instructions. Advise abstaining from intercourse for 24 hours and using tampons for 5 days. Instruct the patient to return if she experiences unusual vaginal odor, discharge, pelvic pain, or fever. Make a specific agreement how the results of the biopsy are to be reported. Unless a problem arises, your patient does not necessarily require a follow-up pelvic examination. Discussing the results of the biopsy sampling and subsequent treatment options on the telephone may be an appropriate follow-up mechanism for some patients; however, most will appreciate a visit to the physician for this important interaction.

HISTOLOGY, CYTOLOGY INTERPRETATION OF DATA

If at all possible, try to have the same pathologist (or at least the same group of pathologists) interpret both the cytology and histology results for a given patient. Be concerned if significant discrepancy is found between the Papanicolaou cytology and your biopsy histology. In general, a report of a greater degree of abnormality from biopsy than from the Pap smear (for example, Pap = CIN 2;

biopsy = CIN 3) is common and acceptable. Be concerned if biopsy-generated histology reports are significantly less advanced than Papanicolaou cytology (two or greater grades of severity less). For instance, a cytology smear indicating carcinoma in situ and biopsy samples of only mild dysplasia might indicate that the worst area was missed on evaluation, and that the patient may have in situ or invasive carcinoma in another site. A good rule of thumb is not to freeze any cervix until you have adequately and sufficiently explained the discrepancy between histology and cytology. Repeating colposcopy and biopsy sampling to reconcile the difference is forgivable, even in the hands of the most experienced clinicians. Freezing invasive cancer is never forgivable.

A negative endocervical curettage sample should indicate strips or fragments of orderly, benign columnar epithelium with mucus and blood. Lack of identifiable endocervical tissue constitutes an inadequate ECC sample. An inadequate ECC sample is not uncommon, and in the overwhelming majority of patients it simply means that the ECC must be repeated before definitive therapy. If the endocervical curettage sample indicates dysplasia, it is a positive ECC and an indication for cone biopsy procedure (see Chapter 82, Cervical Conization). Current protocol does not support freezing the canal with a long narrow probe to treat endocervical dysplasia. Some "positive" ECCs result from contamination with dysplastic lesions at the verge of the os. *Nonetheless, do not assume this!* The beginning colposcopist must remain comfortable referring patients with equivocal or problematic colposcopic, cytologic, and histologic correlation. Know your limitations!

POSTPROCEDURE PATIENT EDUCATION

- Agree on a time to discuss and interpret biopsy findings by phone or follow-up visit.
- Explain that mild vaginal discharge may occur following a cervical biopsy procedure, especially if Monsel's solution was used to control bleeding. This discharge is often grainy and black, which is the result of Monsel's mixing with mucus and blood. This discharge may last approximately 24 hours.
- Advise the patient that she may have spotting for at least 48 hours. Although there may be some spotting, it is safe to resume intercourse after 24 hours.
- Instruct the patient to report passage of clots, onset of fresh profuse bleeding, foul vaginal odor, fever, or pelvic pain. Women with these complaints following a cervical biopsy procedure require evaluation.
- Encourage the patient to continue (or begin) contraception when definitive therapy has been completed.
- Patients rarely require vaginal creams (e.g., triple sulfa) after a cervical biopsy sample has been obtained. Nonetheless, some women may have vaginitis caused by organisms such as yeast, bacteria, or trichomonas, and therapy aimed at these pathogens may be helpful. Women who feel comfortable douching may use a nightly (or morning) dilute povidone-iodine solution as desired.
- *Emphasize the importance of returning for definitive therapy.* Reemphasize the relationship of cervical dysplasia with sexually transmissible disease, poor

diet, smoking, and nonmonogamous sexual practices. Be sure the patient understands the life-long risks of HPV infection.

COMPLICATIONS

- Most postcervical biopsy or endocervical curettage (ECC) bleeding is minimal and handled completely with Monsel's solution. Rarely, the patient may experience a fresh, bloody discharge. Often, a simple reapplication of Monsel's solution is all that is necessary. Very rarely, a simple cervical stitch of 4-0 absorbable suture across a particularly deep biopsy site may be required. Avoid obtaining a cervical biopsy sample immediately before the menses; subsequent bleeding may be confused with menstrual flow, and the uterus may potentially be more prone to infection. Some clinicians will saturate the end of a vaginal tampon with Monsel's solution and insert this to provide pressure and astringent action for persistent cervical oozing. The tampon can then be removed several hours later by the patient. At times, it may be necessary to cauterize the biopsy site. An effective way to control fairly brisk bleeding is to inject 1 to 2 cc of 2% lidocaine with epinephrine into the bleeding site. This will either stop or reduce the bleeding enough to effectively apply Monsel's solution or cauterize the site.
- A foul cervical discharge, fever, or pelvic pain may indicate postprocedure infection. Infection is rare but typically occurs on the third or fourth day after the biopsy sample has been taken. A cervical biopsy sampling should be avoided if there is clinical evidence of invasive cervicitis.
- Despite correct technique, there is the potential risk that the most advanced cervical disease may be missed by the colposcopist at the time of the biopsy sampling or potentially by the histologist at the time of tissue analysis. Careful, timely transport of all samples to a reputable lab is important. Some pathologists prefer all cervical biopsy samples to be placed in the same container, while others prefer separate containers for each, but the ECC sample should remain separate. The colposcopist is well advised to liberally obtain a biopsy sample of all abnormal-appearing areas of the cervix for histologic interpretation. Widespread four-quadrant cervical disease challenges the colposcopist to sample areas most likely to contain cervical carcinoma. Lack of correlation between the Papanicolaou cytology and subsequent histology can suggest situations when potentially the worst area has not been sampled. The main goal of colposcopy is to rule out invasive cervical cancer and to select patients who are candidates for outpatient treatment. When the colposcopist cannot safely accomplish this goal, rarely, but importantly, cervical conization may be the only way of accomplishing this task.
- Some women will experience vaginal discharge after a cervical biopsy sample is obtained. This will typically last 1 or 2 days and should diminish with time.
- Cervical biopsy sampling typically causes brief pain and discomfort. Ordinarily, this pain is very well tolerated by most women. Careful explanation of the procedure, a warm room, and a caring, careful manner all minimize the

discomfort. Topical benzocaine diminishes pain during the procedure and ECC, and is advised in women who demonstrate enhanced cervical sensitivity. Studies have shown preoperative oral nonsteroidal antiinflammatory drugs decrease discomfort associated with the procedure.
- Rarely, vasovagal reactions occur with the procedure, but are much more likely to occur with cervical cryotherapy.

SELECTED RESOURCES FOR COLPOSCOPY

Physician teaching slides and tapes

Physician's Educational Network
3550 Watt Avenue
Suite 6
Sacramento, CA 95821
916-485-9861

Biovision, Inc.
350 Fifth Avenue
Suite 3304
New York, NY 10118
514-354-4277

National society for promotion of quality education and patient care

American Society for Colposcopy and Cervical Pathology (ASCP)
409 12th Street SW
Washington, DC 20024-2188
202-863-2453
800-787-7227

Colposcopy training courses

The National Procedures Institute, Inc.
4909 Hedgewood Drive
Midland, MI 48640
517-631-4664
800-462-2492

American Academy of Family Physicians
8880 Ward Parkway
Kansas City, MO 64114
800-274-2237

American College of Obstetrics and Gynecology
409 12th Street SW
Washington, DC 20024-2188
800-787-7227

Patient education videotapes

Creative Health Communications
809 Elm Street
Essexville, MI 48732
517-892-7614
800-462-2492

Patient education brochures and support groups

American Social Health Association
ASHA/HPV
P.O. Box 13827
Research Triangle Park, NC 27709

Colposcope suppliers

Cabot Medical Co.
2021 Cabot Blvd. W
Longhorne, PA 19047
800-523-6078

Cooper Surgical (Frigitronics)
770 River Rd.
P.O. Box 855
Shelton, CT 06484
800-645-3760

Gyne Tech Instruments
1111 Chestnut St.
Burbank, CA 91506
213-849-1512
800-496-3832

Leisegang Medical
6401 Congree Avenue
Boca Raton, FL 33487
800-448-4450

MedGyn Products
328 N. Eisenhower Lane
Lombard, IL 60148
800-451-9667

Olympus Corporation
4 Nevada Drive
Lake Success, NY 11042
800-645-8160

Wallach Surgical
291 Pepe's Farm Rd.
Milford, CT 06460
203-783-1818
800-243-2463

Zinnati Surgical Instruments (ZSI)
21540-B Prairie St.
Chatsworth, CA 91311
800-223-4740

Editor's note: A complete colposcopy course on videotape (12.5 CME) became available on February 1, 1994. Contact CME Conference Video, Inc., 2000 Crawford Place, Suite 100, Mt. Laurel, NJ 08054; telephone: 800-284-8433.

CPT/BILLING CODES

56605	Biopsy of vulva
56606	Biopsy of each additional
57100	Biopsy of vaginal mucosa
57452	Colposcopy (vaginoscopy)
57454	Colposcopy with biopsy(s) of the cervix and/or ECC
57460	Colposcopy with LEEP
57500	Biopsy of cervix only, single or multiple
57505	Endocervical curettage (not done as part of a dilatation and curettage)

BIBLIOGRAPHY

Allen MH: Primary care of women infected with the human immunodeficiency virus, *Obstet Gynecol Clin North Am* 17(3):557, 1990.

Burke L, Antonioli DA, Ducatman BS: *Colposcopy: text and atlas,* East Norwalk, Conn, 1991, Appleton & Lange

Curry SL, Pfenninger JL, Sarma S: Colposcopy: when? why? how? *Patient Care* 15:167, March 1994.

Felmar E et al: Colposcopy: a necessary adjunct to Pap smears, *Fam Pract Recert* 10(11):21, 1988.

Ferris DG, Willner WA, Ho JJ: Colposcopes: a critical review, *JFP* 34(1):25, 1992.

Hatch KD: Colposcopy of vaginal and vulvar human papillomavirus and adjacent sites, *Obstet Gynecol Clin North Am* 20(1):203, 1993.

Hatch KD: *Handbook of colposcopy diagnosis and treatment of lower genital tract neoplasia and HPV infections,* Boston, 1989, Little Brown.

Nelson JH, Averette HE, Richart RM: Cervical intraepithelial neoplasia and early invasive cervical carcinoma, *Cancer* 39:157, 1989.

Newkirk GR: Teaching colposcopy and androscopy in family practice residencies, *JFP* 31(2):171, 1990.

Pfenninger JL: Colposcopy in a family practice residency: the first 200 cases, *JFP* 34(67):67, 1992.

Reid R: Biology and colposcopic features of human papillomavirus—associated cervical disease, *Obstet Gynecol Clin North Am* 20(1):123, 1993.

Richart R, Pringle P: A state of the art guide to colposcopes and accessories, *Contemp Obstet Gynecol* 30:107, 1988.

Rodney WM et al: Colposcopy and cervical cryotherapy, *Postgrad Med* 81(8):79, 1987.

Staff A, Wilbanks GD: An international terminology of colposcopy: report of the nomenclature committee of the International Federation of Cervical Pathology and Colposcopy, *Obstet Gynecol* 77(2):313, 1991.

Stewart DE et al: The effect of educational brochures on knowledge and emotional distress in women with abnormal Papanicolaou smears, *Obstet Gynecol* 81:280, 1993.

Wright VC, editor: Contemporary colposcopy. In *Obstetrics and gynecology clinics of North America, volume 20,* Philadelphia, 1993, W.B. Saunders.

CHAPTER 82

Cervical Conization

Lydia A. Watson

Proper evaluation of abnormal Pap smears and cervical lesions includes colposcopy, multiple punch biopsy sampling, and endocervical curettage, in most cases. However, conization of the cervix plays an important role in both the diagnosis and the management of abnormalities of the cervix. Cold-knife conization is considered the gold standard by which all other outpatient techniques are critiqued.

Conization of the cervix consists of the removal of a cone-shaped wedge of tissue from the cervix uteri. To be considered an adequate specimen, the tissue removed must include the squamocolumnar junction and the entire lesion surrounded by uninvolved margins. There are several instruments capable of performing this procedure (for example, various lasers, loops, and cautery devices), but this chapter will describe in detail the cold-knife cone. The large-loop electrical excision procedure is described in Chapter 92, Loop Electrosurgical Excision Procedure (LEEP) for Treating CIN.

INDICATIONS

- Inadequate colposcopic evaluation of the cervix: no visualized lesion, but Pap smear is significantly abnormal; lesion that extends into the endocervical canal; or inadequate visualization of the entire transformation zone
- Positive endocervical curettings
- Inconsistencies between cytologic findings, histologic diagnoses, and colposcopic impression (i.e., Pap smear at least two stages worse than colposcopic findings)
- Cytology or biopsy specimen suggestive of microinvasive carcinoma of the cervix
- A therapeutic procedure for high-grade dysplasia
- Large lesion that cannot be treated with cryocautery

CONTRAINDICATIONS

- Pregnancy (*relative contraindication*)

Note: Pregnancy is not an absolute contraindication to conization, but in a pregnant patient the procedure should only be performed by a well-trained obstetrician, gynecologist, or surgeon capable of managing complications. (See Complications.)

- Known invasive carcinoma of the cervix or endocervix
- Patient with contraindications for general or regional anesthesia

PREPROCEDURE PATIENT EDUCATION

- Explain the procedure and complications to the patient, and obtain written informed consent.
- Explain the necessity of general or regional anesthesia.
- Explain all options for treatment and evaluation.

EQUIPMENT

- Povidone-iodine
- Colposcope with green filter
- Acetic acid and full-strength Lugol's solution
- 2-0 chromic or 2-0 Vicryl for hemostatic retraction suture
- Vasopressin 20 units in 20 cc of normal saline for infiltration of the cervix
- Long scalpel handle with No. 11 blade
- Long, fine-tooth forceps
- Kevorkian endocervical curette
- Electrocautery unit
- 0-chromic or 0-Vicryl suture; or Surgicel, Gelfoam, or Avitene for hemostasis
- Large Graves speculum
- Uterine sound

TECHNIQUE

1. *Special considerations:* Most lesions are found on the ectocervix in premenopausal women, so the cone should have a broad base and the top should have a wide angle (Fig. 82-1, *A*). In postmenopausal women, the specimen will be long and narrow, with an acute angle at the cone top. Since the squamocolumnar junction in this subgroup has moved inside the endocervical canal, lesions are more likely to be endocervical, and the transformation zone on the ectocervix is quite small (Fig. 82-1, *B*).
2. Administer general or regional anesthesia to the patient, and obtain adequate exposure of the cervix.
3. Apply full-strength Lugol's solution to the cervix to aid in determining the width of the cone base. All areas that do not stain will be removed. Alternatively, perform colposcopy using acetic acid and the green filter to demarcate the lesion and the transformation zone.

A

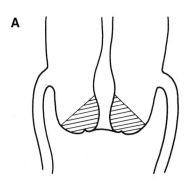

B

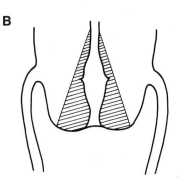

FIG. 82-1.
Variation in size and shape of cervical tissue removed during conization. **A,** Large ectocervical lesion; **B,** Canal lesions.

4. Obtain hemostasis by circumferentially infiltrating the cervical stroma with a solution of 20 units of vasopressin diluted in 20 cc of normal saline (Fig. 82-2).
5. Place hemostatic retraction sutures at the junction of the portio and vagina at the 3 o'clock and 9 o'clock positions (Fig. 82-3).
6. Gently sound the uterine canal to determine position and depth of the uterus.
7. Incise the cervix in a circular fashion, making the incision outside of the Lugol's-negative or acetowhite area. Begin at the 6 o'clock position; this will prevent the blood that runs down from obscuring the incision line (Fig. 82-4, *A* and *B*).
8. Use a fine-toothed forceps to elevate the cone away from the underlying bed. Avoid damaging the cervical epithelium (Fig. 82-4,*C*).
9. Mark at the 12 o'clock position of the specimen with a single suture placed into the cervical stroma.
10. Curette the remainder of the endocervical canal with a small curette to rule out disease above the upper margins of the cone.
11. Perform a dilation and currettage *if indicated* at this time.
12. Obtain hemostasis with superficial electrocoagulation by using a ball electrode or by using individual suture ligatures to control bleeding. The cone site may also be packed with an absorbable gelatin sponge (such as Gelfoam) or similar hemostatic material. Some physicians apply Monsel's solution to the base of the excision after coagulation.
13. Place the cone specimen in fixative to send for pathologic interpretation.

POSTPROCEDURE PATIENT EDUCATION

- Schedule a follow-up appointment for 3 to 4 weeks.
- Instruct the patient to avoid intercourse, douching, and tampon use until follow-up examination confirms healing.
- Ask the patient to notify you of elevated temperature, excessive vaginal bleeding, or purulent discharge.
- Schedule first follow-up Pap smear in 3 to 4 months if all margins are clear.

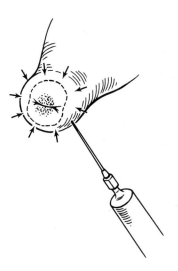

FIG. 82-2.
Intracervical injection.

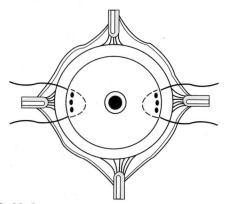

FIG. 82-3.
A cut-away diagram of the cervix showing hemostatic retraction suture placement around vessels.

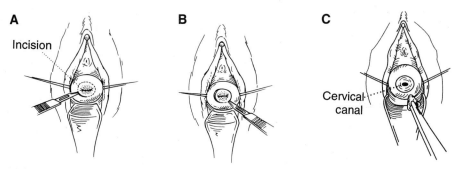

A Incision

B

C Cervical canal

FIG. 82-4.
Example of hemostatic retraction sutures and conization technique. See text for details.

COMPLICATIONS

Nonpregnant Patient (overall rate 10%)

- Hemorrhage, immediate or delayed (Eschar sloughs in 7 to 10 days: delayed hemorrhage can occur at this time.)
- Cervical stenosis (less than 3 mm)
- Uterine perforation
- Pelvic cellulitis or cervicitis
- Damage to the bladder or rectum—usually seen in cases of significant vaginal atrophy with shallow vaginal fornices
- Cervical incompetence
- Infertility due to loss of mucus-producing endocervical glands
- Anesthetic complications

Pregnant Patients

In addition to the complications mentioned for the nonpregnant patient:

- Fetal loss rate of 10% (secondary to rupture of the membranes, premature labor, and excessive hemorrhaging)
- Postoperative hemorrhage rate of 30%

BIBLIOGRAPHY

Parsons, Ulfelder: *An atlas of pelvic operations,* Philadelphia, 1968, W.B. Saunders.

Ryan KJ, Berkowitz R, Barbieu RL, editors: *Kistner's gynecology principles & practice,* Chicago, 1990, Year Book Medical Publishers.

Schaefer G, Graber A, editors: *Complications in obstetrics and gynecologic surgery,* New York, 1981, Harper & Row.

Thompson D, Rock JA, editors: *TeLinde's operative gynecology,* ed 7, Philadelphia, 1992, J.B. Lippincott.

Wheeless CR, editor: *Atlas of pelvic surgery,* ed 2, Philadelphia, 1988, Lea & Febiger.

CHAPTER 83

Cryocone of the Cervix

John E. Hocutt, Jr.

Freezing of the cervix (cryocone) is an important procedure for the primary care physician involved in the treatment of precancerous lesions of the cervix (cervical intraepithelial neoplasia [CIN], squamous intraepithelial lesions [SIL], and dysplasia). It has been proven an effective technique for treatment of most CIN lesions after diagnosis based on tissue biopsy results. It can also be used to treat chronic cervicitis when drug therapy has failed. The technique can be easily mastered by primary care physicians.

For office treatment of CIN lesions, the alternatives to cryosurgery are as follows:

- Laser ablation of the cervix is more difficult, more expensive, and more traumatic. Human papillomavirus (HPV) and human immunodeficiency virus (HIV) particles have been documented in the smoke plumes generated by the equipment. Its effectiveness is approximately equivalent to that of cryocone if the diagnosis is correct. In laser treatments, the advantage over cryocone is that the squamocolumnar junction (SCJ) remains visible on the ectocervix. Cryocones (especially if conical or extended tips are used) can cause the SCJ to migrate up inside the endocervix. The lesions that are more difficult to remove by cryosurgery and that are more easily treated by laser ablation include the anatomically large lesions (CIN I, II, or III), advanced high-grade lesions, and the CIN lesions with glandular extension 5 to 7 mm below the surface.
- Topical chemical treatments for HPV infections of the cervix may involve multiple visits and are not as effective. Topical chemical treatments are not currently indicated and thus generally are not used for CIN.
- Loop electrosurgical excision procedure (LEEP) appears to be quite effective for most CIN lesions, may be easily performed in the primary care physician's office, and is less likely to cause the transformation zone to migrate inside the os than cryosurgery. This procedure may be especially helpful for recurrent cases or cases resistant to cryosurgery (see Chapter 92, Loop Electrosurgical Excision Procedure [LEEP] for Treating CIN).

- Many clinicians are now recommending that low-grade lesions (CIN I and less) be followed closely and not treated. Most lesions will resolve spontaneously or not progress. The lesions should be small and the patient must be extremely compliant with follow-up visits. All criteria for an adequate colposcopy must be met (see Chapter 81, The Colposcopic Examination).

INDICATIONS

- Cryocone after a colposcopic examination is the treatment of choice for most cases of CIN (dysplasia) of the cervix. Criteria include the following: (1) CIN is confirmed by tissue diagnosis; (2) the endocervical curettage is negative for dysplasia; (3) the results of the Pap test correlate adequately with the tissue biopsy and colposcopic appearance of the cervix (The Pap may be negative in biopsy-proven CIN—and often will be—but the Pap should never be *more than* one grade higher in severity than what the biopsy results show); (4) the entire transformation zone is visible by colposcopy (including the squamocolumnar junction); (5) the entire lesion can be seen and can be covered by the cryotip probe; (6) the lesion does not extend more than 4 to 5 mm into the os; and (7) the patient is cooperative and willing to return for frequent follow-up Pap smears.
- Cryocone is often quite helpful in patients who have a chronic culture-negative discharge from cervicitis and who do not respond to antibiotics. Cancer must first be ruled out by colposcopy, endocervical curettage (ECC), and possibly endometrial biopsy (EMB).
- The treatment of biopsy-proven cervical HPV changes without clinical evidence of disease is controversial, with most physicians now deferring treatment until CIN or dysplasia is diagnosed. However, patients with HPV are monitored much more closely than those with negative Pap smears and normal colposcopy.

CONTRAINDICATIONS

- Cervical, endocervical, or endometrial invasive cancer
- Lesion with high-grade dysplasia (moderate or severe) greater than 2 cm in a single diameter or spread over more than two quadrants
- Positive endocervical curettage (ECC) indicating dysplasia
- Pregnancy
- Lack of correlation between Pap smear and biopsies, or between colposcopic impression and biopsy (Pap or colposcopic impression more than one grade higher than abnormality found on biopsy)
- Inability to see entire transformation zone or entire lesion
- Known sensitivity to cryosurgery
- Excessively large lesion (any grade) or any lesion that extends beyond the cryoprobe
- Hysterectomy may be indicated for some cases of CIN III (severe dysplasia, cancer in situ) when future childbearing is not a consideration

- Sexually transmitted disease, especially chlamydia or gonorrhea cervicitis
- Menses within the next 5 to 7 days (Postcryosurgical edema may cause retention of menstrual products.)

RELATIVE CONTRAINDICATIONS

- Immunoproliferative neoplasms, myeloma, lymphoma
- Macroglobulinemia
- Active, severe collagen vascular diseases
- Severe, active ulcerative colitis
- High levels of cryoglobulins
- Acute poststreptococcal glomerulonephritis (Almost 100% of patients have high levels of cryoglobulins.)
- Active, severe subacute bacterial endocarditis (SBE), syphilis, Epstein-Barr virus (EBV), cytomegalovirus (CMV) infections
- Severe, chronic hepatitis B
- High-dose steroid drug therapy

These patients are likely to have an exaggerated response to the freezing of their skin due to high circulating cryoglobulins. If it is appropriate or necessary to use cryosurgery in any of these patients, obtain informed consent and test the axilla or thigh with a brief freeze before treating the cervix.

EQUIPMENT

- Nitrous oxide–powered cryoprobe unit (20-pound tank)
- Cryoprobes: 19 and 25 mm, flat and slightly conical (Do not use long endocervical tips; see Fig. 83-1.)
- Water-soluble lubricant (K-Y Jelly or Cryojel)
- Cotton-tipped swabs
- Timer

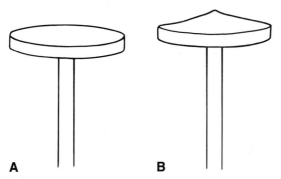

A   **B**

FIG. 83-1.
Diagram of flat (**A**) and slightly conical (**B**) cryoprobes.

- Vaginal speculum
- Vaginal side wall retractors or a condom or glove to place over the speculum (to avoid freezing the vaginal side walls) (See Fig. 79-4 for how to retract sidewalls with a "homemade" vaginal stint.)

SUPPLIERS

Cryomedics (Cabot Medical)
2021 Cabot Boulevard W.
Langhorne, PA 19047
800-523-6078

Wallach Surgical Devices, Inc.
291 Pepe's Farm Rd.
Milford, CT 06460
800-243-2463

GyneTech
1111 Chestnut St.
Burbank, CA 91506
213-849-1554

Spembly—distributed by:
Surgical Medical Instrument Corp
Old Saybrook, CT
203-395-0922

Frigitronics (Cooper Surgical)
770 River Rd.
Shelton, CT 06484
800-243-2974

Leisegang
6401 Congress Ave.
Boca Raton, FL 33487
800-448-4450

PREPROCEDURE PATIENT EDUCATION AND PREPARATION

- Discuss the risks, benefits, and possible complications of cryosurgery. Box 83-1 is a preprocedure handout describing the procedure with instructions.
- Before the procedure, review the indications with the patient.
- Update the menstrual history and do a pelvic examination if one has not been done within the previous few months. Be sure the patient is not pregnant, or postpone the procedure until you are sure. If there is any doubt, a pregnancy test should be performed.
- Confirm the biopsy report and note any area where disease is concentrated to ensure that the cryoprobe readily covers the area.
- Have the office staff premedicate the patient on her arrival to the office (if appropriate) with ibuprofen 800 mg or another nonsteroidal antiinflammatory drug (NSAID) to reduce the cramping that accompanies the procedure. For maximum effectiveness, it should be taken approximately 30 to 60 minutes before the procedure.

TECHNIQUE

1. Select a cryoprobe tip to cover the cervical lesion(s) so that the iceball will extend at least 5 mm beyond the border of the lesion(s).
2. Select a cryoprobe that is completely flat or is only slightly conical to minimize the inward migration of the squamocolumnar junction inside the os. Do not use probes with a long nipple.

BOX 83-1. PATIENT EDUCATION HANDOUT
CRYOCAUTERY OF THE CERVIX

In cryocautery of the cervix, the outer layer of cells on the cervix is frozen using a special flat-tipped instrument about the size of a quarter. This procedure is generally done for several reasons: chronic inflammation of the cervix, an abnormal Pap smear, or venereal warts. Your physician has determined that the best way to treat your lesions is to freeze them.

Cancer of the cervix is highly associated with infection with the human papillomavirus, the same type of virus that causes warts. Just as one of the treatments for warts on fingers, arms, and other parts of the body is freezing, so too is it one of the treatments for the lesions on your cervix. Often the same instrument is used, but with a different type of freezing tip.

Cryocautery is performed in the physician's office. The procedure takes approximately 15 to 20 minutes. You will lie on an examination table with your feet in stirrups. It is best to have this procedure done 5 days *after* your period. The procedure cannot be performed less than *5 days before or during your period.* If you are pregnant or suspect that you might be, please inform your physician. If possible, cryocautery is best avoided during pregnancy.

When the instrument is turned on and inserted, you will hear a small hissing sound. Then you may feel some menstrual-like cramping. The freezing lasts for only three minutes. The cervix is allowed to thaw, then it is frozen a second time. There is no cutting, burning, or bleeding. Taking three or four 200 mg ibuprofen 2 hours before the procedure will help prevent the discomfort of the cramps. *You generally do not experience pain.*

After cryocautery, you can expect a profuse vaginal discharge for 2 to 3 weeks. *This is normal.* Amino-Cerv Creme may greatly reduce this discharge. You may have been given a prescription for this medication. Bring the tube of cream with you for your appointment, and the doctor will insert the first dose before you leave. You will need to use one applicator in the vagina at bedtime every night for 2 weeks. You may resume normal activity, including sexual intercourse, when you feel comfortable, but it is probably best to wait 10 to 14 days. If the cramping persists, you may take ibuprofen three times a day.

Complications of cryocautery of the cervix are rare. Scarring and narrowing of the cervical canal to the degree that it actually blocks the opening and prevents pregnancy is rare. Infection may occur, so if your discharge lasts more than 3 weeks, call your physician. You may also note spotting when you resume intercourse or use tampons. You may want to avoid both for 2 to 3 weeks.

Cryocautery is effective only 85% of the time; that means *15% of patients will need to be retreated.* Cryocautery may be performed again. Sometimes laser or other treatments will be suggested. Follow-up is essential for effective treatment.

After the freezing, you should have a follow-up Pap smear in 4, 8, and 12 months. If any of these Pap smears are abnormal, your physician will discuss further treatment suggestions.

Venereal warts are highly associated with cervical cancer, and they are very contagious. Eighty percent of infected sexual partners will have warts on the penis or in the genital areas. Less than half of these warts will be visible with the naked eye. Staining with vinegar and examining the male with magnification will often identify previously unseen abnormalities. This procedure is called *androscopy,* and it may be recommended for all your male sexual partners. *If you smoke,* you have a much higher chance of developing cervical cancer. Smoking is strongly discouraged. Your partner should also quit smoking. It is very important that you have a high-vitamin diet. The National Institutes of Health recommends at least five helpings of fruit and/or vegetables each day to help boost your immune system.

You are at high risk for developing cervical cancer and should have a Pap smear every year. Even when treated, *you have a 3% chance of developing cervical cancer* in your lifetime. You can spread the virus to new partners, even if you do not see warts.

Should you have any questions or concerns, please feel free to discuss these with your physician. These are only general guidelines and may vary depending on your particular situation.

Used with permission of The Medical Procedures Center, P.C., Midland, Michigan.

3. Moisten the cryoprobe in warm water and apply a thin layer of water-soluble gel to the tip. Cryojel is a little more viscous than K-Y Jelly and may not run as much when applied to a vertical surface (such as that of the cervix when the patient is in the normal pelvic examination position). This difference in viscosity is rarely a significant factor. Lidocaine jelly may also be used if the others are unavailable, unless the patient is allergic to lidocaine.

4. Turn on the gas. Be sure there is sufficient pressure.

5. Position the probe and activate the freezing. Have your assistant start the timer and tell the patient that the procedure has started. After 3 to 5 seconds, the tip will adhere to the cervix and the auto-on feature of the cryogun may be activated. After the tip has adhered to the cervix, apply gentle outward traction to center the cervix in the middle of the vaginal air-space so that the walls of the vagina do not adhere to the cryoprobe. Freezing the vaginal wall is painful and may increase the morbidity of the procedure. Be sure not to pull too hard on the cryoprobe or you may tear tissue.

6. For benign cervicitis, freeze for one 3-minute period. For CIN, freeze long enough to obtain an iceball that extends at least 5 mm beyond the lesions. This generally takes 3 to 4 minutes. Allow the tissue to thaw completely (5 to 10 minutes), then repeat the entire process. Some clinicians have suggested that a single 5-minute freeze may be just as effective as two 3-minute freezes, but most experts use the double 3-minute freeze, and it is what is recommended in the *ACOG Bulletin*. The procedure to follow is freeze, thaw, refreeze. It must be emphasized that the timing of the procedure is not as important as the formation of the iceball. For the treatment of dysplasia, it is crucial that there be a 5 mm iceball extending past the tip.

7. Most units have an active defrost mechanism, and the cryoprobe will detach approximately 10 to 15 seconds after the freezing stops. Do not remove the cryoprobe until it has loosened from the cervix, or the tissue may lacerate. The gas must remain on to have an active defrost.

8. Immerse the cryoprobe tip in warm water between freezings. Effectiveness of contact and efficiency of your cryoprobe are enhanced if the tip is warmed between freezings.

9. Patients experience variable degrees of pelvic and abdominal cramping. This is reduced with preprocedural NSAID administration. They do not generally experience pain. The skin usually flushes during the thaw cycle because of the prostaglandin release.

10. Postcryotherapy discharge may be reduced by Amino-Cerv Creme (one application in the vagina at bedtime for 2 weeks).

POSTPROCEDURE CARE

- Recommended care includes a Pap smear at 4, 8, and 12 months, or at 6, 12, and 18 months. If no recurrence is detected, annual Pap smears are advised. A thorough colposcopy should be done at least at 18 months, if the Pap smears reveal no dysplasia. Many physicians include a colposcopic examination at 6 or 12 months. Follow-up should be yearly once the patient has had three normal Pap tests followed by a normal colposcopy. The goal is to treat the dysplasia and not to try to totally eradicate the HPV virus from the patient.

- A positive Pap smear or abnormal colposcopic examination with positive biopsy means that treatment has failed and a complete reevaluation is indicated.
- Avoid examination and Pap testing until after 4 months; at this time, postcryosurgery healing should be complete. Before this time, reparative changes can be confused with dysplasia.
- If the cryocone treatment is chosen for a CIN III lesion (more advanced dysplasia), most physicians prefer to schedule Pap testing *and* colposcopy at 4, 8, 12, and 18 months.
- Although "atypia" or "HPV changes" need a full workup before cryotherapy, the patient may never have a normal Pap smear after treatment. Any dysplasia on follow-up after cryosurgery is considered abnormal and warrants workup.
- If the patient complains of persistent discharge or pain, examine the vagina for inadvertent injury during the cervical freeze.

POSTPROCEDURE PATIENT EDUCATION

Give the patient written postprocedure instructions and guidelines. Examples of patient instructions are shown in Boxes 83-1 and 83-2. Emphasize that after cryocone, a discharge may be expected for at least 2 to 3 weeks.

COMPLICATIONS

- Cryotherapy may drive the squamocolumnar junction into the os, making a thorough repeat inspection much more difficult.
- Uterine cramping and flushing may occur during and immediately after the procedure.
- Cervical stenosis is very rare unless long nipples are used on the cryoprobe and the procedure is repeated several times.
- Infertility is generally not a problem unless multiple treatments over time are needed.
- Postoperative bleeding is very rare.
- There may be some menstrual irregularity for 1 to 3 months.
- Systemic infection is extremely rare (i.e., pelvic imflammatory disease), although the incidence is perhaps slightly higher in teenage patients.
- Treatment failure is possible even when the patient is properly evaluated and treated (10% to 15%).
- Persistent vaginal discharge or cervicitis lasting more than 3 to 4 weeks can be treated with vinegar or povidone-iodine douches and/or metronidazole.

CPT/BILLING CODE

57511   Cryocone of cervix, initial or repeat

**BOX 83-2. PATIENT EDUCATION HANDOUT
INSTRUCTIONS AFTER CRYOSURGERY OF THE CERVIX**

The cryocautery procedure (freezing of the surface of the cervix) is designed to treat abnormalities of the cervix without doing more extensive surgery. Treatment is often necessary to prevent progression to cancer or worsening of the problem.

Please note:

1. A heavy watery discharge is normal. Wear sanitary pads and change them frequently. Pads are preferred over tampons, but sometimes for the first 3 to 5 days, both are necessary.
2. The watery discharge may be tinged with blood the first few days.
3. If desired, you may insert one suppository of either Betadine (povidone-iodine) or Norform into your vagina daily to decrease odor. Alternatively, your physician may prescribe a cream for the vagina. Follow directions as given.
4. Douching is permissible, if desired. You may use a commercial douch, or mix 1 cup of water with 1 tablespoon of vinegar.
5. Swimming, bathing, and showers are allowed.

Please:

1. Abstain from sexual intercourse for at least 2 weeks. Otherwise you may resume normal activity.
2. Since treatment may fail in 10% to 15% of cases, schedule visits for repeat Pap smear and colposcopy according to the guidelines below:
   CIN I—Pap smear in 4, 8, and 12 months
         Colposcopy in 12 or 18 months (or more often)
   CIN II or III—Pap smear in 4, 8, 12, and 18 months
         Colposcopy in 8, 12, and 18 months
   If these tests are all normal, the treatment of the precancerous lesion is considered successful, but you should have a Pap smear annually for the rest of your life.
3. Call your physician should the discharge last more than 3 weeks or if you should develop any severe cramping or fevers.

BIBLIOGRAPHY

ACOG Committee: Cryotherapy in the treatment of CIN, *ACOG Bulletin* 34: August 1985.

ACOG Committee: Cervical cytology: evaluation and management of abnormalities, *ACOG Bulletin*: 183, August 1993.

Elton RF: The appropriate use of liquid nitrogen, *Prim Care* 10:459, September 1983.

Ferris DG, Ho JJ: Cryosurgical equipment: a critical review, *JFP* 35:185, 1992.

Goode RL, DeGraw JR, Hildebrand WL: Abnormal Pap smear: colposcopy and cryosurgery, *Am Fam Physician* 34(6):99, 1986.

Hocutt JE: Cryosurgery (Parts 1, 2, 3), *Fam Pract Bull* 1(12):1988; 1(16):1989; 1(18):1989.

Hurt WG: Cryotherapy of the cervix, *JFP* 9(1):109, 1979.

Rodney WM et al: Colposcopy and cervical cryotherapy, *Postgrad Med* 81(8):79, 1987.

Yliskoski M et al: Cryotherapy and CO_2 laser vaporization in the treatment of cervical and vaginal human papillomavirus (HPV) infections, *Acta Obstet Gynecol Scand* 68:619, 1989.

CHAPTER 84

Treatment of Vulvar, Perianal, Vaginal, Penile, and Urethral Condyloma Acuminata

Barbara S. Apgar

John L. Pfenninger

Genital human papillomavirus (HPV) infection has become alarmingly prevalent. In HPV infection, acuminate lesions can be either visualized or found as acetowhite epithelium (epithelium that turns white after application of acetic acid). Careful inspection and, if possible, colposcopy of the genital area after application of acetic acid is of great value for locating the areas to be treated. HPV is a multicentric disease: both external and internal lesions may be present. The clinician should be alert to signs of HPV infection, which may involve the entire lower genital system of both men and women. Because the risk of neoplastic transformation is possible with HPV infection, liberal biopsy procedures should be employed for any suspicious lesion (before treatment is initiated). The clinician will decide which treatment modality is best based on clinical skill, extent of disease, and overall chance of success. Because there is no specific "cure" for the HPV virus, reduction of the viral pool by eliminating visible lesions and symptom control are the primary indications for treatment. The patient may harbor HPV-DNA for life; therefore, patient education is very important to prevent unreasonable expectations. Clinical disease can generally be controlled with the methods noted here.

All methods of treating HPV have significant failure and recurrence rates. Common modalities for treatment are noted in Tables 84-1 and 84-2.

INDICATIONS

- Visible, acuminate condylomata
- Symptomatic condylomata

653

TABLE 84-1.

Therapies Currently Recommended for the Treatment of Genital Warts

Therapy	Clearance Rate (%)	Recurrence Rate (%)	Pain	Cost	Number of Doctor Visits	Anesthesia Required?	Can Be Used During Pregnancy?
Podophyllin	22-77	11-74	Mild to moderate	$183	3	No	No
Podofilox	45-50	21-33	Mild	Not available	Not available	No	No
Trichloroacetic acid (TCA)	81	36	Moderate	$183	3	No	Yes
Cryotherapy	63-88	21-40	Moderate Some side effects	$285	3	No	Yes
Surgery	93	29	Moderate	Not available	1	Yes, local	Yes
Electrodessication	94	22	Moderate	$340	2	Yes, local	Yes
Interferon	19-62	21-25	Moderate Some side effects	$1,500	9-18	No	No
Laser	31-94	3-95	Moderate to severe	$2,650	1	Yes, local or general	Yes

Adapted from *HPV News* 2(1): 1992. Used with permission of the American Social Health Association.

CONTRAINDICATIONS

- Any known adverse reactions to the selected treatment modality
- Any lesion that is possibly cancerous (These lesions should be biopsied before ablation.)

PREPROCEDURE PATIENT EDUCATION

Explain the procedure to the patient, along with the risks and benefits of the procedure. If an investigational drug is to be used, such as 5-fluorouracil (Efudex), the experimental nature of the therapy should be explained, and informed consent should be obtained.

CRYOSURGERY

Equipment

Cryosurgery may be carried out with a variety of cryosurgical methods:

- Cryogun with nitrous oxide tank, small dermal tips (see Chaper 17, Cryosurgery, and Chapter 83, Crycone of the Cervix)
- Liquid nitrogen and cotton-tipped applicators

- Liquid nitrogen pressurized sprayer (Brymill Minicryogun)
- Verruca Freeze (see Chapter 17, Cryosurgery)

Suppliers

See Chapter 17, Cryosurgery.

Techniques

No anesthetic is required for the following treatments.

Nitrous Oxide, Cryotip Method

1. Place the patient in the lithotomy position and apply dilute acetic acid or vinegar to the vulva, perineum, and rectum (or scrotum and penis). HPV lesions can be identified by the acetowhite reaction. If the lesions cover a large area, it may be prudent to treat sections at separate visits to prevent excessive post-treatment discomfort. Treatment should be directed at the acuminate warts, rather than at subclinical condylomata that cannot be seen with the naked eye. Staining may make smaller acuminate lesions more prominent. Eventually attempts should be made to treat all of the lesions.
2. Select the proper size of cryotip based on the size of the lesion. The tip should cover small lesions; larger lesions may be frozen in sections or clusters.
3. With the cryotip at ambient temperature, place the tip on an individual lesion. Moisten the lesion with water-soluble gel before positioning the probe to improve tip-to-tissue adhesion. Activate the cryogun to initiate the flow of gas within the probe, which begins the freezing process. Apply gentle traction on the lesion as soon as ice appears on the tissue, creating tip-to-tissue adhesion. This traction isolates the lesion from the surrounding tissue, minimizes discomfort, and ensures cold transfer. Clumped lesions may be frozen in clusters, but will require longer freezing times. Clusters will also require the freeze-thaw-refreeze technique to produce the necessary cryonecrosis. (The tissue is frozen until it appears solid white, then thawed until it turns pink again, and then frozen a second time.) Stop freezing as soon as the ice extends just beyond each lesion's border. Repeat the procedure until all lesions are frozen.
4. Explain to the patient that a tingling or burning sensation is normal.

Liquid Nitrogen Therapy, Brymill Minifreezer, Verruca Freeze

Identify the lesions to be treated.

- Dip the cotton-tipped applicator into the liquid nitrogen and apply immediately to the lesion. Reapply until the lesion blanches. Avoid freezing beyond the border of the lesion.
- With the Brymill Minifreezer, spray a jet of liquid nitrogen on the lesions. (This is a quick and economical way to use liquid nitrogen.) Apply the liquid nitrogen until the lesion blanches. Avoid freezing beyond the lesion.
- Verruca Freeze works similarly to liquid nitrogen. Compressed gas in a can is sprayed into an ear speculum, which is placed over the wart. There is a

variety of speculum sizes, and the selection of speculum should be adapted to the size of the lesion. The compressed gas liquifies with spraying, and rapid evaporation results in freezing of the lesion. Use of this agent obviates the need for maintaining large amounts of liquid nitrogen. The speculum must be positioned so that it is perpendicular to the lesion; in this way, it acts like a funnel. This position requirement may be impractical on the genitalia. Once the material is sprayed into the speculum, it is held in place until the bubbling stops. Care must be taken that the liquid does not leak out from under the speculum and freeze normal tissue. One application may suffice on small lesions. If the lesions are large, a second application may be necessary after thawing.

Postprocedure Care

- Usually no postprocedure medication is needed. Topical anesthetic ointments may be used to minimize discomfort. Sitz baths may aid resolution when large areas are treated; silver sulfadiazine (Silvadene) ointment or antibiotic ointment may not only be soothing, but may also reduce the possibility of superficial infection. No dressing is required, but some patients may request a sanitary napkin. Ice packs are helpful.
- Lesions that are cryonecrosed will progress from erythema to edema, and then will turn black. The lesions will disappear within a few days, and healing should be complete in 7 to 8 days.
- For lesions that are cauterized chemically, the healing process is usually less than one week but may take longer.
- The patient should be counseled to report any signs of infection or excessive discomfort.
- Treated areas should be washed and dried gently each day of the healing process. Postcryotherapy management is similar to a second-degree burn.

Complications

- If the area treated at one visit is too large, extensive necrosis and pain may occur. It is prudent to treat reasonably sized areas over multiple visits.
- Infection may occur at the treatment site if the area is not kept clean by normal hygienic measures.
- Recurrence or persistence of lesions is common.

CHEMICAL CAUTERY

Equipment

- 85% trichloroacetic acid (TCA), podophyllin or 0.5% podofilox
- Cotton-tipped applicators
- Acetic acid (3% to 5%) or household vinegar

Technique

- For chemical cautery, identify the lesions to be treated. For small lesions, use the wooden end of the cotton-tipped applicator to apply TCA directly on the lesion until it whitens. Avoid getting the solution on normal skin. For larger lesions, use the cotton-tipped end of the applicator to apply the TCA, again being careful to avoid getting the solution on normal skin. Continue in the same manner until all the lesions are treated. The patient may experience intense pain, which will subside in about 5 minutes. In one to two days the skin will slough. Patients may need retreatment every 2 weeks until the lesions resolve.

- Patients may apply topical 0.5% podofilox solution themselves at home because podofilox is a pure compound and does not contain the substances in podophyllin that produce local toxicity. Podofilox is indicated for topical treatment of external genital warts, but it is not indicated for the treatment of perianal or mucous membrane (urethra, rectum, vagina) condyloma. Podofilox is applied to the warts with a cotton-tipped applicator supplied with the medication. Treatment should be limited to an area less than 10 cm^2 and no more than 0.5 cc of the solution used each day. The solution is applied in the morning and evening for 3 consecutive days; then a 4-day waiting period, during which the solution is not applied, is observed. This one-week treatment cycle may be repeated six times or until there is no visible wart tissue. Later, the entire treatment can be repeated. There are no established guidelines for usage in pregnancy, pediatrics, and nursing mothers. Burning and pain with use are reportedly more frequent and severe in women than in men. Patient education sheets are supplied by the manufacturer. One bottle, sufficient for 4 one-week cycles, costs approximately $50 to $60.

INTERFERON THERAPY

Indications

- Recalcitrant condyloma unresponsive to other modalities

Equipment

- Recombinant interferon alfa-2b
- Needle and syringe (27- to 30-gauge needle, 1 cc syringe)

Technique

1. The manufacturer recommends that only five warts be treated at one time, making this treatment time-consuming and expensive ($8.00 per dose).
2. The standard dose is one million units of interferon (0.1 cc) three times a week for 3 weeks (total of nine injections).

3. Use a 25- to 30-gauge needle to inject the interferon directly into the center of the wart's base.

4. Maximum response should occur within 4 to 6 weeks. If there is no clinical response after 16 weeks, a second 3-week course should be completed.

Postprocedure Care

The patient may take an analgesic if flulike symptoms develop.

Complications

Patients are less likely to experience flulike symptoms (myalgias, fatigue, headache, chills, fever) with the use of intralesional injection than with systemic injection of interferon.

EXCISIONAL/ABLATIVE THERAPY

Lesions that are small or few in number can be cauterized with a ball or needle electrode. They can also be surgically excised with sharp iris scissors or a knife blade after appropriate anesthesia. However, the penile and vulvar skin is thin, and it is easy to resect too deeply—leaving scars. Warty lesions also tend to be vascular and bleed easily. Although this can be controlled with Monsel's solution, it is often easier to employ radiofrequency surgery. An alternative approach would be laser excision, but it is expensive.

LOOP ELECTROSURGICAL EXCISION (SEE CHAPTER 16, RADIOFREQUENCY SURGERY)

Equipment

- Square or round loop electrodes (Use loop size consistent with the size of the warts. It is easier to use electrodes with shorter shafts than the longer ones used to carry out the LEEP procedure. The shorter shafts allow for better control of depth.)
- Electrosurgical generator (ESU)
- Grounding pad
- Smoke evacuator
- 2% lidocaine with or without epinephrine (Epinephrine should *not* be used on the penis.)
- Syringe with 30-gauge needle
- Ball electrodes, 5 mm
- Macroneedle electrodes
- Silvadene cream
- Mask and nonsterile gloves
- 4 × 4 inch sterile gauze pads

Suppliers

See list of companies in Chapter 92, Loop Electrosurgical Excision Procedure (LEEP) for Treating CIN.

Preprocedure Patient Education

Explain the procedure to the patient, and obtain informed consent.

Technique

1. Turn on the ESU power supply. Check the manufacture's guidelines for proper power settings.
2. Place the grounding pad on the thigh and check the seal.
3. Apply 5% acetic acid (or vinegar) to the warts. Keep the tissue moist by repeated acetic acid application.
4. With a 27- to 30-gauge needle, inject 2% lidocaine under the base of the wart to make a wheal that extends beyond the margin of the wart.
5. Activate the smoke evacuator and place the hose close to the excisional site.
6. Select the cutting or blend mode on the ESU.
7. Use the loop electrode to excise the wart. The loop should not excise deeper than 1 mm to the first surgical plane (looks like chamois cloth). To control the depth of excision, place the fifth finger of the hand holding the pencil wand and electrode on the index finger of the opposite hand that is used to expose the lesion. The loop will travel between the spread index and third fingers (or thumb) of the nondominant hand. For precise excision depth control, it is important to hold the pencil wand close to where the electrode inserts into the wand. Often it is best just to "debulk" the wart on the first pass. Then make fine, superficial "feathering" strokes to remove the remaining tissue. Significant bleeding may be a signal that the excision is too deep.
8. After the loop electrode has been used to excise the wart, the ball electrode or macroneedle may be used to coagulate any bleeders or residual tissue, although this is rarely necessary.
9. Remove the coagulated remnants with cotton-tip applicators or gauze sponges soaked with vinegar or acetic acid (5%).
10. If applicable, inspect the excised area with the colposcope to ensure that the entire wart has been excised and that no coagulated remnants are left on the base of the excised lesion.
11. Apply silver sulfadiazine cream or antibiotic ointment to the excision area, and use gauze pads to cover the excision site.

    Note: Many patients prefer this modality over TCA use because healing is often more rapid and less uncomfortable.

**BOX 84-1. PATIENT EDUCATION HANDOUT
INSTRUCTIONS AFTER ELECTROSURGICAL REMOVAL
OF GENITAL CONDYLOMA (WARTS)**

Although the radiofrequency unit that was used to remove your warts causes very little tissue destruction, the area will be quite sore for the next 4 to 5 days. Minimal scarring or decreased pigmentation (lightening) of the treated skin may occur, but usually the results of the procedure—removal of the warts—are far superior to having the warts themselves.

To obtain the best results, please follow these directions:

1. For the first 7 days, shower or bathe two to three times per day. Wash all treated areas with soap and water.
2. After bathing, apply a thin layer of Mycitracin Plus (an antiobiotic ointment), which can be obtained from your pharmacy over the counter. This aids the healing process, decreases scarring, and is soothing. Your doctor may also prescribe Silvadene. If so, use the Silvadene instead of the Mycitracin.
3. Taking three 200 mg ibuprofen tablets four times per day will minimize any pain or discomfort that you might experience.
4. If you continue to have discomfort, a benzocaine ointment can often provide some relief. This can be mixed with the antibiotic ointment (Mycitracin or Silvadene). Benzocaine ointment can be purchased without a prescription at your local pharmacy.
5. Believe it or not, *warm tea bags* can be applied on the wounds and may provide significant relief. Ice packs may also help.
6. If you have significant redness or discharge, or if the pain has not decreased after 48 hours, please call your physician.
7. Schedule a follow-up appointment about 4 weeks after the procedure.
8. One third of the time, the warts return. At any time, if the warts return, see your physician immediately, rather than waiting until they multiply and enlarge. The smaller the lesions, the easier they are to treat and the less likely you are to have any scars.
9. If you had warts that were treated around the rectal area, keep your stools soft. Use stool softeners and laxatives for 1 to 3 weeks. You may also find that benzocaine or lidocaine ointment applied to the rectal area about 10 to 15 minutes before a bowel movement will help ease pain.

Please feel free to ask any questions.

Used with permission of The Medical Procedures Center, P.C., Midland, Michigan.

Postprocedure Care

- Provide the patient with a patient education handout (see Box 84-1).
- Instruct the patient that postprocedure discomfort may last for up to 2 weeks. However, initial discomfort should resolve in 24 to 48 hours. During the initial recovery period, sitz baths may be taken 2 to 3 times a day. The excision site should be kept clean and dry after the sitz bath. Silver sulfadiazine cream should be applied to the area until the initial discomfort has resolved. Ice

packs may also be used. For those patients who have perianal excisions, stool softeners (docusate sodium) are important throughout the entire recovery period.

- If acute discomfort persists beyond 48 hours, instruct the patient to contact the physician. A mixture of equal parts of 20% benzocaine (Hurricaine) ointment and silver sulfadiazine may be needed.
- Instruct the patient to return to the office in 4 to 6 weeks, and to call if fever, chills, or purulent discharge develop.

Complications

- Hypopigmentation may rarely occur at the excision site. Keloids may form on skin that has a tendency for keloid formation.
- Postprocedure bleeding and wound infections are extremely rare.
- According to Ferenczy, treatment failure at 8 months (average two treatments) is 19%.
- Scarring, if the procedure is performed correctly, is minimal and comparable to that of laser excision.

5-FLUOROURACIL (5-FU) AND THE TREATMENT OF EXTENSIVE CONDYLOMATA

Treatment with 5-FU should be considered only for extensive intractable condyloma resistant to other modalities (e.g., TCA). The Food and Drug Administration has not approved labeling of 5-FU for treatment of condylomata, and the patient should be advised that this is technically an investigational use. Because of the reported teratogenic potential, 5-FU should be used with extreme caution—if at all—in nonsterile women of reproductive age.

Indications

- Extensive vulvar, perianal, penile condyloma
- Vaginal condyloma
- Vaginal intraepithelial neoplasia (VAIN)
- Vulvar intraepithelial neoplasia (VIN)

Equipment

- 5% 5-fluorouracil (5-FU) (Efudex) cream
- Vaginal applicator marked with dosage lines

Preprocedure Patient Education

- Obtain informed consent before initiating treatment.
- Advise the patient of alternative methods of treatment. Frequently when 5-FU is being considered, laser therapy is an option.

- The patient should know that the inflammatory response is delayed by 3 to 4 days. The patient may believe the medication is not working and apply it more frequently, leading to complications.
- Use of 5-FU should be limited to clinicians experienced with managing side effects.

Technique

1. Instruct the patient to use 1.5 gm of 5-FU per week for 10 weeks. A standard ortho-vaginal applicator will hold 10 cc of cream (5 gm of 5-FU). Patients should use one third of an applicator of cream at each treatment. The 5-FU should be inserted intravaginally and/or applied directly to any external lesions at bedtime.
2. Instruct the patient to apply zinc oxide to the vulva (where treatment is not necessary) to protect it in the event that the 5-FU should leak out onto the vulva.
3. The patient may insert a small tampon into the vagina to keep the 5-FU within the introitus.
4. If there is no inflammatory response after 3 weeks, the patient may increase the frequency of application to every 5 days.

   Caution: Those with blond or red hair, or with very light complexions, may be more sensitive to 5-FU.

Postprocedure Care

Instruct the patient to contact the physician if severe inflammation or any hypersensitivity reaction occurs. Intravaginal conjugated estrogens (Premarin) or steroid creams may be used to decrease the inflammatory reaction.

Complications

- Persistent vaginal ulcers may develop in patients who are extremely sensitive to the 5-FU or in patients who overuse the medication.
- For some patients, the vaginal ulcers may fail to heal with time, and they may have persistent vaginal discharge and bleeding. Patients who fail to heal may require surgical excision of the entire ulcer and primary closure of the defect.
- Vaginal stenosis is a rare complication.
- If 5-FU is to be used after cryotherapy of the cervix, wait at least 4 weeks before initiating 5-FU therapy.

PERIANAL AND INTRAANAL LESIONS

Treatment of perianal and intraanal lesions is similar to treatment for vaginal condylomata. Additional guidelines are as follows:

- Podophyllin (if still used) should not be used on mucous membranes (i.e., inside the anus).

TABLE 84-2.

Comparative Costs of HPV Treatment Modalities

Therapy	Cost per Treatment		Average Number of Treatments	Total Cost[1]	Effectiveness[2]	Cost Index[3]
	Medication[4]	Physician's Fees				
Podophyllin	0[5]	50.00[6]	3	150.00	20%	750.00
Podofilox	40.00	90.00[7]	12[8]	130.00	20%	650.00
TCA	0[5]	50.00[6]	3	150.00	40%	375.00
Bleomycin	27.00	90.00[6]	1.5	162.00	?	
5-FU (topical, monotherapy)	30.00	120.00[9]	12	150.00	0 - 50%[10]	
Cryotherapy	0	100.00[11]	3	300.00	65%	461.50
Surgery (electrosurgery or excisional)	0	200.00[12]	1	200.00	70%	285.70
Laser	0	2500.00[13]	1	2500.00	75%	3333.30
Interferon (intralesional)	85.00[14]	65.00[15]	9	670.00	45%	1488.90

[1]Cost per treatment times average number of treatments.
[2]Rough estimate based on literature values: calculated as complete clearance rate × (1-recurrence rate).
[3]Total cost + effectiveness: a rough estimate of the average cost to completely clear a patient of lesions.
[4]Based on average wholesale price in the Atlanta area. Retail prices will run approximately 40% higher.
[5]Cost included in price of physician office visit (medication applied by physician).
[6]Based on chemical destruction of penile condylomata, approximate price plus intralesional injection.
[7]Initial visit plus follow-up visit.
[8]Home treatments done by patient.
[9]Initial visit and two follow-up visits.
[10]Only demonstrated effective for vaginal and intraurethral warts.
[11]Cryotherapy, penile condylomata.
[12]Surgical destruction, penile condylomata.
[13]Based on physician charge, operating room costs, and cost of anesthesia.
[14]10 million unit vial, adequate for one course of treatment.
[15]Office visit plus injection charge.
From Ling MR: Therapy of genital human papillomavirus infections, part II: methods of treatment, *Int J Dermatol* 31(11):774, 1992. Used with permission.

- 85% TCA may be used intraanally.
- Anoscopy should be performed on all patients with perianal lesions to rule out more proximal lesions.
- The risk of rectal carcinoma is increased in homosexual men, and HPV appears to be involved in the process.

CPT/BILLING CODES

11900	Injection, intralesional; up to and including seven lesions
11901	Injection intralesional; more than seven lesions
17100	Destruction by any method, including laser, of benign skin lesions other than cutaneous vascular proliferative lesions on any area other than the face; including local anesthesia; one lesion
17101	Destruction by any method, including laser, of benign skin lesions other than cutaneous vascular proliferative lesions on any area other than the face; including local anesthesia; second lesion

17102	Destruction by any method, including laser, of benign skin lesions other than cutaneous vascular proliferative lesions on any area other than the face; including local anesthesia; over two lesions, each additional lesion up to 15 lesions
17104	Destruction by any method, including laser, of benign skin lesions other than cutaneous vascular proliferative lesions on any area other than the face; including local anesthesia; 15 or more lesions
17105	Destruction by any method, including laser, of benign skin lesions other than cutaneous vascular proliferative lesions on any area other than the face; including local anesthesia; complicated or extensive lesions
17340	Cryotherapy (CO_2 slush, liquid N_2)
46900	Destruction of lesion(s); *anus* (e.g., condyloma), *simple;* chemical
46910	Destruction of lesion(s); electrodesiccation
46916	Destruction of lesion(s); cryosurgery
46922	Destruction of lesion(s); surgical excision
46924	Destruction of lesion(s); *anus, extensive;* any method
54050	Destruction of lesion(s); *penis* (e.g., condyloma), *simple;* chemical
54055	Destruction of lesion(s); electrodesiccation
54056	Destruction of lesion(s); cryosurgery
54060	Destruction of lesion(s); surgical excision
54065	Destruction of lesion(s); *penis, extensive,* any method
56501	Destruction of lesion(s); *vulva, simple,* any method
56515	Destruction of lesion(s); *extensive,* any method
57061	Destruction of *vaginal* lesion(s); *simple,* any method
57065	Destruction of lesion(s); *extensive,* any method

BIBLIOGRAPHY

Baker DA et al: Topical podofilox for the treatment of condylomata acuminata in women, *Obstet Gynecol* 76(4):656, 1990.

Eron LJ et al: Interferon therapy for condyloma acuminata, *N Engl J Med* 315(17):1059, 1986.

Felmar E et al: Primary care office procedures: treatment of genital lesions via cryocautery, *Prim Care Cancer* 6:1, 1988.

Ferenczy A et al: *Loop electrosurgical excision procedure (LEEP) syllabus,* Shelton, Conn, 1991, Cooper Surgical.

Ferenczy A: Diagnosis and treatment of anogenital warts in the male patient, *Prim Care* 10:11, 1990.

Friedman-Kien AE et al: Natural interferon alfa for treatment of condyloma acuminata, *JAMA* 259(4):533, 1988.

Greenberg MD et al: A double blind, randomized trial of 0.5% podofilox and placebo for the treatment of genital warts in women, *Obstet Gynecol:* 735, 1991.

Guidelines for cryosurgery: cryomedics, Langhorne, Pa, 1988, Cabot Medical.

Kling AR: Genital warts—therapy, *Sem Dermatol* 11(3):247, 1992.

Krebs HB: Treatment of vaginal condylomata acuminata by weekly topical application of 5-fluorouracil, *Obstet Gynecol* 70(1):68, 1987.

Krebs HB: Treatment of vaginal intraepithelial neoplasia with laser and topical 5-fluorouracil, *Obstet Gynecol* 73(4):657, 1989.

Krebs HB et al: Chronic ulcerations following topical therapy with 5-fluorouracil for vaginal human papillomavirus-associated lesions, *Obstet Gynecol* 78(2):205, 1991.

Ling MR: Therapy of genital human papillomavirus infections. Part I: Indications for and justification of therapy, *Int J Dermatol* 31(10):682, 1992.

Ling MR: Therapy of genital human papillomavirus infections. Part II: Methods of treatment, *Int J Dermatol* 31(11):769, 1992.

Patsner B: A patient applied topical solution for genital warts, *Contemp Obstet Gynecol* 12:27, 1991.

Richart R et al: Ways of using LEEP for external lesions, *Contemp Obstet Gynecol* 5:138, 1992.

Tyring SK et al: Alpha interferon in the management of genital warts, *Female Patient* 18:33; 1993.

Vance JC et al: Intralesional recombinant alfa-2 interferon for the treatment of the patient with condyloma acuminatum or verruca plantaris, *Arch Dermatol* 122:272, 1986.

Welander CE et al: Intralesional interferon alfa-2b for the treatment of genital warts, *Am J Obstet Gynecol* 162(2):348, 1990.

CHAPTER 85

Postcoital Examination Test or Sims-Huhner Test

Barbara S. Apgar

The postcoital examination test (PCT) is an evaluation of survival and motility of sperm in the cervical mucus. The test is performed just before ovulation, usually between days 12 and 14 of the normal menstrual cycle. In infertility investigations, the incidence of sperm or mucus abnormalities ranges from 20% to 30%.

INDICATIONS

- Investigation of the sperm/cervical mucus interaction to determine whether abnormalities are the cause of infertility

CONTRAINDICATIONS

- Any condition that would preclude unprotected sexual intercourse followed by examination and sampling of the cervix

EQUIPMENT

- Vaginal speculum
- Vaginal swabs
- Tuberculin syringe with cap
- Microscope
- Glass slides and coverslips
- *Optional:* pipelle aspirator

PREPROCEDURE PATIENT EDUCATION

- Explain the proper timing of intercourse (just before ovulation) to the couple. The PCT should be performed 2 to 3 days before ovulation, when the cervical mucus is the most estrogenic. This occurs 2 to 3 days before ovulation. The test is usually performed on days 12 to 14 of an ideal 28-day cycle. Basal body temperature (BBT) charts will help in determining this diagnostic interval.
- Instruct the couple to have intercourse 8 to 12 hours before the office visit. Before performing the PCT, the clinician should determine that the BBT is in accord with the proper timing of the menstrual cycle for the performance of the test. An ovulation kit may also be used to determine the correct testing interval.
- Explain to the couple that vaginal lubricants, medications, and douches should not be used near the time of intercourse or up to the time of the office visit.
- Instruct the woman to come to the office 8 to 12 hours after intercourse.

TECHNIQUE

1. Place the patient in the lithotomy position. Insert a vaginal speculum and visualize the cervix. Gently wipe the cervix with a vaginal swab.
2. Insert a tuberculin syringe (without the needle) into the endocervical canal and retract the plunger to draw the mucus into the syringe. A pipelle aspirator may also be used to obtain the mucus. If the volume of the specimen is inadequate (less than 2 cc), the procedure may be repeated until a sufficient sample is obtained. Place the syringe cap over the hub once the sample is obtained so that the mucus will be stored in an airtight container until it is ready for processing. Note the amount and clarity of the mucus. Record the degree of stretchability of the mucus (spinnbarkeit test). A ring forcep or Kelly clamp may be used to grasp the mucus at the cervical os. The stretch of the mucus may be measured as the forcep is removed from the vagina. The mucus can also be placed between the index finger and thumb. The stretch of the mucus is determined as the fingers are drawn apart. A mucus stretch greater than 10 cm is indicative of a high estrogenic state conducive for ovulation. A spinnbarkeit of less than 3 cm indicates a low likelihood of sperm penetration through the mucus and an unfavorable situation for ovulation.
3. Place a drop of the mucus from the syringe on a glass slide, and immediately place a coverslip over the sample.
4. Examine the cervical mucus under low power for the presence of sperm and other components, such as trichomonads, leukocytes, squamous cells, or Candida. Make a note of the number of sperm. Examine the specimen under high power. The number of sperm in at least five different fields should be averaged. Record an average number or range of numbers of sperm present. Note whether the sperm are mobile, whether they have normal or abnormal morphology,

and whether they exhibit forward progression. For a normal study, if specimens are examined 12 to 14 hours after intercourse, there should be an average of *at least five actively motile sperm per high-power field*.

POSTPROCEDURE CARE

Schedule a repeat examination the following month if the test is inconclusive or abnormal.

COMPLICATIONS

- The validity of the PCT has been questioned because of varying standards for normal results and also because of numerous techniques for obtaining and interpreting the samples.
- Falsely abnormal results can result from poor timing of the menstrual cycle, poor mucus quality due to infection, faulty coital positions not favoring vaginal sperm retention, and low semen volume or low numbers of sperm.

CPT/BILLING CODE

89300   Semen analysis; presence and/or motility of sperm including Huhner test

BIBLIOGRAPHY

Griffith CS, Grimes DA: The validity of the postcoital test, *Am J Obstet Gynecol* 162(3):615, 1990.

Harrison RF: The diagnostic and therapeutic potential of the postcoital test, *Fertil Steril* 36:71, 1981.

Moghissi K: Postcoital test: physiologic basis, technique and interpretation, *Fertil Steril* 27:117, 1976.

Muasher SJ: Infertility. In Rosenwaks Z, Benjamin F, Stone ML, editors: *Gynecology principles and practice,* New York, 1987, Macmillan.

Wentz AC: The cervical factor: evaluation and therapy. In Wentz AC, editor: *Gynecologic endocrinology and infertility for the house officer,* Baltimore, 1988, Williams & Wilkins.

CHAPTER 86

Wet Smear and KOH Preparation

Barbara S. Apgar

The wet smear is an important tool in the office evaluation of vaginitis. It should be performed on all patients with vaginal symptoms, even if the diagnosis seems obvious. The wet smear is an accessory tool to the history, the inspection of the vulvar and vaginal mucosa, and the determination of the pH of the vaginal secretions.

INDICATIONS

- Vaginal discharge
- Vulvar or vaginal pruritus
- Vulvar or vaginal pain
- Malodorous vaginal secretions

CONTRAINDICATIONS

- Recent douching
- Intravaginal medications
- Menses

EQUIPMENT

- Vaginal speculum
- Small cotton-tipped applicators
- Small test tubes
- Normal saline
- 10% KOH (potassium hydroxide) solution
- Glass slides and coverslips
- Microscope
- pH test tape

PREPROCEDURE PATIENT EDUCATION

- Explain the procedure to the patient. Written consent is not required.
- Instruct the patient to avoid vaginal medication, douches, and coitus for 24 hours before the procedure.

TECHNIQUE

1. Place the patient in the lithotomy position and insert a vaginal speculum.
2. Rub a cotton-tipped applicator along the lateral vaginal walls and the lateral fornices to collect the specimen. Put the cotton-tipped applicator in a small test tube (3 to 4 inches long) that contains approximately 1 cc of normal saline. Leave the applicator in the test tube until the wet smear is prepared. Remove the speculum from the vagina.
3. Take the test tube to the laboratory to prepare the wet smear. Remove the cotton-tipped applicator from the test tube, place a drop on the left side of the glass slide, and immediately place a coverslip over the drop. Place another drop from the cotton applicator on the right side of the slide. Add a drop of 10% KOH solution to the drop and immediately place a coverslip over it.
4. Examine the saline- and KOH-prepared samples under low (10×) and high (40×) power of the microscope. Examine the saline preparation for the presence of Lactobacillus species (normal vaginal flora), leukocytes (more than 10 cells per high power field [HPF] may indicate infection), basal cells (may indicate low estrogenic state), trichomonads, and clue cells (bacterial vaginosis). A clue cell is a large epithelial cell with indistinct borders and multiple cocci clinging to it. At least five different microscopic fields should be surveyed to observe an adequate number of representative fields. Scan the KOH-prepared sample for the presence of hyphae or buds (candidiasis).

   Note: Lactobacilli are large, long bacillary rods. Their absence, coupled with an abundance of small cocci, may correlate with the bacterial overgrowth seen in bacterial vaginosis.

5. pH test tape may be used to screen for the specific type of vaginitis. A piece of the pH test tape may be directly applied to the vaginal wall or the tape can be applied to the vaginal secretions adhering to the speculum when it is removed from the vagina. Compare the color of the test tape that has been in contact with the secretions to the color guide on the tape dispenser. The range of values will be determined by the color of the tape.
   Normal flora—pH ≤ 4
   Candidiasis—pH 4 to 5
   Bacterial vaginosis—pH 5 to 6
   Trichomonas—pH 6 to 7
   The pH reading and the microscopic impression combined help make an accurate diagnosis.
6. At the same time that the vaginitis evaluation is performed, specimens from the cervix may be obtained for culture of chlamydia and gonorrhea. The proper sampling devices and proper preparation are important and depend on

the type of test the laboratory uses. If a cotton-tipped swab is used for sample collection, the cervix does not need to be wiped clean before the procedure. Insert the applicator directly into the cervical canal until the cotton tip is completely inside the os. Gently twirl the tip several times in the os. Withdraw the applicator and place it in the proper container. Your laboratory should provide specific directions for obtaining the sample and transporting it to the laboratory.

POSTPROCEDURE PATIENT EDUCATION

Instruct the patient about medication, if needed, and the need for follow-up appointments.

CPT/BILLING CODE

58999   Wet smear and KOH preparation

BIBLIOGRAPHY

Bertholf ME, Stafford MJ: An office laboratory panel to assess vaginal problems, *Am Fam Physician* 32(3):113, 1985.

Eschenbach DA: Vaginal infection, *Clin Obstet Gynecol* 26(1):186, 1983.

Eschenbach DA, Hillier SL: Advances in diagnostic testing for vaginitis and cervicitis, *J Reprod Med* 34(8):555, 1989.

Friedrich EG: Vaginitis, *Am J Obstet Gynecol* 152(3):247, 1985.

Shesser R: Common vaginal infections: a concise work-up guide, *Female Patient* 15:53, 1990.

CHAPTER 87

Dilation and Curettage

Timothy A. Curran

Although newer endometrial biopsy techniques have somewhat lessened the role of classical dilation and curettage (D & C), the procedure is still useful for determining the cause of abnormal uterine bleeding and for therapeutic removal of retained products of conception (see Chapter 89, First Trimester Abortion).

INDICATIONS

- For diagnosis of cause of premenopausal bleeding that has not been corrected by medical management
- For diagnosis of the cause of premenopausal bleeding that occurs in women over 40 years of age with inadequate endometrial biopsies
- For diagnosis of the cause of premenopausal bleeding when submucous myoma or endometrial polyp is suspected
- For diagnosis of the cause of premenopausal bleeding associated with adenomatous hyperplasia with atypia (to rule out cancer)
- For diagnosis of the cause of postmenopausal bleeding when endometrial aspiration is nondiagnostic
- As a prehysterectomy measure in postmenopausal women to exclude the possibility of endometrial or endocervical cancer
- As a part of postmenopausal vaginal surgery without hysterectomy
- To determine the cause of significant uterine bleeding that would contraindicate endometrial biopsy
- For therapeutic removal of retained products of conception associated with postpartum infection or hemorrhaging
- For therapeutic removal of retained products after an incomplete abortion
- For therapy of excessive hemorrhaging

CONTRAINDICATIONS

- Infection, unless cause is thought to be necrotic retained products of conception
- Pregnancy (for therapeutic or elective abortion, see Chapter 89, First Trimester Abortion)
- Lack of facilities to deal with sequelae of uterine perforation in a timely manner
- Lack of resuscitation equipment
- Lack of cooperative patient, if performed in the office

EQUIPMENT (FIG. 87-1)

- Weighted (Auvard) speculum
- Polyp (Stone) forceps/ring forceps
- Hegar cervical dilators
- Uterine sound

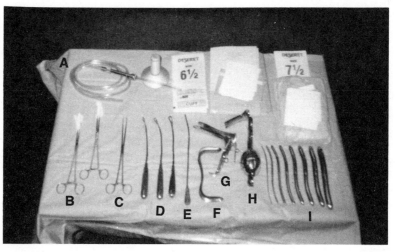

FIG. 87-1.
Instruments used for dilation and curettage. **A,** Vacuum suction and tubing; **B,** Polyp forceps; **C,** Tenaculum; **D,** Sharp uterine curettes; **E,** Uterine sound; **F,** Retractor; **G,** Regular speculum; **H,** Weighted (Auvard) speculum; **I,** Hegar dilators.

- Kevorkian curette for endocervical curettage
- Sharp uterine curette
- Cervical tenaculum
- Vacuum suction apparatus (*optional in some pregnancy-related cases*)
- Paracervical block kit with 10 cc of lidocaine (*optional and not always indicated if patient has light general anesthesia*)
- Sterile preparation pack for vaginal surgery
- Sterile gown and gloves
- Drugs, intravenous solutions and tubing, and mask for administration of inhalants, if used
- Telfa pads

ANESTHESIA

There are many acceptable drug protocols for D & C anesthesia, and each physician has his or her own preference. For many women, a paracervical block alone suffices.

Meperidine, Promethazine, and Benzodiazepine

1. Start an intravenous line and administer 50 to 75 mg meperidine (Demerol) with 25 mg promethazine (Phenergan) intramuscularly.
2. Add 5 to 10 mg diazepam (Valium) intravenously as needed.
3. Have naloxone (Narcan), flumazenil (Romazicon), and resuscitation equipment available.
4. Use a paracervical block if the os is closed or dilation is necessary.
5. Monitor level of intravenous sedation with pulse oximeter.

Benzodiazepine, Alfentanil, and Nitrous Oxide

1. Start an intravenous line and administer 2 mg of midazolam (Versed); increase dose as needed.
2. Add alfentanil (Alfenta) 1 to 2 cc and increase as needed.
3. *Optional:* Administer nitrous oxide and oxygen in 3:2 flow.
4. Use a paracervical block if the os is closed or dilation is necessary.
5. As before, use pulse oximeter (if available) and have flumazenil (Romazicon) and resuscitation equipment available.

TECHNIQUE

Preparatory Steps

1. Blood for complete blood count (CBC), blood type, and screen may be drawn before the procedure.
2. Sedate the patient.

3. Place the patient in the dorsal lithotomy position, and perform sterile preparation with a standard vaginal prep.
4. Put on a sterile gown and gloves.
5. *Optional:* Empty the patient's bladder with a Foley catheter, then remove the catheter.
6. Perform a bimanual examination to determine fundal position.
7. Insert a weighted speculum and administer a paracervical block. Inject 5 cc of lidocaine into the cervix at the 3 o'clock position, making sure you aspirate before injecting. Repeat the injection at the 9 o'clock position. (This is necessary only if dilation of the cervix is indicated, and can be eliminated if the patient has light general anesthesia.) (See Chapter 102, Paracervical Block.)
8. Apply the tenaculum above the os at the 12 o'clock position.

Procedure

1. Sound the uterine cavity to determine its size and confirm its position. The upper limit of normal is 8 cm.
2. Successively dilate the os to 8 or 9 mm with Hagar dilators.
3. If endometrial cancer is to be confirmed or ruled out, use a Kevorkian or Gusberg curette to curettage the endocervix. (A fractional curettage of the endocervix is important to determine the anatomical extensions of endometrial cancer and to rule out an endocervical block.)
   a. Use short firm in-and-out strokes from the internal os to the external os, curetting in a full 360-degree circle twice.
   b. Place the collected tissue on a Telfa pad or lens paper, and send this specimen in a separate container to the pathology laboratory.
4. Place a surgical glove around the handle of the weighted speculum to collect the uterine fragments. Alternatively, place a Telfa pad in the posterior vaginal vault to collect any tissue curetted from the uterus.
5. Insert the sharp uterine curette and scrape the anterior, posterior, and lateral walls of the endometrial cavity gently but firmly. Scrape the top of the cavity with a side-to-side movement. Remove the endometrial scrapings from the glove and place in formalin. If a Telfa pad is used, either submit the entire pad in a formalin container, or scrape the tissue off into a jar with formalin.

   Note: During sharp curettage, the firm stroke should be toward the examiner to lessen the chance of uterine perforation.

6. It is wise as a final step to search the cavity for polyps by systematically opening and closing the polyp forceps while moving across the dome, anterior, and posterior walls of the uterus. Remove any tissue grasped with the forceps with gentle pressure or twisting.

Alternative Method

For suction curettage in incomplete, therapeutic, or elective abortion, see Chapter 89, First Trimester Abortion.

IMMEDIATE POSTPROCEDURE CARE

- 20 units of oxytocin (Pitocin) can be added to a liter of the intravenous solution. Usually when this is added to the solution remaining in the IV bag hung in the operating room, it is adequate to stop bleeding.
- Take the patient to the recovery room and monitor for several hours, if possible, to ensure no complications occur.
- Analgesia, although rarely needed postoperatively, may be achieved with (1) ketorolac (Toradol) 60 mg intravenously or (2) a one-time intravenous or intramuscular dose of meperidine 50 mg with promethazine 25 mg, followed by oral acetaminophen with hydrocodone (Vicodin) or NSAIDs.
- Rhogam should be administered for Rh negative patients, if indicated.

BEFORE DISCHARGE

The patient should be awake, alert, ambulatory, and able to take fluids well. Vital signs should be stable, and if there was significant bleeding, a postprocedure hemoglobin and hematocrit should be determined. If all is well, the patient may not need any medications. The following can be considered:

1. Ergonovine 0.2 mg every 4 hours for 6 doses to diminish bleeding
2. Doxycycline 100 mg twice a day for 7 days
3. Nonsteroidal antiinflammatory drugs (NSAIDs) for pain

POSTPROCEDURE PATIENT EDUCATION

Instruct the patient to avoid sexual activity for at least 2 weeks, and to call if bleeding, fever, purulent discharge, or abdominal pain develop.

COMPLICATIONS

- Hemorrhage (very rare unless pregnancy related; occurrence less than 1%)
- Infection (treat with broad-spectrum antibiotic)
- Perforated uterus:
  1. More likely to occur in presence of uterine infection at time of D & C, in elderly postmenopausal women with a stenotic cervical os, and with sharp as opposed to vacuum curette.
  2. With lateral perforation, there is a risk of injury to uterine artery.
  3. Anterior-posterior perforation is usually not serious if a small curette is used.

  Note: In most cases, treatment for perforation is simple observation. Perforation can be ascertained if the uterine sound or curette passes beyond 9 to 10 cm (unless the uterus actually palpates this large). If perforation occurs, the procedure should be terminated. Before discharging the patient, observe her for unstable vital signs and significant pelvic pain or bleeding. Some physicians provide antibiotic coverage, although this is not always essential.

- Asherman's intrauterine adhesions that may cause secondary amenorrhea, infertility, recurrent abortion, or other menstrual irregularities (This is more common when D & C is performed on the puerperal uterus.)
- Disease may be missed (In most vigorous D & Cs, studies show only 50% to 60% of the endometrial cavity is actually curetted.)

CPT/BILLING CODES

57505	Endocervical curettage (not done as part of a dilation and curettage)
58120	Dilation and curettage, diagnostic and/or therapeutic (non-obstetrical)
59160	Curettage, postpartum (separate procedure)

BIBLIOGRAPHY

Carcinoma of the endometrium, *ACOG Technical Bulletin* 162:1, 1991.

Grimes DA: Diagnostic dilatation and curettage, *Obstet Gynecol* 142:1, 1982.

Hacker NF, Moore JG, editors: *Essentials of obstetrics and gynecology,* Philadelphia, 1986, W.B. Saunders.

Harris GS, Leuchter RS: *Essentials of obstetrics and gynecology,* Philadelphia, 1986, W.B. Saunders.

MacKenzie IZ: Routine outpatient diagnostic uterine curettage using a flexible plastic aspiration curette, *Br J Obstet Gynecol* 92:1291, 1985.

CHAPTER 88

Permanent Female Sterilization (Tubal Ligation)

Gary R. Newkirk

In the United States, voluntary sterilization remains one of the most widely used contraceptive methods, utilized by nearly 20% of married women. Family physicians who are skilled with basic surgical technique are in an ideal position to discuss and perform permanent sterilization procedures for both men and women. Table 88-1 outlines basic terminology related to permanent female sterilization methodology. Minilaparotomy and laparoscopy are abdominal surgical approaches that are considered safe, quick, and readily available. Basic anatomy is outlined in Fig. 88-1.

Despite numerous variations, female sterilization consists of two basic steps: (1) exposing the fallopian tubes, and (2) partially resecting or occluding the tubes to prevent conception. This chapter discusses the minilaparotomy approach to permanent female sterilization, both as an interval and as a postpartum procedure.

Table 88-2 presents advantages and disadvantages of the minilaparotomy and the laparoscopic techniques. Despite the recognized advantages of laparoscopy for certain situations, minilaparotomy—because of its reliance on readily available surgical equipment, fewer technical demands, and its applicability to both interval and postpartum periods—is the method of choice for many primary care physicians. Table 88-3 summarizes the more common methods for ligating the tubes.

This chapter outlines the minilaparotomy approach and the modified Pomeroy or "Parkland" method for ligation. The ideal method is still under debate; however, the modified Pomeroy or Parkland methods (with their variations) remain popular in this country. Prudent physicians should identify patients who may benefit by referral either for alternative methods that they cannot offer because of their lack of skill, training, equipment, or facility, or because of the patient's clinical condition.

TABLE 88-1.

Female Sterilization Terminology

Laparotomy	A relatively large abdominal incision performed to optimize surgical exposure for a variety of intraabdominal surgeries.
Minilaparotomy	Sometimes referred to as minilap; involves a small abdominal incision usually less than 5 cm (2 inches).
Laparoscopy	Involves inserting an illuminated telescope-like instrument into the abdomen that allows visualization of the fallopian tubes to accomplish electrocoagulation, or application of clips or rings. For *open* laparoscopy, a small incision is made within or just below the umbilicus to allow passage of a special cannula, around which the skin makes an airtight seal. The cannula allows for insufflation of the abdomen, passage of the laparoscope and instruments, and occlusion of the tubes. Open laparoscopy is considered safer than traditional *closed* laparoscopy, especially in women with prior pelvic or abdominal surgery or infection. With the closed laparoscopic procedure, the laparoscope is inserted blindly through the abdominal wall.
Postpartum tubal ligation	Tubal ligation performed within 72 hours of delivery.
Interval tubal ligation	Tubal ligation performed at times other than during the immediate postpartum period—generally 6 weeks after delivery or more.
Technical failure	Inability to complete the planned sterilization during the operation, which results in a change of method or failure to perform the sterilization.
Colpotomy	A vaginal approach to tubal ligation through the posterior vaginal fornix.

INTERVAL TUBAL LIGATION

Indications

- Desire for permanent sterilization
- Medical conditions that place the patient at significant risk for irreversible morbidity or death if she should become pregnant
- Known severe inheritable genetic disease where childbearing is not desired

Absolute Contraindications

- Active peritoneal infections
- Severe chronic heart, lung, or metabolic disease (Abdominal insufflation [laparoscopy] and the head-down [Trendelenburg] position can cause acute cardiopulmonary decompensation.)
- Any unstable medical condition
- Lack of informed consent

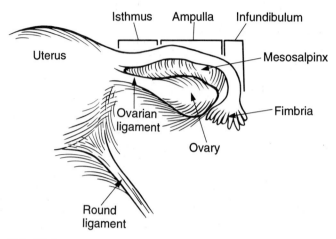

FIG. 88-1.
Basic anatomy of the parauterine structures.

TABLE 88-2.

Advantages and Disadvantages of Minilaparotomy and Laparoscopy

Advantages	Disadvantages
Minilaparotomy	
Easy to learn	Takes longer than laparoscopy
Basic surgical training and skill	Difficult to perform on patients who are obese or who have pelvic scarring or adhesions
Inexpensive instruments	Scar slightly larger
Complications are usually minor	More pain from the abdominal incision
Can be performed as a postpartum or interval procedure	Higher infection rate than laparoscopy
Laparoscopy	
Very low complication rate	Complications may be serious
Quick procedure (10 to 15 minutes)	Requires abdominal insufflation, with its added risk
Very small incision	More difficult to learn; requires specialized training for physician and staff
Useful for other diagnostic and therapeutic purposes	Equipment is more expensive and requires more maintenance and repair
Less painful	Not recommended as a postpartum procedure

Relative Contraindications

- Prior significant pelvic or abdominal infection; minilaparotomy or laparoscopy may be more difficult (Laparotomy may be necessary.)
- Severe obesity, especially with a history of pelvic or abdominal infection

TABLE 88-3.

Common Tubal Ligation Methods

Minilaparotomy ("Open" procedure)	
Pomeroy technique	The most common procedure performed for both interval and postpartum tubal ligations. Absorbable catgut sutures are used to tie the base of a loop of midportion (ampullary) tube. The ligated loop of tube is then removed. As the suture absorbs, the ends pull apart and are obstructed by the healing and scarring process. From 3 to 6 cm of the tube is destroyed (see Fig. 88-2).
Parkland technique	A small length of tube is separated from the mesosalpinx and ligated at each end about 2 cm apart, and the free segment between the ligatures is removed (see Fig. 88-3).
Irving technique	An extremely effective yet more difficult method that cannot easily be reversed. The tube is cut and the uterine end buried beneath the peritoneum within the wall of the uterus. The remaining end is buried within the mesosalpinx.
Uchida technique	A technically demanding yet extremely effective method that is becoming more popular in the United States. The tube is severed and the uterine end is buried within the mesosalpinx.
Fimbriectomy	Accomplished by complete removal of the fimbriated end of the tube. The procedure appears to have a higher pregnancy rate, and reversal is unlikely.
Laparoscopy	
Clips	Under laparoscopic guidance, clips are applied to occlude the tubal lumen. Hulka (spring-loaded) and Filshie clips (titanium/silicone rubber) are commonly used. Clips destroy less than 1 cm of tissue, and reversals are considered much easier.
Electrocoagulation	A bipolar probe is passed through a small segment of tube to cauterize and obstruct the lumen.
Tubal ring	A small silastic ring is stretched and placed over a loop of fallopian tube and then released. The tube is blocked by compression. Usually a 2 to 3 cm segment of the tube is involved. Reversal is more successful than with electrocauterization, Irving, or Uchida techniques.
Vaginal approaches	
Ligation, clips, electrocoagulation rings	Two varieties have been used. *Colpotomy* involves a surgical incision in the posterior vaginal fornix through which the tube is delivered and occluded by ligation, clips, or rings. In *culdoscopy,* a culdoscope is passed through a smaller colpotomy incision to allow identification of the tubes and application of the electroprobe, clips, or rings. Both of these less popular methods share higher complication and failure rates. They are not postpartum methods.
Transcervical	Still considered experimental procedures, these methods of blocking the tubes from a transcervical/intrauterine approach continue to evoke interest. One method is to use silastic "plugs" placed under hysteroscopic guidance.

- Heart disease, irregular pulse, uncontrolled hypertension, pelvic masses, uncontrolled diabetes, bleeding disorders, severe nutritional deficiencies, severe anemia, and umbilical or hiatal hernia (The risks of future pregnancies must be weighed against the risks of permanent sterilization procedures.)
- Inability to tolerate anesthesia
- Patient unsure of desire for permanent sterilization

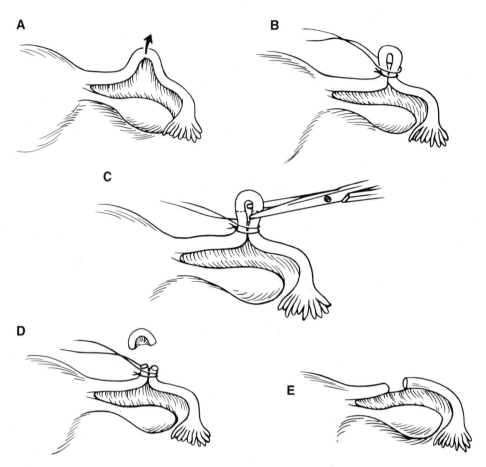

FIG. 88-2.
Modified Pomeroy technique. **A,** Lift loop; **B,** Double ligation 0 or 2-0 plain gut suture, no crushing; **C,** Each limb of tubal loop is cut separately; **D,** Loop is cut off; **E,** Later results.

Equipment

Laparotomy Setup. A laparotomy pack, that contains most of the instruments necessary for basic abdominal surgery is available in most hospital outpatient or inpatient surgical suites. The following are the basics needed for tubal ligation by minilaparotomy:

- Suction catheter (Generally, suction is not used during a routine minilaparotomy tubal ligation. Suction is available on demand at most surgical suites; it is mandatory if complications such as bleeding develop.)
- Coagulation device (Most operative suites have a Bovie or similar coagulation device available. Some surgeons prefer to have this available for all cases; others use this electively, or when complications develop. Since a Bovie requires grounding, it should be set up in advance. A ground plate can be attached before the patient is draped and scrubbed.)
- Sutures

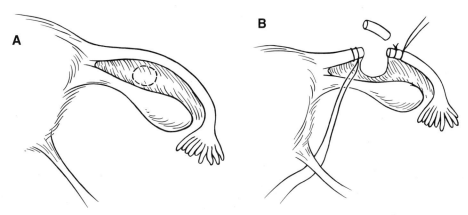

FIG. 88-3.
Parkland method of tubal ligation. **A,** A relatively bloodless area of the mesosalpinx is identified within the isthmic portion of the tube. **B,** A segment of tube is isolated and removed following double ligation with chromic suture.

Anatomical site	Suture
Tubal ligation	0 plain or chromic
Peritoneum	2-0 chromic
Fascia	0 dexon
Scarpa's fascia	2-0 chromic
Skin	metal clips, 4-0 dexon

- 8-inch Babcock forceps to separate and retract fallopian tube (Fig. 88-4, *A*)
- Ring sponge (ring forceps holding a tightly folded gauze pad)
- Small Richardson or Army/Navy retractors for holding the incision open (Fig. 88-4, *B*)

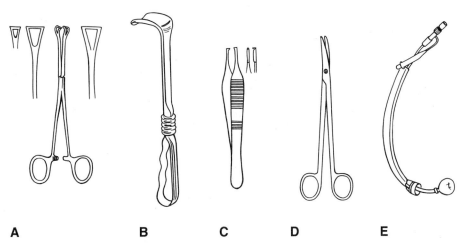

A   **B**   **C**   **D**   **E**

FIG. 88-4.
Instruments for tubal ligation. **A,** Babcock forceps; **B,** Small Richardson retractor; **C,** Adson tissue forceps; **D,** Metzenbaum scissors; **E,** Uterine manipulator.

- Adson tissue forceps for skin manipulation (Fig. 88-4, *C*)
- Metzenbaum scissors for general tissue blunt dissection and incising (Fig. 88-4, *D*)
- Kelly clamps for blunt dissection, and for grasping and tagging suture, bleeders, or tissue planes (fascia, peritoneum)
- Uterine manipulators for use with the cervical tenaculum or the newer uterine manipulators such as Cabot Medical, No. 003276, 4.5 mm uterine manipulator (Fig. 88-4, *E*)
- *Optional:* 5 cc 0.25% bupivacaine (Marcaine)

PREPROCEDURE EVALUATION

Preprocedure Visits

Preprocedure evaluation and counseling for women who want permanent sterilization warrants focused attention. A special visit should be scheduled to discuss contraceptive options, risks, technique, and follow-up demands of sterilization surgery (see Box 88-1). In addition, many insurance companies require preauthorization, which should be obtained at this visit. The counseling session should not be hurried or tacked on to the end of a visit for an acute illness. Written materials should be given to the patient at this time. If federal funding will be utilized, be mindful of the mandatory 30-day wait and age requirements. If the patient is involved in a monogamous relationship, it may be wise to meet with her partner to address his concerns. His written consent is not mandatory, but if he disagrees with his partner's decision, explore his reasons.

A preprocedure examination, which requires a reasonable amount of time, should occur within 10 days (some hospitals require less than 5 days) of anticipated surgery. Review the patient's complete medical history, paying particular attention to prior pelvic or abdominal surgery, or infection. Are there drug allergies or drug intolerances? Is there a history of heart disease (e.g., SBE), diabetes, bleeding disorder, endometriosis, or dysfunctional uterine bleeding? Is other concomitant surgery necessary, for example, dilation and curettage, breast biopsy, or procedure for urinary incontinence? Is the Pap smear normal? Discuss the method of anesthesia that is to be used. Carefully review anticipated postprocedure morbidities (pain, the necessity of limited lifting). Remain mindful of the risk factors for regret. Review current contraceptive methods. Is pregnancy a possibility at the time of surgery? If the patient smokes, can she quit at least several days before surgery?

Preprocedure examination should be thorough. Focus on the heart, lung, breast, and abdominal examinations. During the pelvic examination, assess for the presence of vulvar, vaginal, or cervical disease. Obtain specimens for culture (e.g., gonorrhea, chlamydia) as necessary. Assess the degree of uterine prolapse and urinary incontinence; have the patient bear down and cough. Perform a bimanual examination to assess uterine size, shape, and tenderness. Palpate the ovaries for enlargement. Pay particular attention to uterine mobility. Can the uterus be easily brought out of the pelvis, or is it frozen in a particular direction? Estimate the degree of abdominal wall obesity. Show the patient the location and size of the anticipated abdominal incision and eventual scarring.

BOX 88-1. PATIENT EDUCATION HANDOUT
PERMANENT FEMALE STERILIZATION

Permanent female sterilization is a surgical procedure that women can undergo to prevent ever becoming pregnant. A small incision is made in the abdomen, the fallopian tubes are cut, and a small portion of the tube is removed. This surgery prevents the female's egg from becoming fertilized by the male's sperm. *Minilaparotomy* is the name of a procedure that your doctor offers for performing permanent sterilization on an outpatient or same-day-surgery basis. The surgery is usually performed while you are under general anesthesia (asleep); therefore, you must come to the hospital early in the day following a complete 8-hour fast (nothing taken by mouth). Generally, you will be able to go home within 3 or 4 hours after surgery (a friend or family member is required to drive you home.) You must return for a follow-up visit 2 weeks after your surgery, or at any time a complication develops. Minilaparotomy is a safe, common, and popular way to perform permanent sterilization. You should realize that permanent sterilization, or *tubal ligation* as it is sometimes called, is *permanent.* You should not have this surgery unless you are certain that you do not wish to have any more children. The decision must be made by you. You and your partner must agree that you will never want any more children. Even though reversal is possible for some women, this surgery is very expensive and frequently does not work. You should also understand that there are a number of alternatives to permanent female sterilization, such as barrier methods (condoms, diaphragm), birth control pills (including the newer Norplant System which is placed under the skin and lasts for 5 years), and intrauterine devices (IUDs), which are effective for 8 years. Men can also undergo permanent sterilization, called vasectomy, which is less expensive and safer. It is also possible to check the man after surgery to be sure the surgery was successful. There is no way to do this in the woman. Before having your tubal ligation, you are free to ask questions and express your desires and concerns. You may change your mind about your surgery at any time. You should be aware of the following major risks regarding these procedures:

Pain
All women experience pain from their sterilization surgery. It is felt in the incision, as well as deeper around the fallopian tubes. In general, this pain can be controlled with oral medications, but you should not expect to return to work any sooner than several days after the procedure. Many women prefer to take a week off or to schedule surgery during a vacation. Lifting or twisting will be uncomfortable to some extent for at least 2 weeks. You will benefit from arranging your schedule so that you can take it easy for a reasonable period after your surgery, and at least until you have your follow-up check in the office.

Infection
There is a small chance, less than 1 out of 100, that you may experience an abdominal infection in the fallopian tubes or the skin incision. Inner abdominal infections are very rare; however, they are always serious and may require hospitalization. Skin incision infections are more common, and treatment usually involves skin cleansing, oral antibiotics, and, rarely, a stay in the hospital.

Bleeding
Bleeding in the abdomen from your tubal surgery is uncommon. Most bleeding is controlled during surgery. Bleeding may develop in the skin incision and require drainage. It is very unlikely that you would ever require a blood transfusion to correct the bleeding experienced during or following your surgery.

Continued.

BOX 88-1.—cont'd

Injury

Very rarely (less than 1 chance in 100) other organs may be injured during your sterilization surgery. These organs most commonly are the urinary bladder, the tissues next to the uterus, or the bowel. Prior pelvic or abdominal surgery or infection increase the likelihood of injury to other abdominal organs during sterilization surgery. These injuries may require repair during surgery, and hospitalization may be necessary for initial treatment. In rare instances, the uterus may be injured from the instruments that are used to move or control its position.

Failure

Although tubal ligation is highly successful at preventing future pregnancies, it is not perfect. In other words, there is a small chance (approximately 3 to 10 per 1000) that the tubes may grow back together and that you may become pregnant. Furthermore, if you do become pregnant following tubal ligation, there is an increased chance that your pregnancy would *not* be in the uterus. These are called *ectopic pregnancies*, and they can require emergency surgery.

Regret

Approximately 1% to 2% of women who undergo tubal ligation change their minds and seek reversal surgery so that they can become pregnant again. Women seeking permanent sterilization should base their decision on their free choice and desires. You should be informed about alternatives for birth control and your questions should be answered. If you are not sure about your decision, wait until you are before having surgery.

Other complications

Other complications of tubal ligation are possible, but these are very rare. Death has occurred from sterilization surgery (3 to 11 out of 100,000). However, far more women die from complications of pregnancy than from complications of sterilization surgery. Reactions to the drugs given during surgery are possible. Risks of general anesthesia include allergic reactions, pneumonia, blood clots (pulmonary embolism), heart attacks, and other very rare events. In some instances, your doctor or the anesthesia specialist may advise alternative forms of pain control for your surgery depending upon your medical condition and desires.

Summary

In conclusion, tubal ligation (permanent sterilization) is a very safe, effective form of birth control. It is impossible to discuss every possible risk or complication from this surgery. You should feel comfortable with your decision and free to raise questions you may have.

Note: Permanent sterilization does not eliminate the need for Pap smears. Please consult your physician about the recommended frequency as well as other disease-screening recommendations.

Perform laboratory tests as necessary. Typically, hospitals require hemoglobin levels and a urinalysis as the minimum prerequisites for general anesthesia. Perform a pregnancy test if there is any question of pregnancy. If there is clinical evidence of cervicitis or pelvic inflammation, obtain specimens for culture and treat the condition accordingly. Schedule the surgery only when treatment and clinical response have been adequate. Some hospitals require a copy of the patient's normal, recent Pap smear on the chart.

Many same-day and outpatient surgery services offer preanesthesia counseling. Your patient can meet with the anesthesia clinician to discuss anesthesia, risks, time to arrive at the hospital, how long to fast before surgery, and other issues. This counseling should be utilized whenever available; for many hospitals, this is a requirement.

Call the hospital surgery personnel with any special requests for the anticipated surgery. Will D & C be performed? (If so, it should be done *after* minilaparotomy.) Is a uterine manipulator necessary and what type?

Technique

Check in with the preoperative holding area. Is the operating room schedule on time? Is the patient's chart complete, and informed consent form available and signed? Are the laboratory values within normal range? Does your patient have any questions? Is the family in the waiting room?

Tell the operating room scrub or float nurse what equipment and sutures you will need. Clarify the position that the patient will be placed in for the surgery, (e.g., lithotomy, frog-legged, or standard supine position). Request a specific cleansing agent for patients who are allergic to iodine.

1. Cleanse the vulva and vagina. A vaginal prep is necessary if the bladder is to be catheterized or a uterine manipulator is to be applied.
2. Drain the bladder. Perform a quick, gentle, straight catherization to decompress a distended bladder from the operative field. Catheterization of the bladder is not universally performed. This is particularly true for patients under local anesthesia who can void sufficiently just before anesthesia. However, when the surgeon is new to this technique or when delay is anticipated in completing the abdominal entry (obesity, prior pelvic surgery, or infection), bladder injury is more likely. Draining the bladder helps reduce this risk. The surgeon should remember too that "fluid bolusing" at the time of general anesthesia induction is common and the bladder can fill quickly.
3. Apply the uterine manipulator (for interval minilaparotomy). Traditional devices include acorn or Hulka devices. Newer adaptations, such as Cabot Medical's uterine manipulator (Fig. 88-4, *E*), are easy to apply and are rarely traumatic. Many clinicians use manipulators routinely; others reserve them for anticipated problems with adequate exposure (abdominal obesity, prior pelvic surgery or infection, or retroversion or flexion of the uterus). Less experienced surgeons should use them. The patient must be in either the lithotomy or the frog-leg position, and general anesthesia is required.
4. Sterile gloves may be used without formal gowning for insertion of the uterine manipulator or for straight catheterization of the urinary bladder. In fact, it is advisable for the surgeon not to perform these procedures with the same formal gowning and gloving worn for the minilaporotomy because contamination is likely when the patient is in the lithotomy position.
5. Prepare and scrub the abdomen. Minilaparotomy should not be performed through pubic hair. Depending on patient pubic hair distribution, shaving a small strip of pubic hair over the operative site may be necessary.

6. Perform the procedure following thorough surgical washing and gowning. Wipe any powder from the latex gloves with sterile, saline-soaked sponges.

7. Apply surgical drapes as for abdominal surgery.

8. Palpate three fingerbreadths above the symphysis pubis (Fig. 88-5). With one hand on the abdomen above the symphysis, move the uterine manipulator. Often the uterus can be felt with the abdominal hand, which offers reassurance that the incision will provide ready access to the uterus and adnexa. Using the skin scalpel with a No. 10 blade, make a transverse incision. There is no need to arc this incision. Often the linea nigra, the faint line demarcating the midline, can be visualized. The incision should be no more than 5 cm long, and often a smaller incision will suffice.

9. Switch to the deep knife (No. 10 blade) and progress through Scarpa's fascia (within the fat) until the rectus sheath is encountered. Often, once Scarpa's fascia is divided, the sub-Scarpa's fat can be brushed away with a sponge, using a wiping motion. Bleeders can be cauterized using the electrocoagulator. Do not tunnel the incision, especially in the obese abdomen; this can be prevented by ensuring that the subcutaneous fat has been divided all the way to both edges of the skin incision. The subcutaneous fat presents an excellent opportunity to test the power on the Bovie before entering the

A
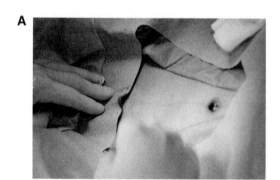

B
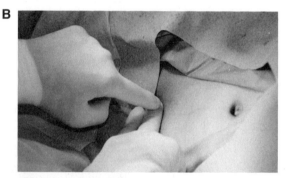

C
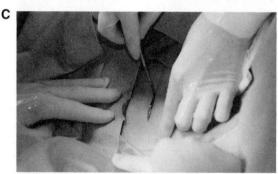

FIG. 88-5.
Locate the abdominal incision. **A,** The top of the upper border of the escutcheon has been shaved. **B,** The area 2 to 3 fingerbreadths above the symphysis pubis is identified. **C,** A 5 cm transverse incision is made. (Photos courtesy of Miltex Instruments Company, Inc.)

abdomen. The Bovie device should never be used for the first time on intra-abdominal tissue, in case the power is set dangerously too high.

10. Once the rectus fascia is identified by its tough, white fibrous appearance, make a small transverse incision on each side of the linea alba. Using a Metzenbaum scissors, carefully extend the fascial incision to the lateral margin of the skin incision and across the midline. Place two Kelly clamps on the incised lower fascial edge and gently retract and elevate the fascia. Gently place the index finger (preferably) or the blunt end of the scalpel along the midline under the incised fascial edge, and gently roll toward the lateral margins, freeing the sheath from the underlying rectus muscle. In the midline, the pyramidalis remains adherent; use the Metzenbaum scissors to carefully cut along the inferior linea alba, freeing the muscle and making more room. Apply Kelly clamps to the upper segment of the anterior rectus sheath, and free the underlying muscles in a similar fashion. You do not need to roll the index finger under the rectus sheath any further than the skin incision. Perforating vessels arise more laterally and can be ruptured. Carefully use cautery to control bleeders.

11. Using blunt dissection with the index finger or the blunt end of the knife, separate the rectus muscles from the transversalis fascia and peritoneum in the midline. A gentle rolling action of the index finger (or the blunt end of the scalpel) under each lateral band of rectus muscles assures adequate room.

12. Using two Kelly clamps or pickups, opposing each other, lift the transversalis and peritoneum, thereby tenting these layers away from underlying abdominal structures. Using either the scalpel or Metzenbaum scissors, make a small buttonhole incision between the two clamps. This incision should be well above the symphysis pubis, favoring the cephalad (toward the umbilicus) portion of the wound to avoid the bladder. At this point, use a Kelly clamp to enter the small incision, and with a combination of blunt dissection and retraction of tissues, enter the abdomen. The key maneuver is to maintain this elevation of the incision edges to expose abdominal viscera. The obese abdomen may contain a significant amount of fat below the peritoneum, which requires special care when dissecting. It may be difficult to distinguish this tissue from omentum or mesenteric fat that may be adherent in the lower pelvis, especially in women with a history of abdominal surgery or infection. The peritoneal incision may be extended either transversely (preferred) or vertically.

13. Place the small Richardson retractors, and with gently opposed and elevating retraction, lift the abdominal wall and inspect the abdominal cavity (Fig. 88-6). If the small intestine obscures the view, place the patient in the reverse Trendelenburg position (head down) to allow the bowel to gravitate cephalad out of view. Use a gauze pad rolled tightly on a ring clamp to brush the bowel and adnexal structures aside if they are obstructing the view. Using Babcock forceps, identify the adnexal structures. Once the fallopian tube is identified, use two Babcock forceps to gently retract the tube until the ovary and fimbriated end are clearly identified. Apply slight traction on the Babcock to deliver the tube through the incision for the ligation procedure

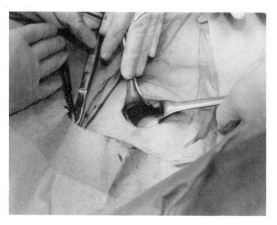

FIG. 88-6.
Small Richardson retractors used in pairs and gently lifted upward offer excellent exposure. (Photo courtesy of Miltex Instruments Company, Inc.)

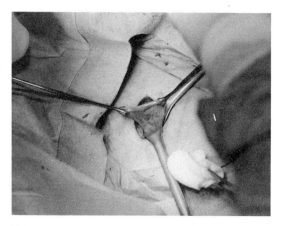

FIG. 88-7.
Using Babcock forceps, gently bring the tube through the incision and identify a portion of the mesosalpinx relatively devoid of vessels. (Photo courtesy of Miltex Instruments Company, Inc.)

(Fig. 88-7). A tube can be avulsed at the uterus with subsequent bleeding, so be careful and avoid forceful retraction. Use the uterine manipulator to help with visualization and exposure.

14. Carefully elevate the fallopian tube and identify a relatively avascular area of the mesosalpinx. Using a Kelly or the Bovie on "coag" (*not "cutting"*), make a small hole through the mesosalpinx (Fig. 88-8). Then, clamp the tube with a Kelly, placing one jaw through this hole and the other across the tube. Place another Kelly clamp 2 cm distal to the first one, isolating a segment of tube. Using a 2-0 chromic suture on a needle, place a stick tie on the uterine

A

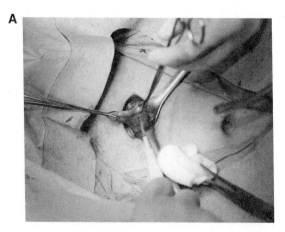

B

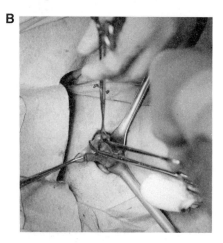

FIG. 88-8.
Using the Bovie on "coagulation," make a 2 to 3 cm incision in the mesosalpinx (**A**) through which two Kelly clamps can be passed to isolate a segment of tube (**B**). (Photos courtesy of Miltex Instruments Company, Inc.)

side of the tube proximal to the Kelly clamp and encircle the tube. Tag this tie (Kelly is placed on the suture to maintain control). Most surgeons place a second tie on the same side and cut (Fig. 88-9). Place a similar tie on the fimbriated side of the tube. Remove the Kelly clamps. Incise through each of the two crush marks made by the Kelly clamps and remove the segment of the tube (Fig. 88-10). Lightly cauterize the exposed mesosalpinx if bleeding is observed. Cut the tags, and repeat this procedure on the other tube. Pouring 2.5 cc of bupivacaine on the cut end of each tube before dropping them back into the abdomen has been said to markedly reduce postoperative pain.

15. Perform a sponge count and, if it is correct, close the abdomen. Identify and hold the edges of the peritoneum with Kelly clamps or pickups (Fig. 88-10, *A*). Use a running 3-0 chromic suture to reapproximate the cut edges. Identify and tag the fascial sheath edges with Kelly clamps. Close this sheath with a running 0 Dexon suture (Fig. 88-10, *B*). Palpate the closure to make sure there are no buttonhole defects in the fascial repair that could later manifest as incisional hernias. If there is more than 1 cm of subcutaneous fat, close Scarpa's fascia with interrupted 2-0 chromic sutures. The skin may be closed with staples or by running a subcuticular stitch of 3-0 chromic suture on a Keith needle.

16. Cleanse the surgical site with normal saline and apply a gauze dressing.

17. Take the patient to the recovery room. She may be discharged when she is awake, is tolerating oral liquids, and is ambulatory.

18. Send the tubal segments for routine pathology; place them in separate bottles marked "right" and "left."

19. Write a brief operative note in the chart. State any complications, blood loss, and other findings. You should also dictate a complete operative report immediately following surgery.

20. The patient should be seen in the office within 7 to 14 days or at any time a complication develops. Review the tubal pathology report.

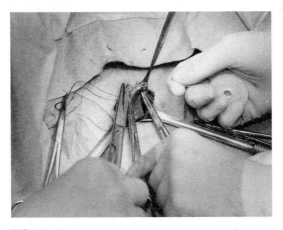

FIG. 88-9.
Tie chromic sutures on each side of the tube next to the Kelly clamps on the portion of the tube that will remain. (Photo courtesy of Miltex Instruments Company, Inc.)

A 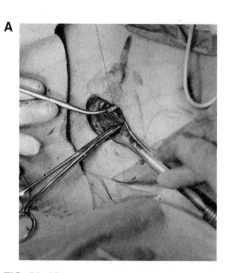   **B**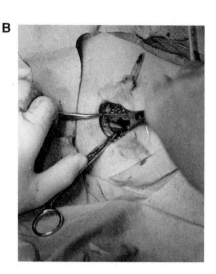

FIG. 88-10.
A, Identify the peritoneum and retract it with Kelly clamps. **B,** Suture the peritoneum with a running 3-0 chromic suture. (Photos courtesy of Miltex Instruments Company, Inc.)

Postprocedure Instructions

Give the patient postprocedure instructions (see Box 88-2) and inform the family of any follow-up instructions.

General Information

- For payment for sterilization, the federal government currently requires that the patient be 21 years old or older and mentally competent, and that a mandatory waiting period of 30 days be observed after signing an informed consent form (or 72 hours if sterilization is desired following a preterm delivery). A government-published patient-education booklet with consent forms can be obtained from health departments.
- Minilaparotomy and laparoscopy are highly effective. Pregnancy rates after one year are usually less than 1 per 100 women. Common reasons for sterilization failure are preexisting pregnancy at the time of sterilization; surgical error in identifying a fallopian tube; spontaneous reanastomosis of the severed tube; and fistula formation, which enables sperm or egg passage.
- Major factors related to the development of complications include clinician inexperience, patient obesity, prior pelvic or abdominal surgery, and other medical problems such as diabetes mellitus, heart disease, asthma, bronchitis, and emphysema.
- Minilaparotomy is the safest sterilization method in the postpartum period, with a complication rate approaching that of interval sterilization. Laparoscopy is not as safe during the immediate postpartum period as at other times.
- Postpartum and postabortion sterilization appears to be somewhat less effective than interval sterilization.

**BOX 88-2. POSTPROCEDURE INSTRUCTIONS
PERMANENT FEMALE STERILIZATION**

Your sterilization surgery was accomplished by entering the tissues of the abdominal wall. This small opening was sutured together by both deep and surface stitches. These stitches will eventually dissolve; you do not need to see the physician to have them removed. The surgery site is normally most painful the first several days after surgery. You may also experience a deeper pelvic discomfort as the tubes themselves begin to heal. The discomfort at both places should gradually improve over 2 weeks. Certain activities such as lifting or bearing down will cause discomfort and should be avoided. It is extremely unlikely that your stitches will come loose, but it is best if you avoid lifting or any activity that causes pain. Acetaminophen will help reduce the discomfort (unless you are allergic to or cannot tolerate this medication).

Bandages have been placed over the surgery site. It is normal for them to become stained with a small amount of blood and tissue fluids. On the day following your surgery, you may remove these bandages and replace them with sterile gauze and paper tape. By the third day after surgery, you may *shower* without bandages (however, do not soak the area by taking a tub bath). You should keep the surgery site covered for about 7 days to reduce irritation by clothing or bedding that may rub this area. It is normal for the skin to itch as healing begins.

Your tubal ligation is immediately effective. You will be able to have intercourse without concern for pregnancy. Most women prefer to wait at least 2 weeks before having intercourse in order to allow their surgery to heal and to become more comfortable. It is also important to remember that your tubal ligation prevents pregnancy but in no way protects you from infections that can be transmitted from sexual intercourse. If at any time you feel you may be exposing yourself to sexually transmitted disease (gonorrhea, AIDS, chlamydia, or herpes) you should avoid intercourse, or at least insist that your partner wear a condom. Also, permanent sterilization does not eliminate the need for Pap smears. Your physician will recommend how frequently you need to have a Pap smear and other disease-screening procedures.

Finally, you should call the doctor's office if you feel you are having problems. Signs of infection include discharge, pus, redness, increasing pain in this area, fever, aches, muscle pains (flulike symptoms), and abdominal pain. Let your doctor know if you experience burning with urination, which may indicate a bladder infection.

Risks for Regret

Of the women who have tubal sterilization, 1% to 2% seek reversal; however, sterility is not easily reversed. Only 30% to 70% of these women are candidates for reversal surgery, and pregnancy occurs in about 50% of those who do undergo it. Reversal is most successful if less than 3 cm of the tube was originally damaged or removed. The most "reversible" techniques include those that do not involve

---

**BOX 88-3. PATIENT EDUCATION HANDOUT
POSTPARTUM TUBAL LIGATION**

Please review the information about permanent sterilization surgery. The postpartum (after delivery) period has become a very popular time for sterilization surgery, which is generally performed within 48 hours of delivery. Postpartum tubal ligation by minilaparotomy is very similar to the sterilization procedure performed on women who have not recently delivered. However, there are some important differences. Often the same anesthetic (epidural, caudal) that you had to deliver your baby can be extended to provide anesthesia for your tubal ligation. Another popular way to undergo postpartum sterilization is by general anesthesia (be put to sleep) the day after delivery.

Remember that although you may plan to undergo postpartum sterilization, a number of things can happen during and after labor to postpone or delay this surgery, such as infection, fever, excessive blood loss, and high blood pressure. If any of these complications occur, sterilization surgery will need to be postponed until at least 6 weeks after delivery. Furthermore, if your newborn is ill, you may wish to wait until your are confident that your baby is healthy.

After delivery, minilaparotomy surgery requires that the abdomen be entered at or near the umbilicus (belly button). The abdominal incision (cut) is usually at the pubic hair line if the surgery is performed at other times. Most women recover quickly after postpartum sterilization surgery, and only rarely is it necessary to stay in the hospital longer than the normal amount of time you would stay for a simple delivery (1 to 2 days). Having help at home is always a good idea with a newborn, but this is especially true if you have undergone postpartum sterilization. Lifting your newborn baby may be quite uncomfortable for at least a week. Finally, if your baby is born by cesarean section, tubal sterilization surgery can easily be performed if desired; but remember, how and when you have your permanent sterilization surgery should be determined by your desires and commitment, not simply because it is convenient.

---

electrocautery and those in which the smallest segment is removed from within the isthmic portion of the tube. Women with the following risk factors for regret should not necessarily be denied surgery; however, the prudent physician should counsel these patients before performing sterilization.

- Marital disharmony at the time of sterilization: Remarriage is the reason 90% of women request reversal.
- Age less than 30 years at the time of sterilization (Some clinicians debate whether this is as significant risk factor).
- Religious, socioeconomic, and educational background show much less correlation with regret. Low parity or number of live children are also less well correlated.
- Regret may be slightly more prevalent following postpartum sterilization procedures; however, as a risk factor, this is less well defined.
- Regret is more likely when sterilization is chosen because of financial difficulties, health, or emotional problems.

POSTPARTUM TUBAL LIGATION

Postpartum tubal ligation (PTL) has many similarities with interval tubal ligation, but there are also major differences. Despite the convenience, cost savings, and ultimate desires of your patient, postpartum tubal ligation remains an elective surgery. Numerous contraindications include maternal fever, pregnancy-related hypertension, uncontrolled diabetes mellitus, and excessive blood loss. Concerns regarding the viability and health of the newborn must be considered as well. Women who must postpone their postpartum sterilization should be reassured that interval tubal ligation as early as 6 weeks' postdelivery is also an excellent method of sterilization surgery. Postpartum tubal ligation can readily be performed during cesarean section; however, *never* assume that PTL remains the patient's desire if the cesarean section was performed because of concern over the condition of the fetus (see Box 88-3).

Technique

1. Often PTL can be performed with the same block (epidural, caudal) that was used during labor. If this is not desirable or possible, there are many advantages to allowing the patient to rest and recover from labor and to schedule the PTL procedure for the next morning. A repeat hemoglobin determination will be much more meaningful after equilibration of fluid, especially if there is concern over blood loss during delivery. This delay also allows more time to observe the condition of the newborn.
2. The bladder should be drained either by having the patient void immediately before surgery or by straight catheterization (preferred method). Prepare the abdomen in the immediate umbilical area. Surgical scrub and draping are required.
3. Make a curved infraumbilical incision in the abdomen with the skin knife (No. 11 blade) (Fig. 88-11). Gentle inferior retraction on the abdominal skin at

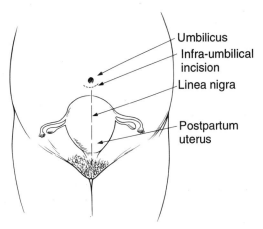

FIG. 88-11.
Postpartum tubal ligation by minilaparotomy requires a small transverse infraumbilical incision.

the time of performing this incision will ensure that the scar will be very close to or within the umbilical crater.

4. Carry the incision deeper with the deep knife (No. 10 blade). Once the skin and subcutaneous fat have been divided, enter the abdomen by favoring the inferior portion of the wound. Dissecting through the substance of the umbilicus can be frustrating since tissue planes are not well defined. Blunt dissection with Kelly clamps, which can probe and spread, is the preferred method for exploring and defining the portal of entry into the abdominal cavity. Some surgeons prefer to grasp each lateral side of the incision with towel clamps and elevate the entire incision away from underlying structures, such as the bowel and the uterus, when entering the peritoneum. Once the abdominal cavity is identified, the incision through the fascia and peritoneum can be extended, but it rarely needs to be longer than 4 to 5 cm.

5. Push the uterus gently to one side to rotate the adnexal structures into view. Use Babcock clamps to identify the fallopian tube, which in the postpartum period is typically swollen and engorged compared to the nonpregnant state. Follow each tube until the fimbriated ends and ovaries are identified. Extremely gentle traction is warranted because vessels within the mesosalpinx can be huge and easily damaged by traction. Tears in these vessels can cause profound bleeding.

6. Once the tube has been clearly identified, perform a tubal ligation as described previously for the interval sterilization technique. If the mesosalpinx is extremely fragile, many clinicians prefer the more traditional modified Pomeroy technique. The loop, tie, and cut features of the Pomeroy render a quick hemostatic procedure that can minimize the traction injuries or raw cut edges of the mesosalpinx produced by other procedures. Remember that if the tube cannot be delivered through the incision for a tubal ligation procedure, clips may be applied to the correctly identified fallopian tube.

7. Close the abdomen in a layered fashion as previously described. With periumbilical incisions, it is sometimes difficult to clearly redefine the peritoneal edges for closure. However, closure of the fascia is crucial and time should be spent clearly identifying the edges of this layer for definitive suturing.

8. Your patient should be seen within 2 weeks of PTL. At this time, the pathology report should be reviewed.

MAJOR COMPLICATIONS

- Major complications occur in less than 2% of all procedures and may require prolonged hospitalization (0.3% requiring 3 or more nights in the hospital) or laparotomy (0.02% to 1.2% in large studies) to resolve complications.
- Delayed complications requiring readmission to the hospital occur after less than 1% of procedures.

- Minilaparotomy and laparoscopy have similar complication rates.
- Female sterilization causes very few deaths, and most are related to anesthetic complications (overdose or drug reaction), infection, and hemorrhage.
- Mortality rates from sterilization are far lower than with childbirth.
- Rare complications of tubal litigations include pregnancy (intrauterine and ectopic) and luteal phase pregancy.

MINOR COMPLICATIONS

- Minilaparotomy appears to have a higher rate of minor complications (12% versus 7%) and a longer average operating time when compared to laparoscopy. Minilaparotomy convalescence appears to be slightly longer, and more painful. Very high complication rates have been reported when laparoscopy is performed by inexperienced physicians.
- Minor minilaparotomy complications include wound infections, slight blood loss, uterine perforation by uterine manipulation instruments, and bladder injury. Most minor injury complications are immediately recognized and managed intraoperatively.
- Laparoscopy complications include those of minilaparotomy, as well as unique problems related to insertion of the instrument and gas insufflation of the abdomen. These include gas embolism, subcutaneous emphysema, or cardiac arrest. Vessel or organ laceration may occur. Open laparoscopy may make some of these complications less likely.
- Pain occurs after both minilaparotomy and laparoscopy. Chest and shoulder pain are common after laparoscopy; this is caused by trapped gas under the diaphragm after insufflation of the abdomen. Most postprocedure and recovery pain can be managed with oral drug therapy, and narcotics are rarely necessary after the third postprocedural day.
- There is no compelling evidence that female sterilization causes long-term complications. Menstrual cycles do not significantly change as a result of sterilization; but abnormalities may persist if they existed before surgery. Among women who do experience menstrual changes, about half observe improvements and half experience irregular cycles or increased bleeding.
- Sterilized women do not appear to have different rates of pelvic inflammatory disease, cervicitis, hysterectomy, or dilation and curettage.
- Sterilized women are no more likely to experience severe psychiatric problems than unsterilized women.

CPT/BILLING CODES

58600	Interval tubal ligation
58605	Postpartum tubal ligation
58982	Laparoscopic tubal ligation

BIBLIOGRAPHY

Chi IC, Potts M, Wilkens L: Rare events associated with tubal sterilizations: an international experience, *Obstet Gynecol Survey* 41(1):7, 1986.

Green LR, Laros RK: Postpartum sterilization, *Clin Obstet Gynecol* 23(2):647, 1980.

Leskin L, Rinehart W: Female sterilization, *Population Reports* 13(9): 1985.

Mattingly RF: Surgical conditions of the fallopian tube. In Linde TE, editor: *Operative gynecology,* ed 5, Philadelphia, 1982, J. B. Lippincott.

McGonigle KF, Huggins GR: Tubal sterilization: epidemiology of regret, *Contemp Obstet Gynecol* 35(10):15, 1990.

Sterilization, *ACOG Technical Bulletin* 113: February 1988.

CHAPTER 89

First-Trimester Abortion

Steven H. Eisinger

Abortion became legal in every state in the United States as a result of the *Roe* v. *Wade* Supreme Court decision in 1973. The *Roe* v. *Wade* decision was based on a person's constitutional right to privacy; thus, abortion of a pregnancy during the first trimester is a private issue to be settled between the woman and her doctor. More than one and a half million elective abortions are now performed in the United States annually. There is now a patchwork of state laws regulating abortion, ranging from highly restrictive to highly liberal. Recent trends have placed increasing legal constraints on abortion, although these are being challenged in the courts. *It is imperative for any physician performing abortion to have an accurate working knowledge of any state and local restrictions governing abortion.*

Abortion differs from other medical procedures because it can generate strong feelings in some people. Before providing abortion services, a thoughtful physician should examine the emotional, ethical, and societal aspects of abortion, and their effects on medical personnel involved and on society as a whole. The decision to perform abortions is complicated; however, those physicians who decide to offer the procedure may take satisfaction in knowing that they are providing an essential service to their patients.

Essentially the same technique explained in this chapter (suction curettage) can be used for a missed or incomplete abortion (see Chapter 87, Dilation and Curettage).

COUNSELING

Usually the woman who requests an abortion has already made her decision. If the physician is supportive, there is usually little conflict; however, counseling is still important—whether the woman *appears* to be ambivalent or confident about her decision. Ambivalent or complicated patients should be referred to a specialist for counseling, especially if the primary physician does not have the specialized skills or time.

- The physician should be nonjudgmental. The physician should not voice a personal bias.
- The counseling should be patient-centered; the final decision made by the patient; and the results should be in the patient's own best interests.
- The patient should be encouraged to seek help in making her decision from whomever in her life she trusts and derives support. This may include her partner, parents, siblings, friends, other medical or mental health professionals, teachers, or spiritual counselor.
- The patient needs to be informed of the different abortion procedures that are available, how they are performed, and what their risks are (Box 89-1).
- Alternatives to abortion should be explored. These include giving birth to the baby and keeping it, or giving the baby up for adoption (alternatives that carry their own risks and costs). Acknowledgment should be made that the decision may be very difficult. If the gestational age is early, there is plenty of time to consider all the possibilities and make a rational decision. On the other hand, if the gestational age is advanced, a decision must be reached quickly.
- The physician should actively support the patient's decision by providing appropriate medical care or referral, and by helping her view her decision in positive terms. Patients who cannot make a decision are, in effect, deciding to keep the pregnancy.
- The patient's feelings about abortion should be elicited—especially doubts and fears, which can be dealt with much more effectively when voiced.
- The patient should be prepared for various feelings and reactions she may experience after the abortion, including relief, guilt, and sadness. Ideally, she should have a support person close by to help her through the experience.
- Short-term follow-up counseling after abortion should be encouraged.
- A contraceptive plan should be offered.

INDICATIONS

Very few strictly medical indications exist for elective first-trimester abortion. Evaluation of these patients is highly individualized and probably would involve the input of consultants. Rarely, a woman may have a life-threatening illness which pregnancy would exacerbate, such as a cancer for which treatment cannot begin until the pregnancy is terminated. Occasionally, a patient may have a progressive life-threatening illness that so limits her life-expectancy that childbearing and child rearing may be unwise or impossible. HIV infection and active AIDS present a special case, since the risk of transmission to the baby is 15% to 40%, and the woman's life expectancy may be low. Abortion is generally considered acceptable for pregnancies resulting from rape or incest, or those in which a major birth defect exists.

BOX 89-1. PATIENT CONSENT FORM
TERMINATION OF PREGNANCY

You have requested that Dr. _____terminate your pregnancy. This will be done by removing the contents of the uterus by suction, a procedure commonly called a suction curettage or suction abortion. The procedure consists of two steps:

1. The evening before the actual procedure, a small fiber cylinder will be inserted into the cervix (opening of the womb). This cylinder is called a laminaria, and it is about the size of a wooden match. It is used to dilate the opening to the uterus.
2. In the morning, the suction abortion will be performed. First, the physician will inject a local anesthetic into the cervix, freezing or numbing the opening to the uterus. Then the doctor will insert a plastic tube through the opening of the cervix and into the uterus; then suction will be applied by a machine to empty the uterus. The whole procedure will take only a few minutes. You can expect some cramping during the procedure, but this usually subsides within 5 to 10 minutes. If no complications occur, you may leave within 1 hour.

Complications of suction curettage are uncommon, but they may occur.

Complications due to laminaria insertion:

- Infection may occur if the laminaria is left in place for more than 24 hours.
- The laminaria may perforate (poke a hole through) the cervix.
- The laminaria may fall out, break into pieces, or be difficult to remove.
- A spontaneous abortion or miscarriage may occur after the laminaria is inserted.

Complications due to local anesthesia:

- An allergic reaction may occur.
- If the anesthetic enters the bloodstream, you may feel its effects: buzzing in the ears, taste in the mouth, etc. This is common and not dangerous.

Complications due to the suction abortion itself:

- Bleeding may occur. This can usually be controlled with medication; however, rarely it may be severe, and you may need to have the procedure repeated, be admitted to the hospital, or have a blood transfusion.
- Infection may occur. This can usually be treated with oral antibiotics; but rarely, intravenous antibiotics, hospital admission, or surgery may be necessary.
- Perforation of the uterus (poking a hole in the wall of the womb) is rare. This may require admission to the hospital and further surgery.
- The abortion may fail to interrupt the pregnancy. If this occurs, the suction curettage will have to be repeated.
- Other very rare complications may occur, including blood clots in the veins which can travel to the lungs, hysterectomy (removal of the womb), or even death. It is impossible to mention every possible complication of this procedure. Serious complications occur very rarely.

I have read this form and I understand how suction abortion is performed, its risks, and its possible complications. All of my questions have been answered.

_____   _____
Date   Signature of Patient

_____   _____
Witness   Signature of Relative or Legal Guardian

CONTRAINDICATIONS

Medical contraindications are quite rare.

- Active pelvic infection
- Any serious medical condition that might complicate surgery (The patient's condition should be stabilized prior to abortion. In such cases, the procedure is probably best performed in the hospital.)

EQUIPMENT

- Method for dilating cervix: Pratt, Hegar, or Denniston cervical dilators; or laminaria, Dilapan, Lamicel, or Dilateria self-expanding cervical dilators (inserted 6 to 12 hours before the procedure)
- Large Graves speculum
- Povidone-iodine or other antiseptic solution
- Ring forceps
- Cotton balls
- 4 × 4 inch gauze pads
- Single-toothed cervical tenaculum
- Uterine sound
- 10 cc of anesthetic (1% lidocaine or 2% chloroprocaine) with 22-gauge spinal needle, or 22-gauge needle on 3-inch needle extender
- Suction curettes in a variety of sizes (from 7 to 12 mm)
- Suction machine with tubing
- Formalin jar
- Roberts, Stone, or small ring forceps to explore uterine cavity
- Intravenous solutions, tubing, and oxytocics (for treatment of excessive bleeding)

PATIENT PREPARATION

1. Perform a standard, accurate pregnancy test. It should be positive, and this should be documented. A home pregnancy test is not adequate.
2. Consider performing a hematocrit or hemoglobin determination.
3. Determine the blood type, including Rh factor (*mandatory*). Rh negative women who have been pregnant less than 13 weeks should receive the 50 µg dose of D immunoglobulin (MICRhoGAM 50 µg); those who have been pregnant longer than 13 weeks should receive the full 300 µg dose. Otherwise, Rh sensitization occurs in 1% to 5% of untreated patients.
4. Optional testing—depending on patient risk factors, the nature of the practice, and financial considerations—includes urinalysis, Pap smear, gonorrhea and chlamydia screening, and blood tests for syphilis and HIV antibodies.
5. Gestational age *must* be determined. This can usually be accomplished by correlating weeks from the last normal menstrual period with a pelvic

examination to size the uterus. Of course, abnormal bleeding in pregnancy, contraception use, menstrual irregularities, poor recall of dates, denial, and even the possibility of falsification may hinder a physician in calculating an accurate gestational age.

Sizing the uterus by examination requires practice and may be complicated when a patient is obese, is uncooperative, has uterine or ovarian tumors, or has a retroverted uterus. As a rough guideline, up to the sixth week of pregnancy, the uterus feels the size of a golf ball or plum in nulliparous women, and slightly larger in parous women. By 8 to 9 weeks, the uterus feels the size of a tennis ball or medium-sized orange, but softer and often asymmetrically enlarged. By 10 weeks, the uterus is the size of a softball or large orange. By 12 weeks, the uterus is as large as a large grapefruit and becomes palpable suprapubically. A retroverted uterus will pop forward out of the pelvis between 12 and 13 weeks. By 14 weeks, the uterus is the size of a cantaloupe.

6. When there is any doubt at all of the gestational age, perform an ultrasound examination. Ultrasound examination is highly accurate in dating a pregnancy and may be accepted as accurate, regardless of historical data or results of the physical examination.

7. A standard brief history and physical examination should be performed; special attention should be given to abortion-related issues.

8. Premedication is optional. Ibuprofen 600 to 800 mg orally or midazolam (Versed) 2 to 5 mg intravenously are commonly used.

9. Establishment of an intravenous line is optional. An intravenous line may be useful for sedatives and oxytocics, but is generally not necessary. However, oxytocin, methylergonovine (Methergine), and other injectable drugs should be readily available should an unexpected hemorrhage occur.

TECHNIQUE

Laminaria Insertion

The patient should be seen the day before the planned abortion for insertion of the laminaria. *Laminaria digitata* is a seaweed stem, 2 to 3 mm wide and several centimeters long, resembling a brown twig with a string attached to one end. It is hygroscopic and in a moist environment, it will swell to five times its original size within 12 hours. Laminaria dilation of the cervix is a common adjunct to abortions, especially for pregnancies 7 weeks and beyond. It accomplishes dilation safely and gently, minimizes trauma to the cervix, and causes less pain than surgical dilation. Insertion of the laminaria is usually an easy and brief procedure, but requires an extra visit, since one visit is required for the laminaria insertion and another for the definitive procedure.

Laminaria insertion is not always necessary. Very early abortions (up to 7 weeks) can usually be performed with a small Karmann cannula (No. 5 or 6) without dilation of any kind (Fig. 89-1). Alternatively, the operator may choose to dilate the cervix surgically with tapered dilators (Pratt or Denniston). This procedure has the advantage of not requiring an additional visit, but the disadvantages of more patient

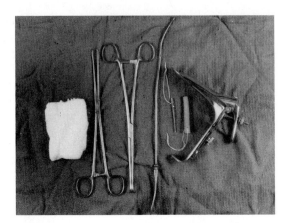

FIG. 89-1.
Laminaria set up.

discomfort and a greater risk of damaging the cervix. Most physicians do not use a laminaria for the vast majority of early abortions because of the extra visit required.

1. Size the uterus with bimanual examination, place the speculum to expose the cervix, and then cleanse the cervix with an antiseptic.
2. Grasp the cervix on the anterior lip with a single-toothed tenaculum. Two to four cc of 1% lidocaine may be instilled submucosally at the 12 o'clock position, so the tenaculum will not be felt. Next, delicately pass a uterine sound through the cervical os. The purpose of sounding is not to determine the depth of the uterus, but rather to determine the axis of the cervical canal and to accomplish slight dilation. Insert the uterine sound just past the internal os and then remove it. By holding the tenaculum steady, the laminaria may be inserted with little difficulty. Grasp the laminaria lightly with a ring forceps and insert it into the cervix, allowing it to pivot in the ring forceps so that the tip "finds" the cervical canal. Push the laminaria all the way into the cervix. It is particularly important to maintain traction on the tenaculum if the uterus is markedly flexed forward or backward, in order to straighten out its axis (Fig. 89-2).
3. Remove the tenaculum and place a sponge against the laminaria to help hold it in position.

A confident and experienced operator may skip the tenaculum and sounding steps and simply slide the laminaria directly into the cervix. Direct insertion is easy if the patient is parous and if the uterus is neither severely retroflexed nor anteflexed.

When the gestational age is more than 11 weeks, a second laminaria—placed along side the first laminaria in the exact same fashion—will permit use of a large suction curette and expedite the procedure.

In most patients, the laminaria is left in overnight. In some patients, it may cause significant cramping, which can be controlled with nonprescription pain medication.

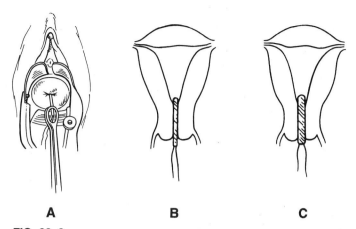

FIG. 89-2.
A, Inserting the laminaria; **B,** Immediately after insertion; **C,** 12 to 24 hours after insertion.

Note: Although the laminaria is inexpensive and has proven itself effective, there are synthetic devices that accomplish the same goal (Dilapan, Dilateria, Lamicel).

Paracervical Block

Paracervical block (see Chapter 102) is a simple, safe, and effective means of providing local anesthesia for abortion in the office setting.

1. Remove the laminaria and sponge, cleanse the cervix and vagina with an antiseptic, and grasp the anterior lip of the cervix with a single-toothed tenaculum.
2. Inject 10 cc of local anesthetic (1% lidocaine or 2% chloroprocaine) with a 22-gauge needle into four sites at the 3 o'clock, 5 o'clock, 7 o'clock, and 9 o'clock positions. (Some prefer to inject in two sites only: the 4 o'clock and 8 o'clock positions.) Ideally the injection should be given submucosally, near the junction of the cervix and vagina. The injection should be superficial enough to raise a bleb or wheal under the mucosa. Since the area is vascular, care must be taken not to inject the anesthetic directly into a vessel. The proper sites for injection can easily be exposed by manipulating the cervix with the tenaculum (Fig. 89-3).
3. Allow a few seconds for the anesthetic to take effect, and continue the procedure.

Suction Abortion

After administering the paracervical block, the operator may perform the actual abortion.

1. Remove the laminaria, if present. Sound gently with a uterine sound, primarily to determine the direction of the canal rather than its depth. Traction on the tenaculum is necessary at all times while one is instrumenting the uterus (Fig. 89-4).

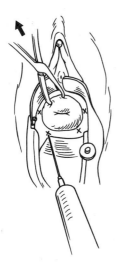

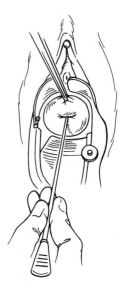

FIG. 89-3.
Paracervical block technique. The tenaculum may be used to elevate the cervix and hold it to either side for better exposure of the injection sites. *X,* locations where submucosal injections can be made.

FIG. 89-4.
Sounding the uterus.

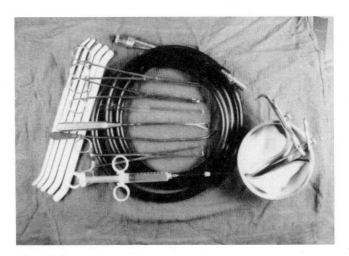

FIG. 89-5.
Suction abortion set up includes cervical dilators, suction tubing, polyp and ring forceps, suction curette, blunt uterine sound, tenaculum, syringe, and speculum.

2. Cervical dilators may be used to assess the adequacy of cervical dilation (Fig. 89-5). Even when the laminaria is used, further dilation may occasionally be useful.

3. Select a suction curette (Fig. 89-6). As a general rule, the size of the curette in millimeters should correspond to the gestational age in weeks. Place the curette into the uterus as far as it will easily go, until it meets resistance (Fig. 89-7).

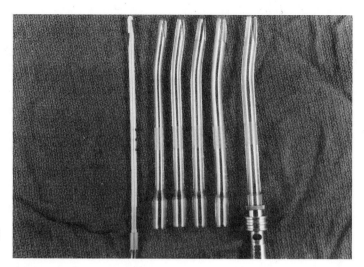

FIG. 89-6.
Suction curettes.

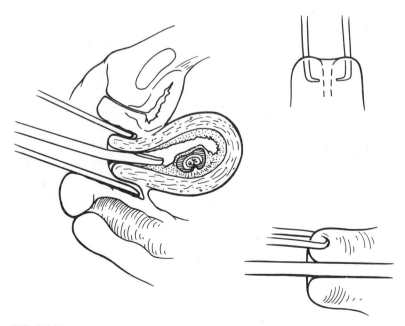

FIG. 89-7.
Initial placement of the suction curette into the uterus. Advance until there is resistance.

4. Attach the curette to the suction machine by means of the tubing. Turn on the machine. Suction pressure of 60 to 65 cm Hg or greater is required to accomplish the procedure. If suction is inadequate, there is probably a leak in the system that should be identified and corrected (Fig. 89-8).

5. Using the rotational device on the tubing, rotate the suction curette vigorously in place, first one way, then the other, several times. Gentle in-and-out piston motions may accompany the rotation.

6. Watch the tissue that appears in the curette and tubing. The products of conception have a characteristic appearance. First, clear fluid is noted, followed by tan "fluffy" appearing material, which is the remnants of the placenta and decidua usually mixed with blood. Fetal parts cannot usually be identified until the pregnancy borders on the second trimester. The appearance of abnormal tissue (such as omental fat or bowel) in the curette is a sign of perforation. Absence of tissue is also important to note.

7. After several rotations in each direction, remove the curette while the suction is still on. Reinsert it into the uterus with the suction off, turn the suction back on, and remove it again, repeating this until no further tissue is seen in the hose. As the uterus is evacuated, it tends to clamp down, bringing additional tissue into the range of the curette portal. Patients will experience more discomfort at this point, and the operator will feel more resistance to rotating the curette.

8. With a medium sharp uterine curette, feel all quadrants of the uterine cavity. A clean uterus will have a firm, slightly gritty or rough feel. Additional tissue

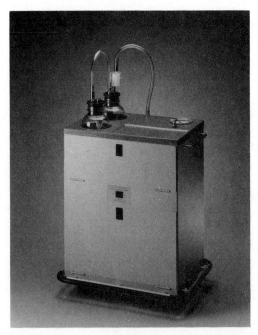

FIG. 89-8.
The Berkeley Synevac vacuum curettage machine.

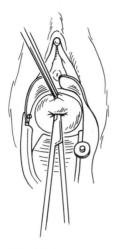

FIG. 89-9.
Exploring the uterus.

that should be removed feels spongy or slippery. Alternatively a Roberts, Stone, or small ring forceps may be used to grasp within the uterine cavity for any additional tissue (Fig. 89-9).*

9. Pass the suction curette once more to remove any debris or blood from the sharp curettage (if done).
10. The procedure is now completed. Remove all instruments and observe the patient for 10 to 15 minutes for bleeding or any unusual reaction. She is then free to leave, with appropriate follow-up information (Box 89-2).
11. Send all tissue for pathological examination.

COMPLICATIONS

The overall complication rate of first-trimester abortion is low, probably less than 5% and certainly lower than that of delivery. However, complications can and do occur, including those resulting in major disability or even death. Careful attention to technique and constant vigilance for complications are mandatory.

Complications of abortion fall into four categories: laminaria complications, paracervical block complications, suction curettage complications, and obstetric and gynecological complications.

Laminaria Complications

• If the laminaria perforates the cervix and creates a false passage, the abortion cannot be subsequently accomplished. Proper placement is essential.

---

*Many operators delete this step.

BOX 89-2. PATIENT EDUCATION HANDOUT AFTER TERMINATION OF PREGNANCY

Resuming normal activities. On the day of the procedure you may wish to rest, avoiding school or work and refraining from vigorous physical activity. On the following day you may return to most normal activities, including work, school, and exercise. Avoid baths and do not place anything in the vagina for 10 days. You may shower any time.

Bleeding. Bleeding is common after abortion and may even last for a few weeks. Light bleeding (lighter than a menstrual period) is normal and will eventually stop. If bleeding becomes heavy—if you are soaking a pad in less than a hour—you should notify your physician or go to the hospital emergency room.

You may be given medication to reduce bleeding. Take one Methergine pill four times a day starting when you get home from the abortion. Take the medication for 3 days.

Some women will pass small fragments of placental tissue after an abortion. This is normal and does not require a visit to the doctor or hospital. Your first period should occur in 4 to 6 weeks. If you do not get your period, notify your physician.

Antibiotics. Your physician may have given you antibiotic pills to treat or prevent any infection. Take them until they are gone. If you cannot tolerate the pills for any reason, please call before you stop taking them.

Cramping. There will be some cramping for a couple of days. You may take three 200 mg ibuprofen tablets four times a day for the cramping.

Sex and fertility. You should avoid intercourse for 10 days after an abortion. When you do resume sexual activity, you should use a method of birth control, because you can become pregnant again 2 weeks after an abortion. The physician will give you a prescription for birth control pills if you wish. Start them the Sunday following the abortion. Other available methods of birth control may be discussed with your physician.

An uncomplicated suction abortion should have no effect on your ability to have children in the future.

Danger signs. If any of these following signs occur, please notify your physician promptly.
Fever of 100.4°F or 38°C or higher
Increasing or severe pain in the lower abdomen
Excessive bleeding
Foul-smelling vaginal discharge
If you believe that there is any other serious problem after your abortion, please call your physician or report to the emergency room at the hospital immediately.

Follow-up visit. You should see your physician in 2 weeks. Your appointment is
Day _____   Time _____ .
There is no additional charge for this visit. If you are unable to see your physician then you should have a follow-up visit with another physician. The follow-up visit is important to make sure everything has returned to normal, and to see that you are comfortable with your birth control method.

Dr._____
Phone #_____
Answering Service #_____
Hospital Emergency Room #_____

- If the laminaria is left in over 24 hours, infection may result.
- The laminaria may fall out, migrate up into the uterus, or fragment. If migration or fragmentation is suspected, a careful search of the uterine cavity must be carried out to remove it.
- Occasionally, the internal os will be stenotic and dilate with difficulty. The laminaria may assume an hourglass configuration, which makes it difficult to remove.
- Some patients may experience a vasovagal reaction, which consists of bradycardia, diaphoresis, nausea, and (rarely) convulsions. Atropine may be administered for treatment and prevention; the patient's legs should be elevated and her head lowered.
- Occasionally, a patient will change her mind after the laminaria has been placed. The laminaria can probably be removed at any time, and in most cases, the pregnancy will continue unaffected. However, the patient must be warned of the risk of miscarriage.

Paracervical Block Complications

- Some bleeding usually results.
- Intravascular injection is common, despite efforts to prevent it. Patients experience dysphoria, tinnitus, an unusual taste in the mouth, and visual disturbances. These sensations are transient.
- More severe reactions, such as convulsions or allergic reactions, are rare.
- Anesthetic effect may not be total, but it is usually adequate to carry out the procedure.

Suction Curettage Complications

- The most feared complication is *uterine perforation*. Perforation is identified by increased pain, hemorrhage, or signs of an acute condition in the abdomen. Fat or bowel tissue observed in the suction apparatus is diagnostic, as is passing a blunt instrument up through the perforation. Culdocentesis may help in diagnosing internal bleeding (see Chapter 77, Culdocentesis [Colpocentesis]).

  Treatment must be individualized and depends on whether the abortion is complete or not and whether there is the likelihood of intraabdominal injury. Minimum treatment includes admission for close observation and antibiotics. If the risk of hemorrhage or visceral injury is great, then laparoscopy or laparotomy may be necessary. If perforation occurs before the uterus is emptied, the procedure may be finished under direct laparoscopic observation.
- *Hemorrhage* that occurs during the procedure suggests laceration or perforation, or, more commonly, uterine atony with incomplete evacuation of the uterus. Oxytocics, such as methylergonovine (Methergine) 0.2 mg intramuscularly, may be helpful, and some clinicians give them routinely when terminating pregnancies of 11 weeks and beyond. Some physicians will also routinely run an oxytocin infusion during the procedure, but this can cause uterine contraction, limiting the ability to readily evacuate the uterus.

If bleeding is severe, repeating the suction curettage under laparoscopic guidance; general anesthesia is recommended. Excessive bleeding in the days or weeks after the abortion suggests incomplete abortion. Carefully repeating the procedure is the best course.

- Postabortal *paraendometritis* is relatively common, but usually is not severe. Symptoms of paraendometritis include uterine tenderness, lower abdominal pain, fever, and elevated white cell count. Oral antibiotics may be prescribed; however, repeat suction curettage may be required. Rarely, a patient will have severe sepsis or septic shock, requiring aggressive treatment, including intravenous antibiotics, fluids, and even hysterectomy.

  Prophylactic antibiotics, such as doxycycline, before or immediately after abortion have been advocated, but their role remains controversial.
- *Incomplete evacuation of uterine contents* can lead to hemorrhage and infection. As noted previously, repeat suction curettage is generally indicated.
- Late sequelae, such as *infertility, premature labor, and incompetent cervix,* have been studied extensively. Most modern studies, especially since laminaria dilation became common, have been very reassuring that serious obstetric and gynecologic consequences are rare.
- About 10% of women will have lasting emotional sequelae—*postabortal depression*. The majority of these women will have been emotionally unstable or highly ambivalent before the procedure. Counseling is recommended.

Obstetric and Gynecologic Complications

- *Ectopic pregnancy* may be unsuspected when a patient requests an early abortion. Pathological examination of the tissue obtained from such a procedure would show only decidua and not the actual products of conception. Thus, pathological examination of tissue is an important means of identifying ectopic pregnancies and is recommended in abortions of pregnancies of durations up to the gestational age at which the products of conception can be identified grossly. The clinician can identify placental tissue by floating the tissue in water. Obviously, prompt action is required when ectopic pregnancy is suspected.
- *Miscarriage.* Patients who request an abortion and who are already bleeding may or may not have passed tissue. Going ahead with the procedure makes sense medically, since eventually the patient would probably require suction completion in the emergency room setting.
- *Scant tissue.* Occasionally, tissue obtained during an abortion is very scant. This may indicate that the patient has already spontaneously aborted, that she has an ectopic pregnancy, that she was not pregnant, or that the procedure failed to interrupt the pregnancy. Ultrasound examination and repeat HCG determinations may be necessary, and clinical follow-up is essential. With a failed abortion, the procedure may be attempted again at a later date.
- *Myomata or fibroids.* These muscular tumors of the myometrium complicate abortion two ways: First, they may disguise the gestational age of a pregnancy by greatly enlarging the uterus. In this case, ultrasound is necessary to reveal

the true age. Second, depending on their location, myomatas may prevent or limit access to the uterine cavity. Performing the procedure under anesthesia and ultrasound guidance may be the only recourse.

- *Ovarian tumors* may also inhibit the accuracy of an examination. Again, ultrasound will clarify the issue. Usually the abortion can be performed, and the ovarian tumor dealt with appropriately at a later time.
- *Duplication anomalies of the female genital tract* result from the failure of the uterus to fuse completely during embryonic development; these anomalies range from arcuate uterus, to total duplication, to a double-barreled vagina. The critical point in abortion is determining which side the pregnancy is on, and gaining access to it.

POSTPROCEDURE INSTRUCTIONS

- Methylergonovine 0.2 mg orally every six hours for 6 to 10 doses may assist in contracting the uterus and prevent bleeding.
- Doxycycline 100 mg orally twice a day for 7 days is advised by some clinicians.
- No sexual activity is advisable for two weeks.
- For additional information, see Box 89-2.

SUPPLIER

All special equipment, including suction machines, hosing curettes, dilators, laminaria, and ancillary instruments can be ordered from:

Berkeley Medevices Inc.
907 Camelia Street
Berkeley, CA 94710
415-526-4046 and 800-227-2388

CPT/BILLING CODE

59840   Suction abortion from 6 to 12 weeks

BIBLIOGRAPHY

Penfield AJ: First trimester abortion. In *Gynecologic surgery under local anesthesia,* Baltimore-Munich, 1986, Urban & Schwarzenberg.

Prevention of D isoimmunization, *ACOG Technical Bulletin* 147: October 1990.

Turk P: Abortion. In Lichtman R, Papera S, editors: *Well-woman care,* Norwalk, Conn, 1991, Appleton & Lange.

Zuspan FP, Quilligan EJ: *Douglas-Stromme operative obstetrics,* Norwalk, Conn, 1988, Appleton & Lange.

CHAPTER 90

Breast Biopsy

Hugh H. Hogle

There is nothing complicated about most breast biopsies. Technically, the removal of a palpable breast mass can be accomplished under local anesthesia with no patient discomfort and minimal bleeding. The surgical skills and training of most primary care physicians should qualify them to do most simple breast biopsies. However, recent changes in the treatment options offered patients with breast cancer—including the prerequisite of complete excision of a cancer, desire for good cosmesis, and the need for obtaining specific information about tumor biology—have complicated this previously simple procedure.

The three most common breast masses are *fibroadenomas* (solid benign tumors most frequently seen in young women), *cysts* (fluid-filled masses most often seen as part of fibrocystic changes during midlife), and *breast cancer* (solid masses that increase in frequency with age, but are not unusual in women in their thirties).

While clinical breast examination and mammography may provide clues whether a mass is benign or malignant, *the only way to establish the diagnosis definitely is to drain a cyst with fine-needle aspiration or to remove a tissue sample for pathologic diagnosis.*

Benign masses are usually smooth, round, and freely movable, but many cancers (e.g., colloid, medullary, expansive intraductal cancers) can feel like benign masses. Most patients whose masses turn out to be cancerous will ultimately be referred to a general surgeon for their definitive cancer care. If it is known in advance that a mass is cancerous or has a high likelihood of being cancerous, it is probably best to refer the patient for biopsy also.

Masses with both "benign" examination and mammographic characteristics are suitable for biopsy by primary care physicians with appropriate experience and training.

All benign-feeling masses should be subjected to fine-needle aspiration (FNA) before surgical excisional biopsy (see Chapter 140, Fine-Needle Aspiration Cytology and Biopsy). This will identify the masses that are cysts, and unnecessary surgery can be avoided. If the mass is solid, a specimen can be removed for cytology; thus, many breast cancers can be identifed in advance. Remember that FNA will have an approximate 10% to 15% false-negative rate.

INDICATIONS

- Palpable dominant or solitary breast mass (in a male or female patient)
- Recurrent cystic mass
- Equivocal fine-needle aspiration
- Unresolved anxiety

CONTRAINDICATIONS

- Coagulation disorder, or anticoagulent drug therapy (until stabilized)
- Bloody discharge from nipple (refer to surgeon)

A definite breast cancer or a mass that has a high probability of cancer should probably be referred directly to a general surgeon.

EQUIPMENT

- Surgical marking pen
- Povidine-iodine or other antiseptic skin preparation solution
- Fenestrated drape
- 5 cc of local anesthetic (1% lidocaine with epinephrine and bupivacaine mixture)
- 4 × 4 inch gauze
- Scalpel with No. 10 and No. 15 blades
- 2 curved and 2 straight hemostats
- Needle holder
- 3-0 or 4-0 Vicryl on large needle
- 5-0 Prolene
- Adson pickups
- Tissue scissors
- Electrocautery unit
- Allis clamp
- Steri-Strips

TECHNIQUE

If an open biopsy is performed, curvilinear incisions following Langer's lines are preferable. When possible, make the incisions along the areolar margin; scarring here is more cosmetically acceptable. Avoid radially oriented incisions except in the most medial portion of the breast. (Should mastectomy be needed later, radially oriented incisions in the medial part of the breast are much easier to deal with than curvilinear Langer's type of biopsy incisions.)

In removing a breast mass, it is important to remove a margin of normal breast tissue around the lump. A radius of 1 to 1.5 cm of tissue will be ample, and if malignancy is identified, the oncologic surgeon will most likely reexcise the biopsy site anyway.

After removing breast tissue, many surgeons do not reapproximate the remaining breast tissue. This "dead space," however, can potentially develop a hematoma. It also creates artifact in later clinical breast examinations. Closing the "dead space" with an absorbable suture (3-0 or 4-0 Vicryl) is usually best.

1. Prepare and drape the breast for surgery, using sterile technique.
2. Use a surgical marking pen to outline the incision, the mass, and the ellipse of tissue to be removed.
3. Infiltrate the area with a local anesthetic (1% lidocaine with epinephrine, mixed 50:50 with 0.5% bupivacaine). Create a wheal of local anesthetic along the incision line and then use this area for needle access while anesthetizing the subcutaneous layer and breast parenchyma. The surgical marking lines for specimen removal will define the area requiring local anesthesia infiltration. If possible do not infiltrate directly over the lesion since this may obscure the nodule, preventing its identification.
4. Make the incision with a No. 15 blade, carrying it vertically through the subcutaneous layer.
5. Use tissue scissors to dissect the subcutaneous layer away from the breast parenchyma at lateral borders.
6. Cauterize bleeders with electrocautery.
7. Apply an Allis clamp to the tissue to be removed and use it for countertraction while excising the specimen. A No. 10 blade is usually best for specimen excision. (Protect the wound edges from the proximal cutting edge of the No. 10 blade to avoid inadvertent nicking of the wound edge.) As the deeper portion of the dissection is approached, more local anesthetic is generally required. Fascia should not be penetrated. If the lesion extends through fascia, it is most likely cancer. After removal of the specimen, use a suture to mark the anterior, superior, and lateral borders of the specimen. This will help the pathologist orient the specimen and also identify the location of inadequate margins should the lesion prove to be an incompletely excised malignancy.
8. Submit the specimen for frozen section evaluation.
9. Obtain hemostasis with electrocautery.
10. If desired, reapproximate the breast parenchyma with absorbable interrupted sutures of 3-0 or 4-0 Vicryl. To prevent deformity, do not use excessively large stitches. Close the subcutaneous layer with absorbable 4-0 or 5-0 Vicryl. Close the skin with running subdermal 5-0 Vicryl sutures or running subcuticular 5-0 Prolene sutures and Steri-Strips.
11. Apply a light pressure dressing.
12. The patient may remove the dressing after 24 hours and may begin showering then. The sutures should be removed in approximately 7 to 8 days.

COMPLICATIONS

- Hematoma
- Infection
- Scarring or skin distortion
- Pain
- Incomplete removal of lesion or not identifying correct nodule for removal
- Unnecessarily penetrating a fascial plane may extend the stage of cancer

CONSIDERATIONS

- Remember that the patient will judge your surgical skill by the scar you leave on her breast. Use careful surgical technique and plastic closures.
- Give the patient some appropriate pain medications for postoperative discomfort.
- Communicate with the oncology surgeon if referral becomes necessary.
- Do not perform a biopsy for lesions requiring needle localization, unless you are specifically trained to do so.
- Do not perform a breast biopsy unless a frozen section is available to establish diagnosis. (Cancers will need to be examined for the presence or absence of endocrine receptors.)
- Do not perform a biopsy for lesions that are likely to be breast cancers. Refer these patients to general surgeons.
- Do not perform breast biopsies unless you are familiar with modern breast cancer treatment options and implications to breast biopsy techniques.
- Do not forget that the entire breast arena is very litigious. Make sure informed consent is obtained and be careful not to overstep you abilities.
- Do not take a biopsy of excessively large or complicated lesions.
- Do not use concomitant sedation unless appropriate patient-monitoring techniques are available.

CPT/BILLING CODES

19100	Biopsy of breast, needle
19101	Biopsy of breast, incisional
19120	Excision of cyst, fibroadenoma, or other benign or malignant tumor, aberrant breast tissue, duct lesion or nipple lesion, male or female, one or more lesions

BIBLIOGRAPHY

Conry C: Evaluation of a breast complaint: is it cancer? *Am Fam Physician* 49:445, 1994.

Donegan WL: Evaluation of a palpable breast mass, *N Eng J Med* 327(13):937, 1992.

Gamble WG: Breast surgery. In Benjamin RB, editor: *Atlas of outpatient and office surgery,* Malvern, Pa, 1994, Lea & Febiger.

CHAPTER 91

Contraceptive Implants (Norplant)

John L. Pfenninger

The Norplant System (levonorgestrel implants), the first and only sustained-release subdermal contraceptive delivery system, provides highly effective contraception for up to 5 years. This progestin-only contraceptive differs from the progestin-only "mini pill" because it maintains a constant level of levonorgestrel. It has two possible mechanisms of action: (1) It suppresses ovulation in the majority of cycles by maintaining a consistent low level of progestin; and (2) It prevents sperm penetration by increasing the viscosity and thickness of cervical mucus.

One significant concern about long-term contraceptive systems is whether women will continue to have their routine Pap smears. Women on birth control pills must return annually for a new prescription, and at this visit, a Pap smear is usually performed. The Norplant System is effective for 5 years, and the intrauterine device (IUD), for 8 years. Clinicians should stress the necessity of annual Pap smears to patients using long-term contraceptive systems—even though they do not need a new prescription.

Although studies of the Norplant System concentrated on women aged 18 to 40, most physicians do not impose a lower or upper age limit.

The Norplant System was introduced and approved in the United States in 1990. However, it has been approved and in use elsewhere since 1986. The system itself consists of six thin, flexible capsules of soft silastic tubing sealed at each end with silicone. The capsules are 34 mm long and 2.4 mm in diameter, and each contains 36 mg of dry, crystalline levonorgestrel. Placement involves a counseling visit, followed by a brief office procedure in which the capsules are inserted in a fanlike pattern just beneath the skin of the medial upper arm.

INDICATIONS

- Female desiring long-term reversible contraception
- Female who is considering sterilization but is not ready to make the final decision

- Female who has difficulty remembering to take birth control pills daily
- Female who cannot tolerate other forms of contraception, such as birth control pills and coitus-dependent techniques (e.g., condoms, diaphragm)
- Female who cannot tolerate estrogen administration
- Female who has contraindications to IUD use (nulliparous, history of ectopic pregnancy, pelvic inflammatory disease, nonmonogamous relationship)

CONTRAINDICATIONS

- Active thrombophlebitis or thromboembolic disease
- Undiagnosed abnormal genital bleeding
- Possible pregnancy
- Acute liver disease
- Benign or malignant liver tumors
- Known or suspected carcinoma of the breast
- Lack of informed consent
- Unwillingness to accept amenorrhea or metrorrhagia for at least 6 to 9 months
- Excessive concern over the minimal scar that will occur at the site of placement
- Patient who is less than 6 weeks postpartum
- Cigarette smokers under 35 years of age (*relative contraindication*)

EQUIPMENT

- The Norplant System, which is obtained from Wyeth-Ayerst Laboratories in Philadelphia, contains the following:
    Set of six Norplant System capsules
    Norplant System No. 10 cannula and trocar
    Scalpel
    Forceps
    Syringe
    Syringe needles (2)
    Package of skin closures
    Package of gauze sponges (3)
    Stretch bandage
    Surgical drapes (2)
    Surgical drape, fenestrated
    Patient booklets (One is informational and the other is a menstrual cycle diary.)
- 5 cc of 1% or 2% lidocaine *without* epinephrine
- Sterile gloves
- Povidone-iodine (Betadine) solution
- Saline solution to wash the area

Note: Some physicians prefer Elastoplast instead of the stretch bandage supplied. Some physicians prefer to use a template to mark the locations for insertion.

PREPROCEDURE PATIENT EDUCATION

Although the patient could be counseled and have the Norplant inserted the same day, it is rare that patients are fully knowledgeable about the implant procedure, risks, benefits, and complications. Consequently, the patient should have a separate counseling visit to inform her of these issues. Many patients assume that birth control pills are "bad" and that they should stop using them. Recent studies have shown that birth control pills actually reduce the risk of ovarian and endometrial cancer. In addition, they may reduce risks for cardiovascular problems in nonsmokers. Patients also need to be informed of other choices for contraception, such as the IUD, surgical contraception, barrier techniques, and bimonthly progesterone injections (Depo-Provera).

When the patient schedules the counseling visit, she should receive an educational handout (see Box 91-1) and possibly several handouts from the manufacturer. Ask her to review these prior to the office visit and to come in early for the counseling visit to review a videotape (provided by Wyeth-Ayerst Laboratories). Before the counseling visit, have the patient complete her portion of the encounter form (see Box 91-2). If there are no contraindications and the patient indicates she still would like to use the Norplant System, then review the method of insertion with her.

Although informed consent is necessary, a consent form is not generally signed for this procedure. However, always document that the patient has read over the patient education handouts, and that you discussed the risks, benefits, possible complications, and alternatives.

Show a model arm from the company, sample capsules, and the site of insertion to the patient. The capsules are usually placed in the inner aspect of the upper nondominant arm.

Review effectiveness of contraception and tell the patient that this method is not absolutely foolproof, but that it is one of the best contraceptive devices available, with a failure rate less than 1%.

Discuss the advantages of the Norplant System, including the absence of estrogen, the long duration, the effectiveness, the reversibility, and the fact that nothing needs to be remembered and it is coitus independent. Although the initial cost is high, compared to the cost of birth control pills for the same duration, it is inexpensive. Overall, after one year, 81% of all patients continue to use Norplant. The capsules do not interfere with activity in any way. It is effective within 24 hours of insertion if inserted within 7 days of the onset of the menstrual period.

Review the side effects and disadvantages of the Norplant system, including the following:

- **Irregular bleeding.** 60% of women can expect to experience an alteration of menstrual patterns during the first year. The menstrual cycle usually becomes more regular within 9 to 12 months.

**BOX 91-1. PATIENT EDUCATION HANDOUT
NORPLANT SYSTEM**

The Norplant system was introduced in the United States in 1991, although it has been used in Europe for many years. The system consists of six thin, flexible capsules that are sealed at each end with silicone. Each capsule contains a hormone called progesterone. This hormone slowly leaks from the capsule, which measures about 1.25 inches long and one-tenth of an inch wide. These capsules are placed under the skin and may remain there for up to 5 years.

The Norplant system is particularly good for women who

- Are considering surgical sterilization but are not ready to make the final decision.
- Want long-term, reversible contraception.
- Want to avoid daily oral contraceptive use or methods that have to be used each time they have intercourse.
- Want to avoid estrogen-containing contraceptives that may have more adverse effects.
- Cannot use an IUD.

The Norplant system should not be used by women who

- Have had blood clots or strokes.
- Have undiagnosed abnormal genital bleeding.
- May be pregnant.
- Have liver disease of any sort.
- Have a history of breast cancer. If there is a family history of breast cancer, discuss this with your physician.

Method of Insertion
It usually takes 10 to 15 minutes to insert the capsules (and 15 to 20 minutes to remove them). A local anesthetic is administered in the skin on the inner side of the left upper arm (for right-handed women). A small incision just big enough to allow the capsule to enter (2 mm or one-tenth of an inch) is made. The six capsules are then placed one at a time just under the skin. The incision site is covered with a small butterfly bandage. Stitches or sutures are not needed.

The insertion should not leave a noticeable scar. The capsules themselves are not visible; however, the outline of the capsules underneath the skin can be felt and sometimes seen.

Effectiveness
A blood level of hormone sufficient to prevent conception is reached within 24 hours. The effectiveness may last up to 5 years. After 5 years, the *capsules must be removed;* however, the capsules can be removed at any time should the user so desire.

The Norplant System is one of the most effective forms of reversible contraception ever developed. The average annual pregnancy rate over 5 years is less than 1%; this is favorable compared to the pregnancy rate of women who use birth control pills and IUDs.

Benefits
The Norplant System has a number of distinct benefits. It is very effective: It provides continuous, long-term protection for up to 5 years. It is estrogen free and delivers an extremely low dose of hormone. It is very convenient and comfortable. It is completely reversible. Upon removal, the user will return to the previous level of fertility. There is nothing a user must do after the capsules are inserted *except have an annual Pap and pelvic examination.*

Continued.

BOX 91-1.–cont'd

Side Effects

The most frequent side effect experienced is a change in the menstrual bleeding pattern. This may include more frequent bleeding, heavier bleeding, spotting, and even a lack of periods. Approximately 60% of women experience one of these conditions. Irregular and prolonged bleeding are more likely to occur during the first year, and less bleeding occurs in subsequent years. Most women can expect to develop a regular menstrual pattern within 9 to 12 months. To keep things in perspective, these side effects should be compared against an unwanted pregnancy.

The most frequently reported side effects (other than menstrual changes) include headache, nervousness, nausea, dizziness, and weight gain.

Infection at the insertion site can occur, but this is very rare. The ovaries can develop *cysts,* but they will usually go away on their own.

Overall, after one year, 81% of all Norplant users continue to use the system. Despite the high rate of changes in menstrual bleeding, only 9% of women had the Norplant removed because of this. Women can perform any activity that they may have been involved in before the insertion.

Even though the Norplant System is extremely effective, there are some women (such as those who are over 150 pounds) who are more likely to get pregnant with this method. If you have any questions about this, please ask the physician.

Breast Feeding

The Norplant may be inserted 6 weeks after delivery and will not affect breast milk.

When to Schedule Your Appointment

You will need to have an initial counseling appointment to discuss the issues about the Norplant. You will be able to either view the videotape available in the office or take it home for your viewing. If there are no reasons you should not have Norplant System inserted, an appointment will be scheduled during the *first seven days of your cycle.* (Day 1 of your cycle is the first day of menstruation.) You may return to work immediately, if you desire. You must have had a breast and pelvic examination, and Pap smear within the previous 6 months. It is suggested that you have this done by your family doctor or gynecologist before the visit so the results can be discussed with the doctor.

If you have any questions, please feel free to discuss them with the physician at the time of the counseling visit.

Used with permission of The Medical Procedures Center, P.C., Midland, Michigan.

- **Headache, nausea, dizziness, nervousness.**
- **Weight gain.** Rare but quite profound in some cases.
- **Ovarian cysts.** Can cause some discomfort but generally resolve on their own. Rarely clinically apparent.
- **Ectopic pregnancies.** Incidence is decreased in the Norplant user.
- **Pregnancy.** Rare, but possible. Patients need to obtain pregnancy tests if they miss their period. After two months of negative pregnancy tests, further pregnancy tests are probably not warranted, since the missed periods are probably the effect of the drug. Should pregnancy occur, the capsules should be withdrawn immediately. There are no long-term studies showing adverse effects on the fetus.

BOX 91-2. PATIENT ENCOUNTER FORM
NORPLANT SYSTEM

Patient To Fill Out:

Name _____ Date _____

Birth date _____ Age ___ Last menstrual period _____

Number of pregnancies _____ Family doctor _____

Miscarriages or abortions _____

Current contraceptive method _____

What contraception have you tried? _____

Did you read and understand the handouts we gave you?   Y   N

Did you see the videotape?   Y   N

How long is your usual period? _____ days

Have you ever had a low blood count?   Y   N

Last Pap smear   date _____ result _____

Last physical/pelvic examination   date _____

When would you like to get pregnant again? _____

Have you ever had

A pregnancy in your tubes?	Y	N	Any liver tumors?	Y	N
Infection in your tubes?	Y	N	A personal or family history		
Any venereal disease?	Y	N	of breast cancer?	Y	N
Any genital warts?	Y	N	Any problems with diabetes?	Y	N
An IUD?	Y	N	Any problems with high		
Blood clots in your			cholesterol?	Y	N
legs or a stroke?	Y	N	Any swelling in your legs?	Y	N
Any type of liver disease?	Y	N	Any unusual vaginal bleeding?	Y	N

For The Doctor:

Model used to show insertion technique   Y   N

Effectiveness reviewed   Y   N

Advantages: Cost (includes counseling, insertion, follow-up), lack of estrogen, good for 5 years, nothing to remember, reversible

Disadvantages/complications:

- Irregular bleeding/lack of periods
- Headache, nausea, weight gain, nervousness
- Insertion
- Removal

- Cysts
- Failure
- Costs

Contraindications: none or _____

Manual reviewed?   Y   N

Impression: _____

Plan: _____

_____

Physician Signature

cc: _____

_____

Date

- **Thromboembolic phenomena.** Low incidence; however, women who will be subjected to prolonged immoblization due to surgery or other illnesses should have the capsules removed prior to surgery or thrombophlebitis prophylaxis.
- **Effect on cholesterol and sugar.** Minimal.

Although cost is an advantage, it is also a disadvantage if the patient must pay the entire price initially. Removal of the capsules is also a disadvantage. Reassure the patient that there is currently no known relationship between this method and any type of genital cancer. However, abnormal bleeding caused by the Norplant itself could mask bleeding from cervical or endometrial cancers.

If the patient has not had a Pap smear and pelvic examination within the past 6 months, then perform these at this time. The patient's Pap smear should be normal prior to insertion of the Norplant.

Give the patient the Wyeth-Ayerst manual, and review it with her. If she still desires placement, then schedule an appointment on a day that falls within 7 days of the start of her menstrual period.

INSERTION

Technique (Fig. 91-1)

1. Use only lidocaine *without* epinephrine. Epinephrine can cause cutaneous ulcerations.
2. Correct subdermal placement of the capsules will facilitate removal. To ensure this, make sure the needle and trocar is inserted with its bevel up. The skin should be visibly tented up at all times during the insertion as the trocar is advanced. *Stay superficial* (subdermal) even though this typically requires more force to insert than subcutaneous insertion.
3. As the trocar is withdrawn, hold the distal tip of the capsule in place through the skin. Proximally, as the trocar is withdrawn to the mark near the tip, you should be able to feel the capsule fall from the tip. Place the index finger over this newly inserted capsule to prevent the trocar from catching on it as you reinsert the trocar (Fig. 91-1). If the trocar catches the capsule, it could damage it or force it back under the skin where it will lie in a **U** position.
4. Before inserting the capsules, always count to be sure that there are indeed six capsules present. After insertion, once again identify the six subdermal implants. If the capsules are dropped or the patient expels a capsule, it can be returned to the company for free replacement.

Complications

- Most patients will have a large ecchymotic area (bruising) around the site of insertion. They can expect this to resolve in approximately 2 weeks. Applying ice to the area immediately after insertion may minimize this.
- Infection around the area of insertion is very uncommon (0.7%); however, if infection does occur, remove the capsules and allow the area to heal. Whether all capsules need to be removed or not is the decision of the physician.

INSERTION PROCEDURE

Insertion should be performed within seven days from the onset of menses. However, NORPLANT SYSTEM capsules may be inserted at any time during the cycle provided pregnancy has been excluded and a nonhormonal contraceptive method is used for the remainder of the cycle. A gynecological examination should be performed before the insertion of NORPLANT SYSTEM capsules, as would be the case before initiating any hormonal contraception. Determine if the subject has any allergies to the antiseptic or anesthetic to be used or contraindications to progestin-only contraception. If none are found, the capsules are inserted using the procedure outlined below. One NORPLANT SYSTEM set consists of six capsules in a sterile pouch. The insertion is performed under aseptic conditions using a trocar to place the capsules under the skin.

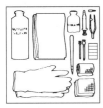

A: The following equipment is recommended for the insertion:
–an examining table for the patient to lie on.
–sterile surgical drapes, sterile gloves (free of talc), antiseptic solution.
–local anesthetic, needles, and syringe.
–No. 11 scalpel, No. 10 trocar, forceps.
–skin closure, sterile gauze, and compresses.

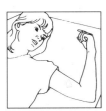

B: Have the patient lie on her back on the examination table with her left arm (if the patient is left-handed, the right arm) flexed at the elbow and externally rotated so that her hand is lying by her head. The capsules will be inserted subdermally through a small 2 mm incision and positioned in a fanlike manner with the fan opening toward the shoulder.

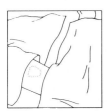

C: Prep the patient's upper arm with antiseptic solution; cover the arm above and below the insertion area with a sterile cloth. The optimal insertion area is in the inside of the upper arm about 8 to 10 cm above the elbow crease.

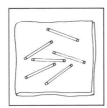

D: Open the sterile NORPLANT SYSTEM package carefully by pulling apart the sheets of the pouch, allowing the capsules to fall onto a sterile cloth. Count the six capsules.

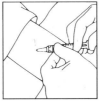

E: After determining the absence of known allergies to the anesthetic agent or related drugs, fill a 5 mL syringe with the local anesthetic. Anesthetize the insertion area by first inserting the needle under the skin and releasing a small amount of the anesthetic. Then anesthetize six areas about 4 to 4.5 cm long, to mimic the fanlike position of the implanted capsules.

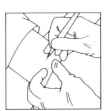

F: Use the scalpel to make a small, shallow incision (about 2 mm) through the skin.

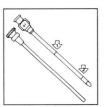

G: The trocar has two marks on it. The first mark is closer to the hub and indicates how far the trocar should be introduced under the skin before the loading of each capsule. The second mark is close to the tip and indicates how much of the trocar should remain under the skin following the insertion of each implant.

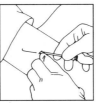

H: Insert the tip of the trocar through the incision beneath the skin at a shallow angle. Once the trocar is inserted, it should be oriented with the bevel up toward the skin to keep the capsules in a superficial plane. It is important to keep the trocar subdermal by tenting the skin with the trocar, as failure to do so may result in deep placement of the capsules and could make removal more difficult. Advance the trocar gently under the skin to the first mark near the hub of the trocar. The tip of the trocar is now at a distance of about 4 to 4.5 cm from the incision. Do not force the trocar, and if resistance is felt, try another direction.

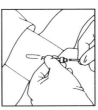

I: When the trocar has been inserted the appropriate distance, remove the obturator and load the first capsule into the trocar using the thumb and forefinger.

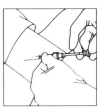

J: Gently advance the capsule with the obturator toward the tip of the trocar until you feel resistance. Never force the obturator.

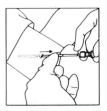

K: Hold the obturator steady, and bring the trocar back until it touches the handle of the obturator.

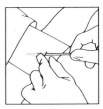

L: The capsule should have been released under the skin when the mark close to the tip of the trocar is visible in the incision. Release of the capsule can be checked by palpation. It is important to keep the obturator steady and not to push the capsule into the tissue.

Continued.

FIG. 91-1.

Norplant insertion and removal technique. (Courtesy of Wyeth-Ayerst Laboratories, Philadelphia, Pa.)

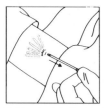

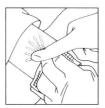

M: Do not remove the trocar from the incision until all capsules have been inserted. The trocar is withdrawn only to the mark close to its tip. Each succeeding capsule is always inserted next to the previous one to form a fanlike shape. Fix the position of the previous capsule with the forefinger and middle finger of the free hand, and advance the trocar along the tips of the fingers. This will ensure a suitable distance of about 15 degrees between capsules and keep the trocar from puncturing any of the

previously inserted capsules. Leave a distance of about 5 mm between the incision and the tips of the capsules. This will help avoid spontaneous expulsions. The correct position of the capsules can be ensured by feeling them with the fingers after the insertion has been completed.

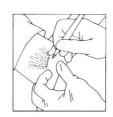

N: After the insertion of the sixth capsule, palpate the capsules to make sure that all six have been inserted.

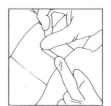

O: Press the edges of the incision together, and close the incision with a skin closure. Suturing the incision should not be necessary.

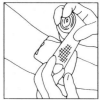

P: Cover the insertion area with a dry compress, and wrap gauze around the arm to ensure hemostasis. Observe the patient for a few minutes for signs of syncope or bleeding from the incision before she is discharged. Advise the patient to keep the insertion area dry for 2 to 3 days. The gauze may be removed after 1 day, and the butterfly bandage as soon as the incision has healed, i.e., normally in 3 days.

REMOVAL PROCEDURE

It is recommended that removals be prescheduled so that preparations for carrying out the procedure can be facilitated. Removal of the capsules should be performed very gently and will take more time than insertion. Capsules are sometimes nicked or cut during removal. The incidence of overall removal difficulties, including damage to capsules, has been 13.2 percent. Less than half of these removal difficulties have caused inconvenience to the patient. If the removal of some of the capsules proves difficult, have the patient return for a second visit. The remaining capsule(s) will be easier to remove after the area is healed. If contraception is still desired, a barrier method should be advised until all capsules are removed. The position of the patient and the asepsis are the same as for insertion.

HINTS
Removal
–The removal of the implanted capsules will take a little more time than the insertion.
–Before removal, apply the anesthetic *under* the capsule ends nearest the original incision site.
–If the removal of some of the capsules proves difficult, interrupt the procedure and have the patient return for a second visit. The remaining capsule(s) will be easier to remove after the area is healed.
–To ensure subdermal placement, the trocar with bevel up should be supported by the index finger and should visibly raise the skin at all times during insertion.

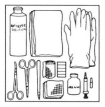

A: The following equipment is needed for the removal:
–an examining table for the patient to lie on.
–sterile surgical drapes, sterile gloves (free of talc), antiseptic solution.
–local anesthetic, needles, and syringe.
–No. 11 scalpel, forceps (straight and curved mosquito).
–skin closure, sterile gauze, and compresses.

This will serve to raise the ends of the capsules. Anesthetic injected over the capsules will obscure them and make removal more difficult. Additional small amounts of the anesthetic can be used for the removal of each of the capsules, if required.

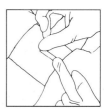

C: Make a 4 mm incision with the scalpel close to the ends of the capsules. Do not make a large incision.

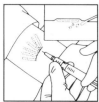

B: Locate the implanted capsules by palpation, possibly marking their position with a sterile skin marker. Apply a small amount of local anesthetic *under* the capsule ends nearest the original incision site.

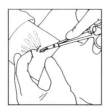

D: Push each capsule gently towards the incision with the fingers. When the tip is visible or near to the incision, grasp it with a mosquito forceps.

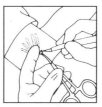

E: Use the scalpel very gently to open the tissue sheath that has formed around the capsule.

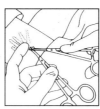

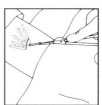

F and G: Remove the capsule from the incision with the second forceps.

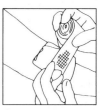

H and I: After the procedure is completed, the incision is closed and bandaged as with insertion. The upper arm should be kept dry for a few days.
Following removal, a return to the previous level of fertility is usually prompt, and a pregnancy may occur at any time. If the patient wishes to continue using the method, a new set of NORPLANT SYSTEM capsules can be inserted through the same incision in the same or opposite direction.

FIG. 91-1.–cont'd

- Expulsion of a capsule can occur. This is more common if the placement is too shallow or if infection occurs at the time of insertion. A new sterile capsule must be placed, since less than 6 capsules may provide inadequate contraception.
- Ulceration over the area is possible and may possibly be more common when the local anesthetic contains epinephrine.

REMOVAL

Removal will take more time—approximately 20 minutes. A local anesthetic does not need to be administered along the full length of the capsules, but rather, just at the site of removal. If the capsules have been in for a while, there will be a fibrous structure encapsulating them. It is often easier just to grasp the Norplant capsule with the curved hemostats and use a blade to cut through this fibrous structure, being careful not to cut the capsule. The capsule will then be easily removed (Fig. 91-1).

Equipment

- Sterile fenestrated drape
- Sterile gloves
- Antiseptic solution
- Local anesthetic with 30-gauge needle and 3 cc syringe
- No. 11 blade
- Straight and curved forceps
- Steri-Strips
- 4 × 4 inch gauze pads
- Elastoplast or a stretch bandage

SPECIAL PROGRAM FOR INDIGENT PATIENTS

The Norplant Foundation (P.O. Box 25223, Alexandria, VA 22314; telephone: 703-706-5933) was formed to assist women in need of contraception. The foundation will provide the Norplant System at no cost to women who meet eligibility requirements (no insurance for reversible contraception; annual income less than 185% of poverty level [$12,247 for a single woman, to $24,790 for head of household]; a sponsor physician who will insert and remove the Norplant at no cost).

CPT/BILLING CODES

11975	Norplant insertion
11976	Norplant removal
11977	Norplant removal with reinsertion

BIBLIOGRAPHY

Ahico NB: Contraception update: oral agents, implants, and investigational methods, *Fam Pract Recert* 14(2):87, 1992.

Bardin CW: Long-acting steroidal contraception: an update, *Int J Fertil* (suppl):88, 1989.

Darney PD et at: Acceptance and perceptions of Norplant among users in San Francisco, USA, *Studies in Family Planning* 2(3):152, 1990.

Flattum-Riemers J: Norplant: a new contraceptive, *Am Fam Physician* 44(1):103, 1991.

Monaghan JC: Norplant insertion and removal, *Patient Care:* 231, March 1992.

Shoupe D, Mishell DR: Norplant: subdermal implant system for long-term contraception, *Am J Obstet Gynecol* 160:1286, 1989.

Zuber TJ, DeWitt DE, Patton DD: Skin damage associated with the Norplant contraceptive, *JFP* 34:613, 1992

Loop Electrosurgical Excision Procedure (LEEP) for Treating CIN

Thomas C. Wright

Ralph M. Richart

A variety of techniques can be used to treat cervical intraepithelial neoplasia (CIN). The appropriateness of a particular technique to treat a particular lesion depends on a number of factors, including lesion size, location, and extension into the endocervical canal. Recently, a new method has been introduced that utilizes modern, solid-state, electrosurgical generators and thin-wire loop electrodes to excise CIN lesions and atypical transformation zones in their entirety. This procedure is known as the loop electrosurgical excision procedure (LEEP). Another term that refers to this procedure is LETZ (large loop excision of the transformation zone). LEEP has a number of advantages over other treatment modalities for CIN including the following:

- It is easy to learn and perform.
- It involves inexpensive equipment.
- It enables the entire lesion to be assessed histologically to rule out an invasive cervical cancer.
- It allows many patients to be diagnosed and treated in a single office visit.
- It results in an excellent pathological specimen with minimal loss of blood and minimal thermal artifact.
- It enables cervical conization to be performed in the office at significantly reduced cost.

INDICATIONS

- Presence of a high-grade squamous intraepithelial lesion (SIL) evidenced on Pap smear together with a colposcopically detected CIN lesion
- Presence of low-grade SIL evidenced on Pap smear together with a clear-cut,

colposcopically visible CIN lesion, or biopsy-proven CIN suitable for conservative management (In this instance, LEEP replaces cryotherapy.)

- When cervical conization is indicated (see Chapter 82, Cervical Conization)

CONTRAINDICATIONS

- Bleeding diathesis
- Severe cervicitis
- Patient exposed *in utero* to diethylstilbestrol
- Pregnancy
- Less than 12 weeks' postpartum
- Clinically apparent invasive carcinoma of the cervix
- Equivocal cervical abnormalities

   Note: It is imperative that the LEEP procedure not be used to excise the transformation zone indiscriminately in women with atypical Pap smears only. The procedure should be reserved to treat CIN lesions, not just atypical Pap smears.

- Lack of expertise to control potential severe cervical bleeding

EQUIPMENT

- Electrosurgical generator (ESU) (Fig. 92-1 and Table 92-1) with the following features:

   Minimum output capability of 50 watts in both cutting and coagulation modes
   Three different waveform outputs—pure cut, blended current, and coagulation current
   Rapid-start features
   Patient-grounding pad monitor (beneficial if the patient is under anesthesia)
   Isolated circuitry

   Editor's note: Although the Ellman Surgitron does not meet some of these qualifications, it has been used extensively for the LEEP procedure (see Chapter 16, Fig. 16-1).

- Loop electrodes of the appropriate size and a ball electrode for fulguration (Fig. 92-2) (These can be either of the disposable or of the sterilizable reusable variety.)

   Authors' note: We recommend using only shallow loop electrodes (i.e., either 0.8 cm or 1.0 cm deep) for LEEP.

- Electrode handle and a patient return electrode (grounding pad or antenna)
- Nonconductive speculum (either coated with a nonconductive material or made of plastic) capable of being used in conjunction with a smoke evacuator
- Smoke evacuator equipped with an adequate viral and odor filter
- Colposcope capable of low magnification (4× to 7.5×)

A

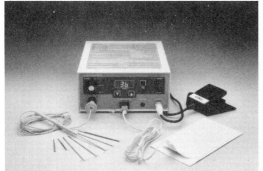

B

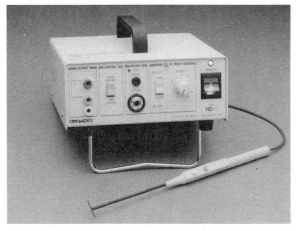

FIG. 92-1.
A, Cooper surgical LEEP unit with handpiece, loop electrodes, disposable return pads, and foot switch; **B,** Cryomedics electrosurgical unit.

TABLE 92-1.

Electrosurgical Generators

	Model No.	Maximum Cutting Current (W)	Maximum Coagulation Current (W)	Cutting Frequency (kHz)	Digital Output Meters	Return Electrode Monitor	List† Price ($)
Aspen (ConMed)*	Sabre 180	100	80	417	Yes	Yes	3,995
Birtcher	4400 Power Plus	300	100	493	—	Yes	6,525
Cabot Medical	110G	120	44	2800	No	No	2,950
Cameron-Miller	26-0375	100	35	500	Yes	No	1,125
	80-1983	85	85	500	No	Yes	1,595
	26-2500	150	75	500	Yes	Yes	2,495
Cooper Surgical	LEEP System 6000	100	80	550	Yes	No	2,990
Ellman	Surgitron FFPF	100	50-80	3800	No	No	2,195
GyneTech	Autolepe 1000	150	150	450	No	Yes	3,495
	Autolepe 2000	150	150	450	No	Yes	3,995
	Autolepe 4000	150	150	450	Yes	Yes	4,395
Leisegang	LM-90	90	45	550	Yes	Yes	3,995
Premier Medical	06301	100	70	2900	No	No	1,535
Utah Medical Products Inc.	Finesse (ESU-100)	99	75	400	Yes	No	5,200
	Finesse II (ESUZ-115)	65	60	400	No	No	3,200
Valleylab, Inc.	Force 2	300	120	500	Yes	Yes	7,550
Wallach Surgical	LEAP 100	100	65	500	Yes	No	2,595

*Other models available. This unit is promoted for LEEP.
†Prices as of October 1993.
Adapted from Wright TC et al: *Contemp Obstet Gynecol:* March 1991. Used with permission.

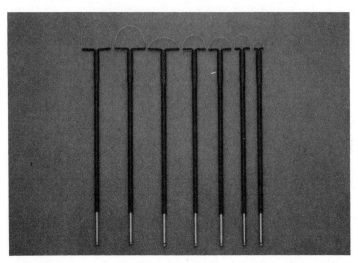

FIG. 92-2.
Wire loop electrodes for LEEP. Loop electrodes come in a variety of sizes and shapes.

- 5% acetic acid and full-strength aqueous Lugol's solution; cotton balls or 2 × 2 inch gauze pads and ring forceps
- Dental type of syringe equipped with a 25- to 27-gauge needle at least 1.5 inches long with two 1.8 cc ampules of 2% lidocaine with 1:100,000 epinephrine or a 5 cc syringe with 4-inch needle extender (can then use the multidose vials of 2% lidocaine with epinephrine)
- Monsel's paste
- Kevorkian endocervical curette
- Containers of histology fixative (usually 10% formalin)
- A 12-inch needle holder and 2-0 Vicryl suture material together with a vaginal pack in the event that large-vessel bleeding occurs
- Vaginal side wall retractor

SUPPLIERS

Aspen (Con Med) (Birtcher)
P.O. Box 3936
Englewood, CO 80155
800-446-1471

Cabot Medical
2021 Cabot Boulevard West
Longhorne, PA 19047
800-523-6078

Cameron-Miller
3949 South Racine Avenue
Chicago, IL 60609
312-523-6360

Cooper Surgical
15 Forest Parkway
Shelton, CT 06484
203-828-8321
800-645-3760

Ellman International, Inc.
1135 Railroad Avenue
Hewlett, NY 11557
516-569-1482
800-835-5355

Gyne-Tech Instrument Corporation
1111 Chestnut Street
Burbank, CA 91506-1688
213-849-1512

Leisegang Medical
6401 Congress Avenue
Boca Raton, FL 33487
800-448-4450

Premier Medical Products
P.O. Box 111
1710 Romano Drive
Norristown, PA 19404-0111
215-277-3800

Utah Medical Products, Inc.
7043 South 300 West
Midvale, UT 84047-1048
801-566-1200

Valleylab, Inc.
5920 Longbow Drive
Boulder, CO 80301
303-530-2300

Wallach Surgical Devices, Inc.
291 Pepe's Farm Road
Milford, CT 06460
203-783-1818

PREPROCEDURE PATIENT EDUCATION

- Provide a patient education handout (see Box 92-1).
- Instruct the patient to take 600 to 800 mg of ibuprofen 1 to 2 hours before the procedure.
- Obtain informed consent.
- The procedure is best performed immediately following menses, so any vaginal bleeding is not confused with menses.

TECHNIQUE

1. Have the patient undress from the waist down and lie on the gynecological examining table. It is important that the patient not move, cough, or change position once the excision is started. Thus, a cooperative patient is essential.
2. Colposcopically evaluate the patient to ensure that a CIN lesion is present.
3. Attach the patient-return electrode grounding pad to the patient's thigh and connect the grounding pad to the ESU.
4. Insert a nonconductive speculum with the smoke evacuator attachment into the vagina and connect the speculum to the smoke evacuator. It is important that the speculum be large enough to allow complete, unobstructed visualization of the cervix. If the vaginal side walls remain in the way, use a vaginal side wall retractor (Fig. 92-3) or vaginal stint.
5. Apply the acetic acid solution and examine the cervix colposcopically.
6. If a clear-cut CIN lesion is identified colposcopically or if the patient has a biopsy-proven CIN, apply full-strength Lugol's solution to the cervix (this lasts longer than acetic acid). Use cotton balls or a large OB-Gyn applicator.
7. Inject approximately 0.5 cc of 2% lidocaine with epinephrine 1:100,000 intracervically (submucosally) at each of the 12, 3, 6 and 9 o'clock positions (to a total of 2 to 6 cc). Take care to inject the cervix superficially, only 3 to 5 mm deep. Additional injections may be needed at intervals between those noted above.

BOX 92-1. PATIENT EDUCATION HANDOUT
LOOP ELECTROSURGICAL EXCISION PROCEDURE

Loop electrosurgical excision procedure (LEEP) is a revolutionary new treatment introduced for the management of precancerous conditions of the uterine cervix, vulva (lips), vagina, and anus. This procedure actually uses radiofrequency waves to remove tissue. The waves are a type of electricity that is similar to AM radio waves. The radio waves cause less destruction of tissue than does electrical current, which was used in the past.

In the past, many abnormalities of the cervix were treated with freezing (cryosurgery). The new LEEP procedure is more effective in treating advanced lesions and very large lesions. For smaller lesions, its cure rate is higher (approximately 95% with just one treatment) than that of cryosurgery (80% to 85% cure rate with one treatment).

Approximately 2 hours before the office visit, you should take three 200 mg ibuprofen tablets. When you come in for the procedure, you will be placed on the examination table with your feet in stirrups. The vaginal speculum will be inserted and mucus will be wiped off the cervix. Vinegar will be used to make abnormalities more visible, and the doctor will then examine the area with the colposcope (essentially a magnifying lens). Iodine will then be placed on the cervix to help identify the abnormal tissue. The cervix will then be numbed with lidocaine. Using a thin wire loop, the physician will remove the abnormal tissue. The procedure only lasts 8 to 10 minutes.

Complications following LEEP may include discomfort, pain, and bleeding. With cryosurgery, many women feel a lot of uterine cramping. Most women who have the LEEP procedure feel that once the anesthetic is placed, there is minimal discomfort, and that it is actually easier than the cryotherapy. There will be discomfort, however, from the speculum and from lying in the pelvic position for up to 15 minutes. The major immediate complication is bleeding. Although rare, it may require suturing or further surgery.

The real advantage of LEEP is that it is quick. In comparison to cryosurgery, it causes less discomfort and eliminates the discharge that lasts 3 to 4 weeks after cryosurgery.

This new technique will most likely replace many of the other treatment methods for your condition, such as cryosurgery, laser, cervical conization (removal of a large cone of cervical tissue), and hysterectomy.

After the LEEP is carried out, please follow these instructions:

- Refrain from sexual intercourse for 3 to 4 weeks.
- Avoid lifting heavy weights (over 20 pounds) for 3 weeks.
- If a smelly discharge develops, use a vaginal douche with half vinegar and half water twice a day for 5 consecutive days. If the odor persists, please call your physician. A brownish-black vaginal discharge for a few days to 2 weeks is normal.
- If spotting or bleeding persists longer than 6 days, call your physician.
- If you develop bleeding with clots, call your physician.
- Return to your physician's office in 4 months for a follow-up Pap smear. A follow-up visit in 6 weeks may also be advised. You will need at least three Pap smears in the first 12 to 18 months.

After you have been treated, you still have an increased lifetime risk of developing cervical, vaginal, and vulvar cancer. You and your partner must refrain from smoking. To prevent the spreading of the wart virus, you should practice monogamy—having sex with the same partner for the rest of your life. Although condoms and nonoxynol-9 spermicidal jelly may help prevent the spread of warts, they are not totally protective. *You must obtain a Pap smear at least once a year for the rest of your life to screen for cervical cancer.*

Please feel free to ask your physician any questions.

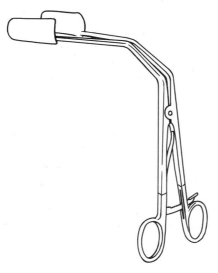

FIG. 92-3.
Vaginal side wall retractor.

8. Although loops of many different sizes are available from various manufacturers, a round loop 2 cm wide by 0.8 cm deep is most frequently used for CIN lesions confined to the portio. For a small, nulliparous cervix use a 1.5 by 0.7 cm loop. For lesions extending into the endocervical canal, a 1 cm by 1 cm square loop electrode can be used to excise the endocervical canal itself. This can be combined with the ectocervical loop to perform a "cowboy hat" type of procedure.

9. The power required for the different sized loops will depend on the ESU used and the diameter of the loop. In general, a 2.0 cm by 0.8 cm loop will require between 35 and 45 watts of power, whereas a 1.0 by 1.0 cm loop will require only 20 to 30 watts of power. For LEEP, the use of blended current with a 20% duty cycle is recommended. (Since the various ESUs differ, check with the manufacturers for their recommended settings.)

10. Three different types of the cervical LEEP excisions can be performed depending on the size and location of the CIN lesion.

    Small lesions confined to the ectocervix. Select a loop electrode 1.5 to 2.0 cm wide and 0.8 cm deep. Place the loop several millimeters lateral to the edge of the CIN lesion and make a test pass over the lesion to ensure that the path is clear. Then activate the loop and push it perpendicularly into the tissue to a depth of 5 to 8 mm, then draw it laterally across and through the endocervical canal and pull it to the other side several millimeters past a lesion or several millimeters beyond the transformation zone, whichever is more lateral. In most instances, the CIN lesion can be entirely removed in a single pass. This produces a donut-shaped specimen with the endocervical canal in the center. The excised tissue should have the proportions of a dome. It is important to remember not to push the loop electrode to a depth greater than 4 to 5 mm at the lateral sides of the cervix, since this is the

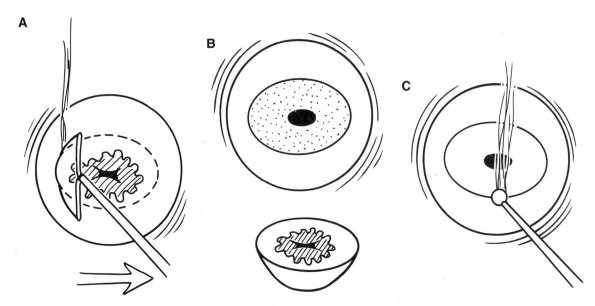

FIG. 92-4.

The standard LEEP procedure for cervical intraepithelial lesions that can be removed in a single pass is as follows: After painting the cervix with Lugol's solution and injecting lidocaine use an exocervical loop (2 cm wide and 0.8 cm deep) to resect the entire lesion (**A** and **B**). Then coagulate the crater base using a 5 mm ball electrode and apply Monsel's paste to the crater base (**C**).

location of cervical arterial supply (3 o'clock and 9 o'clock positions) and significant bleeding can occur if these vessels are cut (Fig. 92-4).

Larger lesions confined to the ectocervix. In some instances, CIN lesions may be too extensive to be removed in a single pass. In this event, remove the central portion of the lesion using a 2 cm wide loop electrode, as previously described. Excise the remaining CIN and transformation zone with additional passes using the same loop electrode, or ablate it using electro-fulguration and a ball electrode (Fig. 92-5).

CIN extending into the endocervical canal. These lesions are removed in a two-step cone biopsy procedure that uses a 2 cm wide exocervical electrode in conjunction with a 1 × 1 cm loop or rectangular endocervical electrode to produce a "cowboy hat" type of excision. For this procedure, two methods can be used. The first, and preferred, approach involves excising the endocervical portion of the lesion first using the 1.0 cm wide by 1.0 cm deep endocervical electrode. Once the endocervical portion of the lesion is excised, the exocervical portion is excised using a standard 2.0 cm by 0.8 cm loop electrode (Fig. 92-6, *A*). In the other approach, the ectocervical portion is excised first, then the endocervical portion is excised. The same-sized electrodes are used. In the outpatient setting, care should be taken not to excise the endocervical canal too deeply. Both approaches leave a "cowboy hat" shape excision on the cervix (Fig. 92-6, *B*). The endocervical and exocervical excisional specimens should be submitted for pathological assessment in separate containers.

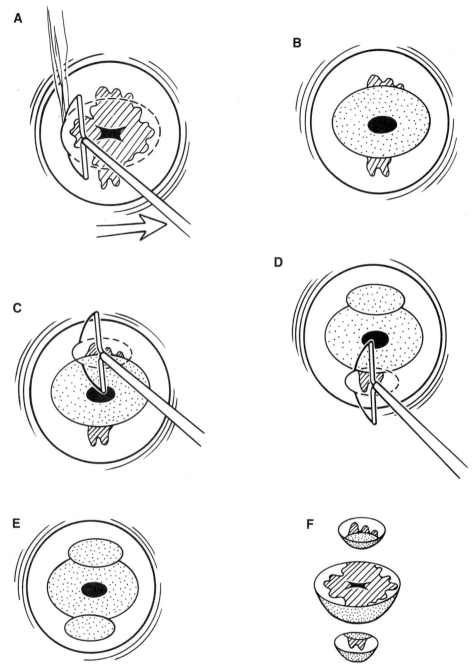

FIG. 92-5.
For lesions too large to be removed in a single pass, use a 2 cm by 0.8 cm leep electrode to resect the central portion of the lesion (**A** and **B**). Then, resect the remaining tissue with additional passes using the same electrode (**C, D,** and **E**). Tissue specimens (**F**) are placed in formalin.

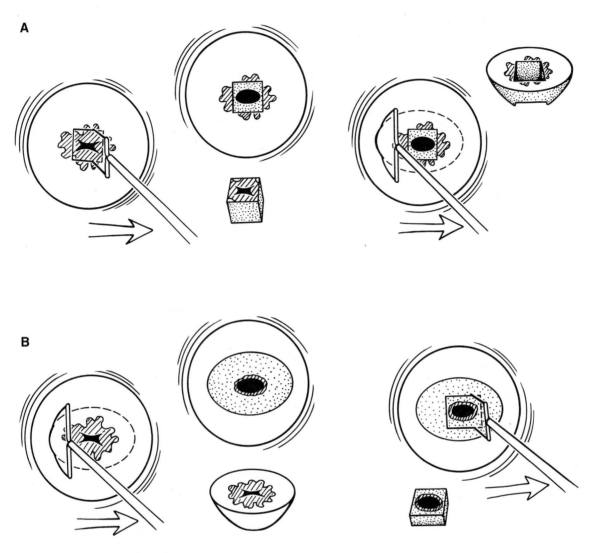

FIG. 92-6.
Two methods for obtaining an endocervical sample with the LEEP procedure: **A**, Resect the endocervical portion of the lesion using a 1 cm by 1 cm loop. Then, use a 2 cm by 0.8 cm loop to resect additional CIN extending on to the portio. **B**, In some cases, it may be necessary to excise the ectocervical portion first. Going more than 1.5 cm into the canal increases the chances of significant bleeding.

Stalling of electrode passage can occasionally occur. This is because the movement is too rapid or because the cutting power is too low or the reusable electrode is not shiny (carbon buildup). If stalling occurs, it is best to remove the electrode and approach from the opposite side. Some pathologists prefer that after the specimen is excised, it be removed from the cervix using forceps, opened along one side, and placed in a plastic holder to allow it to fix in the proper orientation. Some pathologists prefer the specimen be tagged at a certain location. Check with the particular pathologist to determine preferences.

Remember the average cervix is 3 to 4 cm long. Removing 1 to 1.5 cm generally has minimal adverse consequences. It is only after numerous cervical procedures that one begins to see significant long-term complications.

11. After the entire lesion is removed (all tissue that did not stain with iodine as well as the transformation zone should be removed), perform an endocervical curettage above the excisional base and fulgurate any bleeders at the base of the lesion using a ball electrode with the "coagulation" setting on the ESU. For 5 mm ball electrodes, power settings of 40 to 55 watts are usually required to obtain adequate arcing between the electrode and the tissue. (Excessive bleeding is more frequent in patients with severe cervicitis and in those less than 12 weeks' postpartum.) Frequently the entire base of the excision is lightly coagulated. Perform the coagulation up to the endocervical canal, but take care not to insert the electrode into the canal. Apply Monsel's solution.

COMPLICATIONS

- Significant intraoperative bleeding is an uncommon but potentially serious complication. It sometimes occurs when the electrode is inserted too deeply into the tissue at the 3 o'clock and 9 o'clock positions (where the cervical branches of the uterine artery are located) or when the patient has severe cervicitis.
- Postoperative bleeding is minor to moderate persistent bleeding 3 to 6 days post-LEEP. It can usually be managed by electrofulguration or by packing the crater base with Monsel's paste.
- Posttreatment cervical stenosis is an uncommon complication (less than 1%) and occurs predominately in postmenopausal women.
- Electric shock, which is caused by touching the speculum with the electrode during the procedure, is prevented by using a coated, nonconductive speculum.
- Inadvertent burns to the lateral vaginal wall or other sites can occur, but are rare.
- Stalling of the electrode can occasionally occur.
- Pain and discomfort are minimal and generally can be controlled with nonsteroidal antiinflammatory drugs.

- Infection is rare. Metronidazole or doxycyline can be used.
- Recurrence or persistence of disease occurs in 5% to 10% of cases.
- Cervical incompetence is unlikely, unless numerous procedures have been performed on the cervix.
- Infertility is not generally a concern unless stenosis occurs or the majority of the endocervical canal has been removed, reducing the number of mucus-producing glands.

POSTPROCEDURE PATIENT EDUCATION

- Instruct the patient to avoid vaginal intercourse, douching, use of tampons, and heavy exercise (especially weight lifting) for 3 weeks.
- If bleeding persists more than 2 weeks, if the volume is comparable to that of a normal period or greater, or if the vaginal discharge becomes foul smelling, the patient should call the physician or return to the clinic.

FOLLOW-UP CARE

First Protocol

- Reevaluate the patient at 3 to 4 months with colposcopy, cytology, endocervical curettage (if indicated), and colposcopically directed biopsy of any abnormal-appearing areas.
- If no disease is revealed at the 3- to 4-month visit, repeat the Pap smear at 6 months and at 12 months after the LEEP.
- If persistent disease is revealed at the 6-month visit, reevaluate and treat again.

Second Protocol

- Patients are seen 4 to 6 weeks postoperatively for a review of the pathology report and for a brief postoperative check. This helps reassure the patients and decreases their anxiety about how well they have healed. The clinician can also check for cervical stenosis. The remainder of checks are as above.

CPT/BILLING CODES

57460	Colposcopy with loop electrosurgical excision(s) of the cervix (LEEP)
57500	Cervical biopsy
57520	Cervical conization, with or without fulgeration
57505	Endocervical curettage
99070	Supplies and materials for kits and electrodes

BIBLIOGRAPHY

Apgar B, Wright T, Pfenninger J: Loop electrosurgical excision procedure for CIN, *Am Fam Physician* 46:505, 1992.

Bigrigg MA et al: Colposcopic diagnosis and treatment of cervical dysplasia at a single clinic visit: experience of low-voltage diathermy loop in 1000 patients, *Lancet* 336:229, 1990.

Bigrigg MA et al: Efficacy and safety of large-loop excision of the transformation zone, *Lancet,* 343:32, 1994.

Ferenczy A: Management of the patient with an abnormal Papanicolaou test: recent developments. In Wright VC, editor: *Obstetrics and gynecology clinics of North America: contemporary colposcopy,* Philadelphia, 1993, W. B. Saunders.

Luesley DM et al: Loop diathermy excision of the cervical transformation zone in patients with abnormal cervical smears, *Br Med J* 300:1690, 1990.

Mor-Yosef S et al: Loop diathermy cone biopsy, *Obstet Gynecol* 75:884, 1990.

Prendiville W, Cullimore NS: Large loop excision of the transformation zone (LLETZ): a new method of management for women with cervical intraepithelial neoplasia, *Br J Obstet Gynecol* 96:1054, 1989.

Saidi MH et al: Diagnostic and therapeutic conization using loop radiothermal cautery, *J Rep Med* 38(10):775, 1993.

Wright TC et al: Excising CIN lesions by loop electrosurgical procedure, *Contemp Obstet Gynecol:* March 1991.

Wright TC et al: Treatment of cervical intraepithelial neoplasia using the loop electrosurgical excision procedure (LEEP), *Obstet Gynecol,* 79:173, 1992.

Wright TC, Richart RM, Ferenczy A: *Electrosurgical treatment of HPV related diseases of the anogenital tract,* New York, 1992, Arthur Vision.

CHAPTER 93

Barrier Contraceptives: Cervical Cap, Condom, and Contraceptive Sponge

Barry D. Weiss

CERVICAL CAP

The cervical cap is a barrier contraceptive method with efficacy similar to that of the diaphragm. If it is used properly, pregnancy will occur in approximately only 6.5% of cervical cap users at the end of one year. The pregnancy rate rises to about 12% after two years. Because some women do not use the device regularly or properly, the overall pregnancy rate among cervical cap users is about 18% at two years.

Early studies suggested that cervical cap use was associated with development of cervical dysplasia. While subsequent studies have not found cervical dysplasia to be increased, careful monitoring of cervical cytology in cervical cap users is appropriate.

Indications

- Prevention of pregnancy

Contraindications

- Inability of patient to be properly fitted
- Inability of patient to understand instructions for use
- Inability of patient to insert and remove device correctly
- History of toxic shock syndrome
- Known or suspected uterine or cervical malignancy, including unresolved abnormal Pap smear test result
- Congenital or other anatomic abnormalities of the cervix (e.g., polyps) that would preclude proper fitting
- Current vaginal or cervical infection
- Use during menses
- Use during postpartum or postabortal period

Advantages

- Can be used when medical indications or patient intolerance preclude use of birth control pills
- Is often tolerated better in diaphragm users who have recurrent urinary tract infection
- May be worn longer than a diaphragm and requires less spermicide
- Is not affected by weight gain or weight loss

Equipment

A cervical cap fitting set that includes one of each of the four sizes of cervical caps is needed. The four sizes are based on the internal diameter of the rim: 22 mm, 25 mm, 28 mm, 31 mm (Fig. 93-1). Fitting sets are available from the manufacturer (Cervical Cap Ltd., 430 Monterey Ave, Suite 1-B, Los Gatos, CA 95030; telephone: 408-395-2100). The manufacturer also provides an excellent information packet, monograph, and videotape to instruct the clinician on use and fitting of the cervical cap.

After fitting is completed, the cervical cap is dispensed directly by the physician to the patient.

Technique

Before fitting the cervical cap, perform a Pap smear and pelvic examination to exclude cervical or vaginal infection. (Cultures should be obtained, if indicated.) A patient should not be fitted for a cervical cap before 6 weeks' postpartum.

1. Lubricate the cap rim, compress the sides together, and insert it into the vagina. The cavity of the cap should fit over the cervix (Fig. 93-2).

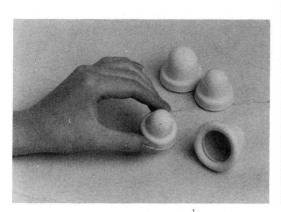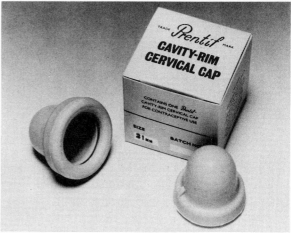

FIG. 93-1.
Prentif cavity-rim cervical cap. (Courtesy Cervical Cap Ltd., Los Gatos, Calif.)

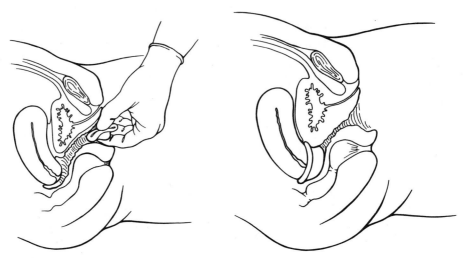

FIG. 93-2.
Properly fitted cervical cap.

2. Try each size of cervical cap until the correct one is identified. The correct size is the smallest that fits satisfactorily. Eighty to ninety percent of women will be fitted with a 22 mm or 25 mm cap.
   a. Ideally the cap should cover the entire cervix.
   b. The cap should adhere firmly to the cervix by its own self-generated suction.
   c. The dome of the cap should be closely applied to the cervix. If there is good suction, squeezing the tip of the rubber cap between the fingers will cause a dent that is maintained for 30 seconds.
   d. The rim of the cap should tuck evenly into the cervicovaginal fornix.
   e. No gaps should exist between the rim of the cap and the cervix itself.
   f. No parts of the cervix should be exposed or palpable below the rim of the cap.
   g. The cap should not be easily dislodged. Light tugging on the dome should not affect it (Fig. 93-3).
3. The correct technique for removing the cap involves pushing the rim away from the cervix to break the suction, then pulling the cap out of the vagina. Do not pull on the dome of the cap. If the cap fits too tightly, it will be difficult to remove.
4. After the correct size has been determined and the techniques have been demonstrated, the patient should satisfactorily perform insertion and removal.
5. Up to 20% of women cannot be fitted properly with the four currently available sizes and should not receive a cervical cap.
6. The manufacturer recommends cleaning fitting caps by soaking them in 70% alcohol for 20 minutes, followed by air drying.

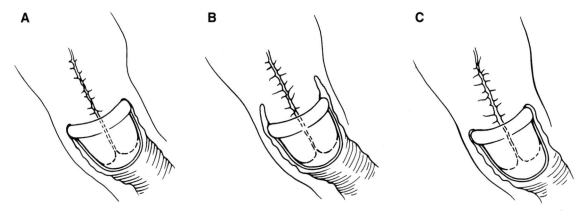

FIG. 93-3.
Properly and improperly fitted cervical caps. **A,** The properly fitted cap is closely applied to the cervix, and the rim of the cap fills the cervicovaginal fornix. **B,** The cap is too small. Although the dome of the cap is closely applied to the cervix, the rim does not reach into the fornix, leaving the base of the cervix exposed. **C,** The cap is too large. Although the dome covers the cervix and the rim extends into the fornix, the cap is not closely applied to the cervix and may be easily dislodged.

Complications

- Dislodgement during intercourse can lead to contraception failure. Dislodgement is the most frequent reason that women discontinue using the cervical cap.
- Vaginal odor or discharge occurs in 5% to 27% of cervical cap users.
- Lacerations and abrasions of the vagina and cervix can occur if the cap is left in place too long.
- The cervical cap causes vaginal discomfort in less than 3% of users.
- Toxic shock syndrome is a theoretical (but unreported) complication.

Patient Education

- Before use, fill the inner side of the dome one-third full with spermicidal jelly. Do not apply jelly to the inner surface of the rim.
- The cap may be inserted any time from immediately before intercourse to 40 hours before intercourse. It is most easily inserted in a squatting or semi-reclining position.
- Allow the cap to remain in place for at least 8 hours after intercourse.
- Do not leave the cap in place longer than 48 hours at a time.
- If intercourse occurs more than once while the cap is in place, no additional spermicide is needed. However, check for correct positioning of the cap.
- Use an additional contraceptive method for the first three times the cap is used, in the event that the cap becomes dislodged during intercourse. If dislodgement occurs, discontinue cap use.
- Do not use the cap during menses.

- Refitting is necessary following abortion or childbirth.
- Do not use in the presence of vaginal infection, discharge, pain, or odor. If these occur, seek medical evaluation.
- If lubrication is needed for intercourse, use only water-based lubricants.
- Generally, the cap should be washed carefully with soap and water. If an odor develops, it can be soaked in vinegar or a cup of water with a teaspoon of lemon juice. Alternatively, clean the cap with a 25% bleach solution for 20 minutes.
- The cap should be replaced yearly. Replace sooner if thin spots or tears occur.

Postprocedure Care

- The FDA-approved labeling states that a Pap smear should be performed after 3 months of cervical cap use. If the test is abnormal, cap use must be discontinued and cytologic abnormality should be evaluated and treated.
- If the 3-month Pap smear is normal, obtain another Pap smear after 12 months of cap use and then yearly thereafter.
- The FDA recommends refitting annually. Have the patient wear the cap into the office so that proper application and fit can be assessed.

CPT/Billing Code

57170   Diaphragm or cervical cap fitting with instructions

CONDOMS

The condom is a male contraceptive device that covers the penis and acts as a barrier to sperm. When used in combination with a spermicide, pregnancy rates range from 2 to 10 pregnancies per user per year. The condom also serves as a barrier to sexually transmissible infectious organisms. The 1991 article in *American Family Physician* by Vinson is an excellent review of use, and *Consumer Reports* has evaluated more than 40 different condoms. The clinician should discuss appropriate use with patients, because condoms are frequently used incorrectly and patients are often reticent about asking questions.

Indications

- For prevention of pregnancy
- For prevention of the spread of sexually transmitted disease

Contraindications

- Allergy or hypersensitivity to latex rubber or spermicides

Complications

- Condom rupture during intercourse can lead to contraception failure. If rupture occurs, intravaginal spermicidal contraceptive jelly or foam should be used immediately.
- Local or systemic hypersensitivity due to latex rubber allergy can occur.

Patient Education

- Only use latex condoms for prevention of disease transmission. Membrane or "natural" condoms do not protect against transmission of hepatitis B or human immunodeficiency virus (HIV).
- Condoms impregnated with spermicide may provide additional protection against sexually transmitted disease. Simultaneous use of spermicidal jellies or foams that contain nonoxynol-9 provide even more protection.
- A condom should be applied to the penis before any genital contact occurs by unrolling it on to the erect penis. Space must be left at the tip of the condom for collection of ejaculate.
- After intercourse, the base of the condom should be held onto the erect penis while the penis is withdrawn. This will prevent the condom from slipping off. Condoms should not be reused.
- Lubrication, if necessary, should be accomplished only with water-soluble lubricants or spermicidal jellies. Oil-based lubricants will damage the latex, predisposing it to rupture.
- Store condoms in a cool, dry place out of the sun, and do not use condoms that appear discolored or stiff.
- Handle condoms carefully to prevent punctures.
- Package inserts generally provide instructions to the patient. After the patient has reviewed the instructions, answer any questions.

VAGINAL CONTRACEPTIVE SPONGE

The sponge is soft polyurethane foam that acts secondarily as a barrier contraceptive and chiefly as a spermicide delivery system (it contains nonoxynol-9) (Fig. 93-4). The sponge provides contraceptive protection for 24 hours. Approximately 10% of sponge users will become pregnant after one year of use. The sponge is available without a prescription.

Indications

- For the prevention of pregnancy

Contraindications

- Hypersensitivity to nonoxynol-9 or polyurethane
- History of toxic shock syndrome

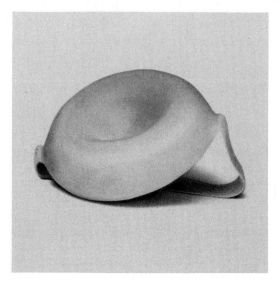

FIG. 93-4.
Vaginal contraceptive sponge. (Courtesy of Whitehall Laboratories, New York.)

- Cannot be used during menstruation
- Should not be used any sooner than 6 weeks' postpartum or immediately after vaginal trauma

Technique

1. After removing the sponge from its package, activate the spermicide by wetting it with clean tap water and squeezing it gently until it is sudsy.
2. Fold the sponge and insert it deeply into the vagina with the string loop dangling toward the outside of the vagina.

Complications

Other than the rare concern about toxic shock syndrome (the same concern exists with cervical caps, diaphragms, and tampons), there are no significant complications from sponge contraceptives. Some patients may be allergic to either the polyurethane or nonoxynol-9.

Patient Education

- Contraceptive protection begins immediately and lasts for 24 to 30 hours.
- Always wait 6 hours after intercourse before removing the sponge.
- If intercourse occurs multiple times, it is not necessary to add additional spermicide. The original sponge can be left in place.

- The maximum recommended time for the sponge to be left in place is 30 hours. However, if intercourse occurs after the sponge has been in place for 24 hours, it must be left in for an additional 6 hours to maintain contraceptive effectiveness.
- For new sponge users, an additional contraceptive method should be used until the user is comfortable with the use of the sponge.

BIBLIOGRAPHY

Can you rely on condoms? *Consumer Reports* 54(3):135, 1989.

Procedures for your practice: fitting a cervical cap, *Patient Care* 25:140, July 1991.

Richwald GA et al: Effectiveness of the cavity-rim cervical cap: results of a large clinical study, *Obstet Gynecol* 74:143, 1989.

Vinson RP, Epperly TD: Counseling patients on proper use of condoms, *Am Fam Physician* 43:2081, 1991.

Weiss BD, Bassford T, Davis T: The cervical cap, *Am Fam Physician* 43:517, 1991.

CHAPTER 94

Diaphragm Fitting

Barbara S. Apgar

The diaphragm is a barrier contraceptive device that mechanically blocks sperm from entering the cervical opening (Fig. 94-1). The diaphragm acts with spermicidal jelly to produce a theoretical contraceptive effectiveness rate of 98%, but has an actual rate of 80% to 93% for new users and 97% for long-term users. In one study, only 45% of users were satisfied with use of the diaphragm for contraception (compared to 57% of birth control pill users).

INDICATIONS

- Desire for reversible contraception without hormonal influences
- Intolerance to normal contraceptives
- Contraception in a nonmutually monogamous relationship
- Desire for sexually transmitted disease (STD) protection even though using another contraceptive method

CONTRAINDICATIONS

- Vaginal stenosis or pelvic abnormalities
- Allergy to spermicidal jelly
- Recurrent urinary tract infections associated with diaphragm use
- Allergy to rubber
- Aversion to touching the genital area
- Fitting sooner than 6 weeks' postpartum or before the uterus has involuted
- Uterine prolapse
- Large cystocele or rectocele

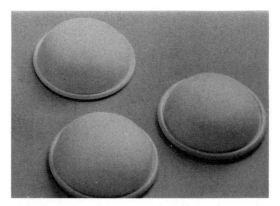

FIG. 94-1.
Vaginal diaphragm. (Courtesy of Ortho Pharmaceutical Company.)

EQUIPMENT

- Diaphragms (sizes 65 to 90) in three types:

  Arching spring: molded one-piece spring and dome with firm rim, which forms an arc when compressed; needs no introducer; recommended for women with decreased pelvic support, cystocele or rectocele, retroverted uterus, or for those who find a firmer rim easier to insert. This is the most popular type in the United States.

  Coil spring: molded one-piece spring and dome with a soft flexible rim; may be used with an introducer; recommended for women with good vaginal support, with no cystocele, rectocele or pelvic floor relaxation, and with a cervix in midplane or anterior position.

  Flat spring: molded one-piece spring and dome with a soft rim and flat plane flexibility; may be used with an introducer; recommended for smaller women with a narrow or shallow pelvic shelf; excellent for nulliparous patients.

- Spermicidal jelly (nonoxynol-9 recommended)
- Set of fitting rings or diaphragms which can be obtained from Ortho Pharmaceutical Company, usually at no cost to practitioners (Rings are measured in millimeters and ordered by size in 5 mm increments.)
- *Optional:* diaphragm introducer

PREPROCEDURE PATIENT EDUCATION

Explain the fitting procedure and diaphragm use to the patient: how the diaphragm will be inserted and fitted, and how the patient will insert the diaphragm herself (Box 94-1). The manufacturer will supply educational handouts for patients at no charge. The patient must understand how to use the diaphragm properly. She must also understand the potential failure rate.

Explain that the fitting rings are cleaned by soaking them in a disinfectant.

BOX 94-1. HOW TO INSERT A DIAPHRAGM

The diaphragm is an effective birth control method when used correctly. The following provides guidelines for its proper insertion.

- The diaphragm can be inserted up to 2 hours before intercourse. If it is in place for longer than 2 hours, you must reapply contraceptive jelly or cream, taking care not to move it.
- Place about 1 tablespoon of contraceptive jelly or cream on the dome of the diaphragm. Spread the jelly or cream around the inside of the dome. You may wish to spread a thin layer on the rim of the diaphragm to help with its insertion.
- Find a comfortable position, such as squatting, standing with one leg raised, or lying down. With one hand, spread the outer lips of the outer part of the *vagina,* or birth canal.
- With your other hand, fold the diaphragm, dome side down, with your thumb and finger and insert it into the vagina: Push the diaphragm as far back into the vagina as possible (see illustration).
- You can check to make sure the diaphragm is placed properly by inserting one finger into your vagina and feeling for the cervix, the narrow lower end of the uterus, which feels similar to the tip of a nose. If the diaphragm covers the cervix and the outer edge is behind the pubic bone, it is in the correct position. *Neither you nor your partner should notice the diaphragm during intercourse.*
- Following intercourse, leave the diaphragm in place for at least 6 hours. Do *not* douche during this time. If you have intercourse more than one time you must reapply contraceptive jelly or cream. Use the plastic applicator to reapply the cream. If you find that this is too messy, you may want to ask your partner to use a condom. Do *not* remove the diaphragm, however.
- Remove the diaphragm 6 hours or longer after intercourse. Do *not* leave it in place for more than 24 hours.
- To remove the diaphragm, insert your finger into your vagina and slide it under the rim of the diaphragm. Pull the diaphragm down and out.
- Wash the diaphragm with mild soap and warm water. Be sure to rinse it well. Pat it dry, especially around the edges where water might remain. You may dust it lightly with cornstarch. Do not use other powders or creams. Place the diaphragm in its container: Sunlight and air can weaken the rubber latex.
- Check your diaphragm each time before you use it for tears or holes, by filling it with water or holding it up to a light and gently stretching it. Never use a diaphragm with tears or holes.
- At each annual checkup, have your doctor check your diaphragm and its fit. You might need a diaphragm of a different size, especially if you have lost or gained 10 pounds, been pregnant, recently had a baby, or had pelvic surgery.
- Be sure to call your doctor if you experience any of the following: signs of allergy to the rubber latex or the contraceptive cream or jelly (itching or discomfort); signs of bladder infection (difficulty urinating when the diaphragm is in place, frequent need to urinate, or burning during urination).
- Be sure to ask your doctor or his or her nurse for help if you have trouble inserting or removing the diaphragm.

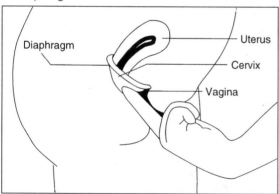

The diaphragm is in the correct position when it covers the cervix, which feels similar to the tip of a nose.

From *Fam Pract Recert* 14(1):65, 1992. Used with permission.

TECHNIQUE

1. Place the patient in the lithotomy (pelvic) position.
2. Measure for the correct size of diaphragm: Hold your index and middle fingers together and straight and insert into the vagina. With the middle finger touching the posterior fornix, raise your hand to bring the surface of the index finger in contact with the pubic arch. Use the thumb to mark the point directly under the pubic bone and withdraw your fingers from the vagina holding the thumb in position (Fig. 94-2,A).
3. To determine the diaphragm size, place one end of the diaphragm rim on the tip of the middle finger with the opposite side of the rim lying just in front of the thumb tip; this is the approximate diameter of the diaphragm needed (common sizes are 75 to 80 mm; Fig. 94-2,B).
4. A lubricant on the fitting rings or diaphragms will aid insertion and make the procedure more comfortable for the patient. Prepare to insert a fitting diaphragm or a ring of the approximate size into the vagina by folding the diaphragm in half: Press the middle of the opposite sides together between the thumb and fingers of one hand (Fig. 94-3). Hold the vulva open with the other hand. Gently slide the folded diaphragm into the vagina and aim toward the posterior fornix (Fig. 94-4). The cervix should be palpable through the dome of the diaphragm (Fig. 94-5,A) and the proximal rim should fit behind the pubic arch without undue pressure (Fig. 94-5,B).
5. When correct fit is completed, remove the diaphragm from the vagina by inserting the index finger into the vagina under the symphysis pubis and hooking it under the proximal rim. Gently pull the diaphragm down and out (Fig. 94-6).

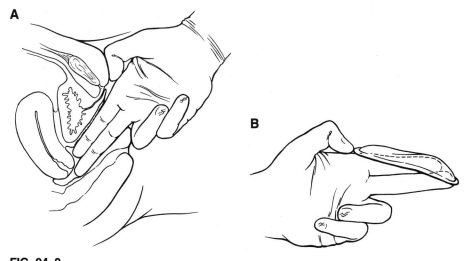

FIG. 94-2.
Clinical examination to measure for appropriate diaphragm size. See text for details. (From Attico NB: *Fam Pract Recert* 14:65, 1992. Used with permission.)

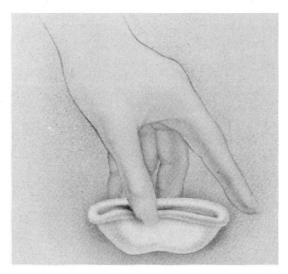

FIG. 94-3.
Fold the diaphragm for insertion. (Courtesy of Ortho Pharmaceutical Company.)

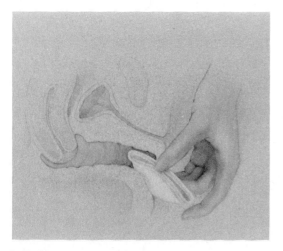

FIG. 94-4.
Inserting the diaphragm. (Courtesy of Ortho Pharmaceutical Company.)

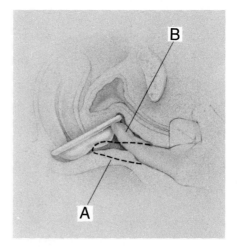

FIG. 94-5.
Proper positioning of the diaphragm. **A,** Cervix is palpable behind the diaphragm. **B,** Rim fits snuggly but without discomfort behind the symphysis pubis.

A

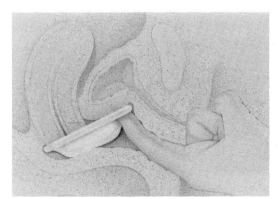

B

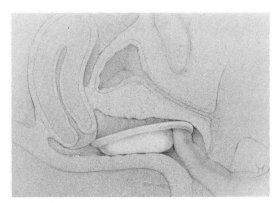

FIG. 94-6.
Removal of the diaphragm. **A,** Hook finger under rim; **B,** Pull diaphragm out through the introitus. (Courtesy of Ortho Pharmaceutical Company.)

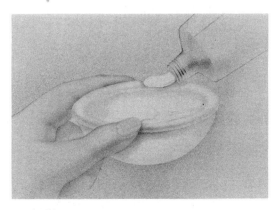

FIG. 94-7.
Proper application of spermicidal jelly to diaphragm and dome. (Courtesy of Ortho Pharmaceutical Company.)

POSTPROCEDURE PATIENT EDUCATION

- Have the patient practice inserting and removing the diaphragm at the clinic. Instruct her on how to apply spermicidal jelly to the rim and the dome (Fig. 94-7). Nonoxynol-9, the spermicidal jelly that is recommended, supplies both contraceptive and STD protection. It should be applied to the concave surface and the rim of the diaphragm so that the uterus is sealed off mechanically and chemically. Place approximately 1 teaspoon of jelly in the dome and apply a thin layer around the rim.
- Instruct the patient to make sure that the diaphragm is firmly in place behind the pubic bone and the distal rim is behind the cervix. She should feel for the cervix behind the dome of the diaphragm.

- Instruct the patient not to douche or remove the diaphragm for 6 hours after intercourse, and to leave the diaphragm in place and insert additional spermicidal jelly into the vagina should additional coitus occur.
- Have the patient walk around the examination room with the diaphragm in place to ensure a comfortable fit.

COMPLICATIONS

- If a diaphragm is too small, it may not completely cover the cervix; if a diaphragm is too large, it may be uncomfortable and not provide a tight seal.
- Toxic shock syndrome has been reported in women who have worn diaphragms continuously for more than 24 hours.
- The pregnancy rate is increased if spermicide is not used with the diaphragm.
- A change in weight (gain or loss of 15 pounds), pregnancy, or pelvic surgery may alter the fit of the diaphragm.
- Pressure ulcerations can occur. These are caused by excessive pressure of the diaphragm against the lateral vaginal walls because of improper fit.
- Increased rates of urinary tract infections have been reported in longstanding diaphragm users, but barrier methods may also decrease the risk of cervical dysplasia.
- Pregnancy may occur.
- A teratogenic effect of nonoxynol-9 is possible.

CPT/BILLING CODE

57170   Diaphragm fitting

BIBLIOGRAPHY

Craig S, Hepburn S: The effectiveness of barrier methods of contraception with and without spermicide, *Contraception* 26:347, 1982.

Fihn SD et al: Association between diaphragm use and urinary tract infection, *JAMA* 254(2):240, 1985.

Gillespie L: The diaphragm: an accomplice in recurrent urinary tract infections, *Urology* 24(1):25, 1984.

Heaton CJ, Smith MA: The diaphragm, *Am Fam Physician* 39(5):231, 1989.

Jackson M, Berger GS, Keith LG: *Vaginal contraception,* Boston, 1981, G.K. Hall.

Jaffe R: Toxic shock syndrome associated with diaphragm use, *N Engl J Med* 305:1585, 1981.

Rosenfelt JA et al: Women's satisfaction with birth control, *JFP* 36(2):169, 1993.

Vessey M, Lawless M, Yeates D: Efficacy of different contraceptive methods, *Lancet* 1:841, 1982.

Widaholm MV: Vaginal lesion: etiology—a malfitting diaphragm? *J Nurse Midwife* 24:39, 1979.

CHAPTER 95

Cervicography

Richard C. Cherkis

The Cervicography system is a universally unified, organized, quality-controlled procedure for the detection of cervical cancer and precancerous conditions. It combines colposcopy with a noninvasive photographic technique that permits quality-controlled expert evaluation of normal and abnormal cervical findings, and provides permanent and objective documentation of these findings. The concept of Cervicography is similar to the concept of cytology.

The Cervicography system lends itself to use in any women's cancer-screening setting, including the private office, the hospital, the family planning clinic, and the mass screening drive. It can be used in conjunction with the Pap smear; it is significantly more sensitive than the Pap smear; it has a high negative predictive value; and, when combined with the Pap smear, it is the best method of screening for cervical cancer available.

A Cerviscope cervical camera (Fig. 95-1) is used to take photographs of the cervix. The Cerviscope standardizes color, depth of field, lighting, and focal length; thus, it results in images that enable uniformity in evaluation. The Cerviscope is handheld and is focused on the cervix by moving it back and forth (Fig. 95-2). When the cervix is in focus, a picture is taken. The film is sent to National Testing Laboratories, where it is developed into photographic slides (Cervigrams). These are projected onto a screen that is at least 6 feet wide, allowing the evaluator to view an image of the cervix with a magnification and resolution comparable to that of colposcopy (Fig. 95-3). Only certified evaluators are used to interpret the films. Certified evaluators are gynecologists specializing in colposcopy who have passed very stringent written and oral examinations given by the Medical College of Wisconsin and National Testing Laboratories.

Cervicography findings are divided into four categories: negative, atypical, positive, and technically defective (Fig. 95-4). A print of the Cervigram with the expert evaluation is returned to the clinician and can be entered into the patient's record. It also provides an excellent medium for patient education.

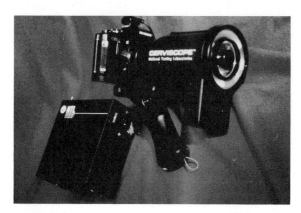

FIG. 95-1.
Cerviscope.

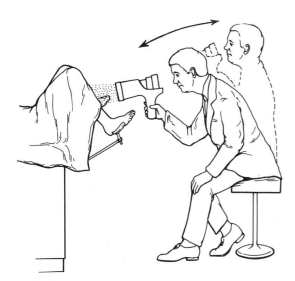

FIG. 95-2.
Focusing the Cerviscope.

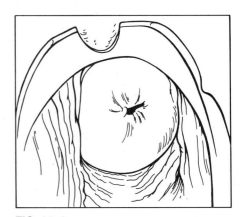

FIG. 95-3.
Cervigram is obtained by focusing through the vaginal speculum.

The Cerviscope, the evaluation method, and the terminology used in the evaluation process are standardized worldwide by National Testing Laboratories. Quality control is strictly maintained in every aspect of the Cervicography system.

RATIONALE FOR CERVICOGRAPHY SCREENING

- The Pap smear has a significant false-negative rate.
- The specificity of the Pap smear is unclear.

☐ NEGATIVE—Routine Cervigram slide and Pap smear recommended.
   1. ____ Squamocolumnar junction and transformation zone are fully visible.
   2. ____ Squamocolumnar junction not fully visible. Components of the transformation zone are visible.
   3. ____ Squamocolumnar junction and transformation zone are not visible.
☐ ATYPIAL—Cervigram slide recommended in ____6 months ____12 months.
   1. ____ Acetowhite lesion outside transformation zone is visible.
   2. ____ Atypical immature squamous metaplasia is visible.
   3. ____ Acetowhite lesion inside transformation zone is visible but of doubtful significance.
☐ POSITIVE—Colposcopy recommended.
   Compatible with: Lesion morphology:
   1. ____Minor grade lesion   ____Acetowhite epithelium
   2. ____Major grade lesion   ____Punctation
   3. ____Cancer ____Exclude cancer   ____Mosaic
                                            ____Atypical vessels
☐ TECHNICALLY DEFECTIVE—Retake Cervigram slide!
   1. ____ View of cervix obscured by:
             ____mucus ____blood ____hair ____vaginal wall ____speculum
             ____acetic acid pool ____position of cervix
   2. ____ Insufficient acetic acid *or* Cervigram slides taken too late after second application of acetic acid
   3. ____ Out of focus   ____ Overexposed   ____ Underexposed

FIG. 95-4.
Cervigram report.

- Colposcopic screening is not always practical because of the time, equipment, and expertise necessary.
- Cervicography identifies high- and low-risk patients for development of cervical neoplasia.
- Cervicography adds an important quality-control dimension to screening.
- A print of the Cervigram is invaluable in minimizing patients' health concerns and sexual apprehensions when an abnormality exists.

INDICATIONS

- Routine screening in conjunction with the Pap smear
- Documentation of ectocervical findings
- Documentation of cervical findings before ablative procedures
- Evaluation of the patient with atypical Pap smears when CIN or cancer is not suspected
- Evaluation of low-grade abnormalities
- Evaluation of the patient with suspicious or positive Pap smears where colposcopy is not available

EQUIPMENT

- Cerviscope, power supply, and patient log sheet
- Speculum
- 5% acetic acid
- Large cotton swabs

TECHNIQUE

1. Insert the speculum for adequate visualization of cervix. Obtain a Pap smear if necessary.
2. Apply the 5% acetic acid. This step requires 15 seconds of swabbing or dabbing.
3. View the cervix with a Cerviscope camera (Fig. 95-2). Do *not* take a Cervigram now. (There would be a 50% false-negative rate.) In this step, look for obstructions of the view: mucus, blood, prolapse of vaginal walls, retroverted or anteverted cervix, and pubic hair across the opening of the speculum. This step is critical because it also allows time for the first application of acetic acid to take effect.
4. Apply a second application of 5% acetic acid. This step requires 15 seconds of swabbing or dabbing.
5. View the cervix with the Cerviscope and eliminate any obstructions as described in Step 3. In addition, also look for acetic acid pooling that obstructs the view of the posterior lip of the cervix. If present, remove any excess with a swab.
6. Take two pictures of the cervix (Cervigrams) now. This should be done within 30 seconds of the second application of acetic acid. If one or both of the Cervigrams are not taken within the 30 seconds, reapply the acetic acid before taking another Cervigram(s).
7. Record the required patient information on the patient log sheet.

SUPPLIER

The clinician who decides to use Cervicography can obtain videotapes and appropriate information from National Testing Laboratories (400 Biltmore Drive, Suite 407, Fenton, MO 63026; fax 314-343-3763 or call 1-800-842-7135). National Testing Laboratories will schedule a full day in-service to explain the various aspects of the system, to train the appropriate office personnel, and to ascertain that the individuals taking the Cervigrams are doing the procedure properly. National Testing Laboratories furnishes the film (as well as the film developing and processing), evaluations, appropriate forms, mailers, and patient educational pamphlets.

COST

National Testing Laboratories' fee to the health care provider for Cervicography screening ($25.00) is comparable to the cost of a Pap smear. The patient cost from the health care provider is approximately $40 to $50. Cervicography costs may be covered by insurance. The cost of a Cerviscope and related equipment is under $3,000.

CPT/BILLING CODE

58999   Miscellaneous gynecologic procedure, "Cervicography" system

BIBLIOGRAPHY

August N: Cervicography for evaluating the "atypical" Papanicolaou smear, *J Reprod Med* 36:89, 1991.

Campion MJ, Reid R: Screening for gynecological cancer, *Obstet Gynecol Clin North Am* 17:695, 1990.

Greenberg MD, Campion MJ, Rutlege LH: Cervicography as an adjunct to cytologic screening. In Wright VC, editor: *Obstetrics and gynecology clinics in North America, volume 20*, Philadelphia, 1993, W.B. Saunders.

Stafl A: Cervicography: a new method for cervical cancer detection, *Am J Obstet Gynecol* 139:815, 1981.

Stafl A: Cervicography in cervical cancer detection, *Postgraduate Obstet Gynecol* 10(3):1, 1990.

Tawa K et al: A comparison of the Papanicolaou smear and cervigram: sensitivity, specificity, and cost analysis, *Obstet Gynecol* 71:229, 1988.

PART SEVEN

Obstetrics

CHAPTER 96

Amniocentesis

Clark B. Smith

Amniocentesis has achieved widespread use in the effort to evaluate the relatively inaccessible patient *in utero*. The primary indication for amniocentesis before 1970 was in the management of Rh factor hemolytic disease. Since then the indications have expanded to include evaluation of fetal lung maturity, genetics, and many others. In some centers, amniocentesis is almost a routine procedure; therefore, it is important to remember the potentially serious, sometimes lethal complications.

INDICATIONS

Prenatal Diagnosis (Second Trimester)

1. Chromosomal studies. Amniotic fluid contains fetal and amniotic cells. The fetal cells include desquamated squamous cells—cells from the gastrointestinal tract, respiratory tract, and urinary system. Although it requires 2 to 3 weeks for results, culture of these cells allows accurate fetal chromosome analysis for chromosomal, sex-linked, and metabolic disorders. Indications include:

    a. Advanced maternal age (≥ 34 years old).

      Note: Some experts are recommending that older mothers be referred to tertiary medical centers for second-trimester amniocenteses and genetic studies. Less fluid is available at this stage, and with proper training there may be less risk of complications if the procedure is performed *through* the placenta. A cell culture is also very fragile, and proper transport, along with assurance against loss or mix-up, is essential. It may be best to perform the study at the institution where the cells will be cultured.

    b. Parent who is a carrier of genetic disease that can be diagnosed by amniotic fluid cell culture.
    c. Mother who is a carrier of X-linked disorder.
    d. History of previous child with chromosomal disorder, neural tube defect, inherited biochemical disorder, or multiple anomalies.
    e. Mother with history of three or more spontaneous abortions.

2. The level of α-fetoprotein in the amniotic fluid, when coupled with careful sonographic fetal evaluation, is helpful in the diagnosis (or exclusion of the diagnosis) of open neural tube defects.
3. Evaluation of amnionitis. In a patient with ruptured membranes and clinical signs of amnionitis, Gram stain and culture of amniotic fluid may be performed before initiation of treatment (antibiotics and prompt delivery of the infant).

Fetal Health (Late Second or Third Trimester)

1. Bilirubin content of the amniotic fluid as measured spectrophotometrically as a $\Delta OD450$ remains the standard for following the Rh-isoimmunized pregnancy, since it shows an excellent inverse correlation with levels of fetal hemoglobin.
2. If the color of the fluid indicates meconium passage by the fetus, this may be an indicator of some degree of fetal distress. Clear fluid, while reassuring, does not completely exclude fetal distress.
3. Amniography may be useful in assessing the fetal gastrointestinal tract, particularly when an anomaly (such as tracheoesophageal fistula or duodenal atresia) is suspected, and may be an indirect indicator of fetal status.

Fetal Maturity (Third Trimester)

The major concern is for fetal lung maturity, and the most commonly used studies are directed toward that determination.

1. Lecithin (L), sphingomyelin (S), and phosphatidylglycerol (PG) are phospholipids in the newborn lung that act as surfactants and lower surface tension in the alveoli. The L/S ratio, the presence of phosphatidylglycerol, and the amniotic fluid creatinine level (which is related to muscle mass of the fetus) together give a physiologic maturation index of the fetus.
2. Phosphatidylglycerol by itself can be used as an indicator of fetal lung maturity. It is not affected by blood or meconium in the amniotic fluid.
3. The "shake test" is a rapid test in which varying dilutions of amniotic fluid are shaken with ethanol. The end point is the stability of bubbles on the surface of the amniotic fluid dilutions. There is a moderately good (not excellent) correlation with the absence of respiratory distress syndrome in the newborn. (Mix 1 ml of amniotic fluid with 1 ml of 95% ethanol. Compare this vial with a second vial of 1 ml of amniotic fluid mixed with 0.5 ml of 95% ethanol and 0.5 ml of normal saline. After 30 seconds of vigorous shaking, a ring of bubbles in the second vial indicates an L/S ratio of 2 or greater. Bubbles in the 1:1 mixture—but not in the second vial—indicate that the fetus is in a bordering stage of development and the pregnancy should be allowed to continue if possible.)

Therapeutic

1. Relief of hydramnios (temporary, since the fluid rapidly reaccumulates).
2. Intrauterine transfusion for Rh-hemolytic disease.

3. Mid-trimester abortion. Agents used include urea, hypertonic saline, hypertonic glucose, and prostaglandins.

CONTRAINDICATIONS

- Infected lesions of abdominal wall where amniocentesis must be done
- Maternal coagulopathy (*relative contraindication*)
- Placental abruption (*relative contraindication*)
- Patient refusal
- Problems not diagnosable by evaluation of the amniotic fluid (teratogen exposure, radiation exposure, drug use early in pregnancy, or history of genetic disorders not diagnosable by amniocentesis)
- When the results of tests will not change the clinical course (e.g., abruptio placentae with brisk bleeding—patient requires cesarean section regardless of laboratory data)

EQUIPMENT

- Real-time diagnostic ultrasound unit
- Commercial amniocentesis tray or sterile tray containing at least three plain sterile specimen tubes (5 to 10 cc each) with caps, standard-length 20-gauge or 22-gauge spinal needle, 20 cc syringe, 5 cc syringe, 1.5-inch 22-gauge or 23-gauge needle, sterile 4 × 4 inch gauze pads, sterile Band-Aids, and sterile towels for drapes
- Skin antiseptic, such as povidone-iodine or chlorhexidine gluconate
- Local anesthetic solution, such as 1% or 2% lidocaine (*without* epinephrine)
- Fetal heart rate monitor
- Sterile gloves

Suppliers: Disposable Amniocentesis Trays

Pharmaceal Division
Baxter Healthcare Corporation
Valencia, CA 91355-8900

Professional Medical Products Division
Seamless Corporation
Ocala, FL 32670

PREPROCEDURE PATIENT EDUCATION

Discuss the procedure with the patient beforehand. Inform her of the risks and explain why the amniocentesis should be performed. Describe alternative modes of evaluation or treatment (if any) and obtain written consent (Box 96-1).

BOX 96-1. CONSENT FOR AMNIOCENTESIS

I, _____ , agree to the performance of an amniocentesis by
Dr. _____ and his or her associates. I understand that amniocentesis involves inserting a needle through my abdominal wall into the fluid that surrounds my baby, and taking a sample of that fluid. I understand that even with
utmost care in performing the amniocentesis, harm may occur to me or to my
baby. While amniocentesis is a commonly done procedure and is relatively safe,
serious complications can occur. While unlikely, it is possible to introduce infection
into the uterus (womb), to puncture the umbilical cord and cause bleeding from
the cord, to cause premature rupture of membranes and/or premature labor, and
to cause the afterbirth (placenta) to separate prematurely with possible death to
me and/or my baby. The alternatives for my care have been explained to me.

I am having the amniocentesis because_____

_____ .

_____   _____
Signed   Date   Witness

TECHNIQUE

1. Have the patient lie on the examining table or bed with head elevated 20 to
   30 degrees. Alternatively, perform the procedure with the patient in the slight
   (15 degree) left decubitus position. Monitor the fetal heart rate for 5 minutes.
2. Locate a pocket of fluid with real-time ultrasound (Fig. 96-1). Try to find a
   pocket that the needle will be able to reach without going through the placenta or near the fetal face. The best locations are usually in the area of the
   fetal extremities (associated with low risk of cord puncture). Sometimes it is
   necessary to elevate the fetal head from the pelvis to insert the needle below
   (associated with increased risk of rupture of membranes or spontaneous abortion). Use the ultrasound calipers to measure the depth of skin that the needle
   must penetrate to enter the pocket. Mark the location of the puncture site on
   the skin using a needle hub.
3. Prepare the abdomen with antiseptic solution.
4. Wearing sterile gloves, raise a skin wheal with the anesthetic at the puncture
   site, then continue to anesthetize along the course of the needle track to the
   parietal peritoneum and serosal surface of the uterus (requires 4 to 5 cc of
   anesthetic solution). Remove the needle.
5. With the stylet in place, insert the 20-gauge or 22-gauge spinal needle along
   the selected track to the previously measured depth (Fig. 96-1, *E*) and remove the stylet.

   Note: You should feel a little "pop" as the needle moves through the fascia, and, when it
   penetrates the amniotic membrane, there is sudden free movement.

   In most cases, the amniotic fluid will flow through the needle. If not, rotate
   the needle to move the tip away from membranes, fetal parts, etc. If there is

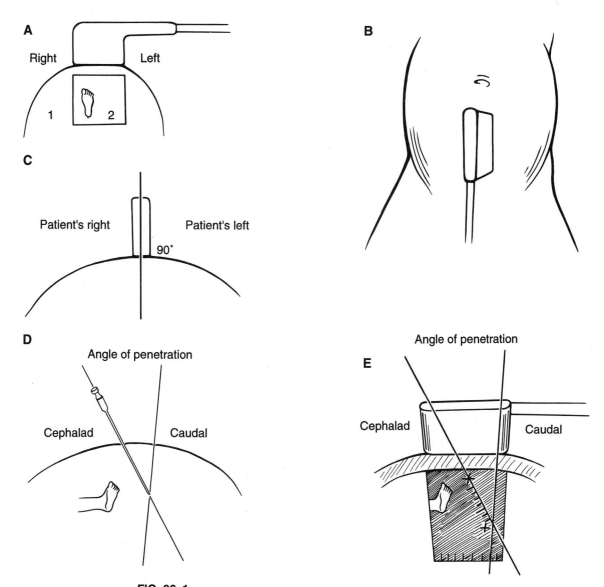

FIG. 96-1.
A, Locating a pocket of fluid with a transverse view. An area near the fetal extremities is usually associated with the lowest risk: *1,* maternal abdomen/pelvis, *2,* intrauterine amniotic fluid and fetal foot. **B,** Turn the probe to a longitudinal position to assess the other dimension of the fluid pocket. If possible, keep the probe perpendicular to the anterior abdominal wall by moving it laterally to position it over the best pocket. Note the angle and measure the depth that it will be necessary to penetrate with the needle to reach the pocket. **C,** Transverse view of the probe turned longitudinal. Note that the probe is held perpendicular to the abdomen. **D,** Longitudinal view. Note the measurements with calipers and direction of needle determined. **E,** Longitudinal view. Needle advanced to previously measured depth (X) at the proper angle.

still no flow of fluid, attach the empty 5 cc anesthetic syringe to the needle hub and apply gentle suction. If there is still no fluid, replace the stylet and insert another 0.5 to 1.0 cm or until resistance is felt. Again, remove the stylet. If there is still no fluid, reattach the small syringe and withdraw the needle slowly with gentle suction, rotating it as you withdraw. Once the fluid pocket is located, withdraw 2 or 3 cc of fluid in the small syringe and discard. This minimizes the amount of blood in the remaining fluid sample, which can affect laboratory results. Then, withdraw 15 to 25 cc of fluid (or the volume needed for the tests planned). Remove the needle, clean the excess antiseptic from the abdominal wall, and cover the puncture wound with a Band-Aid. If the patient is unsensitized Rh-negative, administer 50 to 150 μg of Rh immune globulin.

6. If grossly bloody amniotic fluid is encountered in the specimen, it is important to determine whether it is maternal or fetal blood. If the blood is fetal, use the Kleihauer-Betke technique to estimate the volume in the specimen. Also, monitor the fetal heart rate closely for 1 to 2 hours for the development of tachycardia. If the volume of fetal blood loss is significant for the fetal age, and if the fetus is judged mature enough to survive extrauterine life, fetal tachycardia is an indication for intervention and delivery.

7. If no amniotic fluid is located, repeat the ultrasound examination and again localize the fluid pocket and its distance from the skin, prepare the skin with antiseptic, and repeat the tap.

   Note: It is not recommended that more than two or three attempts be made, since repeated attempts increase the risk of significant fetal injury or induction of labor.

8. With a normal, successful amniocentesis, the fetal heart rate and the mother's response should be monitored for 20 to 30 minutes, after which the patient may leave.

BOX 96-2. PATIENT INSTRUCTIONS AFTER AMNIOCENTESIS

Please rest as much as you can for the rest of the day. If you work outside the home, avoid heavy lifting or prolonged standing for the rest of the day. Otherwise, you may do normal light household activities (but avoid using a vacuum cleaner or wet mop, or moving furniture). Avoid heavy yard or garden work. Do not have intercourse for 24 hours.

REPORT IMMEDIATELY if any of the following occur:

- Abdominal pain or bleeding from the needle mark
- Vaginal bleeding
- Leaking of fluid from your vagina
- Fever or chills
- Feeling of weakness or faintness
- Baby not moving when stimulated

POSTPROCEDURE PATIENT EDUCATION

Printed instructions help patients remember what they are told. Give the patient an instruction sheet for after amniocentesis (Box 96-2).

COMPLICATIONS

A wide variety of complications have been reported, including injuries resulting in fetal death. However, serious complications are uncommon and the procedure is considered relatively safe. Most complications are minor.

- Pain, bruising, or infection at the puncture site
- Uterine contractions, occasionally progressing to labor, but usually self-limited
- Occasional spontaneous abortion after mid-trimester amniocentesis
- Premature rupture of membranes
- Placental separation or abruption
- Fetal injury such as skin scars, dimpling, eye injury, genital injury (Risk increases if volume of amniotic fluid is decreased.)
- Cord or placental blood vessel injury with fetal hemorrhage
- Rh-factor isoimmunization
- Uterine infection
- Fluid leak with resultant oligohydramnios (rare)

DOCUMENTATION

Include a picture of the amniotic fluid pocket from the ultrasound examination (where possible) (Fig. 96-2) and a procedure note (Box 96-3) in your documentation.

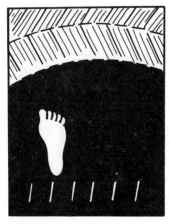

FIG. 96-2.
Example of good image to be photographed to document the site chosen for amniocentesis. Note the large pocket of fluid near an extremity and the absence of the cord.

BOX 96-3. EXAMPLE OF AMNIOCENTESIS PROCEDURE NOTE

The patient was placed in low semi-Fowler's position and the fetal heart tones monitored for 10 minutes. Real-time ultrasound scan then located a collection of amniotic fluid in the area of the fetal extremities at a depth of 5 cm. No loops of cord were noted. The overlying skin was marked, the skin then prepped with povidone-iodine solution and draped with sterile towels. After local anesthesia with 1% lidocaine, a 20-gauge spinal needle was inserted into the fluid pocket and 15 cc of clear (or "meconium stained," "slightly blood tinged," "grossly bloody") amniotic fluid removed without difficulty. Sterile dressing was applied to the puncture site and the fetal heart tones monitored for another 20 minutes. These remained normal and the patient felt well and was discharged home with instructions pending the results of the amniocentesis.

CPT/BILLING CODES

59000	Amniocentesis, any method
59850	Induced abortion by one or more intraamniotic injections
76946	Ultrasonic guidance for amniocentesis, physician supervision and interpretation

BIBLIOGRAPHY

Freda VJ: The Rh problem in obstetrics and a new concept of its management using amniocentesis and spectrophotometric scanning of amniotic fluid, *Am J Obstet Gynecol* 93:341, 1963.

Fuhrmann W: Impact, logistics and prospects of traditional prenatal diagnosis, *Clin Genet* 36(5):378, 1989.

Gluck L et al: Diagnosis of the respiratory distress syndrome by amniocentesis, *Am J Obstet Gynecol* 109:440, 1971.

Jacobs C, Ten Brink HJ, Stellard F: Prenatal diagnosis of inherited metabolic disorders by quantitation of characteristic metabolites in amniotic fluid: facts and future, *Prenat Diagn* 10(4):256, 1990.

McClain CR: Amniography studies of the gastrointestinal motility of the human fetus, *Am J Obstet Gynecol* 86:1079, 1968.

Rodney WM et al: Obstetric ultrasound by family physicians, *JFP* 34:186, 1992.

Schwarz RH, Crombleholme WR: Amniocentesis. In Sciarra JJ, editor: *Gynecology and obstetrics*, Philadelphia, 1988, J. B. Lippincott.

CHAPTER 97

Spontaneous Fetal-Movement Counting

Steve Ratcliffe

Fetal-movement counting is a potentially useful tool for use during the third trimester of the high-risk pregnancy, as well as the low-risk one. Its *primary purpose* is to help identify those pregnancies that without intervention may result in a fetal demise or stillbirth. A recent study evaluated the outcomes of 292 low-risk patients who complained of decreased fetal movement in labor and delivery. Five of these patients had a fetal death upon delivery and 13 of these patients required immediate delivery for both maternal and fetal indications. These outcomes suggest that decreased fetal movement in low-risk patients requires fetal surveillance. This study concluded that a reactive nonstress test (see Chapter 98, The Nonstress Test) and normal amniotic fluid volume should be reassuring in the presence of decreased fetal movement.

Antenatal testing (nonstress tests, contraction stress tests, etc.) is currently reserved for those patients with risks such as pregnancy-induced hypertension, intrauterine growth retardation, and the postdate pregnancy. Unfortunately, 30% to 50% of stillbirths occur in a setting with no identifiable maternal or fetal risk factors.

Fetal-movement counting has not assumed a prominent role in third trimester management in the United States for a number of reasons. This low-technology approach has not been extensively studied, and the studies that have been done have employed different fetal movement protocols and have had varying results. Some of these protocols have required women to do fetal-movement counting for an hour up to three times a day, regimens that result in poor patient compliance. The largest of these studies (*n*=68,000) utilized fetal-movement counting on all women during the third trimester and found no benefit in the treatment versus control group.

The most promising study, by Moore et al, utilized third trimester fetal-movement counting in the evening only, with the patient counting until she perceived 10 fetal movements. The mean time to perceive 10 movements was 20.9 minutes. In the study, 97% of the women perceived these 10 movements within 60 minutes. Those women who did not count 10 fetal movements within 2 hours were referred to the labor unit for monitoring. An astounding 97% of the study participants were compliant with this protocol. The results were a reduction of fetal mortality from 8.7 per 1000 births in the prestudy control period, to 2.1 per 1000 during the study period. Although further studies are needed to replicate these findings before this technique can gain wide acceptance and utilization, there does appear to be additional support in the literature for utilizing a two-hour surveillance period for fetal movement. The following section will detail the fetal-movement technique used in the study.

INDICATIONS

This technique *may* be a useful adjunct for monitoring the status of both the high- and low-risk pregnancy.

CONTRAINDICATIONS

It is unwise to attempt to employ this method for women who have either impaired mental status or significant linguistic or cultural barriers that would prevent adequate communication on the proper utilization of this method.

**BOX 97-1. PATIENT EDUCATION HANDOUT
SPONTANEOUS FETAL-MOVEMENT COUNTING**

It has been shown in one large medical study that you may be able to protect your baby's health by spending some time each evening counting the number of times your baby does any kind of movement. This process is called simply *fetal-movement counting*.

Find a comfortable position on your side. Then begin counting your baby's movements, which may be felt as kicks, flutters, swishes, or rolls. *Continue counting until your baby has moved ten times and then record the time it took for this to happen.* Although this may take up to 1 hour, it will often occur within 20 minutes.

We would like you to do this perhaps two to three times a week. Your doctor will tell you when to start or if you should do it more frequently than that. *Make a chart* and note the *date, time of day,* and the *amount of time* it took you to count the ten movements. Try to start this at the same time each day—when the baby is usually most active.

If 2 hours go by without your counting ten movements, please contact your medical provider or go to your hospital's labor suite for further evaluation.

When you follow these instructions, it may result in a visit to your hospital labor suite. It is hoped that this checking of your baby's movements, however, will result in an increased sense of security for you. It could also alert your doctor to potential problems. Bring your fetal-movement counting chart in with you at each office visit.

TECHNIQUE

Box 97-1 is a sample patient education handout, which describes the method of spontaneous fetal-movement counting.

COMPLICATIONS

This technique produces a large number of false-positive decreased fetal-movement screening tests in order to identify those fetuses that are experiencing real distress. This may at times result in a cascade of false-positive (abnormal) antenatal tests that could result in a decision to induce labor, with its increased risk of fetal distress and cesarean section.

BIBLIOGRAPHY

Ahn MO et al: Antepartum fetal surveillance in the patient with decreased fetal movement, *Am J Obstet Gynecol* 157:860, 1987.

Connors GT et al: Maternally perceived fetal activity from twenty-four weeks' gestation to term in normal and at risk pregnancies, *Am J Obstet Gynecol* 158:294, 1988.

Grant A et al: Routine formal fetal-movement counting and risk of antenatal late death in normally formed singletons, *Lancet* 2(8659):345, 1989.

Moore T, Piacquadio K: A prospective evaluation of fetal-movement screening to reduce the incidence of antepartum fetal death, *Am J Obstet Gynecol* 160:1075, 1989.

Whetty JE et al: Maternal perception of decreased fetal movement as an indication for antepartum testing in a low-risk population, *Am J Obstet Gynecol* 165:1084, 1991.

CHAPTER 98

The Nonstress Test

Steve Ratcliffe

The nonstress test (NST) was introduced in the United States in the early 1970s and has become a mainstay of screening for the fetal health. This test involves the use of fetal monitoring to document fetal heart rate accelerations that occur in conjunction with fetal movements. In a reassuring or *reactive NST* (a "negative" NST), there are at least two accelerations of greater than 15 beats per minute that last for 20 seconds in a 20-minute period. Another method of interpreting NSTs assigns points (0 to 2) to several parameters, including baseline rate, variability, acceleration frequency, deceleration frequency, and fetal movements. A total score equal to or greater than 7 is required for the test to be considered reactive.

Extensive clinical observations have repeatedly shown a strong correlation between absent or decreasing fetal heart rate accelerations and progressive fetal hypoxia. The presence of fetal heart rate accelerations associated with fetal movement (that is, a reactive NST) is a reassuring indicator of good fetal health. A negative or reactive NST has a specificity greater than 90%; that is, a normal test will correctly identify a healthy fetus greater than 90% of the time. Because a reactive NST can occasionally miss an endangered fetus, many recent papers have cautioned providers to evaluate other features of the fetal tracing in addition to its reactivity to decide if further antenatal testing is indicated. Specifically, the presence of baseline abnormalities or decelerations is associated with increased perinatal morbidity and mortality. In addition, many centers are routinely performing ultrasound amniotic fluid assessments when variable decelerations are noted on an otherwise reactive NST to identify those women with decreased amniotic fluid (oligohydramnios).

The sensitivity and positive predictive value of the NST as a screening test are somewhat more problematic. Sensitivity refers to the percentage of patients having a fetus experiencing deteriorating health that will be detected by a nonreactive NST. The predictive value of a *positive test* (nonreactive NST) means it is likely that the patient has a sick fetus. Table 98-1 demonstrates that the sensitivity and positive predictive value of the NST varies with the condition being assessed.

TABLE 98-1.

Use of NST as a Screening Test

Condition	Sensitivity	Positive Predictive Value (%)
Postdatism	0.44	0.15
Intrauterine growth retardation (IUGR)	0.56	0.69
Hypertension	0.31	0.44
Diabetes mellitus	0.53	0.31

Hence, in the setting of confirmed intrauterine growth retardation (IUGR), a nonreactive NST accurately predicts an endangered fetus 69% of the time. The predictive value drops to only 15% in the evaluation of the postdate pregnancy, and it becomes very small when this test is used with a low-risk population. The clinician must therefore take into account the risk status of the patient and the indication for ordering a NST. The low-risk patient at 41 weeks' gestation who has a nonreactive NST (a "positive," abnormal test) most likely has a healthy fetus, and the clinician must undertake further steps to confirm this without subjecting the patient and fetus to unnecessary iatrogenic interventions. The most likely explanation of "false-positive" nonreactive NST is failure to observe the fetus for an adequate period of time. One leading investigator suggests that fetal NST observation for durations up to 90 minutes would decrease the incidence of abnormal tests that require further follow-up to about 5%. Other investigators have suggested using acoustic stimulation to induce a "reactive" tracing, reducing the incidence of false-positive tracings.

Options available to the clinician for evaluating a persistent nonreactive NST include proceeding with an oxytocin challenge or nipple-stimulation contraction test, obtaining a biophysical profile (BPP), or proceeding with induction when favorable conditions exist. A flowchart for the management of NST results as used at the Medical College of Georgia is presented in Fig. 98-1.

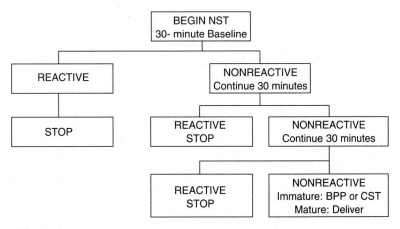

FIG. 98-1.
Flowchart for the management of the nonstress test.

In summary, the NST is an extensively used screening test to assess the health of fetuses judged to be at some increased risk because of underlying medical conditions or prolonged gestational age. Because the NST alone is not a sensitive test, other parameters of the fetal tracing, such as presence of variable decelerations or abnormalities in the baseline, should be assessed. Prolonged observation of the NST reduces the incidence of false-positive NSTs and, at the same time, continues to be highly predictive of fetal compromise.

INDICATIONS

The nonstress test is used extensively to monitor fetal health status of high-risk pregnancies as early as 34 weeks' gestation. Some of these high-risk conditions are:

Suspected or confirmed intrauterine growth retardation
Gestational diabetes
Essential hypertension or preeclampsia
Postdate pregnancy
Decreased fetal movement
Other maternal or fetal condition (renal disease, multiple gestation, substance abuse, prior fetal demise, etc.)

Some investigators have utilized the NST at even earlier stages of pregnancy (28 to 34 weeks). However, they have had to modify some of the criteria for a reactive or reassuring tracing because the premature fetus will have heart rate accelerations that are less pronounced than the more mature fetus.

CONTRAINDICATIONS

There are no specific contraindications to performing a nonstress test other than a gestation less than 28 to 34 weeks. As discussed previously, the clinician must be adept at the proper interpretation of the NST, based upon gestational age and maternal condition, and know whether the patient has taken any medications, including narcotics, that might affect the reactivity of the fetal tracing.

EQUIPMENT

- Fetal monitor (Fig. 98-2)

Major suppliers are Hewlett-Packard and Corometrics.

PREPROCEDURE PATIENT EDUCATION

Give the patient a handout outlining the procedure and the measures to follow before the nonstress test (Box 98-1).

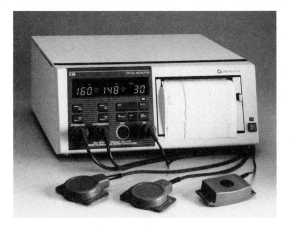

FIG. 98-2.
Intrapartum fetal monitor. (Courtesy of Corometrics Medical Systems, Inc.)

**BOX 98-1. PATIENT EDUCATION HANDOUT
THE NONSTRESS TEST**

Your physician has recommended a nonstress test to check on your baby's health. This test is accomplished using a special monitor that can measure and record your baby's heart rate and any contractions or labor pains that you may experience during this test. It does not hurt you, nor will it harm your baby.

You will be asked to let the nurse know when you feel your baby move, or you may be asked to push a button with each movement. If your baby's heart rate becomes faster shortly after you feel your baby move, this will be regarded as a normal, reassuring nonstress test. Your physician will then determine whether additional nonstress tests are needed.

If your baby's heart rate does not increase shortly after you feel movements, it may mean that your baby is in a sleepy or hungry state. For this reason, you should *not* take any type of pain or sleeping medications starting 6 hours before this test. Make sure you eat within the 4 hours before this test. You may be asked to drink sweetened fruit juice or to extend the time of testing to reach a conclusion that provides you and your physician with accurate, reassuring information. Please do not smoke for at least 2 hours before coming in. The whole test may only take 30 to 40 minutes, but sometimes it may last up to 2 hours.

If the nonstress test does not provide the reassurance the physician is seeking about your baby's health, your physician will discuss additional options, and possibly further testing, to learn more about your baby's health.

TECHNIQUE

Many testing centers attempt to standardize a number of factors to minimize environmental variables. These include encouraging the patient to eat about 2 hours before the nonstress test, not to smoke or take sedative drugs before the test, and to remain sedentary during the hour before testing.

1. Place the patient in a semi-Fowler's position with lateral hip displacement.
2. Apply an external tocodynameter and Doppler to record the fetal heart tracing and any uterine contractions.
3. Ask the patient to record any fetal movements that are corroborated by the observer.
4. Monitor the patient for a 30-minute baseline period. Two additional 30-minute monitoring periods should be considered in the presence of an initial nonreactive tracing. A fetal tracing is considered to be reactive if there are two or more accelerations of more than 15 beats per minute lasting for at least 15 seconds. These accelerations should occur within a 20-minute interval.

COMPLICATIONS

The nonstress test itself poses no known risks to the mother or fetus. However, the improper interpretation of the test may lead to premature interventions that could result in iatrogenic morbidity and mortality. The clinician should extend the observation period for as long as 90 minutes to decrease the incidence of false-positive (nonreactive) tests. When interpretating a nonreactive NST and before proceeding with further interventions, the clinician must consider the maternal-fetal condition being assessed.

CPT/BILLING CODE

59025   Nonstress test

BIBLIOGRAPHY

Bar-Hava I, Barnhard Y: Fetal vibroacoustic stimulation, *Female Patient* 19:63, 1994.

Bourgeois FJ et al: The significance of fetal heart rate decelerations during nonstress testing, *Am J Obstet Gynecol* 150:213, 1984.

Devoe LD: The nonstress test, *Obstet Gynecol Clin North Am* 17:111, 1990.

Hoskins IA et al: Variable decelerations in reactive nonstress tests with decreased amniotic fluid index predict fetal compromise, *Am J Obstet Gynecol* 165:1094, 1991.

Lagrew DC, Freeman RK: Management of postdate pregnancy, *Am J Obstet Gynecol* 154:8, 1986.

Serafini P et al: Antepartum fetal heart rate response to sound stimulation: the acoustic stimulation test, *Am J Obstet Gynecol* 148:41, 1984.

Smith CV et al: Intrapartum assessment of fetal well-being: a comparison of fetal acoustic stimulation with acid-base determinations, *Am J Obstet Gynecol* 155:726, 1986.

CHAPTER 99

Contraction Stress Test

Steve Ratcliffe

The contraction stress test (CST) is a common procedure designed to identify fetuses at risk for either uteroplacental insufficiency or cord compression. This test evaluates whether uterine contractions cause late decelerations in the fetal heart tracing.

It was first recognized in the mid 1960s that late decelerations correlate with stillbirths and low Apgar scores. In 1972, Ray and Freeman began systematic trials of contraction stress testing in the United States. They called this test the oxytocin challenge test because it relied on an infusion of synthetic oxytocin (Pitocin). Contemporary evaluators utilize spontaneously occurring contractions and those induced by breast stimulation or oxytocin administration. Therefore, the procedure is more appropriately referred to as the contraction stress test.

"Negative" test results are reassuring; "positive" or "suspicious" results are cause for concern. A CST is positive if more than 50% of the contractions are accompanied by late decelerations in the absence of uterine hyperstimulation. The reactivity of the fetal tracing (see Chapter 98, The Nonstress Test) is an important factor to weigh when evaluating a positive CST. A *reactive* positive CST is associated with a high incidence of false positives, whereas a *nonreactive,* positive CST has a much higher predictive power in identifying a compromised fetus (Fig. 99-1).

A suspicious CST is one in which less than 50% of the contractions result in late decelerations. Uterine hyperstimulation must again be excluded as the cause of the decelerations.

A negative CST is one in which no late decelerations occur when the contraction frequency is at least three in 10 minutes. In addition, no significant variable decelerations should occur. A negative CST that is nonreactive is uncommon. This test result deserves further scrutiny to determine if the cause is a medication effect (e.g., narcotics or phenobarbital), a fetal central nervous system defect, subtle fetal distress, or prematurity.

A positive or suspicious CST is given careful consideration. Maternal factors (such as dehydration) affecting placental function should be addressed. If improvement in the fetal heart rate tracing cannot be attained, and if fetal pulmonary maturity has been confirmed, labor is often induced.

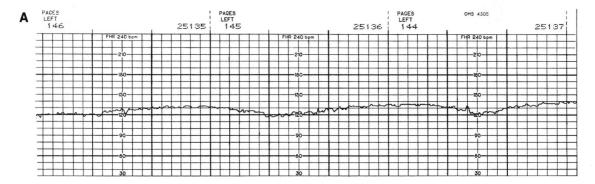

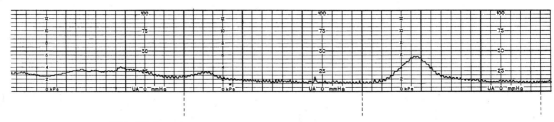

FIG. 99-1.
Nonreactive positive contraction stress test. **A**, Fetal heart rate. **B**, Uterine contractions.

**BOX 99-1. PATIENT EDUCATION HANDOUT
CONTRACTION STRESS TEST**

Your provider has referred you to this center for a test to check out your baby's health. This test, the contraction stress test, evaluates how your baby responds to contractions of your uterus. These contractions may occur naturally, may result from stimulation of your breast nipples, or may be caused by a very small amount of medicine injected into one of your veins. This medicine, oxytocin, closely resembles a natural hormone in your body. It is administered into your vein with a pumping device that carefully controls the amount of medicine you receive. Your baby's heart rate will be followed on a monitor while you have the contractions.

A "negative" or normal contraction stress test occurs if your baby does not experience any slowing of its heartbeat following contractions of your uterus. The test will be regarded as "positive" or "suspicious" if your baby's heartbeat becomes slower after some or all contractions of your uterus. If the test result is positive, your provider will discuss with you what further testing or treatments should be done.

Please tell your medical provider, before undergoing the test, if you are experiencing any illness, because this could lead to a positive or abnormal test result. There is a small risk, about one to three out of a hundred tests, that the test may result in too many contractions of your uterus. If that happens, we may need to give you an injection to slow down these contractions.

INDICATIONS

The contraction stress test, nonstress test (NST), and the biophysical profile (BPP) (see Chapter 104, Obstetric Ultrasound) are utilized when fetal compromise is suspected because of certain conditions, such as intrauterine growth retardation, pregnancy-induced hypertension, or fetal dysmaturity. The CST is a more sensitive test of fetal well-being than the NST. However, it is generally used to follow up abnormal or suspicious NSTs or BPPs because of cost and time. Combining the NST with an assessment of amniotic fluid volume equals the sensitivity of the biophysical profile, approaches that of the CST, and appears to be the emerging screening test of choice.

CONTRAINDICATIONS

Contraction stress tests are contraindicated whenever uterine contractions are to be avoided. Those situations include advanced cases of premature labor, when considerable dilation and effacement have already occurred, and when abnormal anatomical conditions, such as an incompetent cervix, are present.

EQUIPMENT

- Fetal monitor (see Chapter 98, Fig. 98-2; major suppliers are Hewlett-Packard and Corometrics)
- Blood pressure cuff
- Intravenous setup
- Terbutaline

PREPROCEDURE PATIENT EDUCATION

Give the patient a handout explaining the contraction stress test (Box 99-1) and answer any questions she may have.

TECHNIQUE

1. Place the patient in a semi-Fowler's position.
2. Take a baseline blood pressure to assure that supine hypotension, which could cause a false-positive CST, does not exist.
3. Record a baseline fetal heart rate/contraction tracing to assess reactivity and uterine contractions. Provide continuous monitoring. Subcutaneous terbutaline, which relaxes uterine muscle in the event of serious uterine hypersensitivity and hypertonic contractions, should be readily available.
4. After a baseline NST has been obtained, ask the patient to stimulate one nipple by massaging and rolling it until a contraction occurs.

5. Ask the patient to temporarily stop the stimulation until the contraction is over, and then resume. This process is continued until an adequate contraction pattern is achieved. This method has been shown to be effective between 78% and 94% of the time. Uterine hyperstimulation patterns occur in 3% to 4% of these CSTs.

Note: The nipple-stimulation CST is being utilized with increasing frequency because it bypasses the need for an intravenous line placement, and if successful, reduces the testing time.

The CST may also be performed by starting an intravenous infusion of oxytocin at 0.5 mU per minute. This rate may be increased every 15 minutes by increments of 0.5 to 1.0 mU per minute until regular uterine contractions are achieved. An adequate CST has been achieved when there are three contractions lasting from 40 to 60 seconds within a 10-minute period. The majority of patients will achieve this contraction pattern at an infusion level of 4 to 8 mU per minute. Uterine hyperstimulation occurs during this testing modality about 1% of the time and generally responds readily to stopping the oxytocin infusion. If it does not, subcutaneous terbutaline, 0.25 to 0.5 mg, should be administered to stop the hyperstimulation pattern rapidly.

COMPLICATIONS

The major complication of the contraction stress test is uterine hyperstimulation. This often results in a false-positive CST, which may lead to improper management if not correctly identified. Rarely, uterine hyperstimulation may induce sufficient genuine fetal distress to require emergency intervention.

Uterine hyperstimulation almost always resolves if the oxytocin infusion or breast stimulation is stopped. If this is not sufficient, subcutaneous terbutaline may be employed as described above.

CPT/BILLING CODE

59020   Contraction stress test

BIBLIOGRAPHY

Capeless EL, Mann LI: Use of breast stimulation for antepartum stress testing, *Obstet Gynecol* 64:641, 1984.

Copel JA et al: Contraction stress testing with nipple stimulation, *J Reprod Med* 30:465, 1985.

Grundy H et al: Nonreactive contraction stress test: clinical significance, *Obstet Gynecol* 64:337, 1984.

Hoskins IA et al: Variable decelerations in reactive nonstress tests with decreased amniotic fluid index predict fetal compromise, *Am J Obstet Gynecol* 165:1094, 1991.

Pircon RA, Freeman RK: The contraction stress test, *Obstet Gynecol Clin N Am* 17:129, 1990.

CHAPTER 100

Episiotomy

Donald N. Marquardt

Episiotomy, or more correctly, perineotomy, is the second most commonly performed surgical procedure in the United States, surpassed only by circumcision. Episiotomy is used to facilitate the second stage of labor in approximately 60% of all deliveries (and up to 90% of primiparous deliveries) in the United States. Nurse-midwives and physicians in Europe perform the surgery much less frequently (approximately one eighth the frequency), consistent with their view that delivery is a natural process that does not necessarily benefit from intervention. In a comprehensive review, Thacker and Banta conclude that "the widespread use of episiotomy do[es] not withstand scientific scrutiny . . . [and] the risks of episiotomy have been widely ignored."

An episiotomy is made to enlarge the vaginal outlet to facilitate delivery. In a midline or median episiotomy, the incision is made in a direct line posteriorly from the vagina toward the anus, and down to—but not including—the external anal sphincter. Alternatively, in a mediolateral episiotomy, the incision is directed 45 degrees laterally from the midline at the base of the introitus. The latter is generally associated with more bleeding and postoperative pain, has shown no conclusive benefit over the median episiotomy except in limited circumstances, and is performed much less frequently in the United States. This discussion will be limited to the median episiotomy. The reader interested in mediolateral episiotomy is referred to recent texts or the technical review by Varner.

INDICATIONS

Any situation that prolongs the second stage of labor and thereby significantly endangers the life of the mother, the integrity of her perineum, or the brain of the fetus could warrant episiotomy. The fact that episiotomy is a surgical procedure with attendant risks and potentially fatal complications should temper the decision to speed the second stage of labor by a few minutes.

Current obstetric literature suggests that when vaginal delivery is anticipated and one of the following maternal or fetal indications exists, episiotomy may be indicated:

Maternal: • Significant cardiac disease (e.g., mitral stenosis)
   • Prolonged second-stage labor
   • Risk of significant perineal trauma (e.g., large infant, use of forceps)
Fetal: • Significant fetal distress in second stage
   • Prematurity
   • Breech presentation

Several previous indications (e.g., prevention of pelvic relaxation and decreased incidence of perineal morbidity) are not supported by recent clinical trials, and current indications may become less valid as scientific method replaces speculation. Clinical trials are necessary to demonstrate whether surgical episiotomy is indeed superior to less invasive maneuvers (e.g., changes in maternal position, breathing, and pushing) in alleviating second-stage complications or in reducing trauma of a premature or breech infant. Readers are encouraged to remain current with the literature.

CONTRAINDICATIONS

- Patient refusal
- Severe scarring or malformation of perineum (e.g., from inflammatory bowel disease or lymphogranuloma venereum)
- Extensive, large condyloma, which if incised may lead to frank hemorrhage

EQUIPMENT

Episiotomy is usually performed with blunt/blunt surgical scissors, but a scalpel may be used. Equipment for repair includes the following:

- Needle holder
- Nontraumatic forceps
- Allis clamps
- Ring forceps
- Vaginal retractor(s)
- 3-0 and 4-0 glycolic polymer sutures (preferred over chromic, which is associated with more discomfort during healing) on a large, curved needle
- Cutting needle, or a tapered point needle (decision based on physician's preference)

If effective regional (epidural or pudendal) anesthetic has not previously been administered, a 10 cc syringe with a 1.5 inch 27-gauge needle should be available to locally infiltrate the anesthetic of preference (usually 1% lidocaine *without* epinephrine).

PREPROCEDURE PATIENT EDUCATION

Discuss the episiotomy with the patient (and partner) during prenatal care, before that emergent moment of need when neither the physician nor the patient is in position for optimum information exchange. Discuss the potential risks and possible benefits to allow the patient to make an informed decision concerning liberal or restricted use of episiotomy at the time of delivery. Also discuss the specific circumstances in which episiotomy would become absolutely necessary.

TECHNIQUE

Episiotomy

In the second stage of labor, as the fetal cranium begins to distend the maternal perineum, effort should be directed toward assisting with the natural thinning of the perineum and dilation of the introitus. The decision for episiotomy is usually made after the fetal cranium (not just the caput) distends the introitus. Waiting until a minimum of 3 to 4 cm diameter of the fetal scalp is visible and delivery is imminent will prevent excessive blood loss. Insert the index and middle fingers of your nondominant hand between the fetal scalp and the maternal perineum, and direct the perineum toward the maternal anus. Place your thumb on the exterior perineum. Your fingers serve two functions: (1) they protect the fetus; and (2) they palpate the anal sphincter, the thumb defining the bottom of the episiotomy (Fig. 100-1).

If anesthesia is not already present or adequate with a regional block, administer a local anesthetic. Anesthetize the midline of both the perineum (for a median episiotomy) and the floor of the vagina.

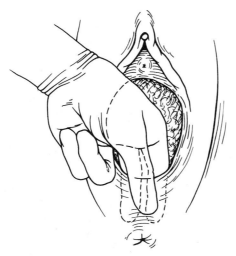

FIG. 100-1.
Palpating the perineum before episiotomy.

Insert the scissors to cut parallel to and between your fingers, and take care to protect the fetal presenting part and to avoid injury to the external sphincter of the anus (Fig. 100-2). Under direct visualization, extend the incision up the vaginal mucosa an additional 2 to 4 cm to prevent tearing. Delivery should proceed expeditiously to minimize blood loss.

Repair

Most physicians prefer to repair the episiotomy only after the third stage of labor, because delivery of the placenta may disturb the episiotomy repair, and the bleeding at separation makes visualization difficult. As with any surgical repair, accurate assessment of the extent of injury (both by palpation and by direct visualization) is crucial to achieve optimal repair. Specifically, closely inspect for "extensions" or tears beyond the episiotomy; this examination may reveal damage (complete or partial) to the anal sphincter (third-degree laceration) or rectal mucosa (fourth-degree laceration). After all deliveries, a rectovaginal examination is important. Palpate the distal 6 cm of the rectal mucosa to determine whether occult damage is present in the absence of damage to the sphincter or anus. An unrecognized buttonhole in the proximal rectum could lead to a rectovaginal fistula later. Change gloves after the rectal examination and before repairing the episiotomy to prevent contamination. Carefully examine the remainder of the lower urogenital tract for lacerations not contiguous with the episiotomy that may also need repair.

Repair of Third- and Fourth-Degree Extensions (Tears)

If the rectal mucosa is no longer intact (fourth-degree laceration), it must be repaired to prevent fistula formation. One method involves approximating the

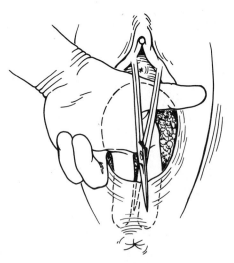

FIG. 100-2.
Performing the midline episiotomy.

submucosa with interrupted 4-0 polyglycolic suture, stitched 3 to 5 mm apart, inverting the mucosa itself into the lumen. (Most physicians try to avoid passing the needle through the mucosa into the rectal lumen.) A second layer of interrupted stitches may be made laterally (horizontally if the patient is in the standard lithotomy delivery position) over the submucosal stitches to decrease the chance of fistula formation between rectum and vagina. After the rectal mucosa and submucosal tissues are repaired, the sphincter is reapproximated as noted below, followed by repair of the episiotomy (Fig. 100-3).

If damage has occurred to the sphincter (third-degree laceration), it must be identified and repaired before closure of the episiotomy or vaginal mucosa laceration (second-degree laceration). Grasp the opposing ends of the sphincter with an Allis forcep (Fig. 100-3, *A*), and repair the rectal *sphincter sheath* by interrupted or figure-eight sutures on the posterior, inferior, superior, and anterior planes to provide adequate sphincter reapproximation and support (Fig. 100-3, *B* and *C*). *The sphincter muscle alone does not have sufficient strength to hold until healing is complete. The fibrous sheath must be included in the repair.*

Repair of the Episiotomy

Once the rectal mucosa and the anal sphincter have been well repaired (if lacerated), carefully examine the wound to optimize reapproximation of vaginal tissue. Use the 3-0 polyglycolic suture to place a stitch above the apex on the vaginal incision and run down in locked sutures to the introitus (Fig. 100-4). It is critical that these stitches (1) provide hemostasis, (2) close all deadspace, and

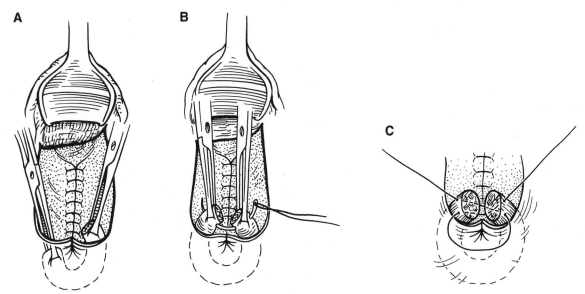

FIG. 100-3.
Repair of fourth-degree extension of a midline episiotomy. The mucosa is repaired then the sphincter is retrieved with Allis forceps (**A**). The ends are approximated with interrupted (**B**) or figure-of-eight sutures (**C**) through the muscle sheath. When the sphincter has been repaired, the remainder of the wound is closed as a median episiotomy.

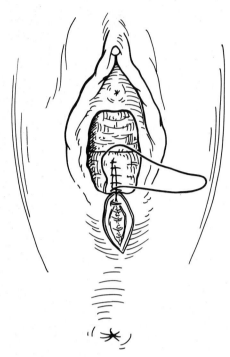

FIG. 100-4.
Closure of the vaginal mucosa. The first stitch is placed *above* the apex of the wound and tied. This stitch is then continued as a running locked stitch down to the introitus. The needle is shown at the level of the bulbocavernosus.

(3) do *not* enter the rectum. One way to accomplish all this is to take wide bites laterally on each side, but bring the needle out at the base of the incision so that it does not go deep into the rectum. The bulbocavernosus should be approximated at the base of the introitus carefully with a crown stitch before the perineum is repaired. With the same or different suture, close the deep perineum with a running stitch down toward the sphincter. Use the remaining suture to close the skin of the perineum with a subcuticular stitch (Fig. 100-5). Alternatively, the deep perineal tissues can be reapproximated with buried interrupted stitches (Fig. 100-6), then closed with a second layer, as in Fig. 100-7, before placing the subcuticulars.

Recent literature indicates that a running nonlocked stitch on the vaginal mucosa (to decrease tissue ischemia and necrosis) and placement of the perineal subcuticular stitches deeply (even leaving the perineal wound gaping 2 to 3 mm) will significantly decrease itching during healing with no loss of cosmesis or function.

Once repair is complete, perform a final rectovaginal examination to verify again that the rectal mucosa is intact, to ascertain that the rectum has not been violated by suture, and to ensure that no gauze sponges or instruments remain in either the rectum or vagina. If either of the first two conditions is not met, immediate correction (by removal of the existing repair and repeat effort with care to avoid the previous offense) is imperative to minimize the risk of infection and fistula formation.

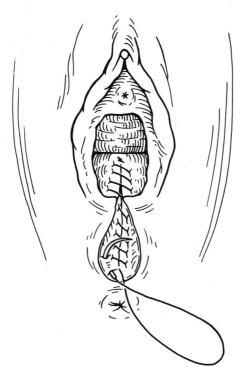

FIG. 100-5.
The repair of the vaginal mucosa has been completed (here with *unlocked* stitches). The bulbocavernosus has been reapproximated and a deep running layer of perineal sutures have been placed, using the same length of suture. The first subcuticular stitch is shown. Finishing the perineal closure would entail running the subcuticular stitches back to the introitus.

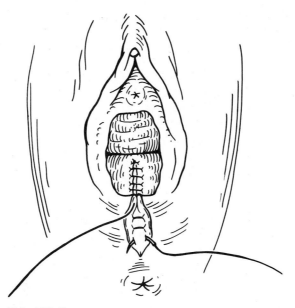

FIG. 100-6.
An alternative method of closing the deep perineal space, using deep interrupted inverted sutures.

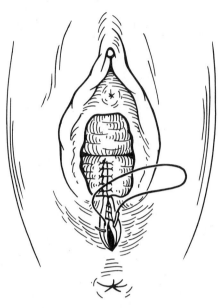

FIG. 100-7.
Closing the second layer of perineum with a continuation of vaginal sutures.

POSTPROCEDURE PATIENT EDUCATION

After delivery, patients with sutures are less comfortable than patients without sutures, and women with episiotomies may experience more pain than women with minor lacerations. Many women will desire analgesia, and nonsteroidal antiinflammatory drugs (e.g., ibuprofen) are increasingly replacing acetaminophen with codeine as the drug of choice. Warm sitz baths and heat lamps aid in comfort and healing, but recently, the use of ice packs to the perineum to reduce swelling and postpartum pain has gained credibility.

It is imperative to discuss with the patient the potential complications so that she is aware of the signs and symptoms for which she must immediately contact the physician should a complication become evident.

COMPLICATIONS

- Blood volume loss is reported to be approximately 300 ml from an uncomplicated median episiotomy, but may easily be more if there is an unexpected delay in delivery or repair. Observe the patient carefully and treat proactively, especially if other conditions threaten to compromise the patient (e.g., intravascular hypovolemia due to preeclampsia or other blood loss). Hematoma formation is unusual but not rare; acute swelling and pain must alert the physician to a possible hematoma that should be opened, the bleeding arrested, and the space either closed or drained to prevent recurrence.

- Infection is probably the most serious threat to episiotomy recovery. A range of wound infections, from a minor exudative wound infection, to a life-threatening septic hematoma, to fatal necrotizing fasciitis are of major concern. Maternal fever and unusual pain or swelling in the perineum must be thoroughly evaluated to rule out serious infections.
- Rectovaginal and urogenital fistulae (vesicovaginal, vesicocervicovaginal, urethrovaginal, and ureterovaginal) may occur from either direct trauma (hence the importance of careful examination of the entire lower genital tract) or from infection or necrosis associated with suturing. Incontinence of either feces or urine starting 10 or more days after delivery should alert the clinician to these complications.
- Pelvic relaxation and poor perineal tone, once thought to be benefited by episiotomy, may actually be exacerbated by the operation. While not life threatening, they may lead to a lifetime of misery and disability for the unfortunate woman.
- Local pain or wound breakdown and dyspareunia are usually self-limited complications. Bartholin's duct cysts, inclusion cysts, and endometriosis at the wound site are rarely encountered and easily corrected surgically.

In addition to maternal complications, episiotomies place another patient in the immediate vicinity in jeopardy: the fetus. Fetal complications may range from minimal abrasions to rare but significant lacerations on the presenting part (e.g., eyelid lacerations and even castration of a male breech infant).

CPT/BILLING CODES

58400	Complete prenatal/labor/delivery with or without episiotomy
59300	Episiotomy or vaginal repair by other than the attending physician

BIBLIOGRAPHY

Fleming N: Can the suturing method make a difference in postpartum perineal pain? *J Nurs Midwifery* 35:19, 1990.

Green JR, Soohoo SL: Factors associated with rectal injury in spontaneous deliveries, *Obstet Gynecol* 73:732, 1989.

Klein M et al: The McGill/University de Montreal multicentre episiotomy trial, *Proceedings of NAPCRG Nineteenth Annual Meeting* 170: 1991.

Thacker SB, Banta HD: Benefits and risks of episiotomy: an interpretive review of the English Language Literature, 1860-1980, *Obstet Gynecol Survey* 38:322, 1983.

Varner MW: Episiotomy: techniques and indications, *Clin Obstet Gynecol* 29:309, 1986.

Pudendal Anesthesia

Donald N. Marquardt

The pudendal nerve supplies both sensory and motor innervation to the perineum. It is composed of parts of the second, third, and fourth sacral nerves, and has three branches:

1. The dorsal nerve of the clitoris, which innervates the clitoris and its erectile tissues
2. The perineal nerve, which innervates the muscles of the perineum and the skin of the labia minora, labia majora, and vestibule
3. The inferior hemorrhoidal nerve, which innervates the external sphincter of the anus and perianal skin (responsible for the anal "wink" reflex)

Pudendal anesthesia attempts to block the nerve as it enters the lesser sciatic foramen, inferior and medial to the sacrospinous ligament insertion on the ischial spine. The pudendal vessels lie lateral to the nerve at this location, so care must be taken to avoid intravascular injection.

Although total block of the pudendal nerve should abolish pain sensation over this entire area, the nerve or its branches may take aberrant pathways. The transvaginal approach to blockade seems more reliable than a transperineal approach, but even then may only be totally effective bilaterally in half the patients.

INDICATIONS

- Obstetrical anesthesia for spontaneous vaginal deliveries, for performing episiotomy and episiotomy repair, for repair of low vaginal lacerations, and when low (outlet) forceps are used
- Minor surgery of the lower vagina and perineum

Note: Because the upper vagina, cervix, and uterus receive separate innervation from the lower thoracic nerves, pudendal anesthesia alone is not sufficient for midforceps application or for high vaginal, cervical, or uterine manipulation. As discussed earlier, pudendal anesthesia is less than 100% reliable, even in the best hands. The patient must

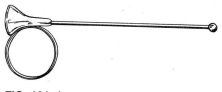

FIG. 101-1.
Iowa trumpet.

be checked bilaterally for loss of the anal "wink" reflex before proceeding with the procedure.

CONTRAINDICATIONS

- Patient refusal
- Sensitivity to local anesthetic agents
- Current infection in the ischiorectal space or neighboring structures, including the vagina and perineum

There is also a relative contraindication for obstetrical use: a successful pudendal block will impair some reflexive maternal pushing. This may prolong the second stage of labor in women who are unwilling to or ineffective at expelling the fetus without reflexive pushing.

EQUIPMENT

- 10 cc syringe with finger ring, filled with anesthetic (usually lidocaine *without* epinephrine*)
- Iowa trumpet (Fig. 101-1) or similar guide to facilitate placement of the needle
- Needle, usually 6-inch 20-gauge (The operator should check before the procedure that the needle is longer than the guiding device and equipped with a "stop" to prevent penetration of tissue deeper than 7 to 10 mm.)
- Resuscitation equipment and medications to support the patient if an adverse reaction to anesthetic is encountered (see Complications)
- Sterile gloves

---

*Volumes and doses are for 1% lidocaine *without* epinephrine, delivering 10 mg lidocaine per cc. Toxicity may occur above 1 mg/kg (70 mg or 7 cc in a 70 kg patient) with rapid absorption or intravascular administration. Maximum dosage should not exceed 4.5 mg/kg or to a maximum of 30 cc of 1% solution (300 mg), and maximum dose should not be repeated in less than 2 hours. See text for usual doses.

PREPROCEDURE PATIENT EDUCATION

Explain the potential risks (see Contraindications and Complications) and the potential benefits to the patient so she may make an informed decision. This discussion should occur before the moment of greatest anesthetic need, when neither the patient nor the physician can communicate optimally.

TECHNIQUE

Appropriate monitoring of the patient (*and, in obstetric cases, the fetus*) is mandatory, with intravenous access readily available. Since a fairly large volume of anesthetic agent is given, there must be provision for speedy resuscitation should toxicity or adverse reaction occur. See Chapter 21, Local Anesthesia, for symptoms of adverse reactions.

1. Timing is important in pudendal anesthesia. Time (5 to 10 minutes) must be allowed for the anesthetic to infiltrate the nerve for effect; however, for obstetric indications, the anesthetic should be administered neither so early that it blocks effective reflex pushing, nor so late that it wears off before delivery. In nulliparous women, it is usually administered after the cervix has completely dilated and the head has descended to a plus 2 to plus 3 station. In multiparous women, the pudendal may be administered earlier when rapid delivery is expected, but never before the cervix has dilated to 5 cm, as it may slow or arrest labor. Anesthesia may last for 20 to 60 minutes depending on the agent used.

2. Prepare and drape the patient in the dorsal lithotomy position; usually no vaginal prep is used. In obstetrical procedures, it is desirable to both minimize the length of time the patient is flat and to monitor the fetus frequently. This is a time of potential fetal compromise due to maternal position.

3. Grasp the guide with your nondominant hand, wrist pronated, with the thumb through the ring and the shaft between the index and middle fingers. Adequately lubricated index and middle fingers protect the vaginal mucosa (and, in obstetric cases, the fetal head) and direct the tip of the guide to the patient's ipsilateral ischial spine (the left hand of the right-handed operator is used to direct the guide to the patient's left ischial spine). Maintain the guide nearly parallel to the patient's back (Fig. 101-2).

4. Careful definition of the anatomy will optimize chances for success. Attempt to delineate the sacrospinous ligament and palpate the pudendal artery. This helps to both prevent injecting the anesthetic directly into the vessels and to define the location of the nerve medial to the vessels.

5. With your dominant hand, grasp the syringe and direct the needle through the guide. *You must aspirate for blood with the syringe before injecting anesthetic each time the needle placement is changed.* If blood is aspirated, intravascular injection is likely; withdraw the needle and redirect away from the vessels. Usually two to three sites are injected on each side: (*a*) posterior to the tip of the ischial spine, (*b*) medial to the tip of the spine, and (*c*) through

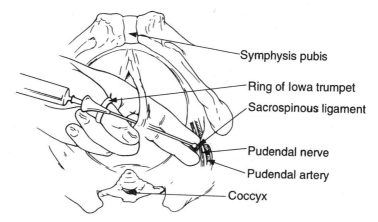

- Symphysis pubis
- Ring of Iowa trumpet
- Sacrospinous ligament
- Pudendal nerve
- Pudendal artery
- Coccyx

FIG. 101-2.
Left hand is directing guide and needle toward the pudendal nerve. This illustration shows the hand directed more laterally to better show the anatomy.

and into the sacrospinous ligament. Inject each site with 2 to 4 cc 1% lidocaine, with a maximum of 10 cc per side.

6. Withdraw the needle, refill the syringe, and inject into the opposite side if bilateral anesthesia is desired. Most operators prefer to use the same hand for the guide; however, some find that switching hands for the opposite side is more effective.

7. After 5 minutes, check anesthesia on *each* side. Using an Allis forceps, gently scratch over the perineum and watch for the anal "wink" reflex. If there is no reflex to mild stimulus, a pinch will confirm effective anesthesia on each side.

8. A smaller repeat dose on a side not demonstrating adequate anesthesia may be used, but care must be taken to avoid doses at which, even with slow absorption from the tissues, toxic serum levels could be reached. Local anesthesia may be used to augment the effect when the regional block is not effective.

POSTPROCEDURE PATIENT EDUCATION

There is little need for specific postanesthesia instruction. Remind the patient of the rare but possible complications so that she will report to her physician if any develop.

COMPLICATIONS

- Systemic anesthetic complications, which usually result from intravascular administration or inappropriate doses, may progress from palpitations, tinnitus, dysarthria, drowsiness, and confusion to loss of consciousness, convulsions, hypotension, and bradycardia. Although complications are usually transient, support of the patient's oxygenation and blood pressure is essential (especially to minimize fetal complications in obstetric cases). See Chapter 21, Local Anesthesia, for management of complication.

- The most frequent complication with pudendal anesthesia is failure to provide adequate anesthesia due to its lack of consistent efficacy. Local or alternative regional (e.g., caudal or epidural) anesthesia should be available.
- Hematomas and infections have been reported, but are rare. Infections may be life threatening (up to 30% mortality in one series), partially because they are difficult to diagnose. Infection frequently travels either superiorly along the psoas muscle or laterally along the obturator internus muscle. Infections must be suspected when there is severe pain in the back or hip, limitation of motion, and, especially, increasing fever. Full evaluation and therapeutic measures are immediately indicated.
- Anesthetic reaches the neonatal bloodstream after regional anesthesia, but studies have failed to demonstrate neonatal neurobehavioral effects or other adverse effects.

CPT/BILLING CODE

64430   Introduction/injection of anesthetic agent (nerve block), diagnostic or therapeutic

BIBLIOGRAPHY

King JC, Sherline DM: Paracervical and pudendal block, *Clin Obstet Gynecol* 24:587, 1981.
Merkow AJ et al: The neonatal neurobehavioral effects of bupivacaine, mepivacaine, and 2-chloroprocaine used for pudendal block, *Anesthesiology* 52:309, 1980.
Scudamore JH, Yates MJ: Pudendal block—a misnomer? *Lancet:* January, 1966.
Svancarek W et al: Retropsoas and subgluteal abscesses following paracervical and pudendal anesthesia, *JAMA* 237:892, 1977.

CHAPTER 102

Paracervical Block

Scott T. Henderson

A paracervical block anesthetizes Frankenhauser's ganglion, which contains the visceral sensory nerve fibers from the uterus, cervix, and upper vagina. By injecting local anesthetic submucosally into the fornix of the vagina, effective anesthesia during the first stage of labor can be attained. A paracervical block can also be used for anesthesia during cervical conization or ablation procedures if desired.

INDICATIONS

- First stage of labor
- Cervical conization or ablation procedures

CONTRAINDICATIONS

- Uteroplacental insufficiency
- Preexisting fetal distress
- Allergy to anesthetic agent
- Presence of infection

EQUIPMENT

- 10 cc syringe with finger rings
- Iowa trumpet with a 6-inch 20-gauge needle (a must during labor) (see Fig. 101-1) or a 3-inch needle extender on the end of a syringe with a 1½-inch 22-gauge needle
- Lidocaine* 1% (or chloroprocaine 1.5% or mepivacaine 1%)

---

*Volumes and doses are for 1% lidocaine (10 mg/cc) *without* epinephrine. Toxicity may occur with doses greater than 1 mg/kg (70 mg or 7 cc in a 70 kg patient), with rapid absorption, or with intravascular administration. Maximum dosage should not exceed 4.5 mg/kg or to a maximum of 30 cc of a 1% solution (300 mg), and maximum dose should not be repeated in less than 2 hours.

- Sterile gloves
- Antibacterial solution and sterile gauze pads
- Fetal heart monitor (if patient is pregnant)

PREPROCEDURE PATIENT EDUCATION

Obtain informed consent, and outline the possible complications, risks, benefits, and alternatives for anesthesia.

TECHNIQUE

1. Place the patient in the lithotomy position.
2. In the gravid patient, assess the cervix and proceed if dilation is 5 to 9 cm. If the cervix is dilated greater than 7 or 8 cm, proceed with caution to preclude injecting the fetal scalp.
3. Prepare the perineal area with an antibacterial solution.
4. Using your lubricated index and middle fingers as a guide, lay the trumpet against them, and insert it into the vagina.
5. Place the 20-gauge needle within the trumpet through the mucosa at the *cervicovaginal junction* at the 3 o'clock position. Use care not to insert the needle deeper than 0.5 cm into the tissue (Fig. 102-1). The positions of the paracervical nerves actually "migrate" superiorly during progressive dilation. In the nonpregnant cervix and in early labor, the nerves are located at the 4 and 8 o'clock positions, respectively. As dilation progresses, they are found more

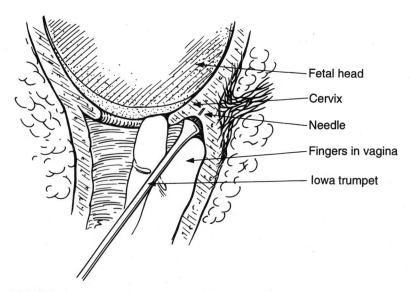

FIG. 102-1.
Technique of administering a paracervical block during labor using an Iowa trumpet.

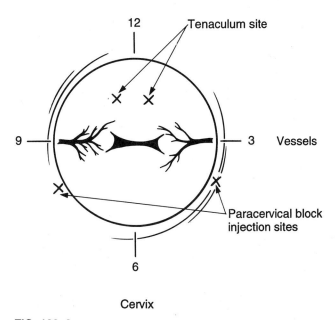

FIG. 102-2.
Paracervical block location in *nonpregnant* cervix.

in the 3 and 9 o'clock areas. Proper location of injection is important to gain maximum effect (Fig. 102-2).

6. After aspirating for blood, inject 5 to 10 cc of 1% lidocaine. (Alternatively, 2 to 3 cc may be placed in two or three locations around the estimated location of the nerve.)
7. Monitor the fetal heart rate for approximately 5 minutes. If no bradycardia is apparent, repeat the procedure on the contralateral side.
8. Monitor the fetal heart rate for 20 to 30 minutes, along with maternal blood pressure and pulse.

It may be necessary to repeat the procedure, depending on the duration of activity of the anesthetic agent. Good response is generally maintained for 45 to 75 minutes. The effect may only last 30 minutes, but it may also last for 90 minutes. If lidocaine is used, use no more than 30 cc of a 1% solution.

COMPLICATIONS

- Intravascular injection
- Intrafetal injection
- Idiosyncratic fetal bradycardia (Generally, there is no adverse outcome unless the child is delivered during the bradycardia. However, patients and physicians often experience significant anxiety for the 3 to 6 minutes it takes for this condition to resolve. This complication is rare but well known among

obstetricians. Despite the fact that it is not associated with adverse outcomes, this is the reason many of them choose not to use paracervical blocks.)
- Inhibits labor if given too soon

CPT/BILLING CODE

| 64435 | Paracervical block |

BIBLIOGRAPHY

Day T: Community use of paracervical block in labor, *JFP* 26:545, 1989.

Ostheimer GW: *Regional anesthesia techniques in obstetrics,* New York, 1980, Breon Laboratories.

Shnider SM, Levinson G: *Anesthesia for obstetrics,* ed 2, Baltimore, 1987, Williams & Wilkins.

CHAPTER 103

Cervical Ripening/Vaginal Prostaglandins

Scott T. Henderson

Various situations warrant the induction of labor, and traditional methods (oxytocin administration and amniotomy) are not always successful. This fact has led to other approaches for preinduction cervical ripening and induction of labor. One proven effective and safe method is the intravaginal application of dinoprostone (prostaglandin E_2 [PGE_2]). It has also been used intracervically.

A hospital protocol for PGE_2 administration should be written and followed. The protocol should include whether the patient should remain hospitalized or can go home if there is no uterine activity. The protocol should also allow the pharmacy to compound the gel.

INDICATIONS

- Postdates with unfavorable cervix (Bishop scoring of 4 or less)
- Chronic hypertension in pregnancy and indications for delivery
- Pregnancy-induced hypertension and indications for delivery
- Gestational or overt diabetes and indications for delivery
- Intrauterine growth retardation and indications for delivery
- Fetal demise

CONTRAINDICATIONS

- Nonreassuring fetal heart tracing
- Hypertonic or hyperactive uterine patterns
- Maternal fever
- Asthma
- Vaginal bleeding
- Allergy to prostaglandins
- Ruptured membranes
- When vaginal delivery is not indicated

EQUIPMENT

- PGE$_2$ gel (1.25 mg/5 cc; see compounding instructions below) in a 10 cc plastic syringe, or commercially available preparation
- Infant endotracheal tube (3 mm inner diameter) with proximal end removed (a normal intravenous catheter without needle works if gel is thin enough) **or** the commercially available Prepidil (Upjohn) 0.5 mg PGE$_2$ per 3.0 g (2.5 ml) in syringe supplied with 2 shielded catheters (10 and 20 mm tip)
- Sterile gloves
- Terbutaline 0.25 mg
- Fetal heart tone and uterine tocographic monitors
- *Optional:* heparin lock

COMPOUNDING INSTRUCTIONS

- Dinoprostone 20 mg suppository
- Sterile lubricating gel (K-Y Jelly) (80 cc)
- Methylene blue 1% solution
- 10 cc plastic syringe

To be done aseptically:

1. Slice the suppository into several pieces and place a drop of methylene blue solution onto each slice.
2. Mix until a smooth, uniform-color paste is formed.
3. Slowly add the lubricating gel to the paste, making a smooth, uniform-color gel without large suppository pieces visible.
4. Store the desired dose of gel in a 10 cc syringe (1 mg/4 cc).
5. Replace the cap of the syringe and store in a freezer for up to 90 days.

PREPROCEDURE PATIENT EDUCATION

Dinoprostone (Prepidil Gel) has recently been approved by the Food and Drug Administration. Review the possible complications with the patient, and be familiar with the package insert information.

TECHNIQUE

1. Thaw the PGE$_2$ for 1 to 2 hours before the procedure.
2. Apply an external fetal monitor. Obtain a nonstress test (NST) and assess for regular uterine contractions. If the NST is nonreactive or a normal uterine contraction pattern is noted, do not proceed.
3. *Optional:* Obtain intravenous access.
4. Connect the modified infant endotracheal tube or the appropriate shielded catheter (20 mm in length if no cervical effacement is present or 10 mm if

greater than 50% effacement on examination) to the filled syringe.

5. To properly administer the gel, the patient should be in a dorsal position with the cervix visualized, using a speculum.

6. *If a compounded gel is used*, attach the filled syringe to the tube. An air-filled syringe will be needed to express all the gel into the vagina or cervix.

   If a *commercial preparation is used*, use a gentle expulsion technique. The gel is easily extruded from the syringe. Use the contents of one syringe for one patient only. Do *not* attempt to administer the small amount of gel remaining in the catheter. The syringe, catheter, and any unused package contents should be discarded after use.

7. Insert the endotracheal tube or catheter into the vagina and express a total of 4 cc (1 mg) of PGE_2-prepared gel onto the exocervix and into the posterior vaginal fornix. (The commercially available preparation is packaged as a single 2.5 cc [0.5 mg] unit dose.) The endotracheal tube or catheter acts as a guide. Alternatively, the tube may be placed approximately 2 cm into the cervical canal with care not to pass beyond the internal cervical os. Instill 0.5 mg of PGE_2 gel into the cervical canal (Fig. 103-1). If the tube becomes disconnected, spread the contents of syringe onto the cervix with your fingers. Only if the prepared gel was used, apply the air-filled syringe, and push any remaining PGE_2 through the tube to make sure all PGE_2 is inserted.

8. The patient should remain supine for at least 15 to 30 minutes to minimize leakage from the cervical canal. Maintain external fetal monitoring for 2 hours following the installation. Monitoring may be discontinued after 2 hours if there is no uterine activity.

9. Have terbutaline 0.25 mg for subcutaneous injection at the patient's bedside in case of hyperstimulation. Reevaluate the cervix after 6 hours. If there is minimal change, the procedure may be repeated with a second dose.

Note: Once applied, PGE_2 cannot be removed or reduced as can oxytocin; therefore, if at all possible, hyperstimulation should be avoided. One method is to start slowly and, only if necessary, repeat the PGE_2 applications. The recommended repeat dose is 0.5 mg dinoprostone with a dosing interval of 6 hours. The maximum recommended cumulative dose for a 24-hour period is 1.5 mg of dinoprostone (6 cc of pharmacy preparation or 7.5 cc of Prepidil), although some clinicians will use up to double this amount.

For practical purposes, this procedure is done in the evening and overnight, with a planned oxytocin and/or amniotomy the following morning.

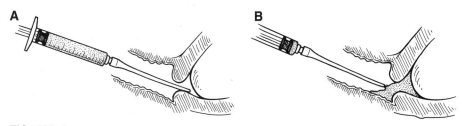

FIG. 103-1.
Application of PGE_2 gel intracervically (**A**) or intravaginally (**B**).

COMPLICATIONS

- Vomiting, fever, diarrhea (0.5% to 8%)
- Uterine hyperstimulation (0.5% to 5%): five or more contractions in 10 minutes or contractions lasting longer than 2 minutes
- Fetal heart rate abnormalities (*Treatment:* Position the patient on her left side. Administer an intravenous fluid bolus, and oxygen by mask. If necessary and not contraindicated, inject 0.25 mg of terbutaline subcutaneously or intravenously; this injection may be repeated once.)

CPT/BILLING CODE

59200   Insertion of cervical dilator (e.g., laminaria, prostaglandin), separate procedure

BIBLIOGRAPHY

Egarter C, Husslein P, Rayburn W: Uterine hyperstimulation after low-dose prostaglandin E$_2$ therapy: tocolytic treatment in 181 cases, *Am J Obstet Gynecol* 163:794, 1990.

Elliott JP, Clewell WH, Rodin TG: Intracervical prostaglandin E$_2$ gel: safety for outpatient cervical ripening before induction of labor, *J Reprod Med* 37(8):713, 1992.

Hayashi RH: Cervical ripening: advances in preinduction of labor (Proceedings from a round table discussion), *J Reprod Med* 1(Suppl): January 1993.

Rayburn W: Prostaglandin E$_2$ gel for cervical ripening and induction of labor: a critical analysis, *Am J Obstet Gynecol* 160:529, 1989.

Reilly KE: Induction of labor, *Am Fam Physician* 49(6):1427, 1994.

Trofatter KF: Preinduction cervical ripening, *Female Patient* 19:15, 1994.

CHAPTER 104

Obstetric Ultrasound

Richard Brunader

Ultrasound is defined as the range of sound waves with frequencies greater than 20,000 hertz, which are undetectable by the human ear. Most ultrasound scanners utilize frequencies of 1 to 10 megahertz, and 3.5 to 5 megahertz is the most commonly employed frequency range for obstetric examinations.

In 1984, the National Institutes of Health sponsored a Consensus Development Conference to evaluate the use of ultrasound in pregnancy and concluded that routine screening was not currently justified. This is supported by the position of the American College of Obstetrics and Gynecology (ACOG). A very recent study also supports this finding (Ewigman). However, other authorities feel this study lacks statistical power or may actually demonstrate *effectiveness* of routine ultrasound. The Royal College of Obstetricians and Gynecologists and the European Committee for Ultrasound Radiation Safety endorse routine prenatal ultrasound examinations. Ultrasound is routinely used in several European countries, including Sweden and Germany.

INDICATIONS

- Estimation of gestational age
- Evaluation of fetal growth
- Vaginal bleeding of undetermined etiology during pregnancy
- Determination of fetal presentation
- Suspected multiple gestation
- Adjunct to amniocentesis
- Significant uterine size–dates discrepancy
- Pelvic mass
- Suspected hydatidiform mole
- Adjunct to cervical cerclage placement
- Suspected ectopic pregnancy

- Adjunct to special procedure:
  In-vitro fertilization
  Embryo transfer
  Chorionic villous sampling
- Suspected fetal death
- Suspected uterine abnormality
- Intrauterine contraceptive device localization
- Ovarian follicle development surveillance for infertility
- Biophysical profile
- Observation of intrapartum events:
  Management of second twin
  Manual removal of placenta
- Suspected polyhydramnios or oligohydramnios
- Suspected abruptio placentae
- Adjunct to external version
- Estimation of fetal weight, fetal presentation in premature rupture of membranes, or in preterm labor
- Abnormal serum α-fetoprotein values
- Follow-up observation of identified anomaly
- Follow-up evaluation of placenta location for identified placenta previa
- History of previous congenital anomaly
- Serial evaluation of fetal growth in multiple gestation
- Evaluation of fetal condition in late registrants for prenatal care
- Evaluation of presenting fetal part

CONTRAINDICATIONS

- Maternal refusal

  Note: After many years, no study of safety has ever indicated more than a theoretical risk to the fetus from routine ultrasound scanning (see Complications). Contraindications may apply with routine scanning if studies fail to indicate improved outcomes.

ULTRASOUND GUIDELINES

Obstetric ultrasound can be performed either transabdominally (TAUS) or transvaginally (TVUS). Transvaginal scanning is performed primarily in the first trimester and generally enables visualization of structures 1 week earlier (gestational age) than transabdominal scanning.

Adequate documentation of the study is essential. This should include a permanent record of the ultrasound images that incorporate the measured parameters and anatomical findings.

The success of ultrasound detection of anomalies in high-risk patients can be excellent, but is technician- or physician-dependent. Even when scanning is performed specifically to detect fetal anomalies, serious birth defects can be missed.

No studies have evaluated the detection rate of anomalies in non–high-risk patients, where the prevalence of major defects is 0.4%. These facts should be kept in mind when discussing the results with the patient.

Obstetric ultrasound studies are defined as either *basic* (survey) or *targeted*. A targeted evaluation is performed to search for fetal anomalies. It should be considered for a patient who is suspected of carrying a physiologically or anatomically defective fetus. Often, basic studies will identify a need for a more-targeted study.

First Trimester Ultrasonography Documentation

1. Document the location of the gestational sac. If possible, identify the embryo and record the crown-rump length.
2. Report the presence or absence of fetal life.
3. Document fetal number. (This portion of the study deserves special attention. It is very easy to overlook a second gestational sac in first trimester scans.)
4. Perform an evaluation of the uterus (including the cervix) and adnexal structures.

Second and Third Trimester Ultrasonography Documentation

1. Document fetal life, number, and presentation.
2. Report an estimate of the amount of amniotic fluid.
3. Record the placental location and determine its relationship to the internal cervical os.
4. Assess gestational age using a combination of biparietal diameter (or head circumference) and femur length. Assess fetal growth (as opposed to age) by considering the abdominal circumference measurements. If previous studies have been performed, give an estimate of the appropriateness of interval growth.
5. Perform an evaluation of the uterus and adnexal structures.
6. The study should include, but not necessarily be limited to, the following fetal anatomy: cerebral ventricles, spine, stomach, urinary bladder, umbilical cord insertion site on the anterior abdominal wall, and renal region.

Note: These guidelines represent antepartum scans as defined by the American Institute of Ultrasound in Medicine (AIUM), American College of Obstetrics and Gynecology (ACOG), and the American College of Radiology (ACR).

TECHNIQUE

Measurements

The biparietal diameter, abdominal circumference, and femur length are measured as the basis of most obstetric ultrasound evaluations. Early in pregnancy, crown-rump length and gestational sac measurements are also important. Early developmental landmarks may offer an additional method of estimating gestational age (Table 104-1).

TABLE 104-1.

Developmental Landmarks by Abdominal Ultrasound

Landmark	Occurence from LMP
Visualization of gestational sac	5-6 weeks
Embryonic pole	6-7 weeks
Fetal heart motion	7-8 weeks
Fetal movement	8-9 weeks
BPD measurable	12-13 weeks

1. Crown-rump length (CRL)
   a. Formula:
      Gestational age [weeks] = (CRL [mm] + 65)/10.
   b. The CRL is the longest length of the fetus, excluding the fetal limbs, and its determination is part of the most accurate sonographic technique for establishing gestational age. One should average crown-rump measurements from three satisfactory images.
   c. Transabdominally, CRL is most accurate between 9 and 13 weeks. Even more accurate is CRL by transvaginal scanning between 7 and 9 weeks. The greatest problem in measurement by transabdominal scanning earlier than 9 weeks lies in knowing whether the maximum longitudinal diameter of the fetus has actually been measured. After 12 to 13 weeks, the fetus no longer is easily measurable in a straight line because it is more likely to flex or extend (Fig. 104-1).
2. Gestational sac (GS) diameter
   a. Formula:
      Gestational age [weeks] = (Avg GS [mm] + 25.43)/7.02.
   b. The GS measurement is not the best value to use for estimating gestational age and it should be used only if no other dating parameters are available.

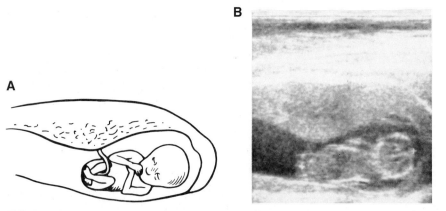

FIG. 104-1.
Measurement of the crown-rump length. **A**, 12- to 13-week fetus. **B**, Ultrasound scan showing the longest length of a 12-week fetus. Measurement is made from the top of the crown (head) to the bottom of the rump.

c. The gestational sac consists of a hypoechogenic area, which corresponds to the chorionic vesicle, and an echogenic rim or ring, which corresponds to the trophoblast. The gestational sac of a *normal* pregnancy may also be characterized by a *double echogenic ring*. The inner ring is the decidua capsularis plus the chorion laevae. The outer ring is the decidua vera. At the implantation site, the hyperechoic rim is thicker, and it comprises the decidua basalis and chorion frondosum (Fig. 104-2).

d. The presence of a true in-utero gestational sac confirms intrauterine pregnancy and indirectly excludes ectopic gestation. In some cases, however, it can be difficult to differentiate between the gestational sac seen with early intrauterine pregnancy and the *pseudogestational sac* (see First-Trimester Scanning) occasionally seen with ectopic pregnancy. A true sac will also contain a yolk sac and display a double echogenic ring sign (Fig. 104-3).

Note: This method of exclusion of ectopic pregnancy may not be helpful for patients taking ovulation-induction medications for fertility (see First-Trimester Scanning).

e. The sac is measured inside the hyperechoic rim, including only the anechoic (dark or fluid-filled) space. If the sac is round, only one dimension is needed; if ovoid, three measurements are taken and an average diameter calculated (Avg GS).

The First Trimester

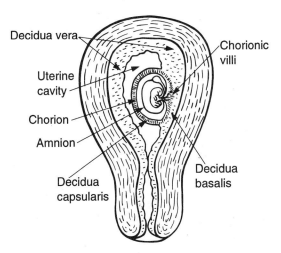
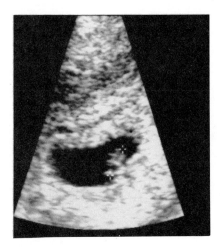

FIG. 104-2.
Medical illustration accompanying a transvaginal photograph detailing an early gestation. The decidua capsularis and the decidua vera form the double echogenic ring. The photograph contains a fetal pole with a 7.0 mm crown-rump length, which corresponds to a 6-week gestation. Pregnancies earlier than 5 weeks by transvaginal scanning and 6 weeks by transabdominal scanning generally do not show a fetal pole. Usually, only a hypoechogenic area corresponding to the chorionic vesicle is seen at this age.

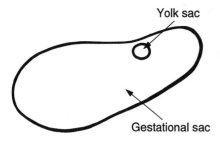

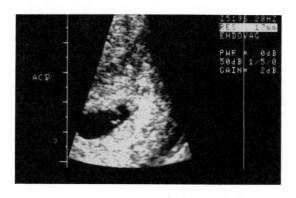

FIG. 104-3.
Gestational sac with yolk sac on transvaginal ultrasound. A yolk sac is generally first seen at about 5 weeks' gestation by transvaginal scanning and 6 to 7 weeks' gestation by transabdominal scanning. Its presence confirms an intrauterine gestation, but does not rule out a concomitant ectopic pregnancy.

3. Biparietal diameter (BPD)
   a. The BPD is ideally measured when the fetus is lying in an occiput transverse position. In this position, it is the distance measured between the outer table of the proximal fetal skull and the inner table of the contralateral side of the skull. The most commonly accepted reference plane is a cross-section parallel to the canthomeatal line and slightly above it. This cross-sectional plane cuts through the falx cerebrei, the thalamus, the cavum septum pellucidum, the medial cerebral artery. The head shape should be oval at this plane.
   b. The BPD is one of the only outer-to-inner diameter measurements utilized in all of sonography because the posterior calvarium causes a lot of artifact and thus tends to distort outer-to-outer measurements (Fig. 104-4).
4. Head circumference (HC)
   a. Formula:
   HC = 1.57 (BPD + occipital-frontal diameter [OFD]).

   Note: Some use HC = 1.57 (BPD + 0.3 cm + OFD) because of the manner in which BPD is measured.

   b. Prenatal molding of the fetal skull is common and may result in an inaccurate determination of the BPD. The cephalic index (CI) (the ratio of the BPD to the OFD) can be used to screen for cranial shape abnormalities. To obtain the ratio, the OFD is measured in the same plane as the BPD. Each diameter measurement should be made from its outer-to-outer aspect. The CI is a constant throughout pregnancy. The normal value is 78.3% ± 8% (±2 SD). Values below this normal range indicate a dolichocephalic head (an ellipse with a BPD that is shorter than expected or "too flat"). Values

A

C-Septi cavum pellucidi
F-Falx cerebrei
T-Thalami

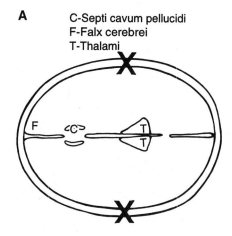

B

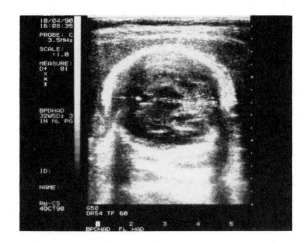

FIG. 104-4.
A, Biparietal diameter (BPD) is measured from outer to inner aspects of the skull. **B,** Ultrasound view of the fetal cranium at the proper level for a BPD, the level of the cavum septum pellucidum and thalamus.

above this normal range indicate a brachycephalic head (an ellipse with a BPD that is longer than expected or "too round").

c. If the CI is significantly above or below the normal range, the BPD might not be a reliable method for estimating gestational age. Instead, the HC should be used for estimating gestational age.

5. Abdominal circumference (AC)

a. Formula:

AC = 1.57 (D_1 + D_2).

(D_1, first diameter; D_2, second diameter)

b. Measurements of the AC are outer-to-outer diameter measurements.

c. Two diameters, the anteroposterior abdominal diameter and the transverse abdominal diameter, are taken at the level of the junction of the umbilical vein and the left portal vein, which appears as an echolucent structure shaped like a hockey stick. These diameters should be at right angles to each other, and the plane in which they are taken should be at a right angle with the fetal spine.

d. For estimating gestational age, the AC is only useful when no clinically apparent maternal or fetal conditions are present that would modify liver growth. It is most useful for establishing gestational age in midgestation and late pregnancy (Fig. 104-5).

6. Femur length (FL)

a. The central diaphysis of the shaft of the femur should be measured. This is not necessarily the largest or longest measurement that can be obtained. The longest measurement may include the femoral neck, which if included would overestimate the true value (Fig. 104-6).

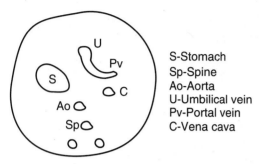
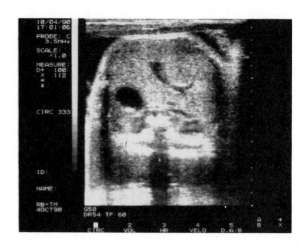

S-Stomach
Sp-Spine
Ao-Aorta
U-Umbilical vein
Pv-Portal vein
C-Vena cava

FIG. 104-5.
Abdominal circumference (AC). This third trimester cross-section of the fetal abdomen shows the junction of the umbilical vein and left portal vein. The stomach is seen on the left side of the fetus.

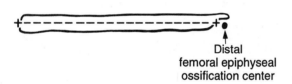

Distal
femoral epiphyseal
ossification center

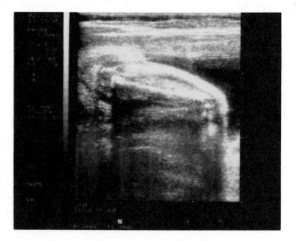

FIG. 104-6.
Femur length. This third trimester femur is measured along the central shaft of the diaphysis. On the right is the echogenic distal femoral epiphyseal ossification center, which indicates a gestational age of 33 weeks or more.

Fetal Body Ratios

1. Cephalic index (CI). See previous discussion.
2. HC/AC. This ratio has a sensitivity of 70% for detecting asymmetric intrauterine growth retardation (IUGR), but has high false-positive results when utilized for screening in a general population. The HC/AC is normally greater than 1 until approximately 36 to 38 weeks' gestation. At that point, it falls to 1 or below and remains at that level until delivery. This method fails to detect symmetric IUGR.

3. FL/AC. The FL/AC ratio will not detect symmetric IUGR, but is sensitive for asymmetric IUGR. This ratio has the further advantage of having normal-range values that do not change after 20 weeks. The normal value for this ratio expressed as a percentage is 22 ± 2% (±2 SD). A value greater than 24% indicates IUGR. A value less than 20.5% is suggestive of macrosomia. However, although this is a very useful ratio, the predictive power for screening a general population is only 25%, and the sensitivity is less than 50%.
4. FL/BPD. After 22 weeks' gestational age, the FL/BPD ratio is almost constant, with a normal range of 79% ± 8% (±2 SD) from 22 to 40 weeks, and a 90% confidence interval. The FL/BPD has three important uses: (1) the evaluation of the ultrasound examination for measurement error, (2) the detection of disease of the fetal head and limbs, and (3) the classification of IUGR.

Ultrasonographic Dating

1. Because of biologic variability, the gestational age can be estimated clinically with only 90% certainty to within 3 weeks by even the best methods (using last menstrual period, date when uterus reaches umbilicus, first-heard fetal heart tones, fundal height, and/or quickening). Ultrasonographic dating early in pregnancy may offer improved estimates over these traditional methods.
2. Ultrasound-determined size of certain measurable body parts correlates with gestational age. In general, growth is quite uniform in the first 20 weeks of gestation. Thereafter, the progressive increase in variability makes estimation of gestational age difficult (Table 104-2).
3. When reporting ultrasound estimates of age, it is very important to understand the variability that can be associated even with these estimates. The variability is usually expressed as plus or minus 2 standard deviations (± 2 SD), which

TABLE 104-2.

Outline of Ultrasonographic Dating of Pregnancy

Weeks of Gestation	Recommended Dating Measurement	Accuracy
3-5	None	
5-6	GS	± 1 week
6-12	CRL	±3-5 days
12-20	BPD	± 1 week
	FL	± 1 week
20-30	BPD	± 2 weeks
	FL	± 2 weeks
	AC	± 3 weeks
30-40	BPD	± 3 weeks
	FL	± 3 weeks
	AC	± 3.5 weeks

For gestational age of 20 to 40 weeks, more accurate data are currently being developed. These measurements can be quite variable and operator-dependent after 20 weeks.

should be applicable to 95% of fetuses in a normal population. Reporting a single age estimate for a given fetal measurement gives a false impression about the accuracy of the method. Thus, the variability of the estimate (in SD) should be given as well.

4. Pregnancy dating often utilizes a method of *averaging estimates of age* based on BPD, AC, HC, and FL. (See Box 104-1 for suggestions as to which parameters to use with each stage of pregnancy). Any of the measurements may be technically incorrect. However, it is unlikely that all four measurements will be incorrectly measured in the same direction. Therefore, using averages, measurement errors tend to be somewhat self-canceling and lead to a more accurate overall estimate of gestational age.

5. In using the multiple-parameter dating approach or when averaging estimates of age, it is critical to avoid using measurements when they might be affected by a pathologic process in the fetus, such as hydrocephaly and microcephaly, macrosomia or IUGR, and fetal dwarfism. After 22 weeks' gestational age, one can minimize potential errors by making certain that the fetal body ratios are within normal limits (see Fetal Body Ratios). If the CI indicates a normally shaped head, the FL/BPD ratio can be measured. If the FL/BPD ratio is below 70%, one should eliminate the FL; and if the ratio is above 86%, one should discard the fetal head measurements. If the FL/BPD ratio is normal, one can measure the FL/AC ratio. If the FL/AC ratio is less than 20%, one should not use the AC because of possible macrosomia; if the ratio is above 24%, one should avoid using the AC because of possible IUGR.

Placental Imaging

1. Maturational changes of the placenta occur in its three basic anatomic areas (the amniochorionic plate, the placental body, and the basal layer) and form the basis for the following grading system of placental maturity (Fig. 104-7):

Grade 0:
Placenta has a chorionic plate that is very smooth. The placental substance is homogenous and without calcifications.

Grade I:
There is some undulation in the chorionic plate, and scattered echogenic areas parallel to the long axis of the placenta represent calcification within the placental substance. These echoes are high-amplitude, bright, white, and linear or comma-shaped.

**BOX 104-1. INDICATED DATING PARAMETERS
BASED ON GESTATIONAL AGE**

From 7 to 10 weeks:	GS and CRL
From 11 to 14 weeks:	CRL, BPD, and FL
From 15 to 28 weeks:	BPD, HC, FL, and AC
After 28 weeks:	BPD (with CI), HC, FL, and AC

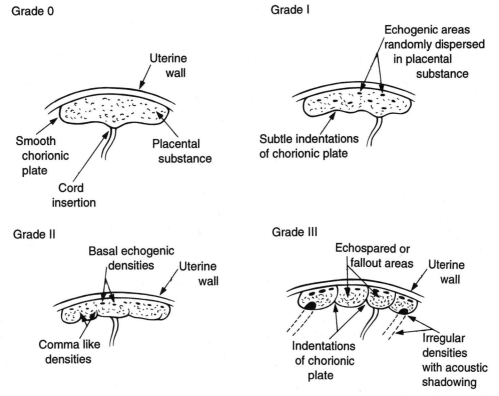

FIG. 104-7.
The four grades of placental maturity.

Grade II:
The chorionic plate has more indentations, but they do not reach the basal plate. The Grade II placenta is characterized by a straight line of echos with calcifications present along the axis of the basal plate.

Grade III:
The chorionic plate indentations reach the basal plate. There is complete compartmentalization of the placenta with extensive echogenic areas representing calcifications. They may cast shadows.

2. Grade 0 is most common in the first trimester; Grade I appears after 14 weeks' gestation and is most common until around 34 weeks. Grade II first appears after 26 weeks' gestation and is most common at around 36 weeks. Grade III most commonly appears beyond 35 weeks' gestation. However, these are very crude measurements. Even with a Grade III placenta, there is a 4% chance of fetal pulmonary immaturity.

3. A Grade II placenta before 26 to 32 weeks or a Grade III placenta before 36 weeks is abnormal.

4. Intrauterine growth retardation, oligohydramnios, and hypertension are associated with accelerated placenta maturation. Diabetes mellitus and Rh factor

sensitization are associated with delayed maturation. Preeclampsia or pregnancy-induced hypertension does not affect placental maturation.

5. The principal purposes of the ultrasound examination for bleeding in the second and third trimesters are to delineate the placental implantation site to exclude placenta previa and to attempt to determine if there has been an abruptia. Placental abruption may be difficult to see on ultrasound.

Amniotic Fluid

1. The American College of Radiology guidelines on amniotic fluid volume (AFV) estimation require only qualitative assessment; however, the reliability and reproducibility of subjective scales are heavily dependent on operator experience.

2. Calculating the amniotic fluid index (AFI) is a quantitative approach to measuring the AFV. The uterus is divided into four quadrants. The ultrasound transducer is then held in a vertical and sagittal alignment (marker dot on the probe on cephalad aspect of probe). The transducer is kept perpendicular to the plane of the floor and aligned longitudinally with the patient's spine. The pocket of fluid with the largest vertical dimension is identified and measured in the vertical dimension. This procedure is repeated in each quadrant and the values summed.

3. Polyhdramnios
   a. In nondiabetic populations, polyhydramnios is defined as an AFI of 24 cm or more.
   b. The most likely etiology is idiopathic (34.6%), followed by diabetes mellitus (24.6%), congenital anomalies (20.1%), erythroblastosis fetalis (11.5%), and multiple gestation (9.2%).
   c. Once identified, a patient with an AFI of 24 cm or more should have a detailed ultrasound examination to rule out fetal anomalies.

4. Oligohydramnios
   a. Oligohydramnios is defined as an AFI less than 5.
   b. Excluding patients with premature rupture of membranes, approximately 83% of patients with oligohydramnios will have fetal IUGR; however, only approximately 16% of patients carrying a fetus with IUGR will have oligohydramnios.
   c. Fetal weight should be calculated whenever oligohydramnios is present.
   d. Premature rupture of membranes can cause severe oligohydramnios or anhydramnios.
   e. Fetal causes of oligohydramnios are usually related to urinary tract anomalies.

Fetal Assessment (Biophysical Profile [BPP])

1. A combination of biophysical variables (the BPP) was first introduced by Manning in 1980. The most important factor in the sensitivity of this testing method is the combination of *acute* (fetal heart rate [FHR] reactivity, fetal movement [FM], fetal breathing movement [FBM], and fetal tone [FT]) and *chronic* (amniotic fluid volume) markers of fetal condition.

2. A normal BPP is indirect evidence that each of the portions of the central nervous system that control particular activities are functioning and, therefore, that the fetus is nonhypoxemic. The absence of a given BPP activity, however, is difficult to interpret because it may reflect either pathologic depression or normal periodicity.

3. In chronic sustained fetal hypoxia, a protective redistribution of the fetal cardiac output may occur, with blood being directed away from nonvital fetal organs (kidney and lung) and toward vital fetal organs (heart, brain, and adrenals). This leads to decreased urine production and oligohydramnios.

4. A fetal BPP score of 8 or more is reassuring of fetal well-being; however, a BPP score of less than 8 is nonreassuring, and repeat testing or delivery is indicated. The presence of oligohydramnios constitutes an abnormal biophysical assessment regardless of the overall score (Table 104-3).

Fetal Size

1. Many formulas are available for prediction of fetal weight. These formulas are based on a variety of combinations of BPD, HC, AC, and FL. The predictive accuracy of these formulas ranges from 14.8% to 20.2% (± 2 SD).

2. Discordancy between size and dates should arouse suspicion of specific disorders, depending on gestational age. In early pregnancy, multiple gestation, a hydatidiform mole, incorrect menstrual history, and genetic or developmental defects should be suspected. Later in pregnancy, fetal malposition, IUGR, fetal

TABLE 104-3.

Fetal BPP Scoring According to Manning

Variable	Score 2	Score 0
FBM	The presence of at least 30 sec of sustained FBM in 30 min of observation	< 30 sec of FBM in 30 min
FM	Three or more gross body movements in 30 min of observation; simultaneous limb and trunk movements are counted as a single movement	Two or fewer gross body movements in 30 min of observation
FT	At least one episode of motion of a limb from a position of flexion to extension and a rapid return to flexion	Fetus in a position of semi- or full-limb extension with no return to flexion with movement; absence of fetal movement is counted as absent tone
Fetal reactivity	The presence of two or more FHR accelerations of at least 15 bpm and lasting at least 15 sec and associated with FM in 40 min	No acceleration or less than two accelerations of the fetal heart rate in 40 min of observation
Qual AF volume	A pocket of amniotic fluid that measures at least 1 cm in two perpendicular planes	Largest pocket of amniotic fluid measures < 1 cm in two perpendicular planes
Maximal score	10	—
Minimal score	—	0

dysmaturity, genetic or developmental defects, multiple gestation, fetal macrosomia, and abnormal amniotic fluid volume should be suspected.

Intrauterine Growth Retardation (IUGR)

1. Clinical signs of IUGR include poor increase in both fundal height and maternal weight gain. However, diagnosis of IUGR by clinical means is only possible in approximately 33% of pregnancies.
2. By comparison, a diagnosis of IUGR by ultrasound is much more accurate than clinical diagnosis. With ultrasound, sensitivities and specificities are variable, so ultrasound information should be correlated with clinical data for patients in whom IUGR is suspected. The combination of information significantly improves a clinician's ability to screen for IUGR.
3. Ultrasound parameters important in evaluation of IUGR are
   a. Oligohydramnios.
      i. For the general population the sensitivity of oligohydraminos in the diagnosis of IUGR is approximately 16%.
      ii. For high-risk populations, the predictive value and sensitivity of oligohydramnios is enhanced. If oligohydramnios is present and there is no evidence of premature rupture of membranes or congenital anomalies, IUGR is the likely etiology.
   b. BPD. Determination of the BPD is not very helpful. With symmetric IUGR, both head and body measurements fall off the growth curve together and result in an erroneous estimate of gestational age. In asymmetric IUGR, the BPD remains normal until late gestation.
   c. HC. The HC is a more shape-independent measurement of fetal head size than the BPD. In cases of cranial shape abnormalities, its inclusion in the growth profile will significantly decrease the high incidence of false-positive results seen when the BPD alone is used. However, because IUGR may not selectively affect brain and head growth, or is relatively "head-sparing," this alone is also not a very useful measurement. The HC is most useful when it is used in combination with another measurement as a ratio.
   d. FL. The FL can also can be misleading. In asymmetric IUGR, FL is more accurate and will parallel gestational age calculated from the last normal menstrual period. In this case, it may be helpful. In symmetric IUGR, all measurements will be small and result in an erroneously early gestational age estimate. FL is most useful for prediction of IUGR when it is used in a ratio.
   e. AC. The AC is very useful for assessing fetal nutritional status. The AC involves measurement of the liver, which is smaller in chronic hypoxia and with low levels of substrate (glycogen); thus, the AC is the best single predictor of IUGR.
   f. Calculation of fetal body ratios (see Fetal Body Ratios).
   g. Placental grade. When fetal growth pattern and estimated weight suggest a small fetus, the finding of a Grade III placenta can be used as adjunctive evidence of IUGR.

4. Suspect IUGR by ultrasound if
   a. AC falls in the lower 15th percentile.
   b. Weight falls in the lower 15th percentile.
   c. FL/AC $\geq$ 23.5%.
   d. HC/AC $\geq$ 95%.
5. When gestational age cannot be established by the menstrual history, the assessment of fetal risk for IUGR must rely on fetal disproportionality for the determination of asymmetric IUGR, and on serial assessments of fetal growth for symmetric IUGR. Symmetric IUGR may be very difficult to diagnose without serial ultrasound studies.
6. Newer techniques being evaluated for identifying IUGR include Doppler ultrasonography of the umbilical artery waveforms, and use of a M-mode echocardiogram of the fetal heart.

Macrosomia

1. Fetal macrosomia is defined in absolute terms as a fetal weight greater than 4000 gm. However, macrosomia is also considered when a fetal weight falls in the upper 90th percentile for any gestational age time during pregnancy.
2. Symmetric macrosomia occurs when the excessive fetal weight is the result of proportionate growth of all fetal parameters, for example, the fetus with weight, length, and head size all above the 90th percentile for age. Symmetric macrosomia is usually the result of prolonged gestation or a consequence of genetic growth. The HC/AC and the FL/AC ratios are usually within the normal range for age.
3. Asymmetric macrosomia generally occurs in patients with class A to C diabetes mellitus. Although the values of HC and FL are higher than average, they usually fall below the 90th percentile for age. The excessive weight results from profound increases in soft tissue mass that are reflected by an AC and estimated fetal weight above the 90th percentile. The HC/AC and the FL/AC ratios usually fall below the 10th percentile for age.

Preterm Labor

1. Preterm labor is defined as the onset of labor prior to a gestational age of 37 weeks. Preterm labor affects 10% of pregnancies and it accounts for 75% of perinatal morbidity and mortality.
2. Ultrasound parameters important in the evaluation of preterm labor include
   a. Fetal number. Multiple gestations have an increased risk of preterm labor.
   b. Estimated fetal weight. Preterm labor is associated with IUGR.·
   c. Amniotic fluid index. Preterm labor is associated with both oligohydramnios and polyhydramnios.
   d. Biophysical profile score. A low BPP may contraindicate tocolysis.
   e. Other possible contraindications to tocolysis:
      i. Fetal malformations.
      ii. Evidence of concealed abruption.
   f. Ultrasonic cervical evaluation.

    i. Cervical shortening (present if the distance from internal os to the leading edge of the portio vaginalis is less than 3 cm).

    ii. Dilation of the endocervical canal (present if the maximal diameter of the endocervical canal exceeds 1 cm).

    iii. Bulging of the fetal membranes into the endocervical canal (conical rather than rounded shape of the isthmic region).

    iv. Thinning of the lower uterine segment (anterior wall thickness less than 0.6 cm).

Postdates Pregnancy

1. Expected date of confinement is defined as 40 weeks (280 days) from the first day of the last normal menstrual period, or 266 days following ovulation, providing cycles are regular and occur at 28-day intervals. Normal term ranges from 38 to 42 weeks.

2. A postdates pregnancy is one with a duration that has exceeded 42 weeks (294 days) from the last normal menstrual period, assuming a 28-day cycle.

3. In a recent study, the incidence of postdates pregnancies was overestimated by 7.5% when gestational age was estimated using the menstrual history; but it fell to 2.6% when using early ultrasound examination, and to 1.1% when only considering patients for whom both menstrual *and* early ultrasound estimations of gestational age exceeded 293 days.

4. Complications detectable by ultrasound include
   a. Physiologic oligohydramnios (detectable by AFV determination).
   b. Macrosomia (detectable by calculation of estimated fetal weight).
   c. Dysmaturity due to chronic uteroplacental insufficiency (detectable by evidence of asymmetric IUGR).
   d. Congenital anomalies (detectable by anatomic survey).
   e. Ill-advised labor induction (preventable by good dating).

5. The contraction stress test is still regarded as the most reliable method of antenatal surveillance for the postdates pregnancy. However, the results of biweekly nonstress tests performed in conjunction with ultrasound scanning of AFV are comparable to those of the contraction stress test. Both are characterized by minimal morbidity and mortality, but high intervention and cesarean section rates.

First-Trimester Scanning

1. The most frequent causes of bleeding in the first trimester are
   a. Unknown causes
   b. Blighted ovum
   c. Threatened/missed abortion
   d. Ectopic pregnancy
   e. Abortion of one member of a multiple gestation
   f. Hydatidiform mole

2. When evaluating for ectopic pregnancy by transabdominal scanning, the classic finding of an extrauterine gestational sac is seen in only 10% to 15%

of cases (rates are higher with transvaginal scanning). Ultrasound is more helpful in *excluding* the diagnosis of ectopic pregnancy by demonstrating an intrauterine gestation, since a simultaneous extrauterine and intrauterine gestation (combination pregnancy) occurs only once in every 7000 to 8000 pregnancies.*

3. The sonographic appearance of a gestational sac can be mimicked by the exfoliation of hyperplastic endometrium associated with an ectopic pregnancy. This sonographic finding, which can appear very similar to a gestational sac, is known as a *pseudogestational sac*. A pseudogestational sac occurs in approximately 10% of ectopic pregnancies. Thus, the unequivocal diagnosis of an intrauterine pregnancy should not be made until two concentric rims, and a fetal pole, a yolk sac, or fetal heart activity can be identified within the sac.

4. In a normal pregnancy, the mean serum human chorionic gonadotropin (HCG) doubling time is 1.98 days. If serial HCG titers show a plateau or fall, an abnormal (ectopic) or nonviable pregnancy is likely.

   There are two common standards for the measurement of HCG activity, the Second International Standard (2nd IS), also known as the 2nd International Reference Preparation (2nd IRP), instituted in 1964, and the International Reference Preparation (1st IRP), instituted in 1974.

   Note: Most hospital laboratories are currently using the 2nd IS.

   It is difficult to convert one standard to the other, but the number of HCG units using the IRP Standard (1st IRP) is approximately twice that of the 2nd IS (2nd IRP). There are many reasons variations can exist between institutions when measuring HCG. Purity differences among test kits (different manufacturers) contribute to variations in measurement. Variations even exist in the same laboratory in different runs, or occasionally in the same run. Thus, with this much variation using a given standard, it is important to be aware of which standard is being employed when correlating the sonographic findings with the quantitative HCG levels. Various studies correlating sonographic findings with quantitative HCG levels have compounded the confusion by referring to misnamed reference standards.

5. With a high-quality machine and an experienced well-trained sonographer, one should lower the threshold (level of HCG) of when to expect to see a gestational sac.

6. Optimally, each institution should correlate its ultrasound equipment and sonographers' skills with quantitative HCG levels obtained from its own reference laboratory. When this is accomplished, externally published quantitative HCG reference levels and expected ultrasound findings should be used only as rough guidelines. Current published quantitative HCG levels and ultrasound correlations are outlined in Tables 104-4 and 104-5.

7. If a gestational sac is absent at an HCG value above the institution's threshold, ectopic pregnancy, recent spontaneous abortion, and early hydatidiform

---

* The rate of combination pregnancies in women on ovulation-inducing drug therapy (clomiphene or human chorionic gonadotropin) can be as high as 1:100.

TABLE 104-4.

Possible Outcomes Based on Ultrasound and Quantitative HCG Correlations (2nd IRP)

HCG Concentration (mIU/ml)*	Detection of Gestational Sac (TAUS Examination)†	Significance
> 1800	+	Intrauterine pregnancy; if fetal pole or yolk sac is identified, no further evaluation is required. Ectopy is ruled out.
< 1800	+	Failed intrauterine pregnancy; ectopic pregnancy with pseudogestational sac; or very rarely, early pregnancy that may continue.
> 1800	–	Suspect ectopic pregnancy.
< 1800	–	Indeterminant. May be due to an intrauterine, ectopic or failed pregnancy. Follow HCG titer every 2 to 4 days. Normal HCG trends occur in 15% of ectopic pregnancies. Thus, as soon as the level crosses the threshold for the facility, repeat the ultrasound examination.

*Actual values will vary from institution to institution based on the particular assay used, quality of TAUS machine, and the skill of the ultrasonographer.
†With transvaginal scanning, the gestational sac can be detected at earlier gestational ages.

TABLE 104-5.

Expected Time of Seeing a Gestational Sac Under Optimal Scanning Conditions

HCG UNITS	TAUS	TVUS
1st IRP	3600 mIU/ml	2000mIU/ml
2nd IRP	1800 mIU/ml	1000 mIU/ml

*Actual level will vary from institution to institution based on the particular assay used, quality of TAUS and TVUS machines, and skill level of the ultrasonographer.

degeneration should be considered. Suspicion of an ectopic pregnancy should be even higher if there is significant fluid in the cul de sac.

8. Ultrasonic examination can be very helpful in evaluating whether tissue is remaining after a spontaneous abortion, in diagnosing the vanishing twin syndrome (abortion of one member of a multiple gestation), and in establishing fetal viability in threatened abortion. It is the procedure of choice for evaluation of gestational trophoblastic disease.

9. With ultrasonic examination alone a normal gestational sac can often be distinguished from an abnormal sac doomed to miscarriage, even before the embryo is visible. The size and appearance of the gestational sac should be evaluated according to certain *major* and *minor* criteria for normalcy. A gestational sac of abnormal size or appearance correlates highly with an abnormal outcome.

   a. Major criteria for a normal-appearing gestational sac:
      i. A sac of 25 mm or more in diameter must reveal an embryo within it.
      ii. The sac must be round in shape.
   b. Minor criteria for a normal appearing gestational sac:
      i. The gestational sac is located in the fundus of the uterus.
      ii. A thick, echogenic, decidual ring surrounds the sac.
      iii. There is evidence of the double ring sign.

10. When a sac with a mean diameter greater than 25 mm lacks an embryo or when the sac is grossly distorted, abnormal pregnancy is almost certain.Using these criteria, 76% of abnormal pregnancies and 93% of normal pregnancies will be correctly classified by only one ultrasound scan. Failure to meet any single major criterion or all three minor criteria will identify 53% of abnormal pregnancies, but will be 100% specific in predicting spontaneous abortion.

11. Once embryonic cardiac motion is seen on ultrasound, the likelihood of spontaneous abortion is reduced to 3% to 10%.

SUPPLIERS

Acuson
1220 Charleston Road
P.O. Box 7393
Mountain View, CA 94039
800-9-ACUSON

Advanced Technology Laboratories
22100 Bothell Highway, S.E.
P.O. Box 3003
Bothell, WA 98041
800-982-2011

Corometrics Medical Systems, Inc
61 Barnes Park Road North
Wallingford, CT 06492
800-243-3952

General Electric Medical Systems
General Electric Company
P.O. Box 414
Milwaukee, WI 53201
800-433-5566

Medison America
5319 Randall Place
Fremont, CA 94538
800-829-7666

Phillips Medical Systems of North America, Inc.
2722 South Fairview
Santa Ana, CA 92704
714-556-7608

Pie Medical, USA
3535 Route 66
Neptune, NJ 07753
800-235-5254

Siemens Burdick, Inc.
5399 Summerwood Court
Frederick, MD 21702
800-289-8688

PATIENT EDUCATION

Issues to be discussed with patients who undergo obstetric ultrasonography include

- Purpose of the examination
- Safety
- Detection of birth defects
- Accuracy of measurements
    Dating
    Estimated fetal weight

Having a handout for the patient to review prior to scanning can be quite helpful. Since fetal anomalies can remain undetected even by the best sonographer with the best equipment, the patient should never be unequivocably assured that the fetus is "fine." However, the patient can be reassured with answers to certain specific questions provided by the scan.

COMPLICATIONS

Although there are theoretical models in which ultrasound is potentially damaging to human fetuses, no proven harm to any human fetus or mother has been documented.

ENCOUNTER FORMS

Fig. 104-8 is a sample patient encounter form.

CPT/BILLING CODES

76805	Echography, pregnant uterus, B-scan and/or real time with image documentation; complete (complete fetal and maternal evaluation)
76810	Complete, multiple gestation, after the first trimester
76815	Limited (gestational age, heartbeat, placental location, fetal position, or emergency in the delivery room)
76816	Follow-up or repeat
76818	Fetal biophysical profile
76830	Echography, transvaginal

BIBLIOGRAPHY

Bowerman RA: *Atlas of normal fetal ultrasonography,* Chicago, 1986, Year Book Medical Publishers.

Callen PW, editor: *Ultrasonography in obstetrics and gynecology,* ed 2, Philadelphia, 1988, W.B. Saunders.

Connor PD, Deutchman ME, Hahn RG: Training in obstetric sonography in family medicine residency programs: results of a nationwide survey and suggestions for a teaching strategy, *J Am Board Fam Pract* 7:124, 1994.

Ewigman BG et al: Effect of prenatal ultrasound screening on perinatal outcome (radius study), *N Engl J Med* 329:821, 1993.

Sabbagha RE, editor: *Diagnostic ultrasound applied to obstetrics and gynecology,* ed 2, Philadelphia, 1987, J.B. Lippincott.

Sauerbrei EE, Nguyen KT, Nolan RL: *A practical guide to ultrasound in obstetrics and gynecology,* New York, 1987, Raven Press.

Table IV						PATIENT IDENTIFICATION:

PATIENT IDENTIFICATION:
Name_____

Age_____ DOB_____

PMD_____

OBSTETRIC ULTRASOUND

LMP_____EDC_____

Age	Gravidity	Term	Preterm	Abortion	Living	Parameter	Measurement	Gestational Age	Indices	
Reason for Exam						GEST SAC			CI	
Requested By						CRL			FL/ BPD	
Estimated Gestational Age at Exam						BPD			HC/ AC	
Number of Fetuses		Presentation				HC			FL/ AC	
Placental Location		Placental Grade				AC			Estimated Fetal Weight	

AFI =

Biophysical Profile Score =
- Movement _____
- Breathing _____
- Tone _____
- Fluid _____
- NST _____

❑ Septum Cavum Pellucidum
❑ Cisterna Magna
❑ Lateral Ventricle
❑ Extremities
❑ 4 Chamber Heart
❑ Stomach
❑ Fetal Kidneys
❑ Fetal Bladder
❑ Normal Abd. Wall
❑ Normal Spine
❑ 3-Vessel Cord

Parameter	Measurement	Gestational Age	Indices
FL			HC/ AC
TCD			AC/ FL
OTHER			AC/ BPD
	Estimated Fetal Age		Other
Estimated Fetal Weight	EFW	Percentile	

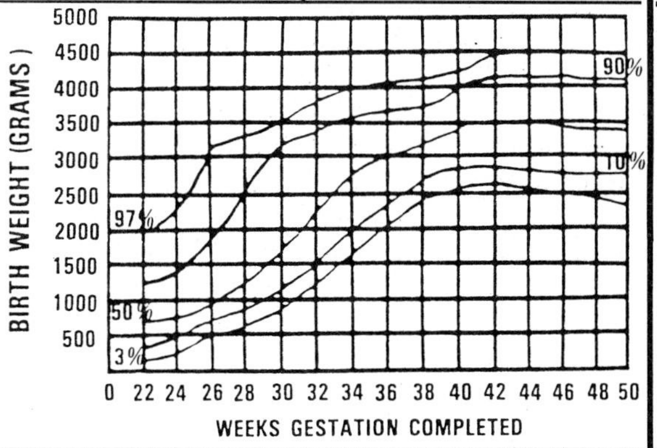

IMPRESSIONS/RECOMMENDATIONS:
_____
_____
_____
_____
_____
_____
_____
_____
_____

PREPARED BY:

(Signature and Title)

DATE OF EXAM:

FIG. 104-8.
Sample patient encounter form.

PART EIGHT

Pediatrics

CHAPTER 105

Intraosseous Venous Access

Kelly T. Locke

When immediate vascular access is needed in young children, intraosseous venous access (IVA) is an extremely low-risk, rapid, and reliable technique. Although IVA should only be considered for temporary measures, some centers use IVA first. IVA involves placement of a needle through the bone cortex into the medullary cavity, through which fluids or drugs may be infused. Originally described in 1922 and utilized during the 1940s, IVA fell into disfavor after improvements in intravenous (IV) catheters. The 1980s saw a resurgence of interest and reevaluation of this technique, and it continues to grow in popularity for pediatric emergencies.

Intravenous access with a catheter may require 10 minutes or more in 24% of children in cardiac arrest. With the proper equipment and training, intraosseous vascular access can usually be obtained in less than 5 minutes. Little training is needed, and IVA can be practiced on raw chicken drumsticks, swine ribs, or piglet tibias. The American Heart Association, the American College of Emergency Physicians, and the American Academy of Pediatrics all recognize and encourage IVA as an alternative to intravenous access in pediatric emergencies.

ADVANTAGES (OVER PERCUTANEOUS INTRAVENOUS TECHNIQUES)

- Rapid needle placement (vascular access in 30 to 60 seconds with 80% success rate)
- Low complication rate
- Immediate absorption of substances into the systemic circulation
- Same dosages, concentrations, and infusion rates for medications and fluids as IV administration (Box 105-1)
- Bone marrow aspirates obtained prior to fluid or drug infusion may be analyzed for chemistries, blood gases, hemoglobin, cross-matching, and cultures
- Serum drug concentrations with IVA remain elevated longer than intravenous administration

---

BOX 105-1. PRODUCTS ACCEPTABLE FOR INTRAOSSEOUS INFUSION

Drugs	**Solutions**
Antibiotics	Calcium gluconate
Atropine sulfate	Colloids
Dexamethasone sodium phosphate	Contrast media
Diazepam	Dextrose (D-glucose)
Diazoxide	Plasma
Digoxin	Ringer's lactate
Dobutamine	Sodium bicarbonate
Dopamine	Sodium chloride
Epinephrine	Whole blood
Heparin	Packed RBCs
Insulin	Parenteral nutrition
Lidocaine	
Morphine sulfate	
Phenytoin	
Succinylcholine	

DISADVANTAGES (OVER PERCUTANEOUS INTRAVENOUS TECHNIQUES)

- Initial peak serum concentration of medications may be less than that achieved with intravenous administration (This difference usually resolves within minutes.)
- Temporary nature of the procedure
- Limited infusion rates
- Rare complications that can be severe
- Patient age limitations

While the flow rate of IVA is slower than flows achieved through peripheral veins, a blood pressure cuff at 300 mm Hg pressure applied to the IV bag can provide rates of more than 24 cc/minute through a 20-gauge needle. The critical limiting factor for infusion rate appears to be marrow cavity size rather than needle size. Unfortunately, IVA is usually limited to young children, because much of red marrow has been replaced by the less vascular yellow marrow by approximately 5 years of age.

Certain physiologic principles make IVA possible. Venous circulation (Fig. 105-1) of blood through the long bones flows rapidly from the medullary venous sinusoids to the central venous sinus, and on to the nutrient and emissary veins. From there, it empties directly and rapidly into the systemic venous circulation. Complementing this circulatory pattern, the marrow cavity functions as a rigid vein that does not collapse with hypovolemia or peripheral circulatory shock, which makes IVA a consistent source of access.

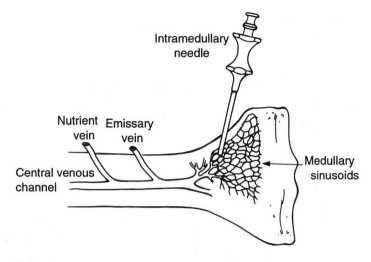

FIG. 105-1.
The intramedullary venous system. Position of intraosseous needle in the medullary sinusoids.

INDICATIONS

- Shock (due to infection, hemorrhage, burns, or severe dehydration)
- Cardiopulmonary arrest
- Lack of endotracheal tube placement for medication administration
- Administration of fluids contraindicated for endotracheal instillation (e.g., blood, sodium bicarbonate, dextrose, Ringer's lactate solution)
- Prolonged life-threatening status epilepticus
- Inability to obtain vascular access (e.g., due to obese or edematous extremities)
- Any emergency condition requiring immediate vascular access for stabilization

CONTRAINDICATIONS

Contraindications for IVA are few, and the risks and benefits should be considered when determining whether to use this route.

Relative contraindications include the following:

- Unsuccessful attempt in one leg (The other leg should then be attempted.)
- Compromised skin over selected site (burn or infection)
- Osteogenesis imperfecta (increased fracture risk)
- Osteopetrosis (increased fracture risk)
- Ipsilateral fracture of an extremity (increased risk of subcutaneous extravasation)
- Bacteremia (increased risk of bacterial seeding of the marrow space when the cortex is punctured)

EQUIPMENT

- Short, large-bore needle (16 to 18 gauge)

  1. Disposable intraosseous needle (preferred) (Fig. 105-2)
  2. 16- or 18-gauge hypodermic needle (Hypodermic needles without a stylet may become plugged with bone marrow. Inserting a second smaller-gauge needle through the lumen of the first needle may clear the obstruction.)
  3. Spinal needle with stylet (Spinal needles may bend or break due to their narrow gauge.)
  4. Bone marrow aspiration needle (Jamshidi)

- Sterile latex gloves
- Sterile drapes
- Antiseptic solution (povidone-iodine, chlorhexidine gluconate [Hibiclens], or alcohol)
- Local anesthetic solution (1% lidocaine)
- Two 5 cc syringes and 25-gauge needles for local anesthetic administration
- 10 cc syringe for aspirating the medullary contents
- Sterile saline (30 cc vial) (*optional:* heparinized saline)
- 10 cc syringe for sterile saline
- One dozen 2 × 2 inch gauze sponges
- Tape
- IV fluids and tubing
- Body or extremity restraint (helpful for uncooperative patients)

As this procedure regains popularity, more companies are marketing needles made especially for intraosseous infusion. Cook Critical Care (P.O. Box 489, Bloomington, IN 47402) offers intraosseous infusion sets.

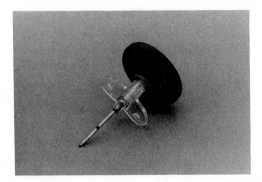

FIG. 105-2.
Intraosseous infusion needle. (Courtesy of Cook Critical Care, Bloomington, Ind.)

SITE PREFERENCE

The proximal tibia (Fig. 105-3) is the preferred site of infusion in children under 5 years of age: The proximal tibia is located away from the areas of ventilation or chest compressions during cardiopulmonary resuscitation; there is broad flat surface close to the skin; there are few intervening muscles, nerves, and vessels; the site has easily recognized landmarks; this injection site has shown efficacy. After age 5 or 6, the proximal tibia becomes less optimal because of thickening of the cortex, which makes penetration difficult.

The distal tibia (Fig. 105-4) and the distal femur are alternative sites for IVA. The distal tibia is a good second choice because the bone and tissues are also thin in this area. The distal tibia is easily penetrated, and penetration does not endanger the saphenous vein or epiphyseal growth plate. The distal femur is generally not a first choice because it is covered with muscles and fat, which often makes palpation of bony landmarks difficult.

The sternum and ileum, although used in the past, are now considered less suitable sites for IVA. The sternum is seldom used because the width of the marrow space is inadequate in children under 3 years of age, and insertion may be technically difficult and dangerous. This site carries a substantial risk of mediastinal puncture.

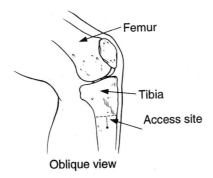

Oblique view

FIG. 105-3.
Proximal tibia site selection.

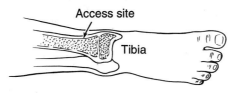

FIG. 105-4.
Distal tibia site selection.

TECHNIQUE

1. Have an assistant restrain the infant and place a small sandbag behind the extremity for support. Do not hold the extremity in your hand.
2. Clean the skin with antiseptic solution using aseptic technique.
3. *Optional:* Drape the area.
4. *Optional:* Administer local anesthestic down to the periosteum (may be unnecessary with depressed mental status).
5. Select a needle insertion site and insert:
   a. Proximal tibia (Fig. 105-5).
      1. Palpate the tibial tuberosity with your index finger.
      2. Select a site below the tibial tuberosity on the flat surface of the proximal anteromedial tibia. (Base site selection on Table 105-1.)
      3. Grasp the medial aspect of the tibia with your thumb.
      4. Insert the needle with a boring or screwing motion at a 0- to 30-degree angle from vertical, parallel to the long axis of the bone, and directed away from the epiphyseal plate.
   b. Distal tibia (Fig. 105-6).
      1. Insert the needle into the distal medial tibia at the broad flat area proximal to the medial malleolus and posterior to the saphenous vein, at an angle perpendicular to the skin.
   c. Distal femur.
      1. Insert the needle 2 to 3 cm above the epicondyles in the anterior midline.
      2. Direct the needle cephalad at an angle of 10 to 15 degrees from vertical.
6. Entry into the marrow space is confirmed by:
   a. Lack of resistance after the needle has passed through the cortex into the softer medulla (The skin-to-cortex distance is rarely more than 1 cm in infants and children.)

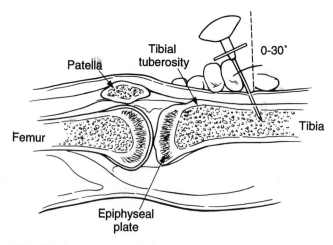

FIG. 105-5.
Proximal tibia needle insertion.

TABLE 105-1.

Insertion Site	Age (months)
At level of tuberosity	3-6
0.5 - 1.0 cm distal to tuberosity	6-12
1.0 - 2.0 cm distal to tuberosity	>12

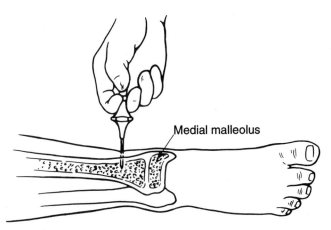

Medial malleolus

FIG. 105-6.
Distal tibia needle insertion.

    b. Needle stands upright without support
    c. Easy aspiration of marrow into a syringe
    d. Fluids infuse freely without extravasation
    e. *Optional:* X-ray confirmation of needle position
  7. Remove the needle stylet.
  8. Flush the needle with saline solution (heparin is optional).
  9. Attach the infusion line.
10. Tape in place a sterile 2 × 2 inch dressing cut to fit around the needle.
11. Tape the IV tubing to the leg (Fig. 105-7).
12. Restrain the limb to avoid inadvertent movement.
13. Observe the infusion site for evidence of extravasation.
14. *Optional:* Obtain a follow-up X-ray of the insertion site to confirm needle placement.
15. Needle removal procedure:
    a. Rotate the needle slightly to loosen its seal.
    b. Withdraw the needle with firm, quick motion.
    c. Place a sterile pressure pad over the puncture site, and apply firm pressure for 5 minutes to allow coagulation.
    d. Apply a sterile dressing. Do not constrict the extremity.
    e. Change the dressing daily. Dressings may be discontinued after 48 hours.
    f. Monitor the site for signs of infection.

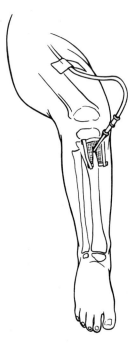

FIG. 105-7.
Completed intraosseous venous access.

PRECAUTIONS

- The needle may be left in the marrow for 72 to 96 hours. If more than one infusion site is needed, rotate the puncture sites (rotate between extremities, if possible). Do not reuse a site for at least 24 to 48 hours.
- After conventional vascular access is gained, the IVA should be discontinued. When rapid, large-volume replacement is necessary, bilateral intraosseous access may be necessary.
- If giving medications by syringe, administer saline through the needle after injecting the medication (i.e., 1 to 2 cc saline in infants, and 5 cc in older children). This improves rapidity of drug dispersement into the circulation. Hypertonic and alkaline solutions should be diluted.
- If the needle becomes obstructed with bone or marrow, occasionally it can be replaced with a second needle passed through the same cannulation site.

COMPLICATIONS

- Unsuccessful placement occurs in approximately 20% of patients because of failure of the technician to adhere to landmarks, a bent needle, dense marrow with a small cavity, replacement of marrow by fat or fibrous tissue, or "through-and-through" placement. Advancement of the needle through the opposite side of the bone can be prevented by placing your index finger approximately 1 cm from the needle bevel to prevent pushing past this mark. (Specially made intraosseous needles may have a preset depth indicator on the shaft.)

- Clotting of marrow in the needle or displacement of the needle may result in loss of access.
- Common complications are subcutaneous or occasionally subperiosteal infiltration of fluid, or leakage from the puncture site. This is most commonly seen with pressurized infusion or long-term use of intraosseous infusion. Extravasated crystalloid is usually not a problem, but solutions containing sodium bicarbonate (or other potentially cytotoxic agents) should be stopped or slowed to minimize extravasation. Muscle/tendon compartment syndrome from excess fluid extravasation may be a concern.
- Slow infusion rates may be due to a small or fibrous marrow cavity. Initially, flow rates may be slow because of plugging of the needle by marrow contents (flushing the needle with 5 to 10 cc of saline often clears the needle).
- No lasting effects have been noted in bone, growth plate, or marrow elements after IVA. The needle is directed away from the growth plate to avoid inadvertent injury to this structure. After successful placement, a small defect is created in the cortex that is visible as a small radiolucency on radiographs. It should resolve in 30 to 40 days.
- Localized cellulitis or subcutaneous abscesses may be seen in less than 1% of cases. Osteomyelitis in a study by Rosetti et al. showed an incidence of 0.6%. Infections usually occurred after prolonged catheter placement, placement in bacteremic patients, or use of hypertonic infusions.
- Hematomas are most likely caused by local trauma from needle insertion.
- Pain is possible when the intramedullary pressure is increased, but is generally not a problem with slow infusions or unconscious patients.
- In one case report, tibial fractures were seen after unsuccessful IVA attempts.
- Creation of a bone embolus when a needle without a stylet is used has not been a documented problem. Fat embolism has not been reported from tibial infusion in humans, probably because the marrow in children is relatively fat free.
- Bone marrow elements (immature white blood cells, including blasts) have been observed in venous blood sampled proximal to the infusion sites of some patients with IVA. In these cases, before more invasive diagnostic measures are undertaken, a repeat complete blood count with differential should be performed, preferably from another intravenous site in another extremity.
- With sternal puncture, death has occurred from mediastinitis, hydrothorax, or injury to the heart or great vessels. This is avoidable if the tibia or femur is used rather than the sternum.

CPT/BILLING CODE

36680   Placement of needle for intraosseous infusion

BIBLIOGRAPHY

Chameides L, editor: *Textbook of pediatric advanced life support,* Dallas, 1988, American Heart Association.

Driggers DA et al: Emergency resuscitation in children: the role of intraosseous infusion, *Postgrad Med* 89(4):129, 1991.

Glaeser PW et al: Pediatric intraosseous infusion: impact on vascular access time, *Am J Emerg Med* 6:330, 1988.

Mofenson HC et al: Guidelines for intraosseous infusions, *J Emerg Med* 6:143, 1988.

Spivey WH: Intraosseous infusions, *J Pediatr* 111(5):639, 1987.

CHAPTER 106

Neonatal Resuscitation

Marvin Dewar

Effective emergency medical care during the newborn period can be the critical factor in preventing a lifetime of adverse sequelae. If emergencies are not managed properly in the first few moments of life, resultant anatomical and physiological abnormalities can be devastating.

Initial resuscitation and assessment measures, including proper positioning, drying, warming, suctioning, and stimulation, should be provided to all newborns.

INDICATIONS

Neonate with:

- Inadequate or ineffective respirations
- Inadequate heart rate
- Central cyanosis
- Other evidence of distress

EQUIPMENT

- Suction equipment, including a bulb syringe, mechanical suction device, suction catheters (6, 8, 10 Fr.), and pediatric feeding tube (8 Fr.)
- Oxygen source with flow meter, infant resuscitation bag ($\leq$ 750 cc) with appropriately sized face masks, laryngoscope with No. 0 and No. 1 straight blades, and sterile newborn endotracheal tubes (2.5, 3.0, 3.5, and 4.0 mm)
- Drugs, including epinephrine 1:10,000 (0.1 mg/ml), naloxone 0.02 mg/ml, normal saline for injection, and sodium bicarbonate 4.2% (0.5 mEq/ml)
- Miscellaneous items, including a radiant warmer, needles (25, 21, and 18 gauge), syringes (1, 3, 10, 20 cc), adhesive tape (½-inch width), and umbilical catheter (3.5 or 5 Fr.)

TECHNIQUE

As with all medical procedures, universal precautions against exposure to blood and other body fluids should be followed.

Positioning, Suction, and Stimulation

1. Prevent heat loss by quickly drying the infant and placing it under a radiant heat source. (Recovery from acidosis is delayed by hypothermia.)
2. Open the airway by positioning the infant on the back with the neck slightly extended. Extreme hyperextension or flexion of the infant's neck may diminish air flow.
3. Clear the airway by suctioning the mouth, then the nose, with a bulb syringe or mechanical suction device. If mechanical suction is used, pressure should not exceed −100 mm Hg. Deep suctioning of the oropharynx may produce a vagal response and cause bradycardia and apnea. Infants with meconium-stained amniotic fluid (particularly when thick or particulate) should have the mouth, pharynx, and nose suctioned as soon as the head is delivered and before the body is delivered, and the hypopharynx and trachea suctioned under direct visualization immediately after delivery. (See Chapter 109, Delee Suctioning.)
4. Initiate respiratory activity by providing tactile stimulation (slap the sole of the foot or gently rub the back).

Initial Assessment

1. Assess the infant's respiratory status, heart rate, and color.
2. Infants with adequate respiratory and cardiac function (good ventilation and heart rate greater than 100 beats per minute), and with no evidence of central cyanosis, can be merely observed. Record Apgar scores (Table 106-1).
3. Infants with depressed respiratory function (shallow, slow, or absent), abnormal heart rate, or central cyanosis should undergo further resuscitation.

Ventilation

1. Ventilatory insufficiency produces the majority of respiratory and circulatory abnormalities in the newborn period. *Rapid* institution of ventilatory support in newborns with abnormalities of respiratory function or heart rate, or central cyanosis, will maximize the chances of a successful outcome.

TABLE 106-1.

Apgar Scores*

Score	0	1	2
Heart rate	Absent	<100	>100
Respiratory effort	Absent, irregular	Slow, crying	Good
Muscle tone	Limp	Some flexion of extremities	Active motion
Reflex irritability (nose suction)	No response	Grimace	Cough or sneeze
Color	Blue, pale	Extremities blue	Completely pink

Adapted from Apgar V: *Anesth Analg* 32:260, 1953. © 1953 International Anesthesia Research Society. Used with permission.
*Rapid clinical assessment of infant performed at 1 and 5 minutes after birth. If infant is compromised, assessment should be repeated at 10 and 20 minutes.

2. Positive pressure ventilation with 90% to 100% oxygen is indicated for infants with inadequate respiratory effort or a heart rate less than 100 beats per minute. Free-flow oxygen administration may be adequate for the infant with central cyanosis if respiratory function is adequate and the heart rate is over 100 beats per minute. (The cause for cyanosis should be sought.) If central cyanosis persists despite oxygen administration, positive pressure ventilation should be applied.

3. Positive pressure ventilation is usually accomplished with bag and mask ventilation alone, using either a self-inflating bag or anesthesia bag. Appropriately sized face masks with cushioned rims should be used.
   a. Anesthesia bag
      i. Inflates only when attached to source of compressed gas.
      ii. Ventilation pressure measured by attached pressure gauge.
      iii. May be used as a free-flow oxygen source.
      iv. Preferred by many experts in neonatal resuscitation (capability of fine-tuned ventilatory control).
   b. Self-inflating bag
      i. Requires oxygen reservoir attachment to obtain necessary high oxygen concentrations.
      ii. Pressure limited pop-off valve usually set at 30 cm H_2O.
      iii. Cannot be used for free-flow oxygen administration.
      iv. Technically easier to operate for clinicians who manage bag and mask ventilation infrequently.

4. Ventilate the infant at a rate of 40 to 60 breaths per minute with a tidal volume of 6 to 8 cc/kg. Adequate ventilation is verified clinically by observing bilateral symmetrical chest expansion and the presence of bilateral breath sounds. Inadequate ventilation may indicate an inadequate face mask seal, a blocked airway, or inadequate ventilation pressure. After initial ventilations, pressures of less than 30 to 40 cm H_2O should be adequate.

5. Perform an endotracheal intubation when prolonged positive pressure ventilation is required, when bag and mask ventilation is ineffective, or when diaphragmatic hernia is suspected. Select an endotracheal tube of appropriate size (Table 106-2), and insert it under direct visualization using the laryngoscope. The tip should rest above the tracheal bifurcation. Appropriate endotracheal tube location is verified clinically by the presence of bilaterally symmetrical breath sounds and is confirmed with a chest X-ray.

TABLE 106-2.

Endotracheal Tube Selection

Infant Weight	Endotracheal Tube Size (Fr.)
< 1000 gm	2.5
1000 - 2000 gm	3.0
2000 - 3000 gm	3.5
> 3000 gm	3.5 - 4.0

6. Oral airways are rarely required during neonatal resuscitation, but are indicated in the following circumstances:
   Bilateral choanal atresia
   Pierre Robin syndrome
   When necessary for adequate ventilation
7. Gastric catheter placement (8 Fr.) is indicated in prolonged resuscitation efforts to prevent stomach distension, a frequent problem in newborns who are being ventilated by mask.

Chest Compression

1. Administer chest compressions if the infant's heart rate is below 60 beats per minute, or below 80 beats per minute and not increasing after adequate positive pressure ventilation with 100% oxygen for 15 to 30 seconds. Chest compressions can be accomplished with the thumbs or the tips of the middle finger and the index finger (Fig. 106-1) and should be repeated 120 times per minute with sufficient pressure to depress the sternum ½ to ¾ inch.
2. Continue the chest compressions until the heart rate is greater than 80 beats per minute without assistance.
3. Apply chest compressions to the midsternum at a point just below an imaginary line connecting the nipples. Chest compressions should always be accompanied by positive pressure ventilation with 90% to 100% oxygen.

Medications

1. Administer medication when the heart rate remains less than 80 beats per minute after adequate positive pressure ventilation and chest compressions for a minimum of 30 seconds. Medication may be administered via the umbilical *vein* through a 3.5 or 5 Fr. umbilical catheter placed just below the skin level. (See Chapter 107, Umbilical Artery Catheterization.) Alternative routes of administration (endotracheal [ET], intramuscular [IM], or subcutaneous [SQ]) are available for some medications.
   a. Epinephrine
      i. Indicated for heart rate below 80 beats per minute despite adequate positive pressure ventilation and chest compressions for 30 seconds.
      ii. Dose: 0.01 to 0.03 mg/kg (0.1 to 0.3 ml/kg) given rapidly. May be repeated every 5 minutes if required.
      iii. Route of administration: IV or ET (may dilute 1:1 with normal saline for ET administration).
   b. Volume expander: normal saline
      i. Indicated for evidence of acute bleeding with signs of hypovolemia.
      ii. Dose: 10 ml/kg given over 5 to 10 minutes. May be repeated if necessary.
      iii. Route of administration: IV.
   c. Sodium bicarbonate
      i. Indicated for documented or likely metabolic acidosis (occurs in prolonged resuscitation). This should not be used for brief arrests or episodes of bradycardia.

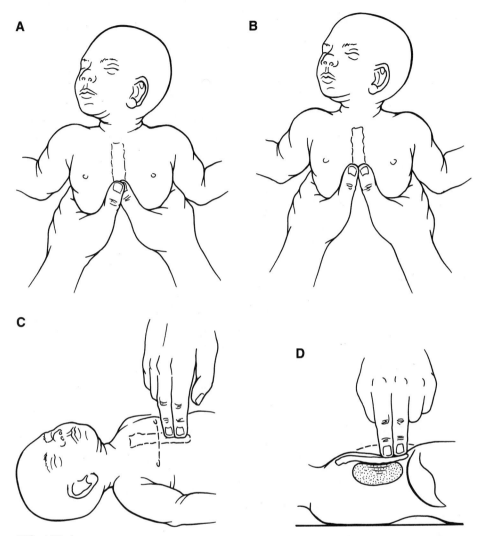

FIG. 106-1.
Chest compression. Two thumb technique with thumb over thumb (**A**) and side by side (**B**). Two finger technique (**C**). Chest compression depth is ½ to ¾ inch (**D**).

      ii. Dose: 2 mEq/kg given over at least 2 minutes.
      iii. Route of administration: IV.
   d. Naloxone hydrochloride
      i. Indicated for neonatal respiratory depression following a history of maternal narcotic administration within 4 hours of delivery.
      ii. Dose: 0.01 to 0.05 mg/kg (0.5 to 2.5 ml/kg) given rapidly.
      iii. Route of administration: IV (preferred), ET (preferred), IM (acceptable), and SQ (acceptable).

POSTPROCEDURE CARE

1. Maintain careful monitoring in an appropriately staffed intensive care unit.
2. Continue evaluation with serial arterial blood gases, frequent determination of fluid and electrolyte status, chest X-rays, and other modalities as indicated by clinical findings.
3. Completely document the resuscitation effort in the medical record.

COMPLICATIONS

Suction

- Vagal response (bradycardia or apnea)
- Hypoxia

Ventilation

- Pneumothorax
- Hypoxia due to inadequate ventilation

Intubation

- See Chapter 59, Endotracheal Intubation—Complications

CPT/BILLING CODE

99440   Newborn resuscitation: care of high-risk newborn at delivery, including for example, inhalation therapy, aspiration, administration of medication for initial stabilization

BIBLIOGRAPHY

American Heart Association: *Neonatal resuscitation,* Dallas, 1991, The Association.
Neonatal advanced life support (part VI), *JAMA* 255:2969, 1986.

CHAPTER 107

Umbilical Artery Catheterization

James A. Sterling

Umbilical artery catheterization (UAC) provides vascular access in the newborn and generally may be performed up to the seventh day of life. Catheterization of one of the umbilical arteries is preferable to umbilical vein catheterization (UVC) in most instances; however, UVC is an alternative in children with difficult to obtain UAC and/or peripheral intravenous access. Easier access to the umbilical vein is the primary advantage of UVC over UAC. It is a relatively simple procedure, and passage of the catheter through either the umbilical artery or vein is easiest if performed in the first 30 to 60 minutes of life.

INDICATIONS

Catheterization of an umbilical artery or vein is indicated in delivery room resuscitation involving

- Need to administer intravenous drugs, blood, or blood expanders
- Continual reassessment of a newborn in cardiorespiratory distress:
    Central venous pressure (CVP) monitoring
    Frequent administration of fluids
    Frequent arterial sampling

In a neonatal intensive care unit (NICU), a UAC is placed for any infant who is

- In respiratory distress and who requires mechanical ventilation
- Under an oxygen hood, and who requires greater than 40% oxygen (FIO_2) and who has an abnormal chest X-ray
- Hypoglycemic and who requires greater than 12.5% dextrose to maintain blood glucose and who is taking nothing by mouth (NPO)
- Requiring pressor drips, total parenteral nutrition (TPN) solution, or medications for a prolonged period of time (usually with weight less than 1000 gm or with critically ill infants)
- Less than 1800 gm, needing an exchange transfusion that can be performed through a UAC or UVC

CONTRAINDICATIONS

For the newborn with normal anatomy, there are no absolute contraindications. Infants with vascular insufficiency of a lower extremity, local infection, and necrotizing enterocolitis should *not* undergo umbilical artery catherization.

EQUIPMENT

- Sterile measuring tape
- 3.5 to 5.0 Fr. umbilical artery catheter
- Surgical cap and mask, sterile gown, and sterile gloves
- 3-way stopcock (sterile)
- Heparin for flush (1 to 2 units heparin/ml of 0.25 normal saline)
- Sterile instrument tray with small clamps, forceps (iris curved), scissors, needle holder, mounted No. 11 scalpel blade, and povidone-iodine or antiseptic solution
- Antibiotic ointment
- 4-0 or 5-0 silk suture with small needle.

A standard rule of thumb for catheter size selection is to use a 5 Fr. for infants greater than 1500 gm and a 3 to 3.5 Fr. for infants less than 1500 gm. An 8 Fr. catheter may be appropriate for term infants (greater than 1800 gm) who require exchange transfusion.

PATIENT PREPARATION

Typically the infant who is a candidate for UAC will demonstrate signs and symptoms of cardiorespiratory distress shortly—if not immediately—after birth. Obtain informed consent from the parent(s) after explaining the possible complications and the necessity for the procedure.

TECHNIQUE

When UAC placement is probable, the umbilical stump should be left at least 4 cm long. The two thick-walled arteries and the single vein are easily identified. The catheter may be inserted for infants up to 7 days of age.

1. Set up the tubing, fluids, fluid chamber, 0.22 µ filter, and infusion pump. Flush and fill the tubing with heparin to remove air from the system.
2. Restrain the infant, if possible.
3. Prepare the periumbilical area, including the umbilical stump, in the standard aseptic fashion, and apply sterile drapes.
4. Measure the distance from the umbilicus to the midsternum to estimate the length of catheter necessary for long-term placement. Alternatively, measure the distance from the shoulder to umbilicus (Fig. 107-1). This should

position the catheter just above the diaphragm when inserted. If the catheter is being placed for a single-exchange transfusion, it may be inserted just below the skin (3 to 5 cm), as long as good back flow is noted. Otherwise, placement must be above or below the renal arteries to avoid thrombosis.

5. Loosely tie the sterile umbilical tape around the proximal stump (the tape will be tightened as needed for bleeding).

6. With the scalpel, transect the cord approximately 1 cm above the umbilical tape (Fig. 107-2, *A*). Correctly identify the artery (or vein if applicable); the umbilical vein is easiest to identify: it is the single vessel with the largest lumen.

7. While gently retracting on the cord, gently dilate the vessel with small curved forceps (Fig. 107-2, *B*). Insert one prong of the iris forceps to partially dilate the lumen, then follow with both prongs. Insert the catheter through the vessel lumen to the length previously measured (Fig. 107-2, *C*). Retraction on the cord usually facilitates this occasionally tedious task. Do *not* advance against resistance. If resistance is met upon insertion, applying continual pressure for 30 seconds may cause the arterial spasm to subside. Alternatively, you may apply lidocaine.

8. Suture the catheter in a purse-string fashion or with a stabilizer (Fig. 107-2, *D*).

9. Apply sterile gauze with antibiotic ointment, and tape the catheter to the abdomen.

10. Obtain X-ray confirmation of placement. If X-ray confirmation is not possible, a UVC should be used instead of UAC. UVCs should never be inserted more than 5 cm.

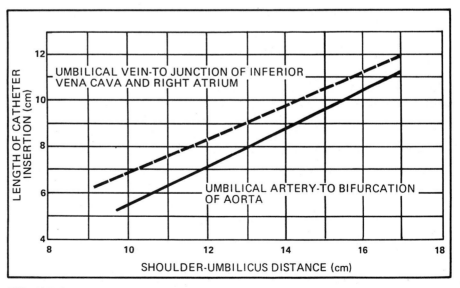

FIG. 107-1.
Determining the length of the catheter for proper position.

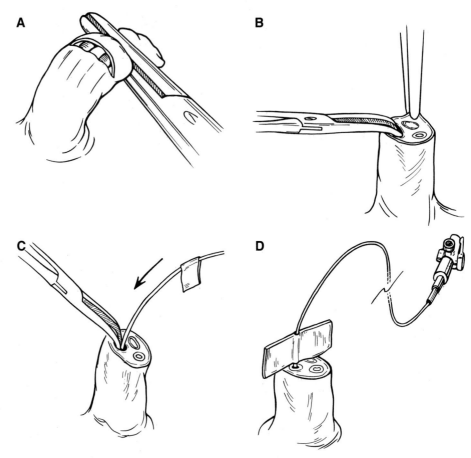

FIG. 107-2.
Umbilical artery placement. See text for details.

POSTPROCEDURE CARE

Check the catheter frequently for patency and for signs or symptoms of infection. If signs or symptoms of infection are noted, take cultures from the catheter. In the face of complications, remove the catheter. If the catheter is located in the vicinity of the liver (probably in the vein), it is better to pull it out. In some NICUs, if peripheral access is extremely critical, the catheter is pulled out enough to place it midline and then used for infusions.

COMPLICATIONS

- Bleeding
- Cellulitis

- Embolization
- Ischemia to bowel or other intraabdominal organ or lower extremity
- Necrotizing enterocolitis (NEC)
- Pelvic exsanguination
- Bacteremia or sepsis
- Vascular perforation
- Hepatic abscess or infarction
- Congestive heart failure (CHF)
- If the catheter is pulled too low, fluid may leak around the umbilicus
- Exsanguination from disconnected tubing

CPT/BILLING CODES

36660	Umbilical artery, for diagnosis or therapy, newborn
36510	Umbilical vein, for diagnosis or therapy, newborn

BIBLIOGRAPHY

American Heart Association: *Advanced cardiac life support,* ed 2, Dallas, 1988, The Association.

Suprapubic Bladder Aspiration

Marvin Dewar

Suprapubic bladder aspiration is often useful in young infants for whom other methods of obtaining sterile urine specimens are unsatisfactory. This technique is most successful in infants less than 2 years old because, up until that age, the bladder is an abdominal organ. After 2 years, the bladder moves into the pelvis as the child grows.

INDICATIONS

- Suspected urinary tract infection
- Exclusion of sepsis

CONTRAINDICATIONS

- Bleeding abnormality or coagulopathy
- Infection at the site of needle insertion
- Anatomical genitourinary tract anomalies
- Bowel distention (ileus, obstructor, etc.)

EQUIPMENT

- Povidone-iodine solution
- 70% alcohol
- Sterile 4 × 4 inch gauze pads
- Sterile gloves
- 3 cc sterile syringe with 1-inch 22-gauge needle
- Sterile urine specimen container

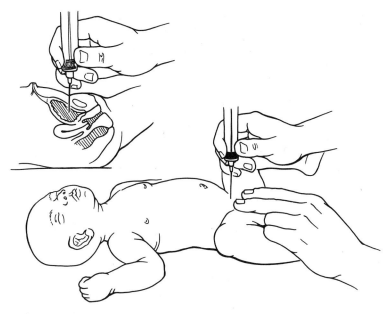

FIG. 108-1.
Proper technique of suprapubic bladder aspiration.

TECHNIQUE

1. Before bladder aspiration, the infant's diaper should be dry, and urination should not have occurred within the previous hour (to ensure a full bladder).
2. Hold the infant in the supine, frog-leg position.
3. Cleanse the lower abdomen with povidone-iodine and 70% alcohol.
4. Direct a 1-inch 22-gauge needle attached to a 3 cc sterile syringe into the mid-line of the abdomen at a point 1 cm above the symphysis pubis (usually there is a transverse skin crease at about the proper location). Hold the needle perpendicular to the abdomen or direct it slightly caudally (Fig. 108-1).
5. Aspirate with the syringe while advancing the needle. To avoid puncturing the posterior bladder wall or retroperitoneal structures, do not advance the needle after urine begins to enter the syringe. If urine is present, it is usually obtained before insertion of the needle to its full depth.
6. If no urine is obtained, withdraw the needle. The bladder is considered empty. The procedure can be repeated in 30 minutes to an hour if the patient is stable.
7. After withdrawing the needle, cover the entry site with a sterile dressing and apply mild pressure.
8. Transfer the aspirated urine to a sterile container and transport to the laboratory for analysis and culture.

An alternative technique is to use ultrasound guidance. See Chapter 144, Emergency Department Ultrasound.

COMPLICATIONS

- Microscopic hematuria (typically transient and resolves without specific treatment)
- Infection (Risk is minimized by the use of sterile technique.)
- Perforation of the bowel (rare and may be managed by close observation and, if necessary, antibiotic administration)
- Retroperitoneal hematoma or damage to retroperitoneal structures (very rare)

CPT/BILLING CODE

51000   Aspiration of bladder by needle

BIBLIOGRAPHY

Gomella TL, editor: *Neonatology,* Norwalk, Conn, 1988, Appleton & Lange.
Greene MG, editor: *Harriet Lane handbook,* St Louis, 1991, Mosby.
Hoekelman RA, editor: *Primary pediatric care,* St Louis, 1992, Mosby.

CHAPTER 109

DeLee Suctioning

David B. Bosscher

Suctioning, using a DeLee suction device, is a means by which the upper airways of the neonate can be cleared and the stomach emptied of meconium-stained secretions. Initially it was felt that DeLee suction carried out before delivery of the neonate's chest would prevent meconium aspiration syndrome (MAS). Although it is now known that some aspiration occurs before delivery, DeLee suctioning before delivery of the shoulder prevents further meconium aspiration with the first breath and still remains a cornerstone in the resuscitation of infants at risk for meconium aspiration.

INDICATIONS

- To minimize meconium aspiration in the neonate when meconium-stained amniotic fluid is present
- To help relieve respiratory distress in the newborn when the stomach is full or when regurgitated stomach contents partially occlude the airway
- To assist in the diagnosis of choanal atresia
- To help exclude certain types of tracheoesophageal fistulae

CONTRAINDICATIONS

- A neonate with choanal atresia should not receive DeLee suctioning via the nasal route.
- Thick, particulate meconium cannot be adequately suctioned with a DeLee suction device alone. DeLee suctioning immediately after the neonate's head is delivered should be followed with more definitive suctioning with an endotracheal tube after completion of the delivery.

EQUIPMENT

- A DeLee suction device or similar suction device, 8 to 10 Fr. (Fig. 109-1)
- A bulb syringe to clear the mouth and nasal openings
- Gloves, facial coverings, and other necessary items for universal blood and body fluid precautions (Many hospitals now use mechanical or wall suction for the DeLee to maintain these precautions.)

TECHNIQUE

1. Prepare the equipment. Be certain that the rolled-up latex on the suction end of the DeLee suction device is *unrolled*. Place this end into your suction source. Make certain the suction is functioning. (If using human suction and wearing a mask, make sure there is an adequate opening in the mask to insert the mouth end.)
2. Quickly clear the mouth and nose of the neonate with a bulb syringe.
3. Gently insert the mouth end of the suction device into the mouth of the neonate. Attempt to keep the catheter sterile.
4. Slowly advance the catheter into the oropharynx, while directing it down into the esophagus (hypopharynx) with your finger.
5. Continue to advance the catheter until approximately 5 cm of its length remains outside the infant's mouth. The distal end is now in the infant's stomach.
6. Using a source of suction which does not exceed −100 mm Hg, apply suction to the suction end of the DeLee device. Occlude the thumb opening on the suction device. After sucking for a few seconds, slowly withdraw the catheter while maintaining suction. If time allows, use the same technique to suction the infant's nose also.

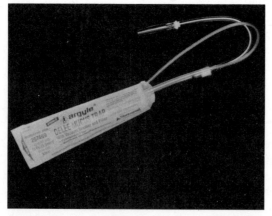

FIG. 109-1.
DeLee suction device.

7. Check for any respiratory distress. Treat minor degrees of distress with proper positioning and oxygen administration if necessary (see Chapter 106, Neonatal Resuscitation).
8. As part of documenting the care of the newborn in the postdelivery period, always mention that DeLee suctioning was performed. Document any complications.

COMPLICATIONS

- Stimulation of the neonatal oropharynx with any suction device during the first few minutes after delivery can evoke a vagal response and induce apnea or bradycardia and resultant fetal distress.
- Vigorous DeLee suctioning could cause trauma to the upper airways, the esophagus, and the stomach.
- In a neonate with a tracheoesophageal fistula, the DeLee suction device could enter the airway below the larynx, causing respiratory distress.
- Older DeLee suction devices and even some of the newer ones that utilize human suction allow aspirated neonatal stomach contents to enter the mouth of the person applying suction. This method has the potential for spreading infectious diseases. *Do not use your mouth to apply suction.* Newer models utilize mechanical or wall suction and are safer for the clinician; however, they are more cumbersome and difficult to use in a sterile field.

CPT/BILLING CODE

99440   Newborn resuscitation; care of the high-risk newborn at delivery, including, e.g., inhalation therapy, aspiration

BIBLIOGRAPHY

Carson BS et al: Combined obstetric and pediatric approach to prevent meconium aspiration syndrome, *Am J Obstet Gynecol* 126:712, 1976.

Falciglia HS et al: Does DeLee suction at the perineum prevent meconium aspiration syndrome? *Am J Obstet Gynecol* 167:1243, 1992.

Guidelines for neonatal resuscitation, Dallas, 1993, American Heart Association.

Katz VL, Bowes WA: Meconium aspiration syndrome: reflections on a murky subject, *Am J Obstet Gynecol* 166:171, 1992.

Textbook of neonatal resuscitation, Dallas, 1993, American Heart Association and American Academy of Pediatrics.

CHAPTER 110

Pediatric Arterial Puncture and Venous Cutdown

Gregg K. Phillips

ARTERIAL PUNCTURE

Arterial blood may be used for blood gas and routine laboratory analysis. In the infant or child, the radial artery is the most appropriate and most common site selected for arterial puncture. The dorsalis pedis, posterial tibial, and brachial arteries are also optional sites for arterial puncture, but each has its own risk of complications. Because of the risk of thrombosis, the femoral artery should not be used for arterial puncture in the infant or child.

Indications

- To evaluate the pediatric patient with respiratory distress
- To guide the medical management of the pediatric patient receiving ventilatory support or undergoing intensive respiratory therapy
- To obtain blood for routine laboratory analysis when venous blood cannot be obtained (This is controversial. The benefit must outweigh the higher risk of obtaining an arterial sample.)

Contraindications

- Infection, burns, or local skin damage at the site of intended puncture

Equipment

- 25-gauge butterfly scalp vein needle or standard 25- or 26-gauge needle
- Alcohol swabs
- Heparin
- *Optional:* lidocaine 1%
- *Optional:* arm or leg board
- *Optional:* fiberoptic light for transillumination of the wrist

Technique

1. Always perform an Allen's test to confirm adequate collateral circulation (see Chapter 51, Arterial Puncture).
2. Draw heparin into a tuberculin syringe, eject the heparin, and attach a 25-gauge butterfly needle (preferred for infants and neonates) or a 25- or 26-gauge needle.
3. Immobilize the upper extremity by taping it to an arm board or by having an assistant manually stabilize it.
4. Identify the radial artery by dorsiflexing the wrist and palpating over the distal volar radius. Grasp the wrist with your nondominant hand. Cleanse the site of intended puncture with an alcohol swab and, as an option, infiltrate with 1% lidocaine *without* epinephrine.
5. Insert the needle at the point of maximum pulsation at a 30- to 40-degree angle (Fig. 110-1). Continuous suction should be applied with the plunger of the syringe because, in a child, arterial blood will not flash into the syringe as in the adult patient. If using the butterfly needle, have an assistant maintain gentle suction while the needle is advanced.
6. If resistance is encountered, it is most likely that the needle has made contact with the underlying radius. At this point, withdraw the needle very slowly while maintaining suction on the plunger until there is blood return. If there is no blood return and the tip of the needle has been withdrawn to a point just beneath the skin, readvance the needle toward the point of maximal pulsation before withdrawing it from the skin. Several attempts can be made in this manner with little trauma to the infant before choosing another site.
7. When arterial blood is encountered, withdraw 0.3 to 0.5 cc of blood into the syringe before removing the needle. Leaving the butterfly needle in place with its extension tubing facilitates changing the syringe to draw more blood for other analyses, if needed.

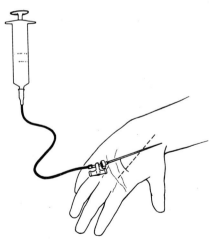

FIG. 110-1.
Arterial puncture using a butterfly needle.

8. After removing the needle, always maintain manual compression at the arterial puncture site for a minimum of 5 minutes to prevent the formation of a hematoma.

Complications

- Bleeding and hematoma formation
- Formation of intraarterial thrombus
- Nerve injury
- Infection

Because the radial artery is not in close proximity to a nerve or vein, its puncture results in fewer complications than puncture of the brachial, posterior tibial, and dorsalis pedis arteries. Repeated punctures at the same site increase the chance of complications, but may not be avoidable.

VENOUS CUTDOWN

Obtaining percutaneous venous access in infants or in hypovolemic children can be a challenge. Venous cutdown can be used to gain vascular access following a failed attempt or simultaneously while trying to place a percutaneous venous line. If the situation is emergent and a percutaneous line cannot be placed in a matter of minutes, venous cutdown can often be performed very rapidly. An additional alternative is placement of an intraosseous line, which may, in fact, be technically less difficult and quicker (see Chapter 105, Intraosseous Venous Access). What follows is a description of how to perform venous cutdown in the pediatric patient to gain vascular access in an emergency situation. Chapter 50, Venous Cutdown, offers additional technical advice on the mechanics of venous cutdown. This chapter offers an explanation of an abbreviated and clinically easier method: the minicutdown. The saphenous vein is the most common site for cutdown in the pediatric patient and minicutdown at this site will be described.

Indications

- Inability to obtain needed percutaneous venous access in a matter of minutes in an emergency situation or inability to maintain a peripheral IV

Contraindications

- Infection or trauma at the site of intended cutdown

Equipment

- Mounted No. 15 scalpel
- Mosquito hemostats
- 4-0 silk sutures
- Skin retractors

Prepackaged venous cutdown trays are available from a number of medical suppliers.

Technique

Standard venous cutdown takes 5 to 15 minutes even in the hands of a skilled physician. Minicutdown is less complicated and can be performed in most cases in less than 5 minutes. The saphenous vein slightly anterior and superior to the medial malleolus is the preferred site for minicutdown in the pediatric patient.

1. Immobilize the lower extremity by securing it to a board or by having an assistant manually hold the patient.
2. The saphenous vein is a consistent anatomical structure and is located a finger-breadth anterior to and a finger-breadth superior to the medial malleolus at the ankle. Cleanse this area with an antiseptic solution and make a 1 cm transverse incision through the dermis, exposing the underlying subcutaneous tissue.
3. Exposure of the vein is accomplished with skin retractors and blunt dissection with a mosquito hemostat, staying parallel to the course of the vein (Fig. 110-2, *A*). When the saphenous vein is identified, pass a 4-0 silk suture

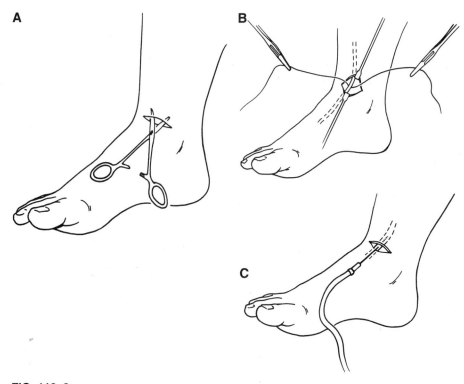

FIG. 110-2.
Venous cutdown. **A,** Blunt dissection after making a transverse incision. **B,** Localizing the vein.
C, Cannulating the vein.

beneath the vessel and clamp both ends of the suture with a hemostat (Fig. 110-2, *B*).

4. Using upward traction on the vein with the sutures to stabilize it, cannulate the vessel in the standard fashion with an intravenous catheter under direct visualization (Fig. 110-2,*C*). Advance the catheter in the usual fashion, then attach intravenous tubing and begin infusing fluid. As with percutaneous line placement, steady fluid flow is indicative of successful cannulation. With the minicutdown technique, the vein is not ligated after cannulation. One advantage is that, although the catheter is not as secure with this technique since the vein can be directly visualized, cannulization can be readily performed when time is crucial. The minicutdown technique does not destroy the vein and, if necessary, standard cutdown can be performed when the clinical situation becomes less emergent.

Complications

- Wound infections and local hematoma
- Phlebitis
- Damage to adjacent structures from incision and dissection

Since this is only a temporary procedure, risk of these complications is minimal.

CPT/BILLING CODES

36420	Venipuncture, cutdown; under 1 year old
36425	Venipuncture, cutdown; over 1 year old
36600	Arterial puncture, withdrawal of blood for diagnosing

BIBLIOGRAPHY

Roberts JR: *Clinical procedure in emergency medicine,* Philadelphia, 1985, W.B. Saunders.
Simon RR: *Emergency procedures and techniques,* Baltimore, 1987, Williams & Wilkins.

CHAPTER 111

Newborn Circumcision

S. Shevaun Duiker

Grant C. Fowler

While there is some disagreement about the medical necessity of routine neonatal circumcision and the associated risks, currently a majority (61%) of newborn boys in the United States undergo this procedure. In fact, circumcision is the most commonly performed surgical procedure in this country. Certain studies indicate that uncircumcised males have an increased risk of balanitis, urinary tract infections, penile cancer, and HIV infection, and that women whose sexual partners are uncircumcised have an increased risk of cervical cancer. However, all of these studies suffer from bias and methodological flaws; therefore, these conclusions may not be valid. The most recent American Academy of Pediatrics (AAP) position is that "circumcision has potential medical advantages as well as inherent disadvantages and risks. When circumcision is being considered, the benefits and risks should be explained to the parents and informed consent should be obtained."

Some physicians are more apt to perform circumcision since improved anesthesia is now available. Methods include dorsal penile nerve block (DPNB) (see Chapter 112), precircumcision oral analgesics, local anesthesia of foreskin, and topical anesthesia such as viscous lidocaine (see Chapter 22, Topical Anesthesia). Studies have shown that infants anesthetized with either DPNB or local anesthesia demonstrate less crying, less tachycardia, less irritability, and fewer behavior changes in the 24 hours following the procedure. They also have lower postprocedure serum cortisol levels than infants circumcised without anesthesia.

INDICATIONS

- Parental desire

CONTRAINDICATIONS

- Hypospadias*
- Unusual appearing genitalia*
- Inability to determine phenotype of child* (ambiguous genitalia)
- Age less than 12 hours (physiologic adaptation requires 12 to 24 hours)
- Severe illness
- Prematurity (until the child is ready for discharge from the hospital)

If there is a family history of bleeding problems, appropriate laboratory studies should be performed before the procedure. Undescended testicles are not necessarily a contraindication; however, they should be noted and evaluated for other reasons. Because of the risk of regurgitation, infants should be at least 1 hour postprandial. Also, document that the child has had at least one void since birth before performing the procedure.

One relative contraindication to circumcision is age greater than 6 to 8 weeks. By this age, adhesions are usually more significant, causing the procedure to be more difficult and time consuming, and frequently it requires a more experienced clinician. The foreskin may develop significant edema after lysis of these adhesion, making it difficult to use the Gomco clamp. By this age, maternal clotting factors have also been metabolized, possibly predisposing the infant to increased blood loss.

PREPROCEDURE PATIENT EDUCATION

Discuss with the parent(s) the risks and benefits of the procedure with and without anesthesia. Informed consent should be obtained.

GOMCO METHOD

Equipment

- Infant restrainer board and padding
- Sterile gloves
- Sterile drape with small opening in the center (fenestrated)
- Alcohol or other skin-sterilizing liquid
- Sterile 2 × 2 or 4 × 4 inch gauze pads
- One 3- to 5-inch flexible probe
- Three small or mosquito hemostats—two curved, one straight
- Small straight scissors
- Gomco circumcision clamp (1.1 to 1.45 cm)

  Note: Clamp sizes most commonly used are 1.1 to 1.3 cm. The 1.1 cm Gomco is usually for a very small child, while the 1.45 cm clamp will usually fit an infant. Larger sizes are available for children and adults.

---

*These patients should be referred to a specialist.

- A large, sterile safety pin
- A mounted No. 10 blade scalpel
- White petrolatum (Vaseline) or white petrolatum gauze
- A diaper
- An adequate light source
- A sterile serrated Adson forceps
- Silver nitrate cautery stick
- Topical epinephrine
- Gelfoam
- A 3-0 absorbable suture (chronic or catgut) on a needle
- Needle holder (in the event of bleeding following circumcision)

Technique

1. Restrain the infant using the infant board.
2. Inspect the penis for abnormalities and the location of the meatus on the glans.
3. If anatomy is normal, anesthetize the penis in a chosen manner, if desired.
4. Using alcohol or other antiseptic solution, cleanse the area, moving from the tip of the glans toward the body. Cleanse an area about 3 inches in diameter around the base of penis, as well as the entire penis.
5. (When describing the penis, use the dorsal direction as the 12 o'clock position.) Attach the curved hemostats to a very small segment of foreskin at a point between the 2 o'clock and 3 o'clock positions and again at the 9 o'clock and 10 o'clock positions, and place gentle traction on the foreskin, taking care not to clamp the hemostats onto the glans. Gently insert the straight hemostat or the flexible probe between the foreskin and the glans to the depth of the corona, at the 12 o'clock position (Fig. 111-1). Open the hemostat and sweep it in both directions toward the ventral attachment of the foreskin to the glans. If using the probe, perform the same maneuver. Care must be taken not to extend beyond the depth of the corona. Caution must also be taken in the ventral aspect of the penis to avoid trauma to the urethra.
6. Lift the foreskin away from the glans to make a tent. With this tenting, ensure that no part of the glans is in the way, and then using the straight

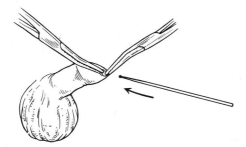

FIG. 111-1.
Insert the hemostat or probe between the foreskin and the glans, carefully avoiding the meatus.

hemostat, firmly clamp the dorsal aspect of the foreskin in the vertical line of the penis to a depth of about one third to one half of the total distance to the corona (one third to one half of the total length of foreskin [Fig. 111-2]). Wait 30 to 60 seconds. Again take care to cause no trauma to the glans.

7. Remove the straight hemostat.
8. Tent the skin and, using the straight scissors, carefully cut along the center of the clamp site (Fig. 111-3), being careful not to extend past the apex of the clamp site. Hemostasis has been achieved using the straight hemostat, and incising beyond this clamp site or lateral to it will result in unnecessary bleeding.
9. Gently retract the foreskin from the glans (Fig. 111-4) and remove any remaining adhesions. (This can be done with gauze.) If at this point, you cannot retract the foreskin, use the straight hemostat again to reclamp it dorsally slightly deeper (more proximally) than the original position, and extend the dorsal cut more proximally. Care must be taken later with placement of the Gomco to remove all of the foreskin *slightly beyond* the apex of the dorsal incision to minimize risk of postprocedure bleeding or an unsightly result.
10. Inspect the glans and foreskin for remaining adhesions. If there are remaining adhesions, gently separate them using either the probe, a hemostat, or a piece of cotton gauze.

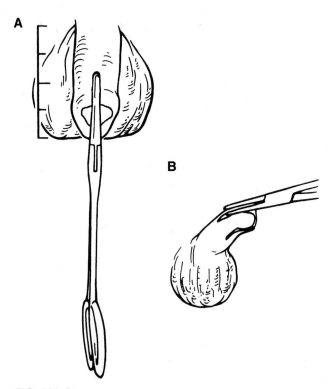

FIG. 111-2.
A, Clamping the dorsal aspect of the foreskin. **B,** Cross section of penis showing depth of hemostat insertion.

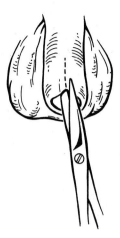

FIG. 111-3.
Incising the dorsal slit.

FIG. 111-4.
Retract the foreskin from the glans, using 4 × 4 inch gauze.

11. Place the bell of the Gomco clamp over the glans.
12. Using the curved hemostats (still attached) to manipulate the foreskin while applying gentle downward pressure on the distal end of the stem or shaft of the Gomco bell, pull the foreskin over the bell. This should reapproximate the foreskin over the bell. The bell should be between the glans and the foreskin and set against the corona.
13. When the Gomco bell is appropriately placed, use the sterile safety pin at the distal corners to reapproximate the dorsal incision (or hold the two sides of the foreskin together.) It should be reapproximated around the shaft of the Gomco bell and above the bell (Fig. 111-5). Insert the safety pin through all the layers of the foreskin of the previous incision to make this reapproximation. Turn the safety pin parallel to the long axis of the Gomco bell.
14. With gentle traction in a distal direction, insert the distal end of the Gomco bell, the safety pin, and the foreskin completely through the opening in the body of the Gomco (Fig. 111-6). Clamp the bell on to the Gomco and tighten slightly.
15. Check for appropriate placement of the Gomco on the foreskin. Make sure that the foreskin has been drawn through the body of the Gomco evenly from all sides. The entire apex of the initial incision should be visible

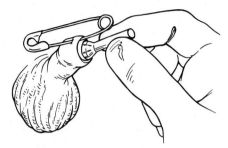

FIG. 111-5.
Placing the Gomco bell.

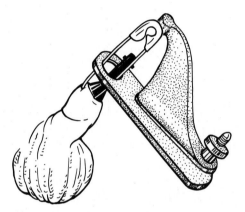

FIG. 111-6.
Bringing the bell and foreskin through the ring. Leave screw very loose until bell stem and safety pin are pulled through opening in body.

and inside the Gomco body. Make sure all of the foreskin that is to be removed is *inside* the Gomco. When the Gomco has been appropriately placed, firmly tighten it.

16. Position the scalpel at an angle slightly above horizontal, place it firmly against the bell of the Gomco, and incise the foreskin to remove the distal portion (Fig. 111-7). Make sure that all skin and mucosal layers are removed. Any remaining tissue above the clamp is necrotic and a possible source of infection.

17. Immediately unclamp the Gomco and remove the body and clamp of the Gomco.

18. To remove the bell, gently tease the avascular tip of the remaining foreskin away from the bell using a piece of cotton gauze.

19. Check for hemostasis. To control any bleeding, apply pressure, topical epinephrine, or silver nitrate to the specific source. In rare cases of persistent bleeding, Gelfoam can be applied with pressure to hasten clotting. Rarely will bleeding require suturing. In the event that it does, use an absorbable suture at the site of the bleeding, which is usually an arteriole. Persistent

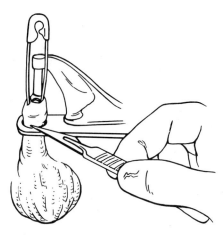

FIG. 111-7.
Trimming the excess foreskin.

bleeding after circumcision is a common sign of factor-deficient bleeding disorders (hemophilia). If bleeding persists following these measures, full clotting studies should be obtained and a hematology consultation considered.

20. Place white petrolatum and gauze (or a piece of white petrolatum gauze) over the site, and rediaper.
21. Document the time of day in the chart and ask that the parents or nurses document the time of next void. The infant should not be discharged until he has voided.

Postprocedure Patient Education

Tell the parents to watch for bleeding or infection; the first urine void time should be recorded on the patient's chart. Remove the white petrolatum the next day, and retract the foreskin with each bathing in the near future. The penis can be washed with soap and water the next day. Occasionally, meatal stenosis (a small membrane over the ventral meatus) forms in the first year of life. If the meatus is less than 2 mm in diameter or less than 25% to 30% of the diameter of the glans, meatectomy should be performed in the office or the patient should be referred to a specialist.

PLASTIBELL METHOD

Equipment

The same equipment as for the Gomco method is used, except the Gomco and the safety pin are replaced with a selection of sizes of Plastibells (1.3 to 1.6 cm is the usual size range needed).

Technique

1. As in Steps 1 and 2 of the Gomco method, restrain the infant and inspect the penis for abnormalities and for the location of the urethral meatus on the glans, and also estimate the size of the glans. Have a Plastibell of this size available.

2. As in Steps 3 through 10 of the Gomco method, cleanse the area, separate the glans and foreskin, tent the tissue, clamp and remove the hemostat, cut along the hemostat line, and retract the foreskin. While the hemostat is clamped, however, place the Plastibell string loosely (2-inch diameter) around the base of the penis and put two turns in the string.

3. Place the Plastibell over the glans (Fig. 111-8).

4. As in Step 12 of the Gomco method, place the Plastibell on the glans and pull the foreskin over it.

5. Remove one curved hemostat and hold both sides of the foreskin in the remaining curved hemostat.

6. Place the Plastibell so that the indentation is below the apex of the incision and at the appropriate place on the foreskin. Use the straight hemostat to clamp across the shaft of the Plastibell and hold the curved hemostat to keep the foreskin in this relationship.

7. Place the string over the indentation in the Plastibell, and tighten the string until it remains in place, but is not firm (Fig. 111-9).

8. Check placement of the string and bell again, making sure that the apex of the foreskin incision is distal to the string, that too much skin is not being removed, and that the Plastibell can move freely on the glans.

9. Tighten the string as much as possible and hold at this tension for 30 seconds. Finish by tying a square knot in the string.

10. Remove the hemostats.

11. Using the scissors, cut the foreskin to within ⅛ to 3/16 of an inch distal to the string. Do not cut too close to the string (Fig. 111-10).

12. Cut the ends of the string to about half an inch long.

13. Holding the body of the Plastibell between the first finger and thumb of one hand, gently bend the shaft of the Plastibell with the other hand until it snaps at the junction of the bell and the shaft (Fig. 111-11).

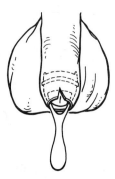

FIG. 111-8.
Plastibell in place over the glans.

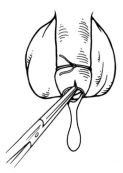

FIG. 111-9.
String is placed over the indentation in the Plastibell. Hemostat holds both ends of incision.

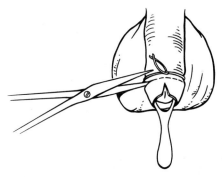

FIG. 111-10.
Excise the foreskin.

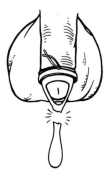

FIG. 111-11.
Snap the Plastibell at the junction of the bell and the shaft.

14. Check that the Plastibell can move up and down on the glans.
15. As in Steps 19 through 21 of the Gomco method, check for bleeding, cover with petrolatum gauze, rediaper, and record the time of the next void.

Postprocedure Patient Education

Inform the parents to keep the area clean and to watch for signs of bleeding or infection. The distal foreskin will turn black and necrotic and fall off within one week, along with the Plastibell. Document the time of day of the first urine void.

MOGEN METHOD

Equipment

The same equipment as the Gomco method is used, except the scissors is unnecessary and the Gomco and safety pin are replaced with a Mogen clamp.

Technique

1. As in Steps 1 through 5 of the Gomco method, restrain the infant, inspect the penis for abnormalities and for the location of the urethral meatus on the glans. Cleanse the area, and separate the glans and foreskin.
2. Inspect to ensure that all adhesions have been disrupted.
3. Use the hemostats to pull the foreskin tight and, with a bright light, transilluminate the tented, liberated foreskin from the side and look for the dark, shadowed curve of the tip of the glans. Place the Mogen clamp over the foreskin in a horizontal direction. Advance proximally until the appropriate amount of foreskin is distal to the clamp. Inspect to be sure the tip of the glans is not within the clamp, and clamp it tight.
4. Use the scalpel to cut the foreskin flush with the distal edge of the Mogen clamp.
5. After 1 minute, remove the clamp. If the clamp remains in place too long, the two sides of the foreskin will be difficult to separate.
6. Gently separate the foreskin to expose the glans; gauze can be used to provide traction. If separation is performed too quickly or too forcibly, the skin layers will separate and there will be bleeding.
7. As in Steps 19 through 21 of the Gomco method, check for bleeding, cover with petrolatum gauze, rediaper, and record the time of the next void.

Postprocedure Patient Education

The postprocedure patient education for the Gomco method applies to the Mogen method also.

COMPLICATIONS (ALL METHODS)

- Bleeding
- Infection
- Trauma to the glans or urethra

- Poor cosmetic result due to remaining adhesions, removal of too much or too little foreskin, or uneven removal of foreskin
- Meatal stenosis in first year of life

CPT/BILLING CODE

54150   Circumcision, using clamp or other device; newborn

BIBLIOGRAPHY

American Academy of Pediatrics: Committee statements: reports of the task force on circumcision, *Pediatrics* 84(2):388, 1989.

Kunz V: Circumcision and meatotomy, *Prim Care Clin Office Pract* 13(3):513, 1986.

Poland L: Sounding board: the question of routine neonatal circumcision, *N Engl J Med* 322(18): 1312, 1990.

Schoen J: Sounding board: the status of circumcision of newborns, *N Engl J Med* 322(18):1308, 1990.

Spach DH, Stapleton AE, Staum WE: Lack of circumcision increases the risk of urinary tract infection in young men, *JAMA* 267(5):679, 1992.

Stang HJ et al: Local anesthesia for neonatal circumcision: effects on distress and cortisol response, *JAMA* 259:1507, March 1988.

Wiswell E: Routine neonatal circumcision: a reappraisal, *Am Fam Physician* 41(3):859, 1990.

CHAPTER 112

Dorsal Penile Nerve Block

Grant C. Fowler

S. Shevaun Duiker

In the past, there has been considerable controversy about whether or not infants should be anesthetized for circumcision: The possibility that the neonatal nervous system is sufficiently developed for the neonate to be truly capable of experiencing pain must be weighed against the risk of anesthesia. As a result of this controversy and because of the lack of training in the techniques available, few physicians currently use anesthesia; however, their number is increasing following studies that demonstrate the minimal risks of some types of anesthesia.

Various methods that have been becoming popular as more evidence suggests that neonates do sense pain include dorsal penile nerve block (DPNB), precircumcision oral analgesics, local anesthesia of foreskin, and topical anesthesia (see Chapter 22). Studies have found that infants anesthetized with either DPNB or local anesthesia show less crying, less tachycardia, less irritability, fewer behavior changes during the 24 hours following the procedure, and lower postprocedure serum cortisol levels than infants circumcised without anesthesia. Administering DPNB adds little time and expense to the overall routine, and no major complications have been reported.

INDICATIONS

- Parental desire in any healthy newborn undergoing circumcision

CONTRAINDICATIONS

- Hypospadias*
- Unusual appearing genitalia*
- Inability to determine phenotype of child* (ambiguous genitalia)

---

*These patients should be referred to a specialist.

- Age less than 12 hours (physiologic adaptation requires 12 to 24 hours)
- Severe illness
- Prematurity (until the child is ready for discharge from hospital)

EQUIPMENT

- 1% lidocaine *without* epinephrine
- 1 cc syringe with 27-gauge needle (tuberculin)
- Alcohol antiseptic solution
- Infant restrainer (papoose board)

PREPROCEDURE PATIENT EDUCATION

Discuss the risks, the benefits, and the controversial issues of neonatal anesthesia with the parents, and obtain informed consent for DPNB. This consent form should be signed separately from the consent form for circumcision.

TECHNIQUE

1. In a warm room, place the infant in restraints. Fold back the diaper to expose the penis.

   Note: As the physician becomes more comfortable using DPNB, time may be saved by performing the procedure *before* the infant is placed in restraints. This allows more time for the anesthetic to take effect while preparations are being made for the circumcision.

2. Using an index finger, palpate the lateral side of the penis to determine the depth of the root of the penis, which is usually about 0.75 to 1 cm beneath the skin surface. Often it is about the size, shape, and consistency of a large blueberry at the base of the penis.

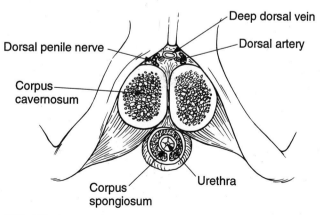

FIG. 112-1.
Anatomy of the penile root (cross section).

3. Before the procedure, note the anatomy as shown in Fig. 112-1. Prepare the skin at the base of the penis with antiseptic solution. Using aseptic technique and stabilizing the penis by gentle, slightly downward or ventral traction, insert the needle at the 2 o'clock position (the dorsal or cephalad direction being the 12 o'clock position, and the ventral direction being the 6 o'clock position) in a posteromedial direction. Insert to a depth of 0.3 to 0.5 cm beneath the skin surface (Fig. 112-2). This depth corresponds to 0.5 to 0.7 cm distal to the penile root, or slightly proximal to where the dorsal nerves branch (Fig. 112-3). The tip of the needle should be freely movable, indicating that it is in loose connective tissue. This prevents injection into the corpus cavernosum. Taking care not to inject into a blood vessel (check by aspirating), inject 0.2 to 0.4 cc of lidocaine. Repeat the injection at the 10 o'clock position. Do not exceed a total of 0.8 cc of lidocaine. Anesthesia will be optimal in 2 to 3 minutes.

4. In the occasional infant whose penile root is not palpable because it is embedded in pubic fat, the anesthetic can be injected at the same locations, depth, and direction, about 0.3 to 0.5 cm superolateral to the penile-suprapubic skin junction (Fig. 112-4).

COMPLICATIONS

- Inadequate response
- Localized bleeding hematoma at the injection site
- Local skin infection or necrosis
- Allergic reaction to lidocaine
- Penile necrosis (theoretical; this has not been reported. Avoid raising a circumferential subcutaneous bleb of anesthetic. Lidocaine *without* epinephrine appears to be the safest anesthetic.)

Note: Two older infants have been reported to have developed transient ischemia of the glans following DPNB (performed in a different manner than described here). Despite many studies, no other major complications have been reported.

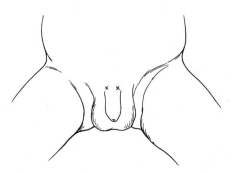

FIG. 112-2.
Injection site for administering dorsal penile nerve block.

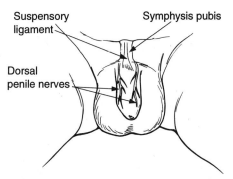

FIG. 112-3.
Location of dorsal penile nerves. Note branching begins after entering penis.

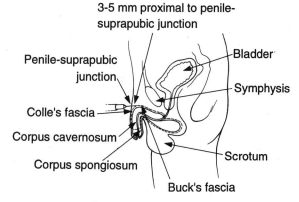

FIG. 112-4.
Sagittal view through the perineum showing anesthetic injection in a posteromedial direction 3 to 5 mm under the skin at or below Buck's fascia. Colle's fascia is superficial to Buck's fascia.

CPT/BILLING CODE

00920   Anesthesia for procedure on male external genitalia; not otherwise specified

BIBLIOGRAPHY

American Academy of Pediatrics: Committee statements: report of the task force on circumcision, *Pediatrics* 84(2):388, 1989.

Fontaine P, Toffler WL: Dorsal penile nerve block for newborn circumcision, *Am Fam Physician* 43(4):1327, 1991.

Kirya C, Werthmann MW: Neonatal circumcision and penile dorsal nerve block—a painless procedure, *J Pediatr* 92(6):998, 1978.

Mintz MR, Ricardo G: Clinical notes: dorsal penile nerve block for circumcision, *Clin Pediatr* 28(12):590, 1989.

Stang HJ, Snellman L: Dorsal penile nerve block for circumcision, *JAMA* 261:702, 1989.

PART NINE

Gastrointestinal

CHAPTER 113

Inguinal Hernia Reduction

George G. Zainea

The indirect inguinal hernia is the most common type of groin hernia. It occurs lateral to the inferior epigastric vessels. The hernia sac passes through the internal inguinal ring. It is associated with patency of the processus vaginalis. This hernia is typically seen in children and young adults.

The direct inguinal hernia occurs medial to the inferior epigastric vessels. It protrudes through the posterior inguinal floor. It is more commonly seen in adults. The risk of incarceration is less than that of indirect inguinal hernia.

Femoral hernias are seen far less commonly. These usually are found in adult women. The protrusion occurs beneath the inguinal ligament just medial to the femoral vessels in the upper thigh.

DIAGNOSIS

Diagnosis involves palpation with the patient both supine and standing. An incarcerated groin hernia manifests as a nonreducible painful groin bulge. Associated intestinal obstruction may also be present.

A Valsalva maneuver will allow the appreciation of a palpable impulse in a true hernia. Auscultation may reveal bowel sounds. Transillumination can be performed to assist with diagnosis.

DIFFERENTIAL DIAGNOSIS

The history and physical examination usually enables exclusion of other disorders that may mimic an incarcerated groin hernia, such as an *inflamed lymph node,* which is usually evident by history and on palpation; a *dilated varicose vein,* which may appear as a bulge in the inguinal region; and a *hydrocele* of the spermatic cord, which is typically not tender, does transilluminate, and rarely is associated with an acute presentation. Other disorders to consider include *testicular torsion,* which manifests as extreme scrotal pain and swelling. However, swelling at the level of the pubic tubercle may not be evident. Pain may be intensified with scrotal elevation. Finally, with a groin bulge an *undescended testicle* should be suspected, especially if the gonad is not present in the scrotal sac.

TECHNIQUE

By definition, a hernia that is nonreducible is incarcerated. Incarceration usually involves either the bowel or the omentum. One may see intestinal obstruction with bowel incarceration; however, the most feared complication of incarceration is strangulation. With strangulation, the blood supply to the intestine is compromised, and ischemic necrosis and gangrene may result.

The decision to reduce incarcerated hernias requires clinical judgment. If one suspects that strangulation exists, then the situation is best dealt with immediately in the operating room. Patients with strangulation typically appear ill. They may be febrile. The bulge is extremely tender, and overlying skin erythema may be present.

If strangulation is not suspected, then the clinician may attempt closed reduction as follows.

1. Place the patient in the supine Trendelenburg position. This allows gravity to assist with hernia reduction.
2. Administer a narcotic for analgesia and intravenous diazepam for muscle relaxation. After sedation, allow for passive reduction of the hernia over a 30- to 40-minute period.
3. If the attempt at passive reduction is not successful, proceed with an attempt at active reduction. Place one hand over the neck of the hernia sac to guide its contents into the peritoneal cavity. Use the other hand to provide gentle and steady distal-to-proximal compression over the hernia.

Using these techniques, the clinician should be able to reduce one third to one half of incarcerated groin hernias. Patients with irreducible groin hernias or incarcerated femoral hernias (one is seldom able to reduce these) should be immediately referred to a surgeon.

Infants and children who successfully undergo closed reduction of inguinal hernias should be admitted to the hospital for surgical repair. An adult patient with suspected compromised bowel in the reduced hernia should be admitted to the hospital for observation. Adults who undergo successful closed reduction and return home should soon thereafter undergo elective hernia repair. A truss should be used only to prevent recurrent protrusion up to the date of surgery.

BIBLIOGRAPHY

Kauffman HM, O'Brien DP: Selective reduction of incarcerated inguinal hernia, *Am J Surg* (119):660, June 1970.

Leape LL, Holder TM: Pediatric surgery. In Sabiston DC, editor: *Davis-Christopher textbook of surgery,* Philadelphia, 1981, W.B. Saunders.

Shandling B: Hernias. In Behrman and Vaughn, editors: *Nelson textbook of pediatrics,* ed 13, Philadelphia, 1987, W.B. Saunders.

Ziegler MM: Lumps and bumps. In Schwartz MW et al, editors: *Principles and practice of clinical pediatrics,* St Louis, 1990, Mosby.

CHAPTER 114

Gastric Lavage

John Harlan Haynes III

Evacuation of undesirable stomach contents using a large-bore flexible catheter has been medically advocated for the past 200 years. Instillation of isotonic solutions with manual or suction-assisted gastric emptying is quite effective in treating ingestion of toxic substances and upper gastrointestinal hemorrhage. Given proper patient selection, the technique may be sanitarily performed with minimal risk.

After a known toxic ingestion, immediate administration of syrup of ipecac (15 ml for children, 30 ml for adults) will induce effective emesis and gastric evacuation. Ipecac should be *avoided* in patients who are semiconscious, obtunded, or who may have seizures (to avoid aspiration), and in cases involving ingestion of the following:

- Caustic or alkali substances
- Petroleum distillates, such as viscous oils that are not absorbed well in the gastrointestinal tract and carry a high risk if aspirated (e.g., mineral, seal, or signal oil in some furniture polishes). Emesis *should* be induced for ingestion of petroleum distillates carrying more toxic substances such as insecticides, heavy metals, aniline, or nitrobenzene, as well as for hydrocarbons that carry a risk of central nervous system toxicity if they are absorbed.
- Chemicals or drugs that are likely to rapidly produce coma or seizures (e.g., sedative-hypnotics, cyanide, tricyclic antidepressants (TCAs), camphor, strychnine)
- Phenothiazines or other antiemetics (high risk of aspiration with jaw dystonia)

Gastric lavage may be the most effective means of rapid gastric evacuation in many cases. However, pulmonary aspiration with subsequent chemical pneumonitis can be a devastating complication of gastric lavage. Precautions—considering risks verses benefits—must be weighed.

INDICATIONS

- Poisoning by recent ingestion of a toxic substance in which attempts at induction of emesis are unsuccessful or contraindicated

Note: The Regional Poison Control Center can be of great help in determining whether gastric emptying by catheter lavage is indicated.

- Upper gastrointestinal hemorrhage
- Poisoning associated with obtunded or comatose patients
- Poisoning associated with rapid onset of seizures, predicted central nervous system toxicity, or respiratory depression in drug overdoses (e.g., TCAs, cyanide, strychnine, camphor)
- Cold gastric lavage for severe hyperthermia

CONTRAINDICATIONS

- Lack of mechanical airway protection in an obtunded patient
- Caustic ingestions (acids, alkalies)
- Ingestion of hydrocarbons, especially those not absorbed (contraindicated in absence of endotracheal intubation)

LAVAGE SYSTEMS

There are various lavage systems available. They may be classified by the action they provide and their type of connection. Open systems may be active or passive in evacuation procedure, while the closed system that is available is primarily active. Open systems are more time-consuming and potentially messy, but are generally less expensive. The closed system is prepackaged, self-contained, easy to use, and provides more protection to the health care provider.

A passive system simply uses gravity to drain the stomach contents once the intragastric tube is in place. An active system uses a syringe to generate pressure, and to aspirate and irrigate the stomach. A single syringe injects and removes the lavage fluid from the stomach through the gastric tube. The syringe must be disconnected from the tube to be filled and emptied after each lavage cycle.

The recently developed closed active system, EASI-LAV, employs a double-barrel syringe with automatic two-way valves. The syringe remains attached to the gastric tube. Its stroke volume of 125 cc allows for rapid fluid movement and the creation of fluid turbulence, resulting in fast, easy removal of toxic substances or clots.

EQUIPMENT

- Large-diameter gastric hose with extra holes cut near the tip (A 32 to 50 Fr. orogastric tube is recommended for adults; a 16 to 32 Fr. orogastric tube is recommended for children. If the practitioner prefers a nasogastric tube, use an 18 Fr. or smaller *open system.*)
- 2% viscous lidocaine gel, or benzocaine; phenylephrine decongestant nasal spray for nasal insertion (*open* and *closed system*)
- 50 cc tube syringe (*open system*)

- Y connector and clamp, with or without suction apparatus (*open system*)
- Endotracheal tube for obtunded patients (*open* and *closed system*)
- 1 liter normal saline for injection with tubing (*open system*)
- Activated charcoal (1 gm/kg) for poisonings (*open* and *closed system*)
- Tape (*open* and *closed system*)
- EASI-LAV kit (Ballard Medical Products, Midvale, Utah), which includes fluid bag and tubing, waste bag and tubing, double-barrel syringe mechanism, gastric tube, sample cup (*closed system*)
- Eye protection, face mask, gloves, and gown (*open* and *closed system*)
- Suction tube with vacuum generator (*open* and *closed system*)

INITIAL SETUP (ALL SYSTEMS)

1. It is extremely important to provide airway protection with a cuffed endotracheal tube for patients whose level of consciousness is depressed or whose airway-protective reflexes are diminished. (The absence of blinking after touching the eyelashes is strong evidence of inability to protect the airway from vomitus.)
2. Position the patient in the left lateral recumbent position with the head lowered approximately 10 degrees. This decreases the risk of aspiration should vomiting occur.
3. Premeasure and mark the length of the tube needed by estimating the distance from the nose to the midepigastrum. Larger holes may be cut in the end of the tube to accommodate larger fragments.
4. If the tube is to be inserted nasally, spray both nostrils with the decongestant nasal spray. Lidocaine gel may be placed into the tube syringe and slowly instilled into one nostril. Ask the patient to "sniff and swallow," if he or she is able to do this. Use an 18 Fr. tube or smaller. (See procedure for nasogastric tube insertion in Chapter 42, Nasogastric Tube and Salem Sump Insertion.) In most cases, nasal intubation for gastric lavage offers no advantage over an orogastric tube and may cause severe hemorrhage and injury to the mucosa and turbinates.
5. For orogastric tube insertion:
   a. If the patient is alert, spray the posterior pharynx with topical benzocaine or Cetacaine aerosol.
   b. Position the patient's head so that it is flexed as far forward as possible, and insert your gloved index and middle finger over the base of the patient's tongue.
   c. Guide the lubricated orogastric tube over the dorsum of your fingers as the patient swallows (Fig. 114-1). If the patient gags, advance immediately after gagging.
   d. Advance the tube to the previously measured distance marked on the tube.
6. Confirm intragastric tube placement by auscultating the stomach while introducing air with the syringe. A large portion of the gastric contents may be removed by careful aspiration. This may be sent for toxicologic analysis. Secure the tube with tape.

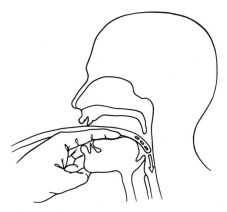

FIG. 114-1.
Orogastric tube insertion.

OPEN SYSTEM

Technique (Fig. 114-2)

1. Introduce the normal saline at a rate of 15 cc/kg per cycle from an IV bag or large syringe attached to the tube with a Y connector in the proximal circuit.
2. During saline infusion, clamp the efferent drainage arm. After instilling approximately 150 to 200 cc (50 to 100 cc in children), clamp the afferent reservoir arm. Then open the drainage arm to allow "passive" gravity evacuation of stomach contents. Intermittent suction may be applied to facilitate gastric emptying. Manual agitation of the stomach by gentle massage of the upper abdominal wall enhances recovery of gastric contents.
3. With active systems, use a syringe and/or vacuum suction instead of gravity to irrigate and evacuate gastric contents
4. Continue gastric irrigation until at least 3 liters of lavage have been accomplished and the return is clear on visual inspection.
5. After gastric lavage has been completed in toxic ingestions, a slurry of activated charcoal may be cleanly administered by adding 1 gm/kg of the powder through an opened upper corner of a partially full, hanging IV bag. This mixture is infused through the nasogastric circuit with the efferent arm clamped.
6. When the procedure is completed, clamp or pinch the gastric tube during removal to prevent contaminating the lung with charcoal and gastric contents. If repeated doses of charcoal are deemed necessary, the large tube may be replaced with a standard, smaller nasogastric tube. In the intubated patient, leave the endotracheal tube in place for at least 15 minutes to prevent aspiration. Confirm adequate spontaneous respirations prior to removing the endotracheal tube.

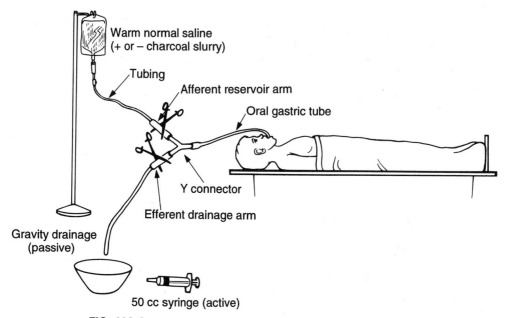

FIG. 114-2.
An open gastric lavage system with components.

CLOSED SYSTEM

Technique (EASI-LAV)

Setup (Fig. 114-3)

1. Hang a waste bag from the bed. Close the sampling port clamp and cap. Close the fluid bag clamp.
2. Fill the fluid bag with normal saline solution. To seal the fluid bag, rest it on the countertop.
3. Hang the fluid bag from an IV pole.
4. Insert an orogastric tube as previously described. Bending or kinking of the gastric tube may cause malfunction of the system. Ensure airway protection.
5. Advance both syringe plungers to the fully forward position.
6. Attach the syringe to the gastric lavage tube and pinch the retaining collar in place.
7. Ensure proper tube placement by locking the red output plunger in the fully forward position, then pump the blue input plunger alone while listening for air bubbles in the stomach.
8. Attach the blue tubing connection from the fluid bag to blue input port on the syringe.
9. Attach the red tubing connection from the waste bag to the red output port on the syringe.

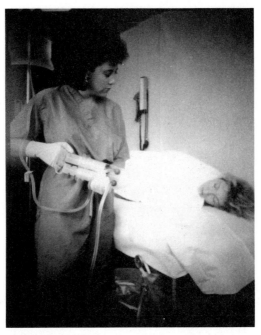

FIG. 114-3.
Performing gastric lavage with the closed double-barrel syringe system. (From Haynes JH: Gastric lavage for serious poisonings, *Fam Pract Recert* 14(10):45, 1992. Used with permission. Photo courtesy of Ballard Medical Products.)

10. Ensure that both syringe plungers are in the fully forward position. Always leave the blue input plunger forward when not in use or fluid will flow into the patient's stomach.
11. Open the clamp on the fluid bag.

Procedure

1. To empty the stomach, pump the red output plunger alone until resistance is encountered or no return is obtained. Confirm that the clamp on the waste bag line is opened. To avoid mucosal injury, never pull the red plunger against stiff resistance.
2. Lock the red output plunger in the forward position by pushing the plunger completely forward and rotating it clockwise 90 degrees.
3. Prime the system by pumping the blue input plunger three times to partially fill the stomach.
4. Unlock the red output plunger by rotating it 90 degrees counterclockwise.
5. Perform the lavage as follows:
   a. Grasp both plunger handles, pull back, and push forward. This will wash out and empty the stomach.
   b. Perform this lavage three times.

BOX 114-1. SUBSTANCES BOUND BY ACTIVATED CHARCOAL

Aspirin
Dextroamphetamine
Strychnine
Chloroquine
Phenytoin
Phenobarbital
Theophylline
Tricyclic antidepressants
Primaquine phosphate
Glutethimide (less effectively bound)

---

    c. With the blue input plunger fully forward, pump the red output plunger three times—or less, if resistance is met.

    d. Repeat Steps a, b, and c until the gastric return fluid is clear.

6. To administer charcoal (see Box 114-1 for substances with which charcoal effectively binds), the following procedure is effective:

    a. Lock the red output plunger in the forward position by pushing it completely forward and rotating it clockwise 90 degrees.

    b. Pour charcoal into the fluid bag and reseal the bag.

    c. Lavage fluid (50 to 75 cc) may be added as a slurry to speed administration.

    d. Pump the blue input plunger until all of the charcoal is in the stomach. Repeat Step 5c above to remove charcoal.

COMPLICATIONS

- Mucosal injury or perforation of the upper gastrointestinal tract
- Fluid and electrolyte disturbances (more common when water is used instead of saline)
- Hypothermia (prevented by using warmed saline)
- Pulmonary aspiration (up to 10% in some studies)
- Hypoxemia
- Laryngospasm
- Cardiac dysrhythmias
- Tracheal intubation instead of gastric placement

CPT/BILLING CODE

91105   Gastric intubation, and aspiration or lavage for treatment (e.g., for ingested poisons)

BIBLIOGRAPHY

Haynes JH: Gastric lavage for serious poisonings, *Fam Pract Recert* 14(10):45, 1992.

Rosen P et al: *Emergency medicine: concepts and clinical practice,* ed 2, St Louis, 1988, Mosby.

Rumack BH: Hydrocarbon management. In Rumack BH, editor: *Poisindex,* Englewood, Colo, 1975, Micromedix.

Tandberg D, Troutman WG: Gastric lavage in the poisoned patient. In Roberts JR, Hedges JR, editor: *Clinical procedures in emergency medicine,* ed 2, Philadelphia, 1991, W. B. Saunders.

Tintinalli J et al: *Emergency medicine: a comprehensive study guide,* New York, 1985, McGraw-Hill.

CHAPTER 115

Abdominal Paracentesis and Peritoneal Lavage

Michael L. Brown

Abdominal paracentesis and peritoneal lavage are useful in a variety of clinical situations. Previously, paracentesis was performed more frequently for relief of increased intraabdominal pressure caused by ascites. Currently, it is most commonly used for diagnostic purposes and only occasionally for relief of discomfort associated with large volumes of ascitic fluid, such as respiratory difficulty.

In abdominal trauma, peritoneal lavage is a useful diagnostic adjunct for hemoperitoneum. Computed tomography (CT) scanning is less invasive, but it is often time-consuming, expensive, and nonspecific. Lavage will distinguish fluid from blood. (Peritoneal dialysis can also be performed using this technique.)

Large volumes of ascitic fluid will tend to float the air-filled bowel toward the midline, where it is then more easily perforated during paracentesis. Additionally, the cecum is relatively fixed and is much less mobile than the sigmoid colon. Hence, bowel perforations are more frequent in the right lower quadrant than in the left.

Ascitic fluid should be sent to the laboratory or pathologist for Gram stain, culture, cytology, protein, and cell count. Grossly bloody fluid in the abdomen constitutes a positive test. Lavage fluid should be tested after 100 cc has returned. The test is positive if the red blood cell count (RBC) is greater than $100,000/mm^3$ or if the physician is unable to read newspaper type through the paracentesis tubing.

INDICATIONS

- Differential diagnosis of ascites
- Intraabdominal pressure causing respiratory distress
- Blunt or penetrating abdominal injury, especially in paraplegics, who may have no other symptoms

- Acute abdomen in patients with altered mental status due to head injury, alcohol intoxication, or drug ingestion
- Acute pancreatitis in those with normal amylase (peritoneal fluid amylase level greater than serum amylase level); peritoneal fluid amylase may also be elevated in perforated peptic ulcer
- Peritoneal dialysis
- Differential diagnosis of acute peritonitis

CONTRAINDICATIONS

- Acute abdomen requiring immediate surgery (*absolute contraindication*)
- Coagulopathy (*relative contraindication*)
- Thrombocytopenia (*relative contraindication*)
- Severe bowel distension (use extra caution or open technique)
- Previous abdominal surgery, especially pelvic surgery
- Pregnancy (necessitates using open technique above umbilicus after first trimester)
- Distended bladder that cannot be emptied with a Foley catheter
- Obvious infection at intended site of insertion (cellulitis or abscess)

EQUIPMENT

Commercially prepared kit or the following equipment:

- Skin cleansing solution (povidone-iodine)
- Sterile gloves and mask
- Sterile marking pen (if area has not been marked indelibly before skin prep)
- Sterile drapes
- 1% or 2% lidocaine (maximum dose: 30 cc of 1%, 15 cc of 2%) with or without epinephrine (Epinephrine helps eliminate unwanted abdominal wall bleeding and false-positives.)
- 12 cc syringe for anesthetic
- 20 cc syringe for diagnostic tap
- 50 cc syringe, if using stopcock technique
- 18-gauge 1½- to 3-inch needle or angiocath, depending on abdominal wall thickness
- 25- or 27-gauge 1½-inch needle
- 20- or 22-gauge spinal needles
- Scalpel, No. 11 blade
- Guide wire with floppy tip (useful if lavage or dialysis is being considered)
- 9 to 18 Fr. peritoneal lavage catheter
- Needle holder
- Mayo scissors and straight scissors
- Sterile IV tubing (without valves) with appropriate sterile connectors for lavage catheter and IV bags
- *Optional:* three-way stopcock (for use with 50 cc syringe)

- 1 liter vacuum bottles, a sufficient number for draining more than 1 liter of fluid if ascites volume is large
- Ringer's lactate (RL) or normal saline (NS) for infusion into abdomen (if necessary for diagnosis of hemoperitoneum)
- Nylon skin suture (4-0 or 5-0) on cutting needle
- Absorbable sutures for peritoneum and fascia, if peritoneum is to be opened

SUPPLIER

For complete commercially prepared kit contact

Arrow Medical Products Ltd.
Unit 20, 150 Britania Road East
Mississauga, Ontario L4Z1S6
Canada

PREPROCEDURE PATIENT EDUCATION AND PREPARATION

- Explain the procedure and its risks to the patient (see Complications).
- Obtain verbal or written informed consent.
- Examine the abdomen, delineate areas of shifting dullness, and find landmarks; mark if necessary.
- Take plain and upright X-rays of the abdomen before performing the procedure. (Air is introduced during the procedure and may confound the diagnosis later.)
- Check for bowel distension.
- Place the patient in the horizontal dorsal decubitus position (may tilt to side of collection slightly for improved fluid positioning).
- Use a Foley catheter and nasogastric (NG) tube if necessary.
- Use wrist restraints, especially in patients with altered mental status.

TECHNIQUE

1. Prepare the abdominal skin at the puncture site with povidone-iodine solution.
2. Apply sterile drapes to outline the area to be tapped. For paracentesis and lavage, the site should be in the midline about one third the distance from the umbilicus to the symphysis (usually 2 to 3 cm below the umbilicus [Fig. 115-1]). You may also use a point about one third the distance from the umbilicus to the anterior iliac crest (with the left side preferred).
3. Infiltrate the skin and subcutaneous tissues with lidocaine (with epinephrine, if possible).
4. Initially direct the needle perpendicular to the skin and infiltrate the peritoneum with anesthetic (resistance will be felt as the needle perforates the peritoneum).
5. Using the No. 11 blade scalpel, create a skin incision large enough to allow threading a lavage catheter (3 to 5 mm), if necessary.

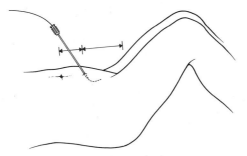

FIG. 115-1.
Insertion of the needle into the peritoneal cavity in the midline, one third of the distance between the umbilicus and the symphysis pubis. A floppy tip guide wire is inserted through the needle.

6. Direct an 18-gauge needle attached to a 22 cc or 50 cc syringe through the anesthetized tract into the peritoneum, applying slight suction to the syringe. You may grasp the needle to prevent accidental thrusting into the abdomen and possible viscus perforation.

7. Once in the cavity, direct the needle toward the center of the pelvic hollow. When fluid returns, fill the syringe and send it off for the desired studies. (It is not recommended to remove more than 2 liters of fluid at one time.)

8. If the tap is dry, perform the lavage technique, if indicated.

9. The guide wire may be introduced through the 18-gauge needle to insert the peritoneal lavage catheter. The wire should insert easily; if there is any resistance, remove the wire and advance the needle until the wire feeds easily.

10. Insert about half of the wire into the pelvis and remove the needle.

11. Slide the peritoneal lavage catheter over the wire, using gentle twisting motions (Fig. 115-2). Always keep a firm hold on the wire to prevent it from slipping into the peritoneal cavity.

12. Remove the wire after the catheter is in the peritoneal cavity. Aspiration may again be attempted, and if the tap is dry, proceed to lavage.

13. Connect the intravenous tubing and infuse about 700 to 1000 cc of Ringer's lactate (RL) or normal saline (NS) into the abdominal cavity. Then connect the tubing to either a 1 liter vacuum bottle or a syringe with stopcock, and remove the fluid just infused. The patient may have to be moved a bit to get an adequate return of as much fluid as possible.

14. After the fluid is removed, gently remove the catheter and apply pressure to the wound; have the first 100 cc of fluid analyzed. If the wound is still leaking fluid after 5 minutes of direct pressure, suture the puncture site using a mattress suture, and apply a pressure dressing.

POSTPROCEDURE PATIENT EDUCATION

Educate the patient about bleeding, pain, infection, hypotension from reaccumulation of fluid, and other complications.

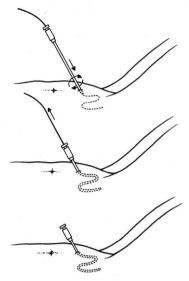

FIG. 115-2.
The plastic catheter is placed over the guide wire and inserted into the peritoneal cavity by means of a twisting motion at the skin level. After the catheter has been advanced, the guide wire is removed.

COMPLICATIONS

- Bladder perforation
- Small and large bowel perforation
- Stomach perforation
- Lacerations of major vessels (mesenteric, iliac, aorta)
- Laceration of catheter or guide wire and loss in peritoneal cavity (might require laparotomy to recover catheter)
- Abdominal wall hematomas and false-positive results
- Incisional hernias
- Wound infection
- Wound dehiscence
- Inability to retrieve majority of instilled fluid

There are no reported deaths.

CPT/BILLING CODES

49080	Peritoneocentesis, abdominal paracentesis, or peritoneal lavage; initial
49081	Peritoneocentesis, abdominal paracentesis, or peritoneal lavage; subsequent

When either procedure is performed at an initial visit (for a new patient) and it is the major service performed, the procedure code 99025 may be used instead of the usual initial visit, as an additional service.

BIBLIOGRAPHY

Brown JS: *Minor surgery, a text and atlas,* Chicago, 1986, Year Book Medical Publishers.

Keating KP, Yeston NS: Diagnostic peritoneal lavage: indications, results, complications, *Res Staff Phys* 37(11):31, 1991.

Mills J et al: *Current emergency diagnosis and treatment,* East Norwalk, Conn, 1985, Lange Medical Publications.

Roberts JR, Hedges JR: *Clinical procedures in emergency medicine,* Philadelphia, 1985, W. B. Saunders.

Wolcott MW: *Ambulatory surgery and the basics of emergency surgical care,* ed 2, Philadelphia, 1988, J. B. Lippincott.

CHAPTER 116

Clinical Anorectal Anatomy and Examination

James A. Surrell

A practical knowledge of anorectal anatomy is necessary for the proper evaluation and treatment of patients with anorectal complaints, such as hemorrhoids and anal fissures. A basic anorectal examination will include inspection of the perianal tissues with digital anorectal examination. Depending on patient complaints, anoscopy and sigmoidoscopy may also be necessary. The purpose of this chapter is to describe the practical and the clinically important features of anorectal anatomy. See Chapter 117, Anoscopy, for more information regarding this topic.

BASIC ANATOMY

Fig. 116-1 is a diagram of the anatomy of the anal canal and lower rectum. The most distal extent of the anal canal at the opening is considered the *anal verge*. Two to three centimeters proximal to the anal verge is a circular row of glands, most commonly referred to as the *dentate line* or *pectinate line*. This dentate line contains anal glands that secrete mucus to lubricate the anal canal. Squamous epithelium is located distal to the dentate line, and columnar epithelium is located proximal to the dentate line in the rectum. There is an area called the *transition zone,* which is composed of mixed columnar and squamous epithelium, and which is where the anal canal merges with the rectum. The distal rectum and anal canal are surrounded by two sleeves of circular muscles. The innermost circular muscle is the *internal sphincter,* and the *external sphincter* is located outside of the internal sphincter as shown in Fig. 116-1. It is important to note that the external sphincter is external to the internal sphincter not only from a medial to lateral aspect, but also from a cephalad to caudad aspect at the anal verge. The *anorectal ring* is located about 1 to 2 cm above the dentate line. This palpable anorectal ring represents the puborectalis muscle, which encircles the very distal rectum from its anterior point of attachment at the pubis. The *rectum* is the distal 10 to 12 cm of the colon.

PATIENT POSITION

A complete anorectal examination can be accomplished with the patient on the examining table in the left lateral decubitus position (Fig. 116-2). The patient's knees are flexed and drawn toward the chest, and the buttocks are drawn toward the examiner to a point just slightly off the table. The patient's head and shoulders should remain well toward the center of the examining table, so that the patient is

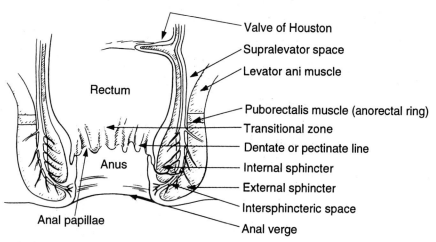

FIG. 116-1.
Anatomy of the anal canal.

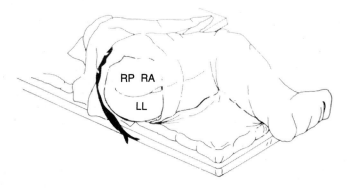

FIG. 116-2.
Placing the patient in the left lateral decubitus position (Sim's position). Digital examination, flexible sigmoidoscopy, and most anorectal procedures can be performed in this position.

confident that he or she will not fall. This position also directs the axis of the anal canal and rectum directly toward the examiner.

EXTERNAL ANAL EXAMINATION

After appropriately advising the patient, visually inspect the external anus. Look for any sign of perianal inflammation that may suggest pruritus ani or other dermatologic conditions. Gently evert the buttocks; this will generally evert the anoderm to a sufficient degree that, if present, a posterior or anterior anal fissure may be directly visualized. If there is a *sentinel skin tag* present in either the posterior midline or the anterior midline, be diligent in evaluation for a fissure, especially if the history is consistent with anal fissure. If present, anal skin tags, perianal abscess, or thrombosed external hemorrhoids should be readily visible at this time. Internal and external hemorrhoids are classically located in the right anterior, right posterior, and left lateral quadrants. *Internal hemorrhoids* are located at and just proximal to the dentate line; *external hemorrhoids* are located distal to the dentate line at the anal verge. Hemorrhoids are collections of arteries and veins that represent normal anatomy and are not considered varicosities.

DIGITAL ANORECTAL EXAMINATION

Inform the patient that the anus will be touched with a lubricated, gloved examining finger. Apply gentle pressure to the anal verge to allow the examining finger to enter the anal canal. If an anal fissure is present, you may feel palpable induration, most commonly in the posterior midline and less commonly in the anterior midline. In males, assess the prostate gland with your gloved examining finger in the anal canal. To assess continence and anal sphincter function, flex your index finger slightly posteriorly and ask the patient to "squeeze down" as if to try to stop a bowel movement. If the patient has normal anatomic sphincter function, you will feel the tightening of the distal extent of the external sphincter at the base of your examining finger. The puborectalis muscle of the anorectal ring will also contract, pulling the tip of the examining finger from posterior to anterior. You should then be able to sweep the examining finger around the circumference of the distal rectum at the level of the anorectal ring and note the point of fixation of the puborectalis muscle at the symphysis pubis. Advise the patient to relax as the examination continues. Generally, internal hemorrhoids and the dentate line are not palpable to the gloved examining finger. However, a large hypertrophic anal papilla present at the level of the dentate line may be palpable. If necessary, obtain a small sample of stool on the tip of the gloved examining finger for occult blood testing.

ANAL CONTINENCE

The external sphincter and puborectalis muscle of the anorectal ring are the two muscles generally thought to afford voluntary anal continence. The external sphincter extends from the anal verge to the anorectal ring. The anorectal ring consists primarily of the puborectalis muscle, which encircles the very distal rectum at the level of the anorectal ring. From a practical standpoint, it is generally accepted that either an intact functional external sphincter or anorectal ring can provide near-perfect anal continence. The internal sphincter plays little role in maintaining voluntary anal continence. This is important when counseling patients when surgical treatment of anal fissures is being considered.

SUMMARY

A practical understanding of the anatomy of the anal canal is essential to conducting an adequate anorectal examination. Lesions commonly seen may include pruritus ani or perianal dermatitis, anal fissures, thrombosed external hemorrhoids, prolapsing bleeding internal hemorrhoids, hypertrophic anal papilla, perianal abscess, pilonidal disease, and others. When anal continence is an issue, you must be able to evaluate the function of the external sphincter and of the puborectalis muscle of the anorectal ring on digital anorectal examination. With appropriate patient preparation and technique, the anorectal examination should not be an uncomfortable or painful experience. See Chapter 117 for a description of the anoscopic examination.

BIBLIOGRAPHY

Corman ML: *Colon and rectal surgery,* Philadelphia, 1989, J.B. Lippincott.
Goligher J: *Surgery of the anus, rectum, and colon,* London, 1984, Bailliere-Tindall.
Gordon P, Nivatvongs S: *Principles and practice of surgery for the colon, rectum, and anus,* St Louis, 1992, Quality Medical Publishing.

Anoscopy

Jay R. Varma

Anoscopy is a common procedure in both ambulatory and emergency medical care. It is used primarily to evaluate the patient with perianal and anal complaints. It is also generally performed just before or after withdrawing the colonoscope or flexible sigmoidoscope. Before performing anoscopy, you should review Chapter 116, Clinical Anorectal Anatomy and Examination.

INDICATIONS

- Initial evaluation of rectal bleeding
- Anal or perianal pain
- Perianal itching (pruritus ani)
- Anal discharge
- Prolapse of the rectum
- External or internal hemorrhoids
- Fissures in ano
- Fistulae in ano
- Painful digital rectal examination
- Perianal condyloma
- Palpable masses on digital examination
- In association with sigmoidoscopy and colonoscopy

CONTRAINDICATIONS

- Unwilling patient
- Severe debilitation
- Acute myocardial infarction or similar cardiovascular condition
- Acute abdomen (*relative contraindication*)
- Marked anal canal stenosis

EQUIPMENT

- Anoscope
- Light source
- Gloves
- Lubricant
- Large-tipped cotton swabs
- Biopsy forceps, if needed
- Monsel's solution

The anoscope is a small cylindrical tool made of disposable plastic or reusable metal (Fig. 117-1). The size varies from 7 to 10 cm in length. They may or may not have handles. Distal diameter is approximately 2.5 cm. Some anoscopes are readily attachable to battery light sources, while others require an external light source (e.g., a goose-neck lamp).

Another type, the Ive's slotted anoscope, provides an unobstructed view of the walls of the anal canal (Fig. 117-2). This instrument is necessary for various techniques used to treat hemorrhoids on an outpatient basis. The advantage of the slotted instrument is that the mucosa is not compressed; thus, small lesions and hemorrhoids may be more easily visible and treated. Rather than looking out the end of the tube, one can visualize the mucosal wall in a more direct fashion.

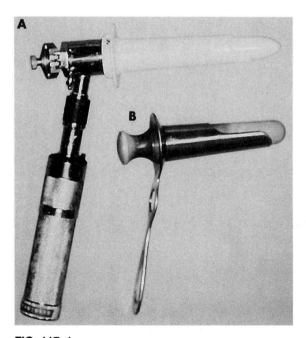

FIG. 117-1.
Two examples of typical anoscopes with obturators in place. **A,** Reusable metal instrument (Ive's slotted anoscope). **B,** Battery light source with disposable plastic tube.

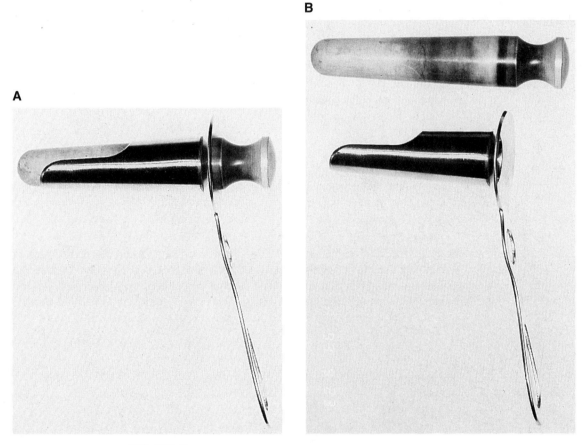

FIG. 117-2.
Ive's slotted anoscope with obturator in place (**A**) and obturator removed (**B**).

PREPROCEDURE PATIENT EDUCATION

Patients dread inspection of the anal canal. They perceive this examination as unpleasant and uncomfortable—short of painful. Their concerns of embarrassment are overwhelming.

This alone mandates that you prepare the patient mentally for what is involved. The patient must be cooperative and relaxed. Frank admission that the procedure will be unpleasant and uncomfortable, but not painful, is helpful. Explain the reasons necessitating the examination and the implications of not performing it. Reassure the patient that there are no significant complications resulting from anoscopy alone. However, if a biopsy sample is obtained or a lesion is removed, there may be some bleeding.

TECHNIQUE

An assistant is helpful. Both physician and assistant must wear gloves on both hands. An enema is generally not needed, but may be helpful.

1. Place the patient in the left lateral position and drape.
2. Have the assistant separate the glutei laterally, allowing full visibility of the perianal area.
3. Inspect the tissue closely. Ask the patient to bear down, and observe for hemorrhoid prolapse.
4. Perform a careful circumferential digital examination with an index finger that has been lubricated with K-Y Jelly or 2% lidocaine jelly. Note the sphincter tone. See Chapter 116, Clinical Anorectal Anatomy and Examination.
5. In male patients, palpate the prostate for size and masses.
6. Lubricate the anoscope well with K-Y Jelly with the obturator in place.
7. Insert the anoscope very gently into the anal aperture, gradually overcoming the resistance of the sphincters. Gently advance the instrument in the direction of the umbilicus until the full length of the anoscope is inserted—subject to patient acceptance and tolerance. The procedure is better tolerated and accomplished by asking the patient to gently take a deep breath in and out a few times at the beginning of the procedure.
8. After inserting the full length of the instrument, remove the obturator so that the mucosa of the anal canal can be visualized. Fecal material is often encountered and can be removed with a large swab. Note the gross appearance of the mucous membrane; the pectinate line; the vasculature; and the presence of blood, mucus, pus, hemorrhoidal tissue, etc.
9. Gradually withdraw the instrument, observing the anal canal as the anoscope is extracted. Often, rotating the scope to the right and to the left improves the examination.
10. If the slotted instrument is used for viewing hemorrhoids or fissures, it must be inserted four times so that each quadrant can be examined. Allowing it to remain in place for a minute or two allows any hemorrhoids that are present to engorge with blood and be more readily visible.
11. If a biopsy specimen is to be obtained, a variety of long-handled biopsy instruments can be used. The instruments used for cervical biopsy work well. Stay superficial—only 3 or 4 mm of tissue is necessary. Control bleeding with Monsel's solution and pressure.
12. Complete the procedure form (Box 117-1).

POSTPROCEDURE PATIENT EDUCATION

Thoroughly explain the findings to the patient, and use pictures and drawings in the explanation. Discuss the etiology, treatment, and course of resolution of each finding as thoroughly as possible.

```
┌─────────────────────────────────────────────────────────────┐
│              BOX 117-1. PROCEDURE FORM                        │
│                    ANOSCOPY                                   │
│                                                              │
│  Patient name _____ B.D. _____ Sex _____ │
│  Patient ID #_____ SS#_____  │
│  Procedure _____ Date_____        │
│  Indication _____ M.D._____        │
│  ICD codes #_____  │
│                                                              │
│  Findings          Normal/Abnormal                           │
│  Sphincters                                                   │
│  Anal canal                                                   │
│  Mucosa                                                       │
│  Tears                                                        │
│  Vasculature                                                  │
│  Tumor/polyps                                                 │
│  Bleeding                                                     │
│  Hemorrhoids                                                  │
│                                                              │
│  Management _____         │
│             _____         │
│             _____         │
│             _____         │
│                                                              │
│  Follow-up date _____                         │
│  Physician _____ Date_____           │
└─────────────────────────────────────────────────────────────┘
```

COMPLICATIONS

This procedure, performed gently, has few complications. Likely or possible complications include tearing of the perianal skin or mucosa, and abrasion or tearing of hemorrhoidal tissue. There may be bleeding after biopsy, but infection almost never occurs.

CPT/BILLING CODES

46600	Anoscopy
46606	Anoscopy with biopsy, single or multiple
46615	Anoscopy with ablation of tumor(s), polyp(s), or other lesion(s)

CHAPTER 118

Flexible Sigmoidoscopy

Jay R. Varma

John L. Pfenninger

The flexible fiberoptic sigmoidoscope (FFS) is an instrument available in 35 cm, 60 cm, and 65 cm lengths. It is highly recommended that only the 60 or 65 cm scopes be considered. The sigmoidoscope has become an essential component in the primary care physician's office as a result of the attempt to detect colorectal cancer. To decrease morbidity and mortality, one must not only detect this cancer earlier, but also identify and remove precursor polyps. Over 150,000 cases of colon cancer occur each year, with 50,000 deaths. In nonsmokers of both sexes, it is the second major cancer killer. The instrument, although intended initially for screening, has also evolved into a valuable tool in evaluating symptomatic patients.

INDICATIONS

The American Society of Gastroenterology (ASGE), the American Cancer Society (ACS), the American College of Physicians (ACP), the National Cancer Institute (NCI), and the American College of Obstetrics and Gynecology (ACOG) recommend routine screening of patients 50 years of age and older for colon polyps and colon cancer. Begin screening at 35 to 40 years of age if the patient has significant risk factors, such as first-degree relatives with colon cancer. The latest revisions in cancer screening guidelines from the ACS state that flexible sigmoidscopy is "preferred" over the rigid scope.

- Surveillance after previous polypectomy
- Surveillance screening in ulcerative colitis/Crohn's disease
- Rectal bleeding
- New onset or persistent constipation
- Protracted diarrhea
- Change in bowel habits

- Abdominal pain
- Hemoccult positive stools (in addition to air contrast and barium enema)
- Unexplained weight loss, fevers
- Anemia

CONTRAINDICATIONS

Absolute

- Patient with acute, severe cardiopulmonary disease
- Inadequate bowel preparation
- Active diverticulitis
- Acute abdomen
- History of subacute bacterial endocarditis (SBE) or prosthetic valves in patients who have not received prophylaxis
- Marked bleeding dyscrasia

Relative

- Recent abdominal surgery (bowel or pelvic)
- Active infection
- Pregnancy

EQUIPMENT

The flexible sigmoidoscope is available in three forms: the self-contained fiberoptic scope, the video endoscope, and the disposable endosheath type. Although the fiberoptic scope is the traditional, most common version, the video sigmoidoscope is state of the art, using computer chip and video technology. The image from the tip of the scope is transmitted to a video monitor. This equipment facilitates videotape recording, sound narration, and other patient information storage. The disposable endosheath has recently been introduced into the market by Vision Sciences for use with its fiberoptic scope. Optics are comparable to other scopes, and the cleaning process is markedly simplified.

The following basic equipment is necessary to carry out routine fiberoptic sigmoidscopy:

- Scope consisting of the body with controls (Fig. 118-1) and the shaft of the scope with tip and apertures (Fig. 118-2)
- Light source (Fig. 118-3)
- Suction apparatus (Fig. 118-4)
- Biopsy forceps
- K-Y Jelly
- 4 × 4 inch gauze pads
- Nonsterile gloves

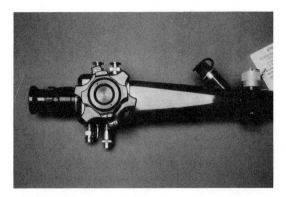

FIG. 118-1.
Control head and body of the fiberoptic sigmoidoscope.

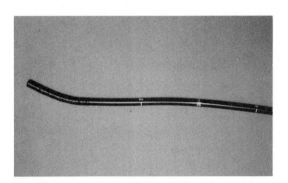 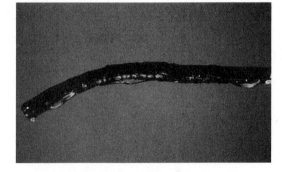

FIG. 118-2.
The tip of the sigmoidoscope. The one on the right has been lubricated with K-Y Jelly.

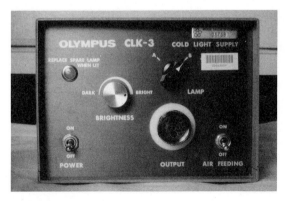

FIG. 118-3.
Light source with air supply.

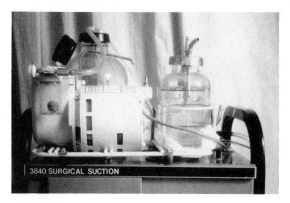

FIG. 118-4.
Suction apparatus.

- Water container (to hold water suctioned through the scope immediately upon completion of the procedure)
- Video unit and monitor (for videoscopy only)
- Anoscope
- Basin of water
- Formalin jars
- Disinfecting cleaner

SUPPLIERS OF SIGMOIDOSCOPES

Fujinon
10 High Point Dr.
Wayne, NJ 07470
201-633-5600
800-872-0196

Olympus
4 Nevada Dr.
Lake Success, NY 11042
516-488-3880
800-222-4554

Pentax FS 34P
30 Ramland Rd.
Orangeburg, NY 10962
914-365-0700

Welch Allyn, Inc.
4341 State Street Rd.
P.O. Box 220
Skaneateles, NY 13153-0220
315-685-4100
800-535-6663

Vision Sciences, Inc.
(video and endosheath models)
6 Strathmore Road
Natick, MA 01760
508-650-9971
800-874-9975

PREPROCEDURE PATIENT EDUCATION

Flexible sigmoidoscopy in most patients is an easy procedure performed in less than 15 minutes. However, for some patients the very thought of a tube in the rectum provokes anxiety, apprehension, and reluctance. This makes it necessary for the physician to reassure the patient and allay apprehension and anxiety with a thorough explanation. Use simple words with the aid of charts and figures. Explain the procedure to be performed, why and how it will be done, and the possible complications. The components of this patient-education process include

1. Bowel cleansing instructions (usually two Fleet enemas)
2. The equipment used
3. Anatomy of the colon
4. The procedure
5. The discomfort experienced during the procedure ("crampy distention")
6. The complications that are remotely likely, e.g., perforation, bleeding
7. Possible diseases likely to be detected
8. Biopsy technique, if needed
9. Whether photography/videotape will be used
10. Management of any findings
11. The need to continue all prescribed medications

See Boxes 118-1, 118-2, and 118-4 for further clarification.

PATIENT PREPARATION

Flexible sigmoidoscopy is well tolerated by the vast majority of patients. Mild analgesia/sedation, whether given orally or intramuscularly, is rarely needed. Oral diazepam and/or ibuprofen can be employed as needed in the individual situation.

Patient Bowel Preparation

Simple enemas (Fleet) administered until clear fluid is passed is all that is needed. This usually entails two enemas (occasionally three) 30 to 60 minutes before the procedure. Patients are allowed to take their medications and eat normally. If the patient tends to be constipated, a laxative should be given the day before the procedure.

It is highly advisable to have the patient (or a family member) sign the informed consent form (Box 118-2).

Antibiotic Prophylaxis (Also See Tables 125-1 and 125-2)

Antibiotic prophylaxis is not recommended for endoscopy procedures with or without biopsies (see Chapter 133, Antibiotic Prophylaxis for Bacterial Endocarditis). However, the physician may choose to administer prophylactic antibiotics to patients with prosthetic heart valves, a history of endocarditis, or surgically constructed systemic-pulmonary shunts or conduits. Prophylactic antibiotics would include parenteral ampicillin (or vancomycin) and gentamicin in most cases.

BOX 118-1. PATIENT EDUCATION HANDOUT
FLEXIBLE SIGMOIDOSCOPY

This information is to help you become informed about a procedure called flexible sigmoidoscopy. If you have any questions after reading this information, please feel free to discuss them with your physician.

Purpose
- To identify and diagnose lesions of the bowel at an early stage to prevent cancer
- To find cancer that may already be developed in earlier stages so that it might be more beneficially treated

Suspicious Symptoms
- Persistent abdominal pain
- A change in bowel habits (constipation or diarrhea that persists)
- Rectal bleeding of any sort
- A stool specimen that tests positive for blood (positive guaiac or Hemoccult)
- Unexplained weight loss or fevers
- Anemia
- Follow-up of previous polyps or cancers
- Any person 50 years of age and older, regardless of symptoms
- A high-risk history before age 50 (previous cancer, history of ulcerative colitis or Crohn's disease, history of female genital cancer, family history of cancer, history of multiple polyps)

The Benefits of Screening
Colon cancer is the second most common cause of cancer death in the United States, surpassed only by lung cancer. Every year, 35,000 lives could be saved by early diagnosis. It has now been fairly well documented that the majority of colon cancers begin in small polyps or growths that are totally benign. It takes 5 to 10 years for these benign polyps to become cancerous. If these polyps can be detected early and removed, cancer may be prevented. Polyps found in the lower part of the bowel may be associated with polyps higher up in the bowel or with other cancers. Therefore, a screening procedure may identify those patients who need a more extensive procedure called colonoscopy. If all polyps are removed and a vigorous screening program is initiated, the chance of colon cancer is decreased to only 15% of what is predicted for an unscreened population.

The Procedure
Flexible sigmoidoscopy is easily carried out in a physician's office. It takes between 15 to 30 minutes. The patient lies on a flat table on his or her left side. The physician performs a rectal examination, trying to feel for any growths, and then inserts the flexible sigmoidoscope instrument. This is a small tube approximately ½ inch in diameter. It is about 24 inches (60 cm) long and is actually quite movable, like a small piece of tubing. The physician can control the movement with some dials at one end, and can make the scope go up and down and to the right or left. The end of the tubing has a small opening for illumination, another for suctioning any fluid that might be left in the bowel, and another one for inserting air. By gently manipulating this tubing, the physician can insert it into the rectum and look at the lower part of the bowel (called the sigmoid colon) and left descending colon.

Continued.

BOX 118-1.—cont'd

Pain
The discomfort is usually minimal. It feels similar to the pain associated with gas cramps, because the physician inflates the colon with air to see inside. Most people compare the pain to a slightly uncomfortable bowel movement. Occasionally, if the bowel really has a lot of loops, pain will be greater, but this is rare. Usually, medication is not prescribed before or after the procedure unless the patient feels particularly anxious and requests it. The patient may take four ibuprofen 200 mg tablets 2 hours before the procedure. One is generally able to come straight from work and return to work after the procedure.

Preparation
Usually, one or two cleansing enemas (Fleet) 30 to 90 minutes before the procedure should be sufficient. If the expelled fluid is not clear, occasionally a third enema is needed. Inactive, elderly, or laxative-dependent patients may need a 24-hour diet restriction of clear liquids and four bisacodyl (Ducolax) tablets the night before. This is rarely recommended, but if you think this may be needed, please discuss it with your physician. If at all possible, no aspirin should be taken for 2 weeks before the procedure. If you have taken aspirin, or if you are on any medication, please notify the doctor.

Reasons for Not Having the Procedure
In some instances, if you are having abdominal pain that is severe enough that you are admitted to the hospital, you should not have the procedure done. Your physician will need to be the guide for this. Likewise, if you are pregnant, have had a recent heart attack, or have some other significant medical disease, you should let your physician evaluate this before going on with the procedure. If you have an artificial heart valve or an artificial joint, you should receive antibiotics before the procedure. Some heart murmurs also require antibiotics. Please discuss these issues with your physician.

Possible Complications
Flexible sigmoidoscopy is relatively safe. Approximately one time out of 10,000 procedures, a tear may be made in the bowel wall. This may require further surgery. Very rarely, there may be some bleeding. Generally, there is little discomfort. Some people who get lightheaded when they see blood or when they are under stress may faint. (If you are one of these, inform your physician who can prescribe medicine to prevent this.)

Possible Biopsy
If your physician sees a lesion, he or she may want to take a small sample of the tissue (biopsy). This will be sent to the pathologist who will look at it under the microscope and define it. This would increase your chance of bleeding a small amount, but it is usually rare.

Costs
The charge for flexible sigmoidoscopy is $ _____ . If it is done totally for the purpose of screening, it is unlikely that your insurance company will cover the charge. However, if you have any symptoms at all, insurance companies generally will provide coverage.

Additional questions and/or concerns should be discussed with your physician.

Used with permission of the Medical Procedures Center, P.C., Midland, Michigan.

**BOX 118-2. PATIENT CONSENT FORM
FLEXIBLE SIGMOIDOSCOPY**

I, _____ , consent of my own free will and
request that Dr. _____ and the doctor's assistants perform the procedure of flexible sigmoidoscopy on me.

If any unforeseen conditions arise in the course of this operation that, in the physician's judgment, require procedures in addition to or different from those now considered, I further request and authorize the physician to do whatever is advisable.

I understand that flexible sigmoidoscopy involves the insertion of a tube into my
rectum. This tube can be inserted up to 60 cm (24 inches) for the purpose of
evaluating the condition of my colon either to help diagnose a symptom I have or
to screen for problems. I understand that, in some instances, a biopsy specimen
may be taken. This means taking a small piece of tissue for further analysis.

I understand the procedure is not without complications, such as (but not limited
to) pain and cramping, bleeding, and possible perforation (causing a small hole in
the bowel). I also understand that at times some lesions are not visible to the physician. The risks involved and the possibility of complications have been fully explained to me.

I have read the previous information above and agree to the terms and conditions.
I understand the risks, the benefits, the procedure itself, and the alternatives. I
hereby release the physician performing the procedure from all and any liability
arising from, or connected with, the performance of the procedure.

_____   _____
Patient   Date

_____   _____
Witness   Date

Used with permission of The Medical Procedures Center, P.C., Midland, Michigan.

TECHNIQUE

The procedure of flexible sigmoidscopy has developed its own vocabulary and
terminology. Table 118-1 summarizes this "language" that must be understood
before learning the procedure.

1. Examine the patient's temperature, pulse, respiration, blood pressure, heart/
   lungs auscultation, and abdomen by auscultation/palpation.
2. Position the patient in the left lateral Sim's position (see Chapter 116, Fig. 116-2).
3. The endoscopist and assistant should wear gloves on both hands. Place the
   body and shaft of the scope alongside the patient. Lubricate the distal 3 to 4
   cm of the shaft tip with K-Y Jelly (avoid the lens). Notice where the dials are
   positioned when the shaft is completely straight.

TABLE 118-1.

Flexible Fiberoptic Sigmoidoscopy Terminology

Tip	Distal end of the shaft of the sigmoidoscope (Fig. 118-2).
Dials	Tip control knobs. Large inner dial moves the tip up and down. Small outer dial moves the tip left and right (Fig. 118-5).
Biopsy channel	The slot through which the biopsy forceps and also the brush wire are passed through the body and shaft of the scope (Fig. 118-5).
Suction control button	When pressed all the way down, this button allows the suction to operate (Fig. 118-5).
Air insufflation/lens cleaner (water) button	This button has a small opening that can be occluded to allow air to pass into the colon (Fig. 118-5). Pressing the button completely down will squirt water across the lens of the tip and will clear away debris.
Suction, air, and water connection ports	The location of tubes connecting on the bottom of the handpiece that go to suction, air, and water sources.
Slide-by	A technique of passing the flexible sigmoidoscope where the advancing tip of the scope is advanced proximally into the colon without the complete visualization of the lumen. This maneuver is often unavoidable but should be used very sparingly, and the scope should be advanced only 5 to 10 cm. If the lumen is not fully visualized or pressure, resistance, or pain is encountered, then pull back.
Pullback	Withdrawing the shaft of the scope to diminish or eliminate whiteout, redout, stretching, or looping.
One-on-one	As the scope is advanced into the rectum, there is an equal advance of the scope into the segment of colon (versus just stretching the colon without true advancement).
Redout	The tip of the scope lies flat on the mucosal surface, resulting in a red appearance through the lens.
Whiteout	The mucosal surface is stretched by the tip of the scope pressing against the mucosal surface. The vessels are thus blanched, giving a white appearance.
Tip deflection	The tip can be directed in four directions by rotating the dials—up ("north"), down ("south"), left ("west"), and right ("east"). The deflection should always be moderate and gentle. Alternatively, the head of the scope can be rotated right and left to turn the tip to the right or left.
Dithering	A to-and-fro advance and withdrawal process performed with an amplitude of 5 to 6 cm and repeated every 2 to 4 seconds, coupled with a clockwise torque on the shaft on the pullback motion and a counterclockwise torque on the inward motion. This maneuver helps straighten the sigmoid colon, allowing it to compress like an accordion over the scope (Fig. 118-6).
Jiggling	A to-and-fro, 5 to 6 cm inward and outward motion of the shaft performed every 2 to 4 seconds. It helps in the visualization of a segment of colon, and can often aid scope advancement (Fig. 118-7).
Alpha manuever	Used only after much practice by the experienced endoscopist to assist in shortening/pleating the segments of the colon. (See text for explanation.)
Torquing	Twisting the distal shaft of the scope either clockwise or counterclockwise.
Retroflexion	Maximally flexing the tip of the scope, enabling it to look back upon the shaft.

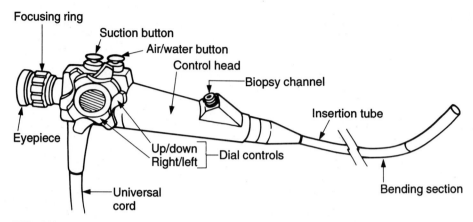

FIG. 118-5.
Schematic diagram of a fiberoptic sigmoidoscope.

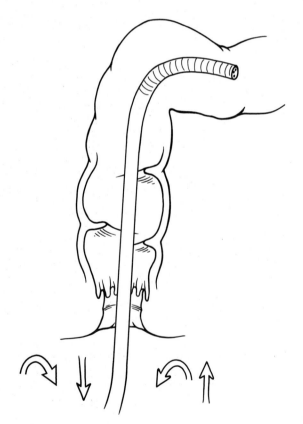

FIG. 118-6.
Dithering maneuver. See text for details.

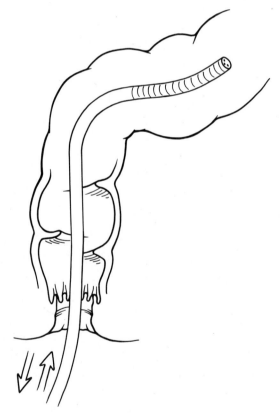

FIG. 118-7.
Jiggle maneuver. See text for details.

4. Have the assistant separate the gluteal folds laterally with the hands to expose the anal area and the anal aperture for inspection. Perform a digital rectal examination with K-Y Jelly or lidocaine ointment to ensure there is no obstruction or stool in the anal canal. Examine the prostate (in males) carefully. A painful examination should alert the endoscopist to a fissure, proctitis, or colitis. The examination is uncomfortable, but should not be painful if it is done gently. This procedure helps to relax the sphincter and also lubricates the anal canal. (See Chapter 116, Clinical Anorectal Anatomy and Examination.)

5. Now hold the body of the scope in your left hand (Fig. 118-8). Hold the tip of the scope shaft in the right hand, and, with the index finger alongside and stabilizing the tip, gently insert it. Hold the tip at an oblique angle pointing posteriorly, and stretch the sphincter as the tip is slipped into the anal canal. The shaft tip can be blindly inserted 8 to 10 cm.

6. With the distal 8 to 10 cm of the scope in the anal canal, switch on the light source and suction, and view at the eyepiece or on the video screen.

7. Keep holding the body of the scope in your left hand so that your thumb controls the large dial and your index finger controls the suction, irrigation, and air valves. Hold the shaft and advance it with your right hand, which is also available to control the small dial. Alternatively, an assistant may advance the scope, and you may use your right hand to manipulate the dials. The assistant must be cautioned never to advance the scope against resistance and to advance the scope only when told to do so.

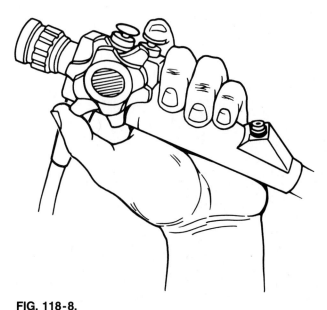

FIG. 118-8.
The control head of the sigmoidoscope should be held in the left hand so that the thumb rests on the up/down control dial and the index finger can regulate the suction and air/water buttons.

8. *Insufflation-Advance Technique.* Air is needed to maintain patency of the lumen and to obtain a clear view adjacent to the tip and a few centimeters beyond. Covering the air port gently with the fingertip will allow insufflation of the bowel. A sufficient amount of air must be used to expand the bowel, but too much air may cause cramping or, in extreme cases, even perforation. Use patient comfort as a guide. With a clear view ahead, gently advance the shaft forward, maintaining a one-on-one motion. The scope is generally advanced up to 15 to 18 cm without difficulty. There are three "valves" that are encountered in the rectum—the valves of Houston (Fig. 118-9). These are semilunar in shape, and are located 6 cm, 9 cm, and 12 cm from the anal verge. Negotiating advancement into the rectosigmoid can at times be hampered by these folds, and the tip needs to be deflected away from the fold and toward the lumen to avoid redout or whiteout. One can get "lost" in the vast arena of the rectal vault and have difficulty in locating the rectosigmoid orifice. This is more likely if too much air is insufflated, which causes the ampulla to expand upward.

At this stage, you do not need to attempt to visualize the entire circumference of the bowel. Rather, the primary goal is to insert the scope as far as possible. It is critical that the complete circumference of the bowel be closely inspected, lest a lesion be missed, but this is generally performed during withdrawal of the scope.

9. Advancing the scope into the sigmoid and descending colon may require utilization of different maneuvers in the presence of redundancy, adhesions, angulation, and loops. At times, especially in young persons, the scope can be advanced all the way up to the transverse colon without any difficulty. In older patients, especially when they have had abdominal or pelvic surgery, the presence of

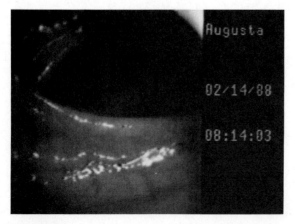

FIG. 118-9.
Semilunar valves of Houston.

adhesions may make further advancement difficult. The rectosigmoid junction is at 15 to 18 cm (Fig. 118-10). Advancement may be hampered here by the angulation of the bowel toward the left into the left iliac fossae. The length of the sigmoid itself varies from 20 to 45 cm. Certain maneuvers individually or in combination can then be attempted in order to advance the scope into the descending colon and into the proximal parts of the splenic flexure.

Advancement by hook and pullback. Deflect the tip of the shaft 30 to 90 degrees behind a mucosal fold (Fig. 118-11, *A-D*), and withdraw the shaft 5 to 10 cm, pulling the segment of the colon downward and creating a pleating and straightening-out effect. You may need to repeat this maneuver several times to achieve the desired goal of compressing the bowel over the shaft of the scope, much like an accordion. It should be done very gently with minimal (if any) resistance.

Dithering-torque maneuver. The dithering-torque maneuver is a to-and-fro advance and withdrawal process performed with an amplitude of 5 to 6 cm every 2 to 4 seconds. It is coupled with a clockwise torque of the shaft of about 45 to 60 degrees on the pullback motion and a counterclockwise torque on the inward motion. This process "accordionizes" the colon onto the shaft of the scope, thereby shortening the colon and enabling a larger length of the colon to be traversed and examined. Gentle tip deflection of 30 degrees with the torque motion is recommended. The clockwise torque tends to loop the sigmoid, whereas the counterclockwise torque tends to straighten it. This is a very effective maneuver in shortening the sigmoid, and it is of greatest use in a redundant

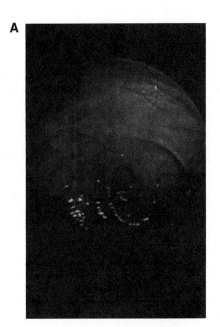

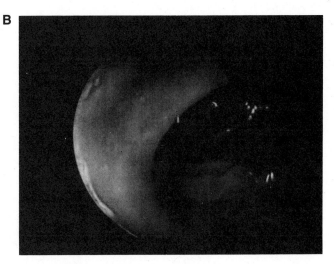

FIG. 118-10.
Rectosigmoid junction. **A,** Sigmoid colon. **B,** Sigmoid colon beyond valves of Houston.

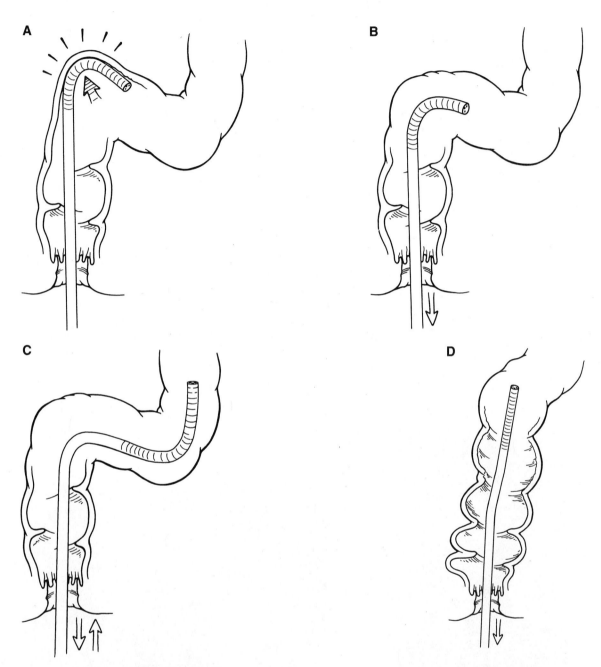

FIG. 118-11.
Method of advancement at the rectosigmoid junction. Various manuevers are needed if, upon advancement, the scope is entering into the anus, but the view from the end of the sigmoidoscope is not changing (**A**). There is no "one-on-one" advancement; rather, the segment of colon is merely being stretched, often causing pain. Try simple hook and pullback technique initially (**B**). If this does not work, attempt dithering and jiggling to negotiate a curve (**C**). Pulling back on the scope causes an accordion effect and straightens the curve (**D**).

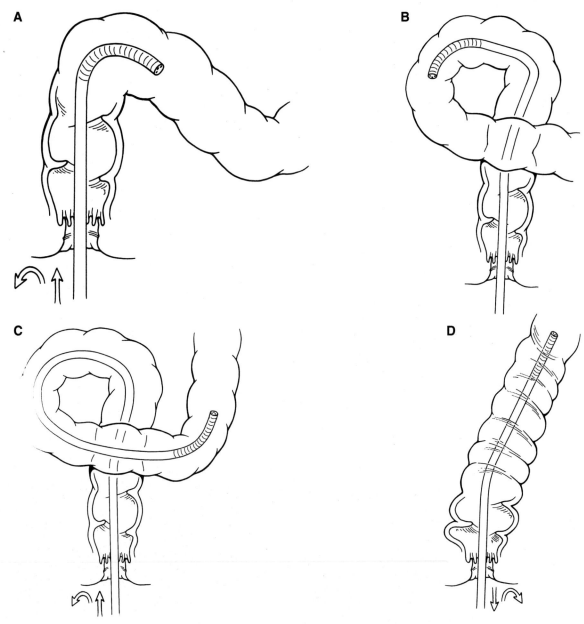

FIG. 118-12.
Alpha maneuver. See text for details.

sigmoid colon. Excessive tip deflection can become a hinderance to further advancement; therefore, it should be kept to the minimum to maintain visualization of the lumen. If the tip needs greater deflection, it should be straightened soon after the lumen is located.

Alpha maneuver (for experienced endoscopist). Advance the scope into the sigmoid. At about 25 to 30 cm deflect the tip to visualize the lumen anteriorly, and then torque the shaft counterclockwise about 145 to 180 degrees (Fig. 118-12, *A*). This swings the proximal part of the sigmoid over the distal part, so that the sigmoid colon forms a loop over itself (Fig. 118-12, *B* and *C*). Here, minimally deflect the tip to locate the lumen and then straighten it as much as possible. Further advancement of the scope will lead it into the descending colon. If resistance is encountered, then rotate the shaft clockwise and withdraw to "accordionize," or shorten, the sigmoid (Fig. 118-12, *D*). The shaft can then be advanced into the descending colon, to the splenic flexure. The area of the splenic flexure can often be recognized by the bluish hue superiorly, which represents the transmitted vascularity of the spleen sitting on the colon exteriorly. The colon takes a turn anteriorly and to the patient's right at this point, and the triangular folds of the transverse colon can easily be identified (Fig. 118-13).

The alpha maneuver is rarely needed, but may be necessary in the redundant bowel. It should be used only by the experienced endoscopist.

10. At this point, the scope is generally advanced with minimal manipulation the remainder of the distance by jiggling, hooking, and pulling back, or just simply by maintaining mild inward pressure on the shaft.

11. Withdrawal of the scope is easy. With the combination of tip deflection and torquing in both directions, gradually withdraw the shaft, visually inspecting the entire circumference of the portion of the intubated colon. Pay careful

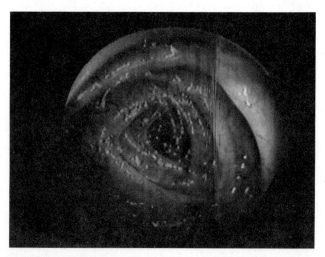

FIG. 118-13.
Transverse colon with triangular folds.

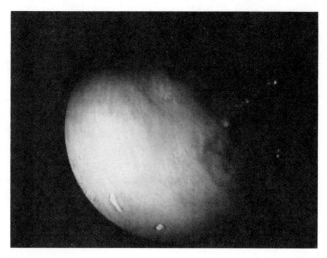

FIG. 118-14.
Retroflection of the tip to examine the anal canal. The scope looks back on itself.

attention to all areas of the mucosal surface, particularly behind mucosal folds. Make note of diverticula and any masses. (See later discussion regarding biopsy.) If any segment is not seen completely, advance and withdraw again. Continue withdrawing until the rectum is reached. Opinions vary as to whether or not changing patient position will improve visualization or aid in advancement of the scope.

12. The anal canal must be thoroughly inspected in one of two ways: by using an anoscope or by completely deflecting the sigmoidoscope tip to hook back on itself. The sigmoidoscope can be simply withdrawn the entire distance, and the anal canal examined with the anoscope. Alternatively, after the first semilunar valve is passed, the tip of the sigmoidoscope can be retroflexed (i.e., deflected to its maximum), and the shaft withdrawn gradually. Essentially, you will be looking up the shaft of the scope (Fig. 118-14). At about 4 to 5 cm, inspect the inner aspect of the anal canal and papillae to detect masses and hemorrhoids. After a 360-degree visual inspection of the entire anal orifice, straighten the tip and withdraw it very slowly. Grasp the tip of the scope as it slips out of the anus so that it does not drop on the table, damaging its delicate construction.

13. Reinsert the scope 5 to 6 cm and remove all the air. Use a to-and-fro motion, rotation, and intermittent suction to prevent the mucosa from being drawn into the suction port, occluding it. After the patient indicates that the air is gone, remove the scope and immediately draw soapy water through the suction port. Also, occlude the air port to "blow out" any accumulated debris. These last two steps will enhance cleaning and preserve proper functioning of the scope.

BIOPSY

There are many opinions about when and if biopsies should be obtained during flexible sigmoidoscopy. Some points of view with countering arguments include the following:

1. Primary care physicians should not biopsy any lesion. (*Counter:* Biopsy technique is simple and virtually without complication when only the biopsy forceps are used. Only sample 2 to 3 mm of the mucosa, and unless the tissue is ulcerated or inside a diverticulum, perforation is almost impossible.)
2. It is useless to obtain a biopsy sample, since the colonoscopist will need to remove the polyp anyway. (*Counter:* If the biopsy returns as a hyperplastic polyp, there is no need for colonoscopy. Documentation of an abnormality aids in categorizing the patient's risk status and reinforces the physician's rationale for the patient to have the often-resisted colonoscopy performed. It also confirms the diagnosis for the colonoscopist and mandates that the lesion be found.)
3. Do not biopsy small polyps (<5 mm). (*Counter:* It is precisely these lesions that are difficult to diagnose accurately. Often a small "diminutive" polyp turns out to be an adenomatous or even a villous lesion.)
4. Doing a biopsy may increase malpractice insurance. (*Counter:* Not doing it may miss a crucial diagnosis.)

Editors' note: It is our practice to biopsy essentially all nonvascular lesions. No complications have been encountered.

Some caveats regarding biopsy:

1. Do not biopsy a vascular lesion.
2. Do not perform electrosurgical removal of a polyp except in a fully prepped bowel (bowel gases in the colon can explode).
3. Upon completion of the procedure, be sure that all bleeding has stopped and document this fact.
4. Document the location from which each polyp was removed, and place each polyp in a separate specimen container.

Biopsy technique is straightforward. The closed forceps are passed down the biopsy channel by the endoscopist. Once they have emerged from the distal tip of the scope, the assistant opens the jaws of the forceps. The operator advances the cable firmly and fixes the forceps on the desired area using the central needle point. The assistant closes the jaws and the endoscopist sharply withdraws the forceps. The biopsy sample is placed in formalin and the site observed for bleeding. Occasionally a second or even a third biopsy sample of the lesion may be indicated.

BOX 118-3. PROCEDURE FORM
FLEXIBLE SIGMOIDOSCOPY

Name: _____ Birthdate: _____ Phone: (H) _____
(W) _____

Your usual doctor: _____ Send a copy of report to him/her?   Y   N
Blood pressure: _____

SYMPTOMS/HISTORY

Change in stools _____   Anemia _____
Diarrhea _____   Weight loss _____
Constipation _____   Fever _____
Blood _____   Polyps _____
Black stools _____   F. H. _____
Hemorrhoids _____   Abdominal pain _____

Hemoccult: Date   positive/negative   not done
Previous sigmoidoscopy: Date _____
                                        Findings _____
Previous barium enema: Date _____
                                        Findings _____

PMH: Bleeding problems?   Yes   No
         Artificial joints?   Yes   No
         Artificial heart valve?   Yes   No
         Heart murmur needing prophylaxis?   Yes   No
         Allergies _____
         Other medical problems? _____
         Medications? _____

PROCEDURE   **Scope: OSF-2**

Abdominal exam:
Preparation: Adequate/Inadequate
Rectal: _____   Depth: _____
Reason for stopping: Limits of scope or _____
Tolerance: _____
Complications: _____   Findings: _____
Biopsy: _____ cm _____ cm _____ cm   Bleeding controlled   Yes   No
Proctoscopy: _____

IMPRESSION: _____

RECOMMENDATIONS: _____
Repeat exam _____
cc: _____   _____   _____
                                  Physician Signature   Date

**BOX 118-4. PATIENT EDUCATION HANDOUT
BOWEL PREPARATION FOR SIGMOIDOSCOPY**

1. Stay on a clear liquid diet after the evening meal the day before your examination. If you have an afternoon appointment, you may eat breakfast, but stay on clear liquids after breakfast until your examination.
2. If you have a problem with chronic constipation, you may take a laxative the night before. You may also take your usual medicines. If you have diabetes, talk to the doctor for special instructions.
3. One-and-a-half hours before the scheduled time of the examination, administer a Fleet enema (which can be obtained at any local pharmacy). Follow the instructions provided in the box.
4. One-half hour before the scheduled time of the examination, administer another Fleet enema.
5. The return from the last enema should be clear. If it is not, it may be necessary to administer a third enema.

CLEAR LIQUID DIET

Only these foods are allowed; avoid *all* others.

Beverages: Carbonated beverages, coffee, Kool-aid, and tea
Desserts: Gelatin dessert (Jello), clear popsicles
Fruit: Apple juice, cranberry juice, and grape juice
Soups: Beef bouillion or clear broth
Sweets: Hard candies or sugar

Used with permission of The Medical Procedures Center, P.C., Midland, Michigan.

DOCUMENTATION

It is important that all findings be noted and documented. A comment should be made on each of the following: scope used, distance inserted, quality of preparation, patient tolerance, vascular and mucosal patterns, size of any polyps identified and depth where they were found, ease of biopsy and control of any bleeding, final impression, and follow-up recommendations (Box 118-3).

SIGNIFICANCE OF VARIOUS POLYPS

It is beyond the scope of this chapter to discuss the significance of various polyps. All adenomatous (neoplastic) polyps (tubular, tubulovillous, and villous lesions) have a malignant potential. Recent articles document the reduction of colorectal cancer if all neoplastic polyps are removed. The significance of hyperplastic polyps is still being debated. Most experts would suggest that their presence has little prognostic significance. Most physicians do not recommend full colonoscopy for hyperplastic polyps, whereas with neoplastic polyps, it is essential.

POSTPROCEDURE PATIENT EDUCATION

After completion of the procedure, explain

- The findings
- Where the biopsy samples have been taken from and the necessity for pathological evaluation
- Further management or referral, and future surveillance plans
- The implications of the presence of cancer or polyps for the patient's siblings and children
- The necessity of reporting any excessive bleeding or abdominal pain

COMPLICATIONS

- Bowel perforation (extremely rare)
- Bleeding (more likely if a biopsy sample was obtained)
- Abnormal distention and pain
- Infection (Although very rare, subacute bacterial endocarditis and transmission of microorganisms between patients may occur.)
- Vasovagal symptoms
- Missed disease

Complications from flexible sigmoidoscopy are very rare. Their incidence is higher in patients with previous bowel or pelvic surgery, or irradiation. These patients have more adhesions, which tether the bowel to a fixed position, predisposing it to perforation. If the scope is advanced blindly, without seeing the lumen, the risk of perforation also increases.

Care must be taken in the presence of diverticulosis. The mouth of the diverticulum can be interpreted as the bowel lumen, and if the scope is inserted, perforation can occur.

CLEANING AND DISINFECTION OF SCOPES

The various instrument representatives will detail the exact cleaning mechanism for each brand of scope. Tremain presents an excellent review, and reading of this article is strongly encouraged. It is essential that the clinician's staff pay meticulous attention to cleaning the scope. The orifices are very small and a small amount of debris can prevent optimal functioning.

CPT/BILLING CODES

45330   Sigmoidoscopy, flexible fiberoptic; diagnostic
45331   Sigmoidoscopy with biopsy and/or collection of specimen by brushing or washing

45332	Sigmoidoscopy with removal of foreign body
45333	Sigmoidoscopy with removal of polypoid lesion(s)
45334	Sigmoidoscopy with control of hemorrhage (e.g., electrocoagulation)
45336	Sigmoidoscopy with ablation of tumor or mucosal lesion
46600	Anoscopy; diagnostic (separate procedure)

BIBLIOGRAPHY

Dajani AS et al: Prevention of bacterial endocarditis: recommendations by the American Heart Association, *JAMA* 264:2919, 1990.

DeCosse JJ, Tsioulias GJ, Jacobson JS: Colorectal cancer: detection, treatment, and rehabilitation, *CA Cancer J Clin* 44:27, 1994.

Fekety R, Kaye D: Does antibiotic prophylaxis help? *Patient Care:*113, June 1992.

Gupta TP et al: Prevention of colon cancer in primary care practice, *Prim Care* 16:157, 1981.

Hocutt JE et al: Flexible fiberoptic sigmoidoscopy, *Am Fam Physician* 26:133, 1982.

Holt WS: Factors affecting compliance with screening sigmoidoscopy, *JFP* 32:585, 1991.

Levine R et al: Prevention and early detection of colorectal cancer, *Am Fam Physician* 45:663, 1992.

Selby JV et al: A case control study of screening sigmoidoscopy and mortality from colorectal cancer, *N Engl J Med* 3(26):653, 1992.

Tremain SC et al: Cleaning, disinfection and sterilization of gastrointestinal endoscopes: approaches in the office, *JFP* 32:300, 1991.

Varma JR, Mills LR: Colon polyps, *JFP* 35:194, 1992.

CHAPTER 119

Office Treatment of Hemorrhoids

George Zainea

Gayle Randall

Daniel A. Norman

John L. Pfenninger

It is estimated that hemorrhoidal disease occurs in 50% to 80% of the U.S. population. Although this disease is rarely fatal, it accounts for a great deal of human pain and suffering. Internal hemorrhoids are the most common cause of lower gastrointestinal (GI) bleeding. Even though most episodes of bleeding will resolve with medical management, this bleeding can mimic or mask the diagnosis of other lesions. Occasionally, bleeding can be severe and is associated with anemia. Although surgery is the accepted definitive treatment for severe symptomatic hemorrhoids, patient acceptance of surgical hemorrhoidectomy is poor. This is because of the need for hospitalization, general anesthesia, postprocedure pain, long recovery time, and loss of time from work or usual activity after surgery.

Rubber-band ligation is a proven alternative method for treating internal hemorrhoids. Several new approaches have been developed in the past decade that make the treatment of hemorrhoids easier in most instances. These include the infrared coagulator (IRC), low amperage direct current (Ultroid), and bipolar electrocoagulator (BICAP).

It is essential to know the anorectal anatomy (see Chapter 116, Clinical Anorectal Anatomy and Examination) and to be able to perform a thorough anoscopic examination (see Chapter 117, Anoscopy) to appropriately assess and treat hemorrhoids.

CLASSIFICATIONS

Hemorrhoids are classified according to their origin above or below the dentate (pectinate) line. Those lying above the dentate line are internal hemorrhoids and those below, external hemorrhoids. It should be clear that classification is dependent on *origin*, not on the location of the most distal portion of the hemorrhoid.

Hemorrhoids above the dentate line, *internal hemorrhoids*, are covered by mucosa and do not have somatic sensory innervation. Those below the dentate line, *external hemorrhoids*, are covered by skin (anoderm) and are extremely sensitive.

Internal hemorrhoids usually occur in three major positions based on the vascular architecture of the anal canal: the right anterior, right posterior, and left lateral positions (Fig. 119-1, *A*). The anoscope divides the anal canal into eight segments, which are usually numbered with the patient lying in the left lateral decubitus position (Fig. 119-1, *B*).

Internal hemorrhoids are also characterized by their size as first through fourth degree, as noted in Table 119-1. With increasing prolapse, the external component becomes more prominent, forming the so-named "mixed hemorrhoid." Symptoms of internal hemorrhoids include bleeding, prolapse, and discharge. The key step in diagnosing and classifying internal hemorrhoids is anoscopic examination (see Chapter 117, Anoscopy).

Approximately 15% to 20% of hemorrhoidal symptoms do not respond adequately to medical treatment and require further therapy.

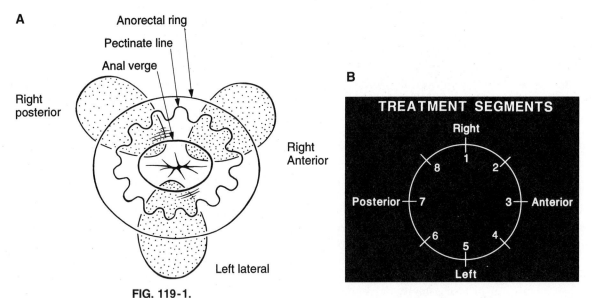

FIG. 119-1.
A, Usual three primary hemorrhoidal groups. **B**, Representation of eight treatment segments in the rectum as seen through a slotted (Ives) anoscope, with the patient in the left lateral decubitus position.

TABLE 119-1.
Classification of Internal Hemorrhoids

1st degree	Small, do not prolapse
2nd degree	Medium, prolapse and return spontaneously
3rd degree	Large, prolapse and reduced manually
4th degree	Largest, prolapsed irreducible

After completing any of these procedures, a medical program to regulate bowel habits should be implemented to prevent recurrence. This is equally as important as the surgical intervention itself.

INDICATIONS

- Bleeding or other symptomatology from internal hemorrhoids that has failed medical management (bulk agents, suppositories or topical preparations, and sitz baths)

  Note: The mere presence of hemorrhoids alone, without symptoms, is not necessarily an indication for treatment.

CONTRAINDICATIONS

- Bleeding diathesis
- Pregnancy or immediate postpartum period (8 weeks)
- Inflammatory bowel disease
- Anorectal fissures
- Active anorectal infections
- AIDS or other immunodeficiency states
- Portal hypertension
- Rectal wall prolapse
- Anorectal tumors

Avoid electrical stimulation in patients with pacemakers or defibrillators. Recommendations for cardiac prophylaxis are not available, but those at high risk for subacute bacterial endocarditis (previous history of SBE, artificial valves, history of rheumatic fever, or very-high-risk murmurs) should be treated with caution. The duration of antibiotic treatment necessary is unknown, and antibiotic therapy may be impractical, since the treated areas may remain irritated and open for 2 to 3 weeks after each treatment.

PATIENT PREPARATION

Give the patient one or two Fleet enemas before the procedure. Although not absolutely necessary, it is aesthetically helpful. Ask the patient to avoid aspirin for 1 week prior to treatment. Provide a patient education handout (Box 119-1) to ensure informed consent.

A complete history and pertinent physical examination are essential. Record these on encounter forms (Boxes 119-2 and 119-3) that summarize the information.

Place the patient in the left lateral decubitus position for examination and treatment. No sedation is necessary for a patient having only anoscopy and hemorrhoid treatment. The patient may take four ibuprofen 200 mg tablets 1 to 2

Text continued on p. 937.

BOX 119-1. PATIENT EDUCATION HANDOUT
HEMORRHOIDS

Hemorrhoids are a very common problem. Hemorrhoids are nothing more than enlarged veins. When they occur in the lower legs, we call them varicose veins. When they occur in the rectum, they are called hemorrhoids or "piles." There are many ways to treat hemorrhoids.

The First Visit
In the past, people would simply tolerate most hemorrhoids until they became so bad that surgery was needed. Modern techniques have eliminated the need for surgical excision (cutting out) of hemorrhoids except in the most advanced cases. You may have heard of the Baron ligation technique, which involves putting a small rubber band around the hemorrhoids. This method has been used for many years. It is less painful than surgery and can be performed in the physician's office. Laser techniques have also been used. More advanced techniques using infrared coagulation, radiofrequency, and low-dose electricity are available. They frequently provide excellent results with even less pain and less complications.

Types of Hemorrhoids
Internal hemorrhoids: Hemorrhoids that start *above* the pectinate line. These hemorrhoids are easy to treat because they start in an area where there are no pain fibers. The "line" is visible to the physician during the examination.
External hemorrhoids: Hemorrhoids that start *below* the pectinate line. These hemorrhoids are more difficult to treat because they start in an area that has pain fibers.
Mixed hemorrhoids: Hemorrhoids that are actually a combination of the previous two types.
Thrombosed hemorrhoids: Hemorrhoids that have developed a small blood clot inside the vein. These clots do not cause any major problems and are not dangerous. Rather, these small clots just cause severe pain. If you develop very severe discomfort, then you probably have a small clotted hemorrhoid. These are easily treated in the office by simply removing the clot.
Prolapsed hemorrhoids: Many times a hemorrhoid will protrude through the anus. Many people will call these external hemorrhoids but that is not technically correct. Hemorrhoids are classified as internal or external, based on *where they start.* Usually hemorrhoids that protrude out through the anus have their base above the pectinate line, so they actually are internal hemorrhoids. Sometimes these prolapsed hemorrhoids will come down and then go back up; and other times, they will stay down.
Skin tags: Oftentimes even after the hemorrhoid or vein is gone, the stretched skin that was over it will remain as a skin tag or an accumulation of loose, stretched out skin. Many people are bothered by skin tags, which are not painful, but make it difficult to keep the area clean.

Each different type of hemorrhoid problem requires a different type of approach. Depending on the problem that you have, a particular instrument will be used for the treatment.

Types of Treatment
Surgery is reserved for only the most advanced cases of hemorrhoids. Surgery is performed in the hospital operating room with the patient under general anesthesia.
Rubber-band ligation is still used frequently by many physicians to treat many types of internal hemorrhoids. It is also known as *Baron ligation.*
Infrared coagulation involves the application of infrared light to the base of the hemorrhoid, which clots the hemorrhoid. There are usually three different areas inside the rectum where hemorrhoids occur, and they are referred to as complexes. One area, or complex, is treated at each office visit. Although the patient will occasionally feel a little warmth, there generally is minimal pain or discomfort. The patient may return to work the same day or the next day. Occasionally a little bleeding will occur between the fourth day and the tenth day after treatment. The patient returns in approximately 1 month for follow-up treatment.

Continued.

BOX 119-1.—cont'd

The *Ultroid unit* is used on the more advanced hemorrhoids. A small probe is inserted into the hemorrhoid and very low levels of electrical power are applied. The probe is left in place for approximately 8 to 10 minutes, which coagulates the enlarged vein. Discomfort is minimal, and the patient may return to work either the same day or the next day. Only one complex is treated at a time, and, as with the radio-frequency surgery or infrared coagulation, approximately three or four visits will be needed to treat all areas.

BICAP treatment involves the administration of an electrical current to resolve the hemorrhoid. A treatment consists of two or three 2-second applications. Generally, it is a painless procedure.

Radiofrequency surgery involves the application of a very high-frequency current to remove external skin tags. The frequency is the same as that of an AM radio. The advantage of this technique is that it will prevent the bleeding that is frequently associated with excision of these tags. Also, very little other tissue is damaged using this technique. It is similar to a laser procedure. Because skin is removed, tenderness in the area will be experienced for a longer period of time (1 to 3 weeks) until the wound is healed. A local anesthetic (to numb the area) is injected before the procedure to minimize pain.

Preparation for the Visit

If infrared coagulation, BICAP, or the Ultroid technique is used, you probably will not need to take time off from work; however, it might be best if you could take it easy for a couple of days after the procedure. Before coming in for the procedure, administer an enema (Fleet enemas are available without a prescription) approximately an hour before the planned surgery. Hold the enema for 5 to 10 minutes and then expel it. After the procedure, expect some weeping from the area and some soreness for up to several weeks. You should be able to do most normal activities within a few days. Often little or no pain medication is needed.

If you would like to play it safe, you may take three ibuprofen 200 mg tablets about an hour before coming to the office. You might want to schedule the procedure later in the day so that you do not have to go back to work. You may want to take a stool softener such as Colace, or a bulk laxative such as Metamucil or Citrucel, for a few days before the procedure. You just need enough to keep the stool soft. Also remember to drink plenty of water. You will probably want to continue this regimen for a week or so after the procedure.

Postprocedure Care

After any hemorrhoid procedure, it is very important that you maintain a high bulk diet (a lot of fruits, vegetables, bran, etc.) so that your stool remains soft. Drink at least four to five glasses of water per day. You may use suppositories, if desired. Sitz baths are beneficial: simply sit in a hot bath for 20 to 30 minutes three or four times per day. It may help to apply an ointment such as Preparation H after bathing and to keep the areas from rubbing together. Your doctor may prescribe some Silvadene cream, benzocaine, or lidocaine ointment. Use them as directed. Ice bags may also help relieve the discomfort.

Complications include pain, bleeding, infection, return of the hemorrhoids, and failure of the treatment itself so that the hemorrhoids persist.

After any of these procedures, if you have extreme pain, excessive bleeding, difficulty urinating, or if you develop fevers, chills, or sweats, call your physician immediately. You should make an appointment for a follow-up visit in 4 weeks.

Special Note

Sometimes hemorrhoids can be caused by a tumor in the bowel. Your physician may suggest a screening test with a flexible sigmoidoscopy either before or after treatment. Be sure to discuss this with the physician.

**BOX 119-2. ENCOUNTER FORM
HEMORRHOIDS**

NAME _____ AGE _____ SEX _____ DATE _____

SUBJECTIVE:

Original onset: _____ Present trouble started: _____

SYMPTOMS:

Anal itching: Fecal incontinence:
Pain—with BM: Protrusion:
  —between BMs: Weight loss:
                                                History: anoscopy
Abdominal Pain: sigmoidoscopy
                                                          barium enema
Bleeding: Other:
  TP/with BMs/dripping

Change in BMs:
Has patient read over and understood handouts?

PRIOR TREATMENT:

  Medical: RP   RL

  Surgical:

  Other:

OBJECTIVE:

Exam (left lateral decubitus position):

External:
  Visual
    redundant tissue
    external hemorrhoidal disease
    prolapse
    fissure
    fistula
    infection
    other
Digital:
  Masses
  Tenderness   LL
  Prostate
Anoscopic:
  Fissure
  Fistula
  Hemorrhoids

Continued.

BOX 119-2.—cont'd

IMPRESSION:

PLAN:

Patient Education —Diet
          —Hygiene
          —Control of symptoms
          —Technique of destruction
          —Risks
          —Benefits
          —Complications

Treatment: IRC   Ultroid   BICAP   Banding

   Surgical:
   Other:

Referral to _____

Flexible sigmoidoscopy indicated?
   Scheduled?

Follow-up:

_____
Physician Signature

Used with permission of The Medical Procedures Center, P.C., Midland, Michigan.

**BOX 119-3. TREATMENT SUMMARY
HEMORRHOIDS**

Patient _____ Date _____

Initial Evaluation Date _____ Referred by _____

Flexible Sigmoidoscopy _____ Barium Enema or Colonoscopy _____

Patient in left lateral decubitus position

Date	Number of Segments Treated	Grade	Technique/Settings	Comments/Symptoms	Sent

_____
Physician Signature

Used with permission of The Medical Procedures Center, P.C., Midland, Michigan.

hours before the office visit. Before anoscopy, peform an external and digital anorectal examination. Ask the patient to perform a Valsalva maneuver (bearing down) to rule out full-thickness rectal prolapse. Only internal hemorrhoids are treated by these methods. Treatment of external hemorrhoids requires excision and is associated with pain; thus, local anesthetics are needed.

TREATMENT

Rubber-band ligation (Barron or McGivney ligation), infrared coagulation (IRC), direct current coagulation (Ultroid), bipolar electrocoagulator (BICAP), sclerotherapy, and treatment of thrombosed external hemorrhoids are discussed below. A summary of techniques and their indications is found in Table 119-2. The treatment of perianal skin tags is dealt with separately in Chapter 120, Perianal Skin Tags. Because of the discharge and poor patient acceptance, cryotherapy is not covered in this discussion for the primary care physician.

RUBBER-BAND LIGATION

This method involves placing a rubber band around an internal hemorrhoid. The ensnared tissue undergoes necrosis and sloughs. Rubber-band ligation is used for treatment of second- or third-degree bleeding or prolapsing internal hemorrhoids.

Equipment

- Slotted Ives anoscope: available from Redfield Corp., 210 Summit Avenue, Montvale, NJ 07645; telephone: 800-628-4472.
- McGivney ligator with bands (or an acceptable alternative device) (Fig. 119-2)
- Alligator forceps (similar to long-handled Allis clamp)

TABLE 119-2.

Comparison of Therapeutic Modalities for Treatment of Internal Hemorrhoids

Method	Grade of internal hemorrhoid				Ease of performing method	Complications
	1	2	3	4		
Infrared coagulator (IRC)	+++	+++	±	-	+++	-
Bipolar coagulator (BICAP)	++	+++	+++	+	+++	-
DC current (Ultroid)	+	++	+++	++	+	+
Rubber band	±	+++	+++	-	+	++
Sclerotherapy	+	+++	±	-	-	+++

Technique (Figs. 119-3 to 119-6)

1. Load the ligating drum with two bands. A small amount of soapy water on the cone will facilitate loading.
2. Insert the anoscope and visualize the hemorrhoid to be ligated. Treat the largest hemorrhoid group first. Have an assistant stabilize the anoscope.
3. With one hand, draw the hemorrhoidal tissue into the ligating drum with an alligator forceps. If the patient experiences pain, grasp the hemorrhoidal tissue more proximally.
4. With the other hand, grasp the handle of the ligator and push forward slightly. Squeeze the handle. The outer drum slides over the inner drum, displacing the rubber bands around the hemorrhoid.
5. Reposition or withdraw the anoscope. Patient tolerance is highest if only one hemorrhoid group is treated per visit.

Postprocedure Patient Education

- Inform the patient that mild aching discomfort may be experienced over the next 2 days (Box 119-4).
- Ask the patient to report any bleeding, fevers, dysuria, inability to urinate (a sign of perineal sepsis), or increasing pain.
- Follow up in 3 to 4 weeks for reexamination and further banding, as needed.

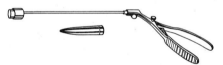

FIG. 119-2.
McGivney ligator. *Top,* Ligator forceps; *Bottom,* Cone to load bands.

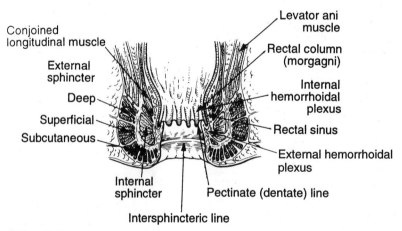

FIG. 119-3.
Anatomy of the anal region. Also see Chapter 116, Clinical Anorectal Anatomy and Examination. Note the location of *origin* of internal and external hemorrhoids.

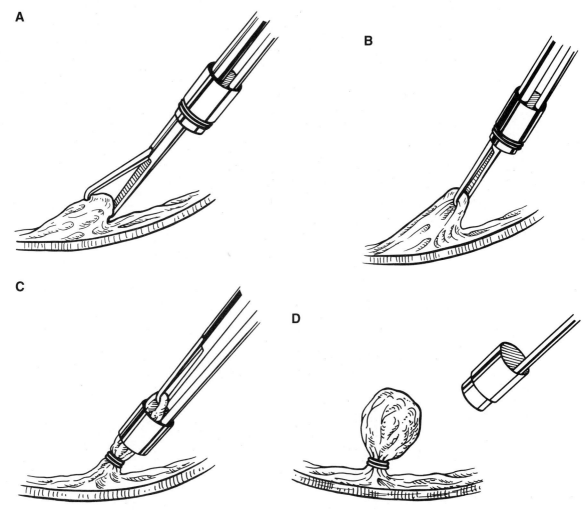

FIG. 119-4.
Rubber-band ligation. **A** and **B,** The hemorrhoid is grasped and firmly tethered. **C** and **D,** The tissue is drawn into the drum and two rubber bands are released. If the patient tolerates the grasping of the hemorrhoid with forceps, ligation can be performed with minimal or no discomfort.

Complications

- Bleeding usually occurs 1 to 2 weeks after the procedure, when the hemorrhoidal tissue sloughs. Bleeding can be very significant.
- Patients may experience a dull ache for 2 days after the procedure. If severe pain is experienced during the procedure, the band will need to be removed with a scissors.
- Thrombosis of external hemorrhoids occurs rarely. Treat symptomatically or with excision.

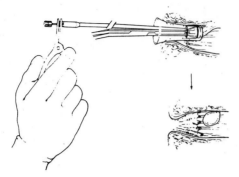

FIG. 119-5.
Above, The internal hemorrhoid is teased into the barrel of the ligating gun. To minimize pain, the point chosen should be well above the dentate line. *Below,* Appearance of a ligated hemorrhoid.

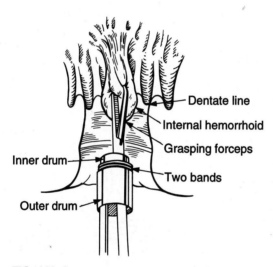

FIG. 119-6.
Rubber-band ligation. An alligator forceps grasps the hemorrhoid. The forceps passes through the drum of the ligator. Squeezing the ligator handle pushes the outer drum over the inner drum, displacing the bands onto the base of the hemorrhoid.

- Sepsis with pelvic cellulitis is a serious complication, but it rarely occurs. Patients complain of fever, perineal pain, swelling, inability to urinate, or dysuria. Treatment requires hospitalization, broad-spectrum antibiotic administration, and debridement.

Advantages

- The instrument itself is inexpensive, and there are no disposable tips to replace.
- Higher grades of hemorrhoids can be treated.
- It is a quick procedure.
- It is a procedure that is easy to learn.

**BOX 119-4. PATIENT EDUCATION HANDOUT
AFTER HEMORRHOID TREATMENTS**

1. Take a *sitz bath* (soaking in a tub) for 20 to 30 minutes three or four times a day for the next 2 or 3 days if needed.
2. You may apply witch hazel or Balneol cream to the rectal area between baths as needed for dryness or local irritation.
3. After you have a bowel movement, clean the area with a moistened tissue or with a Tucks pad. Baby wipes are cheaper and probably just as effective. Blot the area dry, and apply a small amount of Balneol with a tissue.
4. Eat a *high fiber diet* (bran, fresh fruit, and vegetables). Continue this habit forever. *Drink lots of fluids.*
5. Until the rectal area is completely healed, use a *stool bulking agent or a stool softener daily* to keep your bowel movements very soft. Examples include Metamucil, PerDiem Plain, Fibermed, Naturacil, Konsyl, Colace 100 mg capsules, or Surfak 240 mg capsules. Follow the directions on the package.
6. You may have some *swelling and weeping* of the tissues that have been treated. You can use a sanitary pad to absorb the drainage.
7. Note that *slight blood-tinged drainage* is normal. You may actually have some bleeding for 3 to 7 days after the procedure. Unless bleeding is severe, there should really be no worry. Call your physician if you are concerned. Bleeding may also occur 7 to 14 days after the treatment when the scab comes off.
8. Call if you begin running a *fever* or notice redness or swelling past the rectum anytime after the procedure is done. Also call if you are *unable to urinate.*
9. The swollen tissue inside the rectum can often cause a false sensation and an urge to move the bowels. *Avoid prolonged straining* and do not take enemas for at least 10 days after the procedure. The enema tube could damage the tissue and cause bleeding.
10. Use acetaminophen 1000 mg (2 Extra Strength Tylenol) or ibuprofen 600 mg (3 Advil 200 mg) every 6 hours as needed for pain.
11. Please make a *follow-up appointment* for approximately 3 to 4 weeks from the day your procedure was performed.

Used with permission of The Medical Procedures Center, P.C., Midland, Michigan.

Disadvantages

- The procedure is somewhat more uncomfortable than other techniques, and significant complications can occur (e.g., sepsis).
- Two people are needed to perform the procedure (the operator and the assistant, who holds the anoscope).

INFRARED COAGULATION (IRC)

Equipment

- Infrared coagulator (Fig. 119-7): available from Redfield Corp., 210 Summit Ave., Montvale, NJ 07645; telephone: 800-628-4472
- Slotted Ives anoscope (see Chapter 117, Fig. 117-2)

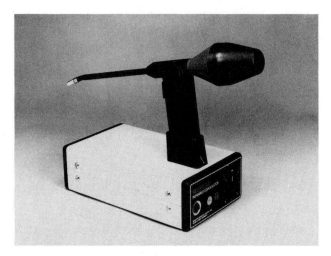

FIG. 119-7.
Infrared coagulator unit, base, and handpiece. (Photo courtesy of Redfield Corporation, Montvale, N.J.)

Infrared light is applied to the base of internal hemorrhoid, forming a white coagulum that ulcerates and then forms a scar. The depth of penetration and diameter of burn correlates with the size of the probe tip (3 to 6 mm). Infrared coagulation is used for first- and second-degree and smaller third-degree internal hemorrhoids. It is a painless procedure that can be used to treat all three hemorrhoid groups at once. However, many clinicians will begin by treating only one complex to determine patient tolerance. Treating more than one complex of hemorrhoids at a time may increase posttreatment discomfort.

Technique

1. Pass a 6 mm probe through the slotted anoscope.
2. Press the tip firmly onto or immediately above the hemorrhoid.
3. Fire the pistol. It has an incorporated time switch that limits exposure. The typical setting is 1.5 seconds. Generally, three to five separate applications are made for each hemorrhoid group. One group is treated per visit at monthly intervals. For the first treatment, select the hemorrhoid that is bleeding or that is the largest. Larger hemorrhoids may require more than one treatment session.

   Caution: Do not overlap treatment sites. Overlapping increases the depth of burn. Place the probe adjacent to a previous site in a linear fashion or in a diamond shape, but do not overlap.

4. Realign the anoscope and apply treatment to another hemorrhoidal group if more than one group is to be treated.
5. Wipe off the tip with saline-soaked gauze between applications. This allows it to cool.

Postprocedure Patient Education

- Follow up in 3 to 4 weeks to treat residual disease or another group.
- Ask the patient to report any severe symptoms of pain, fever, or inability to urinate (see Box 119-4).

Complications

- Patients may experience a mild, dull, aching pain lasting up to 2 days after treatments.
- Minor bleeding may be encountered 1 to 2 weeks after the procedure.

Advantages

- It is an essentially painless procedure.
- There have been no reported cases of perineal sepsis.
- The procedure is quick and simple to learn and is cost-effective.
- The procedure is very well tolerated by patients.

Disadvantages

- The procedure is not very effective for third- and fourth-degree hemorrhoidal disease.

DC CURRENT (ULTROID)

The Ultroid is a simple unit that can be used on all grades of hemorrhoids, although it is best suited for more advanced grades.

The Ultroid current generator provides DC current from 110V AC. The current is delivered by a probe handle and sterile, disposable dual probe tip. Single-hand application is possible because all the controls and the time display are in the handle. The probe is the negative electrode, and the grounding pad is the positive electrode.

By observing patient feedback, the operator can almost be sure that the treatment is painless. As the milliamperage is slowly increased, the patient will report a tingling electrical sensation. Wait several moments until this resolves, then increase the current again. The higher the milliamperage level, the shorter the treatment time needed. Twelve to fourteen milliamperes can be achieved quite readily.

Equipment

- Current generator (Fig. 119-8): available from Cabot Medical Corp., 2021 Cabot Blvd., Longhorne, PA 19047; telephone: 800-523-6078
- Grounding pad and wire to connect pad to generator
- Treatment handle and disposable probe tip

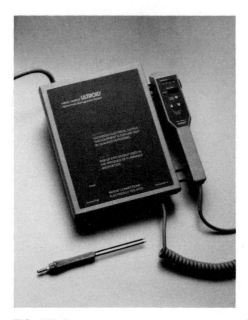

FIG. 119-8.
Ultroid unit for treatment of internal hemorrhoids: base with handpiece and disposable tip. (Photo courtesy of Cabot Medical, Langhorne, Pa.)

- Nonconductive anoscope with operative port
- External light source

Preprocedure Patient Education

Cabot Medical provides a patient education video that explains the risks, benefits, and possible complications of treatment of hemorrhoids with the Ultroid.

The adverse effects of Ultroid treatment have been minor and include discomfort at the site of treatment, bleeding, and scar tissue formation. No perineal sepsis has been reported (see Box 119-1).

Technique

1. Treat the patient in the left lateral decubitus position.
2. Rinse the reusable grounding pad with saline solution, and place it beneath the patient's dependent thigh. Disposable pads are also available.
3. After an external visual, internal digital, and anoscopic examination, isolate the hemorrhoid area to be treated in the anoscope operative port.
4. Secure the disposable probe tip in the treatment handle in the horizontal position for left and right disease, and in the vertical position for anterior and posterior disease.
5. Place the probe tip on (but do not insert into) the uppermost portion of the hemorrhoid, following the longitudinal axis of the vessel and at a slight angle to the anal canal (Fig. 119-9).

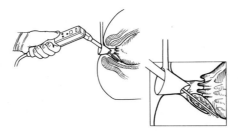

FIG. 119-9.
Direct current probe position on uppermost portion of hemorrhoid (along the longitudinal axis of the vessel and at a slight angle to the anal canal).

6. Then initiate and raise the current to 2 milliamperes (mA). If the patient feels the current, reposition the probe tip more proximally.
7. Advance the probe tip 0.5 cm into the uppermost portion of the hemorrhoid vessel. Insulation covering the probe tip normally prevents further penetration. Stabilize the hand you use to hold the probe. Too much pressure exerted with the tip may force it too deeply into the tissue.
8. Increase the current every 15 to 20 seconds by 2 to 4 mA to a maximum of 16 mA or to patient tolerance. A rapid increase in current may be sensed as a dull ache, and this can often be prevented by a more gradual increase in current. The treatment requirements for resolution of hemorrhoid disease are shown in Table 119-3. First-degree hemorrhoid disease requires about 10 mA applied for 8 minutes, and fourth-degree disease, 12 mA for 14 minutes.
9. When the treatment is completed, slowly decrease the current to zero, and remove and discard the probe. More than one hemorrhoid may be treated per session.

One can judge the adequacy of treatment in several ways. Usually there will be a crackling sound as the current is applied and increased. With sufficient current and duration of application, the hemorrhoid will darken and then turn white. The crackling sound will then stop, which usually indicates sufficient coagulation. As a guideline, the power must be raised at least to 12 mA (go as high as possible

TABLE 119-3.

Hemorrhoid Treatment and Retreatment Requirements Utilizing Direct Current

| Grade of Hemorrhoid Disease | Total Treatment for Resolution (±SD)* | | | | Retreatment Requirements | | | | |
	Current (mA)	Time (Min)	Current × Time (mA × min)	Mean Number of Treatments to Asymptomatic	Number of Segments	%	Number of Treatments of Retreated Segments	Mean Number of Retreatments of Segment
1st degree	9.5 ± 2.3	7.9 ± 4.6	76 ± 52	1.25	23	20	51	2.22
2nd degree	11.0 ± 2.2	9.4 ± 19.5	99 ± 46	1.28	43	19	104	2.42
3rd degree	12.1 ± 2.5	11.0 ± 7.6	128 ± 76	1.38	38	21	105	2.76
4th degree	12.2 ± 3.4	14.3 ± 10.6	158 ± 99	1.80	25	33	86	3.44
Total				1.36	129	22	346	2.68

From Norman DA, Newton R, Nicholas GV: *Am J Gastroenterol* 84:482, 1989. Used with permission.
*Resolution to Grade 0; each grade compared to another is significant at $p<0.01$.

without pain) and be in place at least 8 minutes (usually 10 minutes) to obtain satisfactory results.

Complications

- Care must be taken not to force the Ultroid handle and probe forward, because the tip can penetrate too deeply into the tissue. This not only increases patient discomfort, but also may cause unnecessary deep burns.
- As with all treatment modalities, spotting of blood after treatment occurs.

Advantages

- The equipment is easily controlled to avoid pain.
- It is a simple procedure.
- No major complications occur.
- The procedure works on all grades (first through fourth degree) of internal hemorrhoids.

Disadvantages

- The procedure takes longer than other methods with each visit.
- The disposable probe must be replaced with each visit.

Treat the highest grade of diseased hemorrhoid first. By doing so, significant clinical improvement after the first Ultroid treatment generally occurs. Anatomic resolution of the treated hemorrhoid is delayed for 3 to 10 days. After symptoms have been controlled, minor asymptomatic hemorrhoid disease does not require treatment.

BIPOLAR ELECTROCOAGULATION (BICAP)

The BICAP technique is often referred to as radiofrequency treatment. The rigid hemorrhoid probe used in this technique is 0.6 cm in diameter and 17 cm in length from the handle, which connects to a 50-watt BICAP generator (Circon ACMI, 460 Ward Drive, Santa Barbara, CA 93111; telephone: 800-645-1263) (Fig. 119-10). The positive and negative electrodes aligned at the tip of the probe (the active part of the probe) are 1.7 cm in length and are distributed over 180 degrees of the circumference of the probe tip. The pulses are delivered with a timed trigger button on the handle.

Equipment

- BICAP generator
- Disposable tip
- Slotted Ives anoscope

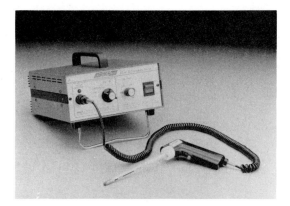

FIG. 119-10.
BICAP hemorrhoid probe and unit. (Courtesy of Circon Corporation, Santa Barbara, Calif.)

Technique

1. With the patient in the left lateral decubitus position, insert the anoscope and identify the group of hemorrhoids to be treated at this visit.
2. Insert the probe into the handle.
3. Set the power level at 6 to 7 or 30 to 35 w.
4. Set the pulse duration at 2 seconds.
5. Place the active part of the probe over the internal hemorrhoid base and deliver energy in time-controlled 2-second pulses. Coagulation is achieved by delivering four to six pulses above the anoderm line at the base of each hemorrhoid segment (Fig. 119-11). The goal is to have an even, horseshoe-shaped coagulum over the hemorrhoid base. Two to three hemorrhoid segments may be treated in this fashion at each session. The patient should return every 3 to 4 weeks until all hemorrhoid segments have been reduced to zero or first degree.

Complications

- Painful ulcer or fissure (rare)
- Prolonged rectal spasm
- Minor bleeding immediately after treatment, or 10 to 14 days after treatment

Complications can be managed with topical corticosteroids for 1 to 2 weeks, stool softeners, and sitz bathes. A painful ulcer may be a result of placing the probe too close to the anoderm line.

Advantages

- The procedure is quick and simple to perform.
- There are rare, minor complications.
- Higher grades and multiple groups of hemorrhoids can be treated at the same time.

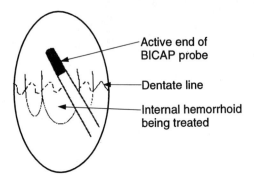

FIG. 119-11.
The BICAP coagulation technique for internal hemorrhoids. Probe placement at hemorrhoid base above the dentate line is indicated by the wavy line. Four to five 2-second pulses are delivered in a line along the hemorrhoid base.

Disadvantages

- The procedure may be slightly more uncomfortable than some other methods if not performed correctly.
- The disposable probe must be replaced with each visit.

SCLEROTHERAPY

Sclerotherapy is used for treatment of first- or second-degree internal bleeding hemorrhoids. Injection of 1 to 2 cc of sclerosant into the internal hemorrhoid results in sclerosis and fixation of the submucosa to the underlying muscularis. This technique is quick, easy, and effective. All three major hemorrhoidal groups can be treated at one sitting.

Equipment

- Anoscope with cutout section (slotted anoscope)
- 5 cc syringe
- 25-gauge spinal needle
- Sclerosant (morrhuate sodium or sodium tetradecyl sulfate)

Technique (Figs. 119-12 and 119-13)

1. Insert the anoscope and visualize the hemorrhoid group to be injected.
2. Insert the spinal needle into or immediately above the hemorrhoid group. Withdraw the plunger of the syringe and aspirate for blood to ensure that the sclerosant will not be injected directly into a vein.

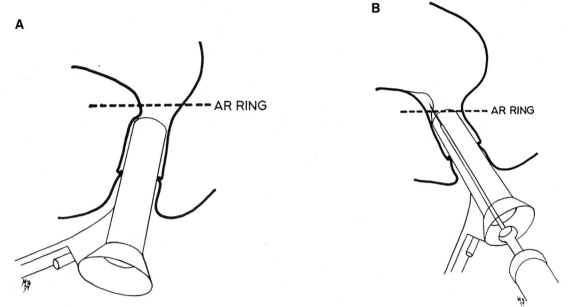

FIG. 119-12.

Proctoscope mechanics of injection for a hemorrhoid. **A,** Proctoscope is withdrawn to a position just below the anorectal ring. **B,** Protoscope is tilted sharply forward to enable clear visualization of the injection site, which is the submucosa at or immediately below the anorectal ring. (From Goligher JC: *Surgery of the anus, rectum and colon*, ed 5, London, 1984, Bailliere-Tindall. Used with permission.)

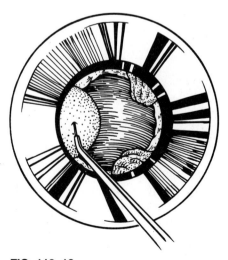

FIG. 119-13.

Sclerotherapy as viewed through the anoscope. If a wheal is not produced, the injection is too deep and the needle should be withdrawn. An injection that is too superficial will produce necrosis of the lining of the anal canal.

3. Inject 1 to 2 cc of sclerosant. A wheal should be noted while injecting. Take care to inject well *above* the level of the dentate line.
4. Document the location of the injection and the amount of sclerosant used.
5. Reposition the anoscope to visualize the next hemorrhoid group to be treated.

Postprocedure Patient Education

- Inform the patient that mild rectal discomfort may occur after treatment, and tell the patient to report any severe symptoms (see Box 119-4).
- Instruct the patient to return to the office in 3 weeks for repeat examination and further treatments if necessary.

Complications

- The procedure is painful if the sclerosant is injected below the level of the dentate line.
- Thrombosis of internal or external hemorrhoids may occur, resulting in pain. Thrombosis is managed with topical creams, analgesics, and sitz baths.
- Bleeding is usually the result of injection into the mucosa rather than the submucosa. Necrosis and ulceration with bleeding occur 2 to 3 weeks after injection. Healing usually occurs in 3 to 6 weeks.
- Abscess occurs very rarely.
- Anaphylaxis from sclerosant is rare.

Advantages

- The procedure is effective.
- The equipment cost is minimal.

Disadvantages

- The procedure is associated with more significant complications.
- The technique is slightly harder to master.

THROMBOSED EXTERNAL HEMORRHOIDS

Patients with thrombosed external hemorrhoids have a painful, tender, swollen, bluish lump at the anal orifice. If the patient is seen within 48 hours of the onset of symptoms, the thrombosed hemorrhoid should be excised. After 48 hours, symptoms have usually improved and symptomatic care is recommended. However, if the patient is still experiencing significant pain, the hemorrhoid can be excised even after 48 hours.

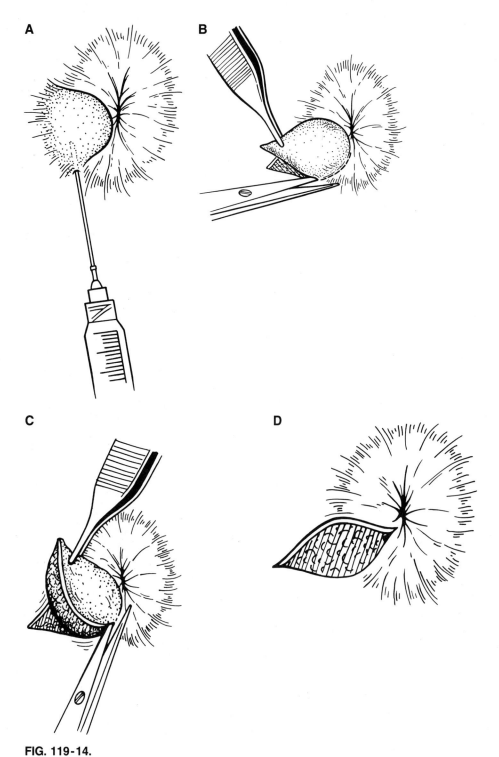

FIG. 119-14.
Excision of a thrombosed hemorrhoid. **A,** The area is infiltrated with 2% lidocaine with epinephrine.
B and **C,** The thrombosed hemorrhoid is excised along with a small wedge of skin. **D,** Skin edges
are sufficiently separated to permit adequate drainage, thereby preventing clot reaccumulation.

Equipment

- No. 11 blade and tissue scissors
- Hemostats
- 2 % lidocaine with epinephrine, 27-gauge 1.5 inch needle, and 3 cc syringe
- Antiseptic solution

Technique (Fig. 119-14)

1. Cleanse the perianal area with antiseptic solution.
2. Infiltrate the base of the thrombosed external hemorrhoid with lidocaine with epinephrine (2 to 5 cc).
3. Excise the hemorrhoid as an ellipse. Be sure to express all clots.
4. Control any bleeding with cautery.
5. Leave the wound open to heal by secondary intention.

Alternatively, some physicians will incise over the thrombus and evacuate the clot. If this is done, it is imperative that *all* clots be removed. After the incision is made, express the clot, and then explore the cavity with hemostats to break down any septae. Frequently more than one clot will be evacuated. Reexpress the area to be sure all clots have been removed.

Postprocedure Patient Education

- Recommend that the patient take sitz baths two to three times per day for 1 week.
- Oral analgesics, topical anesthetic cream, and stool softener are helpful.
- A follow-up examination should be scheduled for 1 week.
- Emphasize that the patient avoid prolonged sitting on the toilet to prevent recurrent thrombosis.
- Explain to the patient that a high-bulk, high-fluid diet is essential.

Complications

- Bleeding
- Pain
- Recurrence
- Chronic fissure
- Infection

CPT/BILLING CODES

46221	Hemorrhoidectomy, by simple ligature (e.g., rubber band)
46230	Excision of external hemorrhoid tags and/or multiple papillae
46320	Enucleation or excision of external thrombosed hemorrhoid
46500	Injection of sclerosing solution, hemorrhoids
46934	Destruction of hemorrhoids, any method; internal

46935   Destruction of hemorrhoids, any method; external
46936   Destruction of hemorrhoids, any method; internal and external

BIBLIOGRAPHY

Bleday R et al: Symptomatic hemorrhoids: current incidence and complications of operative therapy, *Dis Colon Rectum* 35:477, 1992.

Corman ML: *Colon and rectal surgery,* Philadelphia, 1984, J. B. Lippincott.

Dennison AR et al: The management of hemorrhoids, *Am J Gastroenterol* 84:475, 1989.

Devine R, Ory S: Treatment of hemorrhoids in pregnancy, *JFP* 17:65, 1992.

Fazio VW: *Current therapy in colon and rectal surgery,* Philadelphia, 1990, B. C. Decker.

Goligher JC: *Surgery of the anus, rectum and colon,* ed 5, London, 1984, Bailliere-Tindall.

Jensen DM, Randall GM, Machicado GA: Comparison of direct current (DC) vs. BICAP probe for treatment of chronically bleeding internal hemorrhoids (abstract), *Gastrointestinal Endosc* 34(2):196, 1988.

Leibach J, Cerda J: Hemorrhoids: modern treatment methods, *Hosp Med* 53, August 1991.

Norman DA, Newton R, Nicholas GV: Direct current electrotherapy of internal hemorrhoids: an effective, safe, and painless outpatient approach, *Am J Gastroenterol* 84:482, 1989.

Schrock TR: Examination of the anorectum, rigid sigmoidoscopy, flexible sigmodoscopy, and diseases of the anorectum. In Sleisenger MH, Fordtram JC, editors: *Gastrointestinal disease,* ed 4, Philadelphia, 1989, W. B. Saunders.

Schussman LC, Lutz LJ: Outpatient management of hemorrhoids, *Prim Care* 13(3):527, 1986.

Templeton JL et al: Comparison of infrared coagulation and rubber-band ligation for first- and second-degree hemorrhoids, *Br Med J* 286:1387, 1983.

Zinberg SS et al: A personal experience in comparing three non-operative techniques for treating internal hemorrhoids, *Am J Gastroenterol* 84:488, 1989.

CHAPTER 120

Perianal Skin Tags (External Hemorrhoidal Skin Tags)

James A. Surrell

Perianal skin tags represent a stretching and enlargement of the normal perianal skin (Fig. 120-1). As such, they are not true external hemorrhoids. It is generally believed that perianal skin tags occur as a result of the stretching of the perianal skin, secondary to a previously thrombosed external hemorrhoid. Perianal skin tags are not painful; patients most often seek treatment for them when they begin to interfere with anal hygiene. It is important to note that perianal skin tags do not cause pain, bleeding, or itching. If these symptoms are present, then another source must be looked for as the cause of these symptoms.

INDICATIONS

- Large perianal skin tags that interfere with anal hygiene
- Perianal skin tags that annoy the patient

Generally, a conservative approach to the management of perianal skin tags is recommended, as the vast majority of these benign lesions are asymptomatic.

CONTRAINDICATIONS

- If the patient with perianal skin tags also complains of pain, bleeding, or itching, then another source for these symptoms must be sought. Skin tag excision will *not* relieve these symptoms.
- If the perianal skin tags have a fleshy edematous appearance (Fig. 120-2), a diagnosis of anal Crohn's disease must be strongly considered. Nearly all patients with anal Crohn's disease will develop fleshy edematous skin tags and will have associated signs and symptoms of pain, discharge, bleeding, and

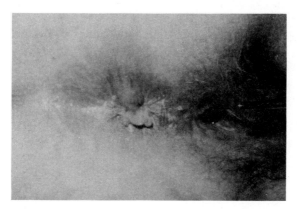

FIG. 120-1.
Perianal skin tags.

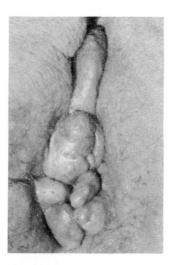

FIG. 120-2.
Crohn's disease: edematous skin tags. (From Thomson J: Disorders of the anus and anal canal. In Misiewicz JJ et al, editors: *Slide atlas of gastroenterology,* London, 1986, Gower Medical Publishing. Used with permission.)

atypical anal fissures (see Chapter 121, Anal Fissure/Lateral Sphincterotomy). Excision of perianal skin tags in Crohn's disease may lead to significant morbidity due to the creation of an indolent, nonhealing wound.

EQUIPMENT

Since the perianal skin tags are external to the anal canal, no anal retractor is needed. Any standard surgical forceps will be adequate to grasp the skin tag, which is generally removed with electrocautery. The electrocautery unit should have both coagulation and cutting capability (see Chapter 16, Radiofrequency Surgery, and Chapter 92, Loop Electrosurgical Excision Procedures for Treating CIN, for listings of manufacturers of various modern electrosurgery units). Alternatively, the lesion can be excised with sharp tissue scissors or a knife blade, but this will increase the likelihood of bleeding.

PREPROCEDURE PATIENT EDUCATION

It is recommended that most patients be discouraged from having their perianal skin tags excised. Perianal skin tags generally cause no significant symptoms. Question the patient in-depth as to his or her reasons for wanting the skin tags excised. The most common indication will be interference with anal hygiene due to the presence of one or more large perianal tags. Advise the patient that there will be some mild to moderate "burning" postoperative pain at the site of the excision. Postoperative bleeding is generally negligible, and infection is rare because the cauterized operative site is generally left open. If sutured (Vicryl, chromic), the chances for infection increase.

TECHNIQUE

1. Position the patient on the procedure table in the left lateral decubitus position.
2. Infiltrate the base of the skin tag with approximately 1 cc of local anesthetic (e.g., 2% lidocaine with epinephrine). To minimize discomfort, inject the anesthetic solution very slowly at the base of the skin tag with a 25- or 30-gauge ½-inch hypodermic needle. Done properly, this injection technique will afford minimal discomfort to the patient.
3. After approximately 1 minute, grasp the skin tag with a 4 × 4 inch gauze pad between the thumb and index finger and compress it to reduce the edema caused from the infiltration of the local anesthetic. This also restores the skin tag to its "normal" anatomy so the site of excision can be properly identified.
4. Grasp the skin tag with forceps (which will confirm that appropriate anesthesia has been induced), and hold perpendicular to its base on the perianal skin. Care must be taken not to put any undue tension on the skin tag, as this will serve to "tent up" and broaden the base of the skin tag and cause a much-larger-than-needed excision site.
5. Excise the skin tag, using the electrocautery unit in the cutting or blend mode. The site of excision should be approximately 3 mm above the normal perianal tissues because there will be electrocautery tissue destruction below the site of excision. If the skin tag is held taut and/or excised right at the level of the perianal skin, the resulting wound defect and patient discomfort will be greater than needed.

6. Cauterize any residual small bleeding sites. It is recommended that no more than three perianal skin tags be excised during any one procedure.
7. Leave the site of excision open, as suture closure of this site will contribute to an increase in postoperative pain and a greater likelihood of perianal abscess.

POSTPROCEDURE PATIENT EDUCATION

Advise the patient to avoid anal creams and ointments. Prescribe a nonconstipating pain medication (ibuprofen). Further advise the patient to follow a high-fiber diet with commercial fiber supplements and four to six glasses of water per day. Time off from work is usually very minimal and would range from 0 to 3 days, depending on the extent of excision. Total healing time may take up to 6 weeks for complete new skin coverage, but perianal discomfort will generally be present for 1 week or less.

COMPLICATIONS

- A perianal abscess can develop at the site of excision of a skin tag, although this is very uncommon and occurs less than 5% of the time. If an abscess does occur, appropriate incision and drainage will be necessary.
- If the skin tag excision site is very close to the anal verge, a chronic fissure may develop, although this is very uncommon. Should a fissure develop and persist, then lateral internal sphincterotomy would be recommended.
- Perianal cellulitis can occur. Should this be diagnosed, appropriate oral antibiotic therapy should be instituted.
- Bleeding/hematoma may occur.

Excision of skin tags should not alter anal continence due to the lack of involvement of this procedure with the anal sphincters.

CPT/BILLING CODE

46230   Excision of perianal skin tag

BIBLIOGRAPHY

Corman ML: *Colon and rectal surgery,* Philadelphia, 1989, J. B. Lippincott.
Goligher J: *Surgery of the anus, rectum, and colon,* ed 5, London, 1984, Bailliere-Tindall.
Gordon P, Nivatvongs S: *Principles and practice of surgery for the colon, rectum, and anus,* St Louis, 1992, Quality Medical Publishing.

CHAPTER 121

Anal Fissure/Lateral Sphincterotomy

James A. Surrell

Anal fissure is defined as a painful linear ulcer of the distal anal canal, located just inside the anal opening (Fig. 121-1). The history of a patient with anal fissure is so characteristic that the diagnosis can usually be made with accuracy based on the history alone. Patients complain of moderate to severe pain during and after bowel movements and have a variable amount of bleeding. Rarely, the patient with an anal fissure will complain of severe and *constant* pain. This is usually seen only with the patient with an acute anal fissure, with significant associated anal spasm causing constant discomfort.

The history must include whether the fissure is acute or chronic. *Chronic fissure* can arbitrarily be defined as one that has been present with signs and symptoms of pain and/or bleeding for more than 3 months. Unless the symptoms are extremely disabling, all fissures should be given a trial of conservative management, as discussed below. If conservative management fails, then lateral internal sphincterotomy is the procedure of choice for the treatment of an anal fissure.

Once the history suggests an anal fissure, the diagnosis can usually be made easily upon visual examination of the external anus and with a gentle digital examination. The left lateral decubitus position is recommended for anorectal examination. With gentle eversion of the anoderm, one can usually directly visualize the fissure. Touching the fissure with a cotton-tipped applicator confirms the diagnosis if this reproduces the painful symptoms experienced with bowel movements.

INDICATIONS

- Patient with an anal fissure that produces severe and constant pain

For most fissures, a 1-month trial of conservative management is indicated. This includes a high-fiber diet of at least 30 gm of dietary fiber per day, 6 to 8 glasses of water per day, and 3 to 6 gm of commercially available fiber supplements per day. If the fissure pain is severe, consider prescribing 5% lidocaine ointment to be applied to the fissure before and after bowel movements. Available nonprescription

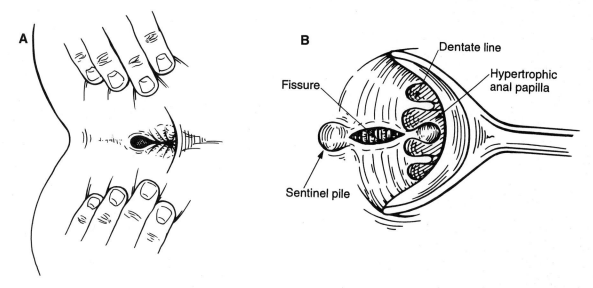

FIG. 121-1.
Anal fissures. Patient in left lateral decubitus position. **A,** External examination. Gentle eversion of the buttocks reveals a posterior midline anal fissure. **B,** Anoscopic examination. Chronic posterior anal fissure with a distal "sentinel pile" (SP) and a proximal hypertrophic anal papilla (HP) at the level of the dentate line (DL).

ointments and creams are minimally effective in the treatment of an anal fissure. They may, however, serve a function to lubricate the anal canal for bowel movements. Tronolane is the recommended cream. Steroid preparations may or may not be helpful, but are not for long-term use. Specifically advise patients *not* to use any ointment or cream with a rectal-tipped applicator, or suppositories, because these products and devices tend to worsen the symptoms of an anal fissure. Advise patients to apply a small amount of any recommended ointment or cream directly to the fissure with the finger, as an anal fissure is always located just inside the anal verge. The application of silver nitrate or electrocautery to the fissure site is *not* recommended, and may even exacerbate the symptoms. Anal dilators should *not* be used because of the unpredictable disruption of the anal sphincters and the potential for causing incontinence.

If conservative management has been recommended and complied with for approximately 1 month, and the symptoms of pain and or bleeding are still present during and after bowel movements, then lateral internal sphincterotomy is necessary.

CONTRAINDICATIONS

Anal fissures occur most commonly in the posterior midline. Approximately 90% of fissures are in this location, and 10% are located in the anterior midline. If the clinician sees an anal fissure in any location other than the anterior or posterior midline, a thorough gastrointestinal workup is necessary to rule out the presence of inflammatory bowel disease. If present, inflammatory bowel disease with an atypical fissure will most commonly be Crohn's disease. Another physical examination feature that should raise the suspicion of perianal Crohn's disease would be the presence of fleshy edematous skin tags (see Chapter 120, Perianal Skin Tags). If the examiner suspects inflammatory bowel disease, upper gastrointestinal and small-bowel X-rays are necessary, as well as colonoscopy or a barium enema X-ray with flexible sigmoidoscopy. Another contraindication to lateral internal sphincterotomy would be preexisting anal incontinence, although the coexistence of an anal fissure and incontinence is uncommon.

EQUIPMENT AND SUPPLIERS

The only special equipment required for lateral internal sphincterotomy is an assortment of various-sized anoscopes and a surgical electrocautery unit. Preferred is the Hill-Ferguson anal retractor, which is available in sizes small, medium, and large. The various anal retractors are available from V. Mueller at 1-800-323-9088. The anoscope product codes are SU180, SU181, and SU182. The Davol Surgical Electrocautery Unit is available from Davol, Incorporated at 1-800-556-6275.

PREPROCEDURE PATIENT EDUCATION

Inform the patient that lateral internal sphincterotomy is a procedure to divide *only* the fibers of the involuntary internal sphincter to allow the anal canal to relax during bowel movements. Warn the patient of an approximate 5% recurrence rate, and a 3% to 5% infection rate. Patients should expect mild to moderate postprocedure pain, usually well controlled with oral analgesics. There will be minimal bleeding and spotting for up to 6 weeks after the procedure. With proper technique, alteration of anal continence is uncommon.

TECHNIQUE

Author's note: My preference is to use IV sedation and local anesthesia. This is an outpatient procedure, generally done in the operating room. It must be emphasized that *this procedure should be undertaken only by a clinician who is thoroughly familiar with the technique and with anorectal anatomy.*

1. Place the patient on the operating table in the left lateral decubitus position, with the buttocks just off the edge of the table and the knees flexed. It is essential that the clinician be able to clearly identify the intersphincteric groove between the internal and external sphincters, so that only the fibers of the internal sphincter are divided to preserve anal continence for both flatus and feces.
2. Use the electrocautery unit to make a 1 cm incision just distal to the palpable intersphincteric groove in the left lateral quadrant of the perianum.

A

B

C

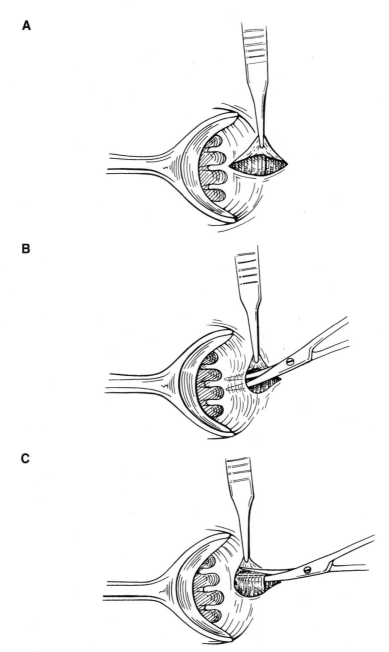

FIG. 121-2.
Lateral internal anal sphincterotomy using the open technique. The patient is placed in the lateral or the prone (jackknife) position. **A,** A radial incision is made across the intersphincteric groove. A narrow Hill-Ferguson retractor is in place. **B,** The internal sphincter is separated from the anoderm by blunt dissection. **C,** The internal sphincter is divided. The wound may be closed or left open.

3. Grasp the proximal skin edge and clearly identify the intersphincteric groove, using the dissecting scissors.

4. Divide the full thickness of the internal sphincter from its distal margin up to the level of the dentate line, which is visible in the anal canal (Fig. 121-2). Because the internal sphincter is immediately subjacent to the internal hemorrhoidal vessels, significant bleeding may be encountered if these hemorrhoidal vessels are divided. If proper hemostasis cannot be obtained by pressure or the use of electrocautery, then figure-of-eight suture ligation of these vessels is necessary.

5. Leave the primary incision site open and allow it to close secondarily. If there is a prominent sentinel skin tag distal to the fissure site or a prominent hypertrophic anal papilla proximal to the fissure site, you may excise the tag or papilla with the electrocautery unit at the time of the sphincterotomy procedure. Generally, no specific operative treatment is performed at the fissure site itself. The average operative time is 15 minutes or less.

POSTPROCEDURE PATIENT EDUCATION

Following lateral internal sphincterotomy, give the patient a prescription for nonconstipating pain medication (ibuprofen). Advise the patient to continue to follow a high-fiber diet of at least 30 gm of dietary fiber per day and to use psyllium-based powder fiber supplements once or twice a day. Instruct the patient to expect some discomfort, slight bleeding, and discharge from the operative site because the wound is generally left open. Bed rest should be 3 days or less, inasmuch as the pain from the sphincterotomy is often minimal, and may be less than that of a severe fissure.

COMPLICATIONS

Approximately 5% of patients will have nonhealing fissures following sphincterotomy and may need repeat sphincterotomy. Various studies have shown a postoperative infection rate of approximately 3% to 5%, and a smaller percentage of these patients will go on to develop an associated anal fistula.

The most morbid long-term complication is a development of anal incontinence, either for flatus or feces. Postoperative anal incontinence can result from technical operative error during the procedure, whereby muscle fibers other than those of the internal sphincter muscle are divided. Other factors that can contribute to postoperative anal incontinence would be unrecognized preexisting anal incontinence.

CPT/BILLING CODE

46080   Anal sphincterotomy

BIBLIOGRAPHY

Corman ML: *Colon and rectal surgery,* Philadelphia, 1989, J.B. Lippincott.

Goligher J: *Surgery of the anus, rectum, and colon,* London, 1984, Bailliere-Tindall.

Goligher J, Duthie H, Nixon H: Anal fissure. In Goligher J, editor: *Surgery of the anus and colon,* ed 5, London, 1984, Bailliere-Tindall.

Gordon P, Nivatvongs S: *Principles and practice of surgery for the colon, rectum, and anus,* St Louis, 1992, Quality Medical Publishing.

Veidenheimer MC: *Seminars in colon and rectal surgery,* Philadelphia, 1990, W.B. Saunders.

Editor's note: I am not aware of family physicians who do internal sphincterotomies. However, because anal fissures are so common it seems we should discuss the procedure in order to be able to better counsel our patients. Treating anal fissures is difficult and frustrating. Surgical outcomes are generally excellent and a great relief to the patient.

CHAPTER 122

Pilonidal Cyst/Abscess Incision and Drainage

James A. Surrell

A pilonidal sinus and/or abscess is located in the gluteal crease, usually within 5 to 10 cm of the anal verge. This lesion was originally described in the mid-1800s, and there has been considerable debate in the literature over whether it is an acquired or a congenital lesion. Most experts now believe that this is an acquired lesion secondary to penetration of the skin at this level from falling shafts of hair. A pilonidal sinus will frequently contain multiple shafts of hair that are microscopically noted to be tapered at both ends like shed hairs. In addition, it has never been conclusively demonstrated that there is a preponderance or even the existence of hair follicles in the wall of the pilonidal sinus tract. Pilonidal sinus and abscess is a disease of the younger population, and 75% of cases are seen in males. Most patients develop symptoms of pilonidal disease between the ages of 20 and 25 years. A typical patient with pilonidal disease develops an abscess or recurrent infection and drainage at the base of the spine. Typical pilonidal disease will be characterized by a recurrence of infection and the development of multiple sinus tracts in this typical location.

Examination of the patient with suspected pilonidal disease will generally reveal an area of inflammation in the midline of the gluteal crease, with one or more sinus openings (Fig. 122-1). The openings may be slightly off the midline. Careful inspection of this site may reveal loose hairs projecting from the sinus openings. If the pilonidal sinus has an associated abscess, the patient will complain of pain and the examiner may note swelling and erythema at this site. Spontaneous and ongoing drainage is the common indicator, however, and if an abscess is present it is usually small. As a general guideline, if the patient gives a history of recurrent infection at the base of the spine, this itself is almost diagnostic of a pilonidal sinus. Some difficulty in diagnosis may occur if the pilonidal sinus is located in the more caudad position closer to the anal canal. This raises the possibility of an anal fistula as the cause of the infection. If, however, hairs are found in the lesion, this offers convincing confirmatory evidence that one is dealing with a pilonidal sinus.

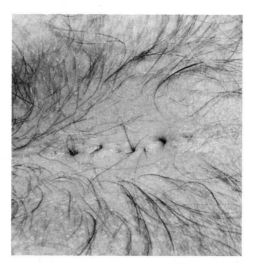

FIG. 122-1.
Multiple (six) pilonidal sinus openings in the natal cleft. (From Thomson J: Disorders of the anus and anal canal. In Misiewicz JJ et al, editors: *Slide atlas of gastroenterology,* London, 1986, Gower Medical Publishing. Used with permission.)

INDICATIONS

- Patients with a history of recurrent infections and drainage at the base of the spine (Antibiotic therapy should only be considered as temporizing and palliative, as recurrence will be the rule until adequate incision and drainage is accomplished.)

CONTRAINDICATIONS

- An immunocompromised patient
- Patient with a paucity of symptoms, such as only minimal drainage with little or no discomfort or inflammation occurring perhaps only once or twice per year or a marked bleeding dyscrasia

EQUIPMENT

Only a minor surgical setup is required. No special equipment is needed to perform incision and drainage for pilonidal disease.

PREPROCEDURE PATIENT EDUCATION

The procedure of choice is incision and drainage, leaving the wound open to heal by secondary intention. With this technique, the patient needs to be informed of a prolonged healing time. The wounds are not at all disabling, and they can be expected to close in 8 to 12 weeks. Various other options for treatment of pilonidal disease must be reviewed to include excision and primary closure, as well as skin flap and other plastic procedures for more extensive and complex pilonidal disease.

TECHNIQUE

Perform an elliptical incision at the site of the pilonidal disease to include the obvious sinus tract(s) (Fig. 122-2). The lateral and deep margins should extend to healthy appearing noninfected tissue. This procedure can be performed under local anesthesia (with intravenous sedation) or under general anesthesia in the operating room. Because of the proximity of the infected site, spinal anesthesia is *not* recommended. Thoroughly inspect the wound during the procedure, and curettage all chronically infected granulation tissue such that the remaining wound defect is lined with healthy appearing tissue with no obvious remaining sinus tracts. If the resultant wound defect is not too deep, depending on the extent of the disease and the body habitus of the patient, then consider marsupialization of the wound by tacking the skin edges to the base of the wound with an absorbable running simple suture (Fig. 122-3). This will tend to prevent premature secondary wound closure. Total procedure time is generally 30 minutes or less.

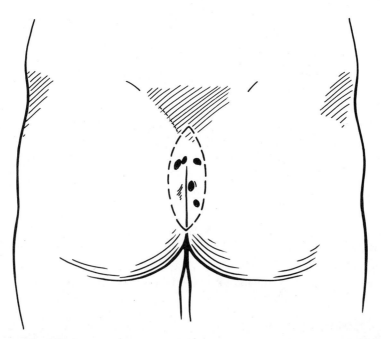

FIG. 122-2.
Area of elliptical excision for pilonidal sinus.

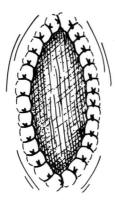

FIG. 122-3.
Marsupialization after excision of pilonidal sinus, closed with interrupted absorbable sutures.

POSTPROCEDURE PATIENT EDUCATION

If the procedure is done with the pilonidal disease excised and the wound left open, instruct the patient as to proper wound management. An open wound should be cleansed daily with water, either by showering or other irrigation.

During the early stages of wound healing, the wound is packed with moistened gauze sponges and changed twice daily. During the early phases of the postprocedure recovery, you should examine the patient on a weekly basis to assess adequate progress. At this time, if hair regrowth is occurring, wound edges may be shaved. Every attempt to prevent loose hairs from entering the healing wound should be made. Clearly instruct the patient in the concept of the wound healing from the inside out so that premature skin bridging does not occur before the entire cavity is obliterated. Usual time off work is approximately 1 week.

COMPLICATIONS

Clearly, the most common complication of surgery for pilonidal disease is recurrence. The results of reported pilonidal disease surgery are variable, but most physicians report that the open technique has less of a recurrence rate than the closed technique. The obvious disadvantage to the open technique is the prolonged healing time, but these wounds generally do not afford significant morbidity to the patient during this longer healing process. Bleeding, excessive pain, and infection are rare.

CPT/BILLING CODE

10080   Incision and drainage of pilonidal cyst

BIBLIOGRAPHY

Corman ML: *Colon and rectal surgery,* Philadelphia, 1989, J.B. Lippincott.

Goligher J: *Surgery of the anus, rectum, and colon,* London, 1984, Bailliere-Tindall.

Gordon P, Nivatvongs S: *Principles and practice of surgery for the colon, rectum, and anus,* St Louis, 1992, Quality Medical Publishing.

Veidenheimer MC: *Seminars in colon and rectal surgery,* Philadelphia, 1990, W.B. Saunders.

CHAPTER 123

Perianal Abscess Incision and Drainage

James A. Surrell

Perianal abscess is clearly one of the most painful anal conditions seen in the outpatient setting. The pain of a perianal abscess is severe, disabling, and progressive, and the only relief these patients obtain is with spontaneous rupture of the abscess, or when they seek medical attention for incision and drainage. The most common etiology of perianal abscess is thought to be an infection originating at the dentate line in the anal crypts (see Chapter 116, Clinical Anorectal Anatomy and Examination). The infection then usually migrates through the path of least resistance to the perianal tissues, where there is a closed-space environment ideal for proliferation of this mixed bacterial infection.

The four locations where abscesses can occur and their relative incidence are shown in Fig. 123-1. The most common site (60%) of a perianal abscess is in the perianal tissues immediately adjacent to the anal verge. If the abscess is located 2 to 3 cm away from the anal verge, then it is most likely in the ischiorectal location (25%) just outside the anal sphincters. A perianal abscess can occur in the intersphincteric plane, between the internal and external sphincters. (An abscess in this location may not be externally visible or palpable in the perianal tissues.) The pain of a perianal abscess will be present with an intersphincteric abscess, but the diagnosis will be confirmed only on digital anorectal examination, where the fluctuant mass is easily palpable. The least common location for a perianal abscess is the supralevator location, and this truly is a peri*rectal* abscess as opposed to a peri*anal* abscess. Most clinicians would agree that if a supralevator abscess is diagnosed, one must look for an intraabdominal or pelvic source. A supralevator abscess may be associated with appendicitis, diverticulitis, pelvic inflammatory disease, or other pelvic or abdominal disease.

Patients with a perianal abscess may develop an associated fever and often have a marked leukocytosis, depending on the severity of the infection. Once the diagnosis of perianal abscess is made, it is essential to proceed with adequate incision and drainage treatment without delay. This is especially important in any patient who may be immunocompromised, on steroids, or who has diabetes or

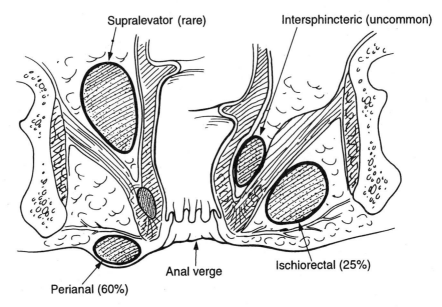

FIG. 123-1.
Various anatomic locations of anorectal abscesses.

any other debilitating comorbidity. The treatment of choice for perianal abscess is clearly incision and drainage—*not* antibiotic therapy. If adequate incision and drainage of a perianal abscess is not done, patients can rapidly develop severe infectious problems such as necrotizing fasciitis, which can become life-threatening.

INDICATIONS

Nearly every perianal abscess should be incised and drained. The only reason not to do this procedure would be if spontaneous drainage of the abscess has occurred and if, in the judgment of the examining clinician, adequate drainage has resulted. It must be remembered that these abscess cavities can have multiple loculations and, if spontaneous drainage has occurred, the abscess cavity must still be explored with a digital examination or hemostats to break down any loculated areas within the abscess.

CONTRAINDICATIONS

Patients with underlying hematologic diseases may have perianal abscesses. The associated hematologic disease may include leukemia, granulocytopenia, and lymphoma. The infecting organisms seen with this type of perianal abscess may be quite different from those seen with an otherwise uncomplicated perianal abscess. In those patients with an associated hematologic disorder and a perianal abscess—for example, with leukemia under poor control—conservative treatment of antibiotics combined with local radiotherapy may be advised. Other clinicians recommend aggressive surgical management of perianal abscess in patients with hematologic disorders, but clearly this is not ever to be attempted in the outpatient setting.

EQUIPMENT

A minor surgical instrument setup is all that is required to perform incision and drainage. A Penrose drain may be needed. Adequate suction should be available, and a surgical electrocautery unit is often helpful to achieve hemostasis at the incision and drainage site of the infected and hyperemic tissue. Various-sized Hill-Ferguson anal retractors, which facilitate visualization, are available from most medical supply companies.

PREPROCEDURE PATIENT EDUCATION

Advise the patient that, in all likelihood, rather dramatic pain relief will follow the procedure. Further advise the patient that, unless adequate incision and drainage is accomplished, further tissue damage may result. Clearly, the most effective way to afford adequate pain relief is to drain the abscess. Recurrence, bleeding, and pain are all possible. Further workup may also be necessary to rule out other disease once the infection is controlled.

TECHNIQUE

Patients with a perianal abscess have a clear need for prompt pain relief. Local anesthesia may be utilized in an attempt to anesthetize the skin at the intended incision and drainage site, but this is often only marginally effective. It must be remembered that these infected perianal tissues usually will not respond well to local anesthetic agents, due to the highly acid environment. Either spinal or general anesthesia for this outpatient procedure may be required, depending on the specific patient circumstances. Before incision and drainage of the abscess cavity, it is appropriate, if not essential, to perform anoscopy to look for an internal opening of a fistula tract feeding the abscess cavity. The advantage of doing the anoscopy before incision and drainage of the abscess is that, with gentle pressure on the abscess cavity, one may see pus expressed from an internal opening at the level of the dentate line. This then clearly establishes the diagnosis of an associated anal fistula. Textbooks of colon and rectal surgery vary widely on the incidence of associated fistula with perianal abscess, but most experts would agree that it is at least in the range of 50%.

1. Make an incision over the fluctuant area near the anal canal in a plane radial to the circumference of the anal canal. The advantage of this type of incision is that it can be easily extended to perform anal fistulotomy if a fistula is

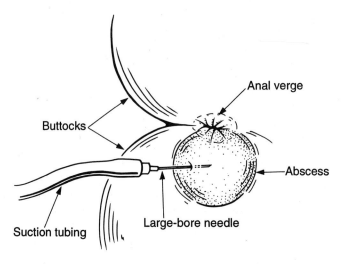

FIG. 123-2.
Needle and suction aspiration of a perianal abscess.

present and fistulotomy is indicated. Another option is to remove an ellipse of tissue such that you can easily place your gloved examining finger into the abscess cavity to break down any loculations and to place drains.

2. Irrigate the abscess cavity and, if deemed necessary, place a Penrose drain loosely into the abscess cavity and suture it at the skin edge level. A Penrose drain will not adhere to surrounding tissue, which makes its subsequent removal generally painless.

3. Remove the drain within 24 to 48 hours. In the office setting, a small perianal abscess can be drained to afford prompt pain relief. Packing with iodoform gauze is used by some clinicians as an alternative to the Penrose drain. This may be removed in 10 to 14 days.

4. In selected patients with a well-defined fluctuant perianal abscess, drainage can be accomplished without anesthesia by placing a large-bore, 16-gauge needle (attached to suction) into the abscess (Fig. 123-2). This can be an effective *temporizing* measure to afford dramatic and prompt pain relief if definitive surgical treatment is not readily available. The disadvantage of this needle suction technique is that evaluation for an associated anal fistula becomes more difficult.

POSTPROCEDURE PATIENT EDUCATION

Following an adequate drainage procedure of a perianal abscess, advise the patient to take sitz baths for 10 to 15 minutes twice a day. Spend some time with the patient and his or her family to reinforce the fact that the infected wound must heal from the inside out. Most patients understand that they must keep the wound from closing with either sitz baths or showering. Explain that daily wound irrigations will prevent the skin edges from closing prematurely before the abscess cavity has resolved, which will help to avoid a secondary infection and a recurrent abscess. These instructions usually serve as adequate motivation to follow the recommended postprocedure care.

COMPLICATIONS

The most common complication following incision and drainage of a perianal abscess is recurrence. The most common cause of recurrence of a perianal abscess is an unrecognized, and therefore untreated, associated fistula. The patient with a recurrent perianal abscess must be thoroughly evaluated for the presence of an associated anal fistula. Another cause of recurrent perianal abscess includes the presence of inflammatory bowel disease, most commonly Crohn's disease. Bleeding, excessive pain, and fasciitis are rare complications.

CPT/BILLING CODE

46050   Incision and drainage of perianal abscess

BIBLIOGRAPHY

Corman ML: *Colon and rectal surgery,* Philadelphia, 1989, J.B. Lippincott.
Goligher J: Surgery of the anus, rectum, and colon. In Gordon P, Nivatvongs S, editors: *Principles and practice of surgery for the colon, rectum, and anus,* St Louis, 1992, Quality Medical Publishing.
Veidenheimer MC: *Seminars in colon and rectal surgery,* Philadelphia, 1990, W.B. Saunders.

CHAPTER 124

Diagnostic Esophagogastroduodenoscopy (EGD)

Donald M. Gelb

John L. Pfenninger

George Villanueva

Elizabeth A. Roaf

The introduction of fiberoptic gastrointestinal endoscopy opened a new vista for the study of diseases of the upper-gastrointestinal tract. Refinements in equipment and technology and advances in pharmacology have brought this valuable technique within the power of primary care physicians, enabling them to evaluate and treat patients with problems of the esophagus, stomach, and duodenum. The entire procedure can be completed in 10 to 20 minutes. One study (Rodney) indicated that esophagogastroduodenoscopy—performed by primary care physicians—was associated with enhanced management or improved diagnostic accuracy in 89% of cases.

The flexible endoscope can be moved in many directions, and it has channels for water, air insufflation, aspiration, and biopsy. The gastroscope is very similar to the flexible sigmoidoscope, which is described in Chapter 118.

The examiner should mentally superimpose the face of a clock on the television monitor, and use this as a reference point.

INDICATIONS

Preexisting Conditions

- Cancer surveillance in high-risk patients (e.g., those with Barrett's esophagus, Ménétrier's disease, polyposis, pernicious anemia)

- Esophageal stricture
- Gastric retention
- Chronic duodenitis
- Chronic esophagitis
- Chronic gastritis
- Symptomatic hiatal hernia
- Gastric ulcer monitoring
- Chronic peptic ulcer disease
- Pyloroduodenal stenosis
- Varices
- Angiodysplasia in other areas of the bowel

Signs

- Abdominal mass
- Unexplained anemia
- Gross or occult gastrointestinal bleeding
- X-ray abnormality on upper gastrointestinal study

Symptoms

(Not improving after 10 days of H_2-blocker therapy, or not resolved after 4 to 6 weeks of H_2-blocker therapy, where appropriate)

- Dyspepsia
- Dysphagia/odynophagia
- Early satiety
- Epigastric pain
- Food sticking
- Meal-related heartburn
- Severe indigestion
- Chronic nausea or vomiting
- Substernal or paraxiphoid pain
- Reflux of food (regurgitation)
- Severe weight loss

CONTRAINDICATIONS

- History of bleeding disorder (platelet dysfunction, hemophilia)
- History of bleeding esophageal varices
- Cardiopulmonary instability
- Suspected perforated viscus
- Uncooperative patient

EQUIPMENT

- Video gastroscope, with an insertion tube diameter of no more than 9.5 mm; channel diameter of 2.8 mm; field of view of 120 degrees; working length of 104 cm; angulation up of 210 degrees, down of 90 degrees, and right and left of 100 degrees, and the standard accessories
- Light source
- Camera source
- Color video printer
- Video monitor
- Video recorder
- Biopsy forceps
- Williams oral introducer
- Endoscopy table
- IV stand and IV sets
- Stool with wheels for endoscopist
- Sphygmomanometer
- Stethoscope
- ECG machine or cardiac monitor
- O_2 saturation monitor (pulse oximeter)
- Dextrose 5% in 0.45% sodium chloride solution, 1 liter
- Suction equipment and tubing
- Specimen jars with formalin solution
- Syringes and needles
- Rubber gloves
- CLO test materials
- Anesthetic, sedative, and narcotic medications
- Oxygen and delivery mask
- Crash cart supplies (see Chapter 135, Anaphylaxis, regarding Banyan kits)

Cleaning Supplies

- Plastic containers for endoscope tube
- Surgical scrub solution and water
- Sporocidin enzyme solution
- 70% isopropyl alcohol
- Manufacturer-supplied cleaning brush
- Glutaraldehyde cleaning solution

PREPROCEDURE PATIENT EDUCATION

Explain the procedure to the patient, including its possible risks and complications. Provide a patient education handout (Box 124-1) and instructions to follow before the procedure (Box 124-2). Obtain informed consent (Box 124-3).

BOX 124-1. PATIENT EDUCATION HANDOUT
ESOPHAGOGASTRODUODENOSCOPY (EGD)

What is an EGD? EGD stands for *esophago-gastro-duodenoscopy.* This procedure allows the doctor to look directly at the lining of your esophagus (food tube), stomach, and the first part of your small intestine, which is called the *duodenum.*

Why do I need this test? An EGD gives your physician specific information that X-rays and other tests do not provide. This test can help your doctor diagnose your problem.

Who performs the test? The test is performed by your physician or your physician's assistant.

How is the EGD done? During an EGD, a flexible tube connected to a light source (called a *flexible fiberoptic endoscope* or *gastroscope*) is inserted into the mouth and advanced into your stomach. As it is slowly withdrawn, the physician will carefully look at the lining of your stomach and esophagus.

Is it uncomfortable? There is usually no pain with this test. You may experience a full feeling. You will be given a sedative prior to the examination. A local anesthetic is sprayed into your throat before the tube is inserted into your mouth. This will numb your gag reflex. Once the tube is in the back of your throat, the doctor will ask you to swallow. This helps to guide the tube into the esophagus. You may feel this tube in the back of your throat. You will be able to swallow and breathe comfortably throughout the test.

How long does the test take? The examination itself takes 10 to 15 minutes. However, you may be in the procedure room approximately 30 minutes, including the time it takes to prepare you for the examination.

Are medications given? Yes. Your doctor will give you a sedative prior to the examination to help keep you comfortable. Some medicines are given by mouth, while others may be given with a needle.

Do I need to do anything before the test? Please read the instruction sheet on what to do prior to the test.

Do I have to do anything special after the test? You may eat 1 hour after the test. The freezing sensation in the back of your throat will usually wear off about 30 minutes after the procedure. You may not drive that day or drink alcohol. You may begin taking your usual medicines 1 hour after arriving home.

When will I get the results? It takes approximately 7 to 10 days to get your biopsy results. After your test, the doctor will briefly discuss the findings of the examination with you and your family. If you do not hear from our office within 2 weeks, call us.

If you have any questions about your test or instructions, please call your doctor.

Used with permission of Tom E. Norris, M.D., Tacoma Family Medicine, Tacoma, Washington.

ANTIBIOTIC PROPHYLAXIS

Antibiotic prophylaxis for endoscopy with or without gastrointestinal biopsy is not recommended according to the latest American Heart Association guidelines (see Chapter 133, Antibiotic Prophylaxis for Bacterial Endocarditis).

BOX 124-2. PREPROCEDURE PATIENT INSTRUCTIONS
ESOPHAGOGASTRODUODENOSCOPY (EGD)

Do not eat or drink *anything* for 8 hours before the procedure.

If you are on any medications, ask your physician if you should take them the day of the procedure. Do not take any aspirin or ibuprofen for 7 days before the test.

If you have any of the following, please be certain your physician knows.

- Diabetes (controlled with insulin or prescription drugs)
- Any history of heart disease or strokes
- History of bleeding or bleeding tendencies
- History of heart infection
- Artificial heart valve
- Joint replacement
- Drug therapy with any blood thinning medications, aspirin, or arthritis medications
- Drug therapy with tranquilizers or sleeping pills

Get a good night's sleep and do not worry about this procedure. It is not usually difficult at all. Most patients have no real discomfort.

Please arrange for a responsible adult to be with you in the office and at home for a few hours after the procedure. This person must drive you home after the test. We recommend *no driving* that day and *no alcohol,* because the medications we use to suppress the gag reflex cause drowsiness and interact with alcohol.

Call immediately if you develop any of the following symptoms after the procedure:

- Dizziness
- Chest pain
- Painful or difficult swallowing
- "Coffee ground" vomit
- Black or bloody stools
- Temperature in the 100s

If biopsies were done, be sure to call in 2 weeks to get the results if you haven't heard from us.

These instructions have been discussed with me.

Patient signature _____

Nurse/Physician signature _____

Date _____   Time _____

One copy to chart/one copy to patient

Used with permission of Tom E. Norris, M.D., Tacoma Family Medicine, Tacoma, Washington.

BOX 124-3. CONSENT FORM
ESOPHAGOGASTRODUODENOSCOPY (EGD)

Esophagogastroduodenoscopy (EGD) is a procedure in which the clinician can look into your esophagus (swallowing tube), stomach, and duodenum (first part of the intestine) with a flexible lighted tube. A small amount of tissue (biopsy) might be removed for examination in the laboratory under a microscope.

The *benefits* of the procedure include the early diagnosis and assistance with treatment of disease. These diseases might include ulcers or cancer.

There are *risks* to this procedure, although we believe that the potential benefits outweigh the potential risks.

- Infection can occur, and you may need to take antibiotic medication after the procedure.
- Bleeding is rare, but it is possible. With severe bleeding you might even need a blood transfusion.
- Perforation (causing a hole in the esophagus, stomach, or duodenum) is rare, but if it happens you may need hospitalization or surgery.
- The medications that we give to prevent pain and discomfort can cause adverse reactions. If these medicines are injected, they can cause redness and swelling of the arm. Any medicine can cause allergic reactions.

There are *alternatives* to EGD, including X-ray studies, but they do not allow us to directly see the areas or to take biopsy samples. If you have questions about this procedure, please ask us. If you want more time to consider this procedure, we can provide it, but you may be subject to the risks of a delayed diagnosis—especially of cancer. If you have questions, please ask us.

INFORMED CONSENT

Having read and understood the above, I feel that the benefits of this procedure outweigh the risks. I have read and understand the patient instruction handout and patient education handout. I agree to allow Dr(s). _____ to perform an EGD procedure with biopsies if needed.

_____   _____
Signature   Date

_____
Witness

Used with permission of Tom E. Norris, M.D., Tacoma Family Medicine, Tacoma, Washington.

SEDATION/MONITORING

Esophagogastroduodenoscopy has traditionally been carried out in a hospital laboratory specializing in gastrointestinal disorders, in an emergency room setting, or in an outpatient surgery facility. Many physicians have performed it in their offices using only topical anesthetic spray. The newer small-diameter scopes allow for a less traumatic examination. Consider the fact that nasogastric tubes are inserted every day by hospital nursing staffs!

The move to office gastroscopy is just beginning, but it will increase as the safety, benefits, and cost savings are documented. The American Academy of Family Physicians is not currently recommending an ECG monitor or oximeter for all low-risk patients. If the procedure lasts more than 30 minutes, a large-bore scope is used. If the patient is at high risk, or if more than "light" sedation is used, oximetry and ECG monitoring should be utilized. All patients should have clinical monitoring of color, degree of sedation, loss of reflexes, blood pressure, pulse, and respiratory rate in a well lighted room.

Table 124-1 provides a summary of the agents usually used for sedation. However, sufficient anesthesia or sedation can often be accomplished *without* intravenous drug administration. The patient can be given diazepam 10 mg orally 2 hours before the procedure, or lorazepam sublingually. An optional intramuscular dose of ketorolac (Toradol) 60 mg may be given 30 to 60 minutes before the procedure. Butorphanol tartrate (Stadol), 1 to 2 sprays (intranasal) generally provides both sedation and analgesia sufficient to carry out EGD.

TABLE 124-1.

Drugs Used with Esophagogastroduodenoscopy

Medication	Dose
Narcotics	
Meperidine (Demerol) iv	10-75 mg (0.5-1 mg/kg)
Fentanyl (Sublimaze) iv	1-2 mg
Butorphanol tartrate (Stadol Nasal Spray)	1-2 mg (1 to 2 sprays in nostril)
Benzodiazepines	
Diazepam (Valium) iv	1-10 mg
Midazolam (Versed) iv	2-7 mg (0.035 to 0.1 mg/kg)
Lorazepam (Ativan) sl (onset in 10 min.)	1-2 mg
Anticholinergic	
Glycopyrrolate (Robinul)	0.2 mg, 30 min preprocedure
Simethicone (Mylicon) drops	0.6 ml (40 mg) in 30 cc water p.o. or flushed through gastroscope with 5 cc of water
Topical local anesthetics	
Lidocaine 2% viscous solution gargle	
Benzocaine 20% (Hurricane) spray	
Benzocaine 14% and tetracaine 2% (Cetacaine)	
Antagonists	
Naloxone (Narcan) iv	0.4-0.8 mg
Flumazenil (Romazicon) iv	0.2-1 mg (Start with 0.2 mg; repeat every 60 seconds to a maximum of 1 mg or until reversal of benzodiazepine effect achieved)

These are the drugs most commonly used. The endoscopist should become familiar with each category and fully understand the common actions, side effects, and dosages. Many physicians do not use an anticholinergic, and it is contraindicated in atony, dysmotility, gastric retention, or tachycardia.

BOX 124-4. HIGH-RISK GROUPS

Greater than 70 years old
Less than 12 years old
Agitated, uncooperative patient
History of angina
History of significant aortic stenosis
History of significant chronic obstructive pulmonary disease
History of cerebrovascular accident
Presence of significant bleeding disorder or coagulopathy
Barium administration within a few hours of procedure

Benzocaine spray often causes significant coughing and gagging. With the "popsicle stick" method of local anesthesia, the patient is given a tongue blade covered with 2% lidocaine jelly and is asked to suck it 10 minutes before the scope is inserted. To increase palatability, flavoring can be added to the lidocaine.

A butterfly IV can be placed if intravenous medications are warranted. Resuscitation equipment and reversal drugs should also be readily available. The use of a benzodiazepine antagonist and a narcotic antagonist makes the entire procedure safer. If intravenous sedation is used, the end point to be titrated is slurred speech with the patient being arousable. Diazepam can occasionally cause paradoxical excitement. If this occurs, use a different medication. It is rarely necessary to supplement initial doses of sedatives.

Patient selection for office-based esophagogastroduodenoscopy is very critical. It would be wise to perform esophagogastroduodenoscopy on the higher-risk patients shown in Box 124-4 in facilities where complications can be handled.

The routine use of oxygen is generally not advocated unless the patient has risk factors or becomes overly sedated. It is essential that oxygen be available if EGD is carried out in the office.

TECHNIQUE

Aspirin and nonsteroidal antiinflammatory agents should be discontinued 7 days before the examination, and the patient should take nothing by mouth after 7 P.M. the evening before the procedure (or at least 8 hours has elapsed since eating).

Have the anesthesiologist or assistant monitor the patient during the procedure, start the IVs (if used), and administer medications. The patient may best be monitored by pulse oximetry and by an ECG. Blood pressure, pulse, and respiration should be monitored as the minimum. Cardiopulmonary complications account for 60% of deaths that occur during esophagogastroduodenoscopy.

1. Examine the oral cavity while the patient is sitting. Remove any dentures.
   Have the patient swallow 40 mg of simethicone in 30 ml of tap water.

Alternatively, simethicone can be used as needed. If gastric bubbles obscure good visualization, inject 0.6 ml of the liquid down the gastroscope, followed by 5 cc of water.

2. Place the patient in the left lateral recumbent position.

3. Spray the back of the throat with 2% lidocaine.

4. Place the Williams introducer in the patient's mouth over the tongue and into the oral pharynx. The Williams introducer, manufactured by the 3M company, was originally intended for use in bronchoscopy, but it is very effective in esophagogastroduodenoscopy. It acts as a guide for the endoscope, obviating the necessity for placing the fingers in the patient's mouth; protecting the patient's tongue, teeth, and oral mucosa; and preventing the patient from inadvertently damaging the endoscope.

5. Insert the lubricated tip of the endoscope down the introducer, and slowly advance it to the first point of resistance, 15 to 17 cm from the patient's teeth, which is the area of the vocal cord and the cricopharyngeus muscle (Fig. 124-1).

6. Ask the patient to swallow repeatedly until a feeling of "give" is obtained; at this point, the endoscope can then be passed naturally into the esophagus (Fig. 124-2).

Note: At no point is force used. Allow the patient's normal swallowing mechanism to advance the endoscope.

7. Once the tip of the scope has entered the esophagus, insufflate just enough air to dilate the esophagus so that you can visualize the mucosa. (Additional air may be needed once the scope is in the stomach or duodenum.)

Note: Identify the channel in front of the scope *before* you attempt to pass the scope to prevent injury to the patient.

8. Gently advance the endoscope down the esophagus. The first landmark will be the bronchoaortic constriction (Fig. 124-3). It is important to visualize the

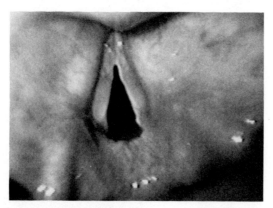

FIG. 124-1.
Open vocal cord.

A

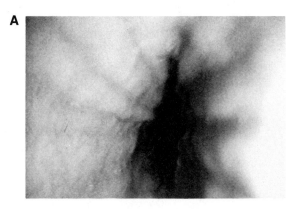

B

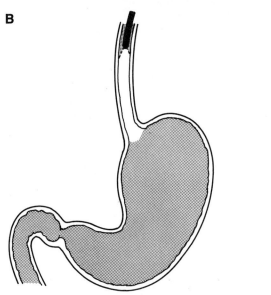

FIG. 124–2.
A, Proximal esophagus. **B,** Unshaded area is seen by lighted scope.

esophagus on the entry approach since the mucosa may become irritated by the passage of the scope. Continue to the squamocolumnar junction between the esophagus and stomach, which is approximately 40 cm from the patient's teeth (Fig. 124-4). The mucosal coloration changes abruptly here from pale to dark pink. This boundary is known as the *Z line*. Ask the patient to sniff. It is important to identify at what level the Z line lies relative to the esophageal hiatus in order to diagnose sliding hiatal hernia. Having the patient sniff constricts the esophagus at the level of the diaphragm. This "sniff" test should also be repeated when viewing the Z line from below.

Note: Use water, air, suction, and "miniwithdrawals" when needed to pass the scope and to help fully examine all surfaces.

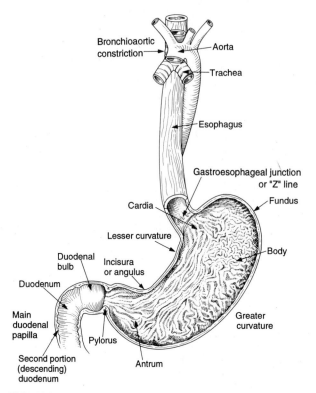

FIG. 124-3.

Relevant anatomy for gastroscopy. The *cardia* is that portion of the stomach immediately surrounding the esophageal opening. The *gastroesophageal junction* is also known as the GE junction, the Z line, ora serrata, or gastric rosette. The upper end or dome of the stomach is the *fundus*. The upturn of the "J" of the stomach is separated from its vertical portion by the *angular notch* (or angulus, angularis, or incisura). The *antrum* lies to the right of the angulus and ends at the *pylorus*, or greatly thickened muscular wall. The *duodenum* lies beyond the pylorus. The *lesser curvature* is the upper, right border of the stomach while the *greater curvature* is the left inferior margin.

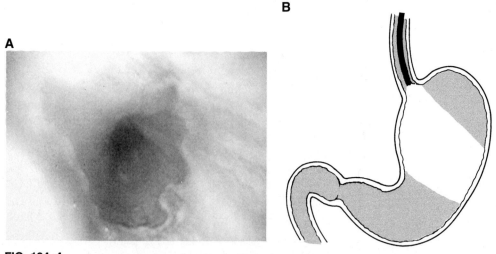

FIG. 124-4.
A, Distal esophagus "Z line." **B,** Unshaded area is seen by lighted scope.

9. After passing the gastroesophageal junction, the endoscope will enter the stomach. The gastric lake and rugae will become visible (Fig. 124-5). Follow the rugae to the angularis, antrum, and prepyloric areas (Figs. 124-6 and 124-7). It may be necessary to suction gastric secretions. Adjust the scope so the small black arrow is at the top of the field and so it corresponds with the incisura. This provides proper orientation with the patient in the left lateral position.

10. Guide the endoscope through the relaxed pyloric sphincter and into the duodenal bulb (Fig. 124-8). The area just distal to the pylorus may be difficult to visualize and several short advancements and withdrawals may be necessary. At this point, complete the examination of the duodenum. It is

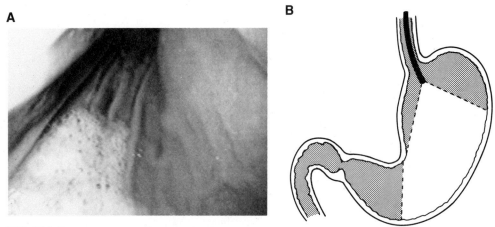

FIG. 124-5.
A, Gastric lake at 8 o'clock and rugae. **B,** Unshaded area is seen by lighted scope.

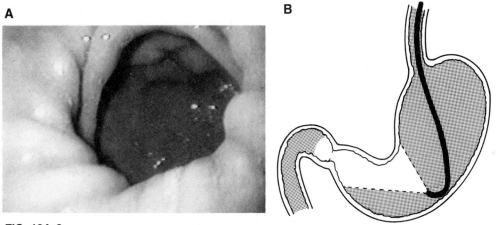

FIG. 124-6.
A, Angularis at 12 o'clock. Closed pylorus. Prepylorus at 6 o'clock. **B,** Unshaded area is seen by lighted scope.

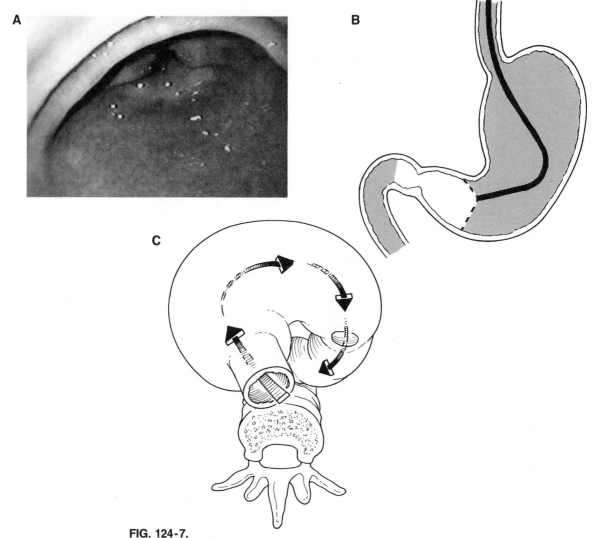

FIG. 124-7.
A, Antrum at 6 o'clock. Pyloric opening and angularis at 12 o'clock. **B,** Unshaded area is seen by lighted scope. **C,** To reach the pylorus, make a clockwise spiral around the vertebral column.

usually not necessary to remove samples for biopsy in the duodenum. The ampulla of Vater may be seen.

11. Withdraw the endoscope past the pyloric sphincter into the antrum. Turn the large wheel 180 degrees so that the scope is looking at itself. Slowly withdraw the endoscope so that the esophagogastric junction can be seen clearly, and fully examine the adjacent cardia (Figs. 124-9 and 124-10).

More air may need to be insufflated to flatten the rugae lest a small ulcer be missed. While the scope is retroverted, examine for a fixed or sliding hiatal hernia.

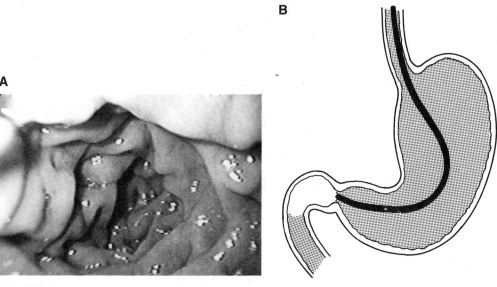

FIG. 124-8.
A, Duodenum. **B,** Unshaded area is seen by lighted scope.

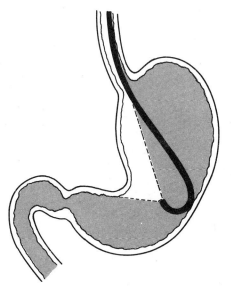

FIG. 124-9.
180-degree angulation retroflexes the tip to see the lesser curve.

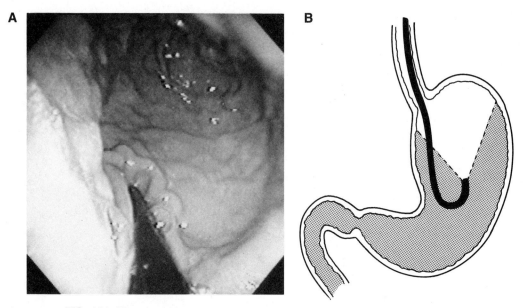

FIG. 124-10.
A, Turn around maneuver (retroflexing) showing the endoscope emerging from a snug esophago-gastric junction at 6 o'clock and the cardia at 12 o'clock. **B,** Unshaded area is seen by lighted scope.

12. Straighten the endoscope by rotating the wheel back to the original position. Slowly withdraw the endoscope through the esophagogastric junction and back through the esophagus.
13. Examine the vocal cords as the instrument is withdrawn.
14. The anesthesiologist or assistant should complete the monitoring process. The physician should reexamine the patient prior to discharge from the facility. A 30-minute observation period is generally sufficient, especially if minimal sedation is used (see Box 124-5).

BIOPSY

Biopsy samples should be taken when visible changes are seen; routine blind biopsy samples should not be taken. A good rule of thumb is to biopsy any gastric or esophageal abnormality unless it appears vascular (pulsating or bluish in color). Biopsy of duodenal ulcers are rarely necessary because the risk of cancer is very small. To remove tissue for biopsy, advance the biopsy forceps out the end of the scope, and biopsy the site under direct observation. For gastric ulcers, remove the tissue from the base and from all four quadrants at the edges. Because the forceps are small, there is generally minimal to no bleeding; however, if bleeding does occur, it must be controlled and noted on the operative report before withdrawing the scope. The acidic medium coagulates bleeding sites. The esophagus has more likelihood of bleeding with biopsy.

BOX 124-5. INTRAVENOUS SEDATIVE ADMINISTRATION AND RECOVERY NURSING DOCUMENTATION PARAMETERS

Note level of consciousness on arrival: response, anxiety level
Note patency of airway: spontaneous respiratory effort
Note status of intravenous access site: redness or edema
Note breathing effort and fall of chest wall
Note vital signs every 5 minutes
Place on cardiac monitor, if indicated
Place on pulse oximeter, and administer oxygen if indicated
Raise head of bed 30 to 45 degrees
Note body temperature
Note skin turgor
Note quality of speech: clearness, ease
Note presence or absence of nausea, gagging, spasmodic coughing, ability to swallow
Note presence or absence of abdominal distention or tenderness
Quality of bowel sounds
Expulsion of flatus
Abdominal cramping

Nursing Assessment
On admission, perform an assessment of the patient's medical conditions that are not included on assessment list above.
Note any untoward symptoms as they occur.
Note the patient's general condition in 15 minutes.
Note discharge status.
Record vital signs every 5 minutes, and post monitor strips with a simple explanation every 15 minutes or when there is an unusual occurrence. Report any abnormal responses immediately.

Gastric biopsies are necessary to perform the CLO test for *Helicobacter pylori*. *H. pylori*–associated gastritis often cannot be diagnosed by endoscopic appearance alone. Even normal-appearing mucosa may exhibit marked histologic gastritis. Warm the CLO test slide by placing it in a pocket before the endoscopy. Antibiotics and bismuth preparations should be discontinued at least 3 weeks prior to the procedure.

Remove tissue from a normal-looking area in the lowest part of the antrum, place it in the CLO test gel, and reseal the slide. A normal-appearing area of mucosa is chosen because *H. pylori* may be scarce in areas where the epithelium is eroded or the mucous layer is denuded. You may read and interpret the test results yourself (it is a simple color change reaction) or the tissue may be sent to the pathologist.

Biopsy samples should be taken from patients with diffuse intestinal metaplasia; however, CLO tests will often be negative from these areas. Because of the often patchy distribution of *H. pylori,* many physicians suggest two gastric biopsies before its presence is ruled out.

Biopsy samples of the esophagus should be taken when the scope is removed, rather than when it is inserted.

COMPLICATIONS

- Perforation
- Hemorrhage, secondary to trauma or biopsy
- Aspiration
- Oversedation and its complications, including cardiopulmonary arrest

The complication rate of endoscopy performed by primary care physicians from eight clinical sites was 0.0014 (1 in 717) (Rodney). All cases were collected sequentially from the beginning of each physician's experience. Six of the physicians were in private practice. Most received their training in short courses. The average hands-on training obtained before independent diagnostic esophagogastroduodenoscopy was eight supervised cases. This complication rate compares favorably with subspecialty complication rates of 0.0013 (1.3 in 1000).

SUPPLIERS

Olympus Medical Instrument Division
8370 Dow Circle
Strongsville, OH 44136
800-627-6264

Pentax
30 Ramland Road
Orangeburg, NY 10962-2699
800-431-5880

Welch Allyn
4341 State Street Rd. Box 220
Skaneateles Falls, NY 13153-0220
800-535-6663

Fuginon
10 High Point Drive
Wayne, NJ 07470
201-633-5600

Tri-Med Specialties, Inc.
P.O. Box 23306
Overland Park, KS 66223
800-874-6331

CPT/BILLING CODES

43200	Esophagoscopy
43234	Simple upper endoscopy
43235	Esophagogastroduodenoscopy
43239	Esophagogastroduodenoscopy with biopsy
94761	Oximetry
99070	Surgical tray—generally reimbursed by Medicare if performed in office

BIBLIOGRAPHY

American College of Physicians, Health and Public Policy Committee: Position paper: endoscopy in the evaluation of dyspepsia, *Ann Int Med* 102:266, 1985.

American College of Physicians, Health and Public Policy Committee: Clinical competence in diagnostic endoscopy, *Ann Int Med* 107:937, 1987.

American Society for Gastrointestinal Endoscopy: *Appropriate use of gastrointestinal endoscopy*, Manchester, Mass, 1992, the Society.

Blackstone MD: *Endoscopic interpretation: normal and pathologic appearances of the gastrointestinal tract*, New York, 1984, Raven Press.

Bremang JA: Neurolept analgesia in ambulatory (nasal) endoscopies, *J Otolaryn* 20(6): 435, 1993.

Brook RH et al: Predicting the appropriate use of carotid endarterectomy, upper gastrointestinal endoscopy, and coronary angiography, *N Engl J Med* 323:1173, 1990.

Coleman WH: Gastroscopy: a primary diagnostic procedure, *Primary Care* 15(1):1, 1988.

Council on Scientific Affairs, AMA: The use of pulse oximetry during conscious sedation, *JAMA* 270(12):1463, 1993.

Crump WJ, Phelps TK: Teaching lower gastrointestinal endoscopy: a comparison of family medicine and internal medicine residencies, *J Am Board Fam Pract* 4:1, 1991.

Dajani AS et al: Prevention of bacterial endocarditis: recommendations by the American Heart Association, *JAMA* 264(22):2919, 1990.

Hacker JF et al: Patient preference in upper gastrointestinal studies: roentgenography versus endoscopy, *So J Med* 80(4):1091, 1987.

Lewis BS, Wayne JD: Upper gastrointestinal endoscopy: state of the art, *Hosp Med:*79, November 1991.

Lieberman DA, Ghormley JM: Physician assistants in gastroenterology: should they perform endoscopy? *Am J Gastroenterol* 7:940, 1992.

Mai HD, Sanowski RA, Waring JP: Improved patient care using ASGE guidelines on quality assurance, *Gastrointest Endosc* 37:597, 1991.

Morrissey JF, Reichelderfer M: Gastrointestinal endoscopy, Part I, *N Engl J Med* 325(16):1142, 1990.

Overholt BF, Chobanian SJ, editors: *Office endoscopy*, Baltimore, 1990, Williams & Wilkins.

Rodney WM et al: Esophagogastroduodenoscopy by family physicians: a national multisite study of 717 procedures, *J Am Board Fam Pract* 3:73, 1990.

Rodney WM et al: Esophagogastroduodenoscopy by family physicians—phase II: a national multisite study of 2500 procedures, *Fam Pract Res J* 13(2):121, 1993.

Sanders LD et al: Comparison of diazepam with midazolam as IV sedation for outpatient gastroscopy, *Br J Anaesth* 63:726, 1989.

Tremain SC et al: Cleaning, disinfection, and sterilization of gastrointestinal endoscopes: approaches in the office, *JFP* 32(3):300, 1991.

Wayne JD et al: *Techniques in therapeutic endoscopy*, Philadelphia, 1987, W.B. Saunders.

Zuber TJ, Pfenninger JL: Interspeciality wars over endoscopy, *JFP* 37(1):21, 1993.

CHAPTER 125

Colonoscopy

James A. Surrell

Colonoscopy is a procedure that enables the visual inspection of the entire large bowel from the distal rectum to the cecum. Colonoscopy is an accepted, safe, and effective means by which the large bowel can be evaluated. A well-trained endoscopist can generally perform a total colonoscopy in 30 to 45 minutes in greater than 90% of attempted procedures. The great advantage of colonoscopy over radiologic evaluation of the large intestine is the ability to perform additional diagnostic and therapeutic measures, such as biopsy, polypectomy, and stool specimen collection. Colonoscopy should not be regarded as a replacement for a well-done air-contrast barium enema study; rather, the two studies should be regarded as complementary. Although traditionally performed in the hospital, colonoscopy can also be performed in free-standing offices or in ambulatory endoscopy centers.

Since the vast majority of colon cancers arise from polyps, the removal of all polyps should greatly reduce the incidence of colon cancer. With colonoscopy, polyps throughout the entire colon can be removed.

INDICATIONS

- Evaluation of abnormal or equivocal barium enema X-ray
- Undiagnosed gross or occult rectal bleeding, where preliminary examinations are negative, or where a strong suspicion of cancer exists
- Biopsy of suspected lesion
- Polypectomy
- Evaluation of inflammatory bowel disease or chronic diarrhea
- Follow-up of previously diagnosed colorectal cancer or polyps
- Full examination of the colon when neoplastic polyps (tubular adenomas, tubulovillous adenomas, or villous adenomas) are found on anoscopy or flexible sigmoidoscopy
- Surveillance of patients at high risk for colorectal cancer (e.g., family history of colon cancer)

- Reduction of sigmoid volvulus
- Prior to surgery for colon cancer to rule out synchronus polyps or cancer in other areas
- Removal of a foreign body
- Therapy of bleeding lesions

CONTRAINDICATIONS

- Suspected peritonitis
- Significant pelvic or abdominal adhesions
- Acute diverticulitis with systemic symptoms
- Acute exacerbation of inflammatory bowel disease
- Suspected bowel perforation
- Unstable cardiopulmonary status
- Recent myocardial infarction or pulmonary embolism
- Blood coagulation abnormalities, including those associated with aspirin use (Aspirin should not be taken within 1 week of colonoscopy.)
- Recent (within 1 week) bowel surgery
- Uncooperative patient

Colonoscopy is often of little benefit in determining the causes of chronic lower abdominal pain, changes in bowel movements *without* rectal bleeding, weight loss, and anorexia.

PATIENT PREPARATION

A clean bowel is essential for colonoscopy, and the most common and most effective preparations for cleansing the bowel include the following:

- Four liters of polyethylene glycol (PEG) solution taken orally (Colyte or Golytely) over a 1- to 3-hour period, *or*
- Ten ounces of magnesium citrate solution taken with four bisacodyl 5 mg tablets, *or*
- Two ounces of castor oil taken with four bisacodyl 5 mg tablets.

One of these bowel preparations should be administered starting at 4:00 P.M. the day before colonoscopy. After the preparation, the patient should only have clear liquids until midnight. It may also be helpful to administer one or two tap-water enemas 1 or 2 hours before the procedure.

It is important to individualize the preparation for each patient and to take time to explain the reasons for the bowel-cleansing preparation. Patients undergoing drug therapy with certain medications may require special adjustments. Optimal examination may be better accomplished if the patient has received an electrolytic purgative solution; however, many physicians claim "less is best." Give the patient information about colonoscopy to review before undergoing the procedure (Box 125-1).

BOX 125-1. PATIENT EDUCATION HANDOUT
COLONOSCOPY

What is colonoscopy?

Colonoscopy is a special test that allows your physician to examine the lining of the colon (large bowel) for abnormal growths such as polyps or cancer.

Who should have a colonoscopy?

Your physician may recommend you have a colonoscopy if you experience:

- A change in bowel habits
- Rectal bleeding
- Unexpected abdominal pain
- Inflammatory bowel disease (colitis)

Also, if polyps or tumors are located with a barium enema X-ray or you have a past or family history of colorectal polyps or cancer, you should have a colonoscopy.

What preparation is required?

The colon must be completely clean for the procedure to be accurate and complete. Your physician will give you detailed instructions regarding the dietary restrictions to be followed and the cleansing routine to be used. Most medications may be continued as usual, but some medications can interfere with the preparation or the examination. Therefore, it is best to inform your physician of your current medications, as well as any allergies to medications, several days prior to the examination.

How is the procedure performed?

Your doctor may give you medication to help you relax during the procedure. During the colonoscopy, your doctor will look through the colonoscope to see the lining of the bowel. If an abnormal area is found, it is possible to obtain a small biopsy or representative specimen of that area. Also, polyps or growths may be removed during colonoscopy.

What are polyps and why are they removed?

Polyps are abnormal growths from the lining of the colon, which vary in size from a tiny dot to several inches. The majority of polyps are benign (noncancerous), but the doctor cannot always tell a benign from a malignant (cancerous) polyp by its outer appearance alone. For this reason, polyps are removed by passing special instruments through the colonoscope and then sent for tissue analysis. Removal of colon polyps is an important means of preventing colorectal cancer.

What happens after colonoscopy?

The examination usually takes less than one hour. After colonoscopy, your physician will explain the results to you. If you have been given medications during the procedure, you will be observed until most of the effects of sedation have worn off (for 30 minutes to 2 hours). You will need someone to drive you home after the procedure.

What are possible complications of colonoscopy?

Although complications after colonoscopy are uncommon, it is important for you to recognize early signs of any possible complications. Contact the physician who performed the colonoscopy if you notice any of the following symptoms: severe abdominal pain, fever and chills, or rectal bleeding of more than one-half cup. Bleeding can occur several days after the removal of a polyp.

Other potential risks may include a perforation or tear through the bowel wall, a reaction to the sedatives used, and complications from heart or lung disease.

Your physician can discuss colonoscopy with you in greater detail.

Used with permission of the Ferguson-Blodgett Digestive Disease Institute, Grand Rapids, Michigan.

ANTIBIOTIC PROPHYLAXIS

The Standards Task Force of the American Society of Colon and Rectal Surgeons has developed practice parameters. It was the consensus of the task force that antibiotic prophylaxis be considered only for the high-risk groups, as listed in Table 125-1. There are several antibiotic prophylaxis regimens for endoscopic procedures (Table 125-2).

TABLE 125-1.

Risk of Infection from Colonoscopy

Condition	Risk
*Cardiac Conditions**	
History of endocarditis	High
Surgically constructed systemic pulmonary shunts or conduits	High
Prostheses	
Prosthetic cardiac valves, including bioprosthetic and homograft valves	High
Vascular graft material	
First year	High
After first year	Low
Orthopedic prosthesis	Low
Central nervous system ventricular shunts	Low
Penile prosthesis	Low
Intraocular lens	Low
Pacemaker	Low
Local tissue augmentation material	Low

*The AHA does not generally recommend preendoscopy prophylaxis for most congenital cardiac malformations, rheumatic and other acquired valvular dysfunction even after valvular surgery, hypertrophic cardiomyopathy, and mitral valve prolapse with valvular regurgitation.

TABLE 125-2.

Antibiotic Prophylaxis Regimens

	Dose	
Drug	Preprocedure	Postprocedure
Ampicillin	2 gms IV or IM	
Gentamicin	1.5 mg/kg (up to 60 mg) IV (over 1 hour) or IM	
Amoxicillin		1.5 gm PO 8 hours later
Vancomycin*	1 gm IV over 1 hour	Repeat initial
Gentamicin	1.5 mg/kg (up to 80 mg)	doses 8 hours later
Amoxicillin†	3 gm PO	1.5 gm PO 6 hours later

*For penicillin allergy
†For low-risk groups

The decision about antibiotic prophylaxis must be made by the individual physician, and must take into account the circumstances presented by the individual patient. If there is any doubt about prophylaxis, seek appropriate cardiology consultation. Further information can also be found in Chapter 133, Antibiotic Prophylaxis for Bacterial Endocarditis.

SEDATION

Optimal examination may be better accomplished if the patient is under sedation. Appropriate equipment must be available to monitor blood pressure, pulse, and respirations. A pulse oximeter is now commonly utilized to monitor oxygen saturation as well. During colonoscopy, it is mandatory to have an assistant available to monitor the patient. Intravenous access should be established and maintained during the entire procedure in patients receiving intravenous sedation. It has been noted by some physicians who use a colonoscope to carry out routine flexible sigmoidoscopy screens that they are able to reach the cecum in 25% to 30% of unsedated patients.

Benzodiazepines are the drugs most commonly used for sedation: midazolam (Versed) 2 to 5 mg or diazepam (Valium) 5 to 10 mg are the benzodiazepines most commonly used. Meperidine 25 to 50 mg may be added, if necessary. Administer these medications slowly through the intravenous route. Dangerous side effects can be reversed with flumazenil (Romazicon) or naloxone (Narcan), and the endoscopist should be thoroughly familiar with the pharmacology of all these drugs. Further discussion can be found in Chapter 124, Diagnostic Esophagogastroduodenoscopy (EGD).

A crash cart should be immediately available in case of cardiopulmonary arrest. See Chapter 135, Anaphylaxis, and the discussion regarding Banyan kits.

TECHNIQUE

Colonoscopy (See Chapter 118, Flexible Sigmoidoscopy)

1. Place the patient on the examining table in the left lateral decubitus position.
2. Following an adequate level of sedation, perform a digital anorectal examination with a well-lubricated, gloved examining finger. Lubricate the shaft of the colonoscope and insert its tip into the anal canal. The lumen of the bowel should be directly visualized at all times during the colonoscopy procedure.
3. With air insufflation into the rectum, the lumen will become readily apparent. The three valves of Houston are often seen as consistent landmarks. The scope can generally be advanced without difficulty as far as the rectosigmoid junction at 15 to 18 cm. Enter the sigmoid colon by passing the scope through the rectosigmoid angle. The sigmoid colon is the most common site of difficulty in passage of the instrument. There may be fixation of the bowel from diverticular disease or adhesions from prior surgery. The sigmoid colon is the

most common site of perforation during colonoscopy. The descending colon can be recognized by a relatively straight passage through the circular-shaped bowel to the splenic flexure. Transversing the angle of the splenic flexure may resemble transversing the rectosigmoid junction. The transverse colon can be recognized by its characteristic triangular appearance, and it generally has a fairly straight configuration. The hepatic flexure is often recognizable by the "liver shadow," which appears as a blue-brown area where the liver is in direct contact with the bowel wall. The hepatic flexure is seen as another angle to traverse with the scope. The ascending colon also appears triangular.

4. Advance the scope into the cecum by pulling back, keeping the tip of the scope in the center of the lumen, and applying full suction. The cecal landmarks, which may or may not be prominent, include the ileocecal valve and the appendiceal orifice. Other methods to ascertain if the cecum has been reached is to check for ballottement above the right inguinal canal or for transillumination.

Polypectomy

Polyps may be sessile or pedunculated. Pedunculated polyps are much more easily removed with the electrocautery snare, and the risk of perforation and bleeding is less than with a sessile polyp. No pain is experienced by the patient.

1. Position the scope so that the polyp can be visualized approximately 2 to 3 cm beyond the tip of the colonoscope.
2. Under direct vision at all times, pass the electrocautery snare through the colonoscope port. Position the tip of the sheath of the snare, advance the wire loop, and open it, *always under direct vision.* Manipulate the snare and maneuver the tip of the colonoscope to place the snare around the polyp. Slowly secure the wire loop around the pedicle or polyp base. Maneuver the colonoscope away from the bowel wall to avoid excess burn injury and possible perforation.
3. Apply the electrocautery current. (The absolute necessity of an adequate prep must be emphasized since residual gas in the colon could cause an explosion with the use of electrocautery.)
4. Retrieve the excised polyp using suction or forceps. Unretrieved polyps may occasionally need to be retrieved later by straining stools after further bowel preparation solutions and cathartics. Large polyps may require multiple snare-resection excisions. Tissue desiccation without prior biopsy should be avoided since it is very important to have pathologic diagnosis of all colonic lesions.
5. Cancerous polyps do not need further resections if the tumor is well differentiated, if there is no lymphatic or vascular invasion, and if there is at least 2 mm between the tumor and the line of resection. With an obvious advanced colon cancer that is friable or ulcerated, biopsies will usually provide sufficient tissue for diagnosis. However, since only tiny samples can be obtained, the cancer may occasionally be missed, and the specimen only reveal benign adenomatous tissue. Strong clinical suspicion of cancer would indicate rebiopsy.

COMPLICATIONS

- Bowel perforation (approximately 1 per 1000 procedures) from mechanical or pneumatic pressure, or from biopsy techniques (Perforations are more common with patients who are oversedated or who are under general anesthesia. It is uncommon for the scope to penetrate the bowel, but it is usually noticed immediately. More frequently the perforation is caused by other factors and goes unrecognized, and the patient later experiences abdominal pain and distention. Radiologically, a flat plate of the abdomen will show pneumoperitoneum. Immediate surgery is indicated. With fecal soiling, a diverting colostomy is needed; however, in the absence of obvious contamination, primary closure is sufficient.)
- Postcolonoscopy/postpolypectomy bleeding (approximately 1 per 1000 procedures) immediately or up to 10 days postprocedure (Most cases of bleeding resolve spontaneously, but some may require repeat colonoscopy with attempts to coagulate the area, or laparotomy.)
- Cardiorespiratory depression or arrest
- Other uncommon complications: thrombophlebitis, vasovagal reaction, postcolonoscopy abdominal distention, sigmoid or cecal volvulus, bacteremia
- Postpolypectomy syndrome (Thermal injury [burn] can cause full-thickness bowel necrosis, which may lead to peritoneal irritation; postpolypectomy syndrome may be accompanied by fever, leukocytosis, and localized and rebound tenderness over the polypectomy site. A conservative approach generally leads to a good outcome.)

LEARNING COLONOSCOPY

For specific endoscopic techniques for the evaluation of the rectum, sigmoid colon, descending colon, transverse colon, ascending colon, and cecum, see Coller, "Technique of Flexible Fiberoptic Sigmoidoscopy," and Chapter 9 of Shinya's textbook on colonoscopy, which contains excellent diagrams, photographs, tips, and techniques. The endoscopic anatomy of the various landmark locations of the colon and rectum are well described and illustrated in Chapter 8 of Shinya's text.

For an in-depth review of colonoscopic polypectomy, see Chapter 15 in Shinya's textbook, Chapter 44 in Bower's textbook, Chapter 3 in Gordon's textbook, and Chapter 1 of Corman's textbook.

Before attempting to perform colonoscopy, one should become proficient and skilled in flexible fiberoptic sigmoidoscopy. The instrument controls and techniques utilized for flexible sigmoidoscopy are identical to those utilized to perform colonoscopy. Formal courses are available to teach colonoscopy concepts, skills, and techniques.

One method often used for obtaining colonoscopy skills in the posttraining environment is to form a teaching relationship with a proficient colonoscopist as a preceptor until adequate proficiency is obtained. Performance of colonoscopy can be mastered without fellowship training. Studies show that high-quality care and complication rates essentially identical to fellowship-trained gastroenterologists can be attained (Rodney) and that physician assistants may also become qualified to perform colonoscopy (Lieberman).

SUPPLIERS

Extensive marketing and technical information about colonoscopy equipment is readily available. When selecting a supplier, consider local availability for education, equipment service, and technical support. It may be desirable to ask for local references from suppliers.

Olympus Corporation
Medical Instrument Division
8370 Dow Circle
Strongsville, OH 44136
800-627-6264

Pentax Corporation
30 Ramland Road
Orangeburg, NY 10962-2699
800-431-5880

Welch Allyn
4341 State Street Rd.
Box 220
Skaneateles Falls, NY 13153-0220
800-535-6663

Most colonoscopies are now carried out with video endoscopes. The colonoscope is similar to that described for flexible sigmoidoscopy, only longer. The outside diameter of the tube varies from 10 to 13 mm, and the length of the shaft from 105 to 185 cm. A light source, suction apparatus, and incidental instruments are needed (see Chapter 118, Flexible Sigmoidoscopy).

Cleaning and disinfecting the instrument and equipment is very important to prevent iatrogenic infections. Tremain presents an excellent overview. Company representatives will also provide excellent guidelines.

CPT/BILLING CODES

45378	Colonoscopy beyond splenic flexure
45379	Colonoscopy with foreign body removal
45380	Colonoscopy with biopsy
45382	Colonoscopy to control bleeding
45383	Colonoscopy with fulguration of tumor
45385	Colonoscopy with polypectomy

BIBLIOGRAPHY

Bauer JJ: *Colorectal surgery illustrated: a focused approach,* St Louis, 1993, Mosby.

Coller JA: Technique of flexible fiberoptic sigmoidoscopy, *Surg Clin North Am* 60:456, 1980.

Colonoscopy by FPs can reduce cancer risk, *Medical Tribune,* November 12, 1992.

Corman ML: *Colon and rectal surgery,* ed 2, Philadelphia, 1989, J.B. Lippincott.

Gordon PH, Nivatvongs S: *Principles and practice of surgery for the colon, rectum, and anus,* St Louis, 1992, Quality Medical Publishing.

Levine R, Tenner S, Fromm H: Prevention and early detection of colorectal cancer, *Am Fam Physician* 45(2):663, 1992.

Lieberman DA, Ghormley JM: Physician assistants in gastroenterology: should they perform endoscopy?, *Am J Gastroenterol* 87:940, 1992.

Lieberman DA, Smith FW: Screening for colon malignancy with colonoscopy, *Am J Gastroenterol* 86(8):946, 1991.

Potter JD: Reconciling the epidemiology, physiology and molecular biology of colon cancer, *JAMA* 268:12, 1992.

Reed DN, Collins JD, Wyatt WJ: Can general surgeons perform colonoscopy safely?, *Am J Surg* 163:257, 1992.

Rex DK et al: Screening colonoscopy in asymptomatic average-risk persons with negative fecal occult blood tests, *Gastroenterol* 100:64, 1991.

Rodney WM, Dabov G, Cronin C: Full-length colonoscopy enhances diagnostic capabilities (abstract), *Am Fam Physician* 44(5 suppl):91, 1991.

Rodney WM, Dabov G, Cronin C: Evolving colonoscopy skills in a rural family practice: the first 293 cases, *Fam Pract Res* 13(1):43, 1993.

Rodney WM et al: Sedation associated with a more complete colonoscopy, *JFP* 36:394, 1993.

Selby JV et al: A case-control study of screening sigmoidoscopy and mortality from colorectal cancer, *N Engl J Med* 326:653, 1992.

Shinya H: *Colonoscopy: diagnosis and treatment of colonic diseases,* New York, 1982, IGAKU-SHOIN.

Standards Task Force of the American Society of Colon and Rectal Surgeons: Practice parameters for antibiotic prophylaxis—supporting documentation, *Diseases of the Colon and Rectum* 35:278, 1992.

Tremain SC, Orientale E, Rodney WM: Cleaning, disinfection and sterilization of gastrointestinal endoscopes: approaches in the office, *JFP* 32:300, 1992.

Varma JR, Nulls LR: Colon polyps, *JFP* 35:194, 1992.

Waye JD: Colonoscopy, *CA-A Cancer Journal for Clinicians* 42:350, 1992.

Weber DJ, Rodney WM, Warren J: Management of suspected perforation following colonoscopy: a case report, *JFP* 36:567, 1993.

Zuber TJ, Pfenninger JL: Interspecialty wars over endoscopy, *JFP* 37(1):21, 1993.

PART TEN

Orthopedics

CHAPTER 126

Ankle Splinting, Taping, and Casting

Jeffrey R. Kovan

Douglas B. McKeag

Treatment of acute and chronic ankle injuries involves an accurate clinical evaluation and often radiographic assessment of potential fractures, avulsions, or instability. Casting and cast-splinting devices are most commonly used in acute situations, whereas splinting and taping best control chronic instabilities and act as adjuncts in rehabilitation.

Despite these mechanisms of bracing, early intervention with rest, ice, compression, and elevation are generally required before acute immobilization is utilized.

INDICATIONS

Casting

- Stable ankle fractures
- Lateral malleolar ankle fractures
- Severe lateral ankle sprains
- Fractures to the calcaneus, talus, navicular, cuboid, cuneiforms, and metatarsals

Splinting (Plaster/Synthetic)

- Unstable ankle fractures requiring surgery
- Severe ankle sprain requiring surgery
- Moderate ankle sprain with inability to bear weight

Splinting (Orthotic Devices)

- Stable lateral ankle sprain
- Stable distal interosseous ligament sprain

- Prophylactic ankle support
- Rehabilitation with increasing activity levels
- Adjunct to athletic participation and chronic stabilization

Taping

- Adjunct to athletic participation with need for additional stabilization
- Prophylactic ankle support

CONTRAINDICATIONS

- Casting of acute injuries prior to cessation of swelling
- Casting, splinting, or taping over open wounds without adequate visualization and inspection

EQUIPMENT

Casting (Fig. 126-1)

- Stockinettes
- Cotton padding
- Synthetic or plaster casting material (3 or 4 inch)
- Rubber gloves
- Bucket with tepid water
- Cast cutter
- Cast separator

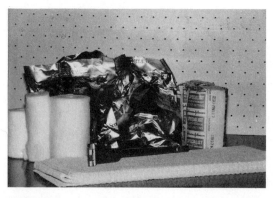

FIG. 126-1.
Materials need for casting: cotton padding, synthetic casting material or plaster rolls, case separator, cast cutter (not shown), and plaster strips.

Splinting

- Posterior cast/splint or stirrup-type splint
- Stockinette
- Cotton padding
- Fiberglass one-step or plaster casting material (8 to 12 strips of 4 to 6 inches in width)
- Rubber gloves
- Bucket with warm water
- Air/gel cast (short or long)
- Swedo/AOA brace
- Ankle ligament protector (ALP)

Taping

- Underwrap
- Pressure pads
- Prepped skin
- 1½- or 2-inch tape

TECHNIQUE

Casting (See Chapter 127, Cast Immobilization)

Immobilization of the ankle joint and metatarsals is achieved by short-leg casting. Despite the lack of joint stability above and often below the involved injury, range of motion is restricted by use of this modality. The cast should extend from the metatarsal-phalangeal joint to just below the knee joint at the level of the proximal fibular head.

1. Seat the patient or place in the prone position with the knee at 90 degrees of flexion. Ninety degrees of flexion at the ankle joint is required to aid in patient ambulation, quicker recovery following cast removal, and ultimately more rapid healing.
2. Place a stockinette over the lower extremity and drape the excess over the toes, extending above the fibular head (Fig. 126-2).
3. Apply cotton padding in an even distribution, overlapping 50% each time to protect the skin from cast irritation. Extra-layered padding can be applied to bony prominences (i.e., malleoli) (Fig. 126-3).

   Caution: Do not fold or "bunch up" the cotton padding; this is both dangerous and uncomfortable.

4. Soak either synthetic or plaster casting material for 5 to 10 seconds in warm water. After excess water is removed, evenly roll the casting material along the distal tibia/fibula and more distally to the metatarsal heads, and apply extra material to the plantar aspect of the foot for added support. Apply a second

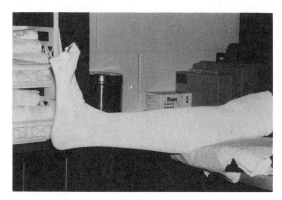

FIG. 126-2.
The first step in the application of a cast is the placement of the stockinette.

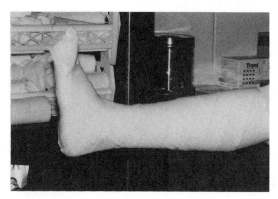

FIG. 126-3.
Application of cotton padding.

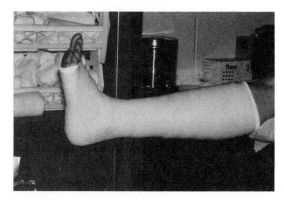

FIG. 126-4.
Placement of synthetic or plaster casting material.

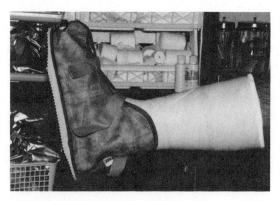

FIG. 126-5.
Use of a walking boot to preserve the cast.

and third roll beginning at the distal lower leg/ankle and extending proximally in an even fashion. If a walking cast is preferred, reinforce the bottom (plantar) portion of the cast. Special care in obtaining 90-degree flexion at the ankle should be obtained prior to hardening of the casting material. While it is still wet, mold the cast to the patient's leg. Using your chest or abdomen to support the foot should allow you to maintain this angle while extending the cast proximally (Fig. 126-4).

5. Once the cast is completed, address your attention to areas of cast irritation on the patient's skin and apply additional padding as needed.
6. Allow 10 minutes for the cast to set and advise the patient to refrain from any weight-bearing for a minimum of 24 hours. Crutches are generally required for the first few days until ease of ambulation increases.
7. A walking boot may be fitted to ease ambulation and improve proximal muscle group strength (Fig. 126-5).
8. Duration of casting varies with injury and patient compliance, but should be minimized. Removal requires use of a cast cutter and separators, cutting along both sides of the cast (Figs. 126-6 and 126-7).

Splinting (Plaster, Synthetic)

Posterior casts/splints provide adequate non–weight-bearing support while allowing the patient to remove the splint for applying ice and taking showers. Generally required for injuries with the potential for much swelling initially, posterior splints provide an initial means of support until a more complete evaluation can be performed.

1. Apply stockinettes and cotton padding as described above, unless one-step material is used (see Figs. 126-2 and 126-3).
2. Use either synthetic one-step (soak in water and secure with Ace wrap once casting material hardens) or plaster casting material. Plaster splints require 8 to 12 strips of 4- to 6-inch plaster sheets. Often two sets are overlapped to maintain greater support and cover a larger surface area. After soaking the casting

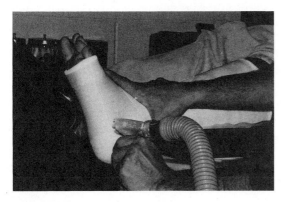

FIG. 126-6.
Using a cast cutter to remove a cast.

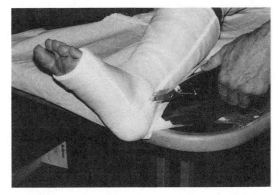

FIG. 126-7.
Cast pliers separate the upper and lower portions of the cast.

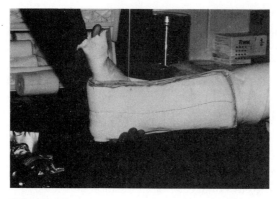

FIG. 126-8.
An ankle splint. The cast material is in the shape of a "U" with the anterior portion being the most open. The splint allows for swelling avoiding neurovascular compromise while still providing support.

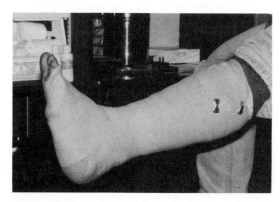

FIG. 126-9.
Securing the splint in place with an Ace wrap.

material in water for 5 to 10 seconds, strip all excess water, then overlap the casting material and apply along the posterior and lateral aspects of the lower leg and ankle and extend to the planter aspect of the foot. The splint assumes a "U" shape. Once the material is hardened, apply an Ace bandage to secure the splint (Figs. 126-8 and 126-9).
3. No weight-bearing should be done with synthetic or plaster splints, and re-evaluation is recommended in 5 to 7 days.

Splinting (Orthotic Devices)

Air/gel casts, Swedo/AOA braces, and the ankle ligament protector (ALP) all require fairly simple application, and they have the ability to control ankle ligament instability.

1. Application generally involves positioning of the brace over the lateral and medial malleoli (air/gel casts), with the calcaneus placed on a well-fitted

cushion at the base. Stabilization is maintained with use of velcro straps and can be adjusted to the patient's comfort. A sock should be worn under the brace, and generally shoes can be applied over the brace to ease patient ambulation (Fig. 126-10).

2. Swedo/AOA braces also require a sock or undergarment to protect the skin and generally are slipped onto the foot much like a sock. Lacing should provide a snug but not constricting fit, and plastic inserts can be applied to the medial and/or lateral surfaces to provide additional support (Fig. 126-11).

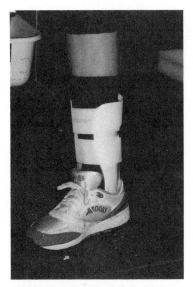

FIG. 126-10.
Splinting using an air cast brace.

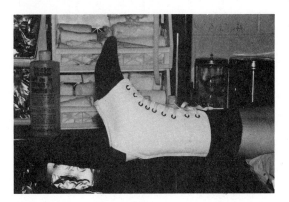

FIG. 126-11.
The Swedo/AOA ankle brace.

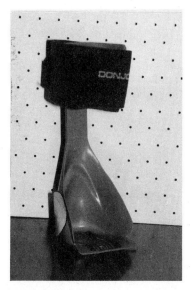

FIG. 126-12.
The ankle ligament protector (ALP) for splinting the ankle.

3. The ALP stabilizes the hind foot as the calcaneus fits into a neatly designed cup (Fig. 126-12). A Velcro strap stabilizes the distal tibia/fibula. Adjustments can be made to improve comfort. Again, this can and should be worn inside a shoe.

Taping

Taping has the disadvantage of requiring considerable skill for application. Taping adds another degree of ankle support, most effective as a prophylactic measure.

1. With the ankle in a 90-degree flexion position, place pressure pads over prepped skin (shaved and sprayed with benzoin-based spray) then cover with a thin elastic underwrap (Fig. 126-13).
2. One-and-a-half to two-inch tape is recommended. Numerous methods are available for taping, with each emphasizing stirrup and anchor strips to secure the ankle joint. Correctly applied tape will limit abnormal motion, but should not restrict normal range of motion. Because the exact sequence of taping varies from examiner to examiner, emphasis on limiting inversion as opposed to plantar/dorsiflexion and eversion is important (Fig. 126-14).

COMPLICATIONS

Casting

- Skin pressure sores over bony prominences (Fig. 126-15)
- Superficial nerve compression (common peroneal nerve at the neck of the fibular head–foot drop) (Fig. 126-16)

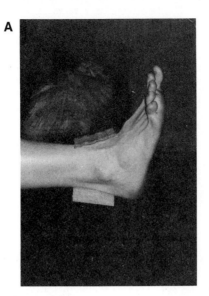

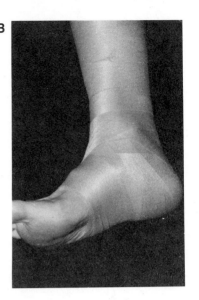

FIG. 126-13.
A, The application of pressure pads before taping. **B,** The second step in taping—the application of a thin elastic underwrap.

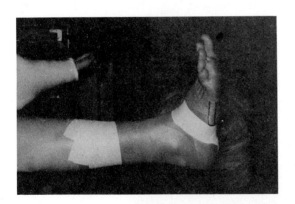

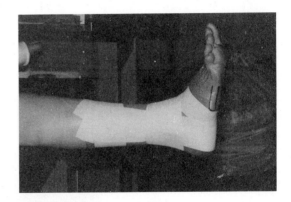

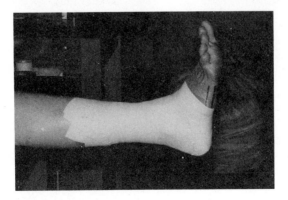

FIG. 126-14.
Adhesive tape (1½ to 2 inch) is used for support. Various techniques are used to stabilize the ankle joint, especially to prevent inversion injuries.

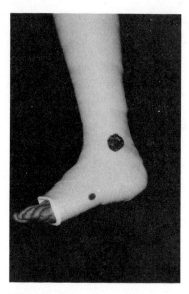

FIG. 126-15.
Common location for pressure sores (noted by ink on cast).

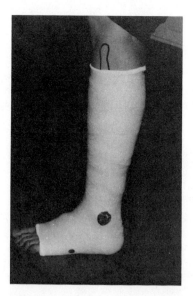

FIG. 126-16.
The outline on the skin denotes the fibular head and indicates where the peroneal nerve is located. Excess pressure in this area leads to paralysis with foot drop.

- Compression/constriction from cast outside or increased swelling of injured joint within (Watch for pain, pulselessness, pallor, and paresthesias and paralysis of toes.)

  Note: Correction of the above involves effective release of pressure (using a cast saw to open one side or bivalve the cast) or removal of cast!

- Maceration of skin secondary to introduction of water/sweat into cast

Splinting

- Excessive compression/constriction from splint (easily adjusted by lightly releasing the Velcro or Ace wrap while maintaining support)
- Prolonged restriction in range of motion (requires additional therapy to obtain previous range and strength)
- Breakage of cast with subsequent pinching of skin

Taping

- Compression/constriction from underwrap or tape (Remove and reapply or use alternative methods.)
- Skin rash due to contact dermatitis from spray, tape, or underwrap

CPT/BILLING CODES

29405	Application of short-leg cast (below knee to toes)
29425	Application of walking or ambulatory type cast
29515	Application of short-leg splint (calf to foot)
29540	Strapping, ankle
99070	Splinting

BIBLIOGRAPHY

Cox JS: Surgical and nonsurgical treatment of acute ankle sprains, *Clin Orthop Related Research* 198:118, September 1985.

Homes DS, Kautman JJ: Plaster splints: techniques and indications, *Am Fam Physician* 30(3):215, 1984.

Hume EL, McKeag DB: Soft-tissue ankle injuries: the need for compulsive assessment and therapy, *Emerg Med Reports* 5(7):45, 1984.

Kuhland DN: *The injured athlete,* ed 2, Philadelphia, 1988, J.B. Lippincott.

Nicholas JA, Hershman EB: *The lower extremity and spine in sports medicine, vol 1,* St Louis, 1986, Mosby.

Smith GF, Madlon-Kay DJ, Hunt V: Clinical evaluation of ankle inversion injuries in family practice offices, *JFP* 37(4):345, 1993.

Smith RW, Reischl SF: Treatment of ankle sprains in young athletes, *Am J Sports Med* 14(6):465, 1986.

CHAPTER 127

Cast Immobilization

Scott W. Eathorne

Douglas B. McKeag

Cast immobilization is a technique often utilized for treating a variety of medical conditions that the primary care physician sees. Although newer technologies have led to an evolution in casting materials, the general principles of this valuable technique have stood the test of time. Having a knowledge of the materials available, understanding the indications and fundamental precepts of cast immobilization, and developing the necessary manual skills can enable the primary care physician to adequately treat the patient who has an injury amenable to such therapy.

HISTORY

The use of immobilization to treat acute fractures dates back to the era of the fifth dynasty (2730–2625 B.C.), when splints made from bark were used to treat fractures of the forearm. Gypsum, from which plaster of paris is derived, was thought to be first used around the sixteenth century in parts of the Turkish Empire.

The year 1927 marked the development of the hard-coated plaster of paris rolls that incorporated a binder, allowing improved adherence of the plaster to the cloth. Since then, various additives have been employed to either accelerate (salicylic acid, zinc, or aluminum) or slow (gums or glue) the setting process.

In the early 1970s, the use of synthetic casting materials, primarily fiberglass, became a more popular alternative to plaster casting. The public perception of a synthetic cast's increased durability and resistance to water, and its availability in an ever-expanding variety of colors and styles, has made it a popular choice among patients. More recently, a moldable, durable rubber casting material (RTV-11) has been developed and is gaining popularity among athletes for whom custom casts can be formed that allow for earlier return to competition following injury.

INDICATIONS

Casts are used to treat (1) a variety of stable, acute fractures, (2) reduced dislocations, (3) injuries to the soft tissues including muscle, tendon, and ligament, (4) congenital and acquired deformities (e.g., correction of talipes equinovarus, or congenital clubfoot), and (5) postoperative vascular, tendon, or nerve repairs following replantation procedures.

The most common diagnosis that the primary care physician makes that requires cast immobilization is the simple, stable, nondisplaced, closed fracture of a long bone, frequently involving the radius or ulna, phalanges, metacarpals, metatarsals, or malleoli. Other conditions include some Grade III ligamentous sprains (e.g., ankle), Achilles tendon disruptions, and tendonitis refractory to other conservative therapies and forms of immobilization.

EQUIPMENT

- Rubber gloves
- Patient drape
- Physician gown and shoe covers
- Stockinette (2-, 3-, and 4-inch widths)
- Soft cotton (e.g., Webril) or synthetic bandages (2-, 3-, 4-, and 6-inch widths)
- Felt padding
- Rubber heels (walking cast)
- Casting material
    Plaster (e.g., plaster of paris)
    Synthetic (e.g., fiberglass, Orthoplast, Scotch)
- Water source
- Elastic (Ace) bandages
- Slings
- Scissors
- Chinese finger traps
- Leg and foot stand

When water is added to the plaster, the water molecules are incorporated into the calcium sulfate hemihydrate molecules with a resultant exothermic reaction. The powdery white substance is converted into a solid, rock-hard material, with a significant amount of heat generated. A curing process then follows over the next few days, characterized by continued water evaporation, a process accelerated by low humidity, high ambient temperature, and increased air circulation.

Synthetic materials require immersion in water to activate the curing process, with generally less heat generated than with plaster. *Attention to water temperature in this process is especially important,* because water that is too warm can lead to rapid curing and significant difficulty in application.

Advantages of plaster casts include low cost, moldability, long shelf life, and low allergenicity as compared to fiberglass. Synthetic cast material is more expensive, has improved in its ease of application, and continues to be superior in strength and durability, weight, water resistance, and drying time. Personal preference continues to play a great role in each physician's choice of material. Both materials are available in common-size rolls, ranging from 2 to 5 inches in width for general, circumferential cast use.

More recent products used for splinting, made of either plaster (e.g., OCL) or *synthetic materials* (3M), are gaining popularity as time-saving alternatives for initial immobilization techniques. These come prefabricated with an outer casing, of which one side is padded and the other covered with casting supplies.

Frequency of use ultimately dictates which equipment is needed by a given physician. Ideally, a single room or area should be dedicated to the application of casts and splints. This room should have a plaster trap in the sink, and all materials should be easily accessible. Rubber gloves, shoe covers, gowns, and drapes should be available to protect against the inevitable exposure to casting materials. A sturdy, easily cleaned examination table and stool can greatly facilitate the process.

COMMON CAST TYPES

Two cast types commonly used by primary care physicians are the short-arm and short-leg casts. *Short-arm casts* are generally indicated in the treatment of stable sprains of the wrist, as well as some stable fractures of the distal radius, carpal bones, and metacarpals. Physicians practicing cast immobilization should be aware of those fractures requiring orthopedic evaluation for possible open reduction and internal fixation. Materials required for short-arm cast application include a 3-inch stockinette, two rolls of 3-inch cast padding, and two to four rolls of either 3- or 4-inch plaster bandage (or 2- or 3-inch fiberglass bandage), depending on preference and size of patient. The patient should be supine or seated, with the arm abducted 90 degrees and the elbow flexed 90 degrees. The wrist should be slightly extended and in a position of function (Fig. 127-1). Chinese finger traps can assist in maintaining this position. The cast extends from the proximal forearm (about 1 inch distal to the flexion crease of the elbow) distally to include the palm and dorsum of the hand, completely covering the forearm. The metacarpal phalangeal joints are allowed complete motion, with the cast stopping just proximal to the distal palmar crease and knuckles. It should be remembered that short-arm casts only partially immobilize the wrist joint, allowing for supination and pronation to occur since the elbow is not included. An adaptation of the short-arm cast is the

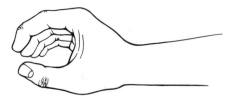

FIG. 127-1.
The position of the wrist in the application of arm casts.

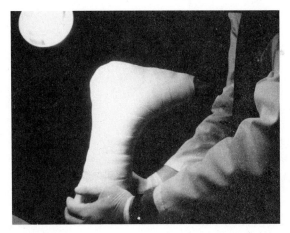

FIG. 127-2.
Short-leg cast applied in the prone position during final molding. Note the position of the ankle postimmobilization. The prone position with knee flexed at 90 degrees facilitates maintaining a 90-degree angle at the ankle.

short-arm thumb spica, in which the thumb is included to the level of the interphalangeal joint. This type of cast may be used in injuries to the scaphoid, trapezium, and first metacarpal as indicated.

Short-leg casts are generally indicated in the treatment of some stable ligamentous injuries to the ankle, and stable fractures of the ankle, calcaneus, tarsals, and metatarsals. Materials include a 4-inch stockinette, three rolls of 4-inch cast padding, and, for fiberglass casts, three rolls of 4-inch fiberglass bandage. A reinforcing strip of heavy-duty fiberglass can also be utilized posteriorly. For plaster casts, used less often, materials will vary widely based on personal preference, but usually include two to three rolls of 6-inch plaster bandage and an adequate number of plaster splint strips, with size based on patient limb size. Application of the short-leg cast is achieved either in the sitting position or prone, with the knee flexed to 90 degrees to help relax the gastrocnemius muscle. The ankle is usually held at a 90-degree angle to the leg, depending on the injury. A foot stand or assistant can provide support to the foot. The cast extends from just below the knee joint, usually including the fibular head, distally to the base of the toes including the metatarsal heads (Fig. 127-2). Again, the ankle joint is only partially immobilized since the cast does not involve both the joint above and below. For *walking short-leg casts,* a posterior reinforcing strip is placed (Fig. 127-7) and molded following application of the second roll of fiberglass bandage, and prior to placing the final roll.

PREPROCEDURE PATIENT EDUCATION

After diagnosing an injury requiring cast immobilization, and prior to its application, discuss the indications for casting, estimated duration of immobilization, and potential impact on activities of daily living with the patient. Typically, discussion of common problems and potential complications from casting occur following application.

TECHNIQUE

Casts are generally applied to immobilize and/or protect an injured part of the body in a position that will facilitate healing. This simplistic view directs the fundamentals of cast immobilization. First, to best approach complete immobilization, *a cast must conform precisely to the anatomy of the region being immobilized*. Failure to accomplish this can lead to unacceptable movement of the injured area, resulting in potential loss of apposition of fracture fragments, malalignment of a reduced dislocation, or persistent inflammation in a refractory tendonitis. Second, *effective immobilization is achieved only by including a sufficient amount of injured area in the cast*. Ideally, this is accomplished by including the joint above and the joint below the area of injury. However, exceptions to this rule are made based on the nature of the injury. Achieving adequate immobilization requires attention to these fundamentals before application of the cast. If these goals cannot be met, the injury may best be served by another means of immobilization.

1. Prior to application of any casting materials, cleanse, dry, and inspect the skin to be included in the cast thoroughly for any lesions such as lacerations, abrasions, or ulcers. If present, they should be noted and, if significant, may contraindicate inclusion in the cast or require special "window" techniques. Also, depending on the acuity of the injury and degree of soft-tissue swelling, immobilization using circumferential casting may be contraindicated, requiring initial splinting of the injury until more definitive care can be given when the swelling has diminished.

2. After this assessment is completed, position the patient such that the injured area can most easily be held in the desired position throughout the application process. This often requires the use of an assistant or assistive device (e.g., leg stand).

   Note: Cast application is performed in a step-wise manner, and development of a systematic approach will help ensure consistency and minimize the potential for error because of a forgotten step.

3. The *first layer* generally applied in casting is the *stockinette*. A poorly fitting stockinette can contribute to skin breakdown, so it must be applied carefully. For adult arm casts, use a 3-inch-wide stockinette, and for legs, a 4-inch-wide, with exceptions based on the extremes of limb size. The material should go well past the toes or fingertips and 4 to 5 inches above the elbow or knee. (Cutting the stockinette too short is a common problem among those learning the procedure.) Some of this "extra" material is ultimately incorporated into the cast or cut off (Figs. 127-3 and 127-4).

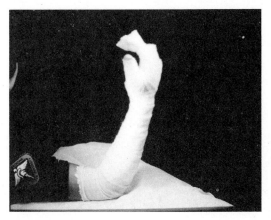

FIG. 127-3.
Short-arm cast application in the seated position, demonstrating adequate length of stockinette and placement of the first roll of plaster bandage. This photograph was taken before folding the extra stockinette over the cast material.

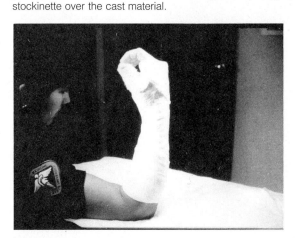

FIG. 127-4.
Demonstration of proper folding of stockinette after application of the first layer of plaster bandage.

4. Remove all transverse wrinkles; they become pressure points after cast application and can cause skin breakdown. This can be achieved by cutting the redundant material, which usually occurs at a joint (Fig. 127-5).
5. After ensuring that the stockinette overlying the area to be immobilized is smooth and free of wrinkles, apply the *second layer, soft cast padding* (Webril). This material comes in rolls. Start at one end and work to the other, overlapping each turn by 50%. Two layers of cast padding can be applied, but care should be taken not to overpad, because this can lead to a loose cast. The goal with padding, as with the stockinette, is to avoid wrinkles, which may contribute to pressure points. Stretch or tear the advancing edge that is to encircle a larger portion of the extremity to avoid wrinkles. Keeping in mind

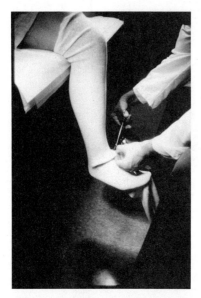

FIG. 127-5.
Application of stockinette for a short-leg cast, demonstrating technique to eliminate transverse wrinkle at ankle. Note the length of the stockinette for a short-leg cast.

the local anatomy, additional padding should be applied to bony prominences and likely areas of increased local pressure (e.g., flexion creases, fulcrum points such as the proximal anterior tibia where short-leg walking casts may rub, and common areas of nerve compression or pressure necrosis, such as over the proximal fibula). Felt pads appropriately fashioned can prevent common complications and improve comfort.

6. Apply the *third layer—the cast material itself.* The type of material used, plaster or synthetic, dictates how the next step will be completed. Although application is quite similar, a few significant differences are worth noting.

When using *plaster-impregnated rolls,* place each roll individually in water at room temperature and submerse until the bubbling stops. Cold water will slow the setting process, whereas warmer water will speed it. A faster setting may be desirable when immobilizing a recently reduced dislocation. Following removal from the water, gently squeeze the roll at both ends to eliminate excess water, and begin the application. Placement of the plaster rolls should follow the direction of the cast padding, with overlapping of approximately 50% with each turn. To avoid transverse wrinkles, plaster rolls can be tucked (folded over) at the edges when redundancy occurs and smoothed using the palm of the hand. Avoid stretching and applying undue pressure with each turn. Apply four to six layers of plaster evenly, with extra reinforcement in areas under increased stress. Apply each roll in a consistent manner, either distal-to-proximal or proximal-to-distal, with the length of the area to be immobilized covered with each layer. Covering only a portion of the extremity and overlapping with the next roll may lead to inherent weakness and future difficulties with the cast.

   Prior to placing the final layers, the ends of the stockinette should be folded over onto the initial layers. Reinforcing strips or cast cushions could be added, depending on the type of cast being applied.

7. Place the final layers of cast material and smooth the cast, using both hands. Make sure that it conforms to the contours of the local anatomy. Position of casting for the injured area is very important. The ankle joint should be at 90 degrees and the hand/wrist in a position of function (slightly extended, relaxed). This position should be closely rechecked prior to hardening of the cast.

Application of *synthetic materials* follows a similar course, with a few noteworthy exceptions. When water is used to activate the curing process, it should be kept no warmer than room temperature to avoid rapid setting of the roll. Normally, this occurs in 2 to 3 minutes. Because of the stretchability of the synthetic bandage rolls, tucking of edges is not necessary to avoid transverse creases. However, care must still be taken to avoid pulling the cast material too tight. Molding should occur between each layer, with most synthetic casts requiring only two to three layers of cast material, depending on the area immobilized (Fig. 127-6). Strips of heavy-duty, reinforcing material are available and frequently applied (e.g., the posterior aspect of a short-leg walking cast) to increase durability (Fig. 127-7). Following application

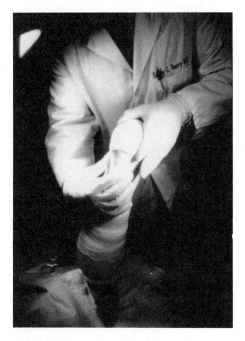

FIG. 127-6.
Method for conforming fiberglass cast bandage to Achilles tendon region during short-leg cast applications.

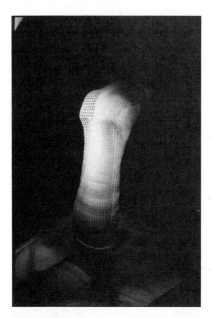

FIG. 127-7.
Placement of posterior fiberglass reinforcing strip during application of short-leg walking cast.

of the last layer, some practitioners wrap the cast with an elastic bandage to further enhance the curing process. This is left on for only a few minutes and removed prior to discharge. In addition to a final check of position, synthetic casts often require trimming of rough edges, which can catch on clothing and ultimately injure the wearer. This can be done with a file, sandpaper, or, depending on the area being altered, even a scissors or the cast saw.

POSTPROCEDURE PATIENT EDUCATION

After cast application, instruct the patient in proper cast care and advise of signs and symptoms that require immediate attention. *For plaster,* avoidance of unnecessary forces to the cast, such as weight bearing, should be advised for at least the first 24 to 48 hours, as the material will still be in the curing process. *Synthetic casts* usually develop sufficient durability to bear increased forces after 12 to 24 hours. Depending on the acuity of injury, elevation for the initial 48 to 72 hours may be recommended to reduce swelling. Crutch walking will obviously be necessary for lower-extremity injuries treated with immobilization until adequate cast strength has been achieved to support weight bearing. Patients requiring crutches should be properly fitted and instructed in correct use of these aides—a step that is frequently overlooked and can lead to great difficulty for the patient. Cast boots and slings can be fitted at this time as well.

Advise patients that, *regardless of the cast material used, care should be taken to avoid getting the cast material wet,* and that submersion of even synthetic casts is unacceptable. If the cast should get wet, the patient may try drying it with an electric blow dryer, being careful not to overheat the cast material. Soaked plaster casts and synthetic casts that have saturated the underlying cast padding require attention by a physician and possible replacement, because of the potential for loss of immobilization, skin irritation, and maceration. The patient must *never introduce foreign objects (e.g., coat hangers) underneath the cast for any reason.*

Instruct cast wearers to contact their physician if they develop increased pain in the immobilized region (potentially more significant if it is unrelieved by prescribed pain medications), *numbness, tingling* or *weakness* in the affected area, *change in skin color* distal to the cast, or *persistent skin irritation,* especially if it progressively worsens then resolves spontaneously (indicating a progressive injury).

CAST REMOVAL

Equipment

- An electric, oscillating, Stryker cast saw
- Cast spreaders
- Bandage scissors

Technique

Removal techniques will differ based on previous experience and training. Patient counseling before starting the procedure, especially in the pediatric population, is likely to be the most effective means of minimizing fear and apprehension. Some practitioners find the solution to this potential problem in allowing ancillary staff, such as nurses or physician assistants, to perform this function. In either case, it is good practice to describe the technique to the patient, including any sensations— such as warmth and vibration—likely to be experienced. Actually turning on the cast saw and applying it briefly to one's own skin is a method sometimes used for demonstrating the relative safety of the procedure. Perhaps more helpful in allaying initial fears would be a warning regarding the loudness of the cast saw which, when first experienced, can be more intimidating than the saw itself. Once the patient is prepared, actual removal of the cast is fairly easy.

1. Stabilize the immobilized limb, with the patient in a comfortable position, with a drape covering any clothing likely to be exposed to cast dust.
2. Determine the cut line before starting and avoid potentially sensitive areas.
3. Hold the cast saw in one hand, and use the thumb and another finger (usually the index) to stabilize the saw against the cast (Fig. 127-8). This technique best allows control of the depth of cut. Constantly changing the area of the blade in contact with the cast and avoidance of prolonged cutting in a single area decreases the heat generated by the procedure and limits the potential for saw-induced burns. Depending on casting material and type of cast, either one (univalve) or two (bivalve) cuts will be required.
4. After full-thickness cuts have been made through the casting material, use the cast spreaders to expose the underlying padding and stockinette, which can then be divided with bandage scissors.

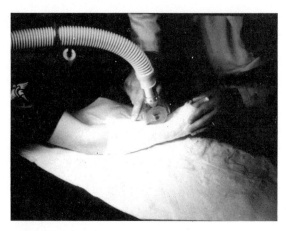

FIG. 127-8.
Method for holding the Stryker cast saw during cast removal.

5. Once all material has been divided, remove the cast and allow the patient to cleanse the skin, providing the injury has healed adequately. Postcast care is injury-specific and geared toward rehabilitation of the affected limb.

COMPLICATIONS

The most well-known and feared complication is the development of a *compartment syndrome*. The process can occur with even a simple, nonthreatening-appearing injury in the absence of arterial or nerve damage, and typically begins as local tissue swelling. If a snug circumferential cast is applied and tissue swelling continues, the conditions are set for compromise of the microcirculation to the immobilized tissue, leading to muscle necrosis and establishing a vicious cycle of further edema and necrosis. If this process continues untreated and compartmental pressures reach a critical level (thought to be 30 to 60 mm Hg between 4 to 8 hours), irreversible damage to the involved tissues may ensue. Ultimately, Volkmann's ischemic contractures may occur, with loss of limb function.

Signs and symptoms of compartment syndrome include *pain* that is out of proportion to the injury or elicited with pressure over the affected compartment or stretching of involved muscle groups, *parasthesias* in the appropriate corresponding dermatome, the *inability to generate a forceful muscle contraction,* and *normal pulses* in the affected limb. Contrary to classical medical school teaching, in the absence of vascular injury, pulselessness and pallor are not characteristics of compartment syndrome, since pressures will never rise high enough in a compartment to completely obstruct the major blood vessels in that area. Patients suffering an acute injury, with any amount of soft-tissue swelling, who require cast immobilization should be made aware of these signs and symptoms. Should they occur, emphasis must be placed on the immediate need to contact the treating physician or to seek care in an emergency department. Delayed diagnosis and treatment can lead to irreversible muscle and nerve damage.

Initial treatment in suspected cases of compartment syndrome is relief of the pressure generated by the cast, either through bivalving or complete removal. Definitive diagnosis rests on characteristic signs, symptoms, and objective measure of compartmental pressure. Treatment of documented compartment syndrome may require surgical intervention in the form of four-compartment fasciotomy.

Less dramatic—yet no less significant—potential complications of cast immobilization include *various skin conditions, nerve palsy, joint stiffness, disuse osteoporosis,* and *thromboembolic events.* Of the skin conditions, cast dermatitis may be the most common, usually resulting in severe, bothersome pruritus from poor ventilation to the underlying skin. Use of absorbent powders may help limit the incidence of this condition, which frequently leads to another complication of casting, the introduction of foreign bodies under the cast. Two problems may result if patients introduce objects under the cast to relieve intense itching. First, the object may become trapped under the cast, producing a pressure point that can cause severe ulceration. Second, such instruments as coat hangers can easily lacerate the skin if used too aggressively, forming a nidus for infection or even requiring suture repair. *Pressure sores* may result from poorly fitting casts that are insufficiently padded over bony prominences or inadequately molded to local anatomic contours. As mentioned, transverse wrinkles in stockinette or cast padding or ridges in the cast material can lead to pressure sores as well. The patient who complains of persistent skin irritation characterized by burning or pain should be seen for evaluation and for possible opening of a window over the symptomatic area to facilitate direct examination.

Any cast used to immobilize an anatomic region where superficial peripheral nerves lie in close proximity to underlying bone may lead to a *nerve palsy.* Long-leg casts and those short-leg casts involving the head of the fibula can produce a common peroneal nerve palsy as the rigid cast compresses the nerve in its course over the fibular head. Symptoms may include loss of sensation over the dorsolateral aspect of the involved foot, and "foot drop," or weakness in the ankle dorsiflexors. Other potential areas of involvement include the ulnar nerve as it passes through the cubital tunnel region, usually seen with long-arm casts, and the median nerve as it passes through the carpal tunnel, possible in both short- and long-arm casts. These neurologic injuries can be complete or incomplete, reversible or irreversible, and should be recognized and treated in a timely fashion.

A nearly universal complaint following cast immobilization is *joint stiffness* and is directly related to duration of immobilization. This fact should be recognized and taken into consideration when determining length of treatment, in addition to the obvious factors influencing healing of the primary injury. Depending on the cause for initial treatment and response to therapy, the physician can initiate fairly aggressive stretching exercises postimmobilization to facilitate the return of normal joint function. Use of simple range-of-motion and other exercises involving nonimmobilized joints in the affected extremity (e.g., straight-leg raising, finger or toe flexion/extension) can minimize the effects of prolonged disuse. Similar programs can also limit the development of disuse osteoporosis, a reversible physiologic process more likely to occur in those populations with preexisting conditions characterized by bone demineralization and requiring prolonged immobilization.

Finally, *thromboembolic complications,* such as deep venous thrombosis with the risk for pulmonary embolism, can occur with cast use (usually of the lower extremity) and must be considered when patients have suspicious symptoms. Diagnosis is difficult because of the presence of the original injury and limitations in examination, and usually requires venography to confirm clinical suspicion.

CPT/BILLING CODES

Selected CPT codes of more common casts are as follows. See special instructions in the CPT code book. Listed procedures include removal of cast or strapping.

Casts

29065	Application, plaster, shoulder to hand (long arm)
29075	Application, plaster, elbow to finger (short arm)
29085	Application, plaster, hand and lower forearm (gauntlet)
29345	Application, plaster, thigh to toes (long leg)
29355	Application, plaster, walker or ambulatory type
29365	Application, plaster, thigh to ankle (cylinder)
29405	Application, plaster, below knee to toes (short leg)
29425	Application, plaster, walking or ambulatory type
29440	Adding walker to previously applied cast

Splints

29105	Application of long-arm splint (shoulder to hand)
29125	Application of short-arm splint (forearm to hand)
29130	Application of finger splint
29505	Application of long-leg splint (thigh to ankle or toes)
29515	Application of short-leg splint (calf to foot)

Removal (use only if casts applied by another physician)

29700	Removal or bivalving, gauntlet, boot, or body cast
29705	Removal or bivalving, full-arm or full-leg cast
29730	Windowing of cast

Miscellaneous

29799	Unlisted procedure, casting or strapping

BIBLIOGRAPHY

Bleck EE, Duckworth N, Hunter N: *Atlas of plaster cast techniques,* ed 2, Chicago, 1974, Year Book Medical Publishers.

Medley ES, Shirley SM, Brilliant HL: Fracture management by family physicians and guidelines for referral, *JFP* 8(4):701, 1979.

Mercier LR: *Practical orthopedics,* ed 3, St Louis, 1991, Mosby.

Salib P: *Plaster casting,* New York, 1975, Appleton-Century-Crofts.

Shirreffs TG, Jr: Compartment syndrome: an extremity at risk, *Emerg Med:* 103, March 1990.

Silfverskiold JP: Fiberglass versus plaster casts: how to choose between them, *Postgrad Med* 86(5):72, 1989.

Wu K: *Techniques in surgical casting and splinting,* Philadelphia, 1987, Lea & Febiger.

CHAPTER 128

Shoulder Dislocations

Fred M. Hankin

The shoulder is uniquely designed to help permit overhead and reaching maneuvers. The proximal humerus and glenoid (scapula) articulate to form the shoulder joint. The glenoid forms a shallow concave surface, which rests against the larger, convex surface of the proximal humerus. The glenoid labrum forms a soft-tissue cuff around the glenoid, which helps to increase its depth and width, thus providing a larger concave surface. Surrounding capsule and ligament structures help to statically hold the humerus against the glenoid. Superficial to this capsule, a cuff of muscles and their tendinous attachments (the rotator cuff) further help to stabilize (statically and dynamically) the proximal humerus against the glenoid (Fig. 128-1).

When the normal static (bone, labrum, capsule, and ligaments) and dynamic (muscles and tendons) restraints are exceeded, the shoulder can slide out of joint. This can result from chronic repetitive attritional injuries, which more frequently result in subluxation of the shoulder. More commonly, a sudden, one-time insult to the shoulder results in frank dislocation of the joint. The shoulder can dislocate in a posterior, anterior, or inferior direction. It may also dislocate in more than one direction, leading to multidirectional instability. Anterior instability occurs when a shoulder dislocates on a frequent basis in the anterior direction. "Dead arm syndrome" refers to the chronic shoulder subluxation syndrome that is seen in persons involved in overhead activities such as baseball pitching or swimming. Posterior dislocations are rare, often misdiagnosed, and should be considered in patients with a loss of external rotation, particularly after a seizure or electroshock therapy.

Most frequently, the physician encounters a subcoracoid, anterior dislocation. This usually results from an abducted, extended, externally rotated upper extremity that has met with resistance, resulting in a lever-arm that forces the proximal humerus anteriorly out of the glenoid socket. This discussion will be limited to anterior dislocations of the shoulder.

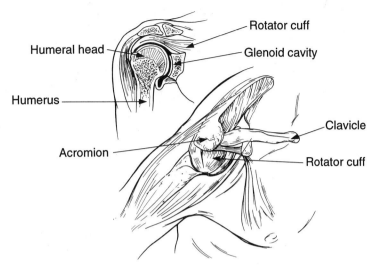

FIG. 128-1.
Anatomy of the shoulder.

DIAGNOSIS

The patient will have a loss of the normal shoulder contour, although this may be hard to detect in heavyset individuals. The acromion becomes very prominent. A prominence (humeral head) may be noted in the anterior chest region. Clinically, a hollow can be appreciated beneath the acromion process, due to the transposed humeral head. The arm will frequently be held in an abducted, externally rotated posture. A neurologic deficit, most frequently the axillary nerve (shoulder abduction and sensation over the deltoid) may be noted on careful examination. All nerves of the brachial plexus can potentially be injured, however, and a careful neurologic examination is warranted. Vascular compromise is uncommon, but proximal and distal arterial flow should be assessed.

RADIOGRAPHIC STUDIES

Radiographic studies are essential prior to attempts to reduce the shoulder. It is important to determine the presence or absence of fractures before the physician's manipulation. Obtain standard radiographs of the shoulder, including an anterior-posterior glenoid fossa projection. The most important projection in this series is the axillary view (Fig. 128-2). In the event of a dislocation, this view will help to determine in which direction the humeral head is dislocated relative to the glenoid. Some authorities prefer the use of a lateral scapular or a Y-type of view. Alternatively, in some obese individuals, a computed tomography (CT) scan may be necessary to help determine the direction of the shoulder dislocation, as well as the presence of concomitant fractures.

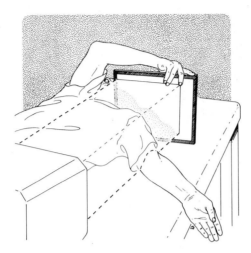

FIG. 128-2.
Radiographs should include an axillary view. This projection helps to document the direction (anterior vs. posterior) of the shoulder dislocation and confirm position following closed reduction maneuvers.

EQUIPMENT

- Stretcher
- Weights
- Analgesia
- Muscle relaxer
- Narcotics
- Benzodiazepines
- Reversal agents

TECHNIQUE

The physician and emergency room staff may pull on the limb to reduce the humeral head back into the glenoid; however, the patient is probably better served by gentle gravity reduction of the joint. Certainly, this is less traumatic for the shoulder, and should help to minimize the chances of developing an iatrogenic fracture related to the reduction process.

1. Adequately sedate the patient. This frequently requires the use of a general anesthetic. Alternatively, under supervised conditions, good sedation can frequently be achieved in the emergency room setting. This procedure is not recommended for the office situation, where adequate respiratory support measures and monitoring may not be present.
2. After adequate levels of sedation are achieved, place the patient in the prone position upon a stretcher (Fig. 128-3). A rolled-up towel or blanket can be placed beneath the coracoid process and pectoralis major muscle. A weight

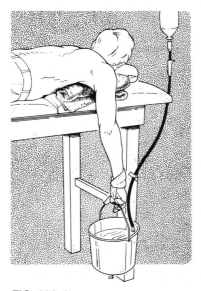

FIG. 128-3.
Gentle, sustained longitudinal traction can provide an effective means for closed reduction of an anterior shoulder dislocation. As the intravenous fluid bag slowly empties into the bucket, a gradual traction force is created.

can be adfixed to the wrist to provide longitudinal, sustained traction. Wrapping a gauze bandage around the wrist, rather than tape, will usually suffice to provide secure fixation of the weights to the limb. A bucket of water can be utilized if weights are not present.

3. With time and relaxation, usually the shoulder will reduce itself. An intravenous fluid bag can be permitted to run into the bucket. This slowly building water volume provides a gradual increase in the longitudinal weight applied to the limb. Occasionally, the physician can help facilitate the reduction by providing gentle, alternating, internal and external rotation to the arm.

   If this reduction maneuver is not successful, then referral to an orthopedic surgeon is recommended.

4. After the shoulder has been reduced, hold the limb in internal rotation against the abdomen and adduction (humerus against the lateral trunk) by a sling and swath device. A careful postreduction neurovascular assessment is required.

5. Obtain appropriate postreduction radiographs to help determine that adequate reduction of the joint surfaces has been achieved. A congruous-appearing joint without significant distraction (interposed tissue) between the glenoid and the humerus must be noted. Occasionally, comparison shoulder radiographs may be required. A repeat axillary view is also required to help confirm location of the proximal humerus in the glenoid. Again, a CT scan may also be utilized to help confirm location of the proximal humerus in the glenoid.

One of the risks following a shoulder dislocation is a redislocation. This is a very common occurrence in the young adult population. If appropriate, postreduction care is not maintained and enforced, the frequency of redislocation increases. Usually, immobilization for a period of 4 to 6 weeks following a successful reduction is warranted. Appropriate follow-up clinical, neurologic, and radiographic examinations are made throughout this time in order to help confirm maintenance of the reduction.

After the designated period of immobilization, assign a gentle strengthening program, with particular emphasis on the shoulder internal rotators. Unrestricted external rotation and lifting activities are usually not permitted for a period of 3 months. With recurrent dislocations, there is a significant incidence of avascular necrosis of the proximal humerus. In patients with frequent dislocations, an arthrogram, CT arthrogram, or arthroscopy might be warranted to help determine the presence of an anatomic variant that might make the patient more prone to redislocation. Patients with peripheral neuropathies, syringomyelia, and psychiatric histories may be more prone to dislocating their shoulders, and these underlying diagnoses should be considered in the patient with repeated dislocations.

CPT/BILLING CODES

23650	Closed treatment of shoulder dislocation, with manipulation, without anesthesia
23655	Closed treatment of shoulder dislocation, with manipulation, with anesthesia

BIBLIOGRAPHY

Rockwood CA et al: Subluxations and dislocations about the glenohumeral joint. In *Fractures in adults,* ed 3, Philadelphia, 1991, J.B. Lippincott.

CHAPTER 129

Nursemaid's Elbow: Subluxation of the Radial Head

Fred M. Hankin

James L. Telfer

The elbow consists of the articulation of the humerus, ulna, and radial head. The radius and ulna flex and extend against the humerus, and the radial head rotates against the ulna and capitellum (humerus), so as to permit forearm pronation and supination. The radial head is held in place against the proximal ulna and capitellum by ligaments and joint capsule.

Often, a child sustains a longitudinal traction injury to the extremity. The radial head is either subluxed from, or soft tissue becomes interposed at, the radial-capitellum joint, resulting in pain, swelling, and immobilization. Several anatomic explanations as mechanisms for this injury have been reported. These include a partial disruption of the orbicular ligament (which holds the radius against the proximal ulna), proximal migration of the orbicular ligament over the radial head, or interposition of capsule or synovium between the articular surfaces.

DIAGNOSIS

Often the history suggests the diagnosis. The child's extended limb has been longitudinally pulled by a parent, sibling, or a caregiver, and acute pain is noted by the child. The child may be reluctant to move the entire extremity. Focal symptoms are noted in the region of the elbow. The child is usually very unwilling to rotate the forearm, and tends to hold it in a pronated and extended posture. Neurovascular compromise is rare with this injury. Careful examination will distinguish pain in the supracondylar humerus region from pain in the radial head region.

RADIOGRAPHIC STUDIES

Take standard elbow radiographs, including three views (anteroposterior, lateral, and an oblique). Comparison radiographs of the other side are essential to help determine the presence of fat pad sign (joint effusion), location of epiphyseal growth centers, and the longitudinal alignment of the radial head with the capitellum. The presence of a fat pad sign is indicative that an injury to the elbow has occurred. It is a nonspecific radiographic finding and simply supports the clinical diagnosis. Usually, with nursemaid's elbow, the radiographs will be normal.

TECHNIQUE

Usually the radial head will reduce with gentle forearm rotation. Supination and flexion are usually required (Fig. 129-1). Sometimes, a snap or a satisfying clunk of the radial head may be felt, indicating reduction. Often, the radial head is reduced by an X-ray technician attempting to obtain satisfactory projections for the radiographic studies. Sometimes, the child will reduce his or her own elbow prior to evaluation by the physician.

If there is concern regarding the possibility of a growth plate injury, generally the best approach is that an orthopedic consultation be obtained. Rarely, an arthrogram can be obtained and an anesthetic is often required to help the child cooperate with such a study. The radiographic contrast can help to outline articular surfaces of the joint and give the examiner a better understanding of the nonossified anatomy.

If there is concern regarding the possibility of more significant trauma or infection in the elbow, an aspiration can be performed. If bloody fluid is obtained,

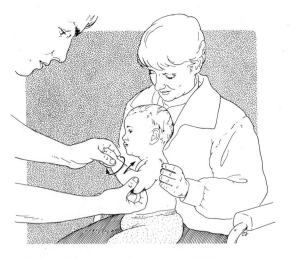

FIG. 129-1.
The reduction manuever for a subluxed radial head (nursemaid's elbow) involves gentle supination of the forearm and flexion of the elbow. The examiner's thumb can be placed over the child's elbow to help palpate the radial head during the reduction process.

this would confirm the presence of a traumatic intracapsular injury, such as a fracture. If purulent material is obtained, this would corroborate the diagnosis of infection. Routine elbow aspiration is not recommended for a nursemaid's elbow. It is an adjunct diagnostic procedure that can be utilized in difficult situations. An anesthetic may be required.

If any of the preceding diagnoses are being considered, consultation with an orthopedic surgeon is recommended.

Following successful reduction of a subluxed radial head, the physician should tell the child to rest the limb for several days and reevaluate the child with follow-up clinical and radiographic studies. Depending upon the age of the child, occasionally splint immobilization is recommended.

> *Authors' note:* For very small children, occasionally we will have them wear a long-sleeved shirt and attach the cuff (wrist area) to the shirt, using a safety pin, to help provide some immobilization.

Generally, children will let their symptoms be their guide in regards to activity level; once they are comfortable, they will resume their activities. It will often take several days for them to resume their normal routines. Follow-up evaluation is recommended to determine that normal joint function is present.

The long-term prognosis following a nursemaid's elbow is usually very favorable. Occasionally, the child will have several episodes of subluxation, but the incidence drops off significantly in the preschool age group. Long-term functional or growth problems are rare following appropriate treatment of this injury. Congenital radial head dislocation is a separate entity and not related to the very common pediatric problem of nursemaid's elbow.

CPT/BILLING CODE

24640   Closed treatment of radial head subluxation in child (nursemaid's elbow) with manipulation

BIBLIOGRAPHY

Salter RB, Zaltz C: Anatomic investigations of the mechanism of injury and pathologic anatomy of "pulled elbow" in young children, *Clin Orthop* 77:134, 1971.

CHAPTER 130

Joint and Soft Tissue Aspiration and Injection

John L. Pfenninger

Aspiration and injection of soft tissues and joints is relatively simple. Steroid injection into joints fell into disfavor for many years because the procedure was overused and abused. When appropriate guidelines are followed, complications are extremely rare. The alternative to focal treatment with injection is usually systemic nonsteroidal antiinflammatory drugs, which have significant toxicity with prolonged use.

Primary care physicians should master the technique of aspiration and injection for many reasons. If the physician aspirates an inflamed joint, a diagnosis can be made immediately. If a joint is distended, pain can be rapidly relieved by aspirating the fluid. Injecting an anesthetic or steroid solution can give focal pain relief without the toxicity of the systemic medications.

INDICATIONS

Diagnostic Indications

- To evaluate synovial fluid and determine whether the cause of effusion is from infectious, rheumatic, traumatic, or crystal-induced etiology
- To perform a therapeutic trial to differentiate various etiologies (e.g., costochondritis from coronary artery disease, trochanteric bursitis from deep hip disease, occipital trigger points from vertebral disease)

Therapeutic Indications

- To remove exudative fluid from a septic joint
- To relieve pain in a grossly swollen joint (e.g., traumatic effusion)
- To inject lidocaine, saline, or corticosteroids into acutely inflamed trigger points or tender joints

Corticosteroids have a marked effect on inflammation. There are no good data to indicate that steroid injections decrease the long-term adverse effects of chronic inflammatory or degenerative diseases, but there is no doubt that they result in acute symptomatic improvement.

Conditions

The conditions that are improved with local corticosteroid therapy are listed in Box 130-1.

CONTRAINDICATIONS

- Cellulitis or broken skin over the intended entry site for the injection or aspiration
- Anticoagulant therapy that is not well controlled
- Severe primary coagulopathy
- Septic effusion of a bursa or a periarticular structure (for injection)
- More than three previous injections in a weight-bearing joint in the preceding 12-month period
- Lack of response to two or three prior injections
- Suspected bacteremia (Unless the joint is suspected as the source of the bacteremia, it should not be tapped. Doing so could inoculate the joint space and actually *cause* infection.)
- Unstable joints (for steroid injection)
- Inaccessible joints (For many primary care physicians, this includes the hip joint proper, the sacroiliac joint, and the joints of the vertebral column.)
- Joint prostheses (If infection is suspected, consider a referral to the orthopedist who placed the prosthesis, if at all possible.)

EQUIPMENT

In the past, joint injections were frequently performed gloveless with only an alcohol wipe. In contrast, some physicians now use an extensive sterile draping procedure. Although the former is grossly inadequate, the latter is probably unnecessary unless the patient is immunosuppressed, diabetic, or is at high risk of infection. Most injections are done after an alcohol or povidone-iodine wipe; sterile or nonsterile gloves are used. When a joint space (as opposed to soft tissue) is entered, sterile gloves are more customarily used. Masks are unnecessary. Required equipment includes the following:

- Povidone-iodine wipes or alcohol wipes
- Sterile or nonsterile gloves
- *Optional:* sterile drapes
- 22- to 25-gauge 1.5-inch needle for injections

**BOX 130-1. CONDITIONS IMPROVED WITH
LOCAL CORTICOSTEROID INJECTION**

Articular Conditions
Rheumatoid arthritis
Seronegative spondyloarthropathies
   Ankylosing spondylitis
   Arthritis associated with inflammatory bowel disease
   Psoriasis
   Reiter's syndrome
Crystal-induced arthritis
   Gout
   Pseudogout
Osteoarthritis

Nonarticular Disorders
Fibrositis
   Localized fibrositis
   Systemic fibrositis
Bursitis
   Subacromial bursitis
   Trochanteric bursitis
   Anserine bursitis
   Prepatellar bursitis
Periarthritis
   Adhesive capsulitis
Tenosynovitis/tendonitis
   De Quervain's disease
   Trigger finger
   Bicipital tendonitis
   Tennis elbow
   Golfer's elbow
   Plantar fasciitis
Neuritis
   Carpal tunnel syndrome
   Tarsal tunnel syndrome
   Costochondritis
   Tietze's syndrome

From Pfenninger JL: Injections of joints and soft tissue: Part 1. General guidelines, *Am Fam Physician* 44:1196-1202, 1991. Used with permission.

- 18- to 20-gauge 1.5-inch needle for aspirations
- 30-gauge 0.5-inch needle, if skin anesthesia is to be given (usually not needed)
- 1 cc to 10 cc syringe for injections (Luer-Lok is recommended.)
- 3 cc to 50 cc syringe for aspirations

Single dose vials of 1% lidocaine or multidose vials of bupivacaine

- Hemostat (to be used if joint is to be aspirated then injected using different syringes but same needle)
- Tubes for culture or other laboratory studies (if aspiration is done)
- Corticosteroid preparation (see Tables 130-1 and 130-2)

PREPROCEDURE PATIENT EDUCATION

Inform the patient of the risks, benefits, and possible complications of injection therapy. This is especially important if steroids are used. Rarely is there ever a

TABLE 130-1.

Relative Potency of Corticosteroids

Corticosteroid	Relative antiinflammatory potency	Approximate equivalent dose (mg)
Short-acting preparations		
Cortisone	0.8	25
Hydrocortisone	1	20
Intermediate-acting preparations		
Prednisone	3.5	5
Prednisolone tebutate (Hydeltra-TBA)	4	5
Triamcinolone (Aristocort, Aristospan, Kenalog)	5	4
Methylprednisolone acetate (Depo-Medrol)	5	4
Long-acting preparations		
Dexamethasone (Decadron-LA)	25	0.6
Betamethasone (Celestone Soluspan)	25	0.6

Adapted from Leversee JH: Aspiration of joints and soft tissue injections, *Prim Care* 13:572, 1986. Used with permission.

TABLE 130-2.

Corticosteroid Dosages

Corticosteroid	Preparation strength (mg/ml)	Common dosages for site (mg)		
		Tendon sheath and bursae	Small joints	Large joints
Cortisone		20-50	10-25	50-125
Hydrocortisone acetate	25,50	8-40	8-20	40-100
Prednisolone tebutate (Hydeltra-TBA)	20	4-10	2-5	10-25
Triamcinolone hexacetonide (Aristospan)	20	4-10	2-5	10-25
diacetate (Aristocort)	40	4-10	2-5	10-25
acetonide (Kenalog)	40	4-10	2-5	10-25
Methylprednisolone acetate (Depo-Medrol)	20,40,80	4-10	2-5	10-25
Dexamethasone sodium phosphate (Decadron)	4	1.5-3.0	0.8-1.0	2-4
acetate (Decadron-LA)	8	1.5-3.0	0.8-1.0	2-4
Betamethasone sodium phosphate and acetate (Celestone Soluspan)	6	1.5-3.0	0.8-1.0	2-4

Adapted from Leversee JH: Aspiration of joints and soft tissue injections, *Prim Care* 13:572, 1986. Used with permission.

TABLE 130-3.

Adverse Effects of Local Corticosteroid Therapy

Complication	Estimated prevalence
Postinjection flare	2 to 5%
Steroid arthropathy	0.8%
Tendon rupture	<1%
Facial flushing	<1%
Skin atrophy, depigmentation	<1%
Iatrogenic infectious arthritis	<0.001 to 0.072%
Transient paresis of injected extremity	Rare
Hypersensitivity reaction	Rare
Asymptomatic pericapsular calcification	43%
Acceleration of cartilage attrition	Unknown

From Gray RG, Gottlieb NL: Intraarticular corticosteroids: an updated assessment, *Clin Orthop* 177:253, 1983. Used with permission.

complication from the use of lidocaine alone. However, with steroids, and especially with repeated injections, there are some adverse consequences (see the section on complications and Table 130-3). Inform the patient that there is always a possibility for infection with the injection, although this is extremely rare. Bleeding into a joint can occur, although this generally does not happen unless the patient has a coagulopathy. The injection may actually cause more pain during the first 24 to 36 hours. This is called *steroid flare*. If the pain lasts for more than 36 hours, evaluate the patient for the possibility of a septic joint. Warn the patient that a second or even a third injection may be needed. Whether or not steroids have significant adverse effects, and the degree of this reaction on the cartilage and bone itself when steroids are injected into the joint space is controversial. Allergic reactions are very rare. Tendon ruptures should be avoidable if the injection is placed peritendonously instead of within the tendon itself. However, rupture is always a possibility. As a final precaution, warn the patient that occasionally a steroid placed too close to the surface of the skin can cause atrophy. This may leave the patient with depigmentation and a slight indentation in the skin.

TECHNIQUE

Before injection therapy, consider the differential diagnosis. If tumor or fracture is possible, radiographs should be obtained. Many times, especially with trigger point injection (see Chapter 26, Technique of Trigger Point Injection), radiographs are not necessary. Other diagnoses may also be fairly straightforward and not require a prior radiograph examination. If the diagnosis is in question, it should be clarified before injection therapy.

Generally, one injects a combination of lidocaine with the steroid of choice. Single-dose vials of lidocaine should be used to avoid the preservative/precipitation problems (see Complications). Using a rather large volume of lidocaine may be beneficial. Not only does it disburse the steroid in a less concentrated solution, but the volume itself may have a therapeutic effect. In some instances, only a minimal amount of lidocaine may be used (e.g., ganglion cysts, trigger fingers). In other sites, larger amounts are recommended (e.g., lidocaine 5 to 10 cc in a shoulder or knee mixed with 0.5 to 1 cc of selected steroid). A good rule of thumb is to use more, not less, when it comes to lidocaine.

The recommended dosages of medications (Table 130-4) and the specific techniques for various injection sites (Figs. 130-1 to 130-22) are included in this chapter. The general approach is as follows:

1. Identify the site of entry and mark it with a thumbnail, ballpoint pen, or indelible marker.
2. Prep the area with an alcohol or povidone-iodine wipe.
3. Draw up the proper amounts of steroid and anesthetic into a single syringe and mix well by tipping the syringe backwards and forward.
4. Using appropriate syringes and needles, either aspirate or inject the site as indicated. After insertion but before injection, pull back the plunger to be sure the needle is not in a blood vessel.
5. If aspiration is to be followed by injection, one can either have two needle/syringe setups and enter the area twice, or enter once, aspirate, grasp the

TABLE 130-4.

Needle Size and Drug Dosage for Injection Therapy

Structure	Needle gauge	Dose of 1% lidocaine (cc)	Dose of methylprednisolone acetate (mg)
Radiohumeral joint	22	3-5	10-20
Lateral or medial epicondyle	22-25	4	10-20
Olecranon bursa	22	2-3	10-20
Finger and toe joints	22-25	0.5-1.0	4-10
Abductor tendon of thumb (de Quervain's disease)	25 (1.5 inch)	3-4	10-20
Flexor tendon sheath (trigger finger)	25 (1 inch)	0.25	4-10
Wrist	22-25	1-2	10-40
Carpal tunnel	25 (1.5 inch)	1	20-40
Ganglion of wrist	18-20	0.25-0.5	4
Subacromial bursa of shoulder	20 (1.5 inch)	5-7	20-40
Biceps tendon	22 (1.5 inch)	5-10	10-20
Acromioclavicular joint	22-25	2-4	4-10
Rotator cuff tendon	18-20 (1.5 inch)	5	20-40
Intraarticular space of shoulder	20 (1.5 inch)	5-7	20-40
Hip joint	20(2.5-3.0 inch)	5	40-80
Trochanteric bursa	22	5-10	20-40
Anserine bursa	22-25	5	20-40
Prepatellar bursa	20	3	20-40
Intraarticular space of knee	20 (1.5 inch)	5	20-80
Calcaneal bursa	22 (1.5 inch)	5	20-40
Trigger point	25	3-5	10-20
Ankle	22	3-5	20-40

From Pfenninger, JL: Injections of joints and soft tissue: Part II. Guidelines for specific joints, *Am Fam Physician* 44:1690, 1991. Used with permission.

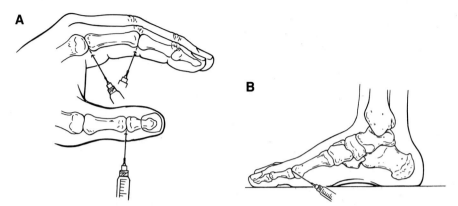

FIG. 130-1.

Finger and toe joints. Any of the finger (**A**) and toe (**B**) joints may be injected in the lateral, medial, or dorsal aspect. Slightly flex the joint to open the joint space. Direct the needle to enter just medial or lateral to the extensor tendon. Avoid going too far laterally or medially where the nerve and vascular structures run.

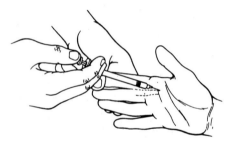

FIG. 130-2.

Trigger finger. Identify the flexor tendon involved. Insert the needle at the distal palmar crease. Attempt to position it peritendinously. When the needle is in position, the syringe will move with flexion of the finger.

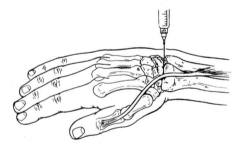

FIG. 130-3.

Wrist joint. Flex the joint 20 degrees to open the joint spaces. The dorsal approach is generally used. Position the needle perpendicular to the skin surface. Enter at a site distal to the radial head and lateral to the extensor pollicis longus tendon (ulnar to the anatomic "snuff box"). If the needle can be easily inserted to 1 or 2 cm, it is correctly positioned in the joint space. The intercarpal joints have interconnecting synovial spaces, and the contents of one correctly placed injection will dispurse into the entire joint complex.

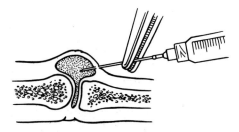

FIG. 130-4.
A ganglion is a manifestation of joint inflammation. Use an 18-gauge needle and a 1 cc to 3 cc syringe to enter the ganglion and aspirate its contents. The contents are often thick, and there may only be minimal return of a gel-like material. Hold the needle in position with the hemostat and remove the syringe. Attach the steroid-containing syringe and inject the contents.

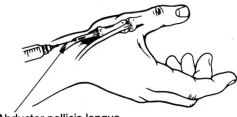

Abductor pollicis longus

FIG. 130-5.
De Quervain's disease. Maximally abduct the thumb to accentuate and identify the tendon. Insert the needle parallel to (but not into) the tendon. Inject at the areas of greatest tenderness. Postinjection splinting may still be necessary.

needle with a hemostat (being careful not to change the position of the needle tip), remove the syringe with the aspirate, then replace it with the lidocaine/steroid syringe, and finally inject the contents.

6. If lidocaine or steroid is to be injected, it is often necessary to inject in two or three areas around the site of tenderness. This is not necessary when the joint space itself has been entered.

7. Although much has been written regarding evaluation of joint fluid aspirates, Schmerling reported that the white blood cell count and polymorphonucleocyte percentage were the only helpful tests to determine the etiology of an exudate. Glucose, protein, LDH, complement fixation, electrolyte, uric acid levels, rheumatoid factor, and antinuclear antibodies were of little benefit. If the exudate is cloudy, then culture is also indicated. If there is any suspicion of gouty arthritis, examine the fluid for crystals under polarized light. A peripheral smear may be helpful when a bloody tap is obtained after trauma. The presence of fat cells indicates a fracture. The Pfenninger articles contain many tables of other characteristics of synovial fluid for differential diagnosis, although the benefit of additional studies is unproven.

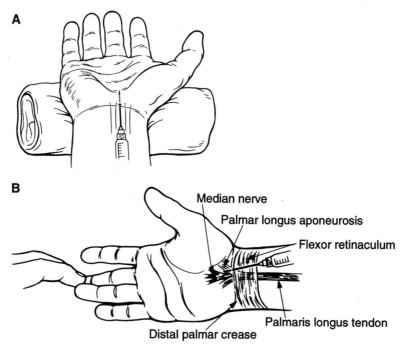

A

B

Median nerve

Palmar longus aponeurosis

Flexor retinaculum

Palmaris longus tendon

Distal palmar crease

FIG. 130-6.
Carpal tunnel syndrome. **A,** Dorsiflex the wrist 30 degrees and rest it on a rolled towel. Insert the needle at the distal crease of the wrist either lateral or medial to the palmaris longus tendon. **B,** Find the tendon by having the patient flex the middle finger against resistance. Angle the needle downward at a 45-degree angle toward the tip of the middle finger. If there is any discomfort in the fingers, withdraw and reposition the needle. Advance 1 to 2 cm until there is no resistance, and then inject the medication. Alternatively, use a perpendicular approach going directly through the flexor retinaculum into the median nerve space (not illustrated).

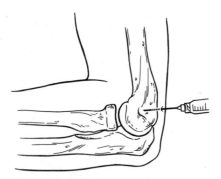

FIG. 130-7.
Lateral epicondylitis (tennis elbow). Find the area of greatest tenderness over the lateral epicondyle. Insert the needle perpendicularly until bone is felt. Withdraw the needle 1 to 2 mm and inject. It may be beneficial to fan out the injections in several directions into the extensor aponeurosis and the radial collateral ligament. Massage the injection site. If distal tenderness is still present after several minutes, another injection in a fanlike pattern may be necessary. Medial epicondylitis (golfer's elbow) is treated in a similiar fashion.

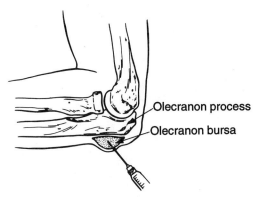

FIG. 130-8.
Olecranon bursa. This bursa is easily identified and entered. Insert the needle directly into the bursa and aspirate until fluid is returned. If the fluid is cloudy, it should be submitted for culture and concurrent infection should be ruled out. If there is a clinical reason to suspect infection, await the culture results before injecting. In a double-blind study comparing focal steroid injection into the olecranon bursa with systemic nonsteroidal antiinflammatory drugs, the most rapid benefit and most lasting effect came from steroid injections.

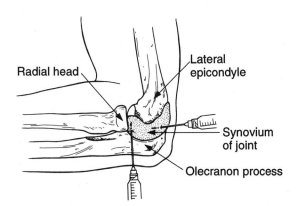

FIG. 130-9.
Elbow joint. Flex the elbow 45 degrees. Identify the lateral epicondyle. Inject into the joint space just inferior to the lateral epicondyle and superior to the olecranon process of the ulna. A slight concavity can be felt just inferior to the radial head and will help identify the proper point of insertion.

POSTPROCEDURE CARE

- A Band-Aid or other dressing should be left on for 8 to 12 hours.
- It is essential that the affected area be rested. Injection therapy is not a cure itself. It is used in conjunction with other modalities. Physical therapy, nonsteroidal antiinflammatories, and hot or cold compresses may all be indicated, depending on the specific problem. If a weight-bearing joint (such as the knee) is injected, rest is indicated for a longer period of time than that for a wrist ganglion cyst injection.

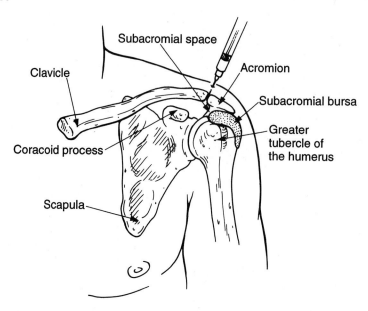

FIG. 130-10.

Acromioclavicular joint. Palpate the clavicle, moving laterally until a prominence is felt. This is the acromioclavicular joint. Insert the needle from an anterior position into the joint and inject.

- The patient should report immediately if he or she develops fever, chills, or any sign of infection. If the discomfort from the injection does not resolve within 72 hours, the patient should be examined to rule out a septic joint.
- The patient may bathe normally.
- A short course of a nonsteroidal antiinflammatory drug is often beneficial at the time of injection; the two modalities combined may have a markedly beneficial effect.

COMPLICATIONS

- Injection into a vein or artery
- Introduction of infection (usually *Staphylococcus*) into joint space (18 infections per 250,000 injections [0.072%])
- Trauma to articular cartilage or injury to nearby nerves
- Pneumothorax (when injecting thoracic trigger points)
- Subcutaneous fatty atrophy
- Adverse drug reaction (see Table 130-3)
- Injection of steroid into a septic joint (If there is any suspicion of infection, do not instill steroids until laboratory studies have ruled it out.)
- Osteoporosis and cartilage damage (This is rare; reported cases have usually occurred after 20 to 30 injections. For joints, especially weight-bearing joints, a limit of three steroid injections per year provides a wide margin of safety.)

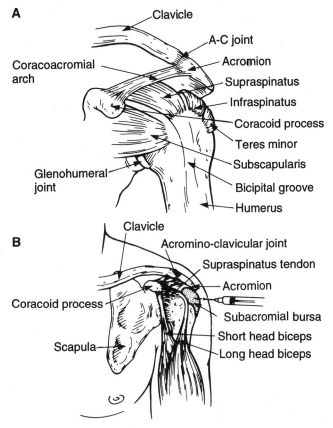

FIG. 130-11.
Subacromial bursa. Most injection procedures involving the shoulder will include an injection into the subacromial bursa. Palpate the superior surface of the shoulder going laterally until there is a slight drop-off. This is the lateral edge of the acromion. The now palpable soft spot above the humeral head is the location of the subacromial, or subdeltoid, bursa. Direct the needle perpendicular to the surface and insert the needle through the deltoid muscle into the bursa. The needle should be free floating since it is within a space, not a muscle or tendon. The tendon of the supraspinatus (**A**), the muscle most commonly involved in a rotator cuff syndrome, is directly medial to this bursa (**B**) and can be entered by directing the needle deeper. If the tendon is calcified, a gritty feeling may be appreciated as it is entered. Inject within the bursa, not within the tendon.

- Tendon rupture (To reduce the possibility of tendon rupture, inject peritendinously instead of intratendinously. Ruptures usually occur after multiple injections and when the patient will not rest the area. Finger tendon ruptures have been reported after steroid injection. Gray recommends setting a limit of five total injections per finger joint.)
- Reactions to lidocaine (Allergies to lidocaine are very rare; however, many physicians believe that the preservatives actually cause the problem. Single-dose vials of lidocaine do not contain preservatives.)

Text continued on p. 1054.

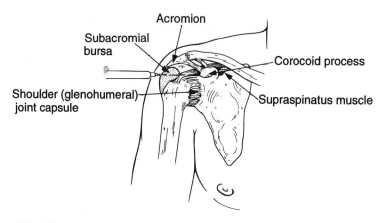

FIG. 130-12.
Rotator cuff (supraspinatus tendonitis). Use the same approach as that used for injecting the subacromial bursa. However, insert the needle deeper to reach the peritendinous area.

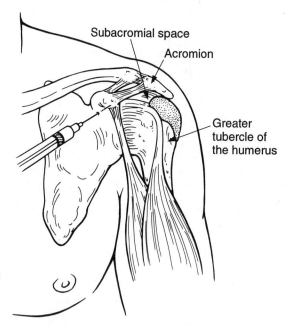

FIG. 130-13.
Short head of the biceps. The short head of the biceps attaches to the coracoid process. This is the palpable bony prominence located inferior to the clavicle and medial to the humerus over the anterior portion of the shoulder. Rarely does this area have to be injected, but should a patient present with pain and discomfort over the coracoid process, insert a needle directly into the point of maximal tenderness until it reaches the bone. Withdraw the needle a millimeter or two and inject. Only a small volume of steroid is needed along with relatively larger amounts of lidocaine. Additional steroid may be injected parallel to the tendon distally (if it is palpable).

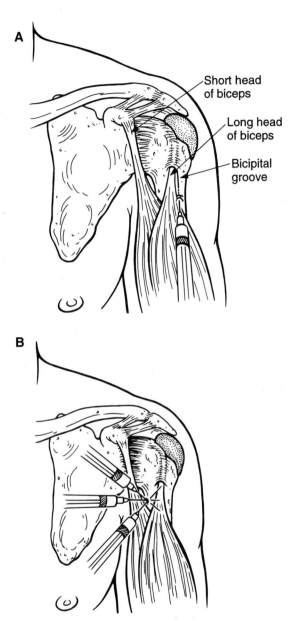

FIG. 130-14.
Injection of the long head of the biceps (bicipital tendonitis). **A,** Identify the biceps tendon by placing your hand on the patient's shoulder with your fingers posteriorly and the thumb anteriorly. Rotate the patient's arm and shoulder outward. The bicipital groove is palpable anteriorly and the tendon rotation can be felt under your thumb. Identify the most tender area of the tendon (usually at the bicipital groove on the humerus). Insert the needle into this groove and attempt to make a peritendinous injection of steroid and lidocaine. Often, a slip of the subacromial bursa surrounds the more proximal portion of the bicipital tendon. Steroid injected into the bursa will also bathe the proximal portion of the tendon. **B,** If pain persists on palpation after the injection, further injection in a fanlike pattern may be needed more distally.

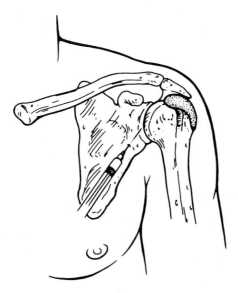

FIG. 130-15.

Intraarticular shoulder joint injection. A posterior or an anterior approach can be used to inject into the space of the shoulder joint (scapulohumeral or glenohumeral joint). In the anterior approach, rotate the shoulder outward. This opens the joint space. Identify the coracoid process. Insert the needle 1 cm inferior and 1 cm lateral to the coracoid process, and direct the needle perpendicularly, or slightly laterally, into the glenohumeral joint. The properly inserted needle should not contact bone.

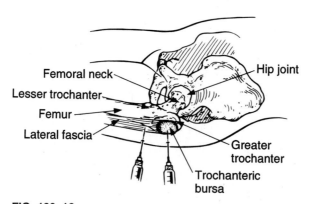

FIG. 130-16.

Trochanteric bursa. The trochanteric bursa is located at the most superior prominent portion of the femur. Tenderness in this area generally denotes a trochanteric bursitis. Direct the needle perpendicular to the femur, and insert until bone is felt. Withdraw the needle 2 to 3 mm and inject. Frequently the pain radiates more distally, as it might with lateral epicondylitis. In this case, the pain radiates down the lateral portion of the femur along the fascia. If the patient is still experiencing discomfort 5 minutes after injection of the bursa and massage of the area, a more distal injection may be necessary at the areas of most tenderness.

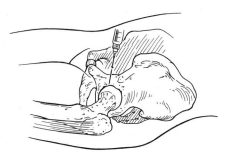

FIG. 130-17.
Hip joint proper. Experience is necessary to inject the hip joint itself. An anterior or posterior approach can be taken. However the anterior approach is most common. Great care must be taken to avoid entering any of the blood vessels or nerves coursing through the inguinal canal area. Position the hip so that the leg is maximally extended and rotated inward. (The hip is placed in extension and internal rotation.) Use a long (2.5-inch) 20-gauge needle to enter 2 to 3 cm below the anterior superior spine of the ilium and 2 to 3 cm lateral to the femoral pulse. The needle should point posteriomedially at a 60-degree angle to the skin, and then should course through the capsule ligaments until it reaches bone. Withdraw the needle slightly and aspirate for fluid. Injection may then be carried out, and there should be little resistance.

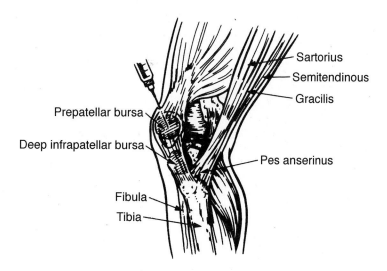

FIG. 130-18.
Prepatellar bursa. Identify the bursa, which is located between the skin and the patella. Insert the needle just above the patella and at the lateral portion of the bursa, and direct it to the center of swelling. Aspirate fluid (for culture), and then inject.

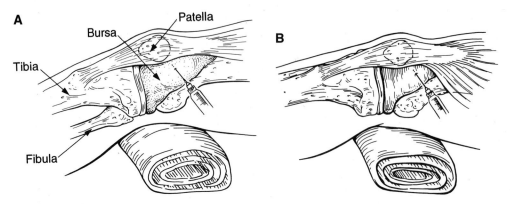

FIG. 130-19.
Knee joint. The knee is one of the easiest joints to enter, and one of the most common joints to aspirate and inject. Position the slightly flexed knee with a towel in the popliteal space on an examination table. Either a lateral (**A**) or medial (**B**) approach may be used. For the lateral approach, palpate the superior lateral aspect of the patella and insert the needle 1 cm superior and lateral to this point. Apply gentle pressure on the contralateral side of the knee to encourage the fluid to pool in the area of aspiration. Direct the needle under the patella at a 45-degree angle to the midjoint area. Aspirate all fluid prior to injection. There should be no resistance.

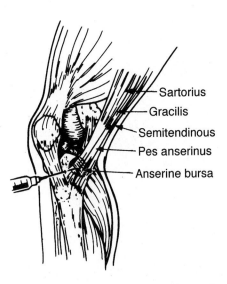

FIG. 130-20.
Anserine bursa. The anserine bursa is located on the upper medial portion of the tibia at the insertion of the sartorius, semitendinous, and gracilis tendons. This bursa frequently becomes inflamed in elderly, somewhat obese women; the symptoms are aggravated by going up and down stairs. Palpate and find the point of maximal tenderness, and insert the needle perpendicular to the tibia. When bony resistance is encountered, withdraw the needle 2 or 3 mm and inject in several areas in a fanlike fashion.

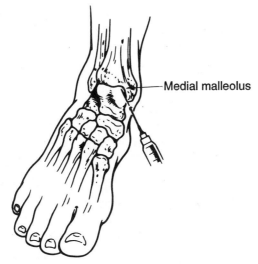

FIG. 130-21.
Ankle joint. The anteriomedial approach is the easiest. Identify the hollow between the medial malleolus and the articulation of the tibia with the talus. The needle must be inserted approximately 3 cm and directed slightly lateral.

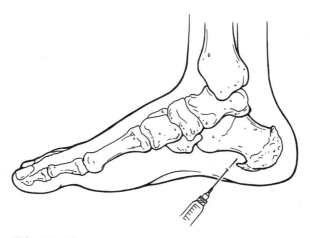

FIG. 130-22.
Calcaneal spur. Two approaches can be used. Many physicians prefer to direct the needle from the lateral side of the foot rather than from the inferior (plantar) side. The adipose tissue of the heel is uniquely segmented to provide cushion for the foot. If the plantar approach is used and steroid leaks out through the track, atrophy could result and thus the patient would have heel pain with walking. Nevertheless, many physicians approach directly from the plantar position to inject steroid right over a calcaneal spur. Using the lateral approach, the physician would direct the needle to enter just below the bony prominence of the calcaneus, and go to the midline until the point of maximal tenderness is reached.

- Steroid flare (Steroid flares occur rarely, but are very painful. The patient actually experiences more discomfort after the injection. It is not associated with fever and resolves spontaneously within 72 hours. It may be controlled with ice and/or nonsteroidal drugs.)

CPT/BILLING CODES

20550	Injection: tendon sheath, ligament, trigger points, or ganglion
20600	Arthrocentesis, aspiration and/or injection; small joint, bursa, or ganglion cyst (e.g., fingers, toes)
20605	Arthrocentesis, aspiration and/or injection, intermediate joint, bursa (e.g., temporomandibular, acromioclavicular, wrist, elbow, ankle, olecranon bursa)
20610	Arthrocentesis, aspiration and/or injection, major joint or bursa (e.g., shoulder, hip, knee, subacromial bursa)

BIBLIOGRAPHY

Anderson B, Kaye S: Treatment of flexor tenosynovitis of the hand ("trigger finger") with corticosteroids: a prospective study of the response to local injection, *Arch Intern Med* 151:153, 1991.

Gray RG, Gottlieb NL: Intraarticular corticosteroids: an updated assessment, *Clin Orthop* 177:235, 1983.

Kolba KS: The approach to the acute joint and synovial fluid examination, *Prim Care* 11:211, 1984.

Leversee JH: Aspiration of joints and soft tissue injections, *Prim Care* 13:572, 1986.

Owen DS, Irby R: Intraarticular and soft-tissue aspiration and injection, *Clin Rheum Pract* 52, March 1986.

Pfenninger JL: Injections of joints and soft tissue: Part I. General guidelines, *Am Fam Physician* 44:1196, 1991.

Pfenninger JL: Injections of joints and soft tissue: Part II. Guidelines for specific joints, *Am Fam Physician* 44:1690, 1991.

Schmerling RH et al: Synovial fluid tests—what should be ordered? *JAMA* 264:1009, 1990.

Smith DL et al: Treatment of nonseptic olecranon bursitis; a controlled, blinded prospective trial, *Arch Intern Med* 149:2527, 1989.

Stefanich RJ: Intraarticular corticosteroids in treatment of osteoarthritis, *Orthop Rev* 15(2): 65, 1986.

Wilke WS, Tuggle CJ: Optimal techniques for intraarticular and periarticular joint injections, *Mod Med* 56:58, 1988.

Zuckerman JD, Meislin RJ, Rothberg M: Injections for joint and soft tissue disorders; when and how to use them, *Geriatrics* 45(4):45, 1990.

CHAPTER 131

Extensor Tendon Repair

Thomas J. Zuber

John L. Pfenninger

Some surgeons recommend that all tendon injuries be immediately referred to a specialist. Flexor tendon lacerations can be complex injuries; these are best repaired in the operating room by an experienced surgeon. Patients with extensor tendon injuries over the forearm, wrist, or fingers may need to be referred to experienced specialist surgeons. Some extensor tendon injuries, however, such as injuries to the tendons over the dorsum of the hand, can be managed by emergency room physicians or by primary care physicians.

PRINCIPLES

For successful tendon repair, the tendons must be covered with healthy, padded skin. Skin grafting should be performed when avulsion or necrosis involves a large area of skin. Tendon injuries that are more than 8 hours old, or that are complicated by conditions such as tissue maceration or contamination, should be debrided in the operating room.

When the tendon is lacerated completely, the cut ends may retract a significant distance from the original site of trauma. Every laceration to the hands, feet, or digits must be carefully examined for underlying tendon injury. A functional deficit of the anatomical part may be the only clue of an underlying tendon injury.

Even with normal finger function on examination, a tendon may be partially lacerated. Unrepaired partial tendon lacerations can result in delayed rupture, which may occur 1 to 2 days after the initial injury. If the tendon cannot be well visualized, extend the skin incision. If the tendon has been more than half way transected, it should be repaired. If only a minimal laceration is discovered, successful results can be achieved by applying a splint for 3 weeks, followed by *passive* motion exercises for 2 to 3 weeks.

A tendon that glides around curves or joints is surrounded by a thin tendon sheath. A lacerated tendon within an intact sheath often makes no effort to heal. If the sheath is severed, the proximal tendon will "reach out" in an effort to reattach itself. The growth from the cut tendon can result in adherence to surrounding structures.

Adhesions invariably form whenever tendons are injured. Patients should be advised that, although adhesions are part of the repair process, they occasionally may interfere with function. Patients that are compliant with instructions and motivated toward rehabilitation have a greater chance of a good outcome following tendon repair.

The specialized elastic fatty tissue that allows tendons to glide over the forearm or dorsum of the foot is called paratenon. Paratenon should be placed around a repaired tendon whenever possible. Smooth, deep fascia can sometimes be used instead to promote the gliding of a repaired tendon.

Repaired tendons must be immobilized to promote healing and to prevent tendon rupture. Following hand extensor tendon repair, a plaster splint can be placed on the palmar surface from the forearm to the fingertips. The wrist is placed in 30 degrees of extension, the metacarpophalangeal joints are flexed 20 degrees, and the fingers are only slightly flexed. Do not allow the fingers to flex when the splint is changed.

A repaired tendon develops a fibroblastic bulbous connection during the first 2 weeks. Tendon *collagen* usually does not begin to form until the third week. At the end of the fourth week, swelling and vascularity will have decreased. Once the junction has become strong, the tendon can begin to perform its gliding motion.

Joint motion during the first 3 weeks often causes excessive tissue reaction and adhesion formation; therefore, 3 weeks of immobilization is generally required. Active motion started after the third week produces a favorable effect on the final strength of the repair. Strong healing can be noted in a repaired tendon as early as 6 weeks from the date of injury.

When dealing with an injury to hand *flexor* tendons, remember that the area between the proximal palmar crease and the proximal interphalangeal joints is known as "No-Man's Land." It consists of a complex series of pulleys and annular ligaments that can be functionally damaged by the original injury or by subsequent scarring.

Flexor tendon lacerations in the upper or lower extremity may best be referred to a specialist for immediate primary closure. A controlled surgical environment, proper instruments, and magnification promote the most beneficial surgical outcome. For most flexor tendon injuries, results of primary repair are better than those of secondary or delayed repair. When suturing, the clinician should avoid compressing the cut ends of the tendon, but sufficient strength should be provided to allow early passive motion of the flexor tendon.

EQUIPMENT

Routine laceration repair setup (see Chapter 3, Laceration Repair)

TECHNIQUE

Lacerations to *extensor* tendons on the dorsum of the hand between the wrist and metacarpophalangeal joints (Verdan classification zone VI) can be repaired in an office setting or emergency department. All hand lacerations should be thoroughly inspected for underlying tendon injury. Since cut tendons may retract from the skin incision, extend the fingers to pull the retracted tendon ends back to the incision site. Extensor tendons are joined to each other by cross ties on the dorsum of the hand; therefore, they usually do not retract to the same degree as flexor tendons.

Most surgeons recommend direct end-to-end repair of extensor tendon lacerations. Frequently, the Kessler technique is employed (Fig. 131-1). Approximate the cut ends of the tendon with a 4-0 nylon or Dacron suture, placing the knot inside the healing tendon. Add a running 6-0 nylon suture to provide additional stability at the laceration site. Do not use the Kessler technique to repair injuries of extensor tendons over the fingers.

When pulling the sutured ends of the tendon together, secure the suture with four knots. The approximated tendon ends should not be buckled or excessively compressed. A flat end-to-end repair promotes proper healing and a return of the proper gliding action of the tendon.

The modified Bunnell technique is often chosen for lacerations to the dorsum of the hand (Fig. 131-2). Another repair technique utilizes 5-0 nonabsorbable interrupted mattress sutures (Fig. 131-3).

All of these techniques promote good healing. Other techniques, such as the double-loop locking suture, provide greater tensile strength at the repair site and allow immediate passive motion exercise, which helps reduce adhesion formation.

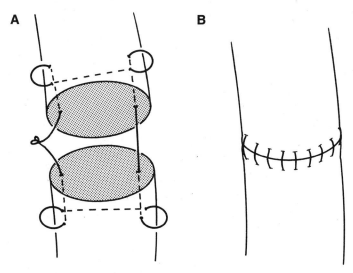

FIG. 131-1.
The Kessler technique of tendon repair. A 4-0 nylon suture is used to approximate the ends of the tendon, and the knot is buried inside the tendon (**A**). A running 6-0 nylon suture can be added to provide additional stability (**B**). The dotted line designates suture *within* the tendon.

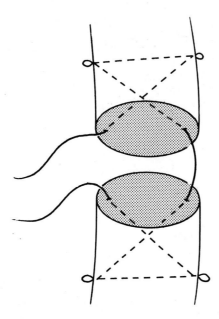

FIG. 131-2.
The modified Bunnell stitch. A nonabsorbable 4-0 suture is passed through the tendon. The suture enters the cut portion of the tendon, exits outside at the opposite side of the tendon, traverses through to the near side, and exits into the cut portion. The other portion of the cut tendon is treated similarly. An additional row of 6-0 nylon suture can be used at the laceration site, similar to the Kessler technique.

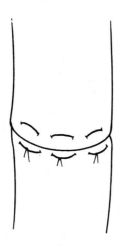

FIG. 131-3.
5-0 nylon is used to place interrupted mattress sutures to close the tendon defect.

Extensor tendon injuries over fingers (Verdan classification zones I through IV) can involve complex anatomical structures. Poorer healing more frequently results from repair over the fingers. Since the tendons lie close to the joint capsule, any complete tendon laceration over a joint should raise suspicion of joint capsule entry. Open lacerations of finger joints should be irrigated and closed in the operating room. Lacerations directly over the metacarpophalangeal joints (Verdan classification zone V) are common, and repair can be attempted in the office by skilled surgeons. Good results often follow proper repair at these sites.

COMPLICATIONS

- Infection
- Finger contracture
- Delayed rupture
- Adhesions

CPT/BILLING CODES

25270	Repair, tendon or muscle, extensor, forearm and/or wrist; primary, single, each tendon or muscle
25272	Same as above only secondary, single, each tendon or muscle
26410	Extensor tendon repair, dorsum of hand, single; primary or secondary, each tendon
26418	Extensor tendon repair, dorsum of finger, single; primary or secondary
28208	Repair or suture of tendon, foot, extensor single; primary or secondary, each tendon

BIBLIOGRAPHY

Ariyan S: *The hand book,* ed 2, Baltimore, 1983, Williams & Wilkins.

Kilgore ES, Graham WP: Hand surgery. In Dunphy JE, Way LW, editors: *Current surgical diagnosis and treatment,* ed 5, Los Altos, Calif, 1981, Lange Medical.

Kinninmonth AWG: A complication of the buried suture, *J Hand Surg* 15A:959, 1990.

Kleinert HE: Report of the committee on tendon injuries, *J Hand Surg* 14A:381, 1989.

Lee H: Double loop locking suture: a technique of tendon repair for early active mobilization, parts I and II, *J Hand Surg* 15A:945, 1990.

Mercier LR: *Practical orthopedics,* ed 2, Chicago, 1987, Year Book Medical.

Newport ML, Blair WF, Steyers CM: Long-term results of extensor tendon repair, *J Hand Surg* 15A:961, 1990.

Trott A: *Wounds and lacerations: emergency care and closure,* St Louis, 1991, Mosby.

Turek SL: *Orthopedic principles and their application,* ed 4, Philadelphia, 1984, J.B. Lippincott.

CHAPTER 132

Orthoses, Plantar Warts, Corns, and Calluses

Joseph Ellis

ORTHOTIC DEVICES

The repetitive and increased stresses placed on the feet and legs during walking and aerobic exercise can cause even mild biomechanical abnormalities to become disease. It is the function of orthotic devices to control abnormal motion and relieve the pressure from abnormal anatomical variations.

A true functional orthotic needs to be custom-made to the patient's foot, with biomechanical measurements and activity incorporated into its manufacture.

Following is a description of the basic materials available for functional orthotic devices and their applications.

Rhoadur

Rhoadur is considered the "old, reliable" material utilized for the past 20 years. Plastic in nature, it is relatively lightweight, thin, and easy to work with. Since it is a hard material, its use is restricted to rigid orthotics. Patients who need maximum control (such as those with extremely flat feet or severe overpronation) are usually placed in this device. It is not designed for most sporting activities, other than walking, because of its hardness and inflexibility—and it has a tendency to break. Rhoadur has been phased out due to a toxic waste problem that occurs during manufacturing, but it should be around a dozen more years.

Polypropylene

Polypropylene or similar material is utilized for the sport orthotics. This material is thicker than rhoadur, so it will not fit easily into dress shoes. Although it does not provide the support or rigidity of rhoadur, it handles the stresses of intense activity well, is significantly more flexible, and rarely breaks. It is used for semirigid devices.

Graphite

Graphite is the newest of the materials used in orthotic manufacture. It can be made either rigid or semirigid, depending on its thickness. It is extremely thin, and fits even into women's dress shoes and men's loafers, as well as tight-fitting shoes such as those for bicycling and ice skating. It is very lightweight and brittle. Thus, graphite has a relatively high frequency of breakage during intense physical activity.

Leather, Plastazote, and Other Soft Materials

Leather, plastazote, and other soft materials are usually used for accommodate devices. They can take pressure off of specific areas of the foot (such as collapsed metatarsals or lesions).

With new manufacturing processes and changing technology, some laboratories are incorporating gels, air, water and a host of other shock-absorbing materials into orthotic devices. These appliances have not yet found their way into the mainstream of medicine, and their effectiveness is anecdotal at this time.

Applications

Most functional orthotics include a rear foot post, and sometimes a forefoot post. These can be hard or soft materials added to the bottom of the back or front of the orthotic to help control or minimize excessive motions. In order to know the amount of correction for these posts, accurate biomechanical measurements need to be taken. There are various methods for accomplishing this, but at minimum, the motion of the subtalar joint and the midtarsal joint need to be determined. Most clinicians will place the patient in a prone position and draw a line bisecting the rear of the calcaneus. By inverting and everting the foot, the total range of motion of the subtalar joint relative to the leg can be determined. When this line is compared to the forefoot, the relative position of the midtarsal joint can be determined.

The method of obtaining the impression of the foot is critical in making a functional orthotic. Although there are differing opinions, the non–weight-bearing method is considered the most biomechanically sound. This method presently involves taking the imprint of the patient's feet while the patient is sitting or lying down. Plaster of paris is usually used to take the impression. The non–weight-bearing method allows the foot to be "captured" as it truly should be, without the abnormal motions or the forces of gravity acting on it, and without the arch collapsing. The negative cast is then filled with more plaster, so that a positive image of the non–weight-bearing foot can be used to make the necessary corrections and the proper material "pressed" or formed over it.

A variation of this method used by doctors and sporting goods retailers involves wrapping the plaster of paris onto the foot and utilizing a vacuum pump to remove the air and force the plaster into the shape of the foot. Within the next few years, computers will be utilized to take the non–weight-bearing imprint of the foot, and the image will be transmitted via modem directly to the laboratories, completely bypassing the casts.

Other semi–weight-bearing and fully weight-bearing methods involve stepping down into a box of foam, tracing the foot onto paper, and stepping onto a sheet of goldenrod or pressure-sensitive paper. Generally, these methods are used by orthotists and people using do-it-yourself kits. They serve to bridge the gap between true, functional orthotics and the over-the-counter inserts.

As a general rule, the more support that is needed, the firmer the material required for the orthotic, and the more important accurate casting and measurements become. Additionally, the more pounding there is in the activity, the more flexible the material should be. This is where clinical experience and a thorough gait evaluation helps decide how the patient will be best helped.

PLANTAR WARTS

Plantar warts are caused by the papillomavirus, which enters the skin by direct contact. The inoculation period is approximately 2 or 3 months, but can be as long as 1 year. The patient is usually 12 to 17 years of age, with women having a higher prevalence than men.

The plantar verruca must first be distinguished from other plantar lesions. The lesion must be pared down to make a diagnosis. Intractable keratoma, corns, and calluses do not have blood supply and will not bleed. Verruca, on the other hand, contain numerous capillary loops, visible as dark "dots," or with significant paring down, points of pinpoint bleeding will be seen. Plantar verruca will also never be found directly beneath a metatarsal head. They tend to be more painful to squeezing than to direct pressure.

Although there are more than 100 documented treatments for plantar warts, they can be unresponsive to any treatment, or completely regress without any treatment. The following treatments appear to have the greatest success.

Forty percent salicylic acid plaster is very effective for treatment of plantar verrucae in children. It should be applied with tape daily and removed at night for 3 to 4 weeks.

If conservative measures fail, the verruca can be bluntly dissected. A sharp blade is initially used to remove the callous tissue covering the wart. After infiltrating the area with local anesthesia, the verruca is then bluntly dissected away from the surrounding tissue. The borders are removed with a scalpel blade or tissue nippers. Because of the vascular nature of the verruca, there tends to be substantial bleeding following surgery, so a thick compression dressing needs to be applied.

Other commonly accepted methods of treatment include surgical dissection, ultrasound (2 watts × 5 minutes daily for 10 days), liquid nitrogen or other cryosurgical modalities, lidocaine injections, laser, electrodesiccation, foraging soaks, and radiofrequency excision. These methods are detailed in other chapters of this book.

CORNS

Corns are caused by pressure from a bony prominence within the foot against the shoe, the ground, or another bony protrubance. Most frequently, it evolves from a bone spur or hammertoe deformity. *Hard corns* are found on the dorsal aspect of the lesser digits, and on the lateral portion of the fifth toe. *Soft corns* are normally interdigital, and usually found in the fourth interspace due to excessive pressure from the fifth digit against the fourth digit. When the lesion is pared down, a white core is found, which will be the area of the greatest pressure. Occasionally, a sinus tract is noted, especially in soft corns.

The treatment consists of reducing the hyperkeratotic tissue and removing the mechanical forces causing the corn. The excessive skin can easily be removed with a scalpel and a sharp No. 15 blade. Care should be taken to avoid cutting into the normal skin. This treatment will give temporary relief. If a sinus tract is noted below the corn, continued debridement at weekly intervals and appropriate antibiotic therapy must be instituted.

Shoes should be evaluated to determine if they are too tight or are causing excessive pressure. If so, they must be modified or changed. Moleskin, accommodative pads, and felt spacers can be used to relieve the pressure on the underlying bone prominence. Occasionally, surgical intervention is necessary to straighten the contracted digit or reduce the underlying bony prominence. As a general rule, acid plasters are not recommended, since they might cause infections or blistering to those who are diabetic or suffer with vascular impairment.

CALLUSES

Calluses are caused by excessive friction and pressure, usually on the plantar aspect of the foot. Rather than being nucleated like a corn, calluses are comprised of diffuse hyperkeratotic tissue. It has been shown that a callus will soften when it absorbs water, but oils and petrolatum jelly have no effect on it.

Calluses are removed by shaving with a scalpel and sharp blade—after being softened with water—or they can be reduced by the patient with a pumice stone or emery board. Because there is not a nucleated section, the underlying normal vascularized tissue is red or pink and is easy to spot when enough hyperkeratotic tissue is removed.

Prevention of the friction can be accomplished with a neoprene (Spenco) innersole. This will help reduce some of the friction between the foot and the shoe. Dual-layered socks will also help absorb some of the friction.

Many times, a collapsing arch or excessive foot motion will cause callus formation. In these cases, an orthotic device will be necessary to control the motion and remove the source of friction.

Calluses on the bottom of weight-bearing areas (such as the metatarsal heads) can be potentially serious to diabetics. They must be debrided regularly and all mechanical causes prevented to decrease the likelihood of their return.

BIBLIOGRAPHY

Dockery, G: *Clinics in podiatric medicine and surgery,* vol 3, Philadelphia, 1986, W.B. Saunders.

McGlamry Ed: *Comprehensive textbook of foot surgery,* Baltimore, 1987, Williams & Wilkins.

Yale I: *Podiatric medicine,* Baltimore, 1980, Williams & Wilkins.

PART ELEVEN

Miscellaneous

Antibiotic Prophylaxis for Bacterial Endocarditis

John L. Pfenninger

The prevention of bacterial endocarditis using prophylactic antibiotics was reviewed in an article in the *Journal of the American Medical Association* by AS Dagani et al. The conclusions are summarized in the following tables, which are reproduced with permission from the American Heart Association, Committee on

TABLE 133-1.

Endocarditis Prophylaxis in Cardiac Conditions

Recommended	Not Recommended
Prosthetic cardiac valves including bioprosthetic and homograft valves	Isolated secundum atrial septal defect
Previous bacterial endocarditis, even in the absence of heart disease	Surgical repair without residua beyond 6 months of secundum atrial septal defect, ventricular septal defect, or patent ductus arteriosus
Most congenital cardiac malformations	Previous coronary artery bypass graft surgery
Rheumatic and other acquired valvular dysfunction, even after valvular surgery	Mitral valve prolapse without valvular regurgitation*
Hypertrophic cardiomyopathy	Physiologic, functional, or innocent heart murmurs
Mitral valve prolapse with valvular regurgitation	Previous Kawasaki disease without valvular dysfunction
	Previous rheumatic fever without valvular dysfunction
	Cardiac pacemakers and implanted defibrillators

*Individuals who have a mitral valve prolapse associated with thickening and/or redundancy of the valve leaflets may be at increased risk for bacterial endocarditis, particularly men who are 45 years of age or older.
From Committee on Rheumatic Fever, Endocarditis, and Kawaski Disease of the Council on Cardiovascular Disease in the Young: Prevention of bacterial endocarditis, *Circulation* 83:1174, 1991. Reproduced with permission. © 1991 American Heart Association.

TABLE 133-2.

Endocarditis Prophylaxis—Dental or Surgical Procedures

Recommended	Not Recommended†
Dental procedures known to induce gingival or mucosal bleeding, including professional cleaning	Dental procedures not likely to induce gingival bleeding, such as simple adjustment of orthodontic appliances or fillings above the gum line
Tonsillectomy and/or adenoidectomy	Injection of local intraoral anesthetic (except intraligamentary injections)
Surgical operations that involve intestinal or respiratory mucosa	Shedding of primary teeth
Bronchoscopy with a rigid bronchoscope	Tympanostomy tube insertion
Sclerotherapy for esophageal varices	Endotracheal intubation
Esophageal dilatation	Bronchoscopy with a flexible bronchoscope, with or without biopsy
Gallbladder surgery	Cardiac catheterization
Cystoscopy	Endoscopy with or without gastrointestinal biopsy
Urethral dilatation	Cesarean section
Urethral catheterization if urinary tract infection is present*	In the absence of infection for urethral catheterization, dilatation and curettage, uncomplicated vaginal delivery, therapeutic abortion, sterilization procedures, or insertion or removal of intrauterine devices
Urinary tract surgery if urinary tract infection is present*	
Prostatic surgery	
Incision and drainage of infected tissue*	
Vaginal hysterectomy	
Vaginal delivery in the presence of infection*	

*In addition to prophylactic regimen for genitourinary procedures, antibiotic therapy should be directed against the most likely bacterial pathogen.
†In patients who have prosthetic heart valves, a previous history of endocarditis, or surgically constructed systemic-pulmonary shunts or conduits, physicians may choose to administer prophylactic antibiotics even for low-risk procedures that involve the lower respiratory, genitourinary, or gastrointestinal tracts.
From Committee on Rheumatic Fever, Endocarditis, and Kawaski Disease of the Council on Cardiovascular Disease in the Young: Prevention of bacterial endocarditis, *Circulation* 83:1174, 1991. Reproduced with permission. © 1991 American Heart Association.

TABLE 133-3.

Recommended Standard Prophylactic Regimen for Dental, Oral, or Upper Respiratory Tract Procedures in Patients Who Are at Risk

Drug	Dose*
Standard Regimen	
Amoxicillin	3.0 g orally 1 hour before procedure; then 1.5 g 6 hours after initial dose
Penicillin-Allergic Patients	
Erythromycin	Erythromycin ethylsuccinate, 800 mg, or erythromycin stearate, 1.0 g orally 2 hours before procedure; then half the dose 6 hours after initial dose
Clindamycin	300 mg orally 1 hour before procedure; and 150 mg 6 hours after initial dose

*Initial pediatric doses are as follows: amoxicillin, 50 mg/kg; erythromycin ethylsuccinate or erythromycin stearate, 20 mg/kg; and clindamycin, 10 mg/kg. Follow-up doses should be one-half the initial dose. The total pediatric dose should not exceed the total adult dose. The following weight ranges may also be used for the initial pediatric dose of amoxicillin: <15 kg, 750 mg; 15 to 30 kg, 1500 mg; and >30 kg, 3000 mg (full adult dose).
From Committee on Rheumatic Fever, Endocarditis, and Kawaski Disease of the Council on Cardiovascular Disease in the Young: Prevention of bacterial endocarditis, *Circulation* 83:1174, 1991. Reproduced with permission. © 1991 American Heart Association.

TABLE 133-4.

Alternative Endocarditis Prophylaxis Regimens for Dental, Oral, or Upper Respiratory Tract Procedures

Drug	Dose*
Patients Unable to Take Oral Medications	
Ampicillin	Intravenous or intramuscular administration of ampicillin 2.0 g, 30 minutes before procedure; then intravenous or intramuscular administration of ampicillin 1.0 g, or oral administration of amoxicillin 1.5 g, 6 hours after initial dose
Penicillin-Allergic Patients Unable to Take Oral Medications	
Clindamycin	Intravenous administration of 300 mg 30 minutes before procedure and an intravenous or oral administration of 150 mg 6 hours after initial dose
High-Risk Patients Not Candidates for Standard Regimen	
Ampicillin, gentamicin, and amoxicillin	Intravenous or intramuscular ampicillin 2.0 g, plus gentamicin, 1.5 mg/kg (not to exceed 80 mg), 30 minutes before procedure; followed by oral amoxicillin 1.5 g, 6 hours after initial dose; alternatively, the parenteral regimen may be repeated 8 hours after initial dose
Penicillin-Allergic Patients Considered High Risk	
Vancomycin	Intravenous administration of 1.0 g over 1 hour starting 1 hour before procedure; no repeat dose necessary

*Initial pediatric doses are as follows: ampicillin, 50 mg/kg; clindamycin, 10 mg/kg; gentamicin, 2.0 mg/kg; and vancomycin, 20 mg/kg. Follow-up doses should be one-half the initial dose. The total pediatric dose should not exceed the total adult dose. No initial dose is recommended in this table for amoxicillin (25 mg/kg is the follow-up dose).

From Committee on Rheumatic Fever, Endocarditis, and Kawaski Disease of the Council on Cardiovascular Disease in the Young: Prevention of bacterial endocarditis, *Circulation* 83:1174, 1991. Reproduced with permission. © 1991 American Heart Association.

TABLE 133-5.

Regimens for Genitourinary/Gastrointestinal Procedures

Drug	Dose*
Standard Regimen	
Ampicillin, gentamicin, and amoxicillin	Intravenous or intramuscular administration of ampicillin, 2.0 g, plus gentamicin, 1.5 mg/kg (not to exceed 80 mg), 30 minutes before procedure; followed by amoxicillin, 1.5 g, orally 6 hours after initial dose; alternatively, the parenteral regimen may be repeated once 8 hours after initial dose
Penicillin-Allergic Patient Regimen	
Vancomycin and gentamicin	Intravenous administration of vancomycin, 1.0 g, over 1 hour plus intravenous or intramuscular administration of gentamicin, 1.5 mg/kg (not to exceed 80 mg) 1 hour before procedure; may be repeated once 8 hours after initial dose
Alternative Low-Risk Patient Regimen	
Amoxicillin	3.0 g orally 1 hour before procedure; then 1.5 g 6 hours after initial dose

*Initial pediatric doses are as follows: ampicillin, 50 mg/kg; amoxicillin, 50 mg/kg; gentamicin, 2.0 mg/kg; and vancomycin, 20 mg/kg. Follow-up doses should be one-half the initial dose. Total pediatric dose should not exceed total adult dose.

From Committee on Rheumatic Fever, Endocarditis, and Kawaski Disease of the Council on Cardiovascular Disease in the Young: Prevention of bacterial endocarditis, *Circulation* 83:1174, 1991. Reproduced with permission. © 1991 American Heart Association.

Rheumatic Fever, Endocarditis, and Kawasaki Disease of the Council on Cardiovascular Disease in the Young.

Those seeking further discussion are referred to the article in the *Journal of the American Medical Association*.

BIBLIOGRAPHY

Antimicrobial prophylaxis in surgery, *Med Letter* 35(906):91, 1993.

Dagani AS et al: Prevention of bacterial endocarditis, *JAMA* 264(2):2919, 1990.

Weitekamp MR, Caputo GM: Antiobiotic prophylaxis: update on common clinical uses, *Am Fam Physician* 48(4):597, 1993.

CHAPTER 134

Informed Consent

Julie Graves Moy

Before the performance of any procedure, the patient and the physician must discuss the reasons for performing the procedure, the treatment options, the possible complications from the procedure, and the possible complications from not having the procedure. Informed consent is often considered to be just a signature on a form before beginning the procedure, and many physicians believe (or hope) that a signed consent form is insurance against a malpractice lawsuit. However, as it is currently interpreted by many courts, a consent form is not sufficient to protect a physician from litigation.

There is no single doctrine of informed consent across the country, and different court decisions have used different standards. Before 1957, physicians accused of not informing patients of potential risk were charged on grounds of battery. In 1957, the emphasis changed to that of deviation from the standard of conduct of a reasonable and prudent physician; a physician was negligent in informing the patient only if the process used was different from that used by most other physicians. The current, most common standard, introduced in 1972, is the "reasonable man" standard of material risk, which means that physicians must tell a patient what a reasonable person in the patient's position would want to know, and that risks that are not serious or are unlikely are not considered material. Most courts expect the disclosure before a procedure to include diagnosis, the nature of the proposed procedure, risks and benefits of the procedure, available alternatives and their risks and benefits, and the consequences of not having the procedure. Courts usually do not require the physician to disclose the risks the patient is already aware of or which an average patient is likely to know. The courts have been criticized for setting standards that do not actually reflect medical practice and may interfere with the doctor-patient relationship. The problem may lie in the implementation, not in the actual concept. The ethical concept of informed consent includes the concepts from the courts, but goes further: the patient must be a partner in the decision-making process (Box 134-1).

The legal development of medical informed consent has not been uniform across states, and some states have codified certain procedures, clarifying the

---

BOX 134-1. ELEMENTS OF INFORMED CONSENT

Disclosure of information
Competency (The patient is not a minor, unconscious, intoxicated, grossly
    psychotic, or senile.)
Understanding
Voluntariness
Decision making
Patient participation

---

responsibility of the physician. Texas, for example, established panels of doctors and lawyers who together write rules for informed consent. Michigan mandates that all women receive a state-approved booklet before mastectomy for breast cancer. All physicians should be aware of the law in their own state, both legislative efforts and court decisions.

PROCEDURE

Just as the laws have evolved in clarifying informed consent, the transition toward involving the patient more in the process has also changed. There are basically four models of medical decision making.

1. Traditional model: The physician decides whether to perform a procedure and which procedure to perform; the patient's trust and confidence in the doctor replace the need for consent.
2. Traditional informed consent: The physician decides whether to perform a procedure and which procedure to perform with the patient's informed consent.
3. Collaboration: The physician and the patient work together to make a joint decision about the procedure.
4. Patient choice: The patient decides with the physician's counsel.

Some patients will choose the traditional model if given the option of one of the four, and a few will choose the last model. Most patients and physicians are more comfortable with either traditional informed consent or collaboration, and physicians should learn to use both of these models as well as how to determine which to use for a specific patient.

All office procedures should be preceded by a discussion that allows the patient to participate in, and perhaps even lead, the decision about whether to have the procedure. The patient should sign a document that summarizes the process. Some states have laws that specify certain language on consent forms for certain procedures. There is rarely an exception to the rule that all procedures should be preceded by the patient's consent. It may be permissible in some cases to obtain verbal consent, but this should be documented explicitly by the physician in the medical record.

Minor children and adults who are not competent to make decisions about their own health may not give consent. For these patients, consent must be obtained from a parent or legal guardian. In emergencies, it is permissible to perform procedures without patient consent, but state law determines the appropriate procedure, such as having two physicians not involved in the case sign the form. Some states also allow the suspension of the informed consent process for reason of therapeutic privilege, the principle under which the physician is excused from disclosure if information given to the patient might have a detrimental effect on the physical or psychological well-being of the patient. This situation can be interpreted differently by different courts, and physicians should use caution before employing the privilege.

In many states, certain procedures are subject to specified forms that list risks for the procedure, and the specific form for that procedure must be used. The legal departments of state medical societies can provide physicians with the laws governing informed consent in that state. In cases that do not require specific forms, a general consent form that allows identification of the patient, the procedure, the indications, and the risks can be used (Box 134-2). Most states require a witness to sign the consent; many offices ask nurses or other office staff to witness, but there are possible conflict-of-interest issues if litigation ensues. If possible, a family member or friend of the patient should serve as a witness to the consent process in addition to office staff.

The process of discussing the procedure with the patient and providing education about the procedure itself, the possible complications, and aftercare responsibilities of the patient should all be considered part of the consent process. The consent form can be used as a patient education tool, with a copy containing the patient's signature to be given to the patient for reference. Patients can be educated during the consent process about the legal requirements for the signed form and the fact that results of medical procedures are not guaranteed. However, bringing the form out at the last minute for signature is thought to produce some anxiety and suspicion on the part of the patient. A better strategy may be to start the process by giving the patient the consent form to read, then using the form to guide the discussion. The consent form can include postprocedure instructions as well as instructions for contacting the physician or an associate if complications occur after hours.

Many liability insurance companies are beginning to advise that patients view videotapes discussing the proposed procedure. This assures that the patient has an opportunity to consider all the pertinent information as well as documents it for liability defense.

The actual process of informed consent can be summarized as follows:

1. Establish responsibility.
   a. The doctor's role.
   b. The patient's role.
2. Establish expected duration of responsibility.
3. Define the problem in negotiation with patient.
4. Set goals for treatment and establish whether cure is a reasonable expectation.

BOX 134–2. PATIENT CONSENT FORM

I came to the office of Dr. _____ on _____ [date] for evaluation and treatment of the following condition:

(description of diagnosis, etiology, and differential diagnosis)

We discussed the different treatments possible, and discussed the risks of not treating the condition. Based upon the advice given by Dr. _____ and my own judgment, I agree to undergo the following procedure:

(description of anesthetic, procedure, and dressing)

We discussed the different outcomes that could occur, and most of the possible complications. I am aware that other complications could occur that we could not foresee. I agree to follow the instructions for self-care after the procedure, and to return for follow-up care on: _____ .

I will call the office or answering service if any problems arise before the scheduled follow-up visit.

_____   _____
Patient signature   Date and time

_____   _____
Witness signature   Physician's signature

One copy for chart, one copy for patient

---

5. Select an approach to treatment; during this step the informed consent form is signed.
6. Perform extended treatment and follow-up.

COMPLICATIONS

"At the core of most lawsuits is either surprise or disappointment."

Elvoy Raines, JD

Physicians must not rely on a signed form for protection in court in the case of a malpractice lawsuit. Courts have imposed a duty-to-warn on physicians, and they do not always consider the patient's role in decision making or causation of injury. The usual method of bringing out a highly technical consent form at the last minute makes patients nervous and insecure and can alienate them. Courts consider consent documents as only one form of evidence, and in lawsuits other evidence is examined as well. The form itself cannot substitute for candid discussion with the patient about the procedure and inclusion of the patient in the decision-making process, or for documentation (in the medical record) of the discussion before signing the form. For some patients, particularly uninformed or anxious patients, knowledge of the risk can dissuade them from undergoing a needed procedure. *Courts do not consider a signed form as evidence that consent was informed.* Many forms use language that is too technical; the forms are often too long to read and interpret during an office visit; and some patients are unable to comprehend the procedure even after explanation. In order to provide the type of documentation most useful in a court case, the physician should include in the patient's chart a narrative of the discussion between doctor and patient during the decision-making process, in addition to the actual consent form.

CPT/BILLING CODES

98900	Medical conference by physician regarding medical management with patient and/or relative or guardian; 30 minutes
98902	Medical conference by physician regarding medical management with patient and/or relative or guardian; 60 minutes

BIBLIOGRAPHY

Green JA: Minimizing malpractice risk by role clarification: the confusing transition from tort to contract, *Am Intern Med* 109(3):234, 1988.

Lidz CW, Appelbaum PS, Meisel A: Two models of implementing informed consent, *Ann Intern Med* 148(6):1385, 1988.

Mazur DJ: What should patients be told prior to a medical procedure? Ethical and legal perspectives on medical informed consent, *Am J Med* 81(6):1051, 1986.

Caterine JM, Miller B: Informed consent: procedure specific, *Iowa Med* 79(5):231, 1989.

Sprung CL, Winick BJ: Informed consent in theory and practice: legal and medical perspectives on the informed consent doctrine and a proposed reconceptualization, *Crit Care Med* 17(12):1346, 1989.

CHAPTER 135

Anaphylaxis

Daniel J. Derksen

Anaphylaxis is an acute and serious allergic reaction in response to antigen exposure in a previously sensitized patient. It can be encountered after administration of intramuscular antibiotics, vaccines, contrast material (IVP or computed tomography contrast), local anesthetics, or allergy injection in the office setting. In addition, patients may come in after an insect bite, pollen exposure, food-product ingestion, or unknown substance exposure with a clinical picture of anaphylaxis. The anaphylactic response is IgE antibody mediated, which results in the release of chemicals from mast cells and basophils.

Since medical procedures frequently require injections or use of foreign materials, the clinician performing various procedures must be prepared to treat the rare but serious complication of anaphylaxis.

DIAGNOSIS

Depending on the severity of reaction, patients may have a variety of symptoms including swelling, rash, urticaria, pruritus, dyspnea, and decreased blood pressure from baseline. As the anaphylaxis proceeds, respiratory compromise may occur with laryngeal edema, bronchospasm, and hypoxia. The patient may progress into shock as manifested by hypotension, bradycardia, peripheral vasodilation, and mental status changes. If steps are not taken quickly to reverse the anaphylactoid reaction in the final stages, vascular collapse and death can occur within minutes.

Vasovagal reactions (fainting and seizurelike activity) and injection of intravascular anesthetic can cause lightheadedness and ringing in the ears, and can be confused with an anaphylactic response.

EQUIPMENT

Any physician or practitioner should be prepared to treat anaphylaxis in the office, especially if any type of injections are given. A collection of medications and equipment, the so-called "crash cart," can be gathered and placed in one area. Alternatively, a fishing tackle box, or similar box or medical bag, can be made. The simplest and best-organized method is to use commercially available Banyan kits. These kits, similar to suitcases, are commercially available and are stocked with various medications and vary in size, contents, and cost ($300 to $800). However, the Banyan Stat Kit 800 is essentially a portable crash cart, lacking only a defibrillator. The Banyan company provides check sheets that can be reviewed regularly to reorder out-of-date stock.

Whether the commercially available kits are used or a do-it-yourself collection is assembled, the entire office staff must know where the kit is stored. One person must be in charge of keeping the medications up to date. Drugs *cannot* be borrowed from this kit for other purposes.

The physician doing office procedures must be prepared for emergencies. Assembling a crash cart or obtaining a Banyan kit may appear expensive, but it is good medicine to have one available and cheap malpractice coverage in the event of an emergency.

The specifics on medications and equipment needed are too extensive to detail here. Refer to the Banyan Kit 800.

TECHNIQUE

Patients who exhibit signs and symptoms of anaphylaxis should be treated immediately. In the earliest stages, anxiety, swelling, urticaria, pruritus, and mild dyspnea will respond very quickly to epinephrine. Dosage can be 0.3 to 0.5 ml of a 1:1000 solution, given subcutaneously every 20 to 30 minutes, as needed to a maximum of three doses. In the milder reactions, antihistamines such as Benadryl (diphenhydramine hydrochloride), 25 to 50 mg by the intravenous (IV), intramuscular (IM) or oral (PO) route every 6 hours can be given. Systemic steroids can be given as a prednisone taper, beginning with 30 to 60 mg the first day and gradual tapering to nothing over a 2-week period. In truly emergent situations, give 100 mg solumedrol intravenously. For life-threatening reactions, 5 ml of a 1:10,000 solution of epinephrine should be given intravenously and repeated every 5 minutes as needed. In addition, an ambulance should be summoned if intubation and resuscitation materials are not available in the clinic. It is important to observe patients with anaphylaxis or anaphylactoid reactions for 4 to 6 hours after treatment of a reaction to ensure that recurrence does not occur.

A quick way to administer epinephrine is to have a preloaded syringe system of epinephrine (e.g., Epi Pen-Epinephrine Auto-Injector, Ana-Kit Anaphylaxis Treatment Kit) available in the office. This eliminates the delay involved in drawing up epinephrine in a syringe before administration. Each examination room should have one of these injection systems taped to a cabinet door for ready access.

SUPPLIERS

Banyan Kits
   Banyan International Corp.
   2118 E. Interstate 20
   P.O. Box 1779
   Abilene, TX 79604-9963
   800-351-4530
Ana-Kit Anaphylaxis Emergency Treatment Kit
   Miles Allergy Pharmaceuticals
   400 Morgan Lane
   West Haven, CT 06516
Epi Pen
   Center Laboratories
   Division of EM Pharmaceuticals, Inc.
   35 Channel Drive
   Port Washington, NY 11050

PREVENTION WITH PREVIOUS HISTORY

Some patients may require tests that necessitate the use of known allergens. For example, patients may require a computed tomography scan with contrast material that previously caused urticaria, dyspnea, or other signs of early anaphylaxis. If an alternative contrast agent cannot be used, and the test is critical to the diagnostic workup, the patient can be counseled about the risks, informed consent obtained, and the patient can be premedicated with Benadryl and steroids to minimize the risk of an anaphylactic reaction. This can be done with 50 to 100 mg of Benadryl taken orally 1 hour before the procedure, and 100 mg hydrocortisone or 50 mg solumedrol given intravenously. The patient should be observed carefully for at least 6 hours following the procedure.

PRECAUTIONS

Procedures and medications that could result in anaphylaxis should not be administered unless the office is equipped to deal with this complication. At a minimum, the office should be able to give subcutaneous epinephrine, give supplemental oxygen, and supply ventilation to the patient until emergency services can arrive. In general, procedures and medications that carry a high risk of anaphylaxis should be followed by an appropriate observation period after the procedure to watch for signs and symptoms.

PATIENT EDUCATION

Sensitized patients should receive detailed patient education. Such patients should be encouraged to wear a medical identification bracelet that identifies the agent that could cause anaphylaxis (e.g., penicillin, a bee sting, IVP contrast). Some patients with recurrent severe anaphylactoid reactions may carry a kit with them (containing 1:1000 epinephrine that can be injected) so that initial treatment can begin without delay. For example, a beekeeper with a known sensitivity to bee stings who refuses to explore a new profession should be encouraged to carry a kit. Patients with previous anaphylaxis should be instructed to seek prompt medical attention for the following symptoms:

Shortness of breath
Swelling (eyes, legs, hands)
Dizziness
Sensation of swelling in the throat
Raised, red rashes (urticaria)
Change in mental status

BIBLIOGRAPHY

Miller TP, Greenberger PA: Anaphylaxis: recognition and management, *Hosp Med*:79, October 1991.

CHAPTER 136

Heimlich Maneuver

Raymond E. Jarris, Jr.

The estimated death rate from swallowed or aspirated objects in the United States is 3000 cases per year. In the event of partial foreign body aspiration, the patient may be able to breathe and speak. The Heimlich maneuver and probing of the oropharynx should then be avoided, and the patient transported to a source of medical care. However, when a patient displays the distress signal for choking (clutching the neck) or becomes cyanotic, unconscious, or unable to effectively cough or breathe—suggesting complete obstruction—efforts to clear the obstruction are warranted. The Heimlich maneuver causes a sudden increase in intrathoracic pressure, forcing an obstructing object from the glottis (Fig. 136-1).

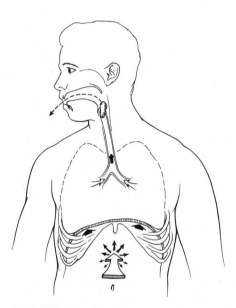

FIG. 136-1.
If the patient is sitting or standing, stand behind the patient and encircle his waist with your arms. Place your fist with the thumb side against the patient's abdomen above the umbilicus, but below the rib cage.

INDICATIONS

- Asphyxiation from foreign body obstruction of the upper airway

CONTRAINDICATIONS

- Infants, small children, and pregnant women (Abdominal thrusts are inappropriate.)

TECHNIQUE

Adults or Children More Than One-Year Old

1. Sitting or standing
   a. Apply three to five abdominal or chest thrusts (Fig. 136-2, *A*).

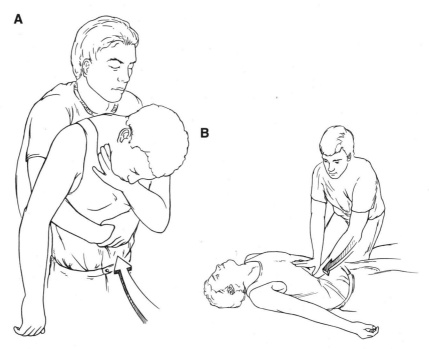

FIG. 136-2.
Abdominal thrusts. **A,** If the patient is sitting or standing, stand behind the patient, wrap your arms around the patient's waist, grasp your fist or wrist of one hand with the other, place your hands against the patient's abdomen between the navel and rib cage, and press your fist into the patient's abdomen with a quick thrust upward. Repeat up to three to five times. **B,** If the patient has collapsed or is unable to be lifted, place the patient in the supine position and kneel at the side of the patient's abdomen or straddle it. Place one of your hands on top of the other, with the heel of the bottom hand in the midline between the patient's navel and rib cage. Lean forward so that your shoulders are over the patient's abdomen, and press toward the diaphragm with a quick thrust inward and upward. Do not press to the right or left of the midline. Repeat up to three to five times if necessary.

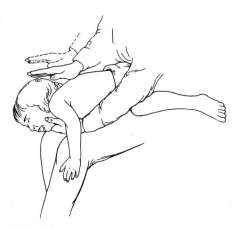

FIG. 136-3.
Back blows for infants and small children. See text for details.

2. Lying
   a. Place the patient in the supine position.
   b. Place one of your hands on top of the other with the heel of the bottom hand positioned in the midline of the patient, between the umbilicus and xiphoid.
   c. Lean forward with your shoulders over the patient's abdomen and quickly press inward and upward three to five times (Fig. 136-2, *B*).
   d. In pregnant or obese patients, use chest thrusts delivered in the same fashion as Step c but with the hands placed over the sternum.
   e. Clear material from the oropharynx with a finger sweep or McGill forceps.

Infants and Small Children

1. Place the child face down on your arm with head directed downward, supporting head and neck with knee and one hand (Fig. 136-3).
2. Deliver three to five gentle back blows between the scapulae with the palm of your hand.
3. If obstruction is still present, roll the child over, lower his or her head, and deliver chest thrusts gently with two to three fingers as in cardiopulmonary resuscitation.
4. Repeat Steps 2 and 3 until the object is cleared or surgical intervention is appropriate.

COMPLICATIONS

- Gastric rupture
- Liver, spleen, or pancreas injury
- Regurgitation
- Rib fracture

BIBLIOGRAPHY

Hedges R: *Clinical procedures in emergency medicine,* Philadelphia, 1991, W.B. Saunders.

Schwartz GR: *Principles and practice of emergency medicine,* Philadelphia, 1986, W.B. Saunders.

CHAPTER 137

Topical Hemostatic Agents

Thomas J. Zuber

John L. Pfenninger

Hemostasis following surgical procedures decreases wound complication rates and improves patient comfort and acceptance. Topical hemostatic agents are useful in controlling bleeding from capillaries and small vessels. Physical measures including direct wound pressure, cold application, or clamping of larger vessels may be employed initially. Topical agents are used whenever rapid hemostasis is desired, or when other measures (such as pressure) fails to control bleeding. Hemostatic agents may be useful in settings where electrocautery or radiofrequency units are unavailable.

Topical hemostatic agents hasten clot formation and provide the structural support necessary for physiologic hemostasis. Most hemostatic agents produce vasoconstriction, vasocclusion, platelet adhesion, or concentrate coagulants.

Table 137-1 describes the commonly used topical hemostatic agents for dermatologic surgery. The products may be divided into three groups: agents with vasoconstrictive, vasocclusive, or denaturing effects; agents producing a physical meshwork; and physiologic agents. The older agents are generally in the first grouping. Each of the products listed in Table 137-1 has also been rated for effectiveness, ease of preparation and application, and cost.

This chapter examines the topical hemostatic agents most frequently considered for controlling bleeding during office surgical procedures.

VASOCONSTRICTIVE, VASOCCLUSIVE, OR DENATURING AGENTS

All the agents noted in this section are applied topically and generally are not used if a wound is closed surgically.

Silver Nitrate

The solid form of silver nitrate is supplied on wooden sticks that have one end coated with the coagulant. This delivery method provides for easy application. Solid silver nitrate is activated when placed on a moist, bleeding wound bed. Silver

TABLE 137-1.

Topical Hemostatic Agents

Generic/Product Name	Effectiveness	Difficulty of Preparation/ Application	Cost
Vasoconstrictive/Vasocclusive/Denaturing Agents			
Silver nitrate sticks	+++	+	++
Ferric subsulfate solution (20%)(Monsel's solution)	+++	++	++
Aluminum chloride (30%)	+++	++	++
Trichloroacetic acid (50% to 85%)	++	++++	++
Zinc chloride paste	++	+++	++
Cocaine hydrochloride	+++	++++	+++
Phenol 50%	++	+++	++
Hydrogen peroxide	+	++	+
Agents Producing a Physical Meshwork			
Absorbable gelatin sponge (Gelfoam)	+++	++++	+++
Oxidized cellulose (Surgicel)	++++	++++	+++
Microfibrillar collagen (Avitene)	+++++	+++++	+++++
Physiologic Hemostatic Agents			
Epinephrine	+++	++	+
Thrombin (Thrombostat)	+++++	++++	+++++
Fibrin sealant (Tissue glue)	+++++	+++++	+++++

Agents rated from
+ Mildly effective   to   +++++ Highly effective
+ Easy to prepare/apply   to   +++++ Difficult to prepare/apply
+ Low cost   to   +++++ High cost

nitrate solutions in strengths of 20% to 50% may also be employed. Silver ions cause proteins to precipitate, resulting in the occlusion of blood vessels. The eschar that forms in wound beds prevents deeper tissue penetration by the hemostatic agent. Silver nitrate is inexpensive, readily available, and has the additional benefit of being a powerful germicidal. However, when multiple sticks are required (e.g., after cervical biopsies), it can be more expensive than Monsel's solution.

Silver salts will stain the tissue beds black due to the deposition of reduced silver. Most of the stain slowly disappears spontaneously, but silver may persist indefinitely, causing a tattooing effect. The use of silver nitrate has decreased because of its slow onset of action and variable depth of tissue destruction. Silver nitrate is caustic, and can be used for tissue destruction in the treatment of pyogenic granulomas or anal fissures. Care must be used with silver nitrate to avoid damaging normal tissue surrounding a wound.

Monsel's Solution (Ferric Subsulfate)

Monsel's solution, or 20% ferric subsulfate, is one of the most commonly used hemostatic agents. First described by Leon Monsel in 1856, the solution is prepared by reacting ferric sulfate with sulfuric and nitric acids. The solution is a very dark brown, almost black. The supernatant solution or precipitate is more effective, and can be obtained by leaving a small bottle open at all times. Evaporation and settling will produce the precipitate at the bottom of the bottle, as well as debris at the mouth of the container. Application of Monsel's solution to a dry wound bed (achieved by drying and stretching the skin) produces good results.

Monsel's solution is applied using a cotton-tipped swab and light pressure. The low pH and the subsulfate group denature protein and occlude blood vessels. Monsel's solution is easily stored, readily available, easily applied, and inexpensive.

Monsel's solution has rarely been noted to cause skin pigmentation and tatooing. While some believe that Monsel's solution should not be used on the face, others feel that the rarity of tatooing should not limit its use. Treatment with Monsel's solution deposits iron that can be incorporated into macrophages and cause hyperpigmentation, thereby causing difficulty in histologic assessment if a wound must be reexcised. Monsel's solution also may delay wound healing.

Aluminum Chloride

Aluminum chloride is usually applied to a wound as a 30% solution, using a swab and light pressure. First, the wound is dried as much as possible. Aluminum chloride hydrolyzes to hydrochloric acid, and the acid is believed to cause hemostasis by tissue coagulation and vasoconstriction. Aluminum chloride is colorless, readily available, easily stored, easy to handle, and inexpensive. This solution is frequently employed following shave excision or curettage techniques.

Aluminum chloride forms a thin layer of coagulum (eschar) over the wound base. As a caustic agent, this solution may produce burning pain and tissue irritation when applied to normal skin. There is concern that aluminum chloride may slow wound healing and may produce larger scars, as compared to using direct pressure for hemostasis. Part of the delay in wound-healing produced by aluminum chloride may be reversed by applying an occlusive dressing (see Chapter 138, Wound Dressing). Aluminum chloride has not been noted to produce tatoos as observed with Monsel's solution. In a wound that is left uncovered (e.g., a shave excision on the face), its use may be more cosmetically pleasing since it is colorless both before and after application.

Trichloroacetic Acid

Trichloroacetic acid (TCA) is readily available, easy to use, and a very effective hemostatic agent. The tissue destruction produced by the acid leaves an eschar at the base of the wound. Some physicians advocate avoiding this agent because of the variable strength of the solution, the unpredictable depth of tissue destruction, and the risk of spillage onto normal tissue. Without anesthesia, it can be painful when it runs onto surrounding skin. Application must be meticulous, since normal tissue may be destroyed. In fact, TCA is frequently employed for the destruction of warts. Solutions of 50% to 85% may be used, but in general, its use for hemostasis is discouraged.

Other Agents

Zinc chloride paste is a mildly effective hemostatic agent that is used by some Mohs micrographic surgeons. The intense vasoconstriction produced by *cocaine* makes this agent useful for hemostasis, especially on mucosal surfaces. The potential for abuse, the cost, and the need for locked storage make the use of cocaine problematic. *Phenol 50%* is effective and readily available, but the caustic effects on normal tissue may enlarge a wound. *Hydrogen peroxide* is often overlooked as a hemostatic agent. Hydrogen peroxide has mild hemostatic and germicidal actions, is inexpensive, is easy to apply, and leaves no residual to serve as a nidus for infection. It also causes some degree of tissue destruction.

AGENTS PROVIDING A PHYSICAL MESHWORK

Absorbable Gelatin Sponge/Powder

Absorbable gelatin is prepared in various forms from purified gelatin solution. Gelatin powder is applied dry to the wound bed with light pressure. Gelatin sponges (such as Gelfoam, available from Upjohn, Kalamazoo, Michigan) can be applied dry or moistened with saline or thrombin. Absorbable gelatin holds blood and allows clot formation and granulation tissue to form. The sponges are moderately priced, convenient, and easy to handle.

Excessive granuloma formation and fibrosis have been reported with absorbable gelatin. Care should be exercised when these agents are used near tendons, which can become excessively fibrosed. The gelatin powder can be difficult to handle. Absorbable gelatin may be less effective than other meshwork agents.

Oxidized Cellulose

Oxidized cellulose is an absorbable fiber prepared from cellulose. Woven strips of cellulose (such as Surgicel, available from Johnson and Johnson, Arlington, Texas) can be cut and held with firm pressure on the wound bed. Oxidized cellulose provides a meshwork for coagulation and causes local vasoconstriction. This preparation is moderately priced, easy to handle, and is mildly bactericidal.

Foreign-body reaction is possible if excessive amounts of cellulose are left in a wound. Cellulose should not be used under grafts or flaps because it separates the graft from the blood supply. Some experts feel that the removal of oxidized cellulose after obtaining hemostasis frequently produces rebleeding.

Microfibrillar Collagen

Microfibrillar collagen is prepared by mechanically breaking down bovine collagen into fibrils. Microfibrillar collagen is available in a fibrous (granular) form (such as Avitene, available from Alcon Laboratories, Fort Worth, Texas) or a web form. The fibrous form is applied directly to the wound and held in place. The highly effective collagen products aggregate platelets on their surface. Collagen matrix applied to skin biopsy sites produces fewer infections, faster healing, and better cosmetic results than Monsel's solution.

Microfibrillar collagen adheres to wet gloves or surfaces, and it must be applied with dry instruments. While the collagen is eventually absorbed, *it cannot be used at skin closure sites* since it impedes the healing of wound edges. The high cost and difficulty in handling make this agent impractical for most office dermatologic surgery.

PHYSIOLOGIC HEMOSTATIC AGENTS

Epinephrine

Epinephrine is a potent activator of adrenergic receptors; the activation of alpha receptors produces vasoconstriction in the skin. Epinephrine is available in local anesthetics such as lidocaine with epinephrine (available from Elkins-Sinn, Cherry Hill, New Jersey) or as adrenalin chloride solution (available from Parke-Davis, Morris Plains, New Jersey). Epinephrine is inexpensive and readily available, and it does not coagulate normal tissue at the base of the wound.

Despite the common belief that epinephrine produces intense vasoconstriction and gangrene when used in digits or the penis, this complication may be very rare. Rebound vasodilation can potentially cause delayed bleeding. Cardiac arrhythmias and other neurologic symptoms have been reported with the use of epinephrine in dermatologic procedures.

Thrombin

Thrombin is a potent physiologic clotting agent produced by the activation of bovine prothrombin. This freeze-dried powder can be either mixed with isotonic saline and sponged or sprayed on the wound bed or applied directly as a powder. The wound bed should be sponged free of excess blood before thrombin is applied. For superficial surgery or plastic surgery involving flaps, dilute solutions of 100 units per ml may be effective. The 5000-unit vial kit of Thrombostat (available from Parke-Davis, Morris Plains, New Jersey) is routinely diluted to 1000 units per ml.

Thrombin does not injure tissue or produce residue on the tissue bed. Once the solution is prepared, it must be used within 6 hours. Thrombin is very expensive, and the high cost prohibits routine use of this agent in office procedures.

Fibrin Sealant (Tissue Glue)

Fibrin sealant is produced by mixing two components of human clotting factors immediately before application. Fibrin clot forms in about 30 seconds; the sealant can be applied with a special spraying device that mixes the components as they are delivered into the wound. Fibrin glue is one of the most effective agents available for hemostasis. The cost, the risk in the use of human blood products, and the cumbersome administration make this therapy undesirable for routine dermatologic surgery.

SUMMARY

Topical hemostatic agents are not a substitute for meticulous surgical technique. Physical measures such as direct pressure, cold application, or suture ligatures should be considered first-line therapy. The ease and speed of topical hemostatic agents make them desirable for many office surgical procedures.

Several of the physical meshwork agents have the advantage of being absorbable, and they may be left in wounds; however, most physicians advocate leaving as little foreign material as possible in a wound. The high cost of some of the meshwork and physiologic agents makes them prohibitive for most office procedures. A small office supply of oxidized cellulose may be beneficial for selected patient use.

Despite the negative reports involving Monsel's solution and aluminum chloride, most physicians still advocate their routine use in dermatologic surgery. Topical agents that prolong healing can be used in conjunction with occlusive dressings to offset this effect. Aluminum chloride may be the preferred agent for facial wounds due to the rare tatooing that can occur with Monsel's solution.

BIBLIOGRAPHY

Armstrong RB, Nichols J, Pachance J: Punch biopsy wounds treated with Monsel's solution or a collagen matrix: a comparison of healing, *Arch Dermatol* 122:546, 1986.

Baden HP: Rapid hemostasis with Monsel's solution, *Arch Dermatol* 120:708, 1984.

Camisa C, Roberts W: Monsel's solution tatooing, *J Am Acad Dermatol* 7:753, 1982.

Duray PH, LiVolsi VA: Recurrent dysplastic nevus following shave excision, *J Dermatol Surg Oncol* 10:811, 1984.

Grekin RC, Auletta MJ: Local anesthesia in dermatologic surgery, *J Am Acad Dermatol* 19:599, 1988.

Landry JR, Kanat IO: Considerations in topical hemostasis, *J Am Podiatr Med Assoc* 75:581, 1985.

Larson PO: Topical hemostatic agents for dermatologic surgery, *J Dermatol Surg Oncol* 14:623, 1988.

Maddin S, Carruthers A, Brown TH: *Current dermatologic therapy,* Philadelphia, 1982, W.B. Saunders.

Raccuia JS et al: Comparative efficacy of topical hemostatic agents in a rat kidney model, *Am J Surg* 163:234, 1992.

Sawchuk WS et al: Delayed healing in full-thickness wounds treated with aluminum chloride solution: a histologic study with evaporimetry correlation, *J Am Acad Dermatol* 15:982, 1986.

Stegman SJ, Tromovitch TA, Glogau RG: *Basics of dermatologic surgery,* Chicago, 1982, Year Book Medical.

CHAPTER 138

Wound Dressing

William Dery

In the past, medical practice dictated that dressings be designed to keep the wound dry. Typically, gauze was secured with tape to protect the wound, without much thought about the physiology of the healing process. Wounds undergo a dynamic process consisting of three stages—inflammation, proliferation, and maturation. Today, superior alternatives exist that promote *moist wound healing*. These newer alternatives include semipermeable films (Opsite, Tegaderm, Biocclusive), semi-occlusive hydrogels (Vigilon, Scherisorb), and occlusive hydrocolloids (Duoderm, Comfeel, Granuflex).

The goal of this chapter is to review the following:

- The characteristics of the ideal dressing
- The standard one- and three-layer dressing techniques
- The advantages, disadvantages, and potential uses of the newer alternative dressing materials

In recent years, dressings have been developed to support the dynamic healing process through its stages of inflammation, proliferation, and maturation. The ideal dressing material would include the following:

- Remove excess exudate and toxic components
- Maintain high humidity at wound/dressing interface
- Allow gaseous exchange
- Provide thermal insulation
- Afford protection from secondary infection
- Be free from particulate or toxic contaminants
- Allow removal without trauma at dressing change
- Have acceptable handling characteristics—size range, resistance to tear, comfort, disposal

On a functional level, dressings can serve other purposes:

- Protection from trauma, temperature, bacteria, drainage
- Antisepsis
- Pressure/hemostasis

- Immobilization
- Debridement
- Absorption of exudate
- Packing
- Support
- Comfort
- Aesthetics

TECHNIQUE

The two basic dressing techniques are the one-layer and the three-layer methods (Table 138-1).

The three-layer method consists of a contact layer, absorbent/intermediate layer, and securing layer. The simplest example is the Telfa bandage—contact layer (perforated plastic) backed by the absorbent layer (cotton) held in place with adhesive tape (securing layer). The three-layer methodology enables one to suit the dressing to the wound by changing the characteristics of each layer. Ideally, the contact layer allows passage of secretions to the absorbent layer, yet acts as a barrier for infection from the external environment. However, dressings may be constructed by layers that make them:

- Nonadhering (Vaseline gauze) vs. adhering (wide-mesh gauze)
- Medicated (Xeroform, scarlet red) vs. nonmedicated
- Permeable vs. nonpermeable vs. occlusive

The absorbent layer may be constructed from gauze, cotton, or cast padding. The outer layer may be constructed from tape, bias-cut stockinette, Ace wrap, Corban wrap, or casting materials.

Example: hand wound—contact: adaptic

intermediate: Kerlex

securing: Kling

The newer environmental dressings are designed to produce a microenvironment conducive to the dynamic healing process. These include semipermeable films, semiocclusive hydrogels, and occlusive hydrocolloids.

TABLE 138-1.

Dressing Techniques for Specific Conditions

	One-Layer	Three-Layer
Drainage	None to slight	Moderate to heavy
Drain	Absent	Present
Depth	Partial thickness or full thickness and sutured	Full thickness and/or left open
Healing	Primary	Secondary, tertiary
Dressing removal	24-48 hours	After 48 hours
Example	Semipermeable polyurethane film (e.g., Tegaderm)	1. Adaptic—contact 2. Kerlix—intermediate 3. Kling—securing layer

SEMIPERMEABLE FILMS

Semipermeable film dressings—including Opsite and Tegaderm (3M), Biooclusive (Johnson & Johnson), and Ensure (Deseret)—are transparent polyurethane films that are permeable to oxygen and water vapor, but impermeable to water and bacteria. They maintain a moist interface to allow moist healing.

Advantages

- Permeable to oxygen, water vapor
- Impermeable to water, bacteria
- Sticks to skin, yet does not adhere to wound
- Flexible, comfortable, has "stretchability"
- Shear resistant
- Patient may shower with the dressing in place
- Hypoallergenic

Disadvantages

- Nonabsorbent—maceration, possible increase in bacterial proliferation
- Transparent—less aesthetic since one can see wound
- Cost—frequent change is necessitated if drainage accumulates; can be expensive

Semipermeable films are promoted to reduce pain, protect fragile tissue, reduce scarring, improve healing time by 35% to 40%, and allow constant monitoring of wound.

Practical Uses

- Covering intravenous catheter sites
- Covering superficial skin tears in elderly after Steri-Strips and reapproximation
- Promoting scab softening to allow debridement
- Covering a Duoderm dressing to decrease pressure and shear forces
- Covering clean, primarily closed incisions
- Protecting abrasions if little drainage is expected

Helpful hints

- Use Skin Prep Wipettes underneath adhesive dressings to prevent skin shearing/abrasion with product removal.
- Shave hair, if excessive.
- Apply to the center first and work outward, trying to avoid wrinkles. Do not stretch.
- Excess fluid accumulation (pooling) under the film can be aspirated with a small-gauge needle.
- If ballooning occurs, change the dressing.
- Leave the dressing in place until reepithelialization is complete, if possible.

- To remove the dressing, pull in the opposite direction and push skin away.
- Remove the dressing if there is any sign of increased inflammation or pus.

SEMIOCCLUSIVE HYDROGELS

Hydrogels, including Vigilon and Scherisorb, are three-dimensional networks of hydrophilic polymers that function as an absorbent mechanism. This provides for a moist healing environment yet adds the advantage of absorbency over the polyurethane films.

Advantages

- Inert
- Moist interface
- Prevents adherence
- Absorbent
- Absorption gradient that assists in removal of toxic components
- Dissolved oxygen permeability
- Clinically decreases pain, gels are cooling

Disadvantages

- Potentially more permeable to bacteria
- Less stretchability
- Cannot observe wound
- Expensive

Practical Uses

- Vigilon—promoted for dermabrasion or similar wounds (i.e., superficial yet not highly exudative)
- Donor sites for skin grafts
- Chronic ulcers
- Superficial operation sites

Contraindications

- Necrotizing ulcerations
- Deeply fissured wounds
- Second-degree burns prior to debridement

Helpful Hints

If one leaves the polyethylene film on the external surface, water vapor transmission is minimal. If removed, wound fluid can be absorbed by placing additional layer of absorbent dressing over Vigilon.

OCCLUSIVE HYDROCOLLOIDS

Hydrocolloids, including Duoderm (Squibb), Comfeel, and Granuflex, contain not only the hydrogels, but also adhesive and elastomeric components. Hydrocolloids have the capability of swelling, filling in, and conforming into a cavity.

Advantages

- Moist environment
- Adhesive
- Impermeable
- Absorbent
- Conformity
- Gel separates when dressing removed, thereby avoiding damage to underlying tissue

Disadvantages

- Less absorbent than Vigilon
- Less stretchable and shear resistant than films

Practical Uses

- Venous stasis ulcers
- Decubitus ulcers
- Ulcers resulting from arterial insufficiency
- Ostomy skin barriers
- Partial and full-thickness wound
- Skin protection from breakdown

TABLE 138-2.

Performance Profile Summary of Films (F), Hydrogels (HDG), Hydrocolloids (HDC)

	F	HDG	HDC
Adhesive	+++	−	++
Conformable	+++	++	+
Elastomeric	+++	+	+
Shear resistant	+++	+	++
Sterilizable	+	+	+
Particle free	+	+	+
Absorbent	−	+++	+
Permeable to water vapor	++	++	−
Permeable to oxygen	+++	−	−
Specific heat	−	+++	+
Impermeable to bacteria	+++	+	++

From Ryan TJ, editor: *An environment for healing: the role of occlusion,* London, 1985, The Royal Society of Medicine. Used with permission.

Contraindications

- Infected wounds
- Narrow wounds with tunnels

A comparison of the performance profiles of films, hydrogels, and hydrocolloids helps emphasize their strengths, weaknesses, and differences (Table 138-2).

SUMMARY

Wound healing is a complex dynamic process involving inflammatory, proliferative, and maturation phases. The dressing chosen should remove excess exudate and toxic components, maintain a moist environment, allow for gaseous exchange, prevent bacterial contamination, be free of toxic contaminants, and allow removal without subsequent trauma. The polyurethane films, hydrogels, and hydrocolloids offer new alternatives and improved healing times as compared to the traditional dry methodologies. The one- and three-layer methodologies have the advantage of using less costly materials. Grossly infected wounds are better managed by dry methodologies, where occulsive dressings should be avoided. As the process of moist healing is accepted by the physician community, the use of polyurethane films, hydrogels, and hydrocolloids will become commonplace.

CPT/BILLING CODE

16020   Burn dressing change

BIBLIOGRAPHY

Pinski JB: Dressings for dermabrasion: occlusive dressings and wound healing, *Cutis* 37:471, 1986.

Ryan TJ, editor: *An environment for healing: the role of occlusion*, London, 1985, The Royal Society of Medicine.

Wysocki AB: Surgical wound healing, *AORN Journal* 49:502, 1989.

CHAPTER 139

Allergy Testing

Gailen D. Marshall

Clinical allergic disease is due to mast-cell–bound immoglobulin (IgE) being cross-linked by allergen exposure. Subsequent mediator release, depending upon the organ system affected, produces the signs and symptoms such as sneezing, itching, congestion, wheezing, urticaria, and, if generalized, hypotension, cardiovascular dysfunction, and possible death. Thus, allergy testing should be reserved for those patients in whom clinical suspicion is sufficient to warrant the risk of testing. In addition, skin testing should only be performed using standardized, commercially available reagents.

INDICATIONS

- Seasonal respiratory symptoms, including nasal and asthmatic
- Perennial respiratory symptoms if history supports exacerbations where mold, dust mite, or animal danders are prevalent
- Children with recurrent upper-respiratory and/or middle-ear infections that occur seasonally
- Adults with recurrent episodes of sinusitis

CONTRAINDICATIONS

- History of anaphylaxis to suspected allergen—particularly stinging insects (These patients should be referred to a board-certified allergist for consultation.)
- Recent use of antihistamines (within previous 72 hours except for astemizole, which is the previous 2 to 4 weeks)
- Dermatographism (In-vitro testing is necessary.)
- Use of any substance (chemical or biological) that is not commercially

identified as an approved test allergen (An irritant response [false-positive] is very high for these reagents.)
- Children under the age of 3
- Patients on beta blocker therapy

PREPROCEDURE PATIENT EVALUATION

- Obtain a thorough patient history to establish the potential atopic nature of the problem. *All rhinitis is not caused by allergies.*
- Perform a thorough physical examination, focusing on the respiratory system. Look for specific evidence of atopic disease such as periorbital edema (allergy shiners), pale nasal turbinates, clear rhinorrhea, oropharyngeal cobblestoning, and a cough and/or expiratory wheezing. Specifically, evidence of infection (purulent drainage, fever) or other metabolic disease (thyroid, adrenal, etc.) should be ruled out.
- Document that the patient has not received antihistamines for the previous 72 hours (2 to 4 weeks if astemizole was used). Oral decongestants and systemic corticosteroids are not absolute contraindications to skin testing.

EQUIPMENT

- Allergen supply should be obtained from commercial sources, of which there are many. The number of allergens should be limited to those necessary to establish sensitivity to the various airborne allergens such as trees, grasses, weeds, molds, mites, and animal danders. As a general rule, testing with food allergens should be reserved for specific clinical suspicions since the false-positive rate for food allergen testing is quite high.
- Alcohol swabs
- 1 cc syringes containing a 26- or 27-gauge 1-inch needle (Tuberculin syringes can be used.)
- Washable marking pen
- Normal saline (negative control)
- Histamine phosphate 2.75 mg/5 cc (positive control)

TECHNIQUE

Epicutaneous Skin Test

This method describes the prick test, whereby allergen is dropped on the skin and a needle is passed through the drop to prick the epidermal layer. Other methods used for epicutaneous testing include the scratch, puncture, and tine test. These are more uncomfortable for the patient or more expensive to perform.

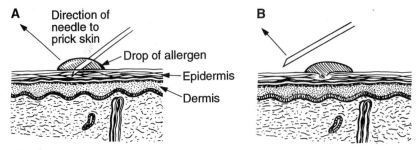

FIG. 139-1.

Method for performing percutaneous skin testing. **A,** The drop of allergen is placed on the skin and a 27-gauge needle (bevel up) placed on the skin through the allergen drop. **B,** The needle pricks the skin, allowing allergen to come in contract with sensitized mast cells located in the epidermis. The dermis is not violated and bleeding at the site is nonexistent or minimal.

1. Expose the volar surface of the forearm (adult) or the upper back (child).
2. Mark the area to be tested with a marking pen based upon the number of allergens to be used. There should be a minimum of 5 mm of space between allergens. The positive (histamine) and negative (saline) controls should be placed as far apart as possible.
3. Place a small drop of allergen on the skin next to the appropriate number. Care should be taken not to let the drop run on the skin.
4. Pass a 26- to 27-gauge 1-inch needle (attached to a tuberculin syringe), bevel up, through the drop on the skin. Gently prick the skin (Fig. 139-1). The skin should *not* bleed after testing.
5. Observe the patient for reactions after 20 minutes. It is common to have a red area around the test site immediately after skin pricking. This will resolve over 3 to 5 minutes and does not reflect allergen sensitivity.
6. After 20 minutes, observe the histamine control for the appearance of a pale, raised, urticarial type of area around the prick site *(wheal)* surrounded by a reddened area that is generally round *(flare)*.
7. Record the greatest diameter of the wheal and flare for each allergen (Fig. 139-2). To be clinically significant, the readings should be at least as large as the histamine control minus any reactivity from the saline site.

Intradermal Skin Test

In selected patients, epicutaneous skin testing will be negative in spite of a clinical history suggesting sensitivity to a given allergen (pollen, mold, etc.). In those in-stances, intradermal testing may be indicated. This form of testing requires com-mercial reagents specifically labeled for intradermal use. Currently, *food allergens are not to be used as intradermal reagents*. This is due to the high false-positive rate and potential for serious systemic reactions in sensitive individuals.

1. On a clear part of skin (typically the posterior aspect of the upper arm), mark the appropriate numbers on the skin.

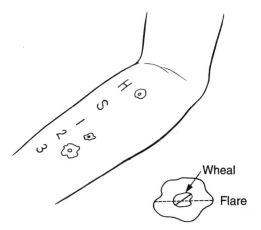

FIG. 139-2.
A valid skin test for interpretation. In this example, the histamine control is positive, the saline control is negative. Thus, the numbered samples can be measured with confidence. The largest diameter of both the wheal (central clear area) and the flair (red area surrounding the wheal) should be measured and recorded. This data is compared to the positive control.

2. Draw a small aliquot of allergen (usually 0.05 cc) into a tuberculin syringe containing a 26- to 27-gauge 1-inch needle.
3. Insert the needle (bevel up) into the skin at a very shallow (<15 degree) angle until the hole of the needle just disappears. Rotate the bevel 180 degrees until it faces down (Fig. 139-3).
4. Inject the smallest volume that raises a skin wheal. This is typically 0.03 to 0.05 cc.
5. Controls should again include saline. If a significant histamine response (>10 mm wheal) was obtained with percutaneous testing, histamine need not be repeated.
6. After 20 minutes, the patient is again observed for the presence of wheal and flare reaction at the injection site. To be considered positive, the test wheals must be at least 5 mm larger at the greatest diameter than the saline controls.

In-Vitro Testing (RAST)

In selected clinical situations (that is, dermatographism, severe dermatitis, excessive patient anxiety about needles, recent use of antihistamines, etc.), selected testing for the presence of allergen-specific serum IgE may be indicated. The most common test available is the radioallergosorbent test (RAST). This is significantly more expensive to the patient than is skin testing but can, under select conditions, be most useful.

This method involves a simple blood draw, with serum sent to specialty laboratories by local reference laboratories. Interpretation of the data typically comes from the laboratory. A major caution is to interpret RAST data in light of clinical history.

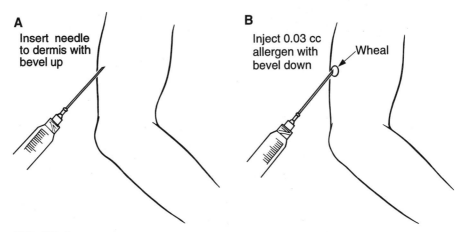

A Insert needle to dermis with bevel up

B Inject 0.03 cc allergen with bevel down — Wheal

FIG. 139-3.
Intradermal skin test. In this procedure, a 1 cc syringe with a 27-gauge needle containing the allergen is used. The needle is inserted (bevel up) just to the point where the hole disappears (**A**). This is intradermal. The bevel is rotated 180 degrees so that it faces down (**B**). Then the allergen is injected into the skin to raise a small wheal. Typical volume necessary to accomplish this is 0.03 cc.

COMPLICATIONS

- False-negative skin responses (The most common reason for this is recent use of antihistamines, particularly the longer-acting nonsedating class. Each patient should be questioned about his or her recent use of antihistamines. A minimum of 72 hours [2 to 4 weeks for astemizole] off all antihistamine should be required before skin testing is performed.)
- Pruritus at the skin test site (This is often intense for 15 to 60 minutes after the wheal and flare appear. The patient can be given an oral antihistamine or have a topical corticosteroid cream applied at the site as needed for comfort.)
- Late phase reactions (In approximately half of positive patients, a delayed reaction to allergens will occur. This may be quite pruritic and represents an inflammatory rather than a direct mast cell–mediated reaction. This is usually successfully treated with topical corticosteroids and resolves overnight.)
- Systemic reactions (Although this occurs relatively infrequently, it can be life threatening. Thus, patients on beta blocker therapy should *not* be skin tested. If a systemic [anaphylactic] response occurs, typical emergency treatment includes subcutaneous epinephrine [1:1000] 0.3 cc [adult] or 0.15 cc [children] every 10 minutes up to three injections. Bronchodilators, antihistamines, cardiovascular support, etc., can be instituted as necessary. It is important to remember that 75% of anaphylactic deaths are primarily respiratory, while only 25% are cardiovascular. Thus, appropriate resuscitative equipment should be immediately at hand when allergy skin testing is performed.)

CPT/BILLING CODES

95004	Percutaneous tests (scratch, puncture, prick) with allergenic extracts; immediate type reaction, specify number of tests
95010	Percutaneous tests (scratch, puncture, prick), sequential and incremented, with drugs, biologicals, or venous; immediate type reaction, specify number of tests
95015	Intracutaneous (intradermal) tests, sequential and incremental, with drugs, biologicals, or venous; immediate type reaction, specify number of tests
95024	Intracutaneous (intradermal) tests with allergenic extracts; immediate type reaction, specify number of tests
95040	Patch or application tests, up to 10 tests
95041	Patch or application tests, 11 to 20 tests
95042	Patch or application tests, 21 to 30 tests
95043	Patch or application tests, more than 30 tests

BIBLIOGRAPHY

Guerin B, Watson RD: Skin tests, *Clin Rev Allergy* 6:211, 1988.
Rodriguez GE, Dyson MC, Mogagheghi HM: The art and science of allergy skin testing, *Ann Allergy* 61:428, 1988.
Shapiro GG: How to administer and interpret allergy skin tests, *J Resp Dis* 3:9, 1982.
Williams PV, Shapiro GG: Avoiding the abuses of allergy skin testing, *J Resp Dis* 10:891, 1990.

CHAPTER 140

Fine-Needle Aspiration Cytology and Biopsy

Lee Green

Fine-needle aspiration (FNA) biopsy is a rapid, safe, relatively painless method of sampling solid and cystic masses in a variety of anatomical sites for cytological examination. Both benign and suspected malignant conditions can be diagnosed with FNA.

Although the procedure is successfully used to sample lesions of the prostate, salivary glands, intraabdominal organs, and intrathoracic organs, the primary care physician will find the technique most useful for masses in the *breast* and *thyroid,* and for *lymph nodes.* For tumors of these sites, positive and negative predictive values for malignancy are typically in the 92% to 98% range, with overall diagnostic accuracy of greater than 70%. However, these rates are highly dependent on the skill of the clinician. It is clear from the literature that FNA should be performed by clinicians who are skillful at technical procedures and well-trained in FNA, in order to obtain adequate diagnostic accuracy. Proper preparation of the smears is as important as the aspiration technique, as is the availability of a cytopathologist skilled in reading FNA specimens.

As implied by the overall diagnostic accuracy rate, as many as a quarter of specimens will return with nondiagnostic results, necessitating repeat aspiration or open biopsy. However, FNA will afford diagnosis in most cases with a procedure that is safer, more comfortable, less invasive, and less costly than open biopsy. These same advantages allow FNA to be employed with less hesitation than open biopsy would be. For example, many breast lesions can be sampled over time in a patient with fibrocystic disease, whereas repeated open biopsy with subsequent scarring would be unacceptable.

INDICATIONS

- Presence of a palpable suspicious mass in the breast
- A thyroid nodule
- A clinically suspicious lymph node or group of nodes

The primary care physician will not ordinarily perform X-ray, ultrasound, or computed tomography–guided FNA of nonpalpable lesions. FNA is probably the procedure of first choice, even over imaging studies, of evaluating thyroid nodules, as well as of detecting the rare parathyroid tumor.

CONTRAINDICATIONS

- Unskilled clinician
- Absence of a cytopathologist capable of proper interpretation of the resulting slides
- Sites of active pyogenic infection, though suspected granulomatous infection (fungal or mycobacterial) of a node does not contraindicate FNA

FNA may be safely performed in the anticoagulated patient if studies are in the therapeutic range, with proper attention to compression of the site afterwards to avoid hematoma, and may be performed in all but the most severely immunocompromised patients. FNA should not be used to evaluate lymph nodes suspected of harboring malignant melanoma, inasmuch as resulting inflammation can make subsequent pathologic diagnosis difficult.

EQUIPMENT

The equipment necessary to perform the procedure is illustrated in Fig. 140-1. The Cameco syringe pistol is available in various sizes from Precision Dynamics Corporation, 3031 Thornton Ave., Burbank, CA 91504. A disposable, spring-loaded

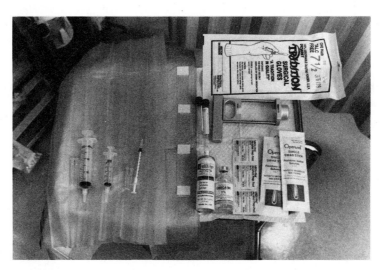

FIG. 140-1.
Setup tray for fine-needle aspiration.

syringe is now available from Euro-Med (15 Forest Parkway, Shelton, CT 06484; telephone: 800-848-0033) that allows single-handed aspiration technique. This frees the other hand for better isolation and stabilization of the mass. Milex also supplies a one-hand breast aspiration biopsy needle (telephone: 1-800-621-1278).

- Two sterile, plain (nonanticoagulant), evacuated blood tubes
- 21-, 22-, or 23-gauge needle (3)
- Syringe of appropriate size
- Slides with frosted ends (3 to 4)
- Fixative if necessary
- Glass cover slips or extra slides for smearing the specimens
- 4 × 4 inch gauze pads
- Sterile gloves
- Isopropyl alcohol pads or povidone-iodine swabs
- Saline or formalin specimen jar (if your pathologist recommends it)
- 1 cc syringe with 30-gauge half-inch needle and 1% plain lidocaine for anesthesia of skin, if desired

PREPROCEDURE PATIENT EDUCATION

Preprocedure patient education should proceed as for any surgical procedure. Advise patients in writing of the risks and benefits of the procedure, the indications, the alternatives, and the comparative risks and benefits of the alternatives. Significant complications of FNA are very rare, but advise patients of the possibility of a mildly sore hematoma forming afterwards, and the likelihood of at least some visible discoloration for a few days (especially from thyroid FNA). You should be certain that the patient understands that nondiagnostic results occur commonly and may require repeat FNA or open biopsy, and that false-negative and false-positive results are possible. Ask patients undergoing FNA of breast lesions to wear a supportive brassiere.

TECHNIQUE

Setup and Preparation

Prep the skin with 70% isopropyl alcohol. Povidone-iodine preparation may be used, but is not required for FNA. Sterile draping is not required, though neither the needle nor the skin entry site should be touched except with a sterile glove after the skin is prepared. Prophylaxis for bacterial endocarditis is not required.

Fig. 140-1 illustrates the typical equipment set up for FNA. The sterile tray contains both a 5 cc syringe for freehand aspiration and a 20 cc syringe for use with the Cameco aspirator handle; ordinarily one or the other is used, not both. Both 21- and 23-gauge needles are illustrated; either size may be used, though 23-gauge may be preferred in the thyroid and 21-gauge for dense masses. The 1 cc syringe with a 30-gauge ½-inch needle may be used for skin anesthesia, if desired. The slides upon which the smears will be made have one frosted end, allowing easy labeling with sequence numbers. The sterile plain (nonanticoagulant) blood specimen tubes are for cyst fluid, if obtained. The spray fixative is that ordinarily used for Pap smears. Not illustrated are 4 × 4 inch gauze pads, which should be ready also, and a saline or formalin jar for a solid-core specimen, if obtained.

Skin anesthesia is often not necessary for FNA, as the needles are small and not painful. If desired, however, excellent anesthesia can be obtained with 1% plain lidocaine by using a 30-gauge needle on a 1 cc syringe. If the lidocaine is injected slowly and in small volume (approximately 0.5 ml) into the subcutaneous tissues without raising a skin wheal, and then allowed to remain for 5 minutes, anesthesia can be achieved painlessly and without obscuring the lesion to be aspirated.

Sampling

Fig. 140-2 illustrates the aspiration of a thyroid nodule using one-handed manual withdrawal of the syringe plunger to create vacuum. The fingers hold the plunger while the thumb exerts pressure on the syringe top flange. Fig. 140-3 illustrates aspiration of a breast cyst using the Cameco syringe holder to withdraw the plunger. Whether FNA is performed freehand, or with the Cameco, use the fingers of the nondominant hand to stabilize the lesion to be aspirated and to provide tactile feedback when the needle has been placed in the lesion.

A

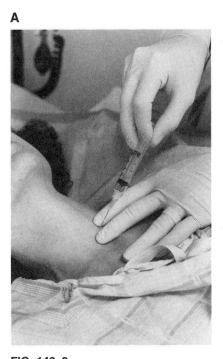

B

Fine Needle Aspiration
FNA-21™

EURO-MED

FIG. 140-2.
A, Thyroid fine-needle aspiration without syringe holder. **B,** Euro-Med FNA-21. (Photo courtesy of Euro-Med, a division of CooperSurgical.)

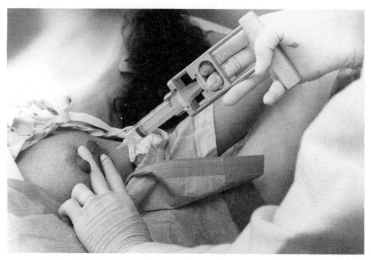

FIG. 140-3.
Breast fine-needle aspiration using syringe holder.

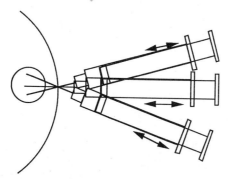

FIG. 140-4.
Fine-needle aspiration technique.

Before the puncture is made, draw air into the syringe, filling approximately one fifth of its volume. Carefully note the position of the plunger against the syringe markings. Then, introduce the needle into the lesion, and fully withdraw the plunger to create vacuum. Fig. 140-4 illustrates the technique of sampling a solid lesion or a cyst that remains palpable after fluid has been drained. Make several (3 to 15) passes through the lesion, filling the needle with cells and sampling all areas of the lesion. Then, return the plunger to its previously noted resting position to avoid drawing the sample up into the syringe when the needle is withdrawn from the tissue. Withdraw the needle from the lesion and skin, and use the air in the syringe to express the sample from the needle onto the slide. Handle the specimen as described below. Remove the needle from the syringe and replace it with a fresh one, and repeat the procedure. Two to three aspirations are typically performed on most lesions.

If a lesion is cystic and fluid is obtained, draw as much as possible into the syringe. Withdraw the needle and empty the syringe, then perform another aspiration if more fluid remains. Alternatively, detach the needle from the syringe and leave it in place, empty the syringe and reattach it, and withdraw more fluid.

Specimen Handling

Preparation of the smears to be submitted for cytological analysis is of crucial importance in obtaining accurate results. The technique is similar to making a blood or bone marrow smear, and may be done in several ways. Clinicians, especially if not well practiced in slide preparation, are strongly urged to make practice slides under the direction of the cytopathologist until good results are consistently obtained, or to have a skilled technician attend FNAs to prepare the slides. The nurse or office assistant who is to prepare slides should be directly and formally trained by the cytopathologist or experienced medical technician. Slides may be stained by the Papanicolau method or the May-Grünwald-Giemsa method; slides destined for the former *must* be alcohol-fixed within 5 to 10 seconds of smearing to prevent drying, and for the latter should be allowed to air-dry completely. The choice of procedure will be determined by the pathologist who will read the slides.

If a solid-core specimen is expressed from the needle, it can be washed from the slide into a vial of saline or formalin and submitted for histologic examination. Consult a pathologist regarding whether to submit cores intact and which solution to use. Fluid obtained from cysts can be smeared on a slide as above, or submitted in bulk in a sterile tube. (Standard evacuated blood tubes are sterile; use those without anticoagulant.) A sterile tube can also be used to submit semisolid material such as that obtained from a lymph node for culture. If infection is suspected, fluid and solid specimens can be submitted in transport media as well.

POSTPROCEDURE CARE

Compression of the site with a gauze pad for 5 to 15 minutes will minimize bruising, especially of the highly vascular thyroid area. A compression dressing of folded gauze pads under elastoplast tape can be applied on suitable sites. In breast biopsies, placement of a stack of folded gauze pads under a snug brassiere forms an effective compression dressing that may be left in place for several hours to prevent hematoma formation. Some physicians apply a small ice pack to the FNA site for 15 to 60 minutes after the procedure.

COMPLICATIONS

Complications of FNA are limited primarily to diagnostic failure, or false-negative and false-positive results. The incidence of failures is strongly operator-dependent. Minor hematoma formation is a frequent occurrence, but seldom of clinical significance. Prior to the widespread use of FNA, concern was often expressed about the possibility of seeding the needle track with malignant cells or releasing malignant cells to spread via lymphatics. Neither of these theoretical complications has been documented to occur, and they should not be considered complications of FNA. Damage to local anatomic structures (e.g., recurrent laryngeal nerve injury with thyroid FNA) is possible but occurs rarely if at all; large case series have not reported such injuries. This is probably due to the small diameter of the needles used for FNA, in contrast to cutting-needle biopsies, which do cause injury with some frequency.

CPT/BILLING CODES

19000	Aspiration drainage of a breast cyst; one cyst
19001	Aspiration drainage of a breast cyst; additional cyst
88170	Fine-needle aspiration of superficial masses; breast, thyroid, or lymph node
90070	Breast biopsy tray

BIBLIOGRAPHY

Bottles K et al: Fine-needle aspiration biopsy: has its time come? *Am J Med* 8 1:525, 1986.

Caruso DR, Mazzaferri EL: Practical evaluation of thyroid nodules, *Hosp Med*:46, January 1992.

Conry C: Evaluation of a breast complaint: is it cancer? *Am Fam Physician* 49:445, 1994.

Erickson R, Shank JC, Gratton C: Fine-needle breast aspiration biopsy, *JFP* 28(3):306, 1989.

Frable W: Thin-needle aspiration biopsy, *Am J Clin Pathol* 6(5):168, 1976.

Hamburger JI: Needle aspiration for thyroid nodules: skip ultrasound—do initial assessment in the office, *Postgrad Med* 84(8):61, 1988.

Hammond S, Keyhani-Rofagha S, O'Toole RV: Statistical analysis of fine-needle aspiration cytology of the breast, *Acta Cytologica* 3(1):276, 1987.

Layfield LJ et al: The palpable breast nodule, *Cancer* 72:1642, 1993.

Lee KR, Foster RS, Papillo JL: Fine-needle aspiration of the breast: importance of the aspirator, *Acta Cytologica* 3(1):281, 1987.

Lever JV, Trott PA, Webb AJ: Fine-needle aspiration cytology, *J Clin Pathol* 3(8):1, 1985.

Stanley, MW: Fine-needle aspiration biopsy: diagnosis of cancerous masses in the office, *Postgrad Med* 85(1):163, 1989.

CHAPTER 141

Lumbar Puncture

John O'Brien

Lumbar puncture (LP) to obtain a sample of cerebrospinal fluid (CSF) is helpful in many neurological diagnoses. The advent of computed tomography and magnetic resonance imaging has superseded lumbar puncture for some diagnoses, but has also improved the safety of its use. Examination of the cerebrospinal fluid remains the most direct and accurate method to determine central nervous system infection.

INDICATIONS

- Central nervous system infection suspected (Cell count, CSF gram stain, and bacterial culture are essential. Countercurrent immunoelectrophoresis is frequently helpful. Fungal culture, acid-fast bacillus, and India ink studies are optional.)
- Subarachnoid hemorrhage suspected (Computed tomography [CT] scan first. Note xanthochromic color and RBC count [$>1000/ mm^3$].)
- Pseudotumor cerebri
- Guillain-Barré syndrome (Very high protein [200 mg%])
- Multiple sclerosis (Elevated IgG amounts and oligoclonal banding present on electrophoresis.)
- Spinal analgesia
- Systemic lupus erythematosus
- Meningeal carcinomatosis
- Intrathecal antibiotics or chemotherapeutics
- Imaging procedures (myelography or cisternography)

CONTRAINDICATIONS

- Local lumbar skin infection (*absolute contraindication*)
- Raised intracranial pressure (except pseudotumor cerebri)

- Supratentorial mass lesions (should be evaluated by CT scan first)
- Severe bleeding diathesis (*relative contraindication*)
- Platelet count less than 50,000/mm^3

EQUIPMENT

Spinal tray (Fig. 141-1) containing:

- Skin swabs
- Povidone-iodine
- Alcohol swab
- Fenestrated drape and sterile gloves
- Manometer, three-way stopcock
- 1% lidocaine
- 3 cc syringe
- 20- and 25-gauge needle
- 20- or 22-gauge spinal needle, plus a spare
- Four numbered, capped test tubes
- Sterile dressing

TECHNIQUE

1. Position the patient near the edge of the bed or the examination table in the lateral recumbent or sitting position. Flex the spine anteriorly. Identify the L3 to L4 interspace at the level of the iliac crests. Lumbar puncture can be performed safely below the level of the conus medullaris, which can be as low as L2 to L3 (Figs. 141-2 and 141-3).

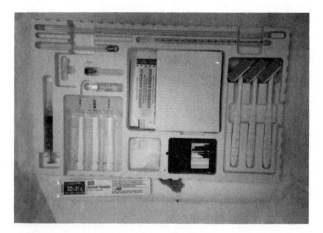

FIG. 141-1.
Lumbar puncture equipment tray.

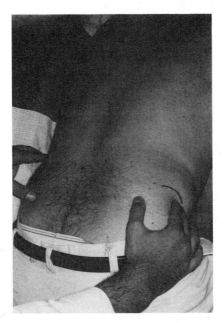

FIG. 141-2.
Black dot over midline at level of iliac crests indicates puncture site.

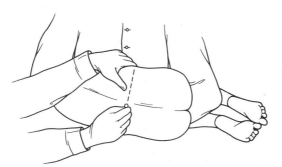

FIG. 141-3.
Diagram showing positioning of infant.

2. Open the spinal puncture tray in a sterile manner. After donning sterile gloves, preassemble the manometer and attach a three-way stopcock. Set this to the side of the tray. Next, open the test tubes and place them in order in an upright position in the slots provided in the plastic tray.
3. Sterilely prepare the skin at the selected interspace, plus the one above and below, with an antiseptic solution such as povidone-iodine. Cover the area with a fenestrated drape.
4. Draw 3 cc of 1% lidocaine up into a syringe. Administer local anesthetic by raising a wheal in the skin with the lidocaine. Inject a small amount into the posterior spinous region.

5. Using the posterior spinous processes and the umbilicus as landmarks, insert a 22- or 20-gauge spinal needle through the skin. Angle the needle about 15 degrees cephalad toward the umbilicus, keeping it level with the sagittal midplane of the body (Figs. 141-4 and 141-5). If bone is encountered, withdraw the needle slightly and change its angle. Depending on the size of the patient, after the needle has advanced about 3 to 4 cm, stop, withdraw the stylus, and check the hub for fluid. If there is no fluid, replace the stylus and advance another fraction before repeating this again. Usually, there is a slight "pop" felt as the spinal needle penetrates the dura. Advance the needle 1 to 2 mm farther.

6. Once fluid is obtained, place the end of the stopcock with the attached manometer onto the hub of the needle. Have the patient straighten the legs and relax his or her position so as not to artificially elevate the opening pressure.

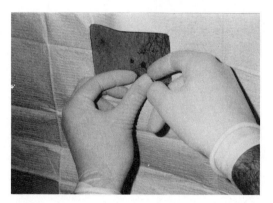

FIG. 141-4.
Proper angle for entering spinal canal. Needle is directed cephalad.

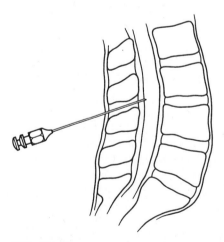

FIG. 141-5.
A drop in resistance will be felt as the needle penetrates the dura.

The cerebrospinal fluid will rise in the manometer to the opening pressure. Note the color of the fluid and the opening pressure.

7. Turn the stopcock to allow the cerebrospinal fluid to flow into the test tubes in order. Fill at least three test tubes with 2 to 3 cc of cerebrospinal fluid each. Label each tube in the order it was collected (Fig. 141-6).

8. Once you have obtained enough cerebrospinal fluid, replace the stylus and withdraw the needle.

9. Cover the puncture site with a sterile dressing. Have the patient turn to the supine position and remain there for the next 2 hours.

Normal Cerebrospinal Fluid Values

Opening pressure . . . . .50-200 mm H_2O
Elevated CSF pressure . . . .>250 mm H_2O

WBC	<5 /mm^3
Glucose	60% to 70% of blood glucose
Protein	15 to 45 mg%

Recommended Cerebrospinal Fluid Tests

Tube #1 Biochemistry	*Tube #2* Bacteriology	*Tube #3* Hematology	*Tube #4* Optionals

glucose
protein
protein electro-
    phoresis*
	gram stain
	culture
	    bacteria
	    fungal*
	    TB*
	    viral*
		cell count
		differential
			VDRL*
			India ink*
			cytology*
			Oligoclonal bands
			myelin basic protein

*If clinically indicated

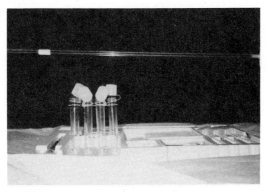

FIG. 141-6.
Test tubes and assembled manometer for doing a lumbar puncture.

COMPLICATIONS

- Postlumbar puncture headache (10% to 25%) is usually self-limiting, lasting for only a few days, but may sometimes last longer. Spinal headache usually occurs 24 to 48 hours following dural puncture. The incidence is reduced when using a 20-gauge or smaller needle and having the patient remain at bed rest following the procedure. Epidural blood patch has been used since 1960 by anesthesiologists for refractory spinal headaches.
- Traumatic or "bloody" tap from inadvertent puncture of the spinal venous plexuses is possible. This is self-limiting in the majority of patients, but could lead to a spinal hematoma in those with bleeding disorders.
- Brain herniation from a supratentorial mass or extreme pressure is another complication. Always check the fundi first for papilledema. If a tumor, an intracranial bleed, or marked increased pressure is suspected, an emergency CT scan should be obtained first to reduce the chances of herniation.
- Shooting pains in the lower extremities are usually transient, but rarely last for more than a year.
- Local pain in the back may be due to injury of periosteum or spinal ligaments.
- Aspiration of nerve roots may be prevented by withdrawing the needle with the stylet in place.
- Meningitis as a result of the procedure is a theoretical complication.

CPT/BILLING CODES

62270	Spinal puncture, lumbar, diagnostic
62272	Spinal puncture, therapeutic, for drainage of spinal fluid

BIBLIOGRAPHY

Marton KI, Gean AD: The spinal tap: a new look at an old test, *Ann Intern Med* 104:840, 1986.

Halliday HL: When to do a lumbar puncture in a neonate, *Arch Dis Child* 64:313, 1989.

Raskin NH: Lumbar puncture headache: a review, *Headache* 30:197, 1990.

Eng RHK, Seligman SJ: Lumbar puncture–induced meningitis, *JAMA* 245:1456, 1981.

Stutman HR, Marks MI: Bacterial meningitis in children: diagnosis and therapy, *Clin Ped* 26:431, 1987.

CHAPTER 142

Bone Marrow Aspiration and Biopsy

John O'Brien

Various techniques are possible to sample bone marrow and assess hemopoietic function. The marrow can be aspirated from the sternum, anterior iliac crest or, in infants, the tibia. The technique using the posterior superior spine (PSS) of the iliac crest is presented here. It has the advantage of being a readily accessible site, plus it allows for obtaining a good bone marrow aspirate and biopsy. The procedure is best performed with an available lab assistant to help with smears and slides.

INDICATIONS

- Unexplained anemia (useful in determining etiology and evaluating iron stores)
- Metastatic disease
- Leukemia or lymphoma (helpful in diagnosis, staging, and determining results of treatment)
- Lymphoproliferative disorders
- Pancytopenia (differentiates relative involvement of red cell, white cell, and platelet lines in the disease)
- Immunodeficiency states
- Fever of unknown origin (may reveal metastatic disease, pyogenic source, or granulomatous disease)
- Thrombocytopenia (differentiates marrow disorders from splenic problems or increased platelet destruction)
- Unusual infections (e.g., tuberculosis, fungi)
- Bone marrow transplantation
- Material needed for chromosomal analysis

CONTRAINDICATIONS

- Hemophilia and other clotting disorders
- Severe osteoporosis (Caution must be exercised.)
- Previous radiation therapy at site

1115

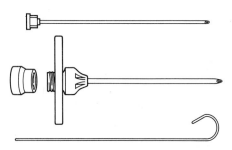

FIG. 142-1.
Jamshidi bone marrow biopsy needles.

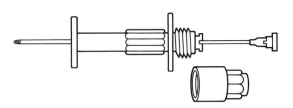

FIG. 142-2.
Bone marrow aspiration needle.

EQUIPMENT

- Povidone-iodine
- 11-gauge Jamshidi needle (Figs. 142-1 and 142-2)
- 25-gauge and 22-gauge needles
- 3 cc syringe
- 1% lidocaine
- 10 cc, EDTA-rinsed syringe
- EDTA (purple top) tube
- Glass slides (10)
- Sterile gloves
- Fenestrated drape
- 4 × 4 inch gauze
- Pressure dressing and tape
- No. 11 blade
- Container with fixative

All of this equipment is generally available in prearranged commercial trays.

PREPROCEDURE PATIENT EDUCATION

It is important to let the patient know there will be discomfort and momentary pain with the procedure. The patient will also need to remain in a supine position for about an hour after the procedure to help keep pressure on the biopsy site. There will be some postprocedure discomfort, so advise the patient to take the remainder of the day off work. The urinary bladder should be emptied before starting the procedure. Written surgical consent should be obtained.

TECHNIQUE

1. Place the patient in the prone position on the bed or examination table. Identify each iliac crest and follow it to its posterior superior spine (PSS). Mark the location of each site (Figs. 142-3 and 142-4).

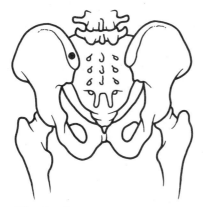

FIG. 142-3.
The iliac sampling site.

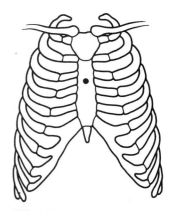

FIG. 142-4.
The sternal sampling site.

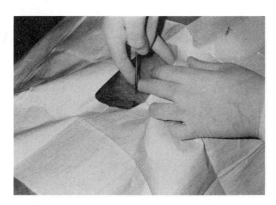

FIG. 142-5.
Insertion of needle.

2. Using sterile technique, prepare the skin with an antiseptic solution, such as povidone-iodine. Put on sterile gloves. Cover the area with a fenestrated sterile drape.

3. In the small syringe, draw up 3 cc of 1% lidocaine. Raise a wheal in the skin with the 25-gauge needle. Switching to a 22-gauge needle, pierce through the soft tissue to the periosteum of the PSS. You should feel a slight grating sensation. Inject 1 cc into the periosteum and the remainder into the soft tissue as you withdraw the needle.

4. Make a small stab wound through the skin using a No. 11 blade.

5. Confirm that the obturator of the Jamshidi biopsy needle is locked into place with the cap secured. Place the capped end in the palm of your hand with the shaft lying between your index and middle fingers (Fig. 142-5). Introduce the needle inside the puncture wound, forcing it through the soft tissue to the periosteum of the PSS. Using a clockwise and counterclockwise rotating maneuver with considerable downward pressure, pierce the cortex of the bone to enter the marrow. This should be about 1 cm thick. As soon as you

feel the cortex "give way," release the downward pressure, inserting the needle only 1 to 2 mm further (Fig. 142-6).

6. Unlock the cap and withdraw the obturator. Immediately attach the 10 cc EDTA syringe to the end of the biopsy needle. Warn the patient that he or she is about to experience pain, then pull up on the plunger of the syringe to aspirate approximately 5 cc of marrow. If no material is aspirated, carefully advance the needle another 1 to 2 mm after the obturator has been replaced. If bone marrow is not aspirated a second time, change sites. A good aspirate is identified by grossly visible bone spiculer on the slides.

7. Detach the syringe and hand it to the assistant to prepare the smears. The smears should consist of:
    a. Thin-spread preparation between two glass slides.
    b. Squash preparation. Flecks of marrow are identified within the aspirate. Drain excess blood off the slide before pressing two glass slides together, in effect, compressing the specimen before rolling the slides apart lengthwise.

8. Marrow biopsies are generally done only from the iliac crest. To obtain a marrow biopsy, keep the obturator locked in place and withdraw the needle about 3 mm so that it rests in the cortex. The needle should be redirected toward the anterior iliac spine. Advance the needle once again through the cortex into the marrow until the resistance decreases (Fig. 142-6, *B*).

9. Remove the obturator. Employ the earlier rotating maneuver to advance the needle about 2 cm (Fig. 142-6, *C*).

10. Rock the needle clockwise five times then counterclockwise five times. Withdraw the needle 2 to 3 mm.

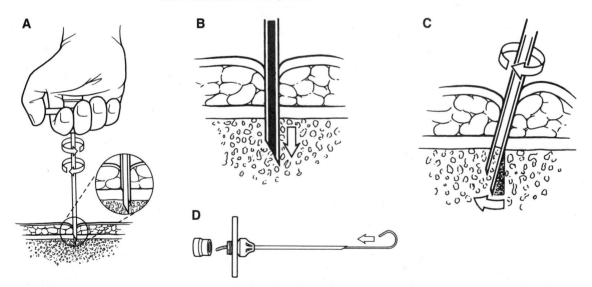

FIG. 142-6.
Technique for obtaining a bone marrow biopsy specimen. **A,** The needle is advanced to the cortical bone. **B,** For a marrow biopsy, the needle is advanced an additional 5 to 15 mm. **C,** The needle tip is redirected, the obturator removed, advanced 2 cm, and rotated 360 degrees to obtain the specimen. **D,** A blunt obturator is used to push the specimen from the needle.

11. Change the angle of the needle about 15 degrees. Advance the needle another 2 to 3 mm, and rock it again in the same fashion. This cuts the specimen loose from the remainder of the marrow.
12. Cover the hub with your thumb and withdraw the needle. Insert the obturator through the distal cutting end of the needle to push the specimen through the hub onto the gauze (Fig. 142-6, *D*).
13. With four glass slides, make light "touch" specimens of the biopsy specimen. Place the sample into the fixative.
14. Apply a pressure dressing over the biopsy site. Have the patient lie supine, with pressure on the biopsy site for at least 1 hour.
15. Ensure that the glass slides, EDTA tube, and container with the biopsy specimen are properly labeled.

POSTPROCEDURE PATIENT EDUCATION

Tell the patient to report any complication promptly to the physician. Supply the patient with telephone contact numbers. The pressure dressing can be removed after 12 hours. Ask the patient to notify you of any pain, drainage, fever, or spreading erythema at the incision site.

COMPLICATIONS

- Retroperitoneal hemorrhage or injury to bowel from breaking through the anterior cortex of the iliac bone (This risk is increased if significant osteoporosis is present.)
- Local infection at the biopsy site
- Hemorrhage at the biopsy site (This is best prevented by use of a pressure dressing.)
- Wound infection
- Dry tap (This may be due to poor site selection or to a disease involving the marrow [myelodysplasia]. Varying the angle of the needle or trying the opposite iliac crest should bring positive results.)

CPT/BILLING CODES

| 85095 | Bone marrow aspiration |
| 85102 | Bone marrow biopsy, needle or trocar |

BIBLIOGRAPHY

Hyun BH, Gulati GL, Ashton JK: Bone marrow examination: techniques and interpretation, *Hem/Onc Clinics North Am* 2:513, 1988.

Knowles S, Hoffbrand AV: Bone marrow aspiration and biopsy, *Br Med J* 281:204, 1980.

Paulman PM: Bone marrow sampling, *Am Fam Physician* 40(6):85, 1989.

CHAPTER 143

Muscle Biopsy

Lori Crago

The muscle biopsy is one of several laboratory methods for identifying disorders of the motor unit. These disorders, which include lesions at the anterior horn cell, peripheral motor nerve, and muscle, are all manifested by flaccid weakness, wasting, and deep tendon reflex depression.

Muscle biopsy is a simple procedure, often performed under local anesthesia. Selection of biopsy site is based on the distribution of weakness, and is case specific rather than disease specific. The muscle chosen should not be so affected that it is largely replaced by fat or connective tissue without trace of the underlying disease process. Acute processes allow selection of a more severely affected muscle to be biopsied. In chronic processes, clinical differentiation is difficult. With proximal muscle weakness, quadriceps or biceps are generally moderately affected and reasonably accessible. With more distal weakness, gastrocnemius is a frequently chosen biopsy site, but care must be taken in patient positioning to keep the muscle extended with the foot dorsiflexed at the ankle. Sites to be avoided include any muscle site of recent electromyogram (EMG) or injection.

INDICATIONS

While some syndromes can be recognized clinically (classic cases of Duchenne dystrophy, Werdnig-Hoffman disease, peripheral neuropathies, myotonia congenita, periodic paralysis, dermatomyositis, myasthenia gravis, and the myoglobinurias), patients may have less well-defined syndromes of proximal limb weakness without clear signs of motor neuron disease (fasciculation) or peripheral neuropathy (sensory loss, high cerebrospinal fluid [CSF] protein). In index cases of familial disorders, muscle biopsy should be performed to confirm diagnosis for genetic counseling.

CONTRAINDICATIONS

- Anticoagulant therapy not reversed before procedure
- Bleeding diathesis

- Infected site
- Recent trauma at intended biopsy site

EQUIPMENT

- Sterile drapes and four towel clamps, if desired
- Povidone-iodine (Betadine)
- Scalpel with No. 10 or No. 15 blade
- Sterile suture scissors, forceps, and tissue scissors
- Two skin retractors
- Two Vicryl sutures (3-0), or other absorbable
- One Ethilon suture (4-0), or other nonabsorbable
- Electrocautery
- Several tongue blades, cut to about 3-inch length, with small wedges cut in each end
- Several 2 × 2 inch gauze sponges
- Dressing tape

PREPROCEDURE PATIENT EDUCATION

Inform the patient that the procedure is relatively painless, but some discomfort may occur when the muscle is handled. For the first 24 hours after the procedure, patients may note a sense of pulling or bruising at the biopsy site. Patients may use the limb immediately after the procedure and should be given routine wound care instructions. Indicate the possible complications, and document the counseling or use of a consent form.

TECHNIQUE

With the muscle in the relaxed (stretched) state, prep and drape the skin. Infiltrate the skin with 1% lidocaine *without* epinephrine. Notably, the muscle should *not* be infiltrated to avoid trauma to the biopsied tissue. Incise the skin approximately 1½ inches over the belly of the muscle parallel to the long axis of the muscle fibers. Retract the skin, and incise and retract the fascia, exposing the muscle fascicles. Place a suture at each end of a strip of muscle 1-inch long and ¼-inch wide to isolate the strip. Then, excise the cylinder of muscle with the sutures attached. Wedging the sutures in the clefts of two ends of a broken tongue depressor allows the biopsy to be sent to the pathology laboratory maintaining the relaxed state. Several biopsies may be taken in this fashion. If oozing is present, cautery may be used to obtain hemostasis. Close the fascia with absorbable suture to prevent muscle herniation, and then close the skin. A pressure dressing may be applied for patient comfort and to minimize ecchymosis.

Best histochemical results are reliably attained if the muscle is frozen within 30 minutes of biopsy. However, proper preparation of the specimen varies greatly, and the primary care physician is advised always to coordinate biopsy timing and preparation with an area pathologist.

COMPLICATIONS

While serious complications are reported very rarely, discomfort is common. Infection at the wound site is uncommon, but slow wound healing may occur in immunocompromised patients. Hematoma occurrence can be limited using a pressure dressing. Sensory loss around the incision site can occur. The biopsy may need to be repeated if studies are negative or inconclusive. There is no definite way to know that the muscle group selected for biopsy is involved in the disease process.

CPT/BILLING CODE

20200   Muscle biopsy

BIBLIOGRAPHY

Adams RD: *Principles of neurology,* ed 4, New York, 1989, McGraw-Hill.
Baker AB, editor: *Clinical neurology,* Philadelphia, 1985, Harper & Row.
Dubowitz: *Muscle biopsy: a modern approach,* Philadelphia, 1973, W. B. Saunders.

CHAPTER 144

Emergency Department Ultrasound

Grant C. Fowler

Dietrich Jehle

Recent advances in the quality of imaging and portability have made real-time sonography a valuable adjunct to the physical examination. Immediately available clinical information from ultrasound is now used in many emergency departments throughout the country. As a result, the American College of Emergency Physicians (ACEP) has released a policy statement encouraging immediate availability of ultrasound examination, interpretation, and clinical correlation 24 hours a day for emergency patients, as well as encouraging research and clinical studies to define the optimal use of ultrasound in emergency medicine. The Society for Academic Emergency Medicine (SAEM) endorsed this policy statement and added its own statement that specific training in the performance and interpretation of emergency ultrasound should be available for both emergency physicians during residency training and for practicing emergency physicians. This chapter will highlight some of the current major applications of ultrasound in the emergency department.

DESCRIPTION OF TECHNOLOGY

Ultrasound technology relies on echoes from pulsed sound waves to provide data for the generation of images. Real-time sonography provides a continuously updated or "live" image while the patient is being scanned. This provides the clinician an excellent opportunity to pursue clinical suspicions while actually obtaining the images. The higher the frequency of ultrasound, the sharper the resolution of the image; however, there is less depth of penetration into the tissue (Fig. 144-1). Frequency is determined predominantly by the choice of the probe, also known as the transducer. High-frequency probes (7.5 to 10 megahertz [MHz]) are used for scanning tissue close to the surface, such as breast and thyroid lumps or testicles. Low-frequency probes (3.5 to 5 MHz) are used to scan deep internal structures such as those of the abdomen, pelvis, and heart. Linear probes utilize parallel sound waves to produce a square or rectangular image (Fig. 144-2). Sound waves from one point source are directed through a field for sector probes, which produce a pie-shaped image (Fig. 144-3).

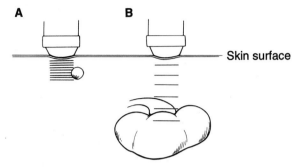

FIG. 144-1.
A, High-frequency probe (7.5 to 10 MHz) provides higher resolution images with less tissue penetration. This is especially useful for tissue near skin surface, such as breast or thyroid. **B,** Low-frequency probe (3.5 to 5 MHz) for deeper tissue such as abdominal (kidney) or pelvic organs.

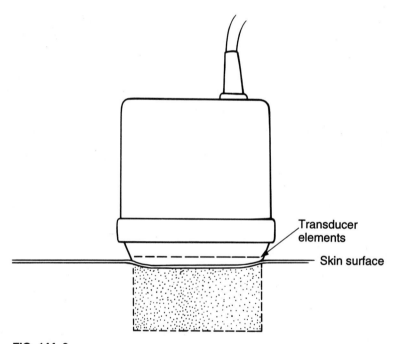

FIG. 144-2.
A linear probe produces a rectangular image and works especially well for obstetric scans.

Sound waves travel more readily through solids and liquids than through air; thus, acoustic gel must be applied between the body surface and the probe to form an interface. By the same principle, any organs that are predominantly air-filled, such as lungs or bowel or those posterior to or surrounded by such organs, are difficult to visualize with sonography. In contrast, the liver, spleen, heart, bladder, and uterus (during pregnancy) are predominantly fluid-filled and therefore provide

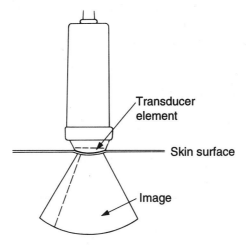

FIG. 144-3.
Wedged-shaped image produced by sector scanning probe may be adequate for most applications, depending on width of image.

excellent "windows" to view those organs or surrounding structures. A window is an area of the body close to the surface through which sound waves can be transmitted to obtain images. Images may be obtained of that particular tissue or of surrounding tissue. For tissue very close to the skin surface such as thyroid, breast masses, and femoral veins, high-frequency probes often have their own windows built into the probe in the form of a stand-off or water path.

Fluid such as amniotic fluid, urine, pus, or blood in the aorta or inferior vena cava appears dark by convention on the ultrasound screen. Predominantly fluid-filled organs such as the liver, spleen, or renal cortex appear grey on the screen with intermittent, bright echoes within their structure. Solid objects such as polyps or gallstones are white or "echogenic." If a solid object (calcified or hardened) such as a gallstone is larger than 3 mm, it should cast a well-defined shadow as well.

INITIAL SCANNING

Most physicians learn anatomy in three dimensions by dissection; ultrasound images require an ability to translate that knowledge into two dimensions. To allow for proper probe placement and angulation, a beginning sonographer should keep in mind that the best image is usually generated when the probe is perpendicular to the tissue being studied (Fig. 144-4). Beginners also want to minimize the planes of anatomy with which they must become familiar and should limit scans at first to transverse and longitudinal planes. Therefore, beginning sonographers should keep the transducer marker dot turned toward either the patient's head or right side, while holding the probe perpendicular to the organ or tissue being scanned. If the probe can also be held perpendicular to the skin surface, it is easier to scan. This probe placement generates the best images and minimizes the number of

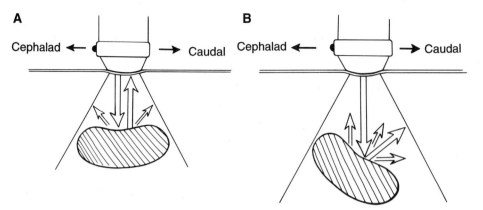

FIG. 144-4.
A, The best image is produced when the sound beam is perpendicular to the organ interface.
B, When the sound beam is not perpendicular to the organ interface, scatter is seen.

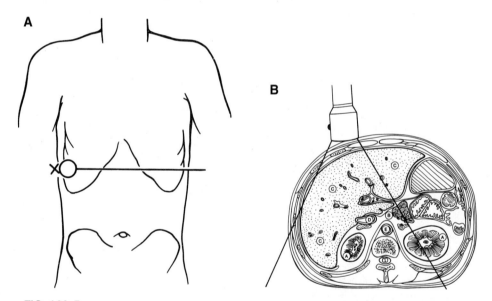

FIG. 144-5.
A, Marker dot toward the patient's right side produces a transverse image of the abdomen.
B, Kidneys (*A*); Pancreas (*B*), Liver (*C*); Inferior vena cava (*D*); Aorta (*E*).

planes. Reviewing these principles may be helpful when getting oriented to the patient's anatomy at the beginning of any scan.

By convention, the marker dot to the patient's right side produces a transverse image similar to computed tomography (CT) orientation (Fig. 144-5). The patient's right side will be to the left of the screen. With the marker dot toward the patient's head, the image is what the physician would see if the patient were dissected longitudinally and viewed looking into the body from the right side with the patient's head to the left of the screen (longitudinal) (Fig. 144-6). A good

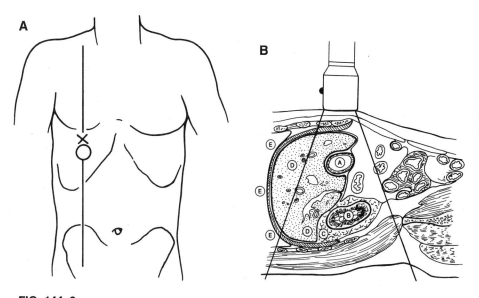

FIG. 144-6.
A, Marker dot toward the patient's head produces a longitudinal view of the abdomen. **B,** Gallbladder (*A*); Right kidney (*B*); Perirenal fat (*C*); Liver (*D*); Diaphragm (*E*).

impression of all of the anatomy and images of most organs can be obtained with longitudinal scanning initially.

Also, when first getting started, it is important to ask what clinical question(s) can be answered while scanning as opposed to attempting to provide an entire survey. This is especially true when scanning the abdomen. Sonographers and radiologists are trained for complete surveys. Emergency department sonography should be brief and goal-oriented to answer specific questions raised by the clinical presentation.

CARDIAC

Suspected Pericardial Effusions

A patient with a significant pericardial effusion can deteriorate rapidly hemodynamically. Echocardiography is the diagnostic procedure of choice for identifying a pericardial effusion. With rapid intervention often a necessity, emergency department echocardiography has saved lives in many cases.

Indications

- Electromechanical dissociation (EMD)—narrow electrical complexes on electrocardiogram without measurable blood pressure or clinical evidence of perfusion
- Unexplained hypotension
- Prominent jugular venous distension

- Pulsus paradoxus
- Enlarged cardiac silhouette
- Electrical alternans on electrocardiogram
- Penetrating wounds to the chest

Equipment

- Acoustic gel
- 2.5 to 5.0 MHz sector or curvilinear transducer and scanner

> *Note:* Since the axis of the heart is directed toward the 4 o'clock position, placing the marker dot of the transducer at about the 4 o'clock position produces the long-axis view of the heart, especially if the probe is located parasternally. The long-axis view is essentially the longitudinal view of the heart if described in the terminology of the remainder of the body. Rotating the marker dot almost 90 degrees to the 8 o'clock position produces the short-axis view of the heart, which is actually a transverse view of the heart (Fig. 144-7).

Technique

1. With the patient in the supine position, place the transducer in the parasternal location (third to fourth intercostal space) or apical location (inferolateral to the left nipple at the point of palpated maximal cardiac impulse). These are the same two traditional auscultatory points used for a stethoscope.
2. With the 12 o'clock position representing cephalad and the 6 o'clock position representing caudal, rotate the marker dot on the transducer toward either the 4 or 8 o'clock positions, in the parasternal space, or the 8 o'clock position when the probe is at the apex. The short-axis view at the level of the mitral valve is often a good view with which to assess adequacy of the window, since the mitral valve is usually prominent and easily located (Fig. 144-8).
3. If you can change the patient's position easily, place the patient on the left side. This allows the lingula of the lung to fall away from the heart and often provides a better window.

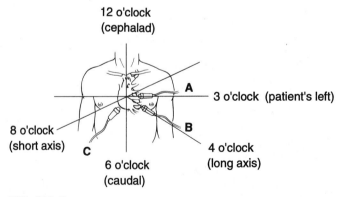

FIG. 144-7.
Typical probe positions (placement) for echocardiogram. *A,* Parasternal position of probe. *B,* Apical position of probe. *C,* Probe in subxiphoid position.

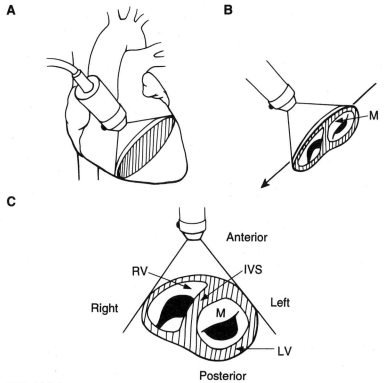

FIG. 144-8.
Short axis view at mitral valve level. Probe is in parasternal position with marker dot at 8 o'clock.
A, Ultrasonic plane transects the short axis of the heart at the level of the mitral valve. **B,** Actual
endocardiac structures connect with probe in this position. **C,** Short axis view as it appears on the
ultrasound screen. The image is displayed as if it is being viewed from the apex of the heart looking
up toward the base. Note "fish mouth" appearance of mitral valve (M) as seen from this view.
RV = Right ventricle; *LV* = Left ventricle; *IVS* = Interventricular septum.

Note: Some ultrasound equipment places the marker dot 180 degrees away from this
standard orientation—that is, the 6 o'clock position = the 12 o'clock position.

4. For unresponsive patients—those who cannot be moved or patients with
   chronic obstructive pulmonary disease—a subxiphoid view may be utilized to
   obtain a good window. Place the transducer directly below the xiphoid and
   angle it toward the patient's head and the marker dot toward the patient's
   right side.
5. Search for fluid posterior to the heart. If present, it will usually appear at the
   bottom of the ultrasound screen. If found, quantify the fluid. Keep in mind
   that, for various reasons (including body habitus), up to 10% of patients cannot be adequately scanned even under optimal conditions. You should scan
   patiently, but not be disappointed if a good window cannot be obtained.
   However, with a significant pericardial effusion, enough fluid is usually
   present to provide an adequate window regardless of body habitus. Any of the

above views should be adequate for visualization of a significant pericardial effusion. After finding a good window with the parasternal short-axis view, many experts suggest using the parasternal long-axis view to search for an effusion (Fig. 144-9), because it provides an image of the entire length of the heart. The parasternal long-axis view is obtained from the short-axis view by simply rotating the probe approximately 90 degrees counterclockwise to the 4 o'clock position.

Note: Even large effusions may develop gradually and not cause EMD.

Interpretation
Effusions (Fig. 144-10)

Small: With the patient in the supine position, pericardial fluid is confined posteriorly without anterior, lateral, or apical spread.
Moderate: Effusion more evenly distributed anteriorly, laterally, and apically.
Large: Effusion extending entirely around the heart.

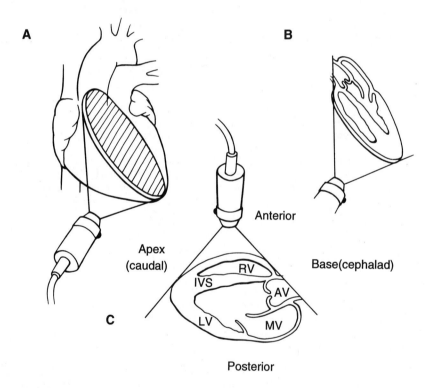

FIG. 144-9.
Parasternal long axis view of the heart. Probe is in parasternal position with the marker dot at 4 o'clock. **A,** Ultrasonic plane transects heart through the long axis. **B,** Actual endocardiac structures viewed. **C,** Image as it appears on ultrasound screen. *AV* = Aortic valve; *MV* = Mitral valve; *IVS* = Interventricular septum; *LV* = Left ventricle; *RV* = Right ventricle.

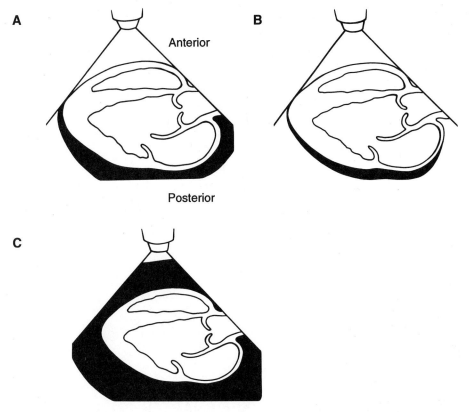

FIG. 144-10.
Effusions: **A,** Small (may be physiologic); **B,** Moderate; **C,** Large.

Clinical Electromechanical Dissociation (EMD)

For those patients found to have EMD, a subjective estimate of organized cardiac activity is made. Patients with poorly organized or absent cardiac activity when viewed on ultrasound have a prognosis similar to that of patients presenting with the ECG pattern of asystole. Patients with no obtainable blood pressure, yet with good cardiac contractility, appear to carry a better prognosis. An aggressive search for reversible etiologies of EMD should be carried out in this group.

Indications

- Electromechanical dissociation (narrow electrical complexes on electrocardiogram without measurable blood pressure or clinical evidence of perfusion)
- Unexplained hypotension

Equipment

- Acoustic gel
- 2.5 to 5.0 MHz sector or curvilinear transducer and scanner

Technique and Interpretation

The technique and interpretation is the same as that for suspected pericardial effusion (see above).

Treatment

Pericardiocentesis should not be performed without sonographic demonstration of an effusion. With experience, the physician should be able to estimate the amount of fluid that can be aspirated and the depth and angle of penetration necessary for pericardiocentesis.

CPT/Billing Codes

93307	Echocardiography, real-time with image documentation (two dimensional) with or without M-mode recording; complete
93308	Follow-up or limited study
76930	Ultrasonic guidance for pericardiocentesis, radiological supervision, and interpretation

OBSTETRIC/GYNECOLOGIC (SEE CHAPTER 104, OBSTETRIC ULTRASOUND)

First-Trimester Vaginal Bleeding

Twenty-five percent of all diagnosed pregnancies experience bleeding during the first half of pregnancy (see Chapter 104, Obstetric Ultrasound, for differential). Ultrasound is recommended as the first test in patients experiencing bleeding or pain beyond 5 to 7 weeks after their last menstrual period. Two frequent causes of first-trimester vaginal bleeding in patients seen in the emergency department are discussed below.

Suspected Ectopic Pregnancy

Ectopic pregnancies vary in prevalence from 1:28 to 1:200 pregnancies. They account for the majority of first-trimester maternal deaths. The incidence has quadrupled since 1970, and there has been a sevenfold increase in maternal mortality.

Emergency department sonography coupled with immediately available sensitive radioimmunoassays for human chorionic gonadotropin (HCG) should help decrease the morbidity and mortality of ectopic pregnancies. It is important to correlate quantitative HCG levels in your laboratory and the type of equipment available to determine at what level of HCG an intrauterine pregnancy should be visible by sonography. This will vary depending on whether transabdominal or transvaginal scanning is performed.

Risk Factors for Ectopic Pregnancy (In order of significance)

Intrauterine device currently in place
Previous tubal surgery
Prior ectopic pregnancy
Prior pelvic inflammatory disease
Infertility

In several large studies, pain (97% to 100%) and amenorrhea (74% to 84%) are more common complaints from patients than vaginal bleeding, although bleeding occurred in the majority of ectopic pregnancies in these studies. HCG values rise predictably, doubling every 2 to 3 days for the first 8 weeks of a healthy intrauterine pregnancy. In contrast, the HCG titer tends to rise at a slower rate in patients with ectopic pregnancies.

When evaluating the medical literature regarding quantitative HCG titers in light of sonographic findings, one must be careful not to confuse the standards being used (Second International Standard equals only about 50% of the International Reference Preparation [IRP]). If the IRP standard of HCG quantities is used, transabdominal sonography should detect an intrauterine pregnancy in 94% of cases when the quantitative HCG reaches 6000 to 6500 mIU/ml (3000 to 3250 mIU/ml for Second Standard). This correlates with about 42 days' gestation. Transvaginal scanning can usually detect an intrauterine gestational sac at 2000 mIU/ml IRP (1000 mIU/ml Second International Standard) or about 35 days' gestation. For a patient with a quantitative HCG above this level and no intrauterine pregnancy visualized, ectopic pregnancy must be considered. It should be noted that most hospital laboratories are currently using the Second International Standard.

Transabdominal Scanning

Equipment

- Acoustic gel
- 3.5 to 5.0 MHz sector, linear or curvilinear transducer, and scanner

Patient Preparation

Scan the patient in the supine position. For an adequate window, the patient's bladder must be full, occasionally to the point of discomfort. If scanning above the pubis does not immediately provide an adequate view, consider the clinical stability of the patient. If she is stable, either a foley catheter infusion or oral or intravenous hydration can be considered to fill the bladder for an adequate window.

Technique

1. Scan the bladder first with the transducer marker dot at the patient's right side to determine the orientation of the uterus behind the bladder (Fig. 144-11).

2. Turn the marker dot cephalad for a longitudinal view (Fig. 144-12). An echogenic line in the midline of the uterus is normal and represents the interface between the anterior and posterior endometria. A pair of dark fluid lines anterior and posterior to the central echogenic line represents endometrium during the proliferative phase. During the secretory phase, the endometrium becomes progressively thicker and echogenic. Occasionally an echogenic line known as the vaginal stripe may be visualized in the vagina distal to the cervix. It represents another interface.

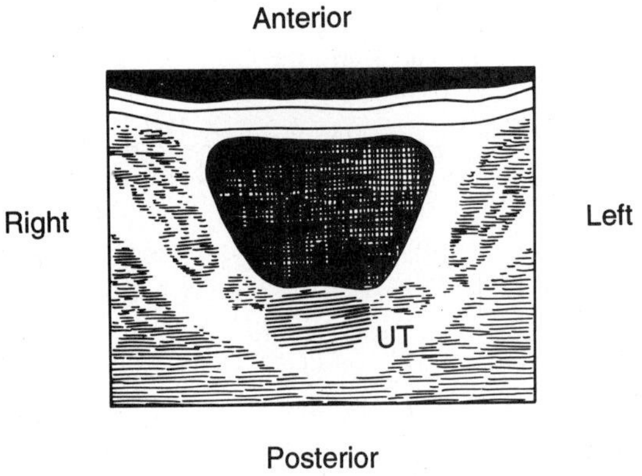

Anterior

Right

Left

UT

Posterior

FIG. 144-11.
Transverse view of the bladder. Note uterus (UT) viewed transversely is found posterior to the bladder.

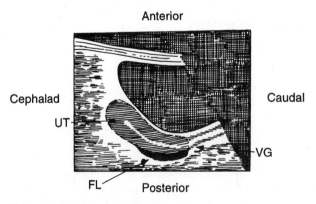

Anterior

Cephalad

Caudal

UT

VG

FL

Posterior

FIG. 144-12.
Longitudinal view of the bladder. Note uterus (UT) viewed longitudinally behind the bladder. Fluid in the cul de sac (FL) is found posterior to the uterus. *VG* = Vagina.

3. Photograph and record any object or fluid accumulation within the uterus or posterior to the uterus. Adnexa should also be scanned and any fluid accumulations or abnormalities noted.

Interpretation

A gestational sac can be described as an anechoic (dark) structure within the uterus with highly echogenic borders. A small echogenic structure within this sac may be a fetal pole. A gestational sac *with* a fetal pole present in the uterus reduces the chance of an ectopic pregnancy to 1:7000 cases. This figure represents the frequency of concomitant ectopic and intrauterine pregnancies or "combination" pregnancies. One exception to this figure is found with patients taking fertility drugs (such as clomiphene) in which the incidence of combination pregnancies may be as high as 1:100.

If no fetal pole is seen within what appears to be a gestational sac, you must consider that 10% of ectopic pregnancies produce pseudogestational sacs in the uterus, and the possibility of an ectopic pregnancy cannot be completely dismissed.

Transvaginal Scanning

Equipment
- Probe cover or condoms with a small amount of acoustic gel placed over the tip (Take care to smooth any bubbles between the transducer and cover.)
- 5.0 to 7.5 MHz sector, linear or curvilinear transducer, and scanner

Patient Preparation

Scan the patient in the supine or lithotomy position. A full bladder is not required for transvaginal scanning; however, some urine remaining can serve as a useful marker to locate the bladder.

Technique

1. Allow the patient to insert the probe while you are out of the room, or you may gently insert the probe with posterior vaginal pressure to a position anterior to the cervix.
2. Locate the midline of the uterus.
3. Obtain both longitudinal and transverse scans of the uterus and adnexa by turning the marker dot anterior to the patient or toward her right side. For longitudinal scanning, the image orientation changes slightly (Fig. 144-13), compared to transabdominal. Transverse orientation remains very similar to transabdominal orientation (Fig. 144-14).
4. Note any evidence of a fetus or fluid accumulations.

Interpretation

The interpretation for transvaginal scanning is the same as for transabdominal scanning except for the correlations with HCG. *Advantages* of transvaginal scanning over transabdominal include:

- Higher frequency probe with higher resolution
- Less tissue layers through which to scan, resulting in less artifact (nine layers on transabdominal)
- Less patient preparation, especially regarding the bladder

   Disadvantages include the necessities of an extra probe and additional training.

Threatened Abortion

Management of a threatened abortion in the emergency department consists of ruling out possible causes, assessing the amount of bleeding, and predicting the prognosis for the pregnancy. If bleeding is minimal and no specific cause is identified, such as infection, the patient is discharged in most cases with instructions for bed rest, minimal stress, and increased hydration. If the evaluation can be

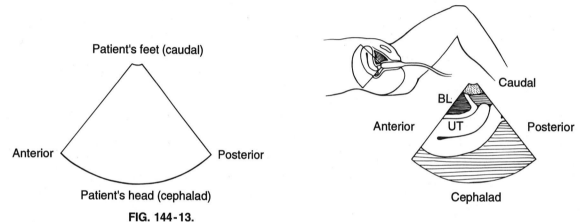

FIG. 144-13.
Longitudinal orientation with transvaginal scanning. *UT* = Uterus; *BL* = Bladder.

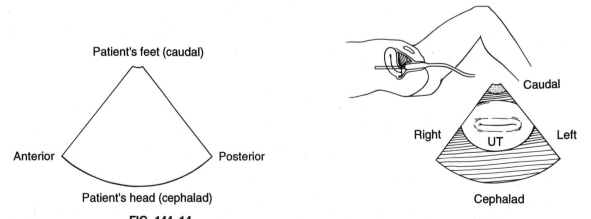

FIG. 144-14.
Transverse orientation with transvaginal scanning. *UT* = Uterus.

completed entirely in the emergency department, treatment goals are more readily accomplished than if the patient must also be evaluated in another department. Using specific sonographic criteria, one may determine which patients need additional ultrasound studies and estimate the prognosis of the early pregnancy. This is a significant improvement for diagnosis/prognosis than without ultrasound, which can only predict that half of all threatened abortions progress to miscarriage.

Patient Preparation and Technique

These are the same as those for suspected ectopic pregnancy above. Frequently, the diagnosis of threatened abortion is decided after ruling out ectopic pregnancy.

Interpretation and Management

Presence of fetal cardiac activity is an encouraging finding with early pregnancies since spontaneous abortion occurs in only 3% to 10% of those pregnancies in which fetal cardiac activity is seen.

With earlier pregnancies (even before the embryo is visible), major and minor criteria are available for evaluating gestational sacs (see Chapter 104, Obstetric Ultrasound). Gestational sacs meeting most or all of these criteria by ultrasound are much less likely to miscarry than the half expected if they are evaluated by clinical means alone.

Failing to meet any one major criteria is 100% specific in predicting spontaneous abortion. Fifty-three percent of abnormal pregnancies are identified by the same criteria. If there is a question about an abnormal sac, the patient should be scanned 7 to 10 days later. As an additional criterion during that time, the mean sac diameter in normal pregnancies should increase by about 1 mm per day.

An example of an abnormality would be a low-lying gestational sac (sac in the cervical region) or an abnormally shaped sac. Both of these are worrisome findings and should be followed with a scan a week later. Frequently, low-lying sacs result in spontaneous abortions, whereas abnormally shaped sacs result in abnormal pregnancies. Failure of the sac to gain 1 cm in mean sac diameter in 1 week or failure to visualize an embryo when the sac reaches 2.5 cm in mean sac diameter are also worrisome findings. They may assist the physician in preparing the patient for the possibility of an abnormal pregnancy, such as one resulting in a spontaneous miscarriage.

Evaluation of Fetal Viability

Detection of fetal heart activity by the second and third trimester of pregnancy should be reliable by transabdominal scanning. Earlier detection may require transvaginal scanning.

Indications

- Maternal demise
- Unable to auscultate fetal heart tones by doppler
- Maternal trauma

Equipment

The equipment is determined by the stage of the pregnancy.

Patient Preparation and Scan Technique

See Chapter 104, Obstetric Ultrasound, for late-trimester scanning. See above for early-trimester scanning.

Interpretation

- Absence of fetal movement over a 5-minute interval in pregnancies of over 20 weeks' gestation is said to be 100% reliable in diagnosing fetal demise.
- For first-trimester pregnancies, if uncertainty exists about fetal heart activity, rescan in 1 to 2 weeks.
- Secondary criteria for fetal demise include fetal anomalies such as hydrops, ascites, and pleural or pericardial effusions. Echogenic gas in the heart and vessels may be early findings. Late findings include morphological changes such as skeletal anomalies and unusual fetal positioning.
- Reaction to external stimulation or uterine manipulation may result in brisk reflexes in viable fetuses as opposed to passive motion in fetal demise.
- Avoid misinterpreting passive motion of the fetus due to uterine contractions as fetal activity.
- Ultrasound studies should be used in conjunction with maternal-fetal monitoring in the pregnant patient with significant abdominal trauma. A monitoring period of 4 hours should be sufficient to identify fetal distress.

Misplaced Intrauterine Device (IUD)

Intrauterine devices are available again after a hiatus, and the most common in recent years is the Paragard IUD. When a string is not palpable on an IUD, several options exist including an extruded IUD, a properly positioned IUD in the uterus that has lost its string, or an IUD that has perforated the uterus and may be lying in the abdomen. IUD users experiencing cramping, pain, or abnormal bleeding also warrant further evaluation. Flat plate X-rays may document the presence of an IUD, but they are unable to determine the exact location. Gynecologic instrumentation puts the patient at risk of infection. In most cases, ultrasound can be used to evaluate the location of an IUD; however, the diameter of recent IUDs is less than 3 mm, and scanning for IUDs in some cases is more difficult than would be expected.

Patient Preparation and Technique

Patient preparation and technique is the same as for ectopic scanning.

Interpretation

- Document location of the IUD in both longitudinal (Fig. 144-15, *A*) and transverse views (Fig. 144-15, *B*). If the posterior wall of the uterus is not easily

A

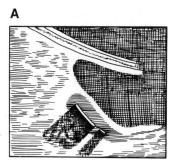

B

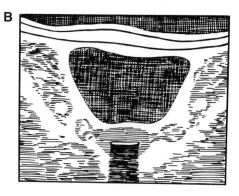

FIG. 144-15.
IUD in longitudinal (**A**) and transverse (**B**) views.

identified, formal scanning may be necessary. IUDs may also be difficult to locate when the uterus is retroverted.

- Decidual reaction may mimic an IUD. IUDs should produce shadowing in at least one plane.
- Perforations should be recorded as either complete or incomplete. Incomplete reveals a portion of the IUD within the uterine wall. Flat plate X-rays may be necessary to document location for complete perforations if not visible by ultrasound.

CPT/Billing Codes

76830	Echography, transvaginal
76856	Echography, pelvic (nonobstetric), B-scan and/or real time with image documentation; complete
76857	Limited or follow-up

See Chapter 104, Obstetric Ultrasound, for coding on gravid uterus.

BILIARY TRACT DISEASE

Acute cholecystitis in the ambulatory setting results from obstruction of the cystic duct by gallstones in approximately 95% of cases. Unfortunately, the diagnosis of acute cholecystitis by purely clinical means has an accuracy of only 50%, even with a positive "Murphy's sign" or pain over the gallbladder with palpation during physical examination. Real-time ultrasound is the preferred screening test for diagnosing cholecystitis. A "sonographic Murphy's sign" combined with gallstones increases the accuracy for diagnosing acute cholecystitis to more than 90%. A "sonographic Murphy's sign" is described as pain elicited with probe compression over a gallbladder. Because early surgical management is now the treatment of choice for acute cholecystitis, early diagnosis is also important. Although laparoscopic cholecystectomy was previously considered a contraindication, more surgeons are now comfortable with performing it in cases of acute cholecystitis. Bedside ultrasound is useful in diagnosing most cases of cholelithiasis and acute cholecystitis; however, more obscure cases may require additional studies.

Indications

- Symptoms suggestive of biliary tract disease
- Right upper-quadrant pain
- Suspected acute cholecystitis

Equipment

- Acoustic gel
- 3.5 to 5.0 MHz sector or curvilinear transducer and scanner

Patient Preparation

If possible, the patient should have been in the fasting state for at least 8 hours; this assures that the gallbladder is fully distended. Early morning scanning may be preferable to minimize bowel gas.

Technique

1. Scan the patient in the supine position longitudinally until you locate the gallbladder. Compared to other abdominal organs, the gallbladder usually has a rather superficial location on the inferior edge of the liver at about the midclavicular line. Prolonged deep inspirations by the patient may bring the liver edge down from under the subcostal margin to facilitate locating the gallbladder. Scanning between ribs may also be necessary to obtain a good window through the liver.
2. After locating the gallbladder with the probe in the longitudinal position, obtain a long-axis view of the gallbladder by rotating the probe out of the longitudinal plane of the body until the maximal length of the gallbladder is visualized.
3. Obtain additional views of the gallbladder with the patient in the decubitus (right side up) position or erect position, to avoid missing stones that may have rolled into a dependent position out of view.
4. Attempt to identify the source of local tenderness. A positive "sonographic Murphy's sign" is focal tenderness over the gallbladder. In conjunction with documented gallstones, this is the most sensitive sonographic criterion for acute cholecystitis.

Interpretation

An echogenic structure with prominent posterior shadowing, for which mobility can be demonstrated when the patient is placed in various positions and which has bile visible circumferentially in at least one view, is diagnostic of cholelithiasis (Fig. 144-16). When coupled with a positive "sonographic Murphy's sign," this is diagnostic of acute cholecystitis. Otherwise, gallstones can have several variations when viewed sonographically:

1. *Nonshadowing:* Gallstones less than 2 to 3 mm in size often do not cast a shadow. Other structures such as polyps or folds can also appear echogenic within the gallbladder. Echogenic structures in the gallbladder that are non-shadowing are calculi in only 50% of cases. If, however, an echogenic structure is noted to have gravity-dependent motion, it is usually a stone (Fig. 144-17).

2. *Intermittent shadowing:* Multiple small stones may form an irregular layer in the most dependant portion of the gallbladder. They may also cast a variable or intermittent shadow. This may be highly suspicious for cholelithiasis, but, without well-defined shadowing, further studies are necessary.

3. *Filled gallbladder:* If the gallbladder is entirely filled with stones, no circumferential bile will be noted. Shadowing may be less prominent or hazy. Since a

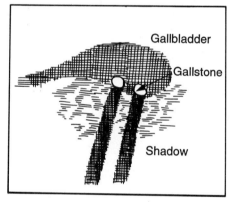

FIG. 144-16.
Acoustic shadowing behind two gallstones.

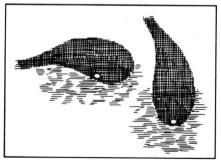

FIG. 144-17.
Stone is small and shadowing is not seen.

gas-filled duodenum can have this same appearance, it must be clearly eliminated from the differential.

4. *Adherent stones:* These could be present as echogenic structures that are not gravity dependent. If no shadowing is seen, further studies may be necessary to exclude other possibilities such as a polyp, tumor, or fold.

5. *Floating stones:* Occasionally stones can float and appear as an echogenic structure or line in a nondependent portion of the gallbladder. If they do not cast a shadow, further studies may be necessary.

6. *Absent gallbladder:* This sonographic appearance (absence) may be present in a nonfasting patient or one with chronic cholecystitis with scarring. A patient with a completely stone-filled gallbladder, with a previous cholecystectomy, or with congenital absence of a gallbladder may also have a nonvisible gallbladder. If the gallbladder is not readily imaged and the patient is clinically stable, scanning should be performed following several hours of additional fasting.

Additional possible findings within and around the gallbladder:

1. *Sludge:* Low-level to mixed echogenic material that takes a while to layer out after the patient has changed positions may be gallbladder sludge. It most commonly represents biliary stasis and may occur in various conditions, including obstructive jaundice, liver disease, sepsis, or in patients receiving hyperalimentation.

2. *Edema:* A thin line of fluid around the gallbladder wall may represent gallbladder edema, which can be found in acute cholecystitis or other conditions such as hypoalbuminemia, hepatitis, or ascites. If the patient has a "sonographic Murphy's sign," discrete pockets of edema may represent small abscesses. This becomes further definitive evidence of acute cholecystitis.

3. *Thickening:* A rim of decreased echogenicity around the gallbladder greater than 3 mm thick may represent chronic cholecystitis, hepatic dysfunction, congestive heart failure, renal disease, or neoplasms (decreased osmotic pressure and elevated portal venous pressures).

CPT/Billing Codes

76700   Echography, abdominal, B-scan and/or real time with image documentation; complete

76705   Limited (e.g., single organ, quadrant, follow-up)

VASCULAR DISORDERS

Suspected Deep Venous Thrombosis

See Chapter 52, Noninvasive Venous and Arterial Studies of the Lower Extremities.

Suspected Abdominal Aortic Aneurysm

The prevalence of abdominal aortic aneurysm (AAA) may be as high as 10% in people over the age of 65 and is the tenth leading cause of death in men more than 55 years old. Unlike coronary artery disease and cerebrovascular disease, the incidence is increasing; the associated mortality rate is increasing as well. Males are predominately affected by a ratio of approximately 5:1 compared to females. To describe normal anatomy, mean abdominal aortic diameters are approximately equal in males and females during the second decade of life: 12.2 mm and 12.3 mm, respectively. However, by the eighth decade, the mean diameter increases to 22.8 mm in males and 16.9 mm in females.

The natural history of an AAA is to expand at a rate of 0.21 to 0.4 cm per year. Over 5 years, an AAA of 4 cm has a 10% chance of rupture, a 5 cm aneurysm an 18% or greater chance, and a 6 cm a 30% or greater likelihood of rupturing. Elective repair in most large centers has a mortality risk of less than 5%, compared to 20% to 80% mortality in those patients who live long enough to reach the operating room after rupture. Therefore, elective resection is indicated for low- to moderate-risk patients with aneurysms that measure more than 5 cm in diameter.

Risk Factors

- Male
- 50 years of age or older
- Use of tobacco
- Hypertension
- Family history of AAA*
- Perhaps other atherosclerotic risk factors as well

The classic triad of ruptured AAA is pulsatile abdominal mass, low back, flank, or abdominal pain, and hypotension. Less than 50% of patients, however, possess this triad and less than 25% are hypotensive on admission. Unfortunately, low back, flank, or abdominal pain is a frequent complaint for patients in the age group at risk for AAA. Patients with AAA may have many other signs and symptoms as well, including chest pain, hematuria, ecchymoses, and scrotal masses. The most common incorrect diagnosis in an elderly patient with symptoms from a clinically significant AAA is left-sided renal colic.

Most aortic aneurysms are found in the midabdomen, just above the iliac bifurcation (about the level of the umbilicus). Physical examination is extremely inaccurate for diagnosing AAA. Aortography may underestimate the size of an aneurysm if it is filled with a thrombus or is dissecting, and lateral radiographs overestimate the possibility and size. Ultrasound is comparable to CT scanning, which is the gold standard for both diagnosis and estimation of size. However, ultrasound may be a difficult study with the presence of a large amount of bowel

---

*Family history is most significant when a female relative has been diagnosed. Elastinolytic enzymes, decreased type III collagen, decreased elastin, and other biochemical variants are being studied to determine what is probably a multifactorial inheritance.

gas, retained barium, or marked obesity. In addition, CT scanning is better than ultrasound for identifying a leaking, although ultrasound may be useful when there is not enough time to perform a CT scan in a emergent situation.

Indications

- Pulsatile abdominal mass
- Unexplained flank or abdominal pain
- Unexplained hypotension in an individual with multiple risk factors

Equipment

- Acoustic gel
- 3.5 to 5.0 MHz sector, linear or curvilinear transducer, and scanner

Technique

1. With the patient in the supine position, attempt to define the general outline of the aorta with longitudinal scanning (Fig. 144-18). If a pulsatile mass is palpated, it should not be difficult to demonstrate that a pulsatile abdominal mass is contiguous with the abdominal aorta.
2. After defining the general outline, measurements should be taken of the largest antero-posterior (AP) diameter on transverse scanning every 1 to 2 cm to a level 3 cm below the umbilicus. The transverse diameter of the aorta on transverse scan may be exaggerated because of unintentional tangential imaging if the aorta makes a lateral turn. Avoid applying too much probe pressure, which can also distort AP measurements.
3. If there is considerable overlying bowel gas, increased surface pressure with the probe may enhance visualization. Turning the patient to the right or left decubitus position may enhance scanning the aorta in the area of the kidney, although the iliac bifurcation may not be visible unless the liver is enlarged.

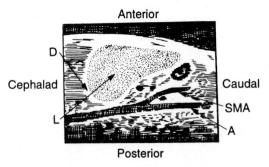

FIG. 144-18.
A longitudinal scan to the left of the midline showing normal structures and orientation. *SMA* = Superior mesenteric artery; *A* = Aorta; *L* = Liver; *D* = Diaphragm.

Interpretation

- An AAA is defined by an aortic diameter of greater than 3 cm in a male and greater than 2.5 cm in a female, or an enlargement of greater than 0.5 cm throughout the length of the aorta. The normal aorta tapers in diameter as it descends to its bifurcation.
- If an AAA is found and the patient is hemodynamically stable, attempt to determine whether branching vessels are involved. Fluid, usually along the left side of the spine or anterior to a kidney, may be a ruptured or leaking aneurysm, and surgical consultation should be obtained immediately. If no fluid is visualized and the patient is hemodynamically stable, a CT scan may be useful to check for retroperitoneal hemorrhage. Consideration should be made for surgery in any patient with persistent abdominal pain and a known AAA.
- Echogenic material in the lumen may represent thrombus or dissection. Alternatively, one should check the gain setting elsewhere on the aorta to make sure it is not artifact.

CPT/Billing Codes

76700   Echography, abdominal, B-scan and/or real time with image documentation; complete
76705   Limited (e.g., single organ, quadrant, follow-up)

PEDIATRIC ULTRASONIC EVALUATION OF THE BLADDER PRIOR TO SUPRAPUBIC ASPIRATION

Up to 8% of infants less than 8 weeks old arriving at the emergency department with a temperature of more than or equal to 100.6° F have a urinary tract infection (UTI). As many as 4.1% of infants younger than 2 years of age with unexplained fever have UTIs. Most studies suggest that bag urine specimens are more likely to yield equivocal results than suprapubic or catheter-obtained specimens. In spite of the fact that suprapubic aspiration (SPA) is inherently invasive, few serious complications have been reported, and numerous studies have demonstrated the superiority of SPA over alternative techniques. Limiting SPA to patients with proven full bladders further minimizes the risk to the infant. See Chapter 108, Suprapubic Bladder Aspiration.

Indications

- Suprapubic aspiration (SPA) in infants younger than 2 years old

Equipment

- Acoustic gel
- 5.0 to 10 MHz sector or curvilinear transducer and scanner

Technique

1. After placing the patient in the supine, frog-leg position, perform the scanning in a transverse manner (transducer marker dot to the patient's right side) slightly above the symphysis pubis to locate the bladder.
2. Angle the probe as needed to locate the maximal diameter of the bladder.
3. Note the angulation of the probe necessary to locate the bladder for future direction of the aspiration needle.

Interpretation and Results

A pocket of fluid larger than 2 cm × 2 cm in the retropubic area measured in the anteroposterior and transverse diameters defines a "full" bladder (Fig. 144-19). Suprapubic aspiration should be attempted at the same angle with which the maximal transverse bladder diameter was measured (Fig. 144-20). One study resulted in obtaining urine in 79% of children meeting these criteria and undergoing aspiration. If the bladder is found to be empty and the patient is clinically stable, repeat scanning to search for a full bladder should be performed from 30 minutes to an hour after the initial scan. If a full bladder cannot be found on the repeat scan, bladder catheterization should be considered.

CPT/Billing Codes

76700	Echography, abdominal, B-scan and/or real time with image documentation; complete
76705	Limited (e.g., single organ, quadrant, follow-up)
76938	Ultrasonic guidance for cyst (any location), or renal pelvis aspiration, radiological supervision, and interpretation

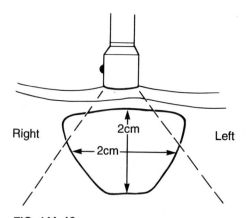

FIG. 144-19.
A transverse view of a full bladder.

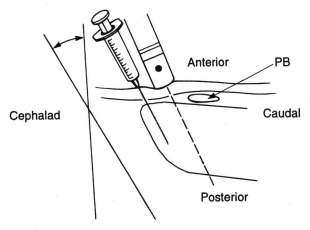

FIG. 144-20.
The needle should be inserted next to the probe and parallel to whatever angle demonstrated the fullest diameters of the bladder. *PB* = Pubic bone.

BIBLIOGRAPHY

Deutchman M: The problematic first-trimester pregnancy, *Am Fam Physician* 39(1):185, 1989.

Gochman RF, Karasic RB, Heller MB: Use of portable ultrasound to assist urine collection by suprapubic aspiration, *Ann Emerg Med* 20:631, 1991.

Jehle D et al: Emergency department sonography by emergency physicians, *Am J Emerg Med* 7(6):605, 1989.

Leach R, Ory S: Management of ectopic pregnancy, *Am Fam Physician* 41(4):1215, 1990.

Sanders RC: *Clinical sonography: a practical guide,* ed 2, Boston, 1991, Little, Brown.

Sarti DA: *Diagnostic ultrasound,* Chicago, 1987, Mosby.

INDEX

Abdomen, transverse/longitudinal ultrasound views, 1126, 1127
Abdominal aortic aneurysm, 143-5, 1144
Abdominal paracentesis and peritoneal lavage, 892-7
Abortion *See also* Culdocentesis (colpocentesis); Dilation and curettage; Obstetric ultrasound; Paracervical block
   amniocentesis, 766-7, 771
   counseling, 699-700, 701
   first-trimester, 699-713
   habitual, 571
   incomplete, 672
   and IUD insertion, 582
   Roe vs. Wade, 699
   threatened, 1136-7
ABPM. *See* Ambulatory blood pressure monitoring
Abrasions, corneal, 221-30
Abscess. *See also* Local anesthesia; Perianal abscess incision and drainage
   Bartholin's, 596-601
   boil, 50
   carbuncle, 50
   and cryosurgery, 104, 115
   furuncle, 50
   hepatic, 850
   incision and drainage of, 50-3
   paronychia, 34, 35, 38, 50
   perianal, 52, 53, 900, 957, 969-73
   perirectal, 970
   pilonidal, incision and drainage, 964-8
   prostatic, 541, 543
   superlevator, 970
   tooth, 52
Absorbable gelatin sponge/powder, topical hemostatic agent, 1087
Acid-base balance, arterial puncture, 340
Acidosis, 842-4
Acne therapy, 54-7
   comedo extractors, use of, 54-5
   comedo removal, 54-5
   cryoslush therapy, 56
   cystic acne, 54-6
   intralesional corticosteroid injection, 55-6
   scar revision, 56
   surgery for pustules and cysts, 55
Acquired immune deficiency syndrome
   IUD insertion and, 579
   abortion, first-trimester, and, 700
   office treatment of hemorrhoids and, 931
Acromioclavicular joint, 1046
Actinic chelitis, CO_2 laser therapy, 84
Actinomycoses, genital, 579
Activated charcoal, gastric lavage, 886, 887, 890
Acupressure, 164
Acute abdomen
   abdominal paracentesis and peritoneal lavage with, 893
   anoscopy for, 902
   flexible sigmoidoscopy for, 908
Adenoma, pituitary, 231
Adenomatous hyperplasia, 672
Adenopathy, 250
Adhesions, endometrial, 571
Adult circumcision. *See* Circumcision, adult
Adult respiratory distress syndrome, 452

Advanced cardiac life support, 416, 418, 419
   cardioversion, 440
   endotracheal intubation, 452
   temporary pacing, 464, 466, 472
Aerobic fitness, 433, 436
AIDS. *See* Acquired immune deficiency syndrome
Alcohol intoxication, abdominal paracentesis and peritoneal lavage, 893
Allen test, 342-3
   pediatric arterial puncture, 859
   percutaneous arterial line placement, 293
Allergy. *See also* Anaphylaxis
   anesthesia, 38, 44, 136, 137, 140, 142, 243, 244
   food, 1097, 1098
   sclerotherapy, 64
   testing, 1096, 1101
Alpha-adrenergic agents, 552, 554
Aluminum chloride, 1086
Alveolar nerve block
   inferior (V_2), 174-6
   posterior superior, 170-1
AMA Drug Evaluations, 159
Ambiguous genitalia, 874
Amblyopia, 225, 226, 231, 235
Ambulatory blood pressure monitoring, 369-77
   interpretation of, 372-6
   limitations of, 370
American Academy of Dermatology, 75
American Academy of Family Physicians, 980
American Academy of Pediatrics, 831, 863
American Cancer Society, 907
American College of Cardiology, 409, 432
American College of Obstetricians and Gynecologists, 578
American College of Obstetrics and Gynecology, 807, 809, 907
American College of Physicians, 907
American College of Radiology, 809, 818
American College of Sports Medicine, 419
American Fertility Society, 577
American Heart Association, 409, 831
   aerobic exercise prescription recommendation, 436
   antibiotic prophylaxis for bacterial endocarditis, 1067-70
   diagnostic esophagogastroduodenoscopy (EGD), 977
   stress testing, 432, 436
American Institute of Ultrasound in Medicine, 809
American National Standards Institute, 179
American Society for Laser Medicine and Surgery, 86
American Society of Colon and Rectal Surgeons, 995
American Society of Gastroenterology, 907
American Speech-Language-Hearing Association (ASHA), 179
American Thoracic Society, 486, 487
Amino amides, 147
Amino esters, 147
Amiodarone, 381, 485
Amniocentesis, 765-72
   obstetric ultrasound and, 807
   oligohydramnios and, 771
Amniography, 766
Amnionitis, 766
Amniotic fluid, 818
Amniotomy, 803, 805
Amoxicillin/clavulanic acid, 248

Anal canal stenosis, 902
Anal continence, 900-1
   anal fissure/lateral sphincterotomy and, 960, 962
Anal examination, external, 900
Anal fissure/lateral sphincterotomy, 958-63
   anoscopy for, 902, 905
   chronic fissure, 958
   conservative management of, 958-9
   continence and, 960, 962
   Crohn's disease, 955
   digital anorectal examination, 900, 901
   external/anoscopic examination, 969
   perianal skin tags, 957
Anal fistula
   anal fissure/lateral sphincterotomy and, 962
   anoscopy and, 902
   perianal abscess, incision and drainage of, 970-1, 973
   pilonidal cyst/abscess, incision and drainage of, 964
Anal papilla, 900, 901
Anal skin tags, 900
Anal sphincter function, 900-1
Anaphylaxis, 1076-9
   allergy testing and, 1096, 1100
   diphenhydramine hydrochloride, 1077, 1078
   sclerotherapy and, 74
Androscopy, 514-9
Anemia
   bone marrow aspiration and biopsy and, 1115
   esophagogastroduodenoscopy (EGD) and, 975
   flexible sigmoidoscopy and, 907
   tubal ligation, interval, and, 680
Anesthesia, 1133-76
   Bier block, 160-3
   for esophagogastroduodenoscopy (EGD), 979-81, 989
   dorsal penile nerve block, 874-7
   local, 135-40
   oral/facial, 168-76
   paracervical block, 799-802
   pediatric sedation, 156-9
   peripheral nerve blocks and field blocks, 145-55
   pudendal, 794-8
   topical, 139-40, 141-4
   trigger point injection, 164-7
Aneurysm
   cranial artery, 231
   dissecting, 416
   percutaneous arterial line placement, 298
Angina, 389
   esophagogastroduodenoscopy (EGD) and, 981
   stress testing and, 414-6
   Swan-Ganz catheterization and, 320
Angiography, pulmonary, 301
Angiotensin-converting-enzyme (ACE) inhibitors, 423
Ankle brace
   air cast, 1008, 1009
   ankle ligament protector (ALP), 1008, 1010
   Swedo/AOA, 1009
Ankle fracture, splinting, taping, and casting, 1003-13
Ankle joint, joint and soft tissue aspiration and injection, 1053
Ankle splinting, taping, and casting, 1003-13
Ankle sprain
   splinting, taping, and casting, 1003-13
   Unna paste boot and, 78, 80
Ankyloglossia, 287-90
Anomalies, congenital. See Birth defects
Anorectal anatomy/examination, clinical, 898-901
   anal continence, 900-1
   digital anorectal examination, 900
   external anal examination, 900

Anorectal fissure
   bipolar electrocoagulation, hemorrhoids, 947
   office treatment of hemorrhoids, 931
   thrombosed external hemorrhoids, 952
Anorectal tumors, 931
Anorectal ulcer, 947
Anoscopy, 902-6. See also Clinical anorectal anatomy and
     examination
   and perianal/intraanal lesions, condyloma acuminata, 663
Antiarrhythmic drug therapy, Holter monitoring, 380-1, 383
Antibiotic prophylaxis
   for auricular hematoma evacuation, 187
   for bacterial endocarditis, 1067-70
   for colonoscopy, 995-6
   for endometrial biopsy, 565
   for esophagogastroduodenoscopy (EGD), 977
   for flexible sigmoidoscopy, 911, 995
   for hysterosalpingography, 574
   for laceration repair, 19
   for lumbar puncture, 1109
Antihypertensive drug therapy, ambulatory blood pressure
     monitoring, 369
Apgar scores
   contraction stress test and, 781
   neonatal resuscitation and, 842
Appendicitis
   culdocentesis and, 594
   perianal abscess incision and drainage and, 970
Arryhthmia monitoring methods
   benefits and drawbacks of, 379-82
   comparison of, 378-9
   Holter monitoring and, 378-407
Arterial and venous studies, noninvasive, of lower extremities,
     348-68
Arterial cannulation. See Percutaneous arterial line placement
Arterial catheterization. See Percutaneous arterial line placement
Arterial laceration, central venous catheter insertion, 317
Arterial line placement. See Percutaneous arterial line placement
Arterial puncture, 340-7
   anatomy, 342-5
   arterial disease and, 340
   assessment of ulnar collateral circulation, 341-3
   Doppler evaluation of, 343-4
   pediatric, 858-60
   site selection for, 341, 345
Arterial studies, noninvasive, of lower extremities, 360-7
   risk factors for peripheral artery disease, 361
Arteries, radial and ulnar, anatomy at wrist and superficial palmar
     arch, 342
Arteriovenous fistula
   central venous catheter insertion and, 317
   percutaneous arterial line placement and, 298, 317
Arthritis, 1038
Arthrogram, 1032
Ascites
   abdominal paracentesis and peritoneal lavage and, 892
   pulmonary function testing and, 492
Asherman's syndrome, 571
Asherman's uterine adhesions, 677
Aspiration and injection, joint and soft tissue, 1036-54
Asthma
   allergy testing and, 1096
   arterial puncture and, 340
   cervical ripening/vaginal prostaglandins and, 803
   colposcopic examination and, 627
   pulmonary function testing and, 485, 492
   sclerotherapy and, 64
   tubal ligation and, 692
Atresia, choanal, 844, 855

Audiometry, 179-83
  audiogram, 179
  audiometer, 181
  Conservationists, 181
  interpretation of, 182
  standardized symbols for recording results of, 180
Auricular hematoma evacuation, 184-7. *See also* Peripheral nerve
    blocks and field blocks
  antibiotic prophylaxis for, 187

Babesiosis, 125
Bacteremia
  abscess and, 53
  endometrial biopsy and, 570
  intraosseous venous access and, 833
  joint and soft tissue aspiration and injection and, 1037
  prostate massage and, 543
  temporary pacing and, 475
  tooth, avulsed, reimplantation of, and, 285
  umbilical artery catheterization and, 850
  venous cutdown and, 339
Bacterial endocarditis
  antibiotic prophylaxis for, 911, 1067-70
  colposcopic examination and, 627
  cryocone of cervix and, 647
  cryosurgery and, 105
  endometrial biopsy and, 570
  fine-needle aspiration cytology and biopsy and, 1104
  flexible sigmoidoscopy and, 908, 927
  IUD insertion and, 580
  office treatment of hemorrhoids and, 931
  Swan-Ganz catheterization and, 331
  tooth, avulsed, reimplantation of, and, 285
Balanitis, circumcision
  in adult, 544
  in newborn, 863
Banyan kit, 1077
Barrett's esophagus, 974
Barrier contraceptives: cervical cap, condom, and contraceptive
    sponge, 742-9
Barron ligation, 937-41
Bartholin's cyst/abscess: Word catheter insertion, 596-601
Basic urodynamic studies for urinary incontinence, 508-13
Behçet's syndrome, 349
Benzocaine, 141
Beta-antagonist, pulmonary function testing, 488
Beta blockers, 390, 395, 423
  allergy testing, 1097, 1100
  silent myocardial ischemia, 384-5
Betamethasone suspension, acne therapy, 56
Bethesda system, Pap smear interpretation, 610, 611
Biceps, joint and soft tissue aspiration and injection
  long head of, 1049
  short head of, 1048
Bier block, 160-3
Biliary tract disease, 1130-41
  interpretation of, 1140-2
Bilirubin, amniocentesis, 766
Biophysical profile, obstetric ultrasound, 808, 818-9, 820, 821
Biopsy
  anoscopy and, 904, 906
  bone marrow, 1115-9
  breast, 714-7
  cervical, 633, 636, 640
  colon cancer and, 997
  colonoscopy and, 992
  colposcopic-directed, 616
  endometrial, 563-670, 646, 672
  esophagogastroduodenoscopy (EGD) and, 988-90

Biopsy—Cont'd
  of esophagus, 988, 990
  fine-needle aspiration and, 1102-8
  flexible sigmoidoscopy and, 924
  of gastric ulcer, 988-9
  of muscle, 1120-2
  of nail plate/nail bed, 44-6
  radiofrequency surgery and, 94-6
  skin, 20-6, 35, 56, 1088
Bipolar electrocoagulation (BICAP), hemorrhoids, 946-8
Birth defects
  abortion, first-trimester, and, 70
  obstetric ultrasound and, 808, 809, 818-20, 821, 822, 825-6
  suprapubic bladder aspiration and, 852
Bladder
  aspiration, suprapubic, 852-4
  catherization of, 495-9
  pediatric evaluation, emergency department ultrasound, 1145-7
  transverse view, full, 1146
  transverse/longitudinal views, emergency department
      ultrasound, 1134
Bleeding
  with gastrointestinal, esophagogastroduodenoscopy (EGD), 975
  with lower gastrointestinal, hemorrhoids, 929
  postmenopausal, 563, 672
  premenopausal, 672
Blepharitis, 215
Blepharoplasties, 98
Blood pressure monitoring, ambulatory, 369-77
Boil, 50
Bone marrow aspiration and biopsy, 1115-9
Bowel perforation, colonoscopy, 993, 998
Bowenoid
  dysplasia, 518
  papulosis, CO_2 laser therapy, 84
BPP. *See* Biophysical profile
Bradyarrhythmia, temporary pacing, 466
Bradycardia
  with cardioversion, 442
  with endotracheal intubation, 463
  Holter monitoring equipment settings and, 385-6
Brain herniation, lumbar puncture, 1114
Breast biopsy, 714-7. *See also* Fine-needle aspiration cytology and
    biopsy
  breast cancer and, 714
  considerations for, 717
  cysts and, 714
  fibroadenomas and, 714
  mammography and, 714
Breech presentation, 786
Bronchitis, 485
Bronchodilators, 486,488
Bronchoscopy, 452
Bruce protocol, 424, 433-5
Brymill Cryogun, 104, 106, 110
Bunnell technique, modified, extensor tendon repair, 1057, 1058
Bupivacaine with/without epinephrine, 135
  maximum dosage, 136, 147
  selection of, 136
  trigger point injection and, 165, 166
Burns
  intraosseous venous access, 833
  wound dressing, semiocclusive hydrogels, 1093
Bursitis, joint and soft tissue aspiration and injection, 1038
  anserine, 1052
  olecranon, 1044
  prepatellar, 1051
  subacromial, 1047
  trochanteric, 1050

Calcaneal spur, joint and soft tissue aspiration and injection, 1053

Calcium channel blockers, 423
  silent myocardial ischemia and, 384-5

Calluses, 1063

Candida
  postcoital examination test or Sims-Huhner test, 666
  west smear and KOH preparation, 670

Carbocaine. *See* Mepivacaine

Carbuncle, 50

Cancer
  abortion, first-trimester, and, 700
  anorectal, 515
  breast, 719
  cervical, 514, 601-12, 617, 635, 640, 641, 646, 724, 757
  colon, 993, 997
  colorectal, 902, 992
  endometrial, 611, 646, 672, 675, 724
  head and neck, 249-50
  penile, 84, 514
  prostate, 511
  rectal, 663
  surveillance, esophagogastroduodenoscopy (EGD), 974
  uterine/cervical hysteroscopy and, 559, 560

Carcinoma, basal cell
  appearance of, 27-8
  approach to, 27-9
  biopsy of, 22, 28-9
  cautery/curettement of, 29
  complete excision of, 29
  cryosurgery for, 104, 106, 114, 118
  Moh's chemosurgery for, 29
  radiofrequency surgery for, 96

Carcinoma, squamous cell, 29-30
  biopsy of, 30
  cryosurgery for, 105
  penis, CO_2 laser therapy, 84

Cardiac
  arrhythmias, 423, 437-45, 452, 554, 1088
  catheterization, 301, 389
  depolarization, cardioversion, 437-43
  drug toxicity, temporary pacing, 475
  dysrhythmia, 309, 310, 318, 340, 373, 416, 890
  ischemia, Swan-Ganz catheterization, 320
  pacing, 320, 321, 464-76
  perforation, Swan-Ganz catheterization, 320
  rehabilitation, stress testing, 413
  tamponade, Swan-Ganz catheterization, 320, 330
  ultrasound, 1127-32

Cardiopulmonary arrest, intraosseous venous access, 833

Cardiopulmonary disease, flexible sigmoidoscopy, 908

Cardiopulmonary instability, esophagogastroduodenoscopy (EGD), 975

Cardiopulmonary resuscitation. *See also* Cardioversion
  arterial puncture and, 340, 341
  central venous catheter insertion and, 318
  internal jugular vein catheterization and, 313
  intraosseous venous access and, 835
  subclavian venipuncture and, 305, 312
  venous cutdown and, 334, 336, 337

Cardioversion, 303, 437-43. *See also* Stress testing
  electrodes and placement with, 437-8
  energy selection for, 438-9
  synchronization, 438

Carpal tunnel syndrome, 1044

Cast immobilization, 1014-27
  cast removal and, 1023-4
  common cast types for, 1016-7

Cast removal, 1023-4
  cast immobilization and, 1023-4

Casting, ankle, 1003-13

Cataract, senile, 231

Catheter
  Bonnano, 503
  Coudé, 496-7
  Foley, 496, 498
  insertion, central venous, 300-18
  Stamey suprapubic, 502

Catheterization
  bladder, 495-9
  umbilical artery/vein, 847-51
  suprapubic, insertion and change, 500-7
  Swan-Ganz, 319-31
  Word catheter insertion, Bartholin's cyst/abscess, 596-601

Cauliflower ear, 184

Cautery, chemical
  curettage biopsy and, 22
  shave biopsy and, 22

Cellulitis
  abscess, incision and drainage of, and, 53
  joint and soft tissue aspiration and injection and, 1037
  perianal, 957
  umbilical artery catheterization and, 850

Cellulose, oxidized, 1087

Central nervous system
  infections, lumbar puncture, 1109
  stress testing, 432
  toxicity, gastric lavage, 885

Central venous catheter insertion, 300-18
  anatomical relationships and, 304, 314
  cardiac catheterization, 301
  hemodialysis and, 301
  hemothorax and, 301, 309, 310, 316
  mastectomy and, 301
  plasmapheresis and, 301
  pneumothorax and, 301, 309, 310, 316
  pulmonary angiography and, 301
  superior vena cava syndrome and, 301
  surface markers on chest wall and, 305
  Swan-Ganz catheter and, 301
  total parenteral nutrition and, 300
  transvenous pacemaker insertion and, 300, 301

Central venous pressure, 30

Cerebral vascular disease, 137

Cerebrovascular accident
  with esophagogastroduodenoscopy (EGD), 981
  with self-injection therapy for treatment of impotence, 555
  with stress testing, 432

Cerumen impaction removal, 192-6. *See also* Removal of foreign bodies from ear and nose

Cerumenex. *See* Triethanolamine

Cervical ablation, 799

Cervical adenocarcinoma, Pap smear, 611

Cervical cap, 742-6
  cervical dysplasia and, 742
  failure of, 745
  vs. diaphragm, 742-3

Cervical cerclage placement, 807

Cervical conization, 640-4. *See also* Loop electrosurgical excision procedure (LEEP) for treating CIN
  biopsy and, 640
  cervical carcinoma and, 640, 641
  colposcopic examination and, 527, 616, 636, 640
  dilation and curettage and, 642
  endocervical curettage and, 640, 642
  loop electrosurgical excision procedure (LEEP) for treating CIN and, 729
  Pap smear and, 640, 642
  pregnancy and, 640, 641
  radiofrequency surgery and, 98, 99

Cervical dysplasia
cervical cap and, 742
CO_2 laser therapy and, 84
colposcopic examination for, 616, 617
HPV-DNA testing of the cervix and, 613
Pap smear and, 601-12
radiofrequency surgery for, 98-100
Cervical incompetence
cervical conization and, 644
hysterosalpingography and, 572
loop electrosurgical excision procedure (LEEP) for treating CIN and, 740
Cervical intraepithelial neoplasia. *See* CIN
Cervical ripening/vaginal prostaglandins, 803-6
Cervical spine disorders, 453
Cervical spine trauma, 453
Cervical stenosis
cervical conization and, 644
endometrial biopsy and, 563
loop electrosurgical excision procedure (LEEP) for treating CIN and, 739, 740
Cervicitis, 685
colposcopic examination and, 623, 636
cryocone of cervix and, 645, 646, 650
endometrial biopsy and, 563
IUD insertion and, 579
loop electrosurgical excision procedure (LEEP) for treating CIN and, 730, 739
permanent female sterilization (tubal ligation) and, 697
Cervicography, 757-61
cervical camera (Cerviscope), 757, 758
cervigram report, 759
colposcopy and, 757, 758
cost of, 761
Pap smear and, 757-61
Cervix, testing for HPV-DNA, 613-5
Cesarean section
obstetric ultrasound and, 822
postpartum tubal ligation and, 695
spontaneous fetal-movement counting and, 775
Cetacaine. *See* Benzocaine
Chalazion and hordeolum therapy, 214-29
chalazion, description of, 214-5
chalazion removal, 215-219
hordeolum, 219-20
Chemical cautery, treatment of vulvar, perianal, vaginal, penile, urethral condyloma acuminata, 656-7
Chemotherapeutics, intrathecal, lumbar puncture, 1109
Chemotherapy
central venous catheter insertion and, 300
Moh's, 29
pulmonary function testing and, 845
Chest compression, neonatal resuscitation, 844-5
Chest tube insertion, 444-51
Chlamydia
abortion, first-trimester, and, 702
cryocone of cervix and, 647
tubal ligation and, 684
wet smear and KOH preparation and, 670-1
Chlorprocaine, 147
Cholecystitis, acute, 1139-42
Cholelithiasis, 1140, 1141
Chorionic villous sampling, 808
Choroiditis, 231
Chromosomal analysis
amniocentesis and, 765
bone marrow aspiration and biopsy and, 1115
Chronic obstructive pulmonary disease, 340
esophagogastroduodenoscopy (EGD) and, 981
management of epistaxis and, 243

Chronic obstructive pulmonary disease—Cont'd
pulmonary function testing and, 485, 486
suspected pericardial effusions and, 1127
Swan-Ganz catheterization and, 320
temporary pacing and, 465
Chylothorax, chest tube insertion, 444
CIN
cryocone of cervix, 105, 645, 646, 650, 651
terminology and definition of, 602
loop electrosurgical excision procedure (LEEP) and, 729-41
Circumcision, adult, 544-9
Circumcision, newborn, 863-73. *See also* Dorsal penile nerve block; Topical anesthesia
Gomco method, 864-9
Mogen method, 872
Plastibell method, 869-73
Cisternography, 1109
Clinical anorectal anatomy and examination, 898-901. *See also* Anoscopy
Clubfoot, cast immobilization, 1015
CO_2 laser therapy, 84-6
Cocaine
description/use of, 139-40, 141
topical hemostatic agent, 1087
Colitis, ulcerative, 105
Collagen injection, acne therapy, 56
Collagen, microfibrillar, 1087-8
Colonoscopy, 992-1000. *See also* Anaphylaxis; Antibiotic prophylaxis; Diagnostic esophagogastroduodenoscopy (EGD); Flexible sigmoidoscopy
anal fissure and, 960
anoscopy and, 902
antibiotic prophylaxis for, 995-6
with barium enema study, 992
learning, 998-9
vs. radioscopic evaluation, 992
Colpocentesis, 588-96
Colposcopic examination, 616-39. *See also* Androscopy; Cervical conization; Cryocone of the cervix; HPV-DNA testing of the cervix; Pap smear: screening for cervical cancer
cervical conization and, 640
cervicography and, 757, 758, 759
colposcopic findings, 617-23
cryotherapy and, 634
histology/cytology interpretation of data, and, 634-5
HPV-DNA testing of the cervix, 613, 614
loop electrosurgical excision procedure (LEEP) for treating CIN and, 729-30, 733
Pap smear and, 623
strong considerations for, 623
terminology, 617, 618
treatment of vulvar, perianal, vaginal, penile, urethral condyloma acuminata, 653
Colpotomy, 679
Comedo
extractors, use of, 54-5
removal of, 54-5
Compartment syndrome, 1024
Compression stockings, sclerotherapy, 70
Computed tomography
abdominal paracentesis and peritoneal lavage and, 892
shoulder dislocations and, 1029, 1031
subarachnoid hemorrhage and, 1109
Condom, 746-7
Condyloma
androscopy and, 514, 515
CO_2 laser therapy and, 84
episiotomy and, 786
perianal, 623, 902

Condyloma acuminata, treatment of vulvar, perianal, vaginal, penile, urethral, 30, 514, 515, 518, 653-5. *See also* Cryosurgery; Cryocone of cervix; Radiofrequency surgery
5-fluorouracil (5-FU)/extensive condylomata, 654, 661-2
  acetowhite epithelium, 653
  chemical cautery and, 656-7
  colposcopy, 653
  comparative costs of treatment modalities, 663
  cryosurgery, 115-7, 654-6
  excisional/ablative therapy for, 658
  interferon therapy for, 657-8
  loop electrosurgical excision and, 658-61
  perianal and intraanal lesions and, 662-3
  radiofrequency surgery and, 96-7
  recommended therapies for, 654
Condylomata, genital
  colposcopic examination and, 623
  Pap smear and, 503, 608, 611, 612
Congenital heart disease, 415
Congestive heart failure, 439
  electrical impedance plethysmography (IPG) and, 351
  endotracheal intubation and, 452
  stress testing and, 342
  Swan-Ganz catheterization and, 320
  umbilical artery catheterization and, 850
Conjunctival foreign bodies, removal of, 221-30
Constipation, 907
Continence, anal, 900-1
Contraception failure, IUD insertion, 582
Contraceptive implants (Norplant), 718-28
  insertion, 724-72
  Pap smears and, 718
  removal of, 726, 727
  side effects of, 720, 722, 724
  special program for indigent patients, 727
Contraceptive methods
  barrier, 742-9, 750-6
  permanent female sterilization (tubal ligation), 678-98
  sponge, vaginal, 747-9
Contraction stress test, 781-4. *See also* Nonstress test; Obstetric ultrasound
  nonreactive, 781-3
  obstetric ultrasound and, 822
  reactive, 781
Convulsions, abortion, first-trimester, 711
Cor pulmonale, Swan-Ganz catheterization, 320
Corneal abrasions and removal of corneal or conjunctival foreign bodies, 221-30. *See also* Pediatric sedation
  fluorescein examination of cornea and conjunctiva, 221-4
  pressure eye patch for, 226
  and removal of residual corneal rust ring, 229
  and removal of superficial foreign body, 228
  treatment of uncomplicated corneal abrasions, 224-7
  Wood's light examination, 82
Corns, 1063
Coronary angioplasty, 414
Coronary arrhythmias, stress testing, 415
Coronary artery disease
  exercise testing for diagnosis of, 432
  stress testing and, 413-5, 432
Coronary artery revascularization, 414, 415
Corticosteroid injection
  hypertrophic scars and keloids and, 50-60
  intralesional, acne therapy, and, 55-6
  joint and soft tissue aspiration and injection, 1036-54
  pulmonary function testing and, 486
Council for Accreditation of Occupational Hearing Conservationists, 181

Counseling
  for abortion, first-trimester, 699-700
  for contraceptive implants (Norplant), 720
  genetics, 1120
CPR. *See* Cardiopulmonary resuscitation
Cricothyroidectomy, emergency, 270-3
  cricothyroid membrane and, 271-2
  needle, 270-1
Cricothyrotomy, 452, 453
Crohn's disease, 954
  anal fissure and, 959-60
  edematous perianal skin tags and, 955
  flexible sigmoidoscopy and, 907
  perianal abscess incision and drainage and, 973
Cryocone of the cervix, 645-52. *See also* Colposcopic examination; Loop electrosurgical excision procedure (LEEP) for treating CIN
  Pap smear and, 646, 650-1
Cryoglobulins, 105
  cryocone of cervix and, 647
Cryoslush therapy, acne, 56
Cryosurgery, 102-20. *See also* Cryocone of the cervix
  areas not recommended for, 106
  biopsies and, 112-4
  cryosurgical tips, 108
  hand gun and unit for, 107
  lesions difficult to treat, 106
  liquid nitrogen, condyloma acuminata, 655-6
  nitrous oxide, condyloma acuminata, 655
Cryotherapy
  colposcopic examination and, 616, 627, 634
  common and plantar warts and, 37
  hypertrophic scars and keloids and, 59
  lentigo and, 31
  seborrheic keratoses and, 31
CST. *See* Contraction stress test
Culdocentesis (colpocentesis), 588-95
  cul de sac mass and, 589, 590
Cyanosis, central, 841, 842, 843
Cyclonine, 141
Cyclopegic drops, 225
Cyst
  breast biopsy and, 714
  nabothian, 608, 610
  pilonidal, 964-8
  sebaceous, 27, 36, 97
Cystocele
  clinical grading system of, 512
  diaphragm fitting and, 750, 751
Cystotomy, 503
Cystourethrogram, 495
Cytology
  fine-needle aspiration, 1102-8
  colposcopic examination, 634-5
Cytomegalovirus
  cryocone of cervix and, 647
  cryosurgery and, 105

D & C. *See* Dilation and curettage
DC current (Ultroid) treatment, hemorrhoids, 943-6
De Quervain's disease, 1043
Dead arm syndrome, 1028
Decubitus ulcers
  Unna paste boot and, 79
  wound dressing, occlusive hydrocolloids, and, 1094
Deep vein thrombosis
  cast immobilization and, 1026
  stress testing and, 416
Dehydration, intraosseous venous access, 833

DeLee suctioning, 855-7. *See also* Neonatal resuscitation
    meconium aspiration and, 855
Dental procedures
    antibiotic prophylactic regimen for bacterial endocarditis in
        patients at risk, 1068
    endocarditis prophylaxis for, 1068, 1069
Depression, first-trimester abortion, 712
Dermabrasion, acne therapy, 56
Dermatofibroma, 30, 106
Dermatological surgery, 1084-9
Dermatomyositis, 1120
Dermatoses, 35
DES. *See* Diethylstilbestrol exposure
Diabetes
    abscess, incision and drainage of, and, 50
    ambulatory blood pressure monitoring and, 370
    arterial studies, noninvasive, of lower extremities, and, 361
    cervical ripening/vaginal prostaglandins and, 803
    corns and calluses and, 1063
    endometrial biopsy and, 563
    gestational, 778
    IUD insertion and, 579
    joint and soft tissue aspiration and injection and, 1037
    local anesthesia and, 135, 137
    perianal abscess incision and drainage and, 970
    peripheral artery disease and, 360, 361
    postpartum tubal ligation and, 695
    segmental pressure measurement, lower extremities, and, 363
    stress testing and, 416
    tonometry and, 237
    tooth reimplantation and, 285
    tubal ligation and, 680, 684, 692
    vasectomy and, 536
Diabetes mellitus
    colposcopic examination and, 627
    macrosomia and, 821
    nonstress test and, 777
    obstetric ultrasound and, 817-8
    tongue-tie snipping (frenotomy) for ankyloglossia and, 288
Diagnostic esophagogastroduodenoscopy (EGD), 974-91. *See also*
    Anaphylaxis; Antibiotic prophylaxis; Flexible sigmoidoscopy
    antibiotic prophylaxis for, 977
    biopsy with, 988-90
    high-risk groups for, 981
    sedation/monitoring with, 979-81, 989
Diagnostic hysteroscopy, 559-62
Diaphragm fitting, 750-6
    vs. cervical cap, 742, 743
Diaphragmatic hernia, 843
Diazepam, 89, 545
    for cardioversion, 442
    for colonoscopy, 996
    for esophagogastroduodenoscopy (EGD), 980
    for hysterosalpingography, 574
    for inguinal hernia reduction, 882
    for temporomandibular joint, dislocated, reduction of, 280
Dibucaine with/without epinephrine, 135, 141
Diethylstilbestrol exposure
    colposcopic examination and, 619, 623, 627
    hysterosalpingography and, 571
    loop electrosurgical excision procedure (LEEP) for treating CIN
        and, 730
    Pap smear and, 603, 612
Digital anorectal examination, 900
Digital nerve block, 148, 149
    anatomy, 138
    ring-block technique of, 39, 45
Digitalis, 415, 431, 440, 442
Digoxin, 416, 432, 442

Dilation and curettage, 672-7. *See also* First trimester abortion;
    Paracervical block
    cervical conization and, 642
    hysterosalpingography and, 572
    tubal ligation and, 684, 697
Dinoprostone, 803-5
Dislocation
    cast immobilization for, 1015
    shoulder, 1028-32
    temporomandibular joint, 279-82
Diverticulitis
    colonoscopy and, 993
    flexible sigmoidoscopy and, 908
    perianal abscess incision and drainage and, 970
Doppler. *See also* Ultrasound
    evaluation, arterial puncture, 343-4
Doppler studies, arterial, lower extremities
    pulse volume waveform analysis, 364-6
    segmental pressure measurement, 361-3
    velocity waveform analysis, 364-6
Doppler studies, venous, lower extremities, 349, 357-60
    interpretation of, 359-60
    Valsalva maneuver and, 359
Doppler ultrasound, radial artery cannulation, 297-8
Dorsal penile nerve block. *See also* Topical anesthesia
Dorsal penile nerve block, 874-7
Doxycycline
    with abortion, first-trimester, 713
    with dilation and curettage, 676
    with hysterosalpingography, 574
    with IUD insertion, 580
    with loop electrosurgical excision procedure (LEEP) for treating
        CIN, 740
Drug ingestion
    abdominal paracentesis and peritoneal lavage, 893
    abnormal Pap smear and, 603
    gastric lavage and, 885
Duodenitis, chronic, 975
Duplex scanning, lower extremities, venous study, 349, 356-7
    interpretation of, 357
Duranest. *See* Etidocaine
Dye laser therapy, 86-9
Dysmenorrhea, 579, 583
Dysrhythmia recognition and management
    Holter monitoring and, 378-407
    office electrocardiogram and, 408-12

Ear
    block, 152
    canal irrigation, 194-6
    infection, 188-91
    lobe, keloid excision and resection, 60-1
    piercing, 202-5
    removal of foreign bodies from, 206-13
ECG. *See* Electrocardiogram
Ectopic pregnancy, 1132-3
    abortion, first-trimester, and, 712
    contraceptive implants (Norplant) and, 719, 722
    culdocentesis and, 588-9, 594
    human chorionic gonadotropin and, 1132, 1133
    hysterosalpingography and, 574
    IUD insertion and, 578, 579, 582
    obstetric ultrasound and, 807, 811, 822-3
    radiofrequency surgery and, 98
    transabdominal scanning for, 1133-5
    transvaginal scanning for, 1135-6
    tubal ligation and, 697
Eczema, 202
Efudex. *See* 5-fluorouracil

Elbow
joint and soft tissue aspiration and injection of, 1045
subluxation of the radial head, 1022-35
Electrical impedance plethysmography (IPG), lower extremities, 349, 351-4
interpretation and sources of error of, 353-4
Electrocardiogram
baseline recommendations for, 409
Holter monitoring and, 391-2, 393
office, 408-12
and rhythm strip, comparison to Holter monitoring, 379
stress testing and, 425
temporary cardiac pacing and, 473
Electrodessication
with curettage biopsy, 22
with shave biopsy, 22
Electromechanical dissociation (EMD), clinical, 1127, 1131-2
interpretation of, 1132
Swan-Ganz catheterization and, 320
Electrosurgery
loop electrosurgical excision procedure (LEEP) for treating CIN, 729-41
sebaceous hyperplasia and, 35
Electrosurgical units/generators, 731
Ellman Surgitron, 730
Embolism
percutaneous arterial line placement and, 298
Swan-Ganz catheterization and, 331
temporary pacing and, 475
venous cutdown and, 339
Embolization, umbilical artery catheterization, 850
Embolus, central venous catheter insertion, 317
Embryo transfer, obstetric ultrasound, 808
Emergency cricothyroidectomy and tracheostomy, 270-8
Emergency department ultrasound, 1123-47. *See also* Noninvasive venous and arterial studies of the lower extremities; Obstetric ultrasound
biliary tract disease and, 1139-41
cardiac, 1127-32
description of technology, 1123-5
initial scanning, 1125-7
obstetric/gynecologic, 1132-9
pediatric evaluation of bladder prior to suprapubic aspiration, 1145-6
vascular disorders, 1142-5
EMLA (eutectic mixture of local anesthetic), 140, 141, 142, 143-4
Emphysema
chest tube insertion and, 450
pulmonary function testing and, 492
tracheostomy and, 277
Empyema, 444
Endocarditis. *See* Bacterial endocarditis
Endocervical curettage
cervical conization and, 640, 642
colposcopic examination and, 617, 632-3
cryocone of cervix and, 646
loop electrosurgical excision procedure (LEEP) for treating CIN and, 739
Endometrial biopsy, 563-70. *See also* Colposcopic examination
Endometrial polyps
dilation and curettage for, 672
hysteroscopy, diagnostic, for, 559
Endometrioma, 589, 594
Endometriosis
radiofrequency surgery for, 98
tubal ligation, interval, and, 684
Endometritis, 580

Endotracheal intubation, 452-63
gastric lavage and, 885, 886, 887
neonatal resuscitation and, 843
Ephedrine sulphate, 552, 554
Epicutaneous skin test, allergy, 1097-8
Epididymitis, congestive, 530
Epiglottitis, 250
Epinephrine, 140, 1077, 1088
Episiotomy, 785-93
Epistaxis, 242-8. *See also* Local anesthesia
anatomy of septal blood supply and, 242
application of pressure for, 244
posterior pack care for, 247-8
rhinolaryngoscopy and, 250, 259
Epstein-Barr infection
cryocone of cervix and, 647
cryosurgery and, 105
Epithelial tags, biopsy, 22
Erythasma, Wood's light examination, 82
Erythroblastosis fetalis, 818
Esophagogastroduodenoscopy, (EGD), 974-91
esophageal stricture and, 975
esophagitis, chronic, and, 975
Ethyl chloride, 142, 144
Etidocaine, 135, 147
European Committee for Ultrasound Radiation Safety, 807
Exanthems, 35
Exercise
physiology of, applied to stress testing, 413-4
prescription/testing, 433-6
Extensor tendon repair, 1055-9. *See also* Laceration repair
Eye
cryosurgery, 118
fishhook removal in, 128
topical anesthesia for, 140
Eye charts
illiterate E or tumbling E, 232, 233, 234
Snellen, 222, 232, 235

5-fluorourcil (5-FU), 30
for treatment of extensive condylomata, 654, 661-2
Facial/oral anesthesia, 168-76
Fasciitis, necrotizing, 793
Ferric subsulfate (Monsel's solution), 1085-6
Fetal
distress, 786, 799
health, amniocentesis, 766
hypoxia, 776, 819, 820
loss, cervical conization, 644
lung maturity, amniocentesis, 765, 766
monitoring, cervical ripening/vaginal prostaglandins, 805
mortality/stillbirth, 773-5, 781, 808
nonstress test, 776
prematurity, episiotomy, 786
size, obstetric ultrasound, 819
tachycardia, 770
viability evaluation, 1137-8
Fibrin sealant (tissue glue), 1088-9
Fibroadenomas, breast biopsy, 714
Fibroids, first-trimester abortion, 712
Fibromyalgia, 164
Fibrosis, absorbable gelatin sponge/powder, 1087
Fibrositis, joint and soft tissue aspiration and injection, 1038
Field blocks and peripheral nerve blocks, 145-55
Fine-needle aspiration cytology and biopsy, 1102-8
wound care for, 1107
Finger, edematous, ring removal, 121-3
string-wrap method, 121-3

Finger/toe joints, joint and soft tissue aspiration and injection, 1041
Fingertip/nail bed hematoma evacuation, 47-9
First-trimester abortion, 699-713
Fishhook removal, 128-32
    angler's string-yank method, 128-9
    barbed, 131
    barb-sheath method, 129-30
    traditional pull-through method, 130-1
Fissure, anal, anoscopy, 902, 905
Fistula
    rectovaginal, episiotomy, 788-90, 793
    urogenital, episiotomy, 793
Fistulectomy, 53
Fistulotomy, anal, perianal abscess incision and drainage, 970-1
Fitness evaluation, exercise testing/prescription, 433-6
Flavivirus, 125
Flexible fiberoptic rhinolaryngoscopy, 240-59, 260, 263
Flexible sigmoidoscopy, 907-8. *See also* Antibiotic prophylaxis;
    Clinical anorectal anatomy and examination
    anal fissure and, 960
    biopsy and, 924
    cleaning and disinfection of scopes, 927
    significance of various polyps and, 926
Flumazenil, 158, 674, 996
Fluorescein examination of cornea and conjunctiva, 221-4
    Wood's light examination and, 82
Fluoroscopy
    hysterosalpingography and, 575
    Swan-Ganz catheterization and, 325, 329
    temporary cardiac pacing and, 469-70
FNA. *See* Fine-needle aspiration cytology and biopsy
Foot blocks, 152-4
    distribution of sensory innervation to foot, 153
    sural nerve block, 152, 154
    tibial nerve block, 152, 154
Forehead block, 150
Foreign bodies, removal
    cornea or conjunctiva, 221-30
    ears and nose, 206-13
Fractures
    ankle splinting, taping, and casting, 1003-13
    ipsilateral, intraosseous venous access, 833
    cast immobilization, 1015
Frankenhauser's ganglion, 799
Freckles. *See* Lentigo
Frenotomy for ankyloglossia, 287-90
Fungus infection, bone marrow aspiration and biopsy, 1115
Furuncle, 50

Gallbladder, 1139-42
Gallstones, 1141-2
Ganglion, joint and soft tissue aspiration and injection, 1043
Gangrene, 53
Gas exchange, arterial puncture, 340
Gastric catheter placement, neonatal resuscitation, 844
Gastric lavage, 884-91. *See also* Nasogastric tube and Salem sump
    insertion
    closed system technique, 888-90
    initial setup (all systems) for, 886
    lavage systems for, 885
    open system technique of, 887, 888
    substances bound by activated charcoal and, 890
Gastric retention, 975
Gastric ulcer
    biopsy of, 988-9
    monitoring for, 975
Gastritis, chronic, 975

Gastrointestinal hemorrhage, upper, 884-91
Gastrointestinal procedures, antibiotic prophylactic regimens for
    bacterial endocarditis, 1070
Gastroscopy, 984
Gelatin sponge/powder, absorbable, topical hemostatic agent, 1087
Genetics
    amniocentesis, 765
    counseling, muscle biopsy, 1120
    disease, interval tubal ligation, 679
Genital anomalies, first-trimester abortion, 713
Genital warts. *See* Androscopy; Condyloma; Human
    papillomavirus
Genitalia, ambiguous, newborn circumcision, 864
Genitourinary procedures, antibiotic prophylactic regimens for
    bacterial endocarditis, 1070
Gestational sac, 1135, 1137
Glaucoma, 231, 232, 237. *See also* Tonometry
Glomerulonephritis, poststreptococcal
    cryocone of cervix and, 647
    cryosurgery and, 105
Gomco method, newborn circumcision, 864-9, 872-3
Gonorrhea
    cervicitis, cryocone of cervix, and, 647
    first-trimester abortion and, 702
    interval tubal ligation and, 684
    wet smear and KOH preparation and, 670-1
Grading system, stress testing, 430-1
Granulocytopenia, 971
Granuloma
    formation, absorbable gelatin sponge/powder, 1087
    pyogenic, 87
Guillain-Barré syndrome, 1109
Gunshot wounds, endotracheal intubation, 453
Gynecologic ultrasound, 1132-9. *See also* Ultrasound

Hand, distribution of cutaneous sensation by radial/ulnar/median
    nerves, 151
Head
    frontal section of, 254
    parasagittal section of, 258
    postlumbar puncture headache, 1144
Heart block
    atrioventricular block, 467
    bifascicular block, 467
    bundle-branch block, 426
    left bundle-branch block, 415, 429
    right bundle-branch block, 415, 430
    temporary pacing parameter settings, 472
Heart disease, interval tubal ligation, 680, 684, 692
Heart valve, prosthetic
    endometrial biopsy and, 565
    Swan-Ganz catheterization and, 321
Heart views, ultrasound, long/short axis, 1129, 1130
Heartburn, 975
Heimlich maneuver, 1080-3
Helicobacter pylori, 989
Hemangiomas
    cherry, 36
    cryosurgery and, 105, 117-8
    pulsed tunable dye laser therapy and, 87
Hematoma evacuation
    auricular, 184-7
    subungual, 47-9
Hematuria
    basic urodynamic studies for urinary incontinence and, 511
    bladder catheterization and, 498
    prostate massage and, 543

Hematuria—Cont'd
  suprapubic catheter insertion and change and, 502
  suprapubic taps or aspirations and, 506
  vasectomy and, 525
Hemoccult positive stool, flexible sigmoidoscopy, 907
Hemodialysis, central venous catheter insertion, 301
Hemodynamic instability, Swan-Ganz catheterization, 320
Hemoperitoneum
  culdocentesis and, 588, 589, 594
  peritoneal lavage and, 892
Hemophilia
  bone marrow aspiration and biopsy and, 1115
  newborn circumcision and, 869
Hemopoietic function, bone marrow aspiration and biopsy, 1115
Hemorrhage
  with abortion, first-trimester, 712
  with intraosseous venous access, 833
Hemorrhoidal skin tags, external (perianal), 954-7
Hemorrhoidectomy, 929
Hemorrhoids, 929-53
  anoscopy and, 902, 903, 905
  bipolar electrocoagulation (BICAP) of, 946-8
  classifications of, 929-31
  CO₂ laser therapy and, 84
  cryosurgery and, 105
  DC current (Ultroid) treatment for, 943-6
  external anal examination and, 900, 901
  infrared coagulation (IRC) treatment for, 941-3
  internal, modalities for treatment of, 937
  radiofrequency treatment for, 946-8
  rubber-band ligation (Barron or McGivney) for, 937-41
  sclerotherapy for, 948-50
  thrombosed external, 950-2
Hemostatic agents, topical, 1084-9
Hemothorax
  central venous catheter insertion and, 301, 309, 310, 316
  chest tube insertion and, 444, 446
  thoracentesis and, 484
Hemotologic disease, perianal abscess incision and drainage, 971
Heparin
  for arterial puncture, 341, 344, 347, 858
  for Swan-Ganz catheterization, 329
  for umbilical artery catheterization, 848
Hepatic abscess/infarction, umbilical artery catheterization, 850
Hepatitis B
  condom and, 747
  cryocone of cervix and, 647
  cryosurgery and, 105
Hernias, incisional, abdominal paracentesis and peritoneal lavage, 896
Herpes zoster, 477
HFG. *See* Hysterosalpingography
Hiatal hernia
  esophagogastroduodenoscopy (EGD) and, 975
  tubal ligation, interval, and, 680
Hidradenitis, 105
Hip, joint and soft tissue aspiration and injection, 1051
Histology, colposcopic examination, 634-6
HIV. *See* Human immunodeficiency virus
Holter monitoring, 378-407. *See also* Office electrocardiograms
  benefits and drawbacks of available monitoring methods, 379-82
  case study of, 391-402, 403-6
  comparison of available arrhythmia monitoring methods, 378-9
  interpretation of, 388-90
  sample Holter monitor, 390-1
  silent myocardial ischemia and, 384-5
  vs. stress testing, 383-4

Hordeolum and chalazion therapy, 214-20
Hormone replacement therapy, 563
HPV-DNA testing of the cervix, 613-5
  cost of, 614-5
  detection tests, 614
  polymerase chain reaction with, 614
Human chorionic gonadotropin
  ectopic pregnancy and, 1132, 1133
  obstetric ultrasound and, 823, 824
Human immunodeficiency virus
  abortion, first-trimester, and, 700, 702
  colposcopic examination and, 623
  condom and, 747
  laser ablation of cervix and, 645
  laser therapy and, 85
  newborn circumcision and, 863
  radiofrequency surgery and, 85
Human papillomavirus. *See also* HPV-DNA testing of the cervix
  laser therapy and, 85
  radiofrequency surgery and, 85
Human papillomavirus lesions
  androscopy and, 514
  colposcopic examination and, 616, 623
  cryocone of cervix, and, 646, 651
  cryosurgery and, 517
  laser ablation of cervix and, 645
  Pap smear and, 601, 609, 611
  penile biopsy and, 517
  radiofrequency surgery and, 517
  rectal carcinoma and, 663
  treatment of vulvar, perianal, vaginal, penile, urethral condyloma acuminata and, 653-65
Hurricaine gel. *See* Benzocaine
Hydatidiform mole, 807, 819, 822, 823
Hydramnios, amniocentesis, 766
Hydrocele of spermatic cord, 881
Hydrocortisone, anaphylaxis, 1078
Hydrocystomas, eccrine, 98
Hydrogen peroxide, 1087
Hydrothorax
  central tube insertion and, 444
  central venous catheter insertion and, 317
Hypercapnia, 452
Hyperlipidemia, 361
Hyperplasia
  adenomatous/endometrial, biopsy and, 563
  sebaceous, 35, 98, 105
Hypertension
  abdominal aortic aneurysm and, 1143
  ambulatory blood pressure monitoring and, 369-77
  arterial puncture and, 341, 346
  cervical ripening/vaginal prostaglandins and, 803
  endotracheal intubation and, 463
  gestational, 777, 778, 818
  obstetric ultrasound and, 817
  office electrocardiogram and, 408
  percutaneous arterial line placement and, 293
  peripheral artery disease and, 361
  portal, 931
  postpartum tubal ligation and, 695
  self-injection therapy for treatment of impotence and, 554
  stress testing and, 415, 416
  tubal ligation, interval, and, 680
  vasectomy and, 536
Hyperthermia, 885
Hyperthyroidism, 231
Hypertrophic anal papilla, 962
Hyperventilation, 340

Hypoglycemia, newborn, 847
Hypokalemia, 442
Hypopigmentation, 661
Hypoproteinemia, 484
Hypospadias
    dorsal penile nerve block and, 874
    newborn circumcision and, 864
Hypotension
    allergy testing and, 1096
    arterial puncture and, 346
    cardioversion and, 439
    endotracheal intubation and, 463
    stress testing and, 432
    suspected pericardial effusions, and, 1127, 1131
    Swan-Ganz catheterization and, 321
    venous cutdown and, 332
Hypothermia
    gastric lavage and, 890
    neonatal resuscitation and, 842
Hypovolemia
    central venous catheter insertion and, 300, 302
    intraosseous venous access and, 832
    neonatal resuscitation and, 844
    thoracentesis and, 484
Hypoxemia, 890
Hypoxia
    endotracheal intubation and, 452, 453, 462
    neonatal resuscitation and, 846
    thoracentesis and, 484
Hysterectomy
    cryocone of cervix and, 646
    permanent female sterilization (tubal ligation) and, 697
Hysterosalpingography, 571-7
Hysteroscopy, diagnostic, 559-62, 587

Ice, topical anesthetic, 142, 144
Immunocompromised patient
    abscess, incision and drainage of, and, 50
    bone marrow aspiration and biopsy and, 1115
    ear piercing and, 202
    fine-needle aspiration cytology and biopsy and, 1103
    IUD insertion and, 579
    joint and soft tissue aspiration and injection and, 1037
    muscle biopsy and, 1122
    myringotomy and, 188
    perianal abscess incision and drainage and, 970
    pilonidal cyst/abscess incision/drainage and, 965
    tooth, avulsed, reimplantation of, and, 285
Impotence, self-injection therapy, 550-6
    alpha-adrenergic agents for, 552
    anatomy, penis and scrotum, 551
    priapism and, 552, 553
    treatment of persistent erection, 554
    vasoactive agents and, 550, 551
In vitro fertilization, obstetric ultrasound, 808
In vitro testing (RAST), allergy, 1099
Incision and drainage of an abscess, 50-3
Incision repair, needle selection, 7-11
Incompetent cervix
    contraction stress test and, 783
    first-trimester abortion and, 712
Incontinence, urinary, basic urodynamic studies for, 508-13
Indigent patients, special program, contraceptive implants
        (Norplant), 727
Indigestion, 975
Indirect laryngoscopy, 260-3
Infants and newborns, visual function examination technique,
        232, 234

Infection. *See* Abscess
Infertility
    cervical conization and, 644
    ectopic pregnancy and, 1133
    endometrial biopsy and, 563
    evaluation for, 559, 563
    first-trimester abortion and, 712
    hysterosalpingography and, 571
    loop electrosurgical excision procedure (LEEP) for treating CIN
        and, 740
    obstetric ultrasound and, 808
    postcoital examination test or Sims-Huhner test and, 666-8
Inflammatory bowel disease
    anal fissure and, 959
    colonoscopy and, 992, 993
    office treatment of hemorrhoids and, 931
    perianal abscess incision and drainage and, 973
Informed consent, 1071-5
Infraorbital nerve block, 171-2
Infrared coagulation, 941-3
Inguinal hernia reduction, 881-3
    direct inguinal hernia and, 881
    femoral hernia and, 881
    incarcerated hernia and, 881, 882
    indirect inguinal hernia and, 881
    strangulated hernia and, 882
Institute of Medicine, 409
Interferon therapy, 657-8
Internal jugular vein
    catheterization technique of, 313-7
    percutaneous arterial line placement for, 302
International Federation of Cervical Pathology and Colposcopy,
        617
Interstitial fibrosis, 492
Intestinal obstruction, 264
Intraatrial thrombosis, cardioversion, 442
Intradermal skin test, allergy, 1098-0, 1100
Intraorbital nerve block, 150-1
Intraosseous venous access (IVA), 831-40
    intramedullary venous system for, 833
    products acceptable for intraosseous infusion, 832
    site preference for, 835
Intraperitoneal fluid, culdocentesis, 588
Intrathecal antibiotics/chemotherapeutics, lumbar puncture, 1109
Intrauterine contraceptive device (IUD)
    insertion, 578-85
    lost, 559, 572
    misplaced, 1138-9
    obstetric ultrasound and, 808
    removal of, 586-7
Intrauterine growth retardation (IUGR)
    cervical ripening/vaginal prostaglandins and, 803
    contraction stress test and, 783
    nonstress test and, 777, 778
    obstetric ultrasound and, 817, 818, 819, 820-1, 822
Intravenous catheter sites, wound dressing, semipermeable films,
        1092
Intravenous regional anesthesia. *See* Bier block
Intubation
    chest tube insertion and, 444-51
    endotracheal, 452-63
    nasogastric tube and salem sump insertion and, 264-9
    rhinolaryngoscopy and, 252-8
IPG. *See* Electric impedance plethysmography
Ischemia
    acute, with angina, 389
    to intraabdominal organ, umbilical artery catheterization, 850
Isopto Hyoscine. *See* Scopolamine HBr

IUD. *See* Intrauterine contraceptive device
IUGR. *See* Intrauterine growth retardation
IVA. *See* Intraosseous venous access

Jaw thrust, endotracheal intubation, 455
Joint and soft tissue aspiration and injection, 1036-54. *See also* Trigger point injection
    corticosteroids with, 1039-141, 1054
Joint stiffness, cast immobilization, 1025-6
Journal of the American Medical Association, 1067

Keloids
    cryosurgery and, 105, 115
    definition of, 58
    formation, ear piercing and, 202, 205
    hypertrophic scars and, 58-61
    loop electrosurgical incision and, 661
Keratoacanthoma, 30
Keratoses
    actinic, 22, 30-1, 98, 104, 113, 118
    seborrheic, 22, 97, 105, 112
Kessler technique, extensor tendon repair, 1057
Ketorolac, 676, 980
Kiesselbach's plexus, 242
Knee, joint and soft tissue aspiration and injection, 1052
KOH preparation and wet smear, 669-71
Kyphosis, pulmonary function testing, 492

Labor
    premature, contraction stress test, 783
    preterm, obstetric ultrasound, 808, 821
Labor, induced. *See also* Cervical ripening/vaginal prostaglandins
    contraction stress test and, 781
    nonstress test and, 777
    obstetric ultrasound and, 822
    spontaneous fetal-movement counting and, 775
Laboratory studies, sclerotherapy, 64-8
Laceration repair, 12-9. *See also* Local anesthesia
    care of sutured lacerations, 18
    concurrent treatment, 19
    initial assessment of, 13
    needle selection for, 7-11
    wound preparation for, 13-4
Lactobacillus, 670
Laminaria digitata. *See* Abortion, first-trimester
Laparascopy
    tubal ligation and, 679, 680, 681, 969-7
    culdocentesis and, 594
Laparotomy, culdocentesis, 594
Large loop excision of the transformation zone. *See* Loop electrosurgical excision procedure (LEEP) for treating CIN
Laryngeal edema, 462-3
Laryngoscopy, indirect, 260-3. *See also* Rhinolaryngoscopy
Laryngospasm
    gastric lavage and, 890
    rhinolaryngoscopy, and, 259
Laser ablation of cervix, 645
Laser therapy, 84-90
    CO_2 laser method, 84-6
    cost of laser units, 85
    pulsed tunable dye laser method, 86-9
    Q-switched ruby laser, 84
Lateral epicondylitis (tennis elbow), 1044
LEEP. *See* Loop electrosurgical excision procedure
Leiomyomata, 571
Lentigo, 31
    cryosurgery and, 105
    maligna (melanoma in situ) and, 31
Lesions, suspicious pigmented/melanomas, treatment of, 33

LETZ. *See* Loop electrosurgical excision procedure (LEEP) for treating CIN
Leukemia
    bone marrow aspiration and biopsy and, 1115
    IUD insertion and, 579
    perianal abscess incision and drainage and, 971-2
Leukoplakia, 608
Levonorgestrel, 718-28
Lidocaine with/without epinephrine, 135, 136, 147
    description and use of, 141
    maximum dosage of, 136, 147
Lipomas, 32
Liquid nitrogen, 104, 110
Liver disease
    contraceptive implants (Norplant) and, 719
    endometrial biopsy and, 563
Liver spots. *See* Lentigo
Local anesthesia, 135-40. *See also* Anaphylaxis; Topical anesthesia
    anaphylaxis, 140
    approaches for the allergic patient, 137
    chest tube insertion and, 446, 447
    commonly used local anesthetics in office setting, 135, 136, 147
    maximum dosages of commonly used local anesthetics, 136, 147
    reducing pain of injection with, 139
    selection of local anesthetics/effects, 136
    topical anesthetics, 139-40
Loop electrosurgical excision procedure
    colposcopic examination, 616
    treatment of vulvar, perianal, vaginal, penile, urethral condyloma acuminata, 658-61
Loop electrosurgical excision procedure (LEEP) for treating CIN, 729-41. *See also* Cervical conization; Radiofrequency surgery
Low cardiac output syndrome, 320
Lower extremities, noninvasive venous and arterial studies, 348-68
Lower extremity venous system, 355
Lumbar puncture, 1109-14
    central nervous system infections, 1109
Lyme disease, 125
Lymph nodes, fine-needle aspiration cytology and biopsy, 1102-8
Lymphoma
    bone marrow aspiration and biopsy and, 1115
    cryocone of cervix and, 647
    cryosurgery and, 105
    perianal abscess incision and drainage and, 971
Lymphoproliferative disorders, bone marrow aspiration and biopsy, 1115
Lytic cocktail, 157

Macroglobulinemia
    cryocone of cervix and, 647
    cryosurgery and, 105
Macrosomia, 820, 821, 822
Malpractice. *See* Informed consent
Mammography, 714
Marcaine. *See* Bupivacaine
Mastectomy, 301
Mastoiditis, 188
Maxillary (V_2) nerve block, 172-3
Mazicon. *See* Flumazenil
McGivney ligation, hemorrhoids, 937-41
Meatal stenosis, 869, 873
Meconium
    aspiration, 855
    passage, amniocentesis, 766
Median nerve block, 148, 150
Medical College of Georgia, 777
Medical College of Wisconsin, 757
Meibomianitis, 215

Melanoma, 32, 33
  acquired nevi, 33, 34
  biopsy, 22, 32
  choroidal, 231
  cryosurgery and, 105, 106
  dysplastic nevi, 34
  fine-needle aspiration cytology and biopsy, 1103
  giant congenital nevi, 34
  in situ (lentigo maligna), 31
  primary subungual, 44
Ménétrier's disease, 974
Meningeal carcinomatosis, 1109
Meningitis, 188
Mental nerve block, 151-2
Meperidine, 157
Mepivacaine, 135, 147
Metabolic disease, stress testing, 416
Metastic disease, 1115
Microfibrillar collagen, topical hemostatic agent, 1087-8
Middle-ear infections, 1096
Milia, 98
Minilaparotomy, tubal ligation, 678
  fimbriectomy and, 681
  Irving technique of, 681
  Parkland method of, 678, 681, 683
  Pomeroy method of, 678, 681, 682, 697
  postpartum tubal ligation and, 695
  Uchida technique of, 681
Miscarriage
  abortion, first-trimester, 711, 712
  hysteroscopy, diagnostic, 559
Mitral regurgitation, acute, 320
Mitral valve prolapse, 430-1
Mogen method, newborn circumcision, 872
Moles. See Nevi
Mulloscum contagiosum, 32
  androscopy and, 518
  cryosurgery and, 105, 117
  removal of, 32
Monsel's solution (ferric subsulfate), 1085-6
Moricizine, 380
Morrhuate sodium, 948
Multiple gestation, 808, 818-20, 821, 822, 824
Multiple sclerosis, 231
  lumbar puncture and, 1109
Murphy's sign, 1139, 1140
Muscle biopsy, 1120-2
  muscular dystrophy, Duchenne, 1120
  myasthenia gravis and, 1120
  myotonia congenita and, 1120
Muscular dystrophy, 1120
Myasthenia gravis, 231, 1120
Mycitracin, 39
Myelography, 1109
Myeloma, 647
Myocardial fibrosis, 475
Myocardial infarction
  anoscopy and, 902
  cardioversion and, 439, 442
  clinical significance of postinfarction ventricular arrhythmias,
    389-90
  colonoscopy and, 993
  Holter monitoring and, 380
  office electrocardiogram and, 408
  self-injection therapy for treatment of impotence and, 555
  ST analysis interpretation and, 430
  stress testing and, 414-6, 426, 432
  Swan-Ganz catheterization and, 320
  temporary pacing and, 475

Myocardial ischemia
  stress testing and, 426
  temporary pacing and, 475
Myocarditis, 416
Myofascial pain syndrome, 164
Myoglobulinuria, 1120
Myoma, submucus, 672
Myomata, first-trimester abortion, 712
Myomectomy
  hysterosalpingography and, 571
  radiofrequency surgery and, 98
Myotonia congenita, 1120
Myringotomy, 188-91. See also Pediatric sedation; Removal of
    foreign bodies from ears and nose
  anatomy of middle ear, 190
  incisions for, 191
Myxedema, 416

Nabothian cysts
  colposcopic examination and, 619
  Pap smear and, 608, 610
Nail bed
  anatomy and terminology, 40
  area to cauterize in toenail removal, 41
  biopsy of, 44-6
  hematoma evacuation, 47-9
Nail care prophylaxis, 43
Nail matrixectomy
  electrode application for, 42
  radiofrequency surgery and, 98
Nail plate
  ablation, 41-2
  definition of, 44
Nail plate and nail bed biopsy, 44-6. See also Skin biopsy
  ring-block technique for digital nerve block for, 45
Nail splitter, 41
Naloxone, 158
Naloxone hydrochloride, 841, 845
Narcan. See Naloxone
Narcotic antagonist, diagnostic esophagogastroduodenoscopy
    (EGD), 981
Nasogastric tube and salem sump insertion, 264-9
Nasopharynx, 255, 256
National Cancer Institute, 907
National Institutes of Health, 807
  melanoma biopsy guidelines, 32
National Testing Laboratories, 757-60
Necrotizing enterocolitis, 848, 850
Necrotizing fasciitis, 971
Needle selection for laceration and incision repair, 7-11
  categories of, 10
  tissue disruption with, 8
Neo-synephrine. See Phenylephrine
Neonatal intensive care, umbilical artery catheterization, 847
Neonatal resuscitation, 841-60. See also DeLee suctioning;
    Endotracheal intubation; Umbilical artery catheterization
Neoplasm, preputial, 544
Nerve blocks, common, 148-54. See also Oral/facial anesthesia
  digital block of finger or toe, 148
  digital nerve block, anatomy and injection technique, 149
  distribution of cutaneous sensation by radial/ulnar/median
    nerves of hand, 151
  distribution of sensory innervation to foot, 153
  ear block, 152
  foot blocks, 152-4
  intraorbital nerve block, 150-1
  locations of various facial nerves and methods to obtain nerve
    block, 152
  median nerve block, 148, 150

Nerve blocks—Cont'd
  mental nerve block, 151-2
  radial nerve block, 149-50, 151
  supraorbital and supratrochlear nerve blocks (forehead block), 150
  sural nerve block, 152, 154
  tibial nerve block, 152, 154
  ulnar nerve block, 148-9, 151
Nerve blocks, oral/facial
  inferior alveolar (V$_2$), 174-6
  infraorbital, 171-2
  maxillary (V$_2$), 172-3
  posterior superior alveolar, 170-1
  trigeminal, 168
Nerve blocks, peripheral, 145-55
Nerve compression, ankle splinting, taping, and casting, 1010, 1012
Nerve palsy, cast immobilization, 1025
Nesacaine. *See* Chlorprocaine
Neural tube defects, amniocentesis, 766
Neuralgia, post herpetic, 142
Neuritis, 1038
Neuroma, 536
Neuropathy, noninvasive arterial studies of lower extremities, 361
Neutra-caine. *See* Sodium bicarbonate
Nevi
  acquired, 33-4
  biopsy, benign intradermal or compound, 22
  cryosurgery, 105
  dysplastic, 34
  giant congenital (bathing trunk), 34
Newborn circumcision. *See* Circumcision, newborn
Newborn distress
  cardiorespiratory, 847, 848
  respiratory, 855, 857
Nitrates, 423
Nitroglycerin, 384-5
Nitrous oxide
  cryosurgery and, 103-4, 110-1
  dilation and curettage and, 674
Noninvasive venous and arterial studies of lower extremities, 348-68
Nonoxynol-9
  diaphragm fitting and, 751, 755, 756
  with condom, 747
  with vaginal contraceptive sponge, 747, 748
Nonstress test (NST)
  cervical ripening/vaginal prostaglandins and, 804
  flowchart for management of, 777
  nonreactive, 776-80
  oligohydramnios and, 776
  oxytocin and, 777
  reactive, 776
  use as screening test, 777
Norplant
  cervical malignancy and, 584
  contraceptive implants and, 718-28
Nose and ear, removal of foreign bodies from, 206-13
Nosebleed. *See* Epistaxis
Novocaine. *See* Procaine
NST. *See* Nonstress test
Nupercaine. *See* Dibucaine
Nursemaid's elbow: subluxation of the radial head, 1022-35

Obesity
  electrical impedance plethysmography (IPG) and, 351, 354
  pulmonary function testing and, 492
  tubal ligation, interval and, 680

Obstetric ultrasound, 807-27, 1132-9
  emergency department, 1132-9
  guidelines for, 808-9
Occlusive hydrocolloids, wound dressing, 1094-5
Office electrocardiograms, 408-12. *See also* Holter monitoring; Stress testing
Office treatment of hemorrhoids, 929-53. *See also* Anoscopy; Clinical anorectal anatomy and examination; Perianal skin tags
Oligohydramnios
  amniocentesis and, 771
  nonstress test and, 776
  obstetric ultrasound and, 808, 817-9, 820, 821, 822
Oligomenorrhea, 563
Onychocryptosis. *See* Toenails, ingrown
Onychogryposis, 38
Onychomycosis, 38
Ophthalmic irrigant, isotonic, 222, 225, 227
Oral contraceptive therapy, risk factor for deep venous thrombosis, 349
Oral procedures
  alternative endocarditis prophylaxis regimens for, 1069
  standard antibiotic prophylactic regimen for bacterial endocarditis in patients at risk, 1068
Oral/facial anesthesia, 168-176. *See also* Local anesthesia
  allergy relating to, 169, 170
  inferior alveolar (V$_2$) nerve block, 174-6
  infraorbital nerve block, 171-2
  maxillary (V$_2$) nerve block, 172-3
  posterior superior alveolar nerve block, 170-1
  supraperiostial injection, 168-70
Orogastric tube insertion, 886, 887, 888
Oropharangeal trauma/obstruction, endotracheal intubation, 453
Oropharynx, 255, 256
Orthoses, plantar warts, corns, and calluses, 1060-4
  calluses, 1063
  corns, 1063
  orthotic devices, 1060-2
  plantar warts, 1062
Orthotic devices, 1060-2
  graphite, 1061
  leather, plastazote, and other soft materials, 1061
  polypropylene, 1060
  rhoadur, 1060
Osteoarthritis, 1038
Osteoenesis imperfecta, 833
Osteomyelitis, 833, 839
Osteoporosis
  disuse, cast immobilization, and, 1025
  bone marrow aspiration and biopsy and, 1115, 1119
Ostomy skin barriers, wound dressing, occlusive hydrocolloids, 1094
Otitis media, 180
  adult, 249
  myringotomy, 188-91
Otoscopy, pneumatic, 197
Ovarian cyst
  contraceptive implants (Norplant), 722
  culdocentesis, 594
Ovarian tumors, first-trimester abortion, 713
Ovulation/anovulation, endometrial biopsy, 563
Oxidized cellulose, topical hemostatic agent, 1087
Oxygen therapy, home, arterial puncture, 340
Oxygen transport assessment, Swan-Ganz catheterization, 320
Oxytocin
  abortion, first-trimester, and, 702, 703
  cervical ripening/vaginal prostaglandins and, 803, 805
  contraction stress test and, 781, 784
  dilation and curettage and, 676
  nonstress test and, 777

Pacemaker PAD. *See* Peripheral artery disease
Pacemaker
  CO_2 laser therapy and, 84
  insertion, transvenous, central venous catheter insertion,
    300
  office treatment of hemorrhoids and, 931
  percutaneous arterial line placement and, 301
  radiofrequency surgery and, 94
  rate-responsive, stress testing, 415
Pain syndrome, myofascial, 164
Pancreatitis, acute, 893
Pancytopenia, 1115
Pap smear
  abortion, first-trimester, and, 702
  cervical cap and, 742, 743, 746
  cervical conization and, 640
  cervicography and, 757-61
  contraceptive implants (Norplant) and, 718, 724
  cryocone of cervix and, 646, 650-1
  HPV-DNA testing of the cervix, 613
  IUD insertion and, 580, 583-4
  loop electrosurgical excision procedure (LEEP) for treating CIN
    and, 729-30, 740
  tubal ligation, interval, and, 684, 685
Pap smear: screening for cervical cancer, 601-2. *See also*
    Colposcopic examination
  abnormal, 603
  appearance of cervix in various age groups, 605
  copolscopy and, 601-3, 608, 608-11
  golden rules of, 609-10
  interpretation of, 610-12
  sampling devices for, 604 606-7
  terminology and definitions of, 602
Papanicolaou smear. *See* Pap smear
Papaverine hydrochloride, self-injection therapy for treatment of
    impotence, 550, 551, 552
Papilloma virus, plantar warts, 1062
Paraben preservatives, 137
Paracervical block, 799-802
  abortion, first-trimester, and, 705, 706, 711
  dilation and curettage and, 674
Paraendometritis, 712
Paralytic ileus, 264
Paraphimosis, 544
Parauterine structures, 680
Parenchymal disease, infiltrative, 492
Parenteral ampicillin, flexible sigmoidoscopy, 911
Paronychia, 34, 35, 38, 50
Pediatric arterial puncture and venous cutdown, 856-62. *See also*
    Arterial puncture; Intraosseous venous access; Venous
    cutdown
Pediatric patients
  pulmonary function testing and, 486
  visual function examination and, 232, 234
Pediatric respiratory distress, pediatric arterial puncture, 858
Pediatric sedation, 156-9
Pelvic infections, diagnostic hysteroscopy, 559
Pelvic inflammatory disease
  colposcopic examination and, 627
  contraceptive implants (Norplant) and, 719
  ectopic pregnancy and, 1133
  endometrial biopsy and, 563
  hysterosalpingography and, 574
  IUD insertion and, 578, 579, 580, 582-3
  Pap smear and, 604
  perianal abscess incision and drainage and, 970
  tubal ligation and, 697
  radiofrequency surgery and, 98

Penicillin
  for tooth abscess, 52
  VK, reimplantation of avulsed tooth, 28
Penile cancer
  newborn circumcision, 863
  squamous cell carcinoma, CO_2 laser therapy, 84
Penile intraepithelial neoplasia, 514-5
Penile nerve block, dorsal, 874-7
Peptic ulcer disease, chronic, 975
Percutaneous arterial line placement, 293-9. *See also* Arterial
    puncture
  artery cannulation, 294-8
  vs. intraosseous venous access, 831-2
Perforation, abdominal organs, abdominal paracentesis/peritoneal
    lavage, 896
Periadnexal adhesive disease, 571
Perianal abscess
  external anal examination and, 900, 901
  perianal skin tags and, 957
Perianal abscess incision and drainage, 909-72. *See also* Clinical
    anorectal anatomy and examination
  perirectal abscess and, 970
  radiotherapy and, 971
  superlevator abscess and, 970
Perianal condyloma, 902
Perianal dermatitis, 901
Perianal skin tags (external hemorrhoidal skin tags), 954-7. *See
    also* Anal fissure/lateral sphincterotomy; Loop electrosurgical
    excision procedure (LEEP) for treating CIN; Radiofrequency
    surgery
  Crohn's disease and, 955
Perianal/intraanal lesions, treatment of condyloma acuminata, 662-3
Periarthritis, 1038
Pericardial effusions, 1127-31
Pericardial tamponade
  central venous catheter insertion and, 317
  Swan-Ganz catheterization and, 320
Pericardiocentesis, suspected pericardial effusions, 1132
Pericarditis, 416
Perichondritis, 184, 187
Perineal sepsis
  DC current treatment, 944
  infrared coagulation, 943
  rubber-band ligation, 938, 940, 941
Perineotomy. *See* Episiotomy
Periodontal fibers, 283
Periodontitis, 284
Peripheral artery disease
  noninvasive diagnostic techniques for, 360
  quantitative screening for, 363
  screening for, 360
  waveform analysis, pulse volume, and, 366
Peripheral circulatory shock, intraosseous venous access, 832
Peripheral nerve blocks and field blocks, 145-5. *See also*
    Oral/facial anesthesia; Local anesthesia
Peripheral neuropathies
  muscle biopsy and, 1120
  shoulder dislocations and, 1032
Peritoneal dialysis, 892, 893
Peritoneal lavage and abdominal paracentesis, 892-7
Peritonitis
  acute, 893
  colonoscopy and, 993
  culdocentesis and, 588, 589
Periungual verrucae, CO_2 laser therapy, 84
Permanent female sterilization (tubal ligation), 678-98
  basic anatomy of parauterine structures, 680
  interval tubal ligation and, 679-94

Permanent female sterilization (tubal ligation)—Cont'd
  minilaparotomy/laparoscopy, 680
  postpartum tubal ligation and, 695-8
  reversal of, 693-4
  risks for regret with, 693-4
  technical failure of, 679
  terminology for, 679
Pernicious anemia, 974
Phenol 50%, 1087
Phenothiazine, 281
Phentolamine mesylate, 550, 551
Phenylephrin, 251
  decongestant nasal spray, gastric lavage, 885
  hydrochloride, 265, 552, 554
Phimosis, adult circumcision, 544
Phlebitis
  abscess, incision and drainage of, and, 50
  septic, 50
  temporary pacing and, 475
  venous cutdown and, 334, 338, 862
Phleborrheograph (PRG), 64
Phospholipids, 766
Photoplethysmography (PPG), 64
Physician's Drug Reference, 159
Pierre Robin syndrome, 844
Pigmentary conditions, Wood's light examination, 82
Pilonidal cyst/abscess incision and drainage, 964-8
Pilonidal disease, 901
Placenta previa, 808, 818
Placental abruption
  with amniocentesis, 767, 771
  with obstetric ultrasound, 808, 817, 821
Plantar warts, 37
  cryosurgery and, 112
  dissection of, 1062
  radiofrequency surgery and, 98
  salicylic acid plaster for, 1062
Plasmapheresis, central venous catheter insertion, 301
Plastibell method, newborn circumcision, 869-72
Plethysmography. See Electrical impedance plethysmography
Pleural adhesions, 478
Pleural effusion
  chest tube insertion and, 444
  pulmonary function testing and, 492
  thoracentesis and, 477
Pleural fluid analysis, thoracentesis, 483
Pleurodesis, chest tube insertion, 444
Pneumonitis, chemical, gastric lavage, 884
Pneumoperitoneum, colonoscopy, 998
Pneumothorax
  central venous catheter insertion and, 301, 308, 309, 310, 316
  chest tube insertion and, 444, 446, 450
  endotracheal intubation and, 462, 463
  joint and soft tissue aspiration and injection and, 1046
  neonatal resuscitation and, 846
  pulmonary function testing and, 492
  Swan-Ganz catheterization and, 328
  thoracentesis and, 483-4
  tracheostomy and, 277
Podofilox, 656, 756
Podophyllin
  for chemical cautery, condyloma acuminata, 656, 657
  for perianal/intraanal lesions, condyloma acuminata, 662
Poison Control Center, 885
Poison ingestion, gastric lavage, 884-91
Polycystic ovarian disease, 563
Polyethylene glycol, 993
Polyhydramnios, 808, 818, 821
Polymerase chain reaction, HPV-DNA testing of the cervix, 614

Polypectomy
  colonoscopy and, 992, 997
  flexible sigmoidoscopy and, 907
  postpolypectomy syndrome and, 998
Polyposis, 974
Polyps
  colorectal, 992, 997
  endocervical, 619
  endometrial, 571
  flexible sigmoidoscopy and, 924
Polysporin, 185
Pontocaine. See Tetracaine
Porphyria cutanea tarda, Wood's light examination, 82
Port-wine stains
  cryosurgery and, 106
  pulsed tunable dye laser therapy and, 87, 88
Postcoital examination test or Sims-Huhner test, 666-8
  spinnbarkeit test and, 667
Postdate pregnancy
  cervical ripening/vaginal prostaglandins and, 803
  nonstress test and, 777, 778
  obstetric ultrasound and, 822
Posthitis, 544
Postpartum bleeding, hysteroscopy, 559
Postphlebitic syndrome, 358
Postpolypectomy syndrome, 998
Preeclampsia, 792
  nonstress test and, 778
  obstetric ultrasound and, 818
Pregnancy. See also Ectopic pregnancy; Abdominal paracentesis
      and peritoneal lavage, 893
  cervical conization, 640, 641
  colposcopic examination, 627
  contraceptive implants (Norplant), 719, 722
  cryocone of cervix, 646, 648
  dilation and curettage, 673
  electrical impedance plethysmography (IPG), 351
  endometrial biopsy, 563
  flexible sigmoidoscopy, 908
  Heimlich maneuver and, 1081, 1082
  hysterosalpingography, 572
  hysteroscopy, diagnostic, 560
  IUD insertion, 578
  loop electrosurgical excision procedure (LEEP) for treating CIN,
      730
  noninvasive venous studies of lower extremities, 351
  office treatment of hemorrhoids 931
  pulmonary function testing, 492
  risk factor for deep venous thrombosis, 349
  sclerotherapy, 64
  tubal ligation, 684, 685, 692, 697
  vaginal diaphragm, 756
Pregnancy termination. See Abortion, first-trimester
Premature labor, 582, 712. See also Labor
Premature ventricular contractions (PVC)
  12-lead electrocardiogram and short rhythm strip and, 379-80
  clinical significance of, 389-90
  evaluation of antiarrhythmic drug therapy for, 383
  Holter recording and, 394, 397
  physical examination and cardiac auscultation, 378, 379
  prevalence in general population, 389
  ST-segment depression, 383-4
  stress (exercise) testing, 379, 428
  trend analysis of abnormal beats, 394-5
Prenatal diagnosis, amniocentesis, 765
Pressure sores
  ankle splinting, taping, and casting, and, 1010, 1012
  cast immobilization and, 1025
Pressure therapy, hypertrophic scars and keloids, 61

Priapism, 552, 553, 554
Principles of extensor tendon repair, 1055-6
Procaine, 137
Prostaglandins
    self-injection therapy for treatment of impotence, 550, 551, 552
    vaginal/cervical ripening, 803-6
Prostate gland, digital anorectal examination, 900
Prostate massage, 541-3
Prosthetic heart valve, 467
Pruritis ani
    anoscopy and, 902
    external anal examination and, 900, 901
Pseudoaneurysm, Swan-Ganz catheterization, 331
Pseudoisochromatic plates, 232
Pseudomonas aeruginosa, 82, 222
Pseudotumor cerebri, 1109
Psychiatric problems, permanent female sterilization (tubal ligation), 697
Pudendal anesthesia, 794-8. *See also* Local anesthesia
Pudendal block, hysteroscopy, 560
Pulmonary artery
    hypertension and, 320, 321
    rupture of, 331
    Swan-Ganz catheterization and, 320, 321, 331
Pulmonary aspiration, gastric lavage, 884, 890
Pulmonary edema, 416
    with cardioversion, 439
    with endotracheal intubation, 452
    with Swan-Ganz catheterization, 320
    thoracentesis, 484
Pulmonary embolism
    with cast immobilization, 1026
    with colonoscopy, 993
    noninvasive venous studies of lower extremities and, 350, 351
    risk factor for deep venous thrombosis and, 349
    with Swan-Ganz catheterization, 320
    with temporary pacing, 475
Pulmonary function testing, 485-92
    errors of, 492
    flow-volume loops and, 490
    interpretation of, 489-90
Pulmonary hemorrhage, 331
Pulmonary infarction, 330, 416
Pulmonary thromboembolism, 340
Pulsus paradoxus, suspected pericardial effusions, 1127, 1131
PVC. *See* Premature ventricular contractions
Pyloroduodenal stenosis, 975

Q fever, 125
Q-switched ruby laser, 84
Quinidine sulfate, 42

Radial artery stenosis/occlusion, 298
Radial nerve block, 149-50, 151
Radiation therapy, bone marrow aspiration and biopsy, 115
Radiation therapy, pulmonary function testing, 485
Radiofrequency surgery, 91-101. *See also* Skin lesions
    electrode tips for Ellman Surgitron, 94
    subungual hematoma evacuation and, 47
Radiography, shoulder dislocations, 1029, 1030, 1031, 1032
Rashes, 35
RAST (radioallergosorbent in vitro) testing, allergy, 1099
Rectal bleeding
    with anoscopy, 902
    with colonoscopy, 992
    with flexible sigmoidoscopy, 907

Rectocele, diaphragm fitting, 750, 751
Rectum, prolapse of
    with anoscopy, 902
    with hemorrhoids, 931
Red reflex, 234
Reduction of dislocated temporomandibular joint, 279-82
Reflectometry, acoustic, 197
Reimplantation of an avulsed tooth, 283-6
Relapsing fever, 125
Removal of foreign bodies from ear and nose, 206-13. *See also* Pediatric sedation; Cerumen impaction removal; Topical anesthesia
Renal disease, 778
Renal failure, 321, 363
Replantations, cast immobilization, 1015
Respiratory compromise, anaphylaxis, 1076
Respiratory distress
    abdominal paracentesis and peritoneal lavage and, 892
    newborn, 766, 847, 848, 855, 857
    pediatric, 858
    syndrome, adult, 320, 321, 452
Respiratory failure, endotracheal intubation, 452
Retin-A. *See* Retinoic acid
Retina, detached, 231
Retinitis pigmentosa, 231
Retinoic acid, actinic keratoses, 31
Retinopathy, hypertensive, 231
Rh factor
    abortion, first-trimester, and, 702
    amniocentesis and, 765, 766, 771
    hemolytic disease and, 765, 766
    sensitization, 818
    negative, 676
Rheumatoid arthritis, 485
Rhinitis, 1097
Rhinolaryngoscopy, 249-59, 260, 263
    acute conditions that may warrant, 250
    anatomic divisions of upper airway, 255
    anatomy of nasopharynx and oropharynx, 255
    ostia of paranasal sinuses and, 253
Rhinophyma, CO_2 laser therapy, 84
Rhogam, 676
Rickettsia, 125
Rocky Mountain spotted fever, 125
Romazicon. *See* Flumazenil
Rosacea, 215
Rotator cuff (supraspinatus tendonitis), joint and soft tissue aspiration and injection, 1048
Royal College of Obstetricians and Gynecologists, 807
Rubber-band ligation, 937-41
    anatomy of anal region, 938

Salpingitis. *See also* Pelvic inflammatory disease
    culdocentesis and, 589, 594
    isthmica nodosa, hysterosalpingography, and, 571, 572, 574
Sampling devices, Pap smear, 604, 606-7
Sarcoidosis, 485, 492
Scabies, Wood's light examination, 82
Scar revision, acne, 56
Scars, hypertrophic, and keloids, treatment of, 58-61
    alternative methods, 61
    corticosteroid injections for, 59-60
    cryosurgery and, 105, 115
    cryotherapy and, 59
    definitions of, 58
    pressure therapy and, 61
    resection of keloid on ear lobe, 60
    surgical excision, 60-1
    telangiectasias, 59

Schiotz tonometry. *See* Tonometry
Sclerosants, 72
Sclerotherapy, 63-76
    anaphylaxis and, 74
    compression stockings and, 70
    laboratory studies of, 64-8
    leg diagrams for, 67
    sclerosants, 72
    spider veins and, 36
Sclerotherapy, hemorrhoids, 948-50
Scopolamine HBr, 225
Seborrheic keratoses, 31
Sedation
    cardioversion, 442
    chest tube insertion, 445
    colonoscopy, 995
    pediatric, 156-9
    monitoring, esophagogastroduodenoscopy (EGD), 979-81, 989
Segmental pressure measurement, lower extremities, 361-3
    interpretation of, 363
    sources of error, 363
Seizures, gastric lavage, 884, 885
Seldinger technique
    central venous catheter insertion, 302-3, 310-2
    percutaneous arterial line placement, 294, 296
Self-injection therapy for treatment of impotence, 550-6
Sellick maneuver, 458-60, 462
Semiocclusive agents, wound dressing, 1093, 1094
Semipermeable films, wound dressing, 1092-3, 1094
Seronegative spondyloarthropathy, 1083
Sexual abuse
    abortion, first-trimester, and, 700
    HPV-DNA testing of the cervix and, 614
    Pap smear and, 603, 612
Sexually transmitted disease
    abnormal Pap smear and, 603
    colposcopic examination, 623
    condoms and, 746, 747
    cryocone of cervix and, 647
    diaphragm fitting and, 750
    hysterosalpingography and, 572, 574
    IUD insertion and, 578, 579, 580
Shock
    anaphylaxis, 1076
    cardioversion, 439
    intraosseous venous access, 833
    percutaneous arterial line placement, 293
    Swan-Ganz catheterization, 320
Shoulder dislocations, 1028-32
    anatomy, 1028, 1092
    computed tomography and, 1029, 1031
    dead arm syndrome and, 1028
    radiographic studies for, 1029, 1030
Shoulder joint, intraarticular, joint and soft tissue aspiration and
        injection, 1050
Sick sinus syndrome, 382
    temporary pacing and, 466
    cardioverison and, 440
Sigmoid volvulus, colonoscopy, 993
Sigmoidoscopy, 902
SIL (squamous intraepithelial lesion)
    cryocone of cervix and, 645
    terminology and definition of, 602
Silent myocardial ischemia
    Holter monitoring and, 379, 383, 384-5
    ST-segment depression and, 384, 395
Silicosis, 492
Silver nitrate, 1084-5
Silver sulfadiazine, 656, 660, 661

Sim's position, 899, 914
Sims-Hubner test or postcoital examination test, 666-8
Sinuses, ostia of paranasal, 253
Sinusitis, 249, 250
    allergy testing and, 1096
    endotracheal intubation and, 463
Skin biopsy, 20-6. *See also* Radiofrequency surgery
    microfibrillar collagen and, 1088
    wound closure and, 23-4, 25
    wound management of, 24
Skin graft
    extensor tendon repair and, 1055
    wound dressing, semiocclusive hydrogels, and, 1093
Skin hooks, laceration repair, 12, 13
Skin lesions, 27-37
    achrochordon (skin tag), 27
    actinic keratoses, 30-1
    basal cell carcinoma, 27-9
    common, surgical diagnosis and management of, 28
    condyloma acuminata, 30
    cysts, sebaceous, 36
    dermafibroma, 30
    hyperplasia, sebaceous, 35
    keratoacanthoma, 30
    lentigo, 31
    lipomas, 32
    melanoma, 32, 33
    mulloscum contagiosum, 32
    nevi, 33-4
    paronychia, 34, 35
    pigmented, suspicious, 33
    pyogenic granulomas, 33
    rashes (exanthems, dermatoses), 35
    seborrheic keratoses, 31
    squamous cell carcinoma, 29-30
    telangiectasias, 36
    warts, 30, 37
    xanthelasma, 37
Skin tags
    approach to, 27
    diagnosis of, 27
    fibroepithelial, and, 97
    perianal (external hemorrhoidal), 954-7
    and polyps, cryosurgery, 105
SMI. *See* Silent myocardial ischemia
Snoring, 250
Society for Academic Emergency Medicine, 1123
Sodium bicarbonate, 137, 139
    neonatal resuscitation and, 841, 844
Sodium pentothal, 454, 455
Sodium tetradecyl sulfate, 98
Soft tissue and joint aspiration and injection, 1036-54
Solumedrol, 1077
Soonawala vasectomy forceps, 528, 534
Sotradecol/aethoxysckerol, 63-4
Sphincterotomy, 958-63
Spinal analgesia, 1109
Spinnbarkeit test, 667
Spontaneous fetal-movement counting, 773-5. *See also* Nonstress
        test
Sports medicine, 184
Sprained ankle, splinting, taping, and casting, 1003-13
Squamous epithelial lesion, loop electrosurgical excision
        procedure (LEEP) for treating CIN, 729-30
Squamous intraepithelial lesion. *See* SIL
ST analysis interpretation, stress testing, 429-30
ST-segment
    depression, 383-4, 395, 429-31
    elevation, stress testing, 428

ST-segment—Cont'd
  level trend analysis, Holter monitoring, 386, 395-6
  slope, stress testing, 426
Staphylcoccus, 50, 51
  chalazion and hordeolum, 215
  joint and soft tissue aspiration and injection, 1046
Static immitance, 197
Status epilepticus, 833
Steinmann pin cutter, 121, 123
Sterilization
  permanent female (tubal ligation), 678-98
  vasectomy, 520-40
Sternal puncture, 835, 839
Steroid drug therapy, cryocone of cervix, 647
Steroid flare, joint and soft tissue aspiration and injection, 1054
Steroids, systemic, anaphylaxis, 1077
Strabismus
  acquired, 231
  concomitant, 231
  esotropia, 235, 236
  exotropia, 235, 236
  noncomitant, 231
  test, 234, 235, 236
Stress testing, 413-36. *See also* Holter monitoring
  controversies, coronary artery disease diagnosis, of, 432
  fitness evaluation and exercise prescription for, 433-6
  general interpretation of, 428, 429, 430
  grading system for, 430-1
  physiology of exercise as applied to, 413-4
  rules of, 428-30
  vs. Holter monitoring, 383-4
  written protocols for, 419, 421
Stroke. *See* Cerebrovascular accident
Subarachnoid hemorrhage, 1109
Subclavian vein
  anatomy/relationships, 304, 314
  venipuncture technique, 303-13
Substance abuse, nonstress test, 778
Subungual hematoma evacuation, 47-9
Suction catheters and pump, cerumen impaction removal, 193
Superior vena cava syndrome, 301
Supraorbital nerve blocks, 150
Supraperiostial injection, 168-70
Suprapubic bladder aspiration, 852-4. *See also* Emergency department ultrasound
  pediatric evaluation, 1145-7
Suprapubic catheter insertion and change, 500-7
Suprapubic taps or aspirations, 504-7
Supraspinatus tendonditis, 1048
Supratentorial mass lesions, 1110
Supratrochlear nerve blocks, 150
Sural nerve block, 152, 154
Surgical/dental procedures, endocarditis prophylaxis, 1068
Surgitron, Ellman
  electrode tips for, 94
  ingrown toenails and, 39, 42
  vari-tip wire electrode for elliptical excision, 95
Sutures
  central venous catheter insertion, 309, 310, 316
  chalazion and hordeolum therapy, 217, 219
  keloid excision, 60
  laceration repair, 14-7
  sebaceous cyst, 36
  selection, dermatology, 3-6
  skin biopsy, 23-4, 25
Swan-Ganz catheterization, 301, 302, 319-31. *See also* Central venous catheter insertion; Temporary pacing
  and catheter care, 329-30

Swan-Ganz catheterization—Cont'd
  temporary pacing, 467, 470
  troubleshooting, 328-29
Syphilis
  and abortion, first-trimester, 702
  and cryocone of cervix, 746
  and cryosurgery, 105
Syringomyelia, 1032
Syrup of ipecac, 884
Systemic lupus erythematosus
  lumber puncture and, 1109
  pulmonary function testing and, 485
Systemic-pulmonary shunt, antibiotic prophylaxis for, 911

TAC (tetracaine-adrenaline-cocaine), 141-3
Tachycardia
  cardioversion and, 437-43
  endotracheal intubation and, 463
  Holter monitor full disclosure strip, 401, 402
  narrative summary of Holter recording, 392-3
  prevalence of, in general population, 389
  stress testing and, 426, 428
  trend analysis, heart rate and ST-segment level trend, 395-6
Tachypnea, 452
Tamoxifen citrate, 563
Taping ankle, 1003-13
Temporary pacing, 464-76. *See also* Central venous catheter insertion; Swan-Ganz catheterization
  external (transcutaneous), 464-5
  internal (transvenous), 465-75
Temporomandibular joint, dislocated, reduction of, 279-82
Tendon, extensor, repair of, 1055-9
Tendon rupture, 1040, 1047
Tennis elbow, 1044
Tenosynovitis, 1038
Terbutaline
  cervical ripening/vaginal prostaglandins and, 804, 805
  contraction stress test and, 783
Testicular torsion, 881-2
Tetanus, 226, 285
Tetracaine, 141, 147
Thoracentesis, 477-84
  pleural fluid analysis in, 483
Thrombin, 1088
Thrombocytopenia
  abdominal paracentesis and peritoneal lavage and, 893
  bone marrow aspiration and biopsy and, 115
Thromboembolism
  cast immobilization and, 1025-6
  contraceptive implants (Norplant) and, 719, 724
Thrombophlebitis, 719
Thrombosed external hemorrhoids, 950-2
Thrombosis
  arterial puncture and, 347
  central venous catheter insertion and, 117
  sclerotherapy and, 950
  Swan-Ganz catheterization and, 331
  temporary pacing, 475
  umbilical artery catheterization, 848
Thrombus
  intraluminal, 356
  pediatric arterial puncture and, 860
Thyroid fine-needle aspiration cytology and biopsy, 1102-8
Thyrotoxicosis, 137, 416
Tibial nerve block, 152, 154
Tinnitus, 180, 192, 196
Tissue glue (fibrin sealant), topical hemostatic agent, 1086-9
Titration, 320
TMJ. *See* Temporomandibular joint

Toe/finger joints, aspiration and injection in, 1041
Toenails, ingrown, 38-43
Tongue-tie snipping (frenotomy) for ankyloglossia, 287-90
  Z-plasty and, 288
Tonometry, 237-41
Tooth, avulsed, reimplantation of, 283-6
  antibiotics and, 285
  storage of tooth, 283
  tetanus toxoid and, 285
Topical anesthesia, 139-40, 141-4
  EMLA (eutectic mixture of local anesthetic), 142-4
  ethyl chloride, 144
Topical hemostatic agents, 1084-9. *See also* Wound dressing
  agents providing a physical meshwork, 1087-8
  physiologic, 1088
  vasoconstrictive, vasocclusive, or denaturing, 1084-7
Toxic shock syndrome
  cervical cap and, 742, 745
  diaphragm and, 748
  tampon and, 748
  vaginal contraceptive sponge and, 747, 748
  vaginal diaphragm and, 756
Tracheal stenosis, 277
Tracheoesophageal fistula
  DeLee suctioning and, 855, 857
  endotracheal intubation and, 463
  tracheostomy and, 277
Tracheomalacia, 463
Tracheostomy, 273-8, 455
  endotracheal intubation and, 453, 455
Transabdominal scanning, suspected ectopic pregnancy, 1133-5
Transfusion
  exchange, umbilical artery catheterization, 847, 848
  intrauterine, amniocentesis, 766
Transtelephonic monitoring, comparison to Holter monitoring,
  379, 381
Transthoracic direct-current electrical shock. *See* Cardioversion
Trichloroacetic acid
  as topical hemostatic agent, 1086
  for chemical cautery, condyloma acuminata, 656
  perianal/intraanal lesions and, 663
Trichomonads
  postcoital examination test or Sims-Hubner test and, 667
  and wet smear and KOH preparation, 670
Triethanolamine, 193, 194
Trigeminal nerve block, 168
Trigger finger, in joint and soft tissue aspiration and injection,
  1042
Trigger point injection, 164-7
Tubal ligation, interval, 678-98
  minilaparotomy and laparoscopy, 680
  postpartum, 695-8
Tubal reanastomosis/reimplantation, 571
Tuberculosis, 1115
Tuboplasty, 571, 574
Tularemia, 215
Tympanocentesis, 188, 189
Tympanotromy, 197-201
  electroacoustic impedance bridge and, 198
  typanogram results and, 200

Ulcerative colitis
  cryocone of cervix and, 647
  flexible sigmoidoscopy and, 907
  and risk factor for deep venous thrombosis, 349
Ulcers
  sclerotherapy and, 74
Ulnar nerve block, 148-9, 151

Ultrasound
  and abortion, first-trimester, 703
  amniocentesis and, 768, 769, 770
  in contraction stress test, 783
  in culdocentesis, 594
  European Committee for Ultrasound Radiation Safety and, 807
  obstetric, 807-27
  pelvic, for IUD removal, 587
  suprapubic catheter insertion and change and, 501, 503
  suprapubic taps or aspirations and, 505, 506
Ultrasound imaging, lower extremities, 349, 354-6
  echogenic matter and, 355
  interpretation, 356
  Valsalva maneuver and, 355, 356
  venous system and, 355
Ultraviolet light, Wood's light examination, 81-3
Umbilical artery catheterization, 847-51
  vs. umbilical vein catheterization, 847
Umbilical vein catheterization. *See* Umbilical artery catheterization
Undermining ski, 14
Undescended testicle, 882
Unna paste boot, 78-80
Upper respiratory tract
  alternative endocarditis prophylaxis regimen for bacterial
    endocarditis, 1068
Upper respiratory symptoms, allergy testing, and, 1096
Urethral stricture
  bladder catheterization insertion and change and, 500
Urinary incontinence, tubal ligation, 684
Urinary system, 493-555
  and basic urodynamic studies for urinary incontinence, 508-13
  bladder catheterization, 495-9
  suprapubic catheter insertion and change, 500-3
  suprapubic taps or aspirations, 504-7
Urinary tract infections, newborn circumcision, 863
Urodynamic studies, basic, 508-13
U.S. Preventive Services Task Force, 432
Uterine bleeding, abnormal
  endometrial biopsy and, 563
  hysteroscopy, diagnostic, 559
  IUD insertion and, 579
Uterine cancer
  cervical cap and, 742
Uterine hyperstimulation, 784
Uterine malignancy, 579
Uterine myomas, submucous, 559
Uterine perforation
  dilation and curettage and, 676
  endometrial biopsy and, 570
  first-trimester abortion and, 711
  hysterosalpingography and, 577
Uterine prolapse, diaphragm fitting, and, 750
Uterine septal resection, hysterosalpingography, and, 571
Uteroplacental insufficiency
  contraction stress test and, 781-4
  obstetric ultrasound and, 822
  paracervical block and, 799

Vagal response
  DeLee suctioning and, 847
  neonatal resuscitation and, 842, 846
Vaginal bleeding, first-trimester, 1132-7
  suspected ectopic pregnancy and, 1132-3
  threatened abortion and, 1136-7
Vaginal contraceptive sponge, 747-9
Vaginitis
  atrophic, 508
  wet smear and KOH preparation and, 669-71

Valium. *See* Diazepam
Valsalva maneuver
    in central venous catheter insertion, 308, 314, 316
    inguinal hernia and, 881
    office treatment of hemorrhoids and, 937
    prostate massage and, 542
    pulmonary function testing and, 489
    ultrasound imaging and, 355, 356
Valvular heart disease
    self-injection therapy for treatment of impotence and, 551
    stress testing and, 415
Valvular lesions, Swan-Ganz catheterization, and, 320
Varicose vein
    dilated, 881
    surgical excision of, 63
Vascular collapse, in anaphylaxis, 1076
Vascular lesion, and cryosurgery, 117
Vasectomy, 520-40
    cautery instrument sterility and, 536
    reversal of, 536, 538
Vasocclusive agents, topical hemostatic, 1084-9
Vasoconstrictive agents, 140
    in nasal solution, 206
    topical hemostatic, 1084-8
Vasospastic arterial disease, percutaneous arterial line placement, 293
Vasovagal reaction
    in abortion, first-trimester, 711
    anaphylaxis and, 1076
    in cervical cryotherapy, 637
    in colposcopic examination, 637
    in endometrial biopsy, 570
    in flexible sigmoidoscopy, 927
    percutaneous arterial line placement and, 298
    rhinolaryngoscopy, flexible fiberoptic, 259
Vein
    basilic, cutdown technique, 336-7
    saphenous, 335
Venipuncture
    internal jugular, 313-7
    subclavian, 303-13
    Seldinger-type guide wire and, 311
Venography, 356, 357
    cast immobilization and, 1026
    contrast, 348, 354, 356
Venous and arterial studies, of lower extremities, 348-68
Venous catheter insertion, central, 300-18
Venous cutdown, 332-9
    cardiopulmonary resuscitation and, 334, 336, 337
    minicutdown, 860-2
    pediatric, 860-2
Venous insufficiency, 351
Venous lakes, radiofrequency surgery, 98
Venous sclerotherapy, 351
Venous stasis ulcers
    Unna paste boot and, 78
    wound dressing for, 1094
Venous studies, noninvasive, 348-60
    for deep venous thrombosis, 350
    duplex scanning and, 356-7
    electrical impedance plethysmography (IPG), 351-4
    ultrasound imaging, 354-6
    venous Dopplers, 357-60
Venous system, lower extremity, 355
Venous thrombosis, deep
    common sites of in the lower body, 350
    Doppler studies and, 358-9
    duplex scanning for, 356

Venous thrombosis—Cont'd
    electrical impedance plethysmography (IPG) and, 351
    ultrasonography and, 356
    ultrasound imaging and, 354
Ventricle
    bigeminy, 387
    dysfunction/infarction, 320, 416
    fibrillation, cardioversion, 437-43
    hypertrophy, 408, 430
    septal defect, 320
    tachycardia, 380-83, 467
Verruca. *See* Warts
Vertigo, 180, 192
Vessel laceration, 896
Visual function examination, 231-6. *See also* Tonometry
    eye charts and, 232-5
Volkmann's ischemic contractures, 1024

Warfarin, 442
Warts
    common (verruca vulgaris), 37
    cryosurgery for, 105, 109
    plantar (verruca plantaris), 37, 1062
    radiofrequency surgery for, 98
    verruca freeze and, 106, 110
Waveform analysis, pulse volume
    arterial studies and, 366
    interpretation of, 366
Waveform analysis, velocity
    interpretation of, 364-66
Werdnig-Hoffman disease, 1120
Wet smear and KOH preparation, 669-71
Wilson's disease, 579, 583
Wolfe-Parkinson-White syndrome, 467
    stress testing and, 429, 430
Wood's light examination, 81-3
    diagnostic uses of, 82
    drugs used with, 82-3
    lamp, 81
    most common findings of, 82
Word catheter insertion, 596-601
World Health Organization, 578
Wound care. *See also* Topical hemostatic agents
Wound closure. *See also* Sutures; Topical hemostatic agents; Wound dressing
    for abdominal paracentesis and peritoneal lavage, 895
    for breast biopsy, 715
    for central venous catheter insertion, 309, 310, 316
    for cervical conization, 642
    for chalazion and hordeolum therapy, 217, 219
    for chest tube insertion and removal, 449, 450
    for circumcision, adult, 548
    for cyst/abscess, 600, 966, 967
    for episiotomy, 788-92
    for keloid excision, 60-1
    for laceration/incision repair, 12-9
    for muscle biopsy, 1121
    for skin biopsy, 23-4, 25
    for suprapubic catheter insertion and change, 502
    for tubal ligation, 691, 692, 696
    for umbilical artery catheterization, 849
    for vasectomy, 534
    for venipuncture, 316
    for venous cutdown, 338, 339
Wound dressing, 1090-5
    for anal/lateral sphincterotomy, 962
    for auricular hematoma evacuation, 185, 186
    for Bartholin's cyst/abscess: Word catheter insertion, 599

Wound dressing—Cont'd
  for bone marrow aspiration and biopsy, 1119
  for breast biopsy, 715
  for chest tube insertion and removal, 450
  for ear piercing, 205
  for endotracheal intubation, 461
  for fine-needle aspiration cytology and biopsy, 1107
  for fishhook removal, 132
  for ingrown toenails, 42
  for intraosseous venous access, 837
  for lumbar puncture, 1113
  moist wound healing, 1090, 1095
  for muscle biopsy, 1121
  occlusive hydrocolloids for, 1094-5
  performance profile, summary of, 1094
  for perianal skin tags, 956
  for pilonidal cyst/abscess incision and drainage, 967
  for sclerotherapy, 73
  semiocclusive hydrogels for, 1093
  semipermeable films, 1092-3
  for temporary cardiac pacing, 473
  for thoracentesis, 479
  for thrombosed external hemorrhoids, 952
  for tick removal, 126
  venous cutdown and, 339
Wound management, skin biopsy, 24
Wound preparation, laceration repair, 13-4
Wrist, joint and soft tissue aspiration and injection, 1042

X-rays
  abnormal, newborn, 847
  abdominal, paracentesis and peritoneal lavage, 894
  central venous catheter insertion, 308, 309, 312, 316
  chest tube insertion, 450
  corneal abrasions and removal of corneal or conjunctival
    foreign bodies, 222
  endotracheal intubation, 462, 843
  intraosseous venous access, 837
  intrauterine device, 537, 1139
  nasogastric tube and salem sump insertion, 268
  neonatal resuscitation, 843, 846
  small-bowel, 960
  Swan-Ganz catheterization, 330
  temporary cardiac pacing, 473
  umbilical artery catheterization, 849
  upper gastrointestinal, 960
Xanthelasma, 37, 97
Xanthoma, 37
Xylocaine. *See* Lidocaine

Z-plasty, 288
Zenker's diverticulum, 264
Zephiran, 71, 72
Zinc chloride paste, 1087